CONTENTS

Congratulations!

You now have access to Mosby's "Get Smart" Bonus Package!

1. MERLIN

Mosby's Electronic Resource Links and Information Network *for* Mosby's Guide to Physical Examination, 4th Edition

Sign on at *http://www1.mosby.com/physexam_seidel*

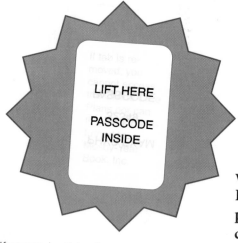

LIFT HERE

PASSCODE INSIDE

If passcode sticker is removed, this textbook cannot be returned to Mosby, Inc.

What you will get

- Content Updates
- Student Forum
- Links to Related Products
- **WebLinks**

WebLinks allow you to directly access hundreds of active web sites keyed specifically to the content of Mosby's Guide to Physical Examination. New sites are continually updated. Simply peel off the sticker on this page and register with the listed passcode.

Merlin
Transforming Nursing Education

2. INTERACTIVE STUDENT CD-ROM

FREE with every copy of Mosby's Guide to Physical Examination

- Provides more than 50 interactive exercises that allow you to test your knowledge and challenge the experts
- Contains 20 patient education guides that may be printed out and used for reference
- Includes examination checklists for each body system chapter that may be printed out and used in the laboratory setting
- Includes a COOL converter calculator that permits you to easily convert Celcius to Fahrenheit, pounds to kilograms, and inches to centimeters

Mosby's Guide to
PHYSICAL EXAMINATION

EXPAND YOUR KNOWLEDGE

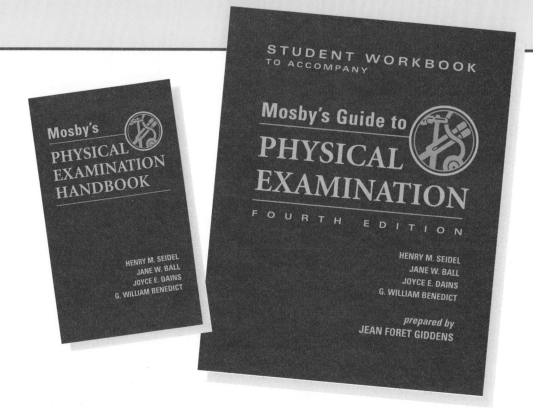

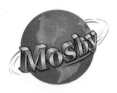

Visit this text online at
http://www1.mosby.com/physexam_seidel

Mosby's Guide to
PHYSICAL EXAMINATION

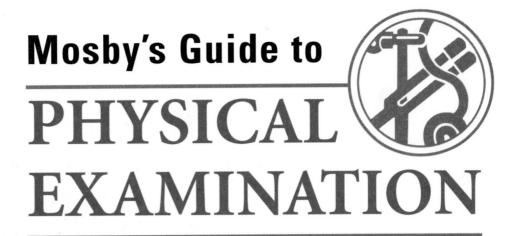

FOURTH EDITION

HENRY M. SEIDEL, MD
Professor Emeritus of Pediatrics
The Johns Hopkins University School of Medicine
Baltimore, Maryland

JANE W. BALL, RN, DrPH, CPNP
Director, Emergency Medical Services for Children
National Resource Center
Children's National Medical Center
Washington, DC

JOYCE E. DAINS, DrPH, JD, RN, CS, FNP
Assistant Professor
Baylor College of Medicine
Houston, Texas

G. WILLIAM BENEDICT, MD, PhD
Assistant Professor, Medicine
The Johns Hopkins University School of Medicine
Baltimore, Maryland

With 1330 illustrations

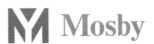 Mosby

St. Louis Baltimore Boston Carlsbad Chicago Minneapolis New York Philadelphia Portland
London Milan Sydney Tokyo Toronto

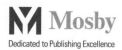

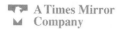

Publisher: Sally Schrefer
Executive Editor: June Thompson
Development Editor: Gail Brower
Project Manager: Deborah L. Vogel
Production Editors: Karen L. Allman and Sarah E. Fike
Designer: Pati Pye
Manufacturing Manager: Linda Ierardi
Senior Composition Specialists: Peggy Hill, Chris Robinson, and Joan Herron

FOURTH EDITION

Lithography/color film by Graphic World, Inc.
Printing/binding by World Color.

Mosby, Inc.
11830 Westline Industrial Drive
St. Louis, Missouri 63146

Library of Congress Cataloging in Publication Data
Mosby's guide to physical examination / Henry M. Seidel . . . [et al.].
    —4th ed.
        p.   cm.
    Includes bibliographical references and index.
    ISBN 0-323-00178-5
    1. Physical diagnosis.   I. Seidel, Henry M.
    [DNLM: 1. Physical Examination—methods.   WB 205M894 1999]
RC76.M63   1999
616.07ˈ54—dc21
DNLM/DLC
for Library of Congress   98-27245
                                                                              CIP

98 99   00   01   02 / 9 8 7 6 5 4 3 2 1

CONTRIBUTORS

Sample Documentation boxes and contributions to Chapter 24, Recording Information, by

Candis Morrison, PhD, CRNP
Associate Professor
Johns Hopkins University School of Nursing
Baltimore, Maryland

Chapter 6, Nutrition, contributed by

Sharon Lechter Smalling, MPH, RD, LD
Clinical Dietitian Specialist
Hermann Wellness Center
Hermann Hospital
Houston, Texas

Pregnant Women variations sections contributed by

Diane Wind Wardell, PhD, RNC
Associate Professor
School of Nursing
The University of Texas-Houston
   Health Science Center
Houston, Texas

Original illustrations by

Barbara Cousins
Newport, Rhode Island

Donald P. O'Connor
St. Peters, Missouri

George J. Wassilchenko
Tulsa, Oklahoma

Photography by

Patrick Watson
Poughkeepsie, New York

PREFACE

Mosby's Guide to Physical Examination has been designed and written for students who are having their first experiences with patients, learning to establish relationships with them, and learning to take histories and do physical examinations. We believe it is a valuable resource for anyone beginning a career in any of the health care professions. The art involved is common to all of these professions, and the need of the patient to be served well is the underlying imperative. We emphasize the patient's needs throughout and stress that this emphasis does not and should not vary, regardless of the specific area of health care being provided. The patient's needs are the common denominator that informs and unifies our individual efforts to serve the patient.

Each patient is unique and not merely a collection of body parts and systems. The whole individual is indeed greater and far more compelling than just the parts. Your relationship with the patient generally begins with conversation and your need to gain information in order to understand and assess the patient. You are asked to consider the patient's reasons for seeking health care at a particular time and also to consider the way in which a problem may be interfering with the patient's life. Although many of the chapters are, by necessity, organized by body parts and systems, that must not detract from your constant consideration of the individual, the whole person. We have written with that goal in mind.

Throughout this edition, there is much that has been refined and embellished in the light of new knowledge developed since the last edition was written.

ORGANIZATION

History taking and physical examination are the core elements of this textbook, but also important is the health care provider's need to establish a sound, trusting, and cooperative relationship with the patient.

Chapter 1 offers guidelines for the development of rapport with the patient. Chapter 2 emphasizes the imperative to learn the context in which the patient lives and his or her cultural background, often quite different from your own. Chapter 3 gives an overview of examination approaches and equipment used during the physical examination. Chapters 4, 5, and 6 address aspects of the overall evaluation of the patient: mental health, growth and development, and nutrition.

Chapters 7 through 20 focus on specific body systems and body parts. The content of each chapter is divided into four major sections: Anatomy and Physiology, Review of Related History, Examination and Findings, and Common Abnormalities. Each of these sections begins with consideration of the adult patient and then follows with variations for other age groups and pregnant women as appropriate.

- The Anatomy and Physiology section of each of these chapters describes the key anatomic landmarks to be noted during the physical examination and provides insight into the physiologic basis of findings.
- The Review of Related History outlines the details of a specific inquiry when a system-related problem is identified during the interview or examination.
- The Examination and Findings section includes a list of needed equipment, the correct approach to the patient, the procedures for the examination in sequence, and the expected findings. This section concludes with a summary of the step-by-step examination and a sample write-up of findings. We have avoided the use of the terms *normal* and *abnormal* in our descriptions of findings whenever possible, because in our view, these terms may suggest a value judgment that may or may not be validated ultimately by experience and additional information.

- Common Abnormalities, disease states generally recognized as being associated with the particular body system or part, appear at the end of each of these chapters. Although the cluster of symptoms and related data given about each of the conditions will be useful to you as you begin the clinical decision-making process, they should be considered only a beginning. You will want to add to your knowledge base with other texts and resources.

The remaining chapters in the textbook will help you put the examination information into practice. Chapter 21 endeavors to help you "put it all together" and offers guidance on integrating the various steps of the examination into a seamless flow, while being always mindful to give respectful attention to what the patient is saying. Chapter 22 offers guidance on organizing and integrating the information you gather. This all-important process of "critical thinking" leads to formulating diagnoses, the setting of priorities, and the institution of management plans. Chapter 23, Emergency or Life-Threatening Situations, provides information on the ABCs of primary assessment and injury assessment, as well as the sequencing of the examination, since urgency mandates a change in approach. It also covers the legal considerations associated with emergency situations. Chapter 24, Recording Information, gives examples of written documentation and stresses the importance of this written record.

The appendix section of this edition has been expanded to include the Denver II Developmental Screening Tool, nutrition screening forms, a language translation guide to help health care providers communicate with Spanish-speaking patients, and a comprehensive sports preparticipation evaluation guide.

FEATURES

- A consistent chapter organization provides easy access to information and facilitates student learning.
- A special feature of this book is the inclusion of approaches, techniques, and findings relevant to infants, children, adolescents, older adults, and pregnant women in each chapter as appropriate.
- Physical findings that distinguish certain groups of patients are highlighted in special sidebar boxes.
- This book is richly illustrated with 1330 photographs and drawings that demonstrate both superficial and underlying anatomic structure, proper examination techniques, and expected and unexpected findings.

- Numerous boxes and tables are provided that summarize information and highlight assessment tools used often in practice. These boxes and tables are listed in the contents for easy access.
- Mnemonics boxes provided in the margins help students remember examination techniques or health-history questions.
- An added bonus in this edition is a free CD-ROM for students with a "toolbox" of over 50 interactive learning activities, patient teaching guides that may be printed out, and laboratory checklists that students can use in the clinical setting.

SUPPLEMENTS

Mosby's Physical Examination Handbook, fourth edition, is a companion text that serves as a comprehensive portable clinical reference on physical examination. It gives brief yet concise descriptions of examination techniques, offers guidelines on how the examination should proceed from one area to the next, and consolidates content related to pediatric patients in separate sections throughout. This text is the only physical examination handbook of its kind in the market with full-color photos and illustrations.

The *Student Workbook to Accompany Mosby's Guide to Physical Examination* includes a variety of activities to help students review and reinforce their comprehension of the history-taking and physical examination processes. The workbook follows the textbook, chapter by chapter, and tests the student on all content areas. Included are critical thinking challenges, key concept application activities, multiple choice questions, matching exercises, fill-in-the blank reviews of terminology, and case studies with follow-up questions.

Every attempt has been made to provide you with a comprehensive guide to the taking of the health history and the performance of the physical examination for patients in all of their variety. The fundamental messages we have done our best to impart in *Mosby's Guide to Physical Examination* are these:

- Respect the patient.
- The relationship with the patient can be indescribably rewarding.
- Strive for the complementary forces of competence and compassion.
- The art and skills essential to history-taking and physical examination are the bedrock of care; technologic resources are but complements.

- The computer cannot replace a competent history and physical examination or provide the pathways to trusting health care relationships.
- There is no such thing as a history without a physical examination, or a physical examination without a history: they are *one*.

It is our hope that you will find this a useful textbook and that it will continue to serve as a reference resource as your career evolves.

Henry M. Seidel
Jane W. Ball
Joyce E. Dains
G. William Benedict

ACKNOWLEDGMENTS

As with each previous edition, there are many people we wish to thank who contributed their efforts to this, our fourth edition. First, we express our profound appreciation for those instructors and students who took the time to offer helpful suggestions and comments that have enhanced the content and style of our textbook. They helped make the planning, preparation, and writing of this edition a rewarding experience.

Many of our colleagues at Mosby worked to make this edition possible. Sally Schrefer, our Publisher, has been with us from the first day of work on the first edition. She continues to be our editorial guide in many respects; she is an extra-special person who has that ineffable quality that enables constructive criticism, the maintenance of a disciplined approach, and friendship. June Thompson, Executive Editor, has been a source of inspiration and innovative ideas. Gail Brower, our Development Editor, weathered the angst of creation with calm competence and compassion and made sure the right steps were taken day by day, assuring the outcome all of us wanted. Gary O'Brien, Editorial Assistant, responded to each of our requests with know-how and good humor. The entire Mosby production team deserves special recognition for the effective editing and design of the book. Karen Allman and Sarah Fike made sure no detail in the manuscript was overlooked. Pati Pye created the visually appealing design that graces this edition. The new photographs taken by Patrick Watson once again confirm his skill and his understanding of our needs. Barbara Cousins adeptly created many of the new illustrations and updated dozens of others. We also want to recognize the remarkable efforts of the Marketing and Sales Representatives who continue to generate great interest in our book and help improve it by reporting comments and suggestions. Without all of these people, there would be no fourth edition.

In addition, we offer many thanks to the following individuals and organizations for their contributions of time, talent, expertise, and resources:

John S. Andrews
Stephen Baylog
Baylor College of Medicine Family Practice Center
Michele Bellantoni
Virginia Berry
Mitchell Blake
Wendy Blake
Charles Bradley
Arlene Butz
Joan Campanaro
Francine Cheese
Sara Chiu
Maureen Clothier
Susan Cummings
Austin Dains
Garvin Davis
John Freeman
Carolyn Harvey
Mary Joyner
Carolyn Kisner
Horace K. Liang
Adriana Linares
James Lord
Keith Loring

Donna Mannello
Andrea Mathias
Wendell Meade
Jeffrey Miller
Deborah Nickles
Mai Phung
Homer Pilgrim
Roberta Preston
Leslie Scott
Richard Smalling
Stephanie Smalling
Patricia Smouse
Evangeline Soulikas
Michelle R. Thompson
Augusta Tucker Townsend
Cornelia Trimble
Rebecca Vickers
Elizabeth Vogler
Robert Vogler
Allen Walker
Jean Wheeler
Lawrence Wissow
Leah Wissow
Nancy Hutton Wissow
Stephen Wissow

The patience, love, and support of our families are the *sine qua non* of all of our effort. We reach out to them with a special "thank you."

CONTENTS

TABLES

BOXES

MNEMONICS BOXES

PHYSICAL VARIATIONS BOXES

CHAPTER 1

THE HISTORY AND INTERVIEWING PROCESS

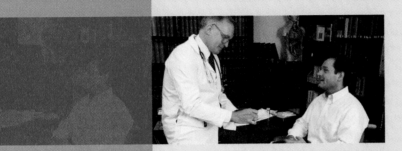

The purpose of this book is to offer instruction in acquiring information about the well and the sick as they seek health and medical care. It is not easy to get the sense of another person or to fully appreciate someone else's orientation in the world. The stimuli we each receive from the external world can often be much the same. However, the way we perceive those images and make them a part of our experience and our base of information varies enormously. If we are to keep our interpretations from being misinterpretations and our perceptions from being misperceptions, we must make every effort to sense the world of the individual patient as that patient senses it; and we must be sensitive to what it is that increases the vulnerability inherent in anyone seeking professional help.

The central objective of interacting with a patient is to find out what is at the root of that person's concern and to help in doing something about it. If you do not keep constant the need to identify the patient's underlying worries, believe them, and try to deal with them, you will probably not be of much help. You need to understand what the patient expects of you and to help define what is to be expected of the patient. You need to understand the power you have.

The history and physical examination begin and are at the heart of the diagnostic and treatment process. They represent the accumulation of information. The subsequent assessment evaluates and integrates that information as the care of the patient proceeds. Your approach must be orderly; random approaches often result in random solutions, seriously limiting the likelihood of successful outcomes. Order, however, does not imply rigidity.

You have to be compulsive as you compile information, giving careful attention to the obvious so that you understand it and record it precisely, while maintaining your sensitivity to the less obvious "soft" clues that are almost always to be found in the history or physical examination. The ability to do this well distinguishes the good

THE POWER OF THE PROFESSIONAL AND THE VULNERABILITY OF THE PATIENT

"We say to you, 'With so much power, walk carefully and humbly. Do no harm: walk carefully so that the granite weight of that power does not crush. Abide with us'."

From Berger, 1996.

clinician. Moreover, since cost containment is essential, the skillfully performed history and physical examination can, in an advantaged society, rationalize the appropriate and cost-effective use of technologic resources and, in a disadvantaged society, compensate in large part for their absence.

ETHICAL CONSIDERATIONS IN PATIENT RELATIONSHIPS

The interview with the patient is an extraordinary event. You can, in a relatively brief time, learn so very much, from the facts of the moment to a patient's deepest feelings. The goals of this communication include:

- Discovering information leading to diagnosis and management
- Providing information to the patient concerning diagnosis
- Negotiating with the patient concerning management; it is not something to be invariably imposed
- Counseling about disease prevention

This interview is the basis for forming a disease prevention and therapeutic "partnership" with the patient based on honesty, empathy, and respect for the individual. Quite obviously, your personality and behavior during the interview will have an impact on its outcome; so, too, will the personality and behavior of the patient, the nature of problem being confronted, the physical setting, and the economic base on which care is provided. These concerns can be given an appropriate context if you remember that at heart, each interaction must be oriented to the patient and not solely to a specific problem or disease. You must make certain to listen very carefully so that you can appreciate what you are told and also what you are not told—perhaps because the patient does not want to tell you, or for some reason, cannot tell you. There are clues in silence. Ultimate satisfaction for the patient and for you requires that you constantly hone your interview skills and that you resist the temptation to allow burgeoning technology to take their place.

The partnership requires the integration of all psychosocial and biologic factors. It requires better personal insights of the patient, as well as a better understanding on all our parts of the many aspects of health care from the technologic to the economic. This partnership recognizes that those of us who offer care are more accountable now than we were in the past.

AN ETHICAL CONTEXT TO THE PARTNERSHIP WITH THE PATIENT

There is an ethical context to the alliance that has been more sharply defined in recent years. Since the principles involved do not always complement each other, the tensions leading to the resolution of problems require sensitivity from all persons involved. You must remember that "ethics" does not provide answers; rather, it offers a disciplined approach to understanding and to determining ultimate behavior. Given a problem, for example, a perceived necessary violation of confidentiality, several concepts must be considered.

- *Autonomy:* the patient's need for self-determination. The definition is clouded when the patient is incompetent or is a child. Parents, family, and other significant persons in the life of the patient must be included, and the boundaries of their participation must be clearly set, often by an advance directive from the patient. The goals for our efforts are better served if there is a clear understanding of the patient's concept of autonomy. The paternalistic professional, acting as parent or priest, can certainly invade autonomy. Although in recent years there has been considerable constraint on paternalism, it may not always be inappropriate. However, the professional must inform and interpret, giving a clear understanding of what the information means. The patient who is well-informed is better able to exercise autonomy. Imbalance in any of these requirements can constrain autonomy.

- *Beneficence:* the care provider's need to do good for the patient. There is always a concern that the need to do good may be too eagerly pursued and may result in a paternalism that might smother autonomy. "Father" or "mother" may *sometimes* know best but, clearly, not always.
- *Nonmaleficence:* the care provider's need to do no harm to the patient: *primum non nocere.*
- *Utilitarianism:* the need to consider the appropriate use of resources for the greater good of the larger community.
- *Fairness and justice:* recognition of the often precarious balance between autonomy and the competing interests of the family and community. Fair treatment is constrained of late, with the advent of managed care and the increased recognition of our limited resources, issues by no means easily resolved.
- *Deontologic imperatives:* the duties of care providers established by tradition and in cultural contexts. Such duties appear to have an ordained existence.

Quite obviously, these principles can come into conflict in any given situation, for example, the use of limited resources in situations thought to be futile. Consideration of each of them, however, can often lead to helpful outcomes. We must understand the patient's major, often decisive contribution and the sometimes competing values and interests of all of us who offer care. Respect for each other's opinions and flexibility in attitudes are key ingredients in the search for answers, and for the preservation of a patient's autonomy that is not constrained by the well-meant but overzealous paternalism of the provider.

Unhappily, however, attention to ethical concepts does not necessarily provide a handy guide to resolution of a problem. Although there is no one correct approach to a seemingly unresolvable issue, we can make sure that in each case we consider the following guidelines:

- The problem at hand is truly one of ethics and not a result of poor communication, legal confusion, or personality conflict
- The facts are as clearly stated as possible
- The substance of ethical conflict and its sources are clearly understood
- The attitudes of patients or their representatives are clearly communicated
- There is a reasonable chance for a satisfactory health or medical care outcome
- External factors such as money, conflict within a family, or conflicting responsibilities outside of the family are properly considered

In the end, despite some recent conflict within the academic community concerning philosophic approaches to the resolution of ethical issues, the patient's point of view should prevail unless there is a compelling argument otherwise. That argument very often derives from cultural influences that must be understood and, whenever possible, respected.

COMMUNICATING WITH THE PATIENT

FACTORS THAT ENHANCE COMMUNICATION

PROFESSIONAL DRESS AND GROOMING

The way you are dressed and groomed will go a long way toward establishing that first impression with the patient. Some personal habits may intrude on the patient's sensibilities. Therefore clean fingernails, modest dress, and neat hair are imperative. Still, you do not have to be stuffy to be neat. Men do not need pinstripes and ties, and women do not need the latest power dress to signify respect for the patient. Health professionals can easily avoid extremes in dress and manner so that appearance does not become an obstacle in the patient's response to care

From the start, there are several points to keep in mind. A stiff, formal demeanor may inhibit the patient's ability to communicate, but a too casual, laid back attitude may fail to instill confidence. Because the patient may search for meaning in everything you say, avoid being careless with words. What may seem innocuous to you may be vital to the patient. You should begin to understand the intellectual and emotional constraints on the way you ask questions and convey information. Similarly, your face need not be a mask, but avoid the extremes of reaction—startle, surprise, laughter, grimacing—as the patient provides information. Your nonverbal demeanor matters fully as much as your words.

Sometimes you will be concerned about the patient's ability to understand what you try to convey and what you are seeking to discover (Box 1-1), but do not allow yourself to discount the patient's experience and the information he or she provides. In addition, it is the patient who should respond to questions if at all possible. Too often a parent, spouse, or other person will answer for the patient unless otherwise counseled.

BOX 1-1 Language Differences

The maintenance of confidentiality is sometimes difficult. For example, you may not speak the patient's language. A family member may be a convenient interpreter but, for reasons unknown to you, a real barrier to a candid response to your questions. A stranger might be more appropriate. Interpreters are also helpful when the patient has an incomplete knowledge of the examiner's language, or vice versa, since idiomatic expression, the "slang" of any language, may need clarification. This is true even in England, where "boot" may not mean "footwear" or a "kick," but rather, an essential part of an automobile.

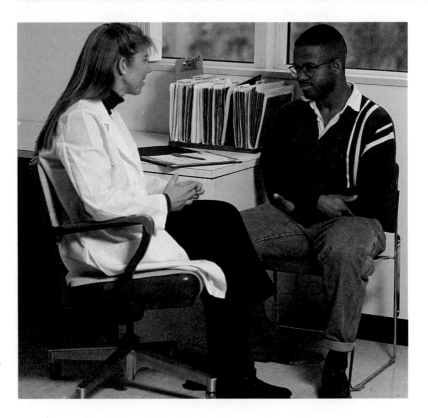

Interviewing a young adult. Note the absence of an intervening desk or table.

Flexibility

The patient's associations may be important, and you must allow freedom for the patient to pursue them. Be flexible! Ask open-ended questions in the beginning (for example, "How have you been feeling since I last saw you?"). Later, as information accumulates, it will be necessary to know precise, measurable details, and you must become more specific. But early in the interview it is entirely appropriate to let the patient tell you what the experience was like. The patient's or observer's description of the experience should be heard and recorded (Box 1-2). This will be helpful in the future for others who are involved with the patient to have a sense of how the patient and the family responded to the experience.

BOX 1-2 | **Listening: The Art of Intelligent Repose**

If we are to be successful in what we do, we must be very skilled listeners and observers with a polished sense of timing and a kind of repose that is at once alert and reassuring, and we must have clear goals for each of our interactions. In Robertson Davies' book *World of Wonders,* an experienced actor gives advice to a very young juggler, tight-rope walker, and would-be actor. From off stage, the two are watching the "star." It is advice you might take to heart as you enter a space with the patient:

Look at the Guvnor—he hasn't a taut muscle in his body, nor a slack one either. He is in easy control all the time. Have you noticed him standing still when he listens to another actor? Have you noticed how still he is? Look at you now, listening to me; you bob about and twist and turn in a scene, you'd be killing half the value of what I say with all that

movement. Just try to sit still. Yes, there you go; you're not still at all, you're frozen. Stillness isn't looking as if you were full of coiled springs. It's repose. Intelligent repose. That's what the Guvnor has. What I have, too, as a matter of fact. What Barnard has. What Milady has. I suppose you think repose means asleep, or dead.

Listen intently. Learn how to listen while being still, achieving "intelligent repose." This will help you be open to *all* the messages in the patient's words and body talk. Ultimately, it will help make the resources you have in all of your senses—touch, smell, and even taste—more acute. If a patient tells you the food is bad, taste it! Every one of your behaviors should contribute to the communication of empathy and the building of the trust essential to a therapeutic partnership.

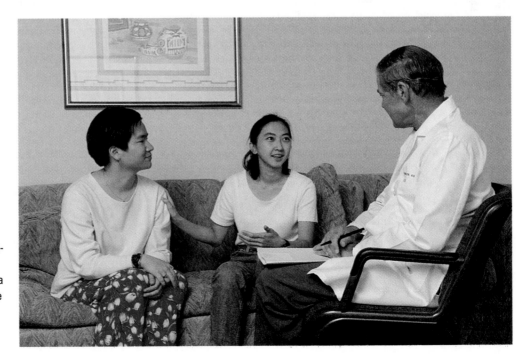

Interviewing a patient with an interpreter. Someone other than a family member may at times be a preferred interpreter when there is a language difference between the examiner and patient.

Open-endedness cannot be allowed to go on forever, of course. Telling the patient at the outset the approximate time available for the interview may be helpful. Gentle guidance is sometimes necessary ("But now let's also talk about . . ."). You cannot assume that a verbose tale is the complete story. You must be certain that you have asked all the questions you need.

Clarity

Your questions must be clearly understood (Box 1-3). Define any words the patient cannot understand, but do not use so many technical terms that the definitions become confusing. Be clear and explicit; use the patient's terms if possible, but you must not be patronizing. Meet the level of your patient's ability to understand. (There can be traps in this, however. A professional colleague who is a patient may not be familiar with the jargon of your particular discipline.)

Resist the tendency to be manipulative. Avoid leading questions. For example, ask how often something happened, allowing the patient to define *often,* rather than asking, "It didn't happen too often, did it?" Pursue the information with short, uncomplicated questions using understandable language. Ask one question at a time, avoiding a barrage of questions that prohibit the patient from being expansive or that limit the patient to simple yes or no answers. It is often better to say, "Tell me about. . . ," rather than, "Is it. . . ?" Always be adaptable to the patient's language. If a patient uses a term to describe an event, adopt that term as you attempt to explore further.

Sometimes you will be confused by what the patient tells you. Recognize the confusion as a piece of information and begin to clarify if you can. The confusion may be a clue to a patient's underlying emotional or organic difficulty, or sometimes it may be due to a momentary loss of attention on your part.

BOX 1-3   Asking Questions

If you are not careful, the phrasing of questions can lead to inaccurate or misleading patient responses:

- The *open-ended question* leaves discretion to the patient about the extent of the answer—"And then what happened?"; "What are your feelings about this?"; "Is that all you wanted to say?"; "Is there anything more you need to talk about?"
- The *direct question* seeks specific information—"How long ago did that happen?"; "Where does it hurt?"; "Please put a finger where it hurts"; "How many pills did you take each time, and how many times a day did you take them?"
- The *leading question* is the most risky, because it may limit the information provided to what the patient thinks you want to know—"It seems to me that that bothered you a lot. Is that true?"; "That wasn't very difficult to do, was it?"; "That's a horrible-tasting medicine, isn't it?"

Questions are, of course, essential tools. Sometimes the patient does not quite understand what you are asking and says so. Recognize the need at different times and in varying circumstances to perform the following functions:

Facilitate	Encourage your patient to say more, with words or with a silence that the patient may break when given the opportunity for reflection.
Reflect	Repeat what you have heard to encourage more detail.
Clarify	Ask, "What do you mean?"
Empathize	Show your understanding and acceptance. Do not hesitate to say, "I understand" or, "I'm sorry" if the moment calls for it.
Confront	Do not hesitate to discuss a patient's disturbing behavior.
Interpret	Repeat what you have heard to confirm the meaning with the patient.

What you ask is complemented by how you ask it. To clarify the patient's point of view:

- Ask often what the patient *thinks and feels* about an issue.
- Make sure you know what the chief *concern* is.
- Make sure that all is well in the family and in the workplace, that nothing major extraneous to the chief complaint and present illness has happened recently.
- Suggest at appropriate times that you have the "feeling" that there is more to say or that things may not be as well as they are reported.
- Suggest at appropriate times that it is all right to be angry, sad, or nervous and it is all right to talk about it.
- Make sure that the patient's expectations in the visit are met and that there are no other questions.

Questions like these can be adapted to persons of any age and circumstance: the elderly, the adolescent, or the parents of an infant or a young child.

> ### BOX 1-4   Gaining Information is not Time Dependent
>
> Just spending more time with a patient isn't always better. Bad habits and poor interviewing skills may only be exacerbated by that investment. Appropriate questions and sensitivity to visual and verbal clues can help you learn a good deal, often quickly:
> - Personalize your approach: know the patient, of course. But also understand the community in which you serve and its resources, and learn as much as you can about the family and other resources available to the patient.
> - Understand the patient's expectations of the visit and do not hesitate to ask if those expectations were met.
> - Evoke unvoiced concerns. Use open-ended questions with a nonjudgmental, empathic attitude.
> - Be alert to nonverbal clues such as demeanor, appearance, and relationship to family members accompanying the patient.
> - Listen alertly. Don't let a charged, meaningful word escape your attention.
> - Support the patient's feelings of competence and self-esteem, and the family's when appropriate. An honest compliment goes a long way!

Modified from Green, Stuy, 1992.

If the patient makes a reference that is not immediately relevant to your purposes, be flexible enough to clarify at least the nature of the irrelevancy. This allows you to make a decision on the need for further exploration. Although too many digressions can lead to the possibility of misspent time, paying attention to a digression of the moment may save a lot of time later on (Box 1-4).

Subtlety

Some apparent irrelevancies may provide important background information. A parent, for example, may have died of cancer. The fact itself may not be important at that moment, but the patient's response to the fact and the intensity of feeling associated with it can give important shape to your approaches. Such an understanding is vital to your pursuit of diagnosis and management. Thus no history is complete without information about the patient's past and present life situation, reaction to earlier events, and coping methods.

Never assume a patient's every question requires an encyclopedic answer. Be sensitive to the extent of an answer that is being sought.

Learn to be sensitive to the subtle as well as the obvious in the question; learn to go far enough but not too far. Your sensitivity must include choosing your words carefully. Most lay people think *tumor* is synonymous with *cancer* and will often interpret your use of the word *nervous* to mean that they have emotional problems. Obviously you can paralyze your spontaneity in a too precise choice of words, but you do need to exercise care. If the patient seems to ask a leading question, one you do not feel prepared to answer at the moment, it is possible to say, "Why do you ask?" to seek better understanding of the direction of the patient's thinking. Children need age-appropriate responses to their questions.

Value Judgment

It is easy to be too directive about certain issues. Avoid that trap! When the patient asks for advice, be sure you understand the patient's experience and attitudes. Try for an interchange that allows the patient to come to a decision as free as possible from the imposition of your value judgment. To the extent that you can avoid this, you remain a health professional and not a preacher. The competent health professional understands that value judgments are not necessarily imbued with wisdom.

The Exploration of Feelings

The American Board of Internal Medicine has suggested the following questions that might be asked by an interviewer who gives full concern to the patient's feelings and needs. We have added one or two. Rarely, if ever, would one patient be asked all of these questions; exactly which ones are appropriate must be determined by each patient's particular situation. For example, questions about a living will would alarm a patient seeking a routine checkup but may relieve a patient hospitalized with a life-threatening disease. In any event, the patient's reactions may appear to be illogical if they are cognitively impaired or if emotion generated by anxiety, depression, genuine fear, or related feelings dominate the ability to reason as we might. The feeling of vulnerability generated by all of this, as well as by racial, gender, ethnic, or other differences may intimidate your effort.

- How are you feeling today?
- What can I do for you today?
- What do you think is causing your symptoms?
- What is your understanding of your diagnosis? Its importance? Its need for management?
- How do you feel about your illness? Frightened? Threatened? As a wage earner? As a family member? Angry that you are afflicted? (Be sure, though, to allow a response without putting words in the patient's mouth.)
- Do you believe treatment will help?
- How are you coping with your illness? Crying? Drinking more? Tranquilizers? Talking more? Less? Changing life-styles?
- Do you want to know all the details about your diagnosis and its effect on your future?
- How important is "doing everything possible"?
- How important is "quality of life"?
- Have you prepared a living will?
- Do you have people you can talk with about your illness?
- Is there anyone else we should contact about your illness or hospitalization? Family members? Friends? Employer? Religious advisor? Attorney?
- Do you want or expect emotional support from the health care team?
- Are there financial questions about your medical care that trouble you? Insurance coverage? Tests or treatment you may not be able to afford? Timing of payments required from you?
- How would you like to be addressed?
- If you have had previous hospitalizations, does it bother you to be seen by teams of doctors, nurses, and medical students on rounds?
- How private a person are you?
- Are you concerned about the confidentiality of your medical records?
- Would you prefer to talk to an older/younger, male/female physician?
- Are there medical matters you do not wish disclosed to others?
- Would you prefer to give your history so no one else can hear?[*]

MOMENTS OF TENSION

Curiosity About You

Patients are aware that you are a person with a life of your own. Most of them will at one time or another have some curiosity about aspects of your experience.

---

[*]From American Board of Internal Medicine, 1985.

Sometimes you will be asked about yourself. You need not violate your personal life. Often a direct answer, unvarnished by detail, will suffice to satisfy the patient's curiosity and prevent great invasion into your personal life but communicate nevertheless that you are not completely isolated. You may find it comfortable to chat about certain, sometimes relevant, aspects of your own experience ("I have trouble remembering to take medicines, too"). Often, reassurance about personal life events (for example, pregnancy and childbirth) can help alleviate fears and—with further exploration—can help in the identification of the patient's concerns. You may, for example, respond to an inquiry that you are married, but you need not give extended details about your spouse.

Anxiety

Anxiety may be defined as a painful uneasiness of mind resulting from an impending or anticipated illness. The intensity can certainly vary. There are some physical disorders that are more likely to have more intense anxiety as a common accompaniment, for example, those associated with crushing chest pain or difficulty in breathing. Just seeing a health professional provokes anxiety in some patients. Still, your approach should be helpful in relieving it. It pays to answer questions forthrightly, never dissembling. You should avoid an overload of information. Pace the conversation. Do not hurry and do not allow the anxiety to be contagious. A calm demeanor, repose, will communicate itself to the patient. That is not necessarily easy to achieve. Pursue it. The patient's vulnerability requires it.

Silence

We are sometimes intimidated by silence, and many of us feel the urge to break it with some kind of chatter. Be patient and do not force. You may have to edge the patient along with an open-ended question ("What seems to worry you?") or a mild nudge ("And after that?"). Remember, though, that the patient's silence may have its uses—a moment of reflection, the summoning of courage. Some issues can be so painful and sensitive that the silence becomes necessary and should be allowed. Most people will begin to talk when they are ready.

As always, the patient's demeanor, use of hands, and facial expression contribute to your interpretation of the moment. The eyes may be brimming with tears, because of emotions so deeply felt that speech is impossible. It may also be cultural; for example, some Native Americans take their time, ponder their responses to questions, and answer when they feel ready. Silence is usually a clue for you to go slower, not to push too hard, and to examine your approach. Learn to be comfortable with silence and to give it reasonable bounds.

Depression

Being sick or thinking that you are sick is enough to provoke at least some depression. Indeed, serious or chronic, unrelenting illness or a variety of drugs (e.g., steroids) often have depression as an accompaniment. A sense of sluggishness in all of the daily experience; disturbances in sleep, eating, and social contact; and feelings of loss of self-worth can be clues. When that happens, it is best to approach your explorations with specific questions, which as they are answered may lead you to the opportunity for a more open-ended approach. First, "When did this problem begin?" Then, "How do you feel about it?" A patient in this circumstance cannot be hurried and certainly cannot be relieved by superficial assurance. It is better to say, "I understand" than to be falsely reassuring.

Crying

People will cry. Let them. Let the moment pass at the patient's pace. Wait to resume your questioning until the patient is ready. If you become aware that the patient needs to cry but is suppressing it, give permission. Offer a tissue or simply say, "I know you're feeling bad. It's all right to cry." Such a moment often generates greater warmth between you and the patient. You have shared something, and you have respected the patient's need. The patient has sensed your feelings of caring, and the relationship has grown.

Manipulations

Patients can be very flattering, often excessively so. Perhaps illness and insecurity invoke a need to have you give extra-special attention, something others are thought not to get. It is sometimes easy to be taken in by such manipulations. Certainly, you should be aware that it happens, and be aware that it should not encourage you to depart from your professional standard of care. We all like to be liked. The complementary danger is that we may too often try to get patients to like us with our own perhaps inappropriate behavior (see below).

Physical and Emotional Intimacy

Most of us have grown up in circumstances that tend to increase the difficulty of dealing intimately with the emotions and the bodies of others. The cultural norms, shadings, and behaviors are at once protective of and barriers to good relationships with the patient. We may have powerful feelings, sometimes attracting us, sometimes repelling us.

The patient most likely shares some of the same feelings and may feel a helplessness in this regard that is induced by the more dependent status. It is all right to acknowledge this and to indicate that you understand. You should then always protect the patient's modesty, using covers appropriately without hampering good examination, and you should always be careful about the ways in which you use words or frame questions. You should not shock the patient.

In particular, you must not be "desensitized" to the issues of intimacy as time goes by. Rather, understanding and accepting your own feelings, and keeping them in context, will help develop a sensitive, empathic relationship with the patient. It is all right to admit that you are both human and to come to positive terms with that admission (Smith, Kleinman, 1989).

Nevertheless, there are boundaries to professional behavior and they must not be crossed. Patients are variably vulnerable; some are not particularly dependent, and others are deeply dependent. As vulnerability increases and professions of intimacy develop, often urged on by the patient's behavior (see Seduction, p. 11, some professionals slide down the "slippery slope" and cross the boundary that should not be crossed. There is no room for sexual misconduct in the patient relationship, and there can be no tolerance for exploitation of the patient in this regard.

Compassionate Moments

Do not hesitate to say that you feel for the patient, that you are sorry for something that happened, and that you know it may have been painful. Be open and direct about a tender circumstance. It is all right to bring things out in the open as long as your guiding hand is gentle and you are not too aggressive or insistent. Sometimes you state the obvious, and you confront it (Box 1-5). Sometimes you make an inference and hope that you guessed right in bringing the patient's feelings to the surface. When you are uncertain, ask without imposing *your* interpretation of what the response might be.

BOX 1-5 Suicide

You may at times sense a patient's contemplation of suicide. Talking about it is essential. In fact, the common error is the failure to ask about suicidal ideation directly. There are clues that can increase your perception of risks:
- Sleep disturbance: a prolonged period, 2 weeks or more, when the patient has difficulty falling asleep, staying asleep, waking too early or sleeping too much
- Mood disturbance: a lengthy period, 2 weeks or more, in which the patient feels sad or blue, uninterested in the daily effort and without pleasure in things that have usually been enjoyed.
- A prolonged period: 2 weeks or more of feeling worthless, sinful, or guilty
- Hopelessness: any period of time when there is a feeling that life is hopeless or that there seems to be a loss of self-esteem

- The successful suicide of a close relative

Given these concerns, it is appropriate to explore the following:
- The patient's understanding of an existing health or medical condition and its implications
- The patient's concern about becoming a burden to others
- Possible fears of nonexisting conditions
- Possible changes in religious beliefs
- Recent loss of support from loved ones: death, divorce, or the end of a relationship
- Unaccustomed anxiety
- Concern about the impact of suicide on those who will survive and the thought given that problem
- Understanding of how to commit suicide

The potential of suicide is to be dealt with forthrightly; consultation with others is helpful and often necessary.

Data from Wagley, 1992; Cooper-Patrick, Crum, Ford, 1994.

Seduction

There are limits to your expressions of warmth and cordiality. Certainly not all touch is sexually motivated. A heartfelt hug is sometimes just right. Still, you are a professional and you must behave professionally. The insecure, dependent patient is sometimes seductive and often too readily susceptible to manipulation. You must not, either intentionally or unintentionally, fall into the trap of responding to the seductive behavior that so often reflects the patient's insecurity and dependence. Such a situation can be averted by being courteously calm and firm from the start, delivering the clear—and immediate—message that the relationship is and must remain professional. It will take skill to do this, to maintain the patient's dignity, and to seek understanding of the behavior.

Anger

Sometimes those patients who are angriest and most hostile are the ones who need you the most. Nevertheless, it may be difficult to understand anger and hostility. We are all to some extent intimidated by it. You can deal with it by confronting it. It is all right to say, "I know you're angry. Please tell me why. I want to hear." You may sometimes be aware that you have made the patient angry by being late for the interview, by taking too long, or by in some way getting in the way of the patient's life or concerns. You will only add to the anger by pretending that it does not exist. Face it head on. Acknowledge it, and if it is appropriate, apologize. The anger generally will not last long. As with crying, the patient should be given the opportunity to express the feeling and to find that you will not shrink away from it. Often, you can continue on better footing after anger is vented. On occasion, nothing will seem to help. It is all right, if the situation allows, to defer to another time or to suggest a different professional. None of us always succeeds, particularly when illness and uncertainty lower the threshold for anger.

Dissembling

Patients may not always tell the whole story. They may be hiding something, either purposely or unconsciously. Demential illness, alcoholism, sexual uncertainties, and child abuse are among the particularly difficult possibilities. Do not push too hard when you think this is happening, but do not neglect it. Allow the interview to go on and then come back to it with gentle questioning. It might become possible to say, "I think that you may be more concerned than you are saying," or, "I think that you're worried about what we might find out." You must be satisfied that you have learned all that is necessary. But satisfaction may not come in one sitting. You may have to pursue it later that day or the next or perhaps with other members of the family, friends, or associates.

Money

The cost of care and the drain on the resources available to the patient are often sources of stress. It is not within the context of this book to discuss these issues, but you must be aware that they are real and that they may often have an impact on the mind-set of the patient. You should be prepared to talk about them with candor and accurate knowledge.

KNOWING YOURSELF

Knowing yourself is important. You must understand what of yourself you bring to each interaction and that you may respond differently to different people. You must know why and how. As an example, if a patient makes you angry, why should that be? Is it your own negative response to some behavior or characteristic of that patient? Is there some underlying frustration in your life? Does your hostile response to someone in need evolve from a conflict of values or an absence of trust? Certainly, we are not always free of prejudice and we are perhaps too often rushed or otherwise harassed for reasons unrelated to the moment. Whatever the reason, you must understand it before you displace anger to the patient and harm the relationship, perhaps making it difficult to continue.

All of us want to be liked by our patients, and if we sense that this is not so, we are apt to react with some degree of hostility. You may even revert to inappropriate techniques to "make" these patients like you. These dangerous moments can be avoided if you understand yourself and if you have the maturity and personal security to respond to that understanding. You are not in "neutral" as you go about your work with the patient. None of us is.

Given all this, there can be barriers to satisfactory outcomes. The words we exchange may not be appropriately interpreted. Our mood may at times be at odds with that of the patient's; individual behaviors can cause discomfort. However, if we explore with candor, expressing our concern, gaining agreement that there may be a problem, and when appropriate, empathizing, we can deal with the barrier. This makes explicit our recognition of the partnership with the patient and the need to give that partnership legitimacy.

CHILDREN

Children are people. They want to have attention paid to them. They do not want to be patronized, and they love it when you get down on the floor and *play with them*. They have anxieties and fears that must be anticipated and eased. Talk with them, hold them, reassure them, include them! And when they are old enough, allow them to be heard fully. The older the child, the more productive it becomes to ask questions directly.

The older child and the adolescent require a particular sensitivity. Their hesitancies or passive, sometimes vaguely hostile silences may suggest that they would prefer to be alone with you, free of a parent. Respect the need for separation. This is more common with adolescents, but the need for privacy may also be evident among older preadolescent children. In general, be aware that it often helps to separate the child from the parent at some point to get a more complete history.

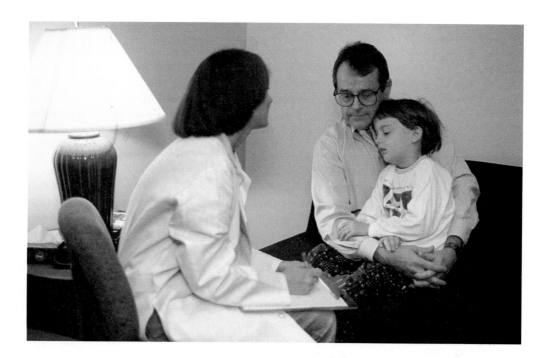

Interviewing a child with his parent. Note that the interviewer is sitting close to the patient and that the child is secure on his father's lap.

The conversation concerning a child (or an infant) can give significant information about the dynamics that prevail within a family and, on occasion, information that may suggest a problem in one of the parents. For example, an excessively tearful mother who doesn't seem to be having much pleasure in her child and who seems self-absorbed, unresponsive and uncommunicative, or even hostile may be telling you to suspect depression and to make appropriate recommendations. Your responsibility goes beyond that for the child. Certainly, in any interaction with any person of any age, clues to possible problems in family, significant others, or friends may become apparent and may demand your action.

ADOLESCENTS

Since adolescents are sometimes reluctant to talk, give clear evidence of your respect for their need for confidentiality and for their impending adulthood. It is helpful in the beginning to talk about what is happening in their day-to-day experiences. It rarely pays to force conversation, because adolescents do not readily respond to confrontation. On the other hand, you will often sense a need to talk and an inability to get the words out. Silences can be long, sometimes sheepish, occasionally angry, and not always leading to constructive talk. Many of us have found it helpful to have a few cards with subjects common to teenagers noted on them (see the Mnemonics box on p. 30.) Simply ask the patient to look at the cards and to indicate silently the ones that note the subjects of present concern. Then you can say the necessary words, phrase the appropriate questions, and make the transition to a verbal discussion reasonably comfortable. In any event, the approach should be open-ended, always indicating a sense of alliance and partnership.

PREGNANT WOMEN

The first interview provides the foundation for the continuing relationship between the woman and her health care provider. Care during the prenatal period involves a personal commitment by the woman to her health and that of the fetus, with direction provided by the health care team. Each woman will manage her pregnancy according to many factors, including previous experiences with childbearing and child-rearing; knowledge, expectations, and perceptions; her relationship with her mother and other significant individuals in her life; her desire for children; and her present life circumstances. It is important to view health care of both the mother and fetus as a complex interactive process. The information obtained during this initial interview includes past history, assessment of health practices, and assessment of knowledge as it affects pregnancy. It provides a unique opportunity during a receptive time for teaching about health care practices.

OLDER ADULTS

Individual variations in knowledge, experience, cognitive abilities, and personality affect the interview process with older adults, just as with the young. Age-related physiologic changes that could be impediments to the interview process may be present in some. Remember, however, that people age at different rates and that chronologic age alone is a poor gauge for determining the presence of those changes. Physiologic age and chronologic age may be disparate.

Some older adults may have sensory losses that make communication more difficult. Some degree of hearing loss is not uncommon. Position yourself so that the patient can see your face. Speak clearly and slowly, taking care not to avert your head while you are talking. (Shouting only magnifies the problem by distorting consonants and vowels.) In some instances, a written interview may ultimately be less frustrating for both you and the patient. If this becomes necessary, tailor the process to include only the most pertinent questions, because this method can be tedious and exhausting for patients.

Conversely, impaired visual perception and light-dark adaptation can adversely affect the interview if written interview forms are used. Provide the patient with a well-illuminated environment and a light source that does not glare or reflect in the eyes.

Some older adults may be confused or experience memory loss, particularly for recent events. Take the extra time needed with these patients. Ask short (but not leading) questions, and keep your language simple. Consult other family members to clarify discrepant information or to fill in the gaps.

Approach each patient as an individual. It is certainly important to be knowledgeable about physiologic, sociologic, and psychologic changes associated with aging, and it is appropriate to anticipate what effect these changes may have on the interview. However, it is equally important to appreciate that not all adults experience the same changes, that such changes do not occur at the same rate, and that some areas do not decline with age. The older patient brings to the interview a lifetime of experience that may be a source of richness, wisdom, meaning, and perspective. Do not discount it.

WATCH YOUR LANGUAGE

Unfortunately, all types of health care providers often lapse into the use of jargon not understood by the patient, the arcane language of their particular profession, and—worse—pejorative words that demean patients. Stress, frustration, fatigue, and anger are common underlying causes. Still, the very use suggests an attitude that does not speak well for the professional health care provider. Know yourself. Understand why you might fall into the habit, and do your best to avoid it.

PATIENTS WITH DISABILITIES

Patients with serious and disabling physical or emotional disorders (for example, deafness, blindness, depression, psychosis, developmental delays, neurologic impairments) require that your approach be adapted to their needs (see Chapter 16). Patients who are emotionally restricted may not be able to give an effective history, but they must be respected and the history must be obtained from them to the extent possible. Their points of view and their attitudes matter. Still, when necessary, the family, other health professionals involved in care, and the patient's record must be queried to get a more complete story. Nevertheless, every patient must be fully involved to the limit of emotion, mental capacity, or physical ability.

Some of the most common communication barriers can be overcome if you keep the following in mind:

■ Families are, happily, often available to make the patient more comfortable and to provide you with information.

- Translators may be found for language barriers most of the time.
- Deaf persons often read, write, and/or read lips, but you must speak slowly and enunciate each word clearly and in full view; a translator who signs may be available.
- Blind persons usually can hear; talking louder to make a point does not help. Remember, however, that you must always make vocal what you are trying to communicate; gestures will not be seen.

THE HISTORY

Taking the history usually begins your relationship with the patient. A first objective is to identify those matters the patient defines as problems. You must be aware of the hidden as well as the obvious concerns, and you need to ensure accuracy to the extent possible. You have to develop a sense of the patient's reliability as an interpreter and reporter of events. Sometimes you will realize that the patient is suppressing some information either intentionally or without realizing it, underreporting other experiences, or giving them a context that is at odds with what you might feel appropriate. You will be in a constant state of subjective evaluation as the history is revealed. Indeed, some circumstances that worry you might not be thought by the patient to be unusual—all the more reason to seek understanding of the patient's perspective. Your attitude of friendliness and obvious respect will go a long way in the pursuit of information and in ensuring your patient's help in obtaining it.

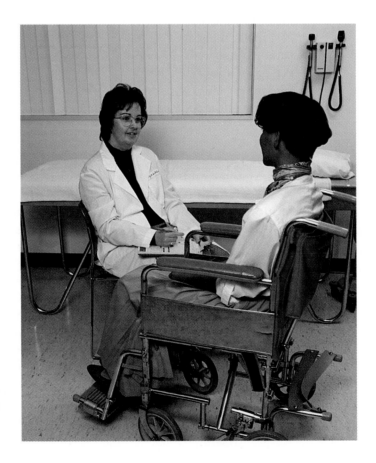

Interviewing a patient with a physical disability. Note the uncluttered surroundings; be sure the patient in a wheelchair has room to maneuver.

SETTING FOR THE INTERVIEW

The large university teaching hospital, the setting in which most health professionals are educated, is in some ways disadvantageous for a first experience with patient care. You must not allow the profusion of technical competence and the variety of skills to obscure the essential interactions that must take place between you and the patient. There are really few extra aids you need to extend your senses. Even in an empty space, the interview can be a rich and positive interchange, an experience that is rewarding to the patient, to those who accompany the patient, and to you.

Obviously, the setting in which you take the history must be as comfortable as possible. Often the space provided is small and rather barren. The colors are often not warm, and the chairs are straightbacked and uncomfortable. No matter; you are the focal point of warmth and attention. You can make sure that there are no bulky desks or tables between you and the patient. If possible, have a clock placed where you can see it without obviously looking at your watch (preferably behind the patient's chair). Sit comfortably and at ease, maintaining eye contact and a conversational tone of voice. Your manner can assure the patient that you care and that relieving the patient's worry or pain is your prime—in fact, your only—concern at the moment.

You can accomplish this only with a discipline that allows you to concentrate on the matter at hand, giving it for that moment primacy in your life, and dispelling both personal and professional distractions.

STRUCTURE OF THE HISTORY

Your purpose in taking the history is to establish a relationship and to learn about the patient, so that you might discover *with* the patient the issues and problems that need attention and the assignment of priority. The process has an organization that has been widely accepted for decades. The structure includes the following areas:

- Chief complaint
- Present problem
- Past medical history
- Family history
- Personal and social history
- Systems review

Do not forget the identifiers: date, time, age, sex, race, occupation, and referral source.

The *chief complaint* is a brief statement of the reason the patient is seeking health care. Directly quoting the patient is helpful. It is always important, however, to go beyond the given reason and to probe for underlying concerns that cause the patient to seek care rather than doing other things (for example, simply going to work). If the patient has a sore throat, why is he or she seeking help about it? Is it the pain and fever, or is it the concern caused by past experience with a friend or relative who developed rheumatic heart disease? Many interviewers include *the duration of the problem* as part of the chief complaint.

Understanding the *present problem* requires a step-by-step evaluation of the circumstances that surround the primary reason for the patient's visit. The medical history goes beyond this to an exploration of the patient's *overall health before the present problem*, including all of the patient's past medical and surgical experiences. Then *the patient's family requires attention*: their health, past medical experiences, illnesses, social experiences, deaths, and genetic and environmental circumstances that have influenced the patient's life. A careful inquiry about the *personal and social experience of the patient* should include work habits and the multiplicity of relationships in the family, school, and workplace. Finally, the *systems review* takes a different tack in that it includes a detailed review of possible complaints in each of the body's systems, looking for complementary or seemingly unrelated symptoms that may not have surfaced during the rest of the history.

Although there must be a structure to the history taking, rigidity is not necessary. You should be flexible, but you must also be compulsive about achieving as many of your goals as possible and sensitive to nuance in pursuing each suggestion, however subtle, that there may yet be information of substance to be found.

Provide opportunity for give and take, for the patient to ask questions and to explore feelings. You need not allow the patient to ramble; gentle constraint is most often recognized and successful.

TAKING THE HISTORY

Introduce yourself to the patient, clearly stating your name and your role in the process. If you are a student, do not mask the fact. Be certain that you understand the patient's full name and that you pronounce it correctly.

Address the patient properly (Mr., Miss, Mrs., Ms.) and repeat the name at appropriate times. Avoid the familiarity of using a first name when you do not expect familiarity in return. Never use a surrogate term for the patient's name; for example, when the patient is a child, do not address the parent as "Mother" or "Father." It is respectful and courteous to take the time to learn a name.

By this time you should *be seated at an easy distance from the patient,* comfortably and without any furniture barriers between you. Unless you have known the patient in the past and know that there is no matter of great urgency, proceed with reasonable dispatch, asking the patient to state the reason for the visit. *Listen; do not be too directive* at this point. *Let the patient spill it all out,* and after the first flow of words, begin to shape the direction of the interview. Begin to probe for what Feinstein calls the "iatrotropic stimulus," the stimulus to seek health care. If, indeed, 100 people wake up with a sore throat and 97 go to work and 3 seek care, what underlying dimension prompted those decisions?

This is the point at which you begin to *give structure to the present problem,* giving it a chronologic and sequential framework, fleshing out the bare bones of the chief complaint, probing for the underlying concerns. Unless there is some obvious urgency, go slowly, hear the full story, and refrain from striking out too quickly on what seems the obvious course of questioning. The patient will take cues from you on the amount of leisure you will allow; you must walk a fine line between permitting this leisure and meeting the many time constraints you are apt to have. You do not need a lot of time to let the patient know that you have *enough* time. Lean back, fix your attention on the patient, and *listen;* avoid interrupting unless you really have to, and do not anticipate the next question before you have heard the complete answer.

Once you have understood the patient's chief complaint and present problem and have obtained a sense of possible underlying concerns, it is time to go on to other segments of the history—the *family and past medical histories, emotional concerns,* and *social accompaniments to the present concerns.* Remember that nothing in the patient's experience is isolated. Aspects of the present illness require careful integration with the medical and family history. Keep in mind that the life of the patient is not constructed according to your outline, that many factors give shape to the present illness, and that any one chief complaint may involve more than one illness.

As the interview proceeds, thoroughly explore each positive response with these *relevant questions:*

- *Where:* Where are symptoms located, as precisely as possible? If they seem to move, what is the range of their movement? Where is the patient when the complaint occurs—at work or play, active or resting, in the city or country?

THE HUMANIZATION OF THE HISTORY

Sadly, the history taking of a patient's health and medical past may follow the routine course we describe so rigidly that little of the patient's substance creeps in, little of that which makes the person unique. It is all right to speak to and write of the patient beyond the constraints of the outline, to describe what you may hear and see in more than technical language, to lend your own style to the fleshing out of the history, and—as a result, perhaps—to give your patient a vibrancy that might otherwise be lost.

- *When:* Everything happens in a chronologic sequence. When did it begin; does it come and go? If so, how often and for how long? What time of day? What day of the week?
- *What:* What does it mean to the patient? What is its impact? What does it feel like? What is its quality and intensity? Has it been bad enough to interrupt the flow of the patient's life, or has it been dealt with rather casually? What happened contemporaneously that might be related? What makes it feel better? Worse?
- *How:* The background of the symptom becomes important in answering the "how" question. How did it come about? What is the ambiance of the complaint? Are other things going on at the same time, such as work, play, mealtime, or sleep? Is there illness in the family? Have there been similar episodes in the past? Is there concern about similar symptoms in friends or relatives? Are there companion complaints? How is the patient coping? Are there social supports? Remember that nothing ever happens in isolation.
- *Why:* Of course, the answer to "why" is the solution to the problem. All other questions lead to this one.

When these questions are kept in mind, you will be able to define what you have heard as clearly as possible. You can place it in a context appropriate to the patient's age and sex. You will also be able to determine the size of a complaint—that is, how intense it is, how frequently it occurs, and how much it affects the patient's life.

As the interview approaches its conclusion, it is possible to return to the more free-flowing, less structured style that might have dominated as the patient first described the present problem. It is a time to review the discussion and ask the patient to supply any missing details, to ask for questions, and to interpret and summarize what you have heard in a way that communicates your wish to devote whatever time is necessary to achieve comfort with regard to a mutual understanding of the issues.

Try to verify that *the patient understands* what has happened and what you have tried to communicate, and that the patient and family seem to be coping. Repeat instructions, if there are any, and ask to hear them back. Always discuss and explain the next step, whether it is the appointment time, methods of keeping in touch, exchange of telephone numbers, or planning for the physical examination that will follow the interview.

CONCLUSIONS

Be sure there is a satisfactory conclusion to the interview. Encourage questions. Interpret. Ensure the patient's understanding of and agreement with your interpretations.

AN APPROACH TO SENSITIVE ISSUES

It is not always easy to question the patient about sensitive issues, for example, sex, drug or alcohol use, or concerns about death. Still, they must not be avoided. Although there is no specific "right" way to deal with these questions, you must feel comfortable with your approach. The suggestions below are common sense guides that are useful at all times in all interviews; they may aid in your discussion of sensitive issues.

- Privacy is essential. Do not forget that this is as true with the older child and the adolescent as it is with the adult.
- Do not waffle; be direct and firm.
- Do not apologize for asking a question. You are doing nothing wrong.
- Do not preach. You are not there to pass judgment.
- Use language that is understandable to the patient, yet not patronizing.
- Do not push too hard. If the patient is defensive, recognize that the patient feels that defense is necessary. Do not demean the behavior; proceed slowly. It is possible to achieve your goals by acknowledging with the patient that you are touching on concerns that are common in society and that therefore need pursuit.

At the start, do not hone in on what the patient is doing or what is happening to the patient with regard to the issue at hand. Begin with open-ended questions. For example, most people find it easier to talk about cigarette smoking than alcohol consumption. You might say, "We've just asked about smoking. Now I'd like to talk about beer and other alcohols." Your questions should not be leading. You should not ask direct questions at the outset (for example, "How much do you drink a day?"). Rather, ask about the person's feelings.

Alcohol

The CAGE questionnaire (Box 1-6), advocated by Ewing, is very helpful as a model. CAGE is an acronym for *Cutting* down, *Annoyance* by criticism, *Guilty* feeling, *Eye-*openers.

The effective use of CAGE does not ensure absolute sensitivity in the detection of a problem. It can be complemented or supplemented by the TACE model (Box 1-7), particularly in the important task of identification of the potential of alcoholism in a pregnant woman.

SCREENING

There is a difference between a screening and an assessment interview. The goal of screening is to find out if a problem exists. This is particularly true of the CAGE, RAFFT, and TACE questionnaires. They are effective, but they are only the start, and assessment goes on from there. Discovering a problem early leads to a better treatment outcome.

BOX 1-6   CAGE Questionnaire

The following questions are included in the CAGE model:
- **C**   Have you ever been *Concerned* about your own or someone else's drinking? Have you ever felt the need to *Cut down* on drinking?
  Probe: What was it like? Were you successful? Why did you decide to cut down?
- **A**   Have you ever felt *Annoyed* by criticism of your drinking?
  Probe: What caused the worry or concern? Do you ever get irritated by others' worries? Have you ever limited what you drink to please someone?
- **G**   Have you ever felt *Guilty* about your drinking? Have you ever felt *Guilty* about something you said or did while you were drinking?
  Probe: Have you ever been bothered by anything you have done or said while you've been drinking? Have you ever regretted anything that has happened to you while you were drinking?
- **E**   Have you ever felt the need for a morning *Eye-opener*?
  Probe: Have you ever felt shaky or tremulous after a night of heavy drinking? What did you do to relieve the shakiness? Have you ever had trouble getting back to sleep early in the morning after a night of heavy drinking?

From Ewing, 1984.

BOX 1-7   TACE Questionnaire

The following questions are included in the TACE model:
- **T**   How many drinks does it *Take* to make you feel high? How many when you first started drinking? When was that? What do you prefer: beer, wine, or liquor? (More than two drinks suggests a tolerance to alcohol that is a red flag.)
- **A**   Have people *Annoyed* you by criticizing your drinking?
- **C**   Have you felt you ought to *Cut down* on your drinking?
- **E**   Have you ever had an *Eye-opener* drink first thing in the morning to steady your nerves or get rid of a hangover?

A positive answer to T alone or to two of A, C, or E may signal a problem with a high degree of probability, and positive answers to all four, with great certainty.

From Sokol, Martier, Ager, 1989.

BOX 1-8   RAFFT Questionnaire

The following questions are included in the RAFFT model:
R   Do you drink or take drugs to *Relax,* feel better about yourself, or fit in?
A   Do you ever drink or take drugs while you are *Alone?*
F   Do any of your closest *Friends* drink or use drugs?
F   Does a close *Family* member have a problem with alcohol or drugs?
T   Have you ever gotten into *Trouble* from drinking or taking drugs?

From Riggs, Alario, 1987.

For adolescents, RAFFT has been proposed (Box 1-8). The questions are quite useful for that age group, although they have not been clinically validated.

There is a certain sameness to all of these questionnaires; as you gain experience, you can adapt them to your style and to the particular patient you are serving, and you can adapt them to concerns about drugs other than alcohol.

Religion

We have made the occasional point that in fulfilling our roles we are not to be priests. That does not deny the patient the positive impact of faith upon a health or medical outcome. It does imply that we must be very careful in approaching the subject and careful not to impose in an area in which some patients may not wish us to tread. It is perfectly all right, if you think the situation calls for it, to ask certain questions:

- How would you characterize your religious or spiritual heritage?
- Do you belong to a formally organized congregation?
- Are the Bible or any associated writings important to you?

Given the responses to these questions, you will learn the patient's perspective and gain a sense of a need to go further. Some physicians, discovering a loss of faith in someone who has previously had a belief in God, do choose to discuss a return to faith, suggesting a complementary power that does not deny what the professional has to offer. Many health care providers cite empiric evidence that prayer aids in healing, and many do not hesitate to pray with a patient. There are studies that validate the use of prayer in the truly faithful. Praying with a patient does not make one a priest; it simply allows the sharing of faith in a circumstance that requires a highly personal decision from each of the participants.

Sexual History

Similarly, questions about the patient's sexual history are best initiated indirectly, addressing feelings rather than facts. The following is a good example of how to address the topic: "Are you satisfied with your sexual life, or do you have worries or concerns? After all, it isn't unusual. Most people do have some." You will recognize in this a trace of a leading question. However, it does not suggest what patients' feelings should be, but rather, if patients do indeed have concerns about sex, can comfort them with the realization that they are not alone.

Given the transition into the discussion, it becomes possible very often to gain more direct information, for example, frequency of sexual intercourse, problems in achieving orgasm, variety and numbers of "partners" (a non–sex-linked term), and particular sexual likes and dislikes. Questions about the possibility of exposure to HIV infection should not be avoided when you believe they are necessary.

Sexual Orientation

The sexual orientation of a patient must be known if appropriate continuity (or any other kind) of care is to be offered (American Medical Student Association, 1991). About 10% of the persons you serve are apt to be other than heterosexual (i.e., gay men, lesbian women, bisexual men and women). Given this knowledge, you are more likely to serve well during times of stress and illness (marshaling the patient's support systems), in the provision of gynecologic care (variable need for Pap smears), in the diagnosis and treatment of sexually transmitted disease, and in counseling about a variety of possible issues (myths about homosexuality, development of meaningful relationships). The risk nonheterosexual patients may feel in revealing their sexual preferences should be recognized. It may take courage, given the possibly unacknowledged and sometimes deep-seated feelings of heterosexism and homophobia in some health professionals. A reassuring, nonjudgmental word helps: "I'm glad you trust me. Thank you for taking the risk you may have felt in telling me." It is also supportive if the health care setting offers some recognition of the patients involved, for example, by making relevant informational pamphlets available in waiting areas.

Trust can be better achieved if questions are "gender neutral":

- "Tell me about your living situation."
- "Are you sexually active?"
- "Are your partners men, women, or both?"

rather than:

- "Are you married?"
- "Do you have a boyfriend/girlfriend?"

With this approach, if you are not judgmental and you have touched an area of need, a variety of questions applicable to *any* patient becomes possible. The questions should be phrased according to the patient's need and understanding. Given a positive response to your first outreach, topics for discussion are apt to flow more easily:

- Sexual behavior or feelings that need discussion
- Concerns with sexual identity
- Sexual behavior that increases the risk of disease or of experiences that involve the harassment of or by others
- Worry about masturbating or even touching the body

Quite obviously, *you must always be ready to explain again why you examine sensitive areas.* A successful approach will have incorporated four steps:

- An introduction, the moment when you bring up the issue
- Questions that first explore the patient's feelings about the issue, whether it be alcohol, drugs, sex, cigarettes, education, or problems at home, and then the direct exploration of what is actually happening
- A period in which you thoughtfully attend to what the patient is saying and then repeat the patient's words or offer other forms of feedback, so that the patient agrees that your interpretation is appropriate; in this way you can confirm what you have heard
- And finally, an opportunity for the patient to ask any questions that might be relevant

OUTLINE OF CLINICAL HISTORY

The following outline is offered as a guide for history taking (Griffith, Seidel, 1996). It should not set limits or indicate a rigid pathway; some ways in which it may be elaborated on are indicated in subsequent chapters. Chapter 24 (Recording Information) offers guidelines for recording the information obtained in the interview.

Chief Complaint

In the briefest terms, the chief complaint is the answer to the question, "What problem or symptoms brought you here?" The duration of the current illness should next be determined ("How long has this problem been present?" or, "When did these symptoms begin?"). The patient's age, sex, marital status, previous admissions at this hospital, and occupation should be noted for the record. Other significant complaints often surface while you are taking the history. These apparently secondary issues may have even greater significance than the original concern, since the driving force for the chief complaint may be found in them. What *really* made the patient seek care? A possibly unexpressed fear or concern? Each hint of a care-seeking reason should be thoroughly explored (Box 1-9).

Present Problem or Illness

No outline for the present problem would be applicable to all cases. You will probably find that it is natural and easiest to question the patient on the details of the current problem immediately after obtaining the chief complaint. Others find it is of more value to obtain the patient's history and family history before returning to the present. The specific order of questioning is not critical. What is important is that you obtain the needed information and organize it before finally recording it. At times it is helpful to let the patient provide an outline of the present problem and then go back to fill in all the pertinent details. This has the advantage of allowing the patient to voice the relative importance of the features surrounding the problem. At other times, experience will dictate that you must obtain the details by specific questions. Nevertheless, leading questions should be avoided. You want the *patient's* version, although you may ultimately write it in your own words. Among the concerns to be explored, you should include:

- Ultimately, a chronologic ordering of events
- State of health just before the onset of the present problem
- Complete description of the first symptoms. The question, "When did you last feel well?" may help define the time of onset and provide a date on which it was necessary to stop work or school, miss a planned event, or be confined to bed (Box 1-10)
- Possible exposure to infection or toxic agents
- If the present problem involves intermittent "attacks" separated by an illness-free interval, ask the patient to describe a typical attack (onset; duration; and associated symptoms, such as pain, chills, fever, jaundice, hematuria, seizures) and any variations; and to define inciting, exacerbating, or relieving factors such as specific activities, positions, diet, or medications
- Impact of the illness on the patient's usual life-style (marriage, leisure activity, ability to perform tasks or cope with stress), an assessment of the ability to function in the expected way with an indication of the limitations imposed by illness
- "Stability" of the problem. Does its intensity vary? Is it getting better, getting worse, or staying the same?
- Immediate reason that prompted the seeking of attention, particularly if the problem has been long-standing
- Compulsive appropriate system review when there is a conspicuous disturbance of a particular organ or system
- Medications: current and recent, including dosage of prescription and home remedies and nonprescription medications

BOX 1-9 | **General Guidelines for History Taking at the Start, Throughout, and at the Finish**

- Be courteous. For example, do not enter an examining room without knocking first. Address the patient formally, as Mr., Ms., Miss, or Mrs. You are engaged in a professional relationship. This does not, however, preclude pleasant inquiry about aspects of the patient's life.
- If more than one person is in the room, such as a spouse, parent, or friend, acknowledge that person, thus not only ensuring comfort, but also indicating that it is appropriate for the other person to remain in the room. While the patient's wishes should prevail, the attention to others is constructive and appreciated. They are to be thought of as partners in care.
- Ensure the physical comfort of the patient and those accompanying the patient, as well as your own. You should be sitting, not standing with one foot in the direction of the door. Try to have as little furniture as possible between you and the patient.
- Look at the patient. Good eye contact facilitates the discussion.
- Provide good lighting.
- Maintain privacy, using available curtains and shades.
- Provide relative quiet. If the setting is a hospital room, turn off the television set (it is distracting to speak with a patient whose eyes are constantly darting up to the television).
- Do not overtire the patient by trying to obtain the entire history at one time. Come back later to finish if possible. If it is during an office or clinic visit, let the circumstance guide the length of the initial interview; it may be appropriate to schedule another appointment to complete the history.
- Always give the patient a chance to state what is primary in his or her mind.
- Do not accept a previous diagnosis as the chief complaint. You need to know exactly what motivated the patient to seek care if you are not the first person to be involved in his or her treatment. You cannot rely on an earlier diagnosis as a firm indicator. The information you gather will be more helpful if you concentrate on what the patient says and not on a diagnosis that may too early lead the interview down a predetermined and inappropriate path.
- Take the patient's history and perform the physical examination before you look at information such as x-ray films and laboratory studies gleaned by other persons at other times. *What the patient has to say* should be considered first.
- Do not pursue the specific, and do not attempt precise descriptions until all of the patient's general concerns have been fully stated. Open-ended questions are necessary, particularly at the start of an interview. They often help get conversation moving.
- Avoid being judgmental. You are not a preacher.
- Avoid questions that may prompt an answer the patient might think you want to hear (leading questions).
- Arrive at a conclusion about the patient's ability to be perceptive and articulate.
- Particularly in the early stages of an interview, you should offer thoughtful, respectful silence with gentle encouragement to talk, and you should listen with obvious interest. Pauses are often productive.
- Be flexible. Remain ready to adapt to the unexpected. A rigid approach seriously limits the potential of the interview.

- Always try to "reach" what is in the patient's mind—the perception of the patient—never forgetting that you contribute by your responses and demeanor to what you are hearing and seeing as you and the patient continually adjust to the contribution each of you makes.
- Save direct approaches for later in the interview. (Ultimately it is essential to be precise about each finding and to establish the sequence of events.)
- If the patient is very talkative or too silent, offer some guidance. Sometimes these verbal behaviors offer a clue to neurologic or emotional need.
- As time goes by, sharpen the skill it takes to constrain a flood of information that may not be useful at the moment. Your ability to define relevance will develop with time and thoughtful experience.
- Symptoms can have multiple causes; do not hone in on one possible cause too quickly.
- A chief complaint or a report of a symptom of any kind very often carries with it a hidden concern. Look for underlying and unstated worries. Never trivialize any finding or concern.
- Define any symptom, concern, or finding by as many of the following dimensions as are appropriate: Where is it? What is it like? How bad is it? How long ago was it noted? Does it come and go? In what situation does it happen? Does anything make it better or worse? What else happens along with it?
- Be mindful of your choice of words. Jargon and medical terminology are often inappropriate. On the other hand, do not be patronizingly simplistic. You want the patient to have accurate information and to understand it. You do not want your words to intimidate or demean the patient.
- When asking direct questions, avoid using a manner that suggests you want only a yes or no answer. If you maintain eye contact, occasionally nod your head, and simply say "Go on" or "Let me hear more," the patient will often continue to talk and give a complete answer.
- Make notes sparingly; jot down enough key words to help you record the history later, but do not be so intent on note taking that it distracts the patient or interferes with listening and observing.
- Take the time to allow the patient to be dressed and comfortably settled after the examination. Saving time by conducting your interaction with the patient still "on the table" indicates a lack of regard and is often felt to be—and often is—demeaning.
- At the end of your meeting, give the patient an opportunity for review and necessary elaboration. You may discover solutions and resources that would not otherwise have become apparent. This takes time, but it provides important clues to understanding and management. It may reveal the psychosocial needs of the patient more clearly, may provide insights that will help your decision making, and leaves the patient more satisfied with the interview.
- The end of an interview should include a summary of what has been discussed and an indication of what is to happen next so that the patient clearly understands and uncertainty is alleviated. The patient, of course, should have the opportunity to express uncertainty; you allow this by asking a question such as, "Is there anything else you need to ask about or you want to bring up?"

BOX 1-10   Factors that Affect the Patient's Perception of Illness

An infinite number of subjective modifications may convert disease into illness or may cause illness without disease.

- Recent termination of a significant relationship because of death, divorce, or other less obvious intrusions such as moving to a new city
- Physical or emotional illness or disability in family members or other significant individuals
- Unharmonious spousal or family relationships
- School problems and stresses
- Poor self-image
- Drug and alcohol misuse
- Poor understanding of the "facts" of a physical problem

- Peer pressure; it occurs among adults as well as adolescents and children
- Secondary gains from the complaints of symptoms, e.g., indulgent family response to complaints, providing extra comforts, gifts; solicitous attention from others; distraction from other intimidating problems

At any age, circumstances such as these can modify perceptions and thus contribute to either the intensity and persistence of symptoms or, quite the opposite, the denial of an insistent, objective complaint. Sometimes, as a result, the patient will be led to seek help and, at other times, to avoid it.

Modified from Green, Stuy, 1992.

- A review, at the end of the interview, of the chronology of events, seeking the patient's confirmations and corrections (if there appears to be more than one problem, the process should be repeated for each problem)
- In the written history, it is helpful to give a specific number and brief title to each problem and, in a summary, to list the problems in the order of apparent importance (always remember that this can change)

Past Medical History

The past history can be of great value in assessing the present complaint.

- General health and strength
- Childhood illnesses: measles, mumps, whooping cough, chicken pox, smallpox, scarlet fever, acute rheumatic fever, diphtheria, poliomyelitis
- Major adult illnesses: tuberculosis, hepatitis, diabetes, hypertension, myocardial infarction, tropical or parasitic diseases, other infections; any nonsurgical hospital admissions
- Immunizations: polio; diphtheria, pertussis, and tetanus toxoid; influenza; cholera; typhus; typhoid; bacille Calmette-Guérin (BCG); last PPD or other skin tests; unusual reactions to immunizations; tetanus or other antitoxin made with horse serum
- Surgery: dates, hospital, diagnosis, complications
- Serious injuries and resulting disability; if the present problem has potential medicolegal relation to an injury, give full documentation
- Limitation of ability to function as desired as a result of past events
- Medications: past, current, and recent medications, including dosage of prescription and home remedies and nonprescription medications, when not mentioned in present problem
- Allergies, especially to medications, but also to environmental allergens and foods
- Transfusions: reactions, date, and number of units transfused
- Emotional status: mood disorders, psychiatric attention

Family History

Ask if there are any blood relatives in the patient's family who have illnesses with features similar to the patient's illness. Determine the ethnicity, health, or cause of death of parents and siblings, including their ages at death. Establish whether there is a his-

---

ETHNICITY

Some conditions are seen more often in certain ethnic groups, for example, thalassemia in those from the Mediterranean, Tay-Sachs disease in Ashkenazi Jews, and sickle cell disease in blacks. On the other hand, other conditions are not often found in some groups, such as cystic fibrosis in blacks.

Many Jewish people do not know if they are Ashkenazi or Sephardic. They may not even have heard the terms. Ask when their parents, grandparents, or remote ancestors emigrated. If it was in the seventeenth or eighteenth century, the patient is probably Sephardic; if it was in the late nineteenth or twentieth century, the patient is probably Ashkenazi.

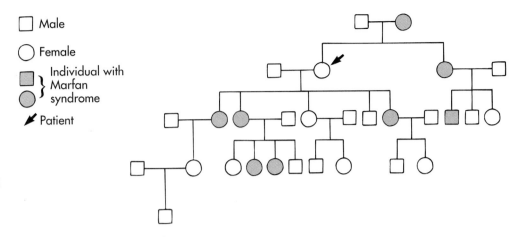

FIGURE 1-1

A Marfan syndrome pedigree. Marfan syndrome is an autosomal (non-sex-linked), dominant, single gene disorder characterized by arachnodactyly, subluxation of the lens, and aortic aneurysm. In this pedigree, the mother had Marfan syndrome and passed it on to her daughters. Because it is not sex-linked and is dominant, we find an affected male in a succeeding generation and inheritance based on the gene contributed by only one parent.

tory of heart disease, high blood pressure, cancer, tuberculosis, stroke, epilepsy, diabetes, gout, kidney disease, thyroid disease, asthma and other allergic states, forms of arthritis, blood diseases, sexually transmitted diseases, or any other familial disease. Determine the age and health of the patient's spouse and children.

If there is a hereditary disease—one that "runs in the family," such as sickle cell disease—inquire into the history of the grandparents, aunts, uncles, siblings, and cousins. It pays to review at least two generations on each side of the patient's family and to probe for consanguinity. A pedigree diagram is often helpful in recording this information (Figure 1-1).

Personal and Social History

- *Personal status:* birthplace, where raised, home environment as youth (e.g., parental divorce or separation, socioeconomic class, cultural background), education, position in family, marital status, general life satisfaction, hobbies, interests, sources of stress, strain
- *Habits:* nutrition and diet, regularity and patterns of eating and sleeping, exercise (quantity and type), quantity of coffee, tea, tobacco, alcohol; illicit drugs (frequency, type, and amount); breast or testicular self-examination
- *Sexual history:* concerns with sexual feelings and performance, frequency of intercourse, ability to achieve orgasm, numbers and variety of partners (it is useful to use the term partner, which does not indicate gender, during the early stages of discussion)
- *Home conditions:* housing, economic condition, type of health insurance if any, pets and their health
- *Occupation:* description of usual work and present work if different; list of job changes; work conditions and hours; physical or mental strain; duration of employment; present and past exposure to heat and cold or industrial toxins (especially lead, arsenic, chromium, asbestos, beryllium, poisonous gases, benzene, and polyvinyl chloride or other carcinogens and teratogens); any protective devices required, for example, goggles or masks
- *Environment:* travel and other exposure to contagious diseases, residence in tropics, water and milk supply, other sources of infection if applicable
- *Military record:* dates and geographic area of assignments
- *Religious preference:* determine any religious proscriptions concerning medical care
- *Cost of care:* resources available to patient, worries in this regard, candid discussion of issues

UBIQUITOUS SOURCES OF CLUES

An indicator of the possibility of acute lymphatic leukemia in a child with suggestive findings is the number of bathrooms in the house. The greater incidence is in the upper social and economic groups, hence this indicator.

Review of Systems

It is probable that all of the questions in each system will not be included every time you take a history. Nevertheless, some questions about each system should be included in every history. The range of these questions is listed in the outline that follows. More comprehensive and detailed questions concerning each system are listed in subsequent chapters and should be included whenever the patient gives positive responses to the first group of questions for that system. Keep in mind that these lists do not represent an exhaustive enumeration of questions that might be appropriate within an organ system. Even more detailed questions may be required, depending on the patient's problem.

- *General constitutional symptoms:* fever, chills, malaise, fatigability, night sweats; weight (average, preferred, present, change)
- *Diet:* appetite, likes and dislikes, restrictions (because of religion, allergy, or other disease), vitamins and other supplements, use of caffeine-containing beverages (coffee, tea, cola); an hour-by-hour detailing of food and liquid intake—sometimes a written diary covering several days of intake may be necessary
- *Skin, hair, and nails:* rash or eruption, itching, pigmentation or texture change; excessive sweating, abnormal nail or hair growth
- *Musculoskeletal:* joint stiffness, pain, restriction of motion, swelling, redness, heat, bony deformity
- *Head and neck*
  - *General:* frequent or unusual headaches, their location; dizziness, syncope, severe head injuries; periods of loss of consciousness (momentary or prolonged)
  - *Eyes:* visual acuity, blurring, diplopia, photophobia, pain, recent change in appearance or vision; glaucoma, use of eye drops or other eye medications; history of trauma or familial eye disease
  - *Ears:* hearing loss, pain, discharge, tinnitus, vertigo
  - *Nose:* sense of smell, frequency of colds, obstruction, epistaxis, postnasal discharge, sinus pain
  - *Throat and mouth:* hoarseness or change in voice; frequent sore throats; bleeding or swelling of gums; recent tooth abscesses or extractions; soreness of tongue or buccal mucosa, ulcers; disturbance of taste
- *Endocrine:* thyroid enlargement or tenderness, heat or cold intolerance, unexplained weight change, diabetes, polydipsia, polyuria, changes in facial or body hair, increased hat and glove size, skin striae
  - *Males:* puberty onset, erections, emissions, testicular pain, libido, infertility
  - *Females*
    - *Menses:* onset, regularity, duration and amount of flow, dysmenorrhea, last period, intermenstrual discharge or bleeding, itching, date of last Pap smear, age at menopause, libido, frequency of intercourse, sexual difficulties, infertility
    - *Pregnancies:* number, miscarriages, abortions, duration of pregnancy, each type of delivery, any complications during any pregnancy or postpartum period or with neonate; use of oral or other contraceptives
    - *Breasts:* pain, tenderness, discharge, lumps, galactorrhea, mammograms (screening or diagnostic), frequency of breast self-examination
- *Chest and lungs:* pain related to respiration, dyspnea, cyanosis, wheezing, cough, sputum (character and quantity), hemoptysis, night sweats, exposure to TB; date and result of last chest x-ray examination
- *Heart and blood vessels:* chest pain or distress, precipitating causes, timing and duration, relieving factors, palpitations, dyspnea, orthopnea (number of pillows

needed), edema, claudication, hypertension, previous myocardial infarction, estimate of exercise tolerance, past ECG or other cardiac tests

- *Hematologic:* anemia, tendency to bruise or bleed easily, thromboses, thrombophlebitis, any known abnormality of blood cells, transfusions
- *Lymph nodes:* enlargement, tenderness, suppuration
- *Gastrointestinal:* appetite, digestion, intolerance for any class of foods, dysphagia, heartburn, nausea, vomiting, hematemesis, regularity of bowels, constipation, diarrhea, change in stool color or contents (clay-colored, tarry, fresh blood, mucus, undigested food), flatulence, hemorrhoids, hepatitis, jaundice, dark urine; history of ulcer, gallstones, polyps, tumor; previous x-ray examinations (where, when, findings)
- *Genitourinary:* dysuria, flank or suprapubic pain, urgency, frequency, nocturia, hematuria, polyuria, hesitancy, dribbling, loss in force of stream, passage of stone; edema of face, stress incontinence, hernias, sexually transmitted disease (inquire what kind and symptoms, and list results of serologic test for syphilis [STS], if known)
- *Neurologic:* syncope, seizures, weakness or paralysis, abnormalities of sensation or coordination, tremors, loss of memory
- *Psychiatric:* depression, mood changes, difficulty concentrating, nervousness, tension, suicidal thoughts, irritability, sleep disturbances

Concluding Questions

At the conclusion of obtaining the history, ask the patient, "Is there anything else that you think would be important for me to know?" If several complaints are mentioned and discussed in the history, it is often useful to ask, "What problem concerns you most?" In certain situations, such as vague, complicated, or contradictory histories, it may be helpful to ask, "What do you think is the matter with you?" or, "What worries you the most about how you are feeling?"

CHILDREN

The history for an infant or child will be modified according to age. It is a good idea to remember that the following is just an outline.

Chief Complaint

The history may be taken from a parent or other responsible adult. However, the child should be included as much as possible as appropriate for his or her age. The latent fears underlying any chief complaint of both parents and children should also be explored. Note the relationship of the person providing the history for the child.

Present Problem or Illness

The degree and character of the reaction to the problem on the part of parent and child should be noted.

Past Medical History

- *General health and strength:* depending on the age of the patient or the nature of the problem, different aspects of the history assume or lose importance; reserve detailed questioning for those aspects most pertinent to the age of the child
- *Mother's health during pregnancy*
  - *General health* as related by the mother if possible, extent of prenatal care
  - *Specific diseases or conditions:* infectious disease (approximate gestational month), weight gain, edema, hypertension, proteinuria, bleeding (approximate time), preeclampsia
  - Medications, hormones, vitamins, special or unusual diet, general nutritional status

- Quality of fetal movements and time of onset
- Emotional and behavioral status (attitudes toward pregnancy and children)
- Radiation exposure
- Use of illicit drugs

■ *Birth*
- Duration of pregnancy
- Place of delivery
- Labor: spontaneous or induced, duration, analgesia or anesthesia, complications
- Delivery: presentation, forceps, vacuum extraction, spontaneous, or cesarian section; complications
- Condition of infant, time of onset of cry, Apgar scores if available
- Birth weight of infant

■ *Neonatal period*
- Congenital anomalies; baby's condition in hospital, oxygen requirements, color, feeding characteristics, vigor, cry; duration of baby's stay in hospital and whether infant was discharged with mother; bilirubin phototherapy, prescriptions (e.g., antibiotics)
- *First month of life:* jaundice, color, vigor of crying, bleeding, convulsions, or other evidence of illness
- *Degree of early bonding:* opportunities at birth and during the first days of life for the parents to hold, talk to, and caress the infant (opportunities for *both* parents to relate to and develop a bond with the baby)

■ *Feeding*
- Bottle or breast, reason for changes, if any; type of formula used, amounts offered and consumed, frequency of feeding and weight gain
- Present diet and appetite; age of introduction of solids; age when child achieved three feedings per day; present feeding patterns, elaborate on any feeding problems; age weaned from bottle or breast; type of milk and daily intake; food preference; ability to feed self

■ *Development:* these are commonly used developmental milestones. The list should be enlarged when indicated. Parents may have baby books, which can stimulate recall; photographs may be helpful
- *Age when able to:*
  - Hold head erect while in sitting position
  - Roll over from front to back and back to front
  - Sit alone and unsupported
  - Stand with support and alone
  - Walk with support and alone
  - Use words
  - Talk in sentences
  - Dress self
- *Age when toilet trained:* approaches to and attitudes regarding toilet training
- *School:* grade, performance, problems
- *Dentition:* age of first teeth, loss of deciduous teeth, eruption of first permanent teeth
- *Growth:* height and weight in a sequence of ages; changes in rates of growth or weight gain
- *Sexual:* present status: in female, development of breasts, nipples, sexual hair, menstruation (description of menses); in male, development of sexual hair, voice changes, acne, nocturnal emissions

■ *Illnesses:* immunizations, communicable diseases, injuries, hospitalizations

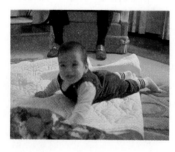

Family History

Obtain a maternal gestational history, listing all pregnancies together with the health status of living children. For deceased children include date, age, cause of death, and dates and duration of pregnancies in the case of miscarriages. Inquire about the mother's health during pregnancies and the ages of parents at the birth of this child. Are the parents cousins or otherwise related? A review of at least two generations on each side of the family is desirable.

Personal and Social History

- *Personal status:* school adjustment, masturbation, nail biting, thumb sucking, breath holding, temper tantrums, pica, tics, rituals; bed wetting, constipation or fecal soiling of pants, and playing with fire; reactions to prior illnesses, injuries, or hospitalization; an account of a day in the life of the patient (from parent, child, or both) is often helpful in providing insights.
- *Home conditions:* father's and mother's occupations, the principal caretaker(s) of child, parents divorced or separated, educational attainment of parents; cultural heritage; food prepared by whom; adequacy of clothing; dependence on relief or social agency; number of rooms in house and number of persons in household; sleep habits, sleeping arrangements available for the child

Review of Systems

In addition to the usual concerns, inquire about any past medical or psychologic testing of the child. Ask about the following:

- Skin: eczema, seborrhea, "cradle cap"
- *Ears:* otitis media (frequency, laterality)
- *Nose:* snoring, mouth breathing, allergic reaction
- *Teeth:* dental care

BOX 1-11   A Child Who Witnesses Violence

The witnessing of violence is a barrier to the smooth evolution of growth and development. It is a fact of life for many children, and it needs to be confronted. Questions should be straightforward, simple, and direct:

- Can you tell me what happened?
- What did you see? What did you hear?
- What scared you the most?
- What were you doing when it happened?
- Do you ever dream about it?
- Do you think about it during the day?
- Do you worry it will happen again?
- Whom do you talk to when you feel worried or scared?
- Why do you think it happened?
- How do you think it changed your life (for the older child and adolescent)?

These questions are not value-laden and are not too constraining. The child is free to talk if you can be comfortable with the frequent silences that may follow your questions. Remember, too, that parents can respond to the same questions in order to fill out the story, and you can then learn how they dealt with the circumstance and what they observed in their child's behavior following the event.

Modified from Augustyn et al, 1995.

ADOLESCENTS

There are many issues that cloud an approach to the adolescent. Essentially, the eternal questions—"Who am I?" and "Where am I going?"—are at the heart of the teenage experience. The problem may be illustrated in the example of a youngster who is deciding to smoke. What are the risk factors (Bradford, 1992)?

- Close associations with friends who smoke
- Less attachment to parents
- Poor school performance
- Lack of involvement in school extracurricular activities
- Poor self-esteem
- Need to appear "mature," leading to apparent rebelliousness
- Tendency of risk-related, often antisocial behavior to be clustered, such as tobacco, alcohol, and sex
- Peer pressure
- Susceptibility to advertising
- Skewed knowledge, attitudes, and beliefs about smoking

The suggested issues, including self-esteem, acceptance by peers, tensions with parents, and inadequate base of knowledge, can make it very difficult to bridge the barriers created by age differences. Those of you who are not too far removed from that somewhat hazardous time may not understand that you are no longer of that culture. Be aware. Make generous use of open-ended questions, and don't force an adolescent to talk. Sometimes allowing an opportunity to write a concern or allowing a choice of concerns presented in written, silent fashion may help. For example, a deck of index cards labeled with topics may be offered with the suggestion to select the ones to consider. The following subjects may be included (Green, 1992: adapted from a form used at Stanford Youth Clinic):

- Bed wetting
- Menstrual pain
- Concern with height or weight: too short, too tall, too thin, too fat
- Concern with breast size: too big, too small
- Concern with penis size: too small
- Worry about pregnancy
- Worry about sexual preference
- Sex? Ready or not?
- AIDS
- Parents' attitudes and demands
- Friends and their pressures
- School: not doing well, excessive work
- What am I going to do in life?
- Thoughts about dying

These are, quite obviously, highly charged issues requiring sensitivity in discussion, knowledge of the language of the adolescent, and an unforced approach if trust is to be established. This may not happen at the first meeting. Your consistent availability for talk will be helpful. In time, you may find that the patient, particularly an adolescent woman (but a man, too), would prefer someone of the same gender.

Flexibility, respect, and confidentiality are key. The adolescent must be aware that the respect is there and that confidentiality is appropriately assured; otherwise little productive discussion will result. The following letter to the editor of the *New England Journal of Medicine* makes the point (Levin, 1990).

MNEMONICS

ISSUES FOR ADOLESCENTS

HEADS

H   *Home*

E   *Education*

A   *Activities, affect, ambitions, anger*

D   *Drugs*

S   *Sex*

                    or

PACES

P   *Parents, peers*

A   *Accidents, alcohol/drugs*

C   *Cigarettes*

E   *Emotional issues*

S   *School, sexuality*

From Goldenring, Cohen, 1988; DiFrancesco, 1992.

BOX 1-12 **The Decade of Adolescence and a Basic Approach to History**

Adolescence continues throughout the years of the second decade of life. At first, the body is beginning to change and a degree of independence from parents develops. The peer group becomes important. In mid-decade, the peer group takes on a dominant role as a fuller independence from parents is established. Late in the decade, adult maturity is approached as the questions concerning personal identity and the ability to establish intimate relationships and career begin to take hold.

The following sequence suggests the structure of exploratory interviews with adolescents:
- How are things going at home? Tell me about your living situation (Don't assume the traditional family structure. Don't ask directly about who else lives in the house). The open-ended question at the start can lead to greater specifics later on.
- How is school going? Are you working? What is it about school that appeals to you? What is it about school that doesn't appeal to you? (Toward the end of the decade you may expect to hear more about jobs outside of school and ideas about the future.)
- Tell me about your friends. Where do you go with them? What do you do with them?

These beginning conversations about home and school and jobs and friends can lead to the many difficult areas that may trouble the adolescent—sex, drugs, and suicidal ideation. The open-ended question is a prelude to the more complex issues in an age period in which talk does not always flow easily as the adolescent moves from dependency to independency, from parents to peer group, and ultimately to self. The process of separation leads to maturity.

To The Editor: I am writing to express concern about what I understand to be a standard practice of physicians in dealing with minors. Recently, I was admitted to the hospital for surgery. Before my operation, my anesthesiologist met with me (16 years old) and my parents to review the procedure. At that time, I was asked if I used recreational drugs, smoked, or drank alcohol. Fortunately, my answers put my parents and my doctor at ease.

This apparent formality could prove to be very dangerous if an adolescent who takes drugs, drinks, or smokes is unable to be frank with the doctor while the parents are listening. Kids have the same right of patient confidentiality as adults. I suggest that doctors review their practices so that minors can speak with them privately, to ensure that appropriate safety precautions can be taken during surgery.

PREGNANT WOMEN

An individualized approach is needed in obtaining information appropriate to the age and concerns of the pregnant patient. For example, the very young adolescent may be concerned with the changes that pregnancy will bring to her body and friendships, whereas the older woman may be concerned about the genetic risks of the pregnancy. However, remember that for most women, pregnancy is an expected physiologic event.

Since pregnancy is a "normal" occurrence, the usual format of the clinical history is modified. Many health care providers and institutions use preprinted history forms (e.g., The American College of Obstetricians and Gynecologists Antepartum Record) on which to record information about the current pregnancy and past pregnancies; medical, contraceptive, family, and psychosocial histories; plans for childbirth; and risk factors for the development of complications.

If no standardized history forms are available, the clinical history format can be used.

Chief Complaint

The following information is included:
- Patient's age
- Marital status
- Gravidity and parity (see the example on p. 32)

Gravity and parity	G	T	P	A	L
	# of Pregnancies	# of Term Pregnancies	# of Preterm Pregnancies	# of Abortions/Miscarriages	# of Living Children

- Last menstrual period (LMP)
- Previous usual menstrual period (PUMP)
- Expected date of confinement/delivery (EDC)
- Occupation
- Father of the baby and his occupation

Present Problem

A description of the current pregnancy is obtained, and previous medical care is identified. Attention is given to specific problems, for example, nausea, vomiting, fatigue, edema.

Obstetric History

Information on each previous pregnancy includes the date of delivery, length of pregnancy, weight and sex of infant, type of delivery (that is, spontaneous vaginal, cesarian section and type of scar—further documentation of the scar is needed for women attempting vaginal birth after cesarian section—or spontaneous or elective abortion), length of labor, and complications in pregnancy or labor, postpartum, or with the infant (see Figure 1-2).

Medical History

The same information as identified previously is obtained, with the addition of risk factors for AIDS, hepatitis, tuberculosis, and exposure to environmental and occupational hazards. A mother who herself had intrauterine growth restriction (IUGR) carries this risk factor for her children (Klebanoff et al, 1997).

Family History

In addition to the information obtained previously, a family history of genetic conditions, twins, and/or congenital anomalies is obtained.

Personal and Social History

Additional information includes feelings toward the pregnancy, whether the pregnancy was planned, preference for sex of child, social supports available, experiences with mothering (of being both mothered and a mother), and history of abuse in relationships.

Date of delivery	Weeks of gestation	Weight	Sex	Type of delivery	Length of labor	Anesthesia	Complications	Condition of infant
10/97	40	7 6	F	SVD	12 hr	None	None	Good
8/95	36	5	M	LT CS	6 hr	Epidural	Fetal distress, preeclampsia	Infant discharged at 4 wks
6/90	8	—	—	SAB	—	IV	D&C	—

SVD, Spontaneous vaginal delivery; *LT*, low transverse; *CS*, caesarian section; *SAB*, spontaneous abortion; *D&C*, dilation and curettage.

FIGURE 1-2
Example of record of an obstetric history.

Review of Systems

The effects of pregnancy are seen in all systems; therefore all are reviewed, but special attention is given to the reproductive and cardiovascular systems. The endocrine system is assessed for signs of diabetes. The urinary tract is assessed for infection, and kidney function is reviewed. Respiratory function is also assessed, because it may be compromised later in pregnancy or with tocolytic therapy for preterm labor.

Risk Assessment

Risk assessment encompasses identifying from the history and physical examination those conditions that threaten the well-being of the mother and/or fetus. Various risk assessment categories exist for such conditions as diabetes, preterm labor, and preeclampsia, eclampsia, or pregnancy-induced hypertension (PIH).

OLDER ADULTS

Older adults can present a special challenge in organizing the information obtained from the history. They may have multiple health problems that are often chronic, progressive, debilitating, and overlapping with the process of aging. Disease symptoms may be less dramatic in older patients, with vague or nonspecific signs and symptoms. Confusion, for example, may be the only symptom of an infection, hypoxia, or a cerebrovascular accident. Pain is often an unreliable symptom, because some older patients seem to lose pain perception and experience pain in a different manner from the classic expectations. The excruciating pain usually associated with pancreatitis, for example, may be perceived by the older patient as a dull ache, and myocardial infarction can occur without the cardinal symptom of pain. Conversely, older patients have a higher risk of developing painful conditions or injuries. Since many conditions may be present simultaneously, the cause of pain may be difficult to isolate.

Some patients fail to report symptoms because they are afraid that the complaint will be attributed to old age or believe that nothing can be done. They may have lived with a chronic condition, such as urinary incontinence (now much more amenable to treatment than customarily believed), for so long that they have incorporated the symptoms as part of their expectation of daily living.

The tendency for multiple problems to be treated with multiple drugs places the older patient at risk for iatrogenic disorders. A complete medication history is essential, with special attention given to interactions of drugs, diseases, and the aging process. This is true for prescription drugs as well as for nonprescription drugs such as laxatives, nonsteroidal antiinflammatory agents, and drugs with anticholinergic side effects such as cough suppressants and hypnotics. It is particularly helpful to have patients bring in medication bottles (patients of all ages), especially patients who have a variety of chronic conditions and a variety of care providers.

Although appropriate at any age when there is apparent disability, functional assessment should be routinely included as part of the older patient's history (see Chapter 20 for additional information). In the review of systems, include questions that address functional capacity as suggested in the box below.

Other dimensions of functional capacity that should also be explored include social resources, economic resources, recreational activity, sleep patterns, environmental control, and use of the health care system. The interrelationship of physical health, mental health, social situation, and the environment is particularly evident in the older population.

In this regard, catastrophic illness is more apt to be a problem among the aged than among others. For all ages, the prospect of an illness that deprives the patient of the ability to join in the decision-making process emphasizes the need for advance directives, a documentation in the medical record of the patient's wishes regarding extraordinary means of life support, such as ventilatory supports and feeding tubes. This documentation should be complemented by the appointment of a surrogate (spouse, child, sibling, or other person with a close relationship) who has a legally executed durable power of attorney for health care. These matters, of course, should be considered whenever possible before the onset of catastrophe.

FUNCTIONAL ASSESSMENT

For All Patients

Quite simply, functional assessment is a disciplined attempt to understand a patient's ability to achieve the basic activities of daily living. This assessment has been best studied and implemented among the aged. However, the same thought should be given to anyone limited not by age but in some way by disease or disability, acute or chronic. It is sometimes difficult to discover just what limits function. A well-taken history and a meticulous physical examination can bring out subtle influences, such as tobacco and alcohol use, sedentary habits, poor food selection, overuse of nonprescription or prescription drugs, and less than obvious emotional distress. Even some physical limitations may not be readily apparent (e.g., limitations of cognitive ability or of the senses).

Whether increasing age or some other factor is the contributor to limitation, your assessment of a patient's response to your questions should be tempered by the knowledge that patients tend to overstate their abilities and, quite often, to obscure reality. You must be cautious in making your judgments.

For the aged, then, and for those limited by disease or other handicap, consider a variety of disabilities: *physical, cognitive, psychologic, social,* and *sexual.* An individual's social support system must be as clearly understood as the physical disabilities.

There are a variety of physical disabilities, including:

- *Mobility*
  - Difficulty walking standard distances: ½ mile, 2 to 3 blocks, ⅓ block, across a room
  - Difficulty climbing stairs, up and down
  - Problems with balance

- *Upper extremity function*
  - Difficulty grasping small objects, opening jars
  - Difficulty reaching out or up over head, such as to take something off a shelf
- *Instrumental activities of daily living (IADLs)*
  - Housework
    - Heavy (vacuuming, scrubbing floors)
    - Light (dusting)
  - Meal making
  - Shopping
  - Medication use
  - Money management
- *Activities of daily living*
  - Bathing
  - Dressing
  - Toileting
  - Moving from bed to chair, chair to standing
  - Eating
  - Walking in home

Limitations, even to a mild degree, in any or many of these areas will affect a patient's independence and autonomy and, to the extent of the limitation(s), increase reliance on other people and assistive devices. The patient's social support system and material resources are then integral to the development of reasonable management plans.

There are a variety of approaches to a finely tuned functional assessment with several available scales and instruments.

Modified from Fried, 1992.

SUCCESSFUL
PATIENT
INTERACTION

Those of us who offer care are
expected to be stunningly successful every time we interact
with the patient. We are not
allowed the privilege of frequent
failure. The expectation of perfec-
tion can most often be realized if
we accept the uncertainty in the
fluid relationship with the patient
and if our flexibility is disciplined
and ever alert.

■ ■ ■

Once the history has been taken, it is necessary to move on to the physical examination—the laying on of hands. Most of the remaining chapters in this book discuss the many parts of the physical examination. The chapters are necessarily segmented and are not meant to reflect the natural flow that you will develop with experience. No matter; in the end, we will bring it all together, and by then you should be ready to move on to the next step of responsibility in your clinical experience.

BOX 1-13   **The Kinds of Histories**

As your experience with interviewing increases, you will find that a "complete" history is not always necessary. One reason may be that you already know the patient very well or because you may be seeing the patient for the same problem over time. Therefore histories should be adjusted to the need at the moment. The following list explains different forms of histories:

- The *complete* history is designed to make you as thoroughly familiar with the patient as possible so that you and the patient can begin to seek solutions to problems or initiate a health supervision and preventive medicine goal. Most often, this history is recorded the first time you see the patient.
- The *inventory* history is related to but does not replace the complete history. It touches on the major points without going into detail. This history is useful when it is necessary to get a "feel" for the situation, and the entire history taking will be completed in more than one session.
- The *problem* (or *focused*) history is taken when the problem is acute, possibly life threatening, requiring immediate attention so that only the need of the moment is given full attention.
- The *interim* history is designed to chronicle events that have occurred since your last meeting with the patient; the substance of this history is of course determined by the nature of the problem and the need of the moment. The interim history should always be complemented by the patient's written record.

BOX 1-14   **The Computer**

The computer is a remarkable resource. It is helpful in recording and providing information. It can remind us about possibilities in diagnosis that we may not have considered and can put at our fingertips, if we have entered it all correctly, the information we have about the patient. Still, it poses a threat. There is an unacceptable temptation to substitute it at times for critical thinking. The computer has no sense of the subtleties of the human dimension; and, a serious threat to confidentiality, it needs to be used with discretion. Confidentiality can be breached not only by random, inadvertent intrusion by any of many users, but also by purposeful invasion. Although it is our responsibility to provide information appropriately and with the knowledge of the patient, we must remain the guardian of what after all belongs to the patient.

More information at *Mosby*   *http://www1.mosby.com/physexam_seidel*

CHAPTER 2

CULTURAL AWARENESS

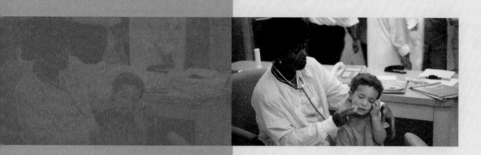

To be culturally aware is to understand those aspects of the human condition that differentiate individuals and groups. These differences sometimes have an overpowering effect on the health and medical care of individuals and groups. They cause a variation in responses to what is sometimes a personal responsibility and at other times a signal to seek out a health care professional. When we as health care providers are sought out, we will serve better if we are culturally aware (Box 2-1).

A DEFINITION OF CULTURE

Culture, in its broadest sense, reflects the whole of human behavior, including ideas and attitudes, ways of relating to each other, manners of speaking, and the material products of physical effort, ingenuity, and imagination. Language is a part of culture. So, too, are the abstract systems of belief, etiquette, law, morals, entertainment, and education of the young. Within the whole, different populations exist in groups and subgroups. Each is identified in some way by a particular body of shared traits; a particular art, ethos, or belief; or a particular behavioral pattern.

Any individual may and probably does belong to more than one group or subgroup. These multiple belongings can be the result of-among others-ethnic origin, religion, gender, occupation, and profession. For example, an Episcopalian, British, white male physician bears to some degree the cultural imprint of each of these groups.

DISTINGUISHING PHYSICAL CHARACTERISTICS

The use of physical characteristics (e.g., gender or skin color) to distinguish a cultural group or subgroup can be a trap. There is a sharp difference between distinguishing cultural characteristics and distinguishing physical characteristics. You should neither confuse the physical with the cultural nor allow the physical to symbolize the cultural. To assume homogeneity in the beliefs, attitudes, and behaviors of all men, or all British, or all physicians is to court error and to miss the mark in the effort to under-

BOX 2-1	Ways to Develop Cultural Sensitivity

- Recognize that cultural diversity exists.
- Demonstrate respect for people as unique individuals, with culture as one factor that contributes to their uniqueness.
- Respect the unfamiliar.
- Identify and examine your own cultural beliefs.
- Recognize that some cultural groups have definitions of health and illness, as well as practices that attempt to promote health and cure illness, that may differ from your own.
- Be willing to modify health care delivery in keeping with the patient's cultural background.
- Do not expect all members of one cultural group to behave in exactly the same way.
- Appreciate that each person's cultural values are ingrained and therefore very difficult to change.

Modified from Stulc, 1990.

stand the individual. The stereotype, a fixed image of any group that rejects the potential of originality or individuality within the group, is *itself* to be rejected. People can and do respond differently to the same stimuli.

This does not minimize the value of understanding the cultural characteristics of groups; it does deny the use of a physical characteristic, such as gender or race, as a metaphor for the culture of a group. Nor does this deny the interdependence of the physical with the cultural. Genetic imprinting, for example, precedes the development of the intellect, sensitivity, and imagination that allow the creation of a Beethoven sonata or a Miles Davis jazz piece, genuine cultural achievements. Similarly, skin color precedes most of the experience of life and the subsequent interweaving of color with cultural experience.

IMPACT OF CULTURE

THE IMPACT OF THE DRUG CULTURE

Almost one in 50 children in the United States has a parent in jail. Fathers in the vast majority, and among both fathers and mothers, about 9 in 10 have used illicit drugs and/or have at least *tried* treatment. If you suspect the possibility, you must ask, albeit discreetly.

Social and economic conditions define many of the subgroups in the United States (Box 2-2). Poverty and inadequate education have a cultural impact that is seriously reflected in health and medical care. Although death rates have declined overall in the United States since 1960, the poorly educated and those in poverty still die at higher rates than those who are better educated and economically advantaged. Furthermore, the disparity increased between 1960 and 1986 (Pappas et al, 1993). Morbidity, too, is greater among the poor. Recent studies also suggest that racial differences can have an impact on the care of individuals even in the absence of financial differences. Whites, for example, are more apt to be subjected to invasive cardiac procedures and tests than are blacks, suggesting that social, cultural, and clinical factors may be weighed differently in different cultural groups (Whittle et al, 1993). These rather stark facts are but the tip of the iceberg; they are, however, sufficient to underscore the need for cultural awareness in health and medical care professionals.

THE BLURRING OF CULTURAL DISTINCTIONS

Cultural differences are malleable in a way that physical characteristics may not be. For example, one nation can be distinguished from another by language. However, change and necessity mandate more and more that we learn one another's languages, beginning in that way to override political divisions. Modern technology and economics will slowly but inevitably ensure the achievement of universality in language.

BOX 2-2   **A Lexicon of Cultural Considerations**

Acculturation: The process by which an individual assumes the traits and behaviors of another culture, adapting to it, adopting its values, and shedding those of the group to which the person has been previously enculturated. The degree of acculturation can vary. The past is rarely, if ever, completely rejected.

Culture: A complex, integrated system reflecting the whole of human behavior and experience.

Custom: The habitual activity of a group or subgroup; patterned responses to given occasions, generally passed on from one generation to the next.

Enculturation: The process by which an individual assumes the traits and behaviors of a given culture, adapting to it, adopting its values, and taking on that particular cultural identity.

Ethnocentrism: The belief in the superiority of one's own group and culture, combined with disdain and contempt for other groups and cultures. Any degree of ethnocentrism in any health care provider impairs that person's effort and impairs the ability to understand patients within the context of their individual cultures.

Ethnos (Ethnic group): A group of the same race or nationality, with a common culture and distinctive traits.

Minority: A group that is different from the majority of a population, as with religion, race, or ethnic origin. When the difference is deep-seated in the historical relationships of the past or is obvious (e.g., because of skin color), the minority group may be treated unjustly, sometimes obviously, sometimes more subtly.

Norm: A prescribed standard of behavior within a group or subgroup. A norm indicates the allowable behavior expected within the group. To the extent that individuals adopt the positive values of their group or groups, and to the extent that they measure up to the norms, they are judged favorably or unfavorably by the other members of the group.

Race: A physical, not a cultural, differentiator based on a common heredity, using as identifiers characteristics such as skin color, head shape, and stature.

Rite: A prescribed, formal, customary observance (e.g., ceremonial religious acts, graduation ceremonies).

Ritual: A stereotypic behavior regulating religious, social, and professional behaviors (e.g., the expected use of "please" and "thank you") in a variety of circumstances.

Stereotype: A simplified, generally inflexible conception of the members of a group or subgroup.

Subculture: A group or subgroup having values and behavioral patterns or other distinctive traits that differentiate it from other groups or subgroups within a larger culture. Individuals may share the traits of more than one group or subgroup and may, with adaptation, shed some traits and adopt others.

Values: The ideals, customs, institutions, and behaviors within a group or subgroup for which the members of the group have a respectful regard. Values may be positive or negative and desirable or undesirable (e.g., with regard to charitable donation or criminal behavior, consensual sexual relationships or rape).

The changes may be imperceptible, spanning generations, but they are also relentless. However, the resistance to change, driven for better or worse by our culturally derived territorial need to protect individual space, is at the root of social, political, and economic tragedy. This worldwide resistance to develop a true "awareness" of each other is keenly evident. Still, as health care providers, we must not resist or we will not serve well.

THE PRIMACY OF THE INDIVIDUAL IN HEALTH CARE

THE IMPACT OF GENDER

If a *female* internist or family practitioner serves a woman, that patient is more apt to be screened with Pap smears and mammograms.

The individual patient may be visualized as being at the center of an indefinite number of concentric circles. The outermost circles represent constraining universal experiences, for example, death. The circles closest to the center represent the various cultural groups or subgroups to which anyone must, of necessity, belong. The constancy of change forces adaptation and acculturation. The circles are constantly interweaving and overlapping. For example, a common experience in the United States has been the economic gain at the root of the assimilation of many ethnic groups, with greater homogeneity dominating, but not necessarily excluding, earlier ethnic behaviors. However, predicting the individual's character merely on the basis of the common cultural behavior is not appropriate; understanding and taking the common cultural behavior into account are. The stereotype cannot prevail. The individual at the center is unique (Box 2-3).

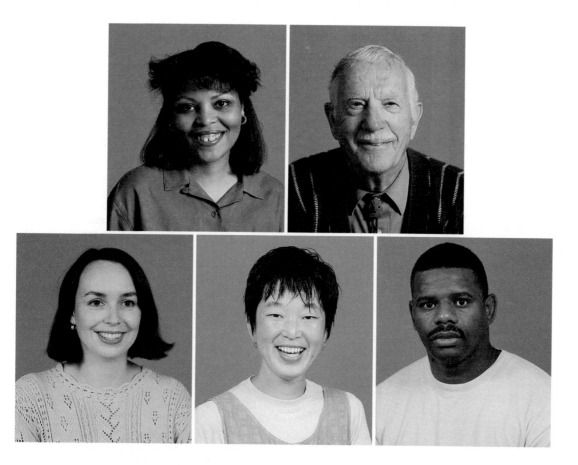

BOX 2-3 | **Questions that Explore the Patient's Culture**

- What do you think caused your problem?
- Why do you think it started when it did?
- What does your sickness do to you?
- How does it work?
- How bad is your sickness?
- How long do you think it will last?
- What should be done to get rid of it?
- Why did you come to me for treatment?
- What benefit will you get from the treatment?
- What are the most important problems your sickness has caused for you?
- What worries you and frightens you the most about your sickness?
- Who else or what else might help you get better?
- Has anyone else helped you with this problem?

Modified from Kleinman, Eisenberg, Good, 1978.

Nevertheless, ethical issues often arise when the care of an individual comes into conflict with the needs of the larger community, particularly with the recognition of limited resources, and in the United States, the imposition of managed care. The resolution of such issues is a matter of cultural disposition. Cultural dispositions, often vague and poorly understood, may constrain our professional behavior and may confuse the context in which we serve the individual. Understanding the patient's beliefs and practices can relieve confusion (Box 2-4).

BOX 2-4   **Cultural Assessment Guide: The Many Aspects of Understanding**

Health Beliefs and Practices

How does the patient define health and illness? How are feelings concerning pain, illness in general, or death expressed?

Are there particular methods used to help maintain health, such as hygiene and self-care practices?

Are there particular methods being used by the patient for treatment of illness?

What is the attitude toward preventive health measures such as immunizations?

Are there health topics that the patient may be particularly sensitive to or that are considered taboo?

Are there restrictions imposed by modesty that must be respected; for example, are there constraints related to exposure of parts of the body, discussion of sexual matters in male/female relationships, and attitudes towards various procedures such as termination of pregnancy or vasectomy?

What are the attitudes toward mental illness, pain, handicapping conditions, chronic disease, death, and dying? Are there constraints in the way these issues are discussed with the patient or with reference to relatives and friends?

Is there a person in the family responsible for various health-related decisions, such as where to go, whom to see, and what advice to follow?

Does the patient prefer a health professional of the same gender, age, ethnic and racial background, or is this not a significant issue?

Religious Influences and Special Rituals

Is there a religion that the patient adheres to?

Is there a significant person that the patient looks to for guidance and support?

Are there any special religious practices or beliefs that may affect health care when the patient is ill or dying?

What events, rituals, and ceremonies are considered important within the life cycle, such as birth, baptism, puberty, marriage, and death? What is the culturally appropriate way to respond to these life events? To what extent is an overt expression of emotion and spirituality inherent in that response?

Language and Communication

What language is spoken in the home?

How well does the patient understand English, both spoken and written?

Are there special signs of demonstrating respect or disrespect?

Is touch involved in communication?

Are there culturally appropriate ways to enter and leave situations, including greetings, farewells, and convenient times to make a home visit?

Is an interpreter needed? Should that person be a relative, friend, or a presumably objective stranger? Certainly, whoever it might be should be acceptable to the patient.

Parenting Styles and Role of Family

Who makes the decisions in the family?

What is the composition of the family, how many generations are considered to be a single family, and which relatives compose the family unit?

When the marriage custom is practiced, what is the attitude about separation and divorce?

What is the role of and attitude toward children in the family?

When do children need to be disciplined or punished, and how is this done (if physical means are used, in what way)?

Do the parents demonstrate physical affection toward their children and each other?

What major events are important to the family, and how are they celebrated?

Are there special beliefs and practices surrounding conception, pregnancy, childbirth, lactation, and child rearing?

Sources of Support Beyond Family

Are there ethnic or cultural organizations that may have an influence on the patient's approach to health care?

Are there individuals in the patient's social network who can influence perception of health and illness?

Is there a particular cultural group with which the patient identifies? Can this be clarified by where the patient was born and has lived?

What is the patient's need for relationships with others?

Is the patient socially gregarious or a loner, and is the preference indicated by behavior before illness?

Dietary Practices

What does the family like to eat, and does everyone in the family have similar tastes in food?

Who is responsible for food preparation?

Are any foods forbidden by the culture, or are some foods a cultural requirement in observance of a rite or ceremony?

How is food prepared and consumed?

Are there specific beliefs or preferences concerning food, such as those believed to cause or to cure an illness?

Are there periods of required fasting? How are those periods defined?

Modified from Stulc, 1990.

RELATIONSHIPS WITHIN THE HEALTH PROFESSIONS

There is a harmony—a unity—in the care of patients that is not hemmed in the cultural and administrative boundaries of the individual health professions. Caring and curing in a practical and a deeply emotional sense are not the sole province of any of them. To the extent that we stake out territories of care by allowing individual professional cultures and needs to take precedence over patient needs, we impede the

TABLE 2-1	Comparison of Value Orientations Among Cultural Groups
Value Orientation	**Cultural Group**
Time Orientation	
Present oriented: accepts each day as it comes; future unpredictable	Black, Hispanic, Native American
Past oriented: maintains traditions that were meaningful in the past; worships ancestors	Eastern Asian
Future oriented: anticipates "bigger and better" future; places high value on change	Dominant American
Activity Orientation	
"Doing" orientation: emphasizes accomplishments that are measurable by external standards	Dominant American
"Being" orientation: spontaneous expression of self	Black, Hispanic, Native American
"Being-in-becoming": emphasizes self-development of all aspects of self as an integrated whole	Eastern Asian
Human Nature Orientation	
Human being basically evil but with perfectable nature; constant self-control and discipline necessary	Black, dominant American, Hispanic
Human being as neutral, neither good nor evil	Eastern Asian, Native American
Human-Nature Orientation	
Human being subject to environment with very little control over own destiny	Black, Hispanic
Human being in harmony with nature	Eastern Asian, Native American
Human being master over nature	Dominant American
Relational Orientation	
Individualistic: encourages individualism: interpersonal relationships occur more with outsiders and less with family	Dominant American
Lineal: group goals dominant over individual goals; ordered positional succession (father to son)	Eastern Asian
Collateral: group goals dominant over individual goals: more emphasis on relationship with others on one's own level	Black, Hispanic, Native American

Modified from Kluckhohn, 1976.

achievement of harmony. The blurring of professional cultural borders works to the advantage of the patient, provided the blurring is motivated by the best interest of the patient. Each of us must understand our professional role and must be adaptable as cultural shifts suggest greater homogeneity in a number of those roles. In addition, each of us must recognize that there are health beliefs and practices that are different from the long-institutionalized Judeo-Christian, Western perspective that dominates health education in the United States (Table 2-1). Your ability to seek understanding, to respect differences, and to allow for the blurring of borders will be a measure of your ability to form mutually reinforcing relationships with other professionals and to care for a wide variety of individuals.

CULTURAL IMPACT ON DISEASE

Disease is shaped by illness, and illness—the full expression of the impact of disease on the patient—is shaped by the totality of the patient's experience. Cancers are diseases. The patient dealing with, reacting to, and trying to live with a cancer is having an illness-is "ill" or, in personal terms, is "sick." The definition of "ill" or "sick" is based on the individual's belief system and is determined in large part by his or her enculturation. If we do not consider the substance of illness, the biologic, emotional, and cultural aspects, we will too often fail to offer complete care. To make the point, imagine that while taking a shower you have done a self-examination and, still young, still looking ahead to your career, you have discovered an unexpected mass in a breast or a testicle. How will you respond? What contributes to the components of your response?

THE COMPONENTS OF A CULTURAL RESPONSE

The pattern of a culture can be shared with others and understood. When differences exist, you must be sensitive to that and certain that you understand exactly what the patient means and exactly what the patient thinks you mean in words and actions. Ask if you are not sure; this is far better than making a damaging mistake. Avoid making assumptions about cultural beliefs and behaviors without validation from the patient.

Those cultural beliefs and behaviors that will have an impact on your assessment of the patient include the following:

- Health beliefs and practices that may vary from the Judeo-Christian, Western model
- Diet and nutritional practices
- The nature of relationships within a family
- Modes of communication: the uses of speech, body language, and space

In particular, there can be a wide variety of ethnic attitudes toward autonomy. The patient-centered model, still firmly respected in the United States (although subject now to some critical discussion), is at odds with a more family-centered model that is more likely dominant, for example, among patients with Mexican or Korean roots. Many cultures believe that a patient should not be told of a diagnosis of a metastatic cancer or a terminal prognosis for any reason, attitudes not likely to be shared by Americans with European or African traditions. The desire to avoid dis-

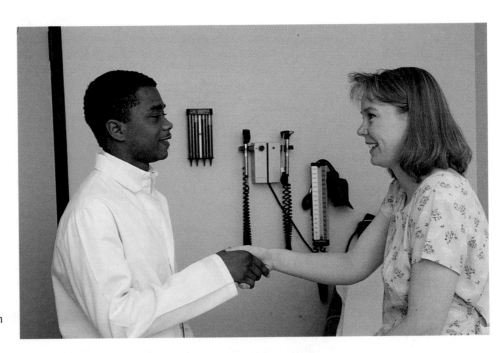

Being sensitive to cultural differences that may exist between you and the patient can help avoid miscommunication.

cussing such negative information is particularly strong among the Navajo Native Americans. Traditionally, the Navajo culture holds that thought and language have the power to shape reality. Talking about a possible outcome is thought to ensure the outcome. It is important, then, to avoid thinking or speaking in a negative way. It is important to think and talk "in the Beauty Way" (Carrese, Rhodes, 1995). The situation can be dealt with by talking in terms of a third person or an abstract possibility. Obviously, the conflicts that may arise from differing views of autonomy, religion, and information sharing need first, understanding, and second, an effort that is dominated by a clear understanding of the patient's goals.

COMMUNICATION

Communication and culture are interrelated, particularly in the way feelings are expressed verbally and nonverbally. The same word may have different meanings for different people. For example, in the United States, a "practicing physician" is an experienced, trained person. "Practicing," however, suggests inexperience and the status of a student to an Eskimo or to some Western Europeans. Similarly, touch, facial expressions, eye movement, and body posture all have varying significance.

Americans, for example, tend to talk more loudly and to worry less about being overheard than others do. The English, on the other hand, tend to worry more about being overheard and to speak in modulated voices, at a level that might be considered conspiratorial by Americans. Americans are very direct in conversation and are eager to be "logical," preferring to avoid the subjective and to come to the point quickly. The Japanese tend to do the opposite, using indirection, talking around points, and emphasizing attitudes and feelings.

Many groups use firm eye contact. The English look right at you and tend to blink the eyes rather than bob the head to indicate understanding. The French, too, have a very firm gaze and often stare openly at others. Americans are more apt to let the eyes wander and to grunt, nod the head, or say, "I see," or "uh huh," to indicate understanding. Americans also tend to avoid touch and are less apt to pat you on the arm in a reassuring way than are, for example, Italians.

These are but a few examples of cultural variation in communication (Hall, 1969). They do, however, suggest a variety of behaviors within groups, and as with any example we might use, they are not to be thought of as rigidly characteristic of the indicated groups. Still, the generalizations can at times provide insight to particular situations and can help avoid misunderstanding and miscommunication. If you are an American, you might feel disconcerted by an Englishman who is almost whispering, staring you in the eye, and blinking. Perhaps you need not be.

The cultural and physical characteristics of both patient and practitioner may therefore significantly influence communication. Social class, as well as age and gender, are variables that characterize everyone, and they can intrude on successful communication if there is no effort for mutual knowledge and understanding. The young student or practitioner and the elderly patient may have an important bridge to cross if they are to work together successfully. If that practitioner is a young woman and that patient is an old man, the crossing may be even more difficult. Recognizing the possible problem and talking about it, evoking feelings sooner rather than later, makes it easier. It is all right to ask if the patient is uncomfortable with any aspect of your person and to talk about it. Also, when any aspect of the patient's person disturbs you, you must try to understand why.

HEALTH BELIEFS AND PRACTICES

The patient may have a view of health and illness and an approach to cure that are shaped by a particular cultural and/or religious belief or paradigm. If that view is "scientific" in the sense that a cause can be determined for every problem in a very precise way, the patient is more apt to be comfortable with Western approaches to health and medical care.

However, the scientific view is reductionist and looks to a very narrow, specific cause and effect. A more naturalistic or "holistic" approach broadens the context. It views our lives as part of a much greater whole, the entire cosmos, that must be in harmony. If the balance is disturbed, illness can result. The goal, then, is to retrieve balance and harmony. Aspects of this concept are evident among the beliefs of many Hispanics, Native Americans, Asians, and Arabs, and they are increasingly evident in the United States today (Box 2-5). There are also those who believe in the "supernatural," or forces for good and for evil that determine individual fate. In such a context, illness may be thought of as a punishment for wrongdoing.

Clearly, there can be a confusing ambivalence in many of us, patient and provider alike, since our heartfelt and genuine religious or naturalistic beliefs may conflict with the options available for the treatment of illness. Consider, for example, a child with a broken bone, the result of a careless accident that occurred while the child was under the supervision of a baby-sitter. The first need is to tend the fracture. That done, there is a need to talk with the mother about the guilt she may feel because

---

BOX 2-5   The Balance of Life: The "Hot" and the "Cold"

A naturalistic or holistic approach often assumes that there are external factors, some good, some bad, that must be kept in balance if we are to remain well. The balance of "hot" and "cold" is a part of the belief system in many cultural groups, such as the Arab, Chinese, Filipino, and Hispanic. To restore a disturbed balance, that is, to treat, requires the use of opposites, for example, a "hot" remedy for a "cold" problem. Different cultures may define "hot" and "cold" differently. It is not a matter of temperature, and the words used might vary, for example, the Chinese have named the forces *yin* (cold) and *yang* (hot). Western medicine cannot ignore the naturalistic view if many of its patients are to have appropriate treatment for illness as well as disease.

Hot and Cold Conditions and Their Corresponding Treatments

Hot Conditions	Cold Foods	Cold Medicines and Herbs	Cold Conditions	Hot Foods	Hot Medicines and Herbs
Fever	Fresh vegetables	Orange flower water	Cancer	Chocolate	Penicillin
Infection	Tropical fruits	Linden	Pneumonia	Cheese	Tobacco
Diarrhea	Dairy products	Sage	Malaria	Temperate-zone fruits	Ginger root
Kidney problem	Meats such as goat, fish, chicken	Milk of magnesia	Joint pain	Eggs	Garlic
Rash	Honey	Bicarbonate of soda	Menstrual period	Peas	Cinnamon
Skin ailment	Cod		Teething	Onions	Anise
Sore throat	Raisins		Earache	Aromatic beverages	Vitamins
Liver problem	Bottled milk		Rheumatism	Hard liquor	Iron preparations
Ulcer	Barley water		Tuberculosis	Oils	Cod-liver oil
Constipation			Cold	Meats such as beef, water-fowl, mutton	Castor oil
			Headache	Goat's milk	Aspirin
			Paralysis	Cereal grains	
			Stomach cramps	Chili peppers	

Modified from Wilson, Kneisl, 1988.

she was away working, despite her husband's disapproval. She might think this accident must be God's punishment. It is important to be aware of, to respect, and to discuss *without belittlement* a belief that may vary from yours, in a manner that may still allow you to offer your point of view. This can apply to the guilt of a parent and to the use of herbs, rituals, and religious artifacts. After all, the pharmacopeia of Western medicine is replete with plants and herbs that we now call drugs. Our inability to understand the belief of another does not invalidate its substance. Nor does a patient's adherence to a particular belief preclude concurrent reliance on allopathic health practitioners. They can be complementary.

DIET PRACTICES

Beliefs and practices related to food, as well as the social significance of food, play an obvious vital role in everyday life. There may be a cultural and/or religious significance that will have an impact on your care. An Orthodox Jewish patient will not take some medicines, particularly during a holiday period like Passover, because the preparation of a drug does not meet the religious rules for food during that time. The Muslim woman must respect Halal (prescribed diet) even throughout pregnancy. A Chinese person with hypertension and a salt-restricted diet may need to consider a limited use of monosodium glutamate (MSG) and soy sauce. Attitudes toward vitamins vary greatly, with or without scientific "proof," in many of the subgroups in the United States. It is still possible to work out a mutually decided care or management plan if the issues are recognized and freely discussed.

FAMILY RELATIONSHIPS

Family structure and the social organizations to which a patient belongs (churches, clubs, and schools) are among the many imprinting and constraining cultural forces. This needs emphasis in America today, with its shift toward dual-income families, single-parent families, and an increased number of teenage pregnancies. The prevalence of divorce, roughly one for every two marriages, and the increasing involvement of fathers in child care suggest cultural shifts that need to be recognized.

One type of already known behavior may predict another type of behavior. For example, mothers who take advantage of appropriate prenatal care generally take advantage of appropriate infant care, regardless of educational level, marital status, family relationships, or maternal drug use (Butz et al, 1993). Adolescents who are unsupervised after school are more apt to smoke, use alcohol and marijuana, perform poorly in school, be depressed, and take risks than are those who are well supervised (Richardson et al, 1993). Being aware of this sequence of related behaviors is especially important because it often appears unrelated to the integrity of the family structure, gender, or racial or ethnic background. This is particularly true with the American cultural addiction to mass media. Adolescents who spend large amounts of time watching television and listening to heavy metal music are more apt to engage in risky behaviors than are those who do not; this too is regardless of race, gender, or parents' education (Klein et al, 1993). These examples remind us that one individual may belong to many groups and that the behaviors and attitudes of one of those groups, including pregnant women or adolescents, can override or modify the impact of the cultural values of other groups to which that person belongs.

> ### BOX 2-6 | Syncopation
>
> Think of the songwriter's success with syncopation: placing the accents on beats that are not ordinarily accented. Think then of the flexible approach suggested in syncopated history taking. Just as song writing requires the positive union of words and music, the union of two artistic expressions to create a third, the productive interaction with the patient requires the positive union of two cultures, one usually serving, one usually needing. The two join under emotional and practical pressures, mingling and achieving a result. The relationship and balance must be freshly resolved in every encounter, regardless of the past history of encounters. When the outcome is mutually supportive and satisfying, the process has to have had a fascinating rhythm and there must have been variation in the accents in the history and physical examination, in syncopation, from time to time (Rosenberg, 1991).

SUMMING UP

A compelling need exists to meet each patient on his or her own terms and to resist forming a sense of the patient based on prior knowledge of the culture or cultures from which that patient comes. That knowledge should not be formative in arriving at conclusions; rather, it should be drawn on to help make the questions you ask more constructively probing. Otherwise, you will see the patient as a stereotype, a risk you must avoid.

You need to understand yourself well. There is no denying that your involvement with any patient gives that interaction a character that is unique, and that you bring a substance that makes it to some extent different from what it might have been with anyone else. If you do not understand this well, your attitudes, largely culturally derived, may be so insistent as to overwhelm your better understanding of the patient, and that increases the probability of stereotypic judgment. You must constrain your prejudices and your likes, as well as your tendencies to preach and to be judgmental.

CHAPTER 3

EXAMINATION TECHNIQUES AND EQUIPMENT

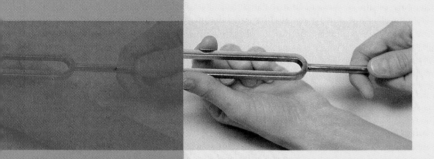

This chapter provides an overview of the techniques of inspection, palpation, percussion, and auscultation that are used throughout the physical examination. In addition, general use of the equipment for performing these techniques is discussed. Specific details regarding utilization of each of the techniques and the equipment as they relate to specific parts of the examination can be found in the appropriate chapters.

PRECAUTIONS TO PREVENT INFECTION

Because persons of all ages and backgrounds may be sources of infection for the examiner, it is important to take proper precautions. In 1985, largely because of the human immunodeficiency virus (HIV) epidemic, isolation practices in the United States were altered dramatically by the introduction of a new strategy, which became known as Universal Precautions (UP). The UP approach applies blood and body fluid precautions universally to all persons, regardless of their presumed infection status. In addition to emphasizing prevention of needle-stick injuries and the use of traditional barriers such as gloves and gowns, UP expands the precautions to include use of masks and eye coverings to prevent mucous membrane exposures during certain procedures, as well as the use of individual ventilation devices when the need for resuscitation is predictable. UP applies to blood, to body fluids that have been implicated in the transmission of bloodborne infections (semen and vaginal secretions), to body fluids from which the risk of transmission is unknown (amniotic, cerebrospinal, pericardial, peritoneal, pleural, and synovial fluids), and to any other body fluid visibly contaminated with blood. UP does not apply to feces, nasal secretions, sputum, sweat, tears, urine, or vomitus unless they contain visible blood.

In 1987, a new system of isolation, called Body Substance Isolation (BSI), was proposed. BSI focuses on the isolation of all moist and potentially infectious body substances (blood, feces, urine, sputum, saliva, wound drainage, and other body fluids) from all patients, regardless of their presumed infection status, primarily through the use of gloves.

BOX 3-1   Guidelines for Standard Precautions

Standard Precautions apply to all patients receiving care in hospitals, regardless of their diagnosis or presumed infection status. Standard Precautions apply to (1) blood; (2) all body fluids, secretions, and excretions except sweat, regardless of whether or not they contain visible blood; (3) nonintact skin; and (4) mucous membranes. Standard Precautions are designed to reduce the risk of transmission of microorganisms from both recognized and unrecognized sources of infection in hospitals.

Standard Precautions

Use Standard Precautions or the equivalent, for the care of all patients.

Handwashing

- Wash hands after touching blood, body fluids, secretions, excretions, and contaminated items, whether or not gloves are worn. Wash hands immediately after gloves are removed, between patient contacts, and when otherwise indicated to avoid transfer of microorganisms to other patients or environments. It may be necessary to wash hands between tasks and procedures on the same patient to prevent cross-contamination of different body sites.
- Use a plain (nonantimicrobial) soap for routine handwashing.
- Use an antimicrobial agent or a waterless antiseptic agent for specific circumstances (e.g., control of outbreaks or hyperendemic infections), as defined by the infection control program.

Gloves

Wear gloves (clean, nonsterile gloves are adequate) when touching blood, body fluids, secretions, excretions, and contaminated items. Put on clean gloves just before touching mucous membranes and nonintact skin. Change gloves between tasks and procedures on the same patient after contact with material that may contain a high concentration of microorganisms. Remove gloves promptly after use, before touching noncontaminated items and environmental surfaces, and before going to another patient, and wash hands immediately to avoid transfer of microorganisms to other patients or environments.

Mask, Eye Protection, Face Shield

Wear a mask and eye protection or a face shield to protect mucous membranes of the eyes, nose, and mouth during procedures and patient-care activities that are likely to generate splashes or sprays of blood, body fluids, secretions, and excretions.

Gown

Wear a gown (a clean, nonsterile gown is adequate) to protect skin and to prevent soiling of clothing during procedures and patient-care activities that are likely to generate splashes or sprays of blood, body fluids, secretions, or excretions. Select a gown that is appropriate for the activity and amount of fluid likely to be encountered. Remove a soiled gown as promptly as possible, and wash hands to avoid transfer of microorganisms to other patients or environments.

Patient-Care Equipment

Handle used patient-care equipment soiled with blood, body fluids, secretions, and excretions in a manner that prevents skin and mucous membrane exposures, contamination of clothing, and transfer of microorganisms to other patients and environments. Ensure that reusable equipment is not used for the care of another patient until it has been cleaned and reprocessed appropriately. Ensure that single-use items are discarded properly.

Environmental Control

Ensure that the hospital has adequate procedures for the routine care, cleaning, and disinfection of environmental surfaces, beds, bedrails, bedside equipment, and other frequently touched surfaces, and ensure that these procedures are being followed.

Linen

Handle, transport, and process used linen soiled with blood, body fluids, secretions, and excretions in a manner that prevents skin and mucous membrane exposures and contamination of clothing, and that avoids transfer of microorganisms to other patients and environments.

Occupational Health and Bloodborne Pathogens

- Take care to prevent injuries when using needles, scalpels, and other sharp instruments or devices; when handling sharp instruments after procedures; when cleaning used instruments; and when disposing of used needles. Never recap used needles, or otherwise manipulate them using both hands, or use any other technique that involves directing the point of a needle toward any part of the body; rather, use either a one-handed "scoop" technique or a mechanical device designed for holding the needle sheath. Do not remove used needles from disposable syringes by hand, and do not bend, break, or otherwise manipulate used needles by hand. Place used disposable syringes and needles, scalpel blades, and other sharp items in appropriate puncture-resistant containers, which are located as close as practical to the area in which the items were used, and place reusable syringes and needles in a puncture-resistant container for transport to the reprocessing area.
- Use mouthpieces, resuscitation bags, or other ventilation devices as an alternative to mouth-to-mouth resuscitation methods in areas where the need for resuscitation is predictable.

Patient Placement

Place a patient who contaminates the environment or who does not (or cannot be expected to) assist in maintaining appropriate hygiene or environmental control in a private room. If a private room is not available, consult with infection control professionals regarding patient placement or other alternatives.

From Garner J, 1996.

The guideline for Standard Precautions, subsequently developed, synthesizes the major features of UP and BSI into a single set of precautions to be used for the care of all patients in hospitals regardless of their presumed infection status. These precautions are designed to reduce the risk of transmission of bloodborne and other pathogens in hospitals.

The Standard Precautions are summarized in Box 3-1. Although the precautions are intended for the care of hospitalized patients, the need for such precautions extends to the primary care areas as well. Remember that precautions can be used not only to protect health care workers, but also to protect patients with compromised immune systems.

A second tier of precautions, named Transmission-Based Precautions, is designed only for the care of specified patients who are known or suspected to be infected by epidemiologically important pathogens that are spread by airborne or droplet transmission or by contact with dry skin or contaminated surfaces. Further information regarding the recommendations for Transmission-Based Precautions can be obtained from the Centers for Disease Control (CDC: http://www.cdc.gov/ncidod/hip/isolat/isopart2.htm, updated Feb. 18, 1997).

LATEX ALLERGY

The incidence of serious allergic reaction to latex has increased dramatically in recent years. Latex allergy occurs when the body's immune system reacts to proteins found in natural rubber latex. Latex products also contain added chemicals such as antioxidants, which can cause irritant or delayed hypersensitivity reactions. See Box 3-2 for a description of the types of latex reactions.

Health care providers are at risk for developing latex allergy because of their exposure to latex through gloves and other equipment and supplies. Sensitization to the latex proteins occurs through direct skin or mucous membrane contact or through airborne exposure. Table 3-1 lists examples of workplace and home products that may contain latex. The National Institute for Occupational Safety and Health (NIOSH) has issued an alert and recommendations for both employers and workers to prevent latex allergy in the workplace. See Box 3-3 for a summary of the recommendations that you should follow to protect yourself from latex exposure in the workplace. Also be aware that some patients, such as children with spina bifida who have had multiple procedures or surgeries performed, are at higher risk for the development of latex allergy.

BOX 3-2   Types of Latex Reactions

- *Irritant contact dermatitis*—chemical irritation that does not involve the immune system. Symptoms are usually dry, itching, irritated areas on the skin, usually the hands.
- *Type IV dermatitis (delayed hypersensitivity)*—allergic contact dermatitis that involves the immune system and is caused by the chemicals used in latex products. The skin reaction usually begins 24 to 48 hours after contact and resembles that caused by poison ivy. The reaction may progress to oozing skin blisters.
- *Type I systemic reactions*—true allergic reaction caused by protein antibodies (IgE antibodies) that form as a result of interaction between a foreign protein and the body's immune system. The antigen antibody reaction causes release of histamine, leukotrienes, prostaglandins, and kinins. These chemicals cause the symptoms of allergic reactions. Type I reactions include the following symptoms: local urticaria (skin wheals), generalized urticaria with angioedema (tissue swelling), asthma, eye/nose itching and gastrointestinal symptoms, anaphylaxis (cardiovascular collapse), chronic asthma, and permanent lung damage.

TABLE 3-1 Examples of Products Containing Latex and Nonlatex Substitutes

This list is intended to provide examples of products. It is not an exhaustive list.

Products Containing Latex	Nonlatex Substitutes
Medical Equipment	
Disposable gloves	Vinyl, nitrile, or neoprene gloves
Blood pressure cuffs	Covered cuffs
Stethoscope tubing	Covered tubing
Intravenous injection ports	Needleless system, stopcocks, covered latex ports
Tourniquets	Cloth-covered tourniquets
Syringes	Glass syringes
Adhesive tape	Nonlatex tapes
Oral and nasal airways	Nonlatex tubes
Endotracheal tubes	Hard plastic tubes
Catheters	Silicone catheters
Eye goggles	Silicone eye goggles
Anesthesia masks	Silicone masks
Respirators	Nonlatex respirators
Rubber aprons	Cloth-covered aprons
Wound drains	Silicone drains
Medication vial stoppers	Stoppers removed
Household Items	
Rubber bands	String
Erasers	Silicone erasers
Automobile tires	(No substitute)
Motorcycle and bicycle handgrips	Handgrips removed or covered
Carpeting	Other types of flooring
Swimming goggles	Silicone sealers
Racquet handles	Handles covered
Shoe soles	Leather shoes
Expandable fabric (waistbands)	Fabric removed or covered
Dishwashing gloves	Vinyl gloves
Hot water bottles	Bottles covered
Condoms	Nonlatex condoms
Diaphragms	Synthetic rubber diaphragms
Balloons	Mylar balloons
Pacifiers and baby bottle nipples	Silicone, plastic, or nonlatex pacifiers and nipples

BOX 3-3 Summary of Recommendations for Workers to Prevent Latex Allergy

- Use nonlatex gloves for activities not likely to involve infectious materials. Hypoallergenic gloves are not necessarily latex-free, but they may reduce reactions to chemical additives in the latex.
- For barrier protection when handling infectious materials, use powder-free latex gloves with reduced protein content.
- When wearing latex gloves, do not use oil-based hand creams or lotions unless they have been shown to reduce latex-related problems.
- After removing gloves, wash hands with mild soap and dry thoroughly.
- Use good housekeeping practices to remove latex-containing dust from the workplace.
- Take advantage of all latex allergy education and training provided.
- If you develop symptoms of latex allergy, avoid direct contact with latex gloves and products until you can see a health care provider experienced in treating latex allergy.

From NIOSH, 1997.

EXAMINATION TECHNIQUES

INSPECTION

Inspection is the process of observation. Your eyes and nose are sensitive tools for gathering data throughout the examination (Box 3-4). Take time to practice and develop this skill. Challenge yourself to see how much information can be collected through inspection alone. As the patient enters the room, for example, observe the gait and stance and the ease or difficulty with which undressing and getting onto the examining table are accomplished. These observations alone will reveal a great deal about the patient's neurologic and musculoskeletal integrity. Is eye contact made? Is the demeanor appropriate for the situation? Is the clothing appropriate for the weather? The answers to these questions provide clues to the patient's emotional and mental status. Color and moisture of the skin or an unusual odor can alert you to the possibility of underlying disease. These preliminary observations require only a few seconds, yet they provide basic information that can influence the rest of the examination.

Unlike palpation, percussion, and auscultation, inspection can continue throughout the history-taking process and during the physical examination. With this kind of continuity, what you see about the patient and the patient's demeanor is constantly subject to confirmation or dispute. Be aware of both the patient's verbal statements and body language right up to the end of the appointment. At that point, the stance, stride, strength of a handshake, and eye contact can tell you a great deal about the patient's perception of the consultation.

Some general guidelines will be helpful as you proceed through the examination and inspect each area of the body. Adequate lighting is essential. The primary lighting can be either daylight or artificial light, as long as the light is direct enough to re-

---

BOX 3-4 | **The Sense of Smell: The Nose as an Aid to Physical Examination**

On occasion, a first observation when entering an examining room may be an odor, obvious and pervasive. A foreign body that has been present in a child's nose may do this. Indeed, many problematic conditions can be characterized in this way, but the presentation is rather subtle more often than obvious. Distinctive odors provide clues, occasionally the first one, leading to the diagnosis of certain conditions, some of which need early detection if life-threatening sequelae are to be avoided. Some examples of odor "clues" are given below.

	Source of Odor	Kind of Odor
Inborn errors of metabolism	Phenylalanine hydroxylase defect	Mousy
	Tyrosinemia	Fishy
Infectious diseases	Tuberculosis	Stale beer
	Diphtheria	Sweetish
	Rubella	Freshly plucked feathers
Ingestions of poison or intoxication	Cyanide	Bitter almond
	Chloroform and salicylates	Fruity
Physiologic nondisease states	Sweaty feet	Cheesy
Foreign bodies (e.g., in the nose or vagina)	Organic material (e.g., bean in a child's nose)	Foul-smelling discharge

The odors may range from objectionable to bland to rather pleasant. The descriptors include *fishy, putrid, fetid, alcoholic, bitter almond,* and on and on. The examiner often is the one to determine the characterization of the odor.

In years past, practiced clinicians noted that certain breath and body odors were indicative of a variety of conditions or diseases. Some examples follow:

Condition or Disease	Odor
Yellow fever	Butcher shop
Typhoid fever	Fresh-baked bread
Diabetic coma	Fruity smell
Small pox	Zoo-like smell
Scurvy	Putrid smell
Pellagra	Sour, musty bread

These lessons from the past remind us that the nose, fully as much as our other sensors, is portable equipment that we must train and educate if it is to be of value to us as competent examiners.

Suggested by a Grand Rounds presentation, Rebecca Vickers, MD, May 28, 1997.

BOX 3-5 **Examination Techniques: Cultural Considerations**

Nonverbal communication, which includes touch, posture, space, and facial expression, is an integral part of physical examination. Nonverbal communication may have different meanings in different cultures. For example, in North American middle-class culture, direct eye contact is important, whereas in some other cultures (Asian, Native American, Indochinese, Arab, Appalachian) looking directly at another person may be a sign of disrespect or aggression. Touch is also subject to varied cultural interpretations. Some groups, such as those of Mediterranean descent, use touch to communicate feelings, while other groups view touch as an invasion of privacy. As you become sensitive to cultural variations, remember that individuals are just that—individual—and avoid the pitfall of making decisions based on stereotypes rather than on specifics of the patient and the circumstances.

veal color, texture, and mobility without distortion from shadowing. Secondary, tangential lighting from a lamp that casts shadows is also important for observing contour and variations in the body surface. Inspection should be unhurried. Give yourself time to tune in to what you are inspecting. Pay attention to detail and note your findings. An important rule to remember is that you have to expose what you want to inspect. All too often, exposure is compromised for modesty at the cost of important information. Part of your job is to look and observe critically.

Knowing what to look for is, of course, essential to the process of focused attention. Be willing to validate inspection findings with your patient. The ability to narrow or widen your perceptual field selectively will come with time and experience, but the process must begin right now and will develop only through practice.

PALPATION

Palpation involves the use of your hands and fingers to gather information through the sense of touch. Certain parts of your hands and fingers are better than others for specific types of palpation (Table 3-2). The palmar surface of the fingers and finger pads is more sensitive than the fingertips and is used whenever discriminatory touch is needed for determining position, texture, size, consistency, masses, fluid, and crepitus. The ulnar surface of the hand and fingers is the most sensitive area for distinguishing vibration. The dorsal surface of the hands is best for estimating temperature. Of course, this estimate provides only a crude measure and is best used to detect temperature differences in comparing parts of the body.

Specific techniques of palpation are discussed in more detail as they occur in each part of the examination. Palpation may be either light or deep and is controlled by the amount of pressure applied with the fingers or hand. For light palpation press in to a depth up to 1 cm, and for deep palpation press in about 4 cm. Light palpation should always precede deep palpation, since the latter may elicit tenderness or disrupt tissue or fluid, thus interfering with your ability to gather information through light

RIGHT-SIDED EXAMINATION?

It is the convention, at least in the United States, to teach students to examine patients from the right side and to palpate and percuss with the right hand. We have generally continued with this convention, if only to simplify description of a procedure or technique. We feel no obligation to adhere strictly to the right-sided approach. Our suggestion is that students learn to use both hands for examination and that they be allowed to stand on either side of the patient, depending on both the patient's and examiner's convenience and comfort. The important issue is to develop an approach that is useful and practical and yields the desired results.

TABLE 3-2	Areas of the Hand to Use in Palpation
To Determine	**Use**
Position, texture, size, consistency, fluid, crepitus, form of a mass, or structure	Palmar surface of the fingers and finger pads
Vibration	Ulnar surfaces of hand and fingers
Temperature	Dorsal surface of hands

palpation. Short fingernails are essential to avoid discomfort or injury to the patient. In keeping with current concerns about bacterial or viral transmission, most practitioners now recommend that you wear gloves while examining a patient.

Touch is in many ways therapeutic, and palpation is the actuality of the "laying on of hands." It is the moment at which we begin our physical invasion of the patient's body. Our much repeated advice that your approach be gentle and your hands be warm is not only practical but symbolic of your respect for the patient and for the privilege the patient gives you.

PERCUSSION

Percussion involves striking one object against another, thus producing vibration and subsequent sound waves. In the physical examination your finger functions as a hammer, and the vibration is produced by the impact of the finger against underlying tissue. Sound waves are heard as percussion tones (called resonance) that arise from vibrations 4 to 6 cm deep in the body tissue. The degree of percussion tone is determined by the density of the medium through which the sound waves travel. The more dense the medium, the quieter the percussion tone. The percussion tone over air is loud, over fluid less loud, and over solid areas soft. The degree of percussion tone is classified and ordered as shown in Table 3-3 and in the following list:

- Tympany
- Hyperresonance
- Resonance
- Dullness
- Flatness

Tympany is the loudest, and flatness is the quietest. Quantification of the percussion tone is difficult, especially at first. As noted in Table 3-3 for points of reference, the gastric bubble is considered to be tympanic, air-filled lungs (as in emphysema) to be hyperresonant, healthy lungs to be resonant, the liver to be dull, and muscle to be flat. Degree of percussion is more easily distinguished by listening to the sound change as you move from one area to another. Since it is easier to hear the change from resonance to dullness rather than from dullness to resonance, proceed with percussion from areas of resonance to areas of dullness. A partially full milk carton is a good tool for practicing percussion skills. Begin with percussion over the air-filled space of the carton, appreciating its resonant quality. Work your way downward and listen for the change in sound as you encounter the milk. This principle applies in percussion of body tissues and cavities.

TABLE 3-3	Percussion Notes				
Tone	**Intensity**	**Pitch**	**Duration**	**Quality**	**Example Where Heard**
Tympanic	Loud	High	Moderate	Drumlike	Gastric bubble
Hyperresonant	Very loud	Low	Long	Boomlike	Emphysematous lungs
Resonant	Loud	Low	Long	Hollow	Healthy lung tissue
Dull	Soft to moderate	Moderate to high	Moderate	Thudlike	Over liver
Flat	Soft	High	Short	Very dull	Over muscle

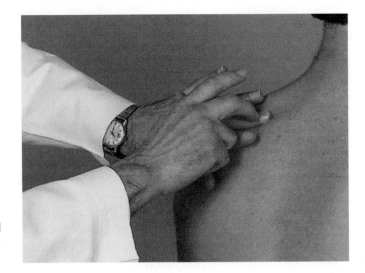

FIGURE 3-1

Percussion technique: tapping the interphalangeal joint. Only the middle finger of the examiner's nondominant hand should be in contact with the patient's skin surface.

The techniques of percussion are the same, regardless of the structure you are percussing. Immediate (direct) percussion involves striking the finger or hand directly against the body. A more refined variant of the technique, called mediate or indirect percussion, is used by most clinicians. In this technique the finger of one hand acts as the hammer (plexor) and a finger of the other hand acts as the striking surface. To perform indirect percussion, place your nondominant hand on the surface of the body with the fingers slightly spread. The distal phalanx of the middle finger should be placed firmly on the body surface with the other fingers slightly elevated off the surface. Snap the wrist of your other hand downward, and with the tip of the middle finger sharply tap the interphalangeal joint of the finger that is on the body surface (Figure 3-1). You may tap just distal to the interphalangeal joint if you choose, but decide on one and be consistent because the sound varies from one to the other.

Several points are essential to note in developing the technique of percussion. The downward snap of the striking finger originates from the wrist and not the forearm or shoulder. The tap should be sharp and rapid; once the finger has struck, the wrist snaps back, quickly lifting the finger to prevent dampening the sound. The tip and not the pad of the plexor finger is used (hence short fingernails are again a necessity). Percuss one location several times to facilitate interpretation of the tone. Like other techniques, percussion must be practiced to obtain the skill needed to produce the desired result (Box 3-6). In learning to distinguish between the tones, it may be helpful to close your eyes to block out other sensory stimuli, concentrating exclusively on the tone you are hearing.

BOX 3-6 **Common Percussion Errors**

Percussion requires practice, but practice of incorrect techniques will not assist in obtaining the desired results. In learning percussion, beginning practitioners often make the following errors:

- Failing to exert firm pressure with the finger placed on the skin surface
- Failing to separate the hammer finger from other fingers
- Snapping downward from the elbow or shoulder rather than from the wrist
- Tapping by moving just the hammer finger rather than the whole hand
- Striking with the finger pad rather than the fingertip of the hammer finger

The fist may also be used in percussion. Fist percussion is most commonly used to elicit tenderness arising from the liver, gallbladder, or kidneys. In this technique, use the ulnar aspect of the fist to deliver a firm blow to the area. Too gentle a blow will not produce enough force to stimulate the tenderness, but too hearty a blow can create unnecessary discomfort even in a well patient. The force of a direct blow can be mediated by use of a second hand placed over the area. Practice on yourself or a colleague until you achieve the desired middle ground.

AUSCULTATION

Auscultation involves listening for sounds produced by the body. Some sounds, such as speech, are audible to the unassisted ear. Most others require a stethoscope to augment the sound. Specific types of stethoscopes, their use, and desired characteristics are discussed in the section on stethoscopes in this chapter.

Although what you are listening for will depend on the specific part of the examination, there are some general principles that apply to all auscultatory procedures. Auscultation should be carried out in a quiet environment. Place the stethoscope on the naked skin, because clothing obscures the sound. Listen not only for the presence of sound but also its characteristics: intensity, pitch, duration, and quality. The sounds are often subtle or transitory, and you must listen intently to hear the nuances. Closing your eyes may help you focus on the sound and narrow your perceptual field to prevent distraction by visual stimuli. Try to target and isolate each sound, concentrating on one sound at a time. Take enough time to identify all the characteristics of each sound. Auscultation should be carried out last, except with the abdominal examination, after other techniques have provided information that will assist in interpreting what you hear. Too often the temptation is to rush right in with the stethoscope, thus missing the opportunity to gather other data that would be useful.

One of the most difficult achievements in auscultation is learning to isolate sounds. You cannot hear everything all at once. Whether it is a breath sound or a heartbeat or the sequence of respirations and heartbeats, each segment of the cycle must be isolated and listened to specifically. After the individual sounds are identified, they are put together. Do not anticipate the next sound; concentrate on the one at hand. Auscultation of the lungs is discussed in Chapter 12, the heart in Chapter 13, and the abdomen in Chapter 15.

MEASUREMENT OF VITAL SIGNS

The triad of pulse, respiration, and blood pressure is often considered to be the baseline indicator of a patient's health status, which is why they are called vital signs. They may be measured early in the physical examination or integrated into separate aspects of the examination.

PULSE

The pulse may be palpated in several different areas. However, the radial pulse is most often used as the screening measure for heart rate, which is the number of cardiac cycles per minute. With the pads of your second and third fingers, palpate the radial pulse on the flexor surface of the wrist laterally. Count the pulsations, also noting the rhythm, amplitude, and contour. A detailed discussion of evaluation of arterial pulses is found in Chapter 13, Heart and Blood Vessels, in the section on the peripheral vascular system.

RESPIRATION

Respirations are counted and evaluated by inspection. Observe the rise and fall of the patient's chest and the ease with which breathing is accomplished. Count the number of respiratory cycles (inspiration and expiration) that occur in 1 minute to determine the respiratory rate. In infants the rise and fall of the abdomen with respiration facilitates the count. Also observe the regularity and rhythm of the breathing pattern. Note the depth of respirations and whether the patient uses accessory muscles. A more thorough evaluation of respiration is detailed in Chapter 12, Chest and Lungs.

BLOOD PRESSURE

CHOOSING THE RIGHT SIZE BLOOD PRESSURE CUFF FOR CHILDREN

Since children (even those of the same age) vary markedly in build, choosing the correct cuff is more than a matter of size-for-age recommendations. The following guidelines will assist you in choosing an appropriate size cuff to obtain the most accurate blood pressure reading:
The bladder width should not exceed two thirds the length of the upper or lower arm.
The bladder length should not completely wrap around or overlap the extremity used to take the measurement, but it should ideally cover three fourths of the circumference of the extremity.

Blood pressure is a peripheral measurement of cardiovascular function. Indirect measures of blood pressure are made with a stethoscope and an aneroid or mercury sphygmomanometer. Electronic sphygmomanometers, which do not require the use of a stethoscope, are also available. Each sphygmomanometer is composed of a cuff with an inflatable bladder, a pressure manometer, and a rubber hand bulb with a pressure control valve to inflate and deflate the bladder. The electronic sphygmomanometer senses vibrations and converts them into electrical impulses. The impulses are transmitted to a device that translates them into a digital readout. The instrument is relatively sensitive and is also capable of simultaneously measuring the pulse rate. It does not, however, indicate the quality, rhythm, and other characteristics of a pulse and should not be used in place of your touch in assessing pulse.

Cuffs are available in a number of sizes; the appropriate size is determined by the size of the patient's limb (Figure 3-2). For adults, choose a width that is one third to one half the circumference of the limb. The length of the bladder should be twice the width (about 80% of the limb circumference), not quite enough to completely encircle the limb. For children, the cuff width should cover approximately two thirds of the upper arm or thigh. For both adults and children, cuffs that are too wide will underestimate blood pressure, and those that are too narrow will give an artificially high measurement. The correct cuff size ensures that equal pressure will be exerted around the artery, thus resulting in an accurate measurement.

Other pointers for using blood pressure equipment are as follows:
- If you are using a mercury sphygmomanometer, keep the manometer vertical and make all readings at eye level, no more than 3 ft away.
- If you are using an aneroid instrument, position the dial so it faces you directly, no more than 3 ft away. An aneroid manometer becomes inaccurate with repeated use and needs periodic calibration.

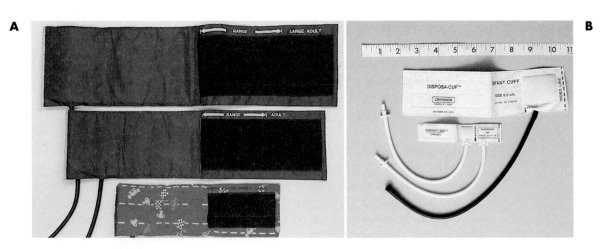

FIGURE 3-2
Select the appropriate size blood pressure cuff. **A,** *Top to bottom:* large adult, adult, and child cuffs.
B, Infant cuff *(top)* and neonatal cuff for use with Dinamap vital signs monitor *(bottom)*.
A from Thompson, Wilson, 1996.

■ If the patient has an obese arm, substitute a larger cuff, using the cuff size principles to choose the appropriate size. If a sufficiently large cuff is unavailable, a standard cuff can be wrapped around the forearm and a stethoscope placed over the radial artery. The size of the cuff and the site of auscultation should be recorded.

■ If the adult patient is very thin, a pediatric cuff may be necessary.

■ Avoid slow or repeated inflation of the cuff, which can cause venous congestion and result in inaccurate readings. If repeated measurements are needed, wait at least 15 seconds between readings, with the cuff fully deflated. You can also remove the cuff and elevate the arm for 1 or 2 minutes.

The specific technique for measuring blood pressure is described in Chapter 13, Heart and Blood Vessels.

TEMPERATURE

The assessment of body temperature may often provide an important clue to the severity of a patient's illness. In cases of bacterial infection, especially with infants, toddlers, and the elderly, it may well be the most critical diagnostic indicator. Temperature measurement can be accomplished through several different routes, most commonly oral, rectal, and axillary. A fourth route of measurement, the tympanic membrane, is becoming widely used because of its ease, speed, and noninvasive nature.

Electronic temperature measurement has decreased the time required for accurate temperature readings (Figure 3-3, *A*). One piece of equipment that contains an electronic sensing probe can be used for measurement of rectal, oral, and axillary temperatures. The probe, covered by a disposable sheath, is placed either under the tongue with the mouth tightly closed, in the rectum, or in the axillary space with the arm held close to the torso. A temperature (either Fahrenheit or Celsius) is revealed on a liquid crystal display (LCD) screen within 15 to 60 seconds, depending on the model used.

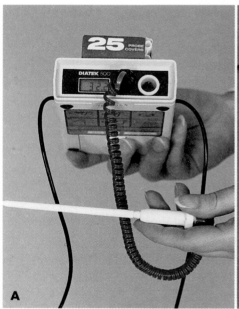
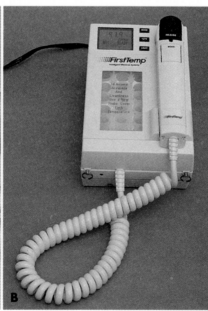
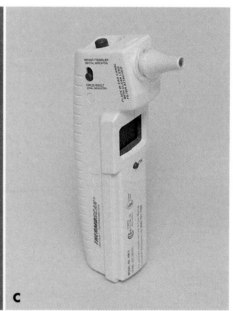

FIGURE 3-3
Devices for electronic temperature measurement. **A,** Rectal, oral, or axillary thermometer. **B** and **C,** Tympanic membrane thermometers.

Tympanic thermometers are becoming increasingly popular, although their measurements vary somewhat from those obtained by oral or rectal routes (Figure 3-3, *B* and *C*). In some situations, as with very young infants, traditional routes of measurement may be more accurate, and in other situations the tympanic route is preferred. Although tympanic thermometers are simple to use, accurate measurement depends on correct technique, so be sure to follow the manufacturer's instructions.

For tympanic membrane temperature measurement, a specially designed probe similar in shape to an otoscope is required. Gently place the covered probe tip at the external opening of the ear canal. Do not try to force the probe into the canal or to occlude it. Infrared technology provides a temperature reading on the LCD screen in approximately 2 seconds. Ear temperature reflects the body's temperature, because the tympanic membrane shares its blood supply with the hypothalamus in the brain.

Infrared axillary thermometers for neonates are now available. Axillary measurements correlate well with core temperatures of newborns because of the infant's small body mass and uniform skin blood flow. A recessed reflective cup on the probe protects the measurement from the effects of external heat sources, making these thermometers suitable for use in incubators and under radiant warmers or phototherapy lights.

MEASUREMENT OF HEIGHT AND WEIGHT

Height and weight of adults are measured with a standing platform scale with a height attachment. The scale uses a system of adding and subtracting weight in increments as small as 0.25 lb or 0.1 kg to counterbalance the weight placed on the scale platform. The scale is calibrated each time it is used.

Calibrate the scale to zero before the patient mounts the platform by moving both the large and small weights to zero. The balance beam should be made level and steady by adjusting the calibrating knob. The height attachment is pulled up, and the head piece is positioned at the patient's crown (Figure 3-4). The height attachment should be pulled up before the patient steps on the scale to avoid a jab with the horizontal piece. Place a paper towel on the platform before the patient steps on it to avoid the potential transmission of organisms from bare feet.

Electronic scales are becoming more common. The weight is electronically calculated and provided as a digital read-out. These scales are automatically calibrated each time they are used.

The infant platform scale is used for measuring weights of infants and small children (Figure 3-5). It works the same as the adult scale but can measure in ounces or grams. The scale has a platform with curved sides in which the child may sit or lie. Place paper under the child.

Infant heights can be measured by using an infant measuring device that comes with a rigid headboard and movable footboard. The measuring board is placed on the table so that the headboard and footboard are perpendicular to the table. The infant lies supine on the measuring board with the head against the headboard. The footboard is moved until it touches the bottom of the infant's feet.

An alternative to the rigid measuring device is a commercially available measure mat, consisting of a soft rubber graduated mat attached to a plastic headboard and footboard (Figure 3-6). The measure mat is lightweight and folds up for storage or portability. To use it, fully unfold the mat on a hard flat surface, smoothing it out.

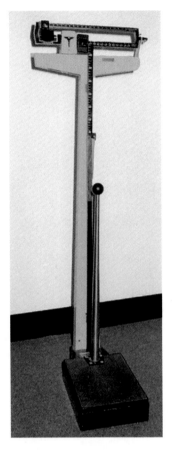

FIGURE 3-4
Platform scale with height attachment.

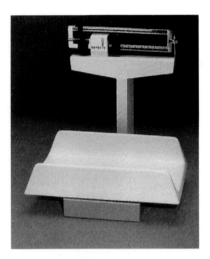

FIGURE 3-5
Infant platform scale.

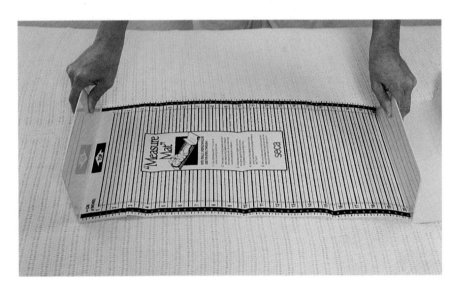

FIGURE 3-6
Measure mat to determine length of infant.

Place the baby on the mat with the top of the head touching the headboard of the mat. Holding the baby's knees together and pressing them gently against the mat with one hand, bring the footboard up against the baby's heels. The baby's length can be read in either inches or centimeters. Be sure to clean the mat between uses.

An infant can also be measured by placing the baby on a pad, putting one pin into the pad at the top of the head and another at the heel of the extended leg. The length is then measured from pin to pin.

Once a child is able to stand erect without support, a stature measuring device is used to measure height. The device consists of a movable headpiece attached to a rigid measurement bar and platform. A tape measure attached to the wall and a movable headpiece can also be used (Figure 3-7, *A* and *B*).

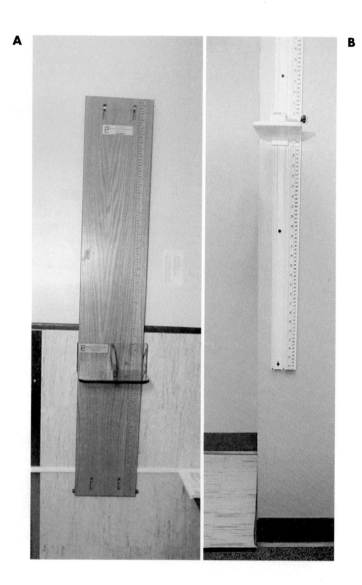

FIGURE 3-7
Devices used to measure height of child.

INSTRUMENTATION

STETHOSCOPE

Auscultation of most sounds requires a stethoscope. Three basic types are available: acoustic, magnetic, and electronic. The acoustic stethoscope is a closed cylinder that transmits sound waves from the source along its column to the ear (Figure 3-8). The rigid diaphragm has a natural frequency of around 300 Hz. It screens out low-pitched sounds, and best transmits high-pitched sounds such as the second heart sound. The bell endpiece, with which the skin acts as the diaphragm, has a natural frequency varying with the amount of pressure exerted. It transmits low-pitched sounds when very light pressure is used. With firm pressure, it converts to a diaphragm endpiece. The chestpiece contains a closure valve so that only one endpiece, either the diaphragm or bell, is operational at any one time (thus preventing inadvertent dissipation of sound waves).

The magnetic stethoscope has a single endpiece that is a diaphragm. It contains an iron disk on the interior surface behind which is a permanent magnet. A strong

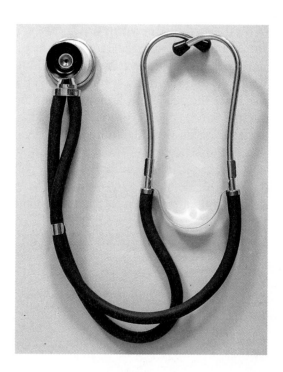

FIGURE 3-8
Acoustic stethoscope.

spring keeps the diaphragm bowed outward when it is not compressed against a body surface. Compression of the diaphragm activates the air column as magnetic attraction is established between the iron disk and the magnet. Rotation of a frequency dial adjusts for high, low, and full frequency sounds.

The electronic stethoscope picks up sound vibrations transmitted to the surface of the body and converts them into electrical impulses. The impulses are amplified and transmitted to a speaker where they are reconverted to sound.

The most commonly used is the acoustic stethoscope, which comes in several models. The ability to auscultate accurately depends in part on the quality of the instrument, so it is important that the stethoscope have the following characteristics:

- The diaphragm and bell are heavy enough to lie firmly on the body surface.
- The diaphragm cover is rigid.
- The bell is large enough in diameter to span an intercostal space in an adult and deep enough so that it will not fill with tissue.
- A rubber or plastic ring is around the bell edges to ensure secure contact with the body surface.
- The tubing is thick, stiff, and heavy, which conducts better than thin, elastic, or very flexible tubing.
- The length of the tubing is between 30.5 and 40 cm (12 to 18 in) to minimize distortion.
- The earpieces fit snugly and comfortably. Some instruments have several sizes of earpieces and some have hard and soft earpieces. The determining factors are how they fit and feel. The earpieces should be large enough to occlude the meatus, thus blocking outside sound; if they are too small they will slip into the ear canal and be painful.
- Angled binaurals point the earpieces toward the nose so that sound is projected toward the tympanic membrane.

To stabilize the stethoscope when it is in place, hold the endpiece between the second and third fingers, pressing the diaphragm firmly against the skin (Figure 3-9). The diaphragm "piece" should never be used without the diaphragm. Since the bell functions by picking up vibrations, it must be positioned so that the vibrations are not dampened. Place the bell evenly and lightly on the skin, making sure there is skin contact around the entire edge. To prevent extraneous noise, avoid touching the tubing with your hands or allowing the tubing to rub against any surfaces.

A fourth type of stethoscope, the stereophonic stethoscope, is becoming more widely available (Figure 3-10). With a single tube, diaphragm, and bell, it looks and functions like an acoustic stethoscope. However, a two-channel design allows the stethoscope to differentiate between the right and left auscultatory sounds. The right

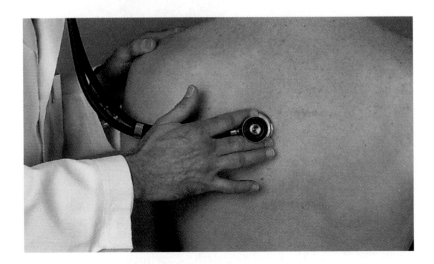

FIGURE 3-9
Position the stethoscope between the index and middle fingers.

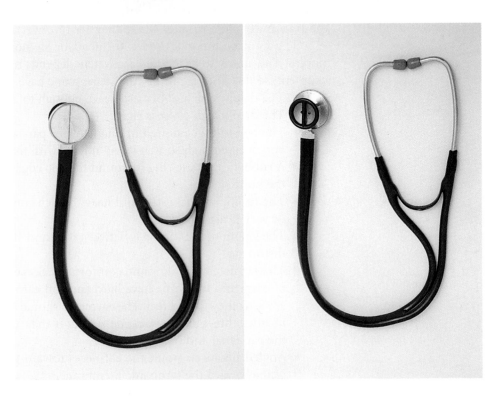

FIGURE 3-10
Stereophonic stethoscope. Note divided bell and diaphragm.

and left ear tubes are independently connected to right and left semicircular microphones in the chestpiece.

Many pediatric specialists have found that a tiny, virtually weightless doll clinging to the structure of a stethoscope provides a diversion for the young child without interfering with the examination. Decoration and color will not interfere with what you hear.

DOPPLER

Some sounds are so difficult to auscultate that a regular stethoscope will not suffice. Dopplers are useful at these times (Figure 3-11). Dopplers are ultrasonic stethoscopes that detect blood flow rather than amplify sounds, and they vary in frequency from 2 MHz to 10 MHz. The use of a Doppler requires that you first place transmission gel on the skin over the area where you will be listening. Then place the tip of the instrument directly over the area being examined. Tilt the tip at an angle along the axis of blood flow to obtain the best signal. Arterial flow is heard as a pulsatile pumping sound, and venous flow resembles the sound of rushing wind. When using a Doppler, do not press so hard as to impede blood flow.

The mechanism of action for a Doppler is known as the "Doppler shift" principle. A low-power sound wave of very high ultrasonic frequency is directed into the body. Reflections occur at the various tissue interfaces; if an object is moving relative to the instrument, these reflections will have their frequency shifted slightly, resulting in audible sounds.

The Doppler has many uses. It can be used to detect systolic blood pressures in patients with weak or difficult-to-hear sounds, such as patients in shock, infants, or obese persons. It is used to auscultate fetal heart activity, locate vessels, take weak pulses, and assess vessel patency. Other uses include localization of acute and chronic arterial occlusions in the extremities, assessment of deep vein thrombosis and valvular incompetency, and assessment of testicular torsion and varicocele.

FETAL MONITORING EQUIPMENT (FETOSCOPE, LEFF SCOPE, STETHOSCOPE, AND ELECTRONIC VERIFICATION OF THE FETAL HEARTBEAT)

The fetal heart rate is determined by use of specially designed instruments called the fetoscope and Leff scope, the clinical stethoscope addressed previously, or an electronic instrument that uses the Doppler effect. The fetoscope has a band that fits against the head of the listener and makes handling of the instrument unnecessary (Figure 3-12). The metal band also aids in bone conduction of sound, so that the heart tones are heard more easily. The Leff scope has a weighted end that, when placed on the abdomen, does not need stabilization by the practitioner. These instruments can pick up the fetal heart rate at 17 to 19 weeks' gestation.

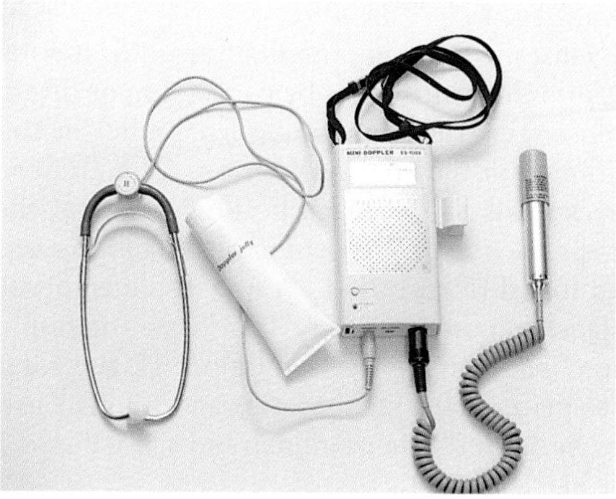

FIGURE 3-11
Doppler.

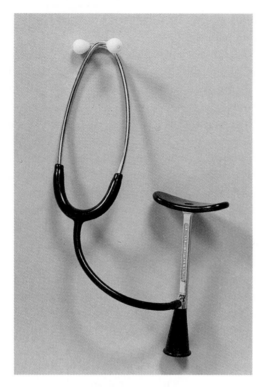

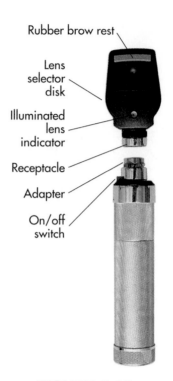

FIGURE 3-12
Fetoscope.

FIGURE 3-13
Ophthalmoscope.

The Doppler method employs a continuous ultrasound that picks up differing frequencies from the beating fetal heart. It is a more sensitive method and can detect the fetal heart at 10 to 12 weeks' gestation, and earlier in some individuals. These instruments are often supplied with amplifiers, so that both the practitioner and mother can hear the fetal heartbeat at the same time.

OPHTHALMOSCOPE

The ophthalmoscope has a system of lenses and mirrors that enables visualization of the interior structures of the eye (Figure 3-13). A light source in the instrument provides illumination through various apertures while you focus on the inner eye. The large aperture, which is used most often, produces a large round beam. The various apertures, described in Table 3-4, are selected by rotating the aperture selection dial.

The lenses in varying powers of magnification are used to bring the structure under examination into focus by converging or diverging light. On the front of the ophthalmoscope is an illuminating lens indicator that displays the number of the lens positioned in the viewing aperture. The number, ranging from about −20 to +40, corresponds to the magnification power of the lens (diopter). The positive numbers (plus lenses) are shown in black, and the negative numbers (minus lenses) are shown in red (Figure 3-14). A way to remember this is that when you are using a *minus* lens, you are in the *red*. Clockwise rotation of the lens selector brings the plus sphere lenses into place. Counterclockwise rotation brings the minus sphere lenses into place. The system of plus and minus lenses can compensate for myopia or hyperopia in both the examiner and the patient. There is no compensation for astigmatism.

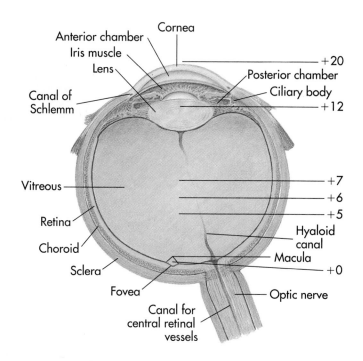

FIGURE 3-14
Longitudinal cross-section of eye showing lens diopters to focus eye structures.

Labels in figure: Anterior chamber, Iris muscle, Lens, Cornea, Canal of Schlemm, Posterior chamber, Ciliary body, +20, +12, Vitreous, +7, +6, +5, Retina, Choroid, Hyaloid canal, Macula, Sclera, +0, Fovea, Optic nerve, Canal for central retinal vessels

TABLE 3-4	Apertures of the Ophthalmoscope
Aperture	**Examination Use**
Small aperture	Small pupils
Red-free filter	Produces a green beam for examination of the optic disk for pallor and minute vessel changes. Also permits recognition of retinal hemorrhages, with blood appearing black.
Slit	Examination of the anterior eye and determination of the elevation of lesions
Grid	Estimation of the size of fundal lesions

The ophthalmoscope head is seated in the handle by fitting the adapter of the handle into the head receptacle and pushing downward while turning the head in a clockwise direction. The two pieces will lock into place.

Turn on the ophthalmoscope by depressing the on/off switch and turning the rheostat control clockwise to the desired intensity of light. Turn the instrument off when you have finished using it to preserve the life of the bulb.

A more detailed discussion of the actual ophthalmoscopic examination is provided in Chapter 10, Eyes.

STRABISMOSCOPE

The strabismoscope is used for detecting strabismus and can be used as part of routine eye testing in children (Figure 3-15). Instruct the child to focus on an accommodative target. Turn on the strabismoscope and place it over the patient's eye. Because of a one-way mirror, you are able to see in but the patient is not able to see out. As a result, subtle eye movements associated with strabismus are more easily detected. With the strabismoscope in place, watch for movement in both the covered and uncovered eyes. Repeat with the other eye. The instrument comes with a wall poster with test instructions and a guide to interpretation of test results.

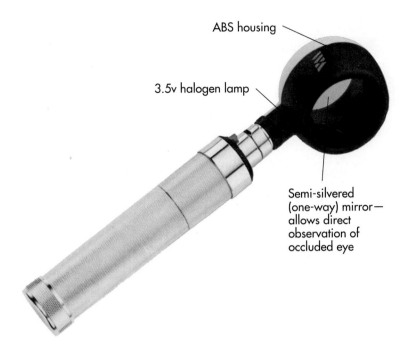

ABS housing

3.5v halogen lamp

Semi-silvered
(one-way) mirror—
allows direct
observation of
occluded eye

FIGURE 3-15
Strabismoscope.

Courtesy Welch Allyn, Skaneateles Falls,
New York.

SNELLEN VISUAL ACUITY CHART

The Snellen alphabet chart is used for a screening examination of far vision (Figure 3-16, *A*). The chart contains letters of graduated sizes with standardized numbers at the end of each line of letters. These numbers indicate the degree of visual acuity when read from a distance of 20 ft. The "E" chart can be used in the same way for illiterate or non-English-speaking patients and for children (Figure 3-16, *B*). Ask these patients to show you which way the "table legs" are pointing. Variations of the chart with geometric patterns or pictures rather than letters are also available.

Test visual acuity for each eye, using the standardized numbers on the chart. Visual acuity is recorded as a fraction, with the numerator of 20 (the distance in feet between the patient and the chart) and the denominator as the distance from which a person with normal vision could read the lettering. The larger the denominator, the poorer the vision. The standard used for normal vision is 20/20. Measurement other than 20/20 indicates either a refractive error or an optic disorder. Record the smallest complete line that the patient can read accurately without missing any letters. If the patient is able to read some but not all letters of the next smaller line, indicate this by adding the number of letters read correctly on that next line, for example, 20/25 +2. This would indicate that the patient read all of the letters in the 20/25 line correctly and also two of the letters of the 20/20 line correctly.

NEAR VISION CHARTS

To assess near vision a specially designed chart such as the Rosenbaum or Jaeger chart can be used, or simply use newsprint. The Rosenbaum chart contains a series of numbers, Es, Xs, and Os in graduated sizes (Figure 3-17). Test and record vision for each eye separately. Acuity is recorded as either distance equivalents such as 20/20 or Jaeger equivalents such as J-2. Both these measures are indicated on the chart. If newsprint is used, the patient should be able to read it without difficulty.

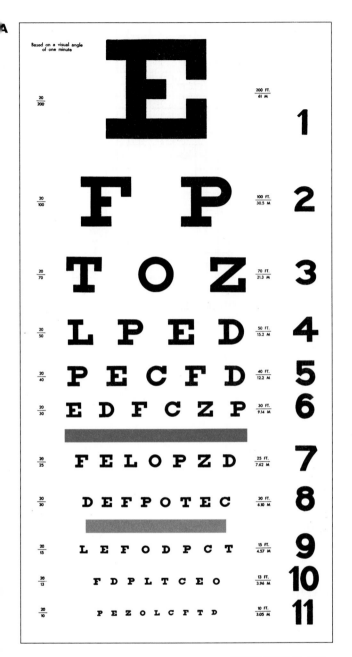

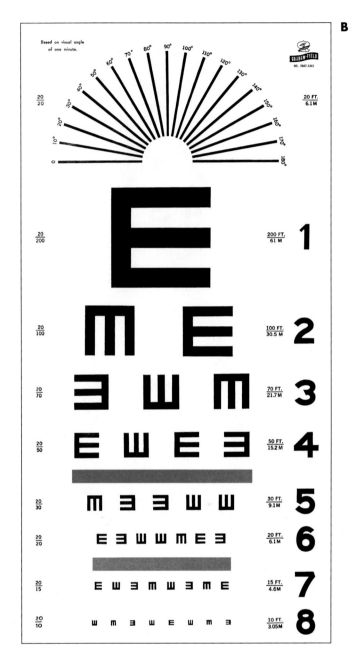

FIGURE 3-16
A, Snellen and, **B,** E charts for testing distant vision.

AMSLER GRID

A screening test for use with individuals at risk of macular degeneration is provided with the Amsler grid (Figure 3-18). The grid is used when retinal drusen bodies are seen during an ophthalmologic examination or when there is a strong family history of macular degeneration. The grid consists of straight lines that resemble graph paper. At the center of the grid is a black dot that acts as a fixation point. About 10 degrees of central vision is monitored. The patient views the grid with one eye at a time and notes the occurrence of line distortion or actual scotoma (see Chapter 10).

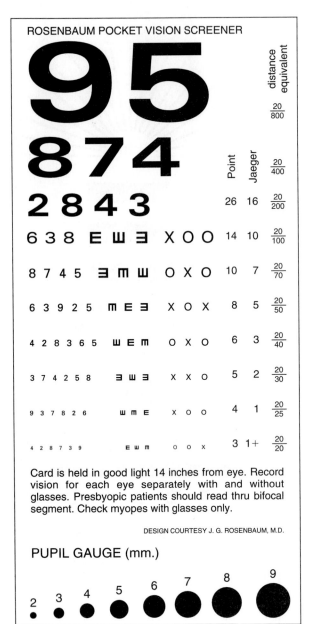

FIGURE 3-17
Rosenbaum chart for testing near vision.

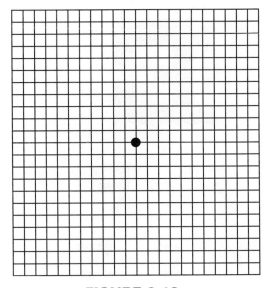

FIGURE 3-18
Amsler grid.
From Palay, Krachmer, 1997.

OTOSCOPE

The otoscope provides illumination for examining the external auditory canal and the tympanic membrane (Figure 3-19). The otoscope head is seated in the handle in the same manner as the ophthalmoscope and is turned on the same way. An attached speculum narrows and directs the beam of light. Select the largest size speculum that will fit comfortably into the patient's ear canal. A glass plate magnifies and acts as a viewing window. In many models the glass plate slides aside, allowing insertion of a cerumen spoon or forceps while the otoscope remains in place. Chapter 11 (Ears, Nose, and Throat) discusses the specific techniques of examination.

The otoscope can also be used for the nasal examination if a nasal speculum is not available. Use the shortest, widest speculum and insert it gently into the patient's naris.

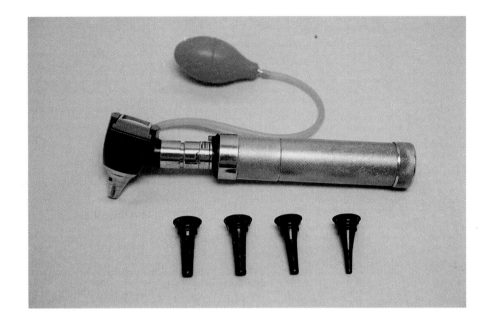

FIGURE 3-19
Otoscope with various sizes of specula and a pneumatic attachment.

Pneumatic Attachment

The pneumatic attachment for the otoscope is used to evaluate the fluctuating capacity of the tympanic membrane. A short piece of rubber tubing is attached to the head of the otoscope. A handbulb attached to the other end of the tubing, when squeezed, produces puffs of air that cause the tympanic membrane to move. If no handbulb is attached, place the open end of the tubing in your mouth and alternately puff into and suck gently through the tubing to produce the same effect.

TYMPANOMETER

Various instruments are available for performing screening tympanometry. Tympanometry is a simple, reliable, and objective means of assessing the functions of the ossicular chain, eustachian tube, and tympanic membrane, and the interrelation of these parts.

Position the probe at the opening of the ear canal (Figure 3-20). When a tight seal is obtained, a known quantity of sound energy is introduced into the ear. A measurement of the energy not transmitted to the middle ear is recorded. The amount of the sound energy transmitted is the amount of sound energy introduced minus the amount of sound energy that returns to the probe microphone. The amount of energy transmitted is directly related to the compliance of the system. Compliance (measured in milliliters or cubic centimeters of equivalent volume) indicates the amount of mobility in the middle ear. Low compliance measurement indicates that more energy has returned to the probe, with less energy admitted to the middle ear. A high compliance reading indicates a flaccid or highly mobile system.

At this point, the probe introduces a pressure of +200 daPa (dacaPascals) to the middle ear canal. DacaPascals is a measurement of air pressure. This positive pressure forces the tympanic membrane inward, and the approximate ear canal volume is recorded. This volume gives a baseline from which the compliance curve is drawn. The pressure is then varied in the negative direction, constantly monitoring the compliance of the system. The pressure continues toward the negative direction, until a pressure peak has been detected or until a pressure of −400 daPa is present in the ear canal, whichever comes first. Once the pressure is equalized on both sides of the tympanic membrane, the point of peak compliance occurs.

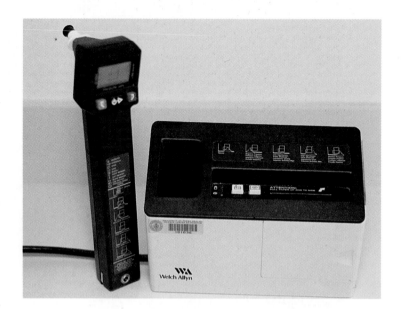

FIGURE 3-20
Tympanometer.

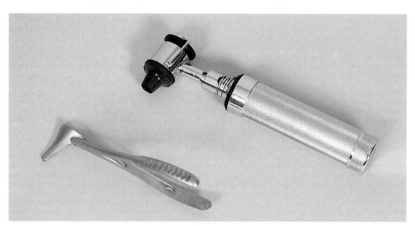

FIGURE 3-21
Nasal specula.

A tympanogram is a graphic representation of the change in compliance of the middle ear system as air pressure is varied. The tympanogram results are displayed on the probe monitor or can be printed out for a hard copy.

NASAL SPECULUM

The nasal speculum is used with a penlight to visualize the lower and middle turbinates of the nose (Figure 3-21). Be sure that the patient is in a comfortable position. The head may need to be supported, or you can have the patient lie down. You will need to tilt the patient's head at various angles for a complete nasal examination. Stabilize the speculum with your index finger to avoid contact of the blades with the nasal septum, which can cause discomfort. The blades are opened by squeezing the handles of the instrument.

TUNING FORK

Tuning forks are used in screening tests for auditory function and for vibratory sensation as part of the neurologic examination (Figure 3-22). As tuning forks are activated, vibrations are created that produce a particular frequency of sound wave, expressed as cycles per second (cps) or Hertz (Hz). Thus a fork of 512 Hz vibrates 512 cycles per second.

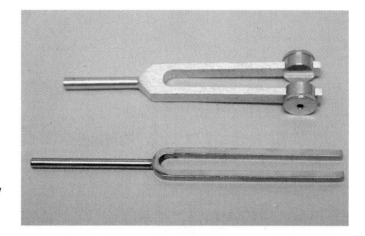

FIGURE 3-22

Tuning forks for testing vibratory sensation *(top)* and auditory screening *(bottom)*.

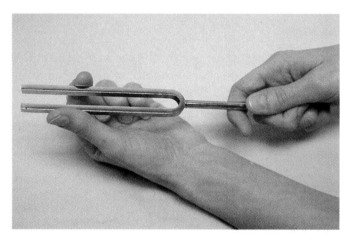

FIGURE 3-23

Squeezing and stroking the tuning fork to activate it.

For auditory evaluation use a fork with a frequency of 500 to 1000 Hz, because it can estimate hearing loss in the range of normal speech, approximately 300 to 3000 Hz. Forks of lower frequency can cause you to overestimate bone conduction and can be felt as vibration as well as heard. Activate the fork by gently squeezing and stroking the prongs or tapping them against the knuckles of your hand, so that they ring softly (Figure 3-23). Because touching the tines will dampen the sound, the fork must be held at the base. Hearing is tested at near-threshold level, which is the lowest intensity of sound at which an auditory stimulus can be heard. Striking the prongs too vigorously results in a loud tone that is above the threshold level and requires time to quiet to a tone appropriate for auditory testing. The specific tuning fork tests for hearing are described in Chapter 11, Ears, Nose, and Throat.

For vibratory sensation, use a fork of lower frequency. The greatest sensitivity to vibration occurs when the fork is vibrating between 100 and 400 Hz. Activate the tuning fork by tapping it against the heel of your hand and apply the base of the fork to a bony prominence. The patient feels the vibration as a buzzing or tingling sensation. The specific areas of testing are described in Chapter 20, Neurologic System.

PERCUSSION (REFLEX) HAMMER

The percussion hammer is used to test deep tendon reflexes. Hold the hammer loosely between the thumb and index finger, so that as you tap the tendon, the hammer moves in a swift arc and in a controlled direction. Use a rapid downward snap of the wrist, tap quickly and firmly, and then snap your wrist back so that the hammer

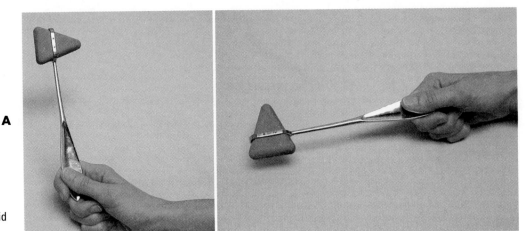

FIGURE 3-24
A, Reflex hammer. **B,** Use a rapid downward snap of the wrist.

does not linger on the tendon (Figure 3-24). The tap should be brisk and direct. Practice this action to achieve smooth, rapid, and controlled motion. You can use either the pointed or flat end of the hammer. The flat end is more comfortable when striking the patient directly; the pointed end is useful in small areas, such as on your finger placed over the patient's biceps tendon. Chapter 20 (Neurologic System) contains a detailed discussion of evaluation of deep tendon reflexes.

Your finger can also act as a reflex hammer, which can be particularly useful when you are examining very young patients. Certainly it is less threatening to a child than a hammer. There are many pediatric specialists who let the child hold the hammer while they use their fingers.

NEUROLOGIC HAMMER

A variant of the percussion hammer is the neurologic hammer, which is also used for testing deep tendon reflexes (Figure 3-25). The hammer has two additional features that make it a multipurpose neurologic instrument. The base of the handle unscrews, revealing a soft brush. A tiny knob on the head also unscrews, to which is attached a sharp needle. These additional implements were intended to be used to determine sensory perception as part of the neurologic examination. The brush can still be used for that purpose. However, because of the possibility of cross infection, the needle should not be used at all. Instead, use a disposable needle, pin, or sharp end of a broken tongue blade each time. The procedure for testing sensory perception is described in detail in Chapter 20, Neurologic System.

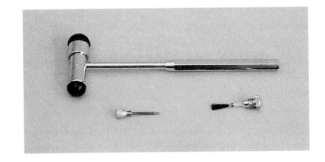

FIGURE 3-25
Neurologic hammer. Note the brush and needle. Remember that the needle should not be used.

TAPE MEASURE

A tape measure 7 to 12 mm wide is used for determining circumference, length, and diameter. It may be helpful to have one that measures in both inches and metric units. Tape measures are available in a variety of materials, including paper (disposable) and cloth. The tape measure should be nonstretchable for accuracy and pliable for circumference measurement. Since it is placed against the skin, beware of edges that are sharp and can cut.

When measuring make sure that the tape is not caught or wrinkled beneath the patient. Pull the tape closely but not tightly enough to cause depression of the skin when measuring circumference.

When monitoring serial measures, such as head circumferences or abdominal girth, it is important to place the tape measure in the same position each time. If serial measures are made over a period of days, an easy way to ensure accurate placement is to mark with pen the borders of the tape at several intervals on the skin. Subsequently, the tape can be placed within the markings. Accurate placement of the tape for specific measurements is described in Chapter 5 and related chapters.

TRANSILLUMINATOR

TRANS-ILLUMINATION

Compared to radiologic imaging technology, transillumination may seem archaic and imprecise. Radiologic imaging is to be used when necessary, of course, but transillumination maintains its value as a clinical tool and is far less expensive.

A transilluminator consists of a strong light source with a narrow beam. The beam is directed to a particular body cavity and is used to differentiate between various media present in that cavity. Light is differentially transmitted by air, fluid, and tissue, which allows you to detect the presence of fluid in sinuses, the presence of blood or masses in the scrotum, and abnormalities in the cranium of infants.

Specific transilluminating instruments are available, or a flashlight with a rubber adapter can be used (Figure 3-26). It is fine, when situations demand, to use a plain flashlight or penlight. Do not use a light source with a halogen bulb, because you can burn the patient's skin. In any case, transillumination should be performed in a darkened room. Place the beam of light directly against the area to be observed, shielding the beam with your hand if necessary. Watch for the red glow of light through the body cavity. Note the presence or absence of illumination and any irregularities.

VAGINAL SPECULUM

A vaginal speculum is composed of two blades and a handle. There are three basic types of vaginal specula, which are used to view the vaginal canal and cervix. The Graves speculum is available in a variety of sizes with blades, ranging from 3.5 to 5 inches in length and 0.75 to 1.25 inches in width. The blades are curved with a space between the

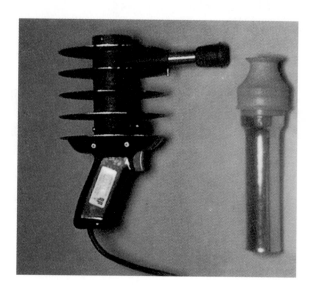

FIGURE 3-26
Transilluminators. Watch for the red glow. *Left,* Chun gun. *Right,* Flashlight with transilluminator attachment.

closed blades. The bottom blade is about 0.25 inch longer than the top blade to conform with the longer posterior vaginal wall and to aid in visualization. The Pederson speculum has blades that are as long as those of the Graves speculum but are both narrower and flatter. It is used for women with small vaginal openings. Pediatric or virginal specula are smaller in all dimensions, with short, narrow, flat blades (Figure 3-27).

Specula are available in either disposable plastic or reusable metal. The metal speculum has two positioning devices. The top blade is hinged and has a positioning thumbpiece lever attached. When you press down on the thumbpiece, the distal end of the blade rises, thus opening the speculum. The blade can be locked in an open position by tightening the thumbscrew on the thumbpiece. The degree of opening of the proximal end of the blades is controlled by moving the top blade up or down; it is locked in place by another thumbscrew, which is on the handle.

The plastic speculum operates differently from the metal one. The bottom blade is fixed to a posterior handle, and the top blade is controlled by an anterior lever handle. As you press on the lever, the distal end of the top blade elevates. At the same time the base of the speculum also widens. The speculum is locked into position with a catch on the lever handle that snaps into place in a positioning groove.

You will need to become familiar with and practice with both types of specula to feel comfortable with them. Do not wait until you are in the process of doing your first examination, or you are likely to be embarrassed and cause discomfort to the woman because of your initial clumsiness in handling (or mishandling) the instrument.

The procedure for performing the speculum examination is described in detail in Chapter 16, Female Genitalia.

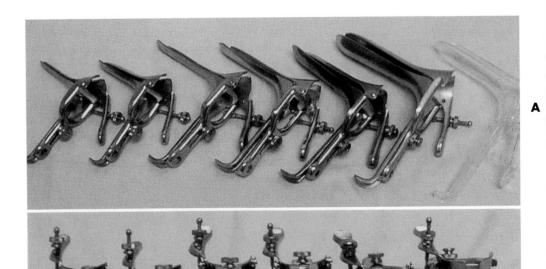

A

B

FIGURE 3-27

Vaginal specula. *From left to right:* **A,** Short-billed pediatric, pediatric, small Pederson, Pederson, small Graves, large Graves, plastic Graves. **B,** Short-billed pediatric, pediatric, small Pederson, Pederson, small Graves, large Graves.

GONIOMETER

The goniometer is used to determine the degree of joint flexion and extension. The instrument consists of two straight arms that intersect and can be angled and rotated around a protractor, which is marked with degrees (Figure 3-28). Place the center of the protractor over the joint, and align the straight arms with the long axis of the extremity. The degree of angle flexion or extension is indicated on the protractor. The specific joint examinations are discussed in Chapter 19, Musculoskeletal System.

WOOD'S LAMP

The Wood's lamp contains a light source with a wavelength of 360 nm (Figure 3-29). This is the black light that causes certain substances to fluoresce when exposed to the light. It is used primarily to determine the presence of fungi on skin lesions. Darken the room, turn on the Wood's lamp, and shine it on the area or lesion you are evaluating. Yellow-green fluorescence indicates the presence of fungi.

Darkening the room can sometimes be intimidating, particularly to children. Children and their parents react positively when they know what to expect. You can accomplish this by shining the lamp on something fluorescent (such as a nondigital watch) to give them the sense of what you are looking for.

EPISCOPE

The episcope is a skin surface microscope that utilizes the technology of epiluminescence microscopy (ELM)—the application of oil on a skin lesion while performing surface microscopy (Figure 3-30). The oil renders the epidermis translucent, which allows for a more detailed inspection of the surface of pigmented skin lesions.

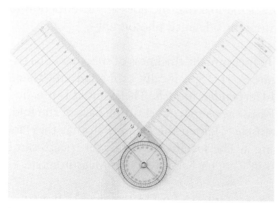

FIGURE 3-28
Goniometer.

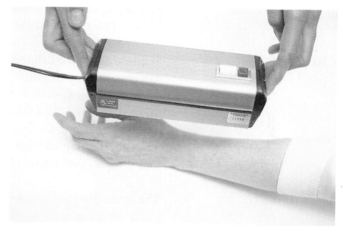

FIGURE 3-29
Wood's lamp. The purple color on the skin indicates no fungal infection is present.
From Thompson, Wilson, 1996.

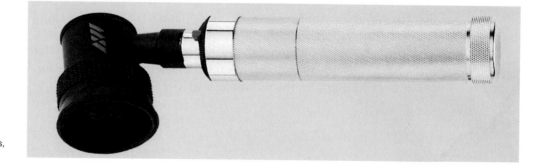

FIGURE 3-30
Episcope.
Courtesy Welch Allyn, Skaneateles Falls, New York.

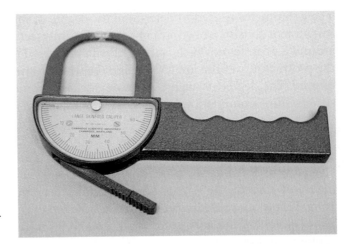

FIGURE 3-31
Triceps skinfold caliper. Grasp the handle and depress the lever with thumb.

Locate the lesion and examine its surface. To reduce the glare from the stratum corneum, moisten the lesion with oil (mineral oil, petroleum jelly). Turn on the skin surface microscope and gently rest it over the lesion so that the lesion is in the center of the contact plate. Adjust for optimal focus while your eye is resting on the eye guard. Observe the illuminated and magnified lesion, making note of its general appearance, surface, pigment pattern, border, and depigmentation. Remove the contact plate for examination of raised moles or lesions. Clean the contact plate after each use. The instrument comes with an owner's manual that includes an introduction to ELM, tables of diagnostic criteria, and numerous detailed photographs.

CALIPERS FOR SKINFOLD THICKNESS

Skinfold thickness calipers are designed to measure the thickness of subcutaneous tissue at certain points of the body (Figure 3-31). Specifically calibrated and tested calipers are used, such as the Lange and Herpenden models. The skinfold is pinched up so the sides of the skin are parallel. Place the caliper edges at the base of the fold, being careful not to capture bone or muscle. Tighten the calipers so that they are grasping the skinfold but not compressing it. The specific technique for triceps skinfold thickness measurement is described in Chapter 5, Growth and Measurement.

MONOFILAMENT

The monofilament is a device designed to test for loss of protective sensation, particularly on the plantar surface of the foot (Figure 3-32). It bends at 10 g of linear pressure. Patients who cannot feel the application of the monofilament at the point it bends have lost their protective sense and are at increased risk for injury.

Test intact skin on the plantar surface of the foot at various areas, as shown in Figure 3-33, including the great toe, heel, and ball of the foot. Lock the monofilament in its handle at a 90-degree angle. With the patient's eyes closed, apply the monofilament perpendicular to the surface of the skin. Press hard enough to allow the monofilament to bend. Application at test sites should be in random order and last approximately 1.5 seconds. Have the patient indicate whether the monofilament is felt. Note the response at each location in the patient record. Clean the monofilament with alcohol. See Chapter 20, Neurologic System, for further discussion of skin testing with the monofilament.

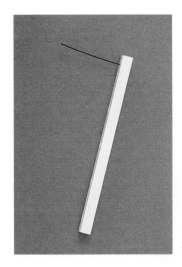

FIGURE 3-32
Monofilament.

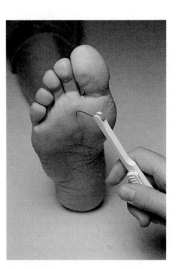

FIGURE 3-33
Press the monofilament against
the skin hard enough to allow it
to bend.

BOX 3-7   **What Equipment Do You Need to Purchase?**

Students are confronted by a large number and variety of pieces of equipment that are necessary to perform physical examination. A frequently asked question is, "What do I really need to buy?" The answer to that depends somewhat on where you will be practicing. If you are in a clinic setting, for example, wall-mounted ophthalmoscopes and otoscopes are provided. This is not necessarily true in a hospital setting.

The following list is intended only as a guideline to the equipment that you will use most often and should personally own. The price of stethoscopes, otoscopes, ophthalmoscopes, and blood pressure equipment can vary markedly. Different models, many with optional features, can affect the price. Since these pieces of equipment represent a significant monetary investment, evaluate the quality of the instrument, consider the manufacturer's warranty and support, and decide on the features that *you* will need.

- Stethoscope
- Ophthalmoscope
- Otoscope
- Blood pressure cuff and manometer
- Centimeter ruler
- Tape measure
- Reflex hammer
- Tuning forks: 500-1000 Hz for auditory screening, 100-400 Hz for vibratory sensation
- Penlight
- Near vision screening chart

Check it out— 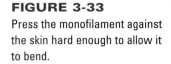 *http://www1.mosby.com/physexam_seidel*

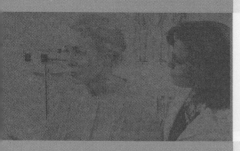

CHAPTER 4

MENTAL STATUS

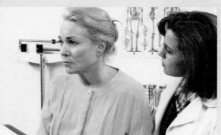

Mental status is the total expression of a person's emotional responses, mood, cognitive functioning, and personality. It is closely linked to the individual's executive functioning that involves motivation and initiative, goal formation, planning and performing work or activities, self-monitoring, and integration of feedback from multiple sources to refine or redirect energy. The mental status portion of the neurologic system examination is performed constantly throughout the entire interaction with a patient. A major focus of the examination is identification of the individual's strengths and capabilities for interaction with the environment.

ANATOMY AND PHYSIOLOGY

The cerebrum of the brain is primarily responsible for the individual's mental status. Many areas in the cerebrum contribute to the total functioning of a person's mental processes. Two cerebral hemispheres, each divided into lobes, form the cerebrum. The gray outer layer, the cerebral cortex, houses the higher mental functions and is responsible for perception and behavior (Figure 4-1).

The *frontal lobe* contains the motor cortex associated with speech formation (Broca area). The associated areas related to emotions, affect, drive, and awareness of self and the autonomic responses related to emotional states also originate here. Goal-oriented behavior and short-term recall memory are also associated with this section of the brain.

The *parietal lobe* is primarily responsible for processing sensory data as it is received.

The *temporal lobe* is responsible for perception and interpretation of sounds and determination of their source. It contains the Wernicke speech area, permitting comprehension of spoken and written language. It is also involved in the integration of behavior, emotion, and personality. Long-term memory is associated with this area.

The *limbic system* mediates certain patterns of behavior that determine survival, such as mating, aggression, fear, and affection. Reactions to emotions such as anger, love, hostility, and envy originate here. Expression of affect is mediated by connections between the limbic system and the frontal lobe.

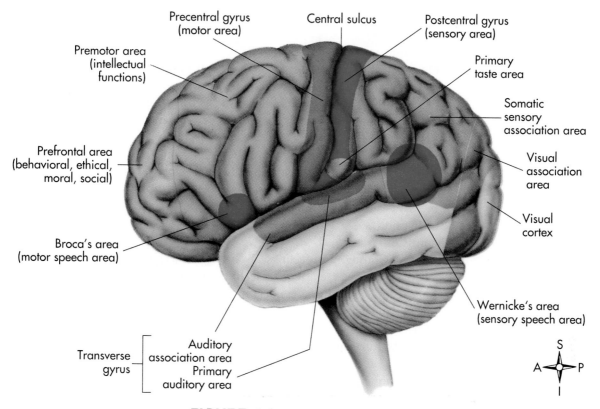

Precentral gyrus
(motor area)

Central sulcus

Postcentral gyrus
(sensory area)

Premotor area
(intellectual
functions)

Primary
taste area

Somatic
sensory
association area

Prefrontal area
(behavioral, ethical,
moral, social)

Visual
association
area

Visual
cortex

Broca's area
(motor speech area)

Wernicke's area
(sensory speech area)

Transverse
gyrus

Auditory
association area
Primary
auditory area

S
A ◆ P
I

FIGURE 4-1

Functional subdivisions of the cerebral cortex.

Modified from Thibodeau, Patton, 1996.

INFANTS AND CHILDREN	The brain cells are all present at birth, but it takes the first years of life for all the brain cells to fully develop and myelinize. Insults such as infection, trauma, or chemical imbalance can damage the brain cells, leading to potentially serious dysfunction in mental status. Environmental influences may promote or impair intellectual development.
ADOLESCENTS	Intellectual maturation continues with greater capacity for information and vocabulary development. Abstract thinking—the abilities to develop theories, use logical reasoning, make future plans, use generalizations, and consider risks and possibilities—all develop during this period. Judgment begins to develop with education, intelligence, and experiences. A set of values eventually is reflected in thinking and action.
OLDER ADULTS	No decline in general intelligence is evident unless a systemic or neurologic disorder develops. Problem-solving skills may decline, probably from disuse, but vocabulary skills and inventories of available information do not significantly change. Remote memory may be more efficient than recent memory, but that may be a function of the individual's overall health. With aging, there is a decline in synthesis and metabolism of neurotransmitters. In times of stress, the metabolism is inadequate to respond to heightened pressures. This often results in an increased risk of delirium with acute illness or metabolic derangement.

REVIEW OF RELATED HISTORY

PRESENT PROBLEM

- Disorientation and confusion
  - Onset: abrupt or insidious, associated with physical condition, time of day
  - Duration: hours, days, or persistent
  - Associated problems: loss of vision or hearing, neurologic disorder, head injury, systemic infection, withdrawal from alcohol, metabolic or electrolyte disorder, vascular occlusion
  - Associated symptoms: delusions, hallucinations, mood swings, anxiety, sadness, lethargy or agitation, insomnia, change in appetite, drug toxicity
  - Medications: anticholinergics, benzodiazepines, opioid analgesics, tricyclic antidepressants, levodopa or amantadine, diuretics, digoxin, antidysrhythmics, sedatives, or hypnotics
- Depression
  - Troubling thoughts or feelings, always worried; change in outlook on life; change in feelings or always feel this way; feelings of hopelessness; inability to control feelings
  - Energy level; agitation; feel best in the morning or at night
  - Recent cause of grief; changes in life-style or neighborhood; death or relocation of friends or family members
  - Feels like hurting self; any plans for harming self, any thoughts about dying; any plans for the future
  - Medications: antidepressants, prescription or nonprescription

PAST MEDICAL HISTORY

- Neurologic disorder, brain surgery, residual effects
- Psychiatric counseling or hospitalization

FAMILY HISTORY

- Psychiatric disorders, mental illness, alcoholism
- Mental retardation
- Alzheimer disease
- Learning disorders

PERSONAL AND SOCIAL HISTORY

- Emotional status: feelings about self; ability to cope with current stressors in life; level of stress; anxiety or irritability; restlessness; appetite; weight loss or gain; decreased sexual activity; problems with money, job, marriage, or children
- Discouragement, life goals, frustrations, attitudes, relationship with family members
- Intellectual level: educational history, any cognitive changes, communication pattern (understand questions, speech is coherent and appropriate), change in memory or thought processes, access to information
- Sleeping or eating patterns; weight loss or gain; anxiety
- Use of alcohol
- Use of street drugs, especially mood-altering drugs

CHILDREN

- Speech and language: first words, intelligibility, quality of sounds, progression to phrases and sentences
- Behavior: temper tantrums, breath-holding, hyperactivity, limited attention span, ability to separate from family and adjust to new situations
- Performance of self-care activities: dressing, toileting, feeding
- Personality and behavior patterns: changes related to any specific event, fever of unknown origin, trauma
- Learning or school difficulties: associated with attention, interest, activity level, or ability to concentrate

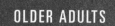

OLDER ADULTS

- Changes in mental functions: cognitive, thought process, memory, sudden or gradual confusion
- Depression

EXAMINATION AND FINDINGS

Mental status (cerebral function) is assessed throughout the physical examination by evaluating the patient's awareness, orientation, cognitive abilities, and affect (Box 4-1). Observe the patient's physical appearance, behavior, and responses to questions asked during the history (Figure 4-2). Note any variations in response to questions of differing complexity. Speech should be clearly articulated. Questions should be answered appropriately with ideas expressed logically, relating current and past events.

BOX 4-1   Procedures of the Mental Status Screening Examination

The shorter screening examination is commonly used for health visits when no known neurologic problem is apparent.
Information is generally obtained during the history in the following areas (pp. 82-88):

Appearance and Behavior

Grooming
Emotional status
Body language

Cognitive Abilities

State of consciousness
Memory
Attention span
Judgment

Emotional Stability

Mood and feelings
Thought processes

Speech and Language

Voice quality
Articulation
Comprehension
Coherence
Aphasia

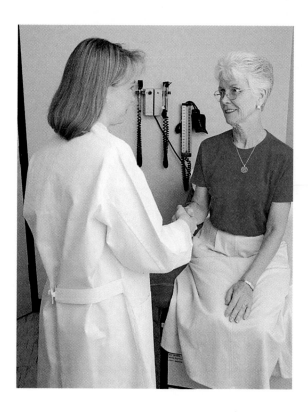

FIGURE 4-2

Observe the patient during initial greeting for behavior, emotional status, grooming, and body language.

PHYSICAL APPEARANCE AND BEHAVIOR

If you have concerns about any of the patient's responses or behaviors, it is important to interview a family member or other independent observer, especially if this is your first visit with the patient.

Grooming

Poor hygiene; lack of concern with appearance; or inappropriateness of dress for season, gender, or occasion in a previously well-groomed individual may indicate an emotional problem, psychiatric disturbance, or organic brain syndrome.

Emotional Status

The patient should behave in a manner expressing concern with the visit appropriate for the emotional content of topics discussed. Consider cultural variations when assessing emotional responses. Note behavior that conveys carelessness, indifference, inability to sense emotions in others, loss of sympathetic reactions, unusual docility, rage reactions, or excessive irritability.

Body Language

Posture should be erect, and the patient should make eye contact with you (Figure 4-3). Slumped posture and a lack of facial expression may indicate depression or a neurologic condition such as Parkinson disease. Excessively energetic movements or constantly watchful eyes suggest tension, anxiety, or a metabolic disorder.

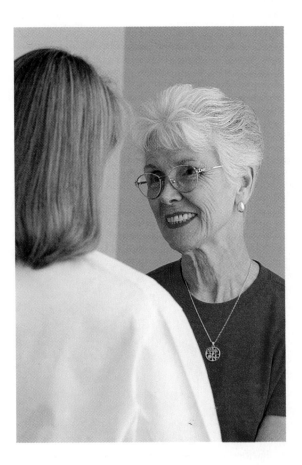

FIGURE 4-3

Note the patient's body posture and ability to make eye contact.

COGNITIVE ABILITIES

Cognitive functions are evaluated while the patient responds to your questions during the history-taking process. Specific questions and specific tasks can provide detailed assessment of cognition. The Mini-Mental State Examination (MMSE) is a standardized tool that may be used to quantitatively estimate cognitive function or to serially document cognitive changes (Figure 4-4). It is a good screening tool for detecting organic disease. The 11 questions take approximately 5 to 10 minutes to administer. Figure 4-5 shows testing the "copying" skill under the language portion of the MMSE.

Signs of possible cognitive impairment include the following: significant memory loss, confusion (getting lost in familiar territory or at night), impaired communication, inappropriate affect, personal care difficulties, hazardous behavior, agitation, and suspiciousness.

State of Consciousness

The patient should be oriented to time, place, and person and be able to appropriately respond to questions and environmental stimuli (Box 4-2). Time disorientation is associated with anxiety, depression, and organic brain syndrome. Place disorientation occurs with psychiatric disorders and organic brain syndromes. Person disorientation results from cerebral trauma, seizures, or amnesia.

Analogies

Ask the patient to describe simple analogies first and then those more complex:
- What is similar about these objects: peaches and lemons; ocean and lake; pencil and typewriter?
- Complete this comparison: An engine is to an airplane as an oar is to a ____.
- What is different about these two objects: a magazine and a telephone book; a bush and a tree?

Correct responses should be given when the patient has average intelligence. An inability to describe similarities or differences may indicate a lesion of the left or dominant cerebral hemisphere.

Abstract Reasoning

Ask the patient to tell you the meaning of a fable, proverb, or metaphor, for example:
- A stitch in time saves nine.
- A bird in a hand is worth two in a bush.
- A rolling stone gathers no moss.

BOX 4-2	Unexpected Levels of Consciousness
Confusion	Inappropriate response to question Decreased attention span and memory
Lethargy	Drowsy, falls asleep quickly Once aroused, responds appropriately
Delirium	Confusion with disordered perceptions and decreased attention span Marked anxiety with motor and sensory excitement Inappropriate reactions to stimuli
Stupor	Arousable for short periods to visual, verbal, or painful stimuli Simple motor or moaning responses to stimuli Slow responses
Coma	Neither awake nor aware Decerebrate posturing to painful stimuli

Patient ....

Examiner ....

Date ....

MINI-MENTAL STATE EXAMINATION

Maximum
Score   Score

ORIENTATION

Max	Score	
5	( )	What is the (year) (season) (date) (day) (month)?
5	( )	Where are we: (state) (county) (town) (hospital) (floor).

REGISTRATION

3   ( )   Name 3 objects: 1 second to say each. Then ask the patient all 3 after you have said them. Give 1 point for each correct answer. Then repeat them until he learns all 3. Count trials and record.

Trials

ATTENTION AND CALCULATION

5   ( )   Serial 7's. 1 point for each correct. Stop after 5 answers. Alternatively spell "world" backwards.

RECALL

3   ( )   Ask for the 3 objects repeated above. Give 1 point for each correct.

LANGUAGE

9   ( )   Name a pencil, and watch (2 points)

Repeat the following "No ifs, ands, or buts." (1 point)

Follow a 3-stage command:

"Take a paper in your right hand, fold it in half, and put it on the floor" (3 points)

Read and obey the following:

CLOSE YOUR EYES (1 point)

Write a sentence (1point)

Copy design (1 point)

_____   Total score

ASSESS level of consciousness along a continuum _____

Alert   Drowsy   Stupor   Coma

INSTRUCTIONS FOR ADMINISTRATION OF MINI-MENTAL STATE EXAMINATION

ORIENTATION

(1) Ask for the date. Then ask specifically for parts omitted, e.g., "Can you also tell me what season it is?" One point for each correct.

(2) Ask in turn "Can you tell me the name of this hospital?" (town, county, etc.). One point for each correct.

REGISTRATION

Ask the patient if you may test his memory. Then say the name of 3 unrelated objects, clearly and slowly, about one second for each. After you have said 3, ask him to repeat them. The first repetition determines his score (0-3) but keep saying them until he can repeat all 3, up to 6 trials. If he does not eventually learn all 3, recall cannot be meaningfully tested.

ATTENTION AND CALCULATION

Ask the patient to begin with 100 and count backwards by 7. Stop after 5 subtractions (93, 86, 79, 72, 65). Score the total number of correct answers.

If the patient cannot or will not perform this task, ask him to spell the word "world" backwards. The score is the number of letters in correct order. E.g. dlrow = 5, dlorw = 3.

RECALL

Ask the patient if he can recall the 3 words you previously asked him to remember. Score 0-3.

LANGUAGE

Naming: Show the patient a wrist watch and ask him what it is. Repeat for pencil. Score 0-2.

Repetition: Ask the patient to repeat the sentence after you. Allow only one trial. Score 0 or 1.

3-Stage command: Give the patient a piece of plain blank paper and repeat the command. Score 1 point for each part correctly executed.

Reading: On a blank piece of paper print the sentence "Close your eyes", in letters large enough for the patient to see clearly. Ask him to read it and do what it says. Score 1 point only if he actually closes his eyes.

Writing: Give the patient a blank piece of paper and ask him to write a sentence for you. Do not dictate a sentence, it is to be written spontaneously. It must contain a subject and verb to be sensible. Correct grammar and punctuation are not necessary.

Copying: On a clean piece of paper, draw intersecting pentagons, each side about 1 in., and ask him to copy it exactly as it is. All 10 angles must be present and 2 must intersect to score 1 point. Tremor and rotation are ignored.

Estimate the patient's level of sensorium along a continuum, from alert on the left to coma on the right.

FIGURE 4-4

The MMSE is a standardized screening tool of mental status. The maximum score is 30. Depressed patients without dementia usually score between 24 and 30. A score of 20 or less is found in patients with dementia, delirium, schizophrenia, or an affective disorder.

From Folstein et al, 1985.

A 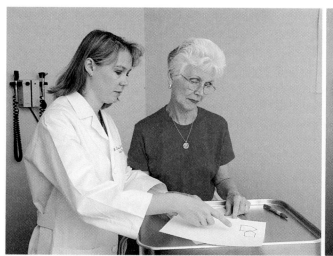 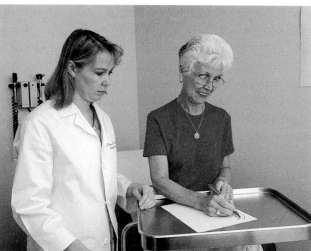 **B**

FIGURE 4-5
Copying is one of the tasks on the MMSE. **A,** Draw intersecting pentagons, and **B,** have the patient copy them.

An adequate interpretation of the phrase should be given when the patient has average intelligence. An inability to give adequate explanation may indicate organic brain syndrome, brain damage, or lack of intelligence.

Arithmetic Calculations

Ask the patient to do simple arithmetic without paper and pencil:

- Subtract 7 from 50, 7 from that answer, and so on until the answer is less than 10.
- Add 8 to 50, 8 to that total, and so on until the answer is near 100.

The calculations should be completed with few errors within a minute when the patient has average intelligence. Impairment of arithmetic skills is associated with depression and diffuse brain disease.

Writing Ability

The patient should write his or her name and address, or you can dictate a phrase. Omission or addition of letters, syllables, words, or mirror writing may indicate aphasia. If the patient cannot write, ask him or her to draw simple geometric figures (triangle, circle, square) and then more complex figures such as a house or flower. Uncoordinated writing or drawing may indicate a cerebellar lesion or peripheral neuropathy.

Execution of Motor Skills

Ask the male patient to comb his hair or the female patient to put on her lipstick (Figure 4-6). Apraxia, an inability to complete a task—unrelated to paralysis or lack of comprehension—may indicate a cerebral disorder.

Memory

Immediate recall is tested by asking the patient to listen and then repeat a sentence or series of numbers. Five to eight numbers forward or four to six numbers backward can usually be repeated. Test recent memory by showing the patient four or five test objects, saying you will ask about them in a few minutes (Figure 4-7). Ten minutes later, ask the patient to list the objects. All objects should be remembered. Remote memory is tested by asking the patient about verifiable past events, such as his or her mother's maiden name, high school attended, or a subject of basic knowledge.

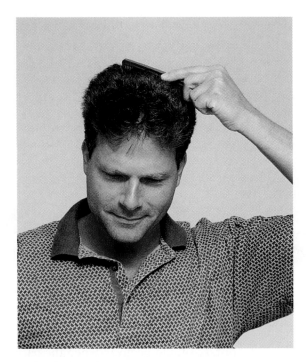

FIGURE 4-6
Ask the patient to complete a simple task such as combing the hair.

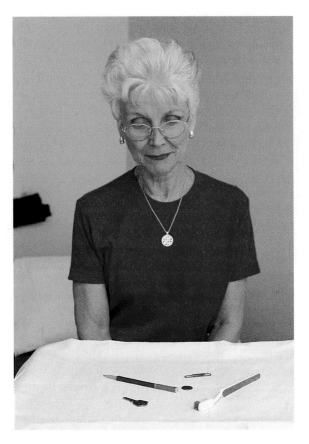

FIGURE 4-7
Show the patient four or five test objects for later recall to test memory.

When the patient is visually impaired, recent memory is tested by using unrelated words rather than test objects. Pick four unrelated words that have distinct sound differences, such as *green, daffodil, hero,* and *sofa,* or *bird, carpet, treasure,* and *orange.* Tell the patient to remember these words. After 5 minutes, ask the patient to list the four words. The patient can be asked to repeat the words again after 30 minutes to test longer term memory.

Impaired memory occurs with various neurologic or psychiatric disorders, such as anxiety and depression. Loss of immediate and recent memory with retention of remote memory suggests dementia.

Attention Span

Ask the patient to follow a series of short commands or repeat a short story you relate. The patient should respond to directions appropriately. Easy distraction, confusion, negativism, and impairment of recent and remote memory may all indicate a decreased attention span. This may be related to fatigue, anxiety, or medication in an otherwise healthy patient.

Judgment

Determine the patient's reasoning skills by exploring these areas:
- How is the patient meeting social and family obligations?
- What are the patient's plans for the future? Do they seem appropriate?

- Have the patient provide solutions to hypothetical situations, such as: What would you do if you found a stamped envelope? If a policeman stopped you after you drove through a red light?
- Have the patient explain fables (such as *The Tortoise and the Hare*) or metaphors.

The patient should be able to evaluate the situations presented and provide appropriate responses. If the patient is meeting social and family obligations and adequately dealing with business affairs, judgment is considered intact. Impaired judgment may indicate mental retardation, emotional disturbance, or organic brain syndrome.

EMOTIONAL STABILITY

Emotional stability is evaluated when the patient does not seem to be coping well or does not have resources to meet his or her personal needs.

Mood and Feelings

Observe the mood and emotional expression from the patient's verbal and nonverbal behavior during the physical examination. Note any mood swings or behaviors indicating anxiety or depression.

Ask the patient how he or she feels right now, if feelings are a problem in daily life, and if there are times or experiences that are particularly difficult.

The patient should express appropriate feelings that correspond to the situation. Unresponsiveness, hopelessness, agitation, euphoria, irritability, or wide mood swings indicate disturbances in mood, affect, and feelings.

Thought Process and Content

During the examination, observe the patient's patterns of thinking, especially the appropriateness of sequence, logic, coherence, and relevance to the topics discussed. You should be able to follow the patient's thought processes, and the ideas expressed should be logical and goal directed.

Illogical or unrealistic thought processes, blocking (an inappropriate pause in the middle of a thought, phrase, or sentence), or disturbance in the stream of thinking (repetition of a word, phrase, or behavior) indicates an emotional disturbance or a psychiatric disorder.

Disturbance in thought content is evaluated by asking the patient about obsessive thoughts related to making decisions, fears, or guilt. Does the patient ever feel like he or she is watched or followed, is controlled or manipulated, or loses touch with reality? Does the patient compulsively repeat actions or check and recheck something to make sure it is done? Obsessive thoughts, compulsive behaviors, phobias, or anxieties that interfere with daily life or are disabling indicate mental dysfunction or a psychiatric disorder.

Perceptual Distortions and Hallucinations

Determine whether the patient perceives any sensations that are not caused by external stimuli (hears voices, sees vivid images or shadowy figures, smells offensive odors, feels worms crawling on skin). Find out when these experiences occur.

Auditory and visual hallucinations are associated with psychiatric disorders, organic conditions, and psychedelic drug ingestion. Tactile hallucinations are most commonly associated with alcohol withdrawal.

SPEECH AND LANGUAGE SKILLS

Detailed evaluation of the patient's communication skills, both receptive and expressive, should be performed when the patient has difficulty communicating during the history. The patient's voice should have inflections, be clear and strong, and be able to increase in volume. Speech should be fluent and articulate, with clear expression of thoughts.

FUNCTIONAL ASSESSMENT

Mental Status

Instrumental activities of daily living (ADLs) are dependent on the patient's mental status. When talking with patients, attempt to determine the patient's ability to perform the following ADLs:

- Manage personal finances and business affairs
- Shop, cook, and prepare balanced meals
- Use problem-solving skills
- Manage medications
- Understand spoken and written language
- Speak and write
- Remember appointments, family occasions, holidays, household tasks

Voice Quality

Determine if there is any difficulty or discomfort in making laryngeal speech sounds. Dysphonia, a disorder of voice volume, quality, or pitch, suggests a problem with laryngeal innervation or disease of the larynx.

Articulation

Evaluate spontaneous speech for pronunciation, fluency, rhythm, and ease of expression. Abnormal articulation includes imperfect pronunciation of words, difficulty articulating a single speech sound, rapid-fire delivery, or speech with hesitancy, stuttering, repetitions, or slow utterances. Dysarthria, a defect in articulation, is associated with a motor deficit of the lips, tongue, palate, or pharynx. Cerebellar dysarthria, which is poorly coordinated, irregular speech with unnatural separation of syllables (scanning), is associated with multiple sclerosis.

Comprehension

The patient should follow simple instructions during the history and physical examination.

Coherence

The patient's intentions or perceptions should be clearly conveyed to you. Circumlocutions and perseveration (repetition of a word, phrase, or gesture) should not be present. Words or sentences that proceed in disorderly fashion (flight of ideas or loosening of associations), gibberish, neologisms, echolalia, or utterances of unusual sounds are associated with psychiatric disorders.

Aphasia

Listen for an omission or addition of letters, syllables, and words or the misuse or transposition of words. Indications of aphasia include hesitations, omissions, inappropriate word substitutions, circumlocutions, creation of new words, and disturbance of rhythm of words in sequence. Aphasia can result from facial muscle or tongue weakness or neurologic damage to brain regions controlling speech and language.

ADDITIONAL PROCEDURES

Glasgow Coma Scale

When a patient has an altered level of consciousness because of head trauma or another hypoxic event, the Glasgow Coma Scale is often used to quantify consciousness. This instrument assesses the function of the cerebral cortex and brainstem through the patient's verbal response, motor response, and eye opening to specific stimuli (Box 4-3).

BOX 4-3   **Glasgow Coma Scale**

Level of consciousness can be evaluated and quantified when the patient has an acute brain injury.

Assessed Behaviors	Criteria for Scoring	Scores
Eye opening response	Spontaneous opening	4
	To verbal stimuli	3
	To pain	2
	None	1
Most appropriate verbal response	Oriented	5
	Confused	4
	Inappropriate words	3
	Incoherent	2
	None	1
Most integrated motor response	Obeys commands	6
	Localizes pain	5
	Withdraws from pain	4
	Flexion to pain (decorticate)	3
	Extension to pain (decerebrate)	2
	None	1

Add the numbers from each category. Maximum score = 15, minimum score = 3.

From Teasdale, Jennett, 1974.

This assessment can be repeated at intervals to detect improvement or deterioration in the patient's level of consciousness. The instrument was initially developed to predict mortality associated with head injuries, but it is now widely used in coma assessment.

The patient's best response in each category is matched to the criteria for scoring. Appropriate verbal stimuli are questions eliciting the patient's level of orientation to person, place, and time. Painful stimuli are used when necessary to obtain eye opening and motor responses. Begin with less painful stimuli such as pinching the skin and progress to squeezing muscle mass or tendons if there is no response. See Table 4-1 for a description of postures found in unresponsive patients.

Three scores are added to produce the Glasgow Coma Score. The maximum score of 15 indicates the optimal level of consciousness. The lower the score, the more severe the impairment in consciousness. The lowest score possible is 3, indicating deepest coma. See Box 4-4 for common causes of unresponsiveness.

BOX 4-4   **Common Causes of Unresponsiveness**

Type of Disorder	Cause
Focal structural lesions of the brain	Hemorrhage, hematoma, infarction, tumor, abscess, trauma
Diffuse brain disease	Drug intoxications
	Metabolic disorders such as hypoglycemia, ketoacidosis, hypernatremia or hyponatremia, renal failure, myxedema, hypercalcemia or hypocalcemia, pulmonary insufficiency
	Hypothermia, hyperthermia
	Hypoxemia—strangulation, drowning, cardiopulmonary arrest, pulmonary embolism
	Encephalitis, meningitis
	Seizures
Psychogenic unresponsiveness	Dementia

TABLE 4-1	Postures Often Found in Unresponsive Patients
Posture and Site of Lesion	**Characteristics**
Decorticate Corticospinal tracts above the brainstem	Rigid flexion; upper arms held tightly to the sides of body; elbows, wrists, and fingers flexed; feet are plantar flexed, legs extended and internally rotated; may have fine tremors or intense stiffness 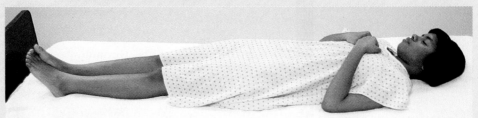
Decerebrate Brainstem	Rigid extension; arms fully extended; forearms pronated; wrists and fingers flexed; jaws clenched, neck extended, back may be arched; feet plantar flexed; posturing may occur spontaneously, intermittently, or in response to a stimulus 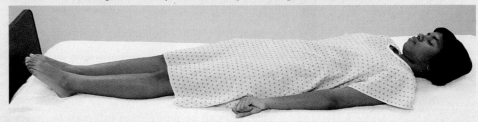
Hemiplegia Corticospinal tract	Unilateral flaccidity or spasticity; voluntary movement on unaffected side 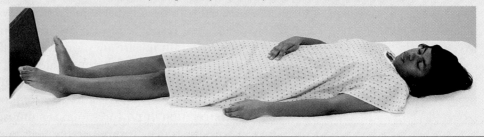

INFANTS AND CHILDREN

The infant's general behavior and level of consciousness are evaluated by observing the level of activity and responsiveness to environmental stimuli. Note whether the baby is lethargic, drowsy, stuporous, alert, active, or irritable (Figure 4-8). By 2 months of age, the infant should appear alert, quiet, and content and should recognize the face of a significant other (Figure 4-9).

By the time an infant is 2 to 3 months old, it is reasonable to expect that a careful examiner who devotes time to developing a relationship with the baby could coax a smile. If it is difficult or impossible to elicit a social smile, there should be concern about the child's immediate health and neurologic competence.

Drooling babies are ubiquitous. In the first year of life, drooling is frequently attributed to teething. Past the age of 1 year, drooling becomes much less common; by age 2 it generally disappears. If it persists, the examiner should be concerned about some neurologic handicap, perhaps mental retardation, or anomalies of the teeth or the upper gastrointestinal tract.

Because language has not yet developed, crying and other vocal sounds are evaluated. The infant's cry should be loud and angry, not high pitched or hoarse. A shrill

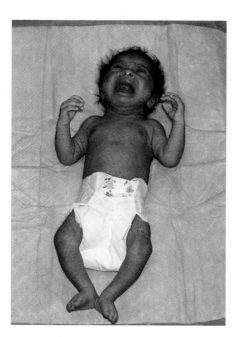

FIGURE 4-8
Note the level of irritability and posturing expressed by this newborn with cocaine withdrawal.

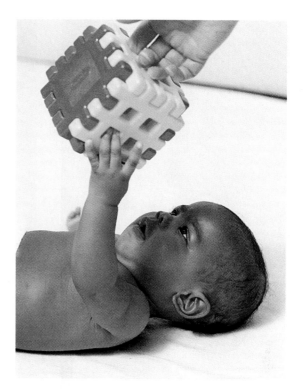

FIGURE 4-9
Note the level of alertness and interest in various objects and people.

or whiny high-pitched cry or catlike screeching cry suggests a central nervous system deficit. Cooing and babbling are expected after 3 and 4 months of age, respectively. One or two words (mama, dada, bye-bye) should be distinct by 9 to 10 months of age.

The Denver II is a useful tool to determine whether the child is developing as expected with fine and gross motor skills, language, and personal-social skills. Older children can be asked to draw a picture of a person to assess cognitive development with the Goodenough-Harris Drawing Test (Figure 4-10).

Observe the child's mood, communication pattern, preferences, and responsiveness to the parent. Evaluate the types of words and speech patterns used. The child's language and speech should be appropriate for age. Table 4-2 describes expressive language milestones. Articulation is a fine motor skill, and speech should be more clearly understood with advancing age. Articulation milestones may be evaluated with the Denver Articulate Screening Exam (DASE).

Memory testing may be attempted at about 4 years of age, if the child pays attention and is not too anxious. Expected memory skills vary with the age of the child. Test immediate recall by asking the child to repeat either numbers or words. A 4-year-old can repeat three digits or words, a 5-year-old can repeat four digits or words, and a 6-year-old can repeat five digits or words. Recent memory is not usually tested in children but may be done with modification. Show the child only familiar objects, and wait no longer than 5 minutes to ask the child to recall what objects were shown (Figure 4-11).

Older preschoolers will be more skilled with this test. Test remote memory by asking the child what he or she had for dinner the previous night, his or her address, or to recite a nursery rhyme.

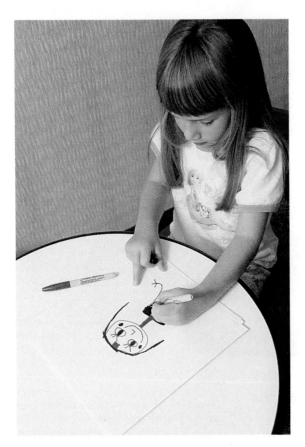

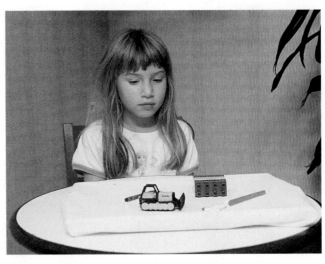

FIGURE 4-11
Test memory recall using familiar objects.

FIGURE 4-10
Ask the child to draw a picture of a man or woman. The presence and form of body parts provide a clue about the child's development.

TABLE 4-2	Expressive Language Milestones for the Toddler
Age (months)	**Expressive Language Milestones**
12 to 15	Says 3-4 words appropriately, including names; uses flow of connected sounds that have inflection and seem like a sentence
15 to 18	Uses 10 words including names; makes requests by naming objects; begins to repeat words heard in adult conversations
18 to 24	Uses short sentences (3-4 words); uses pronouns but some syntax errors; tells full name; echoes last 2-3 words of a rhyme
24 to 36	Caregiver understands 90% of speech; uses noun-verb combinations with correct verb tense; repeats 3 numbers, given intervals

Modified from Krajicek, Tomlinson, 1983.

There is little evidence that the individual's personality changes with age, in the absence of other health problems; however, existing personality traits may become exaggerated. Paranoid thought is the most striking alteration in personality. Attempt to determine whether the thought process is accurate or a paranoid ideation, keeping in mind that the incidence of abuse of the elderly is increasing.

Deterioration of intellectual function should not be found until 70 years of age unless the patient has a disease of the central nervous system or a disease affecting it. Determine whether any changes in cerebral function could be the consequence of cardiovascular, hepatic, renal, or metabolic disease. Medications can also impair central nervous system function, causing slowed reaction time, disorientation, confusion, loss of memory, tremors, and anxiety. Problems may develop because of the dosage, number, or interaction of medications prescribed or purchased over the counter.

Some problem-solving skills deteriorate with age, but this may be related to disuse. Skills involving vocabulary and inventories of available information are expected to remain at younger adult levels of performance. Recent memory deteriorates before remote memory. Most older adults comment that their remembrance of distant events actually improves. Since the ability to perceive spatial relationships and to reason abstractly declines with age, some patients may have a problem understanding new concepts by 80 years of age.

Mental function as a whole may be evaluated with the Set Test in about 5 minutes. The patient is asked to name 10 items in each of four groups: *fruits, animals, colors,* and *towns*/cities (FACT). Do not prompt or rush the patient. The patient's ability to respond demonstrates motivation, alertness, concentration, short-term memory, and problem solving. In addition, the patient has had to categorize, count, name, and remember the items listed. Each of these skills is important for older persons to adapt to a new environment and learn new self-care skills.

To score, give each item 1 point. A maximum of 40 points is possible. Scores under 15 are associated with dementia. Scores above 25 are not associated with dementia. Scores between 15 and 24 need further investigation to distinguish between mental changes and cultural, educational, or social factors.

Facial expressions that are masklike or overly dramatic, or a stance that is stooped and fearful may indicate a progressive disease.

SAMPLE DOCUMENTATION

Appropriate dress and behavior. Oriented to time, place, and person. Reasoning and arithmetic calculation abilities intact. Immediate, recent, and remote memory intact. Appropriate mood and feelings expressed. Speech clearly and smoothly enunciated. Comprehends direction.

SUMMARY OF EXAMINATION   Mental Status

1. Observe physical appearance and behavior (p. 82).
2. Investigate cognitive abilities by assessing the following (pp. 83-87):
   - State of consciousness
   - Response to questions
   - Reasoning
   - Arithmetic ability
   - Memory
   - Attention span
3. Evaluate emotional stability from the following (p. 87):
   - Signs of depression or anxiety
   - Disturbance in thought content
   - Hallucinations
4. Observe speech and language by the following (pp. 87-88):
   - Voice quality
   - Articulation
   - Coherence
   - Comprehension

COMMON ABNORMALITIES

DISORDERS OF ALTERED MENTAL STATUS

DEPRESSION

Depression is a common psychiatric illness with symptoms that range from mild to psychotic. Mood and affect are affected with extreme sadness or anxiety and agitation expressed. Somatic complaints may include altered appetite, constipation, headache, and fatigue. The disorder may result from grief, reaction to medical or neurologic diseases, or a psychoneurosis. Characteristics are described in Table 4-3.

TABLE 4-3 Comparison of the Characteristics Associated with Various Causes of Altered Mental Status

Characteristic	Delirium	Dementia	Depression
Onset	Sudden	Insidious, relentless, or sporadic	Sudden, related to specific events
Duration	Hours, days	Persistent	Episodic or persistent
Time of day	Worse at night and when drug levels peak, sleep-wake cycle disturbed	Stable, no change	Insomnia, sleeps during the day
Cognitive impairment	Memory, attentiveness, consciousness, calculations	Abstract thinking, judgment, memory, thought patterns, calculations, agnosia, permanent and progressive	Complains of memory loss, forgetfulness, inability to concentrate
Activity	Increased or decreased, may fluctuate; tremors, spastic movements	Unchanged from usual behavior	Lack of motivation, lethargic; restless or agitated
Speech/language	Slurred or rapid and manic, rambling, incoherent	Disordered, rambling, incoherent; struggles to find words	Slow, sluggish speech; slow processing and response to verbal stimuli
Mood and affect	Rapid mood swings; fearful, suspicious	Depressed, apathetic, uninterested	Extreme sadness, anxiety, irritability
Delusions/hallucinations	Visual, auditory, tactile, hallucinations, delusions	Delusions, no hallucinations	Delusions about worthlessness, paranoid ideation
Associated factors or triggers	Physical condition, drug toxicity, head injury, change in environment, vision or hearing problems	Chronic alcoholism, vitamin B_{12} deficiency, Huntington chorea, arterial disease, HIV* infection, Alzheimer disease	Loss of friends, family, health, life-style
Reversibility	Potential	No, progressive	Potential

*HIV, Human immunodeficiency virus

DELIRIUM

MNEMONICS

CAUSES OF DELIRIUM:
"DELIRIUM"

D Drugs: ethanol, bromism

E Electrolyte imbalance

L Low Po_2

I Injury to brain

R Relapsing fever (malaria)

I Infection

U Uremia

M Metabolic (liver damage)

Delirium is a confusional state in which there is a disorder of perception. It is accompanied by intense agitation, frenzied excitement, trembling, hallucinations, vivid dreams, an inability to sleep, absurd fantasies, and delusions. It may be associated with a withdrawal from an excessive intake of alcohol over time, age-related impairment of drug metabolism, or diminished reserves in responding to physiologic stress. Other characteristics are described in Table 4-3.

DEMENTIA

MNEMONICS

CAUSES OF DEMENTIA:
"DEMENTIA"

D Drugs and toxins

E Endocrine

M Metabolic and Mechanical

E Epilepsy

N Nutritional and Nervous system

T Tumor and Trauma

I Infection

A Arterial

Dementia is a clinical syndrome of failing memory and impairment of other intellectual functions, behavioral abnormalities, and personality changes resulting from a chronic progressive deterioration of the brain. It is usually related to obvious structural diseases of the brain tissue. Other characteristics are described in Table 4-3.

KORSAKOFF AMNESIC STATE

Korsakoff amnesic state (Korsakoff psychosis) is a syndrome often associated with chronic alcoholism and malnutrition, but it may also occur with brain tumors of the thalamus and other toxic conditions. It is characterized by amnesia for recent events and disorientation in space and time. Recent memory is most affected, but immediate memory is usually intact. Long-standing habits, automatic motor skills, and words and visual impression are unimpaired. The patient may use confabulation to fill in gaps in memory related to events.

INFANTS AND CHILDREN

MENTAL RETARDATION

Significant subaverage general intellectual functioning, existing concurrently with deficits in adaptive behavior, is manifested during the developmental period. Signs and symptoms include delayed developmental milestones, inability to discriminate between two or more stimuli, impaired short-term memory, and lack of motivation.

ATTENTION DEFICIT HYPERACTIVITY DISORDER

A combination of behavior problems that interfere with the child's ability to learn, including developmentally inappropriate inattention, impulsivity, and hyperactivity. Onset occurs before 7 years of age and is not related to mental retardation or a psychiatric disorder.

AUTISTIC DISORDER

Autistic disorder is a pervasive developmental disorder of unknown cause with a combination of behavioral traits and communication deficits that begins before age 3. The child has a deficit in at least one of three areas: social interaction; language for social purposes; or symbolic and imaginative play. Language is delayed or does not develop. Echolalia or parrot speech is common. Behavioral traits of this condition may include a lack of awareness of others, an aversion to touch or being held, odd repetitive behaviors, or preoccupation with parts of objects. Motor development often progresses normally. The majority of autistic children are mentally retarded. This condition is more common in boys than girls with a ratio of 4:1. Only 1% to 2% of affected children progress to function independently as adults.

OLDER ADULTS

DEMENTIA OF ALZHEIMER TYPE

This type of dementia accounts for approximately 35% to 50% of dementia cases. There is severe progressive deterioration in mental functions with a subtle, insidious onset. The duration and rate of progression varies. Impaired ability to learn new information or to recall previously learned information is present. At least one of the following signs are also present: aphasia, apraxia, agnosia, or a disturbance in executive functioning. The disorder leads to profound disintegration of personality and eventual complete disorientation. Cognitive deficits are not caused by other central nervous system or systemic conditions. It is present in approximately 5% of persons over 65 years and 20% of persons over 85 years. Women, especially those with a positive family history, are at greatest risk.

VASCULAR DEMENTIA (MULTI-INFARCT DEMENTIA)

Vascular dementia has a rapid onset with deterioration in cognitive ability, often related to a series of cerebrovascular accidents (CVAs). The patient has impaired memory, leading to an inability to learn new information or to recall previously learned information. In addition, the patient has either aphasia, apraxia, agnosia, or a disturbance in executive functioning. Other focal neurologic signs are usually present. Patients have a history of cerebrovascular disease.

http://www1.mosby.com/physexam_seidel

CHAPTER 5

GROWTH AND MEASUREMENT

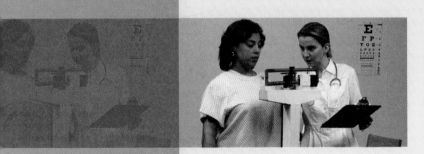

Weight and body composition offer much information about an individual's health status and often provide a clue to the presence of disease when they are out of balance. The care of children is exciting because of the constancy of change that is explicit in growth and development. Children just do not stay the same. Measuring their weights and heights and giving careful attention to the sequence of their achievements is gratifying as you get to know a child over time. When all goes well and the child grows and develops as expected, there is great pleasure. But when all is not well, your careful attention and early detection can often correct or at least ameliorate a problem.

The focus of this chapter is the evaluation of an individual's anthropometric parameters and the examination for growth, gestational age, and pubertal development. Nutritional assessment is discussed in Chapter 6. Neurologic and motor development of children are discussed in Chapters 19 (Musculoskeletal System) and 20 (Neurologic System). For specific age-related milestones, see Tables 19-3 and 20-13.

ANATOMY AND PHYSIOLOGY

Growth, the increase in size of an individual or single organ, is dependent on a sequence of endocrine, genetic, constitutional, environmental, and nutritional influences. Through the biologic process of development and maturation, individual organ systems acquire function.

ENDOCRINE INFLUENCES

The growth process requires the interaction and balance of many hormones for normal growth and development to proceed (Figure 5-1).

Growth hormone is secreted by the pituitary gland under the neuroendocrine control of two hormones of the hypothalamus. Growth hormone-releasing hormone (GHRH) stimulates the pituitary to release the growth hormone. Somatostatin inhibits the secretion of both GHRH and thyroid-stimulating hormone.

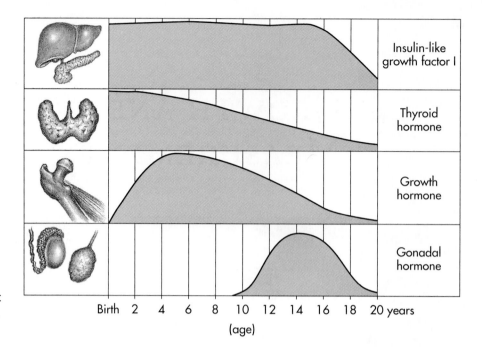

FIGURE 5-1

Hormones affecting growth during childhood and the age at which they are most influential.

Redrawn from Hughes, 1984.

Growth hormone needs the insulin-like growth factor I (IGF I), produced by the liver, to stimulate skeletal growth. The production of IGF I is regulated by growth hormone, the thyroid hormones, and possibly insulin. IGF I acts by stimulating target cells that control ossification. Growth hormone also has a direct effect on the growth of other tissues. IGFs act primarily as local regulators of cell growth and differentiation.

The gonads begin to secrete testosterone and estrogen during puberty. Testosterone enhances muscular development and sexual maturation and promotes bone maturation and epiphyseal closure. Estrogen stimulates the development of female secondary sexual characteristics and linear growth by the acceleration of skeletal maturation and epiphyseal fusion. It also stimulates the growth and differentiation of the genitalia during the fetal period. Androgens, secreted by the adrenal glands, promote masculinization of the secondary sex characteristics and skeletal maturation.

The developmental changes of puberty are caused by the interaction of the hypothalamus, pituitary gland, and gonads. Gonadotropin-releasing hormone, secreted by the hypothalamus, stimulates the pituitary to secrete follicle-stimulating hormone (FSH) and luteinizing hormone (LH). These hormones, in turn, act on the gonads to stimulate germ cell maturation and the synthesis of sex steroid hormones.

Growth at puberty is dependent on the interaction of growth hormone, IGF I, and the sex steroids. The sex steroids stimulate an increased secretion of the growth hormone, which in turn mediates the dramatic increase in IGF I. This leads to the adolescent growth spurt. Thyroid hormones play a central role in skeletal maturation by stimulating growth hormone secretion and controlling the effect of growth hormone on IGF I production. Thyroid hormones are also likely to have a direct effect on stimulating bone maturation.

DIFFERENCES IN GROWTH BY ORGAN SYSTEM

Each organ or organ system has its particular period of rapid growth, marked by rapid cell differentiation and changes in form, that is influenced by the physical and environmental factors to which it is exposed. As individuals, each of us has a unique growth timetable and final growth outcome. However, the sequential patterns are consistent for all of us, unless some external environmental or inherent pathophysiologic process intervenes (Figures 5-2 and 5-3).

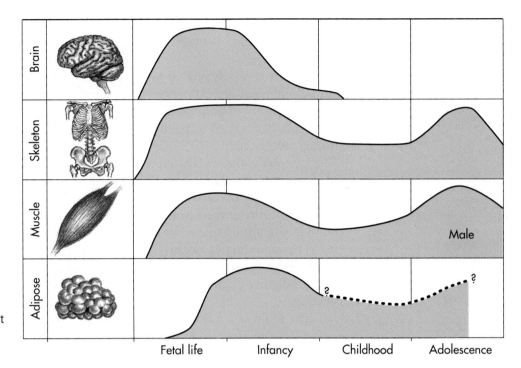

FIGURE 5-2

Rates of growth in various tissues between fetal development and adolescence.

Redrawn from Smith, 1977.

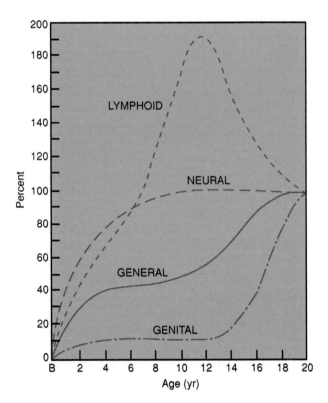

FIGURE 5-3

Growth rates for body as a whole and three types of tissues. **Lymphoid type:** thymus, lymph nodes, and intestinal lymph masses. **Neural type:** brain, dura, spinal cord, optic apparatus, and head dimensions. **General type:** body as a whole; external dimensions; and respiratory, digestive, renal, circulatory, and musculoskeletal systems. **Genetal type:** includes the reproductive organ system.

From Wong, 1995. Modified from Harris et al, 1930.

General growth encompasses most body measurements and organ growth, specifically the musculoskeletal system, liver, and kidneys. Their growth approximates the growth curves described for stature.

Skeletal growth is considered complete when the epiphyses of long bones have completely fused. The mean age for this event (±2 years) in males is 17.5 years and in females is 15.5 years, 2 years after menarche. However, skeletal growth continues until 30 years of age with the apposition of bone to the upper and lower surfaces of the vertebral bodies. The increase in stature is only 3 to 5 mm during this time. Stature is stationary between the ages of 30 and 50 years and then begins to decline (Tanner, 1990).

Weight is closely related to growth in stature and organ development. Growth and development are influenced by nutritional adequacy, which contributes to the number and size of adipose cells. The number of adipose cells increases throughout childhood. Sex-related differences in fat deposition appear in infancy and continue through adolescence.

Lymphatic tissues (lymph nodes, spleen, tonsils, adenoids, and blood lymphocytes) are small in relation to total body size but are well developed at birth. These tissues grow rapidly to reach adult dimensions by 6 years of age. By age 10 to 12 the lymphatic tissues are at their peak, about double adult size. During adolescence they decrease in size until stable adult dimensions are reached.

The reproductive organs, both internal and external, have a slow prepubertal growth. With the interaction of the hypothalamus, pituitary, and gonadal hormones, the reproductive organs double in size during adolescence, achieving maturation and function.

The brain is a marvelous organ, so fully developed at an early age that it provides infants and young children opportunities to sense and appreciate the world and to learn an enormous amount. We often fail to appreciate the sophistication of that brain in the body of a baby or a toddler. At some subconscious level we do not expect it to do all that it can, and we tend to underestimate the ability of the very young to sense their environment.

The brain, with the skull, eyes, and ears, completes physical development more quickly than any other body part. The most rapid and critical period of brain growth occurs between conception and 2 years of age. Most of the neurons are present by 18 to 20 weeks' gestation, and two thirds of brain cells are present at birth. Glial cells and myelin continue to develop after birth, and by 10 months of age, new cell development is complete. Cell size continues to increase, and at 2 years of age, 80% of the brain growth is completed (Trauner, 1979). During adolescence the size of the head increases because of development of air sinuses and thickening of the scalp and skull, not because of brain growth.

INFANTS AND CHILDREN

As the child grows from infancy to adulthood, the change in body proportion is related to the pattern of skeletal growth (Figure 5-4).

Growth of the head predominates during the fetal period. Fetal weight gain naturally follows growth in length, but weight reaches its peak during the third trimester with the increase in organ size. The birth weight of the infant is in large part determined by the mother's prepregnancy weight and the weight the mother gained during pregnancy, placental function, and gestational age (Figure 5-5).

During infancy the growth of the trunk predominates, and weight gain velocity proceeds at a rapid but decelerating rate. The fat content of the body increases slowly during early fetal development and then rapidly accelerates during infancy until approximately 9 months of age.

The legs are the fastest growing body part during childhood, and weight is gained at a steady rate. Fat tissue increases slowly until 7 years of age, at which time a prepubertal fat spurt occurs before the true growth spurt.

The trunk and the legs elongate during adolescence. During this period about 50% of the individual's ideal weight is gained, and the skeletal mass and organ systems double in size. It is during adolescence that males develop broader shoulders

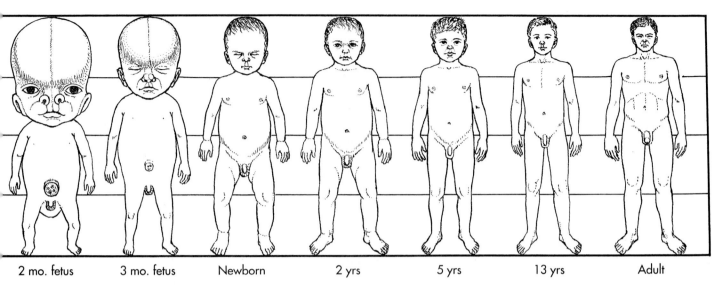

FIGURE 5-4

Changes in body proportions from 8 weeks of gestation through adulthood.

Redrawn from Crouch, McClintic, 1976.

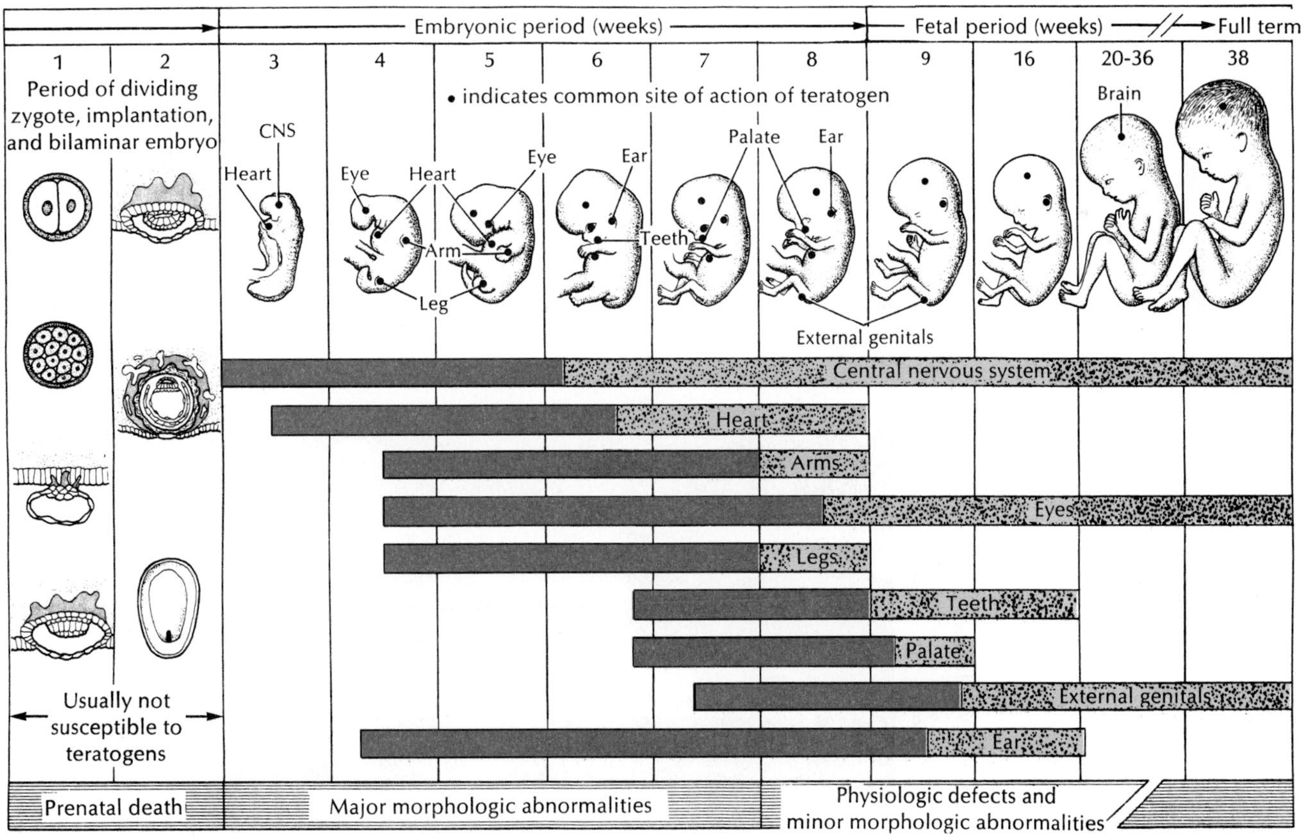

FIGURE 5-5

Sensitive or critical periods in human development. Solid red denotes highly sensitive periods; stippled red indicates stages that are less sensitive to teratogens.

From Moore, 1977.

and greater musculature than females, whereas females develop a wider pelvic outlet. Males have a slight increase in body fat during early adolescence, and then they have a proportionate gain in lean body tissue. Females have a persistent increase in fat tissue throughout adolescence, occurring after the peak growth spurt (Peck, Ullrich, 1985).

PREGNANT WOMEN

Progressive weight gain is expected during pregnancy, but the amount varies among women. The growing fetus accounts for only 5 to 10 lb of the total weight gained. The remainder results from an increase in maternal tissues (placenta, amniotic fluid, uterus, blood and fluid volume, breasts, and fat reserves) (Figure 5-6).

Desirable weight gain follows a curve through the trimesters of pregnancy. The rate of weight gain is slow during the first trimester, rapid during the second trimester, and less rapid during the third trimester. Maternal tissue growth accounts for most of the weight gained in the first and second trimesters, whereas fetal growth accounts for weight gained during the third trimester.

OLDER ADULTS

Stature declines in the older adult, beginning at approximately 50 years of age. This is caused by a thinning of the intervertebral disks and by the development of kyphosis with osteoporotic vertebral compression.

Muscle mass decreases by up to 30% between 30 and 80 years of age; however, exercise contributes to a slower reduction of muscle mass (McCance, Huether, 1994). This decline in lean body mass is accompanied by an increase in body fat, so that the total body weight tends to remain constant with aging. There is a reduction in size and weight of various organs associated with aging, especially the liver, lungs, and kidneys.

REVIEW OF RELATED HISTORY

PRESENT PROBLEM

- Weight loss and weight gain (See Chapter 6, Nutrition, Review of Related History).
  - Undesired weight loss: anorexia; vomiting or diarrhea, frequency, consistency, time period; excessive thirst, frequent urination; change in life-style; activity and stress levels

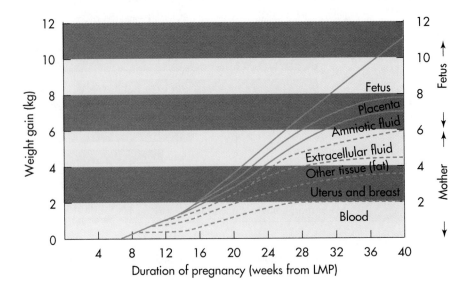

FIGURE 5-6

Weight gain during pregnancy and tissue growth contribute to the total weight gained.

From Schneider, 1977.

- Medications: chemotherapy, diuretics, insulin, fluoxetine (Prozac); nonprescription diet pills, laxatives, steroids, oral contraceptives
■ Changes in body proportions
- Coarsening of facial features, enlarging of hands and feet, moon facies
- Change in fat distribution: trunk-girdle versus generalized
- Medication: steroids

PAST MEDICAL HISTORY

■ Chronic illness: gastrointestinal, renal, pulmonary, cardiac, cancer, infections, or allergies
■ Previous weight loss or gain efforts: weight at 21 years, maximum body weight

FAMILY HISTORY

■ Obesity
■ Constitutionally short or tall stature, precocious or delayed puberty
■ Genetic or metabolic disorder: cystic fibrosis, dwarfism, mucopolysaccharidosis

PERSONAL AND SOCIAL HISTORY

■ Usual weight and height
■ Use of alcohol
■ Use of street drugs

INFANTS

■ Estimated gestational age, birth weight
■ Following an established percentile growth curve
- Unexplained changes in length, weight, or head circumference
- Poor growth: falling one or more standard deviations off growth curve pattern; below fifth percentile for weight and height; infant small for gestational age; quality of mother-infant interaction
■ Development: achieving milestones at appropriate ages
■ Congenital anomaly or chronic illness: heart defect, hydrocephalus, microcephalus, malabsorption syndrome, urinary tract infection, and others
■ See Chapter 6, Nutrition.

CHILDREN & ADOLESCENTS

■ Sexual maturation of girls: early (before 8 years) or delayed (beyond 13 years) signs of breast development and pubic hair, age at menarche
■ Sexual maturation of boys: early (before 9 years) or delayed (beyond 14 years) signs of genital development and pubic hair
■ Short stature: not growing as fast as peers, change in shoe and clothing size in past year, extremities short or long for size of trunk, size of head disproportionate to body, height of parents
■ Tall stature: growing faster than peers, height of parents, signs of sexual maturation
■ Medications: steroids, growth hormones

PREGNANT WOMEN

■ Pregnancy weight, dietary intake
■ Date of last menstrual period, weight gain pattern, following established weight gain curve for gestational course

OLDER ADULTS

■ Chronic debilitating illness: problems with meal preparation, problems eating, poorly fitting dentures, ability to follow prescribed diet, difficulty chewing or swallowing
■ See Chapter 6, Nutrition.

EXAMINATION AND FINDINGS

EQUIPMENT

- Standing platform scale with height attachment
- Skinfold thickness calipers
- Measuring tape, nonstretching
- Infant scale
- Recumbent measuring device (for infants)
- Stature measuring device (for children)

WEIGHT AND STANDING HEIGHT

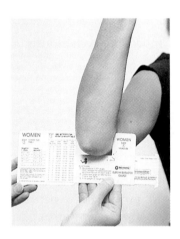

FIGURE 5-7
Measurement of elbow breadth using sliding calipers.

To measure weight, have the patient stand in the middle of the scale platform while you balance the scale. Move the largest weight to the 50-lb or 10-kg increment under the patient's weight. Adjust the smaller weight to balance the scale. Read the weight to the nearest 0.1 kg or ¼ lb. Weight variations occur during the day and from day to day with changes in fluid and intestinal contents of the body. When monitoring a patient's weight daily or weekly, weigh the patient at a consistent time of day.

To measure height, have the patient stand erect with his or her back to the scale. Pull up the height attachment and position the headpiece at the patient's crown. Make the reading at the nearest centimeter or half inch.

Measurement of the elbow breadth provides an estimate of frame size. Have the patient extend the right arm and flex the elbow to 90 degrees. The patient's thumb should be pointing up with the palm turned laterally. Facing the patient, place the elbow-breadth measuring device or skinfold calipers, held on the same plane as the upper arm, on the two most prominent bones of the elbow to measure the elbow breadth (Figure 5-7). (Sliding calipers may be needed if the skinfold calipers do not extend to the breadth of the elbow.) Read the patient's measurement in centimeters and compare it with the table of elbow breadth measurements for age and sex (Table 5-1).

Another method for determining frame size when calipers are not available is to measure the patient's wrist circumference. This measurement is used with the patient's height to create a ratio. Place the measuring tape around the smallest part of the wrist distal to the styloid process of the radius and ulna. Obtain the measurement in centimeters to the nearest millimeter. The wrist circumference ratio = the patient's height in centimeters divided by the wrist circumference in centimeters. Refer to Table 5-2 to determine the body frame size based on the wrist circumference ratio.

TABLE 5-1	Elbow Breadth Measurements (Medium Frame)[*†]		
Men		**Women**	
Age (yr)	**Elbow Breadth (cm)**	**Age (yr)**	**Elbow Breadth (cm)**
18-24	>6.6-<7.7	18-24	>5.6-<6.5
25-34	>6.7-<7.9	25-34	>5.7-<6.8
35-44	>6.7-<8.0	35-44	>5.7-<7.1
45-54	>6.7-<8.1	45-54	>5.7-<7.2
55-74	>6.7-<8.1	55-74	>5.8-<7.2

Modified from Frisancho, 1984.
*Data from National Center for Health Statistics, 1981.
†Measurements lower than ranges given indicate a small frame, whereas higher measurements indicate a large frame.

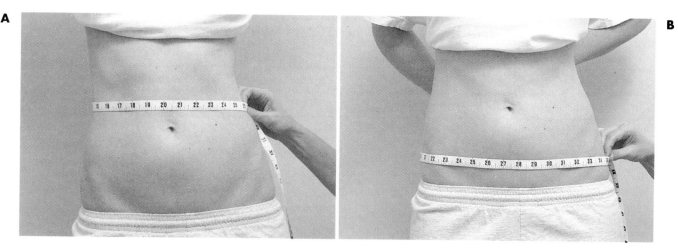

FIGURE 5-8
Measurement of **(A)** waist circumference and **(B)** hip circumference to calculate the waist-to-hip circumference ratio.

TABLE 5-2	Determining Body Frame Size from the Wrist Circumference Ratio*	
Frame Size	**Ratio for Men**	**Ratio for Women**
Small	>10.4	>10.9
Medium	10.4 to 9.6	10.9 to 9.9
Large	<9.6	<9.9

*Height (cm) ÷ wrist circumference (cm)

Once the frame size has been determined, the appropriateness of the patient's weight for height and frame can be evaluated (Tables 5-3 and 5-4). It will be necessary to convert the patient's weight to kilograms to utilize the tables.

Severe weight loss and wasting are usually associated with a debilitating disease or self-starvation.

Waist-to-Hip Circumference Ratio

The waist-to-hip circumference ratio is a measure of fat distribution by body type. It is not as helpful as the body mass index in assessing total body fat (Chapter 6). An excess proportion of trunk and abdominal fat (ovoid or apple-shaped body) has a higher risk association with diabetes mellitus, hyperlipidemia, stroke, and ischemic heart disease than does a larger proportion of gluteal fat (pear-shaped body). Using a tape measure with millimeter marks, measure the waist at or 1 cm above the umbilical midline. Then measure the hip at the level of the superior iliac crest (Figure 5-8). Divide the waist circumference by the hip circumference to obtain the ratio. Ratios over 0.9 in men and 0.8 in women indicate increased risk of disease. This measurement is an indicator of central fat distribution and seems predictive of certain disease risk for both whites and blacks.

TRICEPS SKINFOLD THICKNESS

The measurement of skinfold or fatfold thickness provides another parameter to evaluate the nutritional status of the patient. The jaws of skinfold thickness calipers must be correctly placed to get an accurate reading.

| TABLE 5-3 | Selected Percentiles of Weight and Triceps Skinfold Thickness for U.S. Men Ages 25 to 54 Years* |

Height		Weight (kg)					Triceps (mm)						
In	Cm	5th	15th	50th	85th	95th	5th	10th	15th	50th	85th	90th	95th
Small Frames, Men													
62	157	46	52	64	71	77				11			
63	160	48	53	61	70	79			6	10	17		
64	163	49	55	66	76	80		5	5	10	16	18	
65	165	52	58	66	77	84	4	5	6	11	17	19	21
66	168	56	59	67	78	84	5	6	6	11	18	18	20
67	170	56	62	71	82	88	5	6	6	11	18	20	22
68	173	56	62	71	79	85	5	6	6	10	15	16	20
69	175	57	65	74	84	88		6	6	11	17	20	
70	178	59	67	75	87	90			7	10	17		
71	180	60	70	76	79	91			7	10	16		
72	183	62	67	74	87	93				10			
73	185	63	69	79	89	94							
74	188	65	71	80	90	96							
Medium Frames, Men													
62	157	51	58	68	81	87				15			
63	160	52	59	71	82	89				11			
64	163	54	61	71	83	90		6	6	12	18	20	
65	165	59	65	74	87	94	5	7	8	12	20	22	25
66	168	58	65	75	85	93	5	6	7	11	16	18	22
67	170	62	68	77	89	100	5	7	7	13	21	23	28
68	173	60	66	78	89	97	4	5	7	11	18	20	24
69	175	63	68	78	90	97	5	6	7	12	18	20	24
70	178	64	70	81	90	97	5	6	7	12	18	20	23
71	180	62	70	81	92	100	4	5	7	12	19	21	25
72	183	68	74	84	97	104	5	7	7	12	20	22	26
73	185	70	75	85	100	104	6	7	8	12	20	24	27
74	188	68	77	88	100	104		6	9	13	21	23	
Large Frames, Men													
62	157	57	66	82	99	108							
63	160	58	67	83	100	109							
64	163	59	68	84	101	110							
65	165	60	69	79	102	111				14			
66	168	60	75	84	103	112			9	14	30		
67	170	62	71	84	102	113		7	10	11	23	27	
68	173	63	76	86	101	114		9	10	14	22	23	
69	175	68	74	89	103	114	6	7	8	15	25	29	31
70	178	68	74	87	106	114	7	7	7	14	23	25	30
71	180	73	82	91	113	123	6	8	10	15	25	27	31
72	183	73	78	91	109	121	5	6	7	12	20	22	25
73	185	72	79	93	106	116	5	6	7	13	19	22	31
74	188	69	82	92	105	120			8	12	19		

Modified from Frisancho, 1984.
*Data from National Center for Health Statistics, 1981.

TABLE 5-4   Selected Percentiles of Weight and Triceps Skinfold Thickness for U.S. Women Ages 25 to 54 Years[*]

Height		Weight (kg)					Triceps (mm)						
In	Cm	5th	15th	50th	85th	95th	5th	10th	15th	50th	85th	90th	95th
Small Frames, Women													
58	147	37	43	52	58	66		12	13	24	30	33	
59	150	42	44	53	63	72	8	11	14	21	29	36	37
60	152	42	45	53	63	70	8	11	12	21	28	29	33
61	155	44	47	54	64	72	11	12	14	21	28	31	34
62	157	44	48	55	63	70	10	12	14	20	28	31	34
63	160	46	49	55	65	79	10	11	13	20	27	30	36
64	163	49	51	57	67	74	10	13	13	20	28	30	34
65	165	50	53	60	70	80	12	13	14	22	29	31	34
66	168	46	54	58	65	74			12	19	30		
67	170	47	52	59	70	76				18			
68	173	48	53	62	71	77				20			
69	175	49	54	63	72	78							
70	178	50	55	64	73	79							
Medium Frames, Women													
58	147	41	50	63	77	79			20	25	40		
59	150	47	52	66	76	85	15	19	21	30	37	40	40
60	152	47	52	60	77	85	14	15	17	26	35	37	41
61	155	47	51	61	73	86	11	14	15	25	34	36	42
62	157	49	52	61	73	83	12	14	16	24	34	36	40
63	160	49	53	62	77	88	12	13	15	24	33	35	38
64	163	50	54	62	76	87	11	14	15	23	33	36	40
65	165	52	55	63	75	89	12	14	15	22	31	34	38
66	168	52	55	63	75	83	11	13	14	22	31	33	37
67	170	54	57	65	79	88	12	13	15	21	29	30	35
68	173	58	60	67	77	87	10	14	15	22	31	32	36
69	175	49	60	68	79	87		11	12	19	29	31	
70	178	50	57	70	80	87				19			
Large Frames, Women													
58	147	56	67	86	105	117							
59	150	56	67	78	105	116				36			
60	152	55	66	87	104	116				38			
61	155	54	66	81	105	115		25	26	36	48	50	
62	157	59	65	81	103	113	16	19	22	34	48	48	50
63	160	58	67	83	105	119	18	20	22	34	46	48	51
64	163	59	63	79	102	112	16	20	21	32	43	45	49
65	165	59	63	81	103	114	17	20	21	31	43	46	48
66	168	55	62	75	95	107	13	17	18	27	40	43	45
67	170	58	65	80	100	114	13	16	17	30	41	43	49
68	173	51	66	76	104	111		16	20	29	37	40	
69	175	50	68	79	105	111			21	30	42		
70	178	50	61	76	99	110				20			

Modified from Frisancho, 1984.
[*]Data from National Center for Health Statistics, 1981.

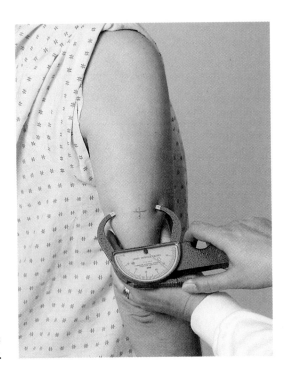

FIGURE 5-9

Placement of calipers for triceps skinfold-thickness measurement.

To determine the site of the triceps skinfold thickness measurement, have the patient flex the right arm at a right angle. Position yourself behind the patient and make a horizontal mark halfway between the tips of the olecranon and acromial processes on the posterior aspect of the arm. Then draw a line along the vertical plane of the arm to cross the midpoint. Allowing the patient's arm to hang relaxed, use your thumb and forefinger to grasp and lift the triceps skinfold about ½ in (1.27 cm) proximal to the marked cross. Make sure you feel the main bulk of the triceps muscle, identifying the muscle's subcutaneous interface between your fingers deep to the skinfold. (If you do not feel the muscle bulk, you may be too medial or lateral to the muscle mass and need to reposition your fingers.) Place the caliper jaws at the marked cross on each side of the raised skinfold, but not so tight as to cause an indentation (Figure 5-9). With the gauge at eye level, make two readings to the nearest millimeter at the same site and derive an average.

Since approximately 50% of the body fat is present in the subcutaneous tissue layers, a correlation exists between the triceps skinfold thickness and the body's fat content. Therefore the triceps skinfold measurement may be used in the diagnosis of obesity. Compare the patient's measurement with the percentiles of triceps skinfold thickness by age and sex (Tables 5-3 and 5-4).

Measuring skinfold thickness in the very obese is difficult because calipers are not large enough for some skinfolds. The thickness of adipose tissue in the obese also makes it more difficult to raise the skinfold with parallel sides for the measurement.

INFANTS

A baby born at term who is the size and proportion expected (e.g., not too big and not too small) and is free of a history of prenatal or perinatal difficulty has the best chance to be a healthy neonate and infant. Unexpected deviations during the first few days of life must always be given serious attention, since they may be clues to potential problems. This is true whether the deviation is one of measurement or is suspected because of a subjective impression on physical examination of the baby's vibrancy and interest in life, particularly in feeding.

PHYSICAL VARIATIONS

Black infants generally weigh 181 to 240 g less than white infants at birth. Oriental, Filipino, Hawaiian, and Puerto Rican babies generally also weigh less than white infants. But the birth weights of Native American infants vary a great deal: as much as 362 g separates the mean birth weights of various tribes.

Data from Hulsey, Levkoff, Alexander, 1991; National Center for Health Statistics, 1981; Yip, Li, Chong, 1991; Crowell et al, 1992; Adams, Niswander, 1973; Thomson, 1990.

Most babies born to the same parents weigh within 6 oz of each other at birth. If the baby has a lower birth weight than earlier siblings, suspect an undisclosed congenital abnormality or intrauterine growth retardation. Babies with a larger birth weight than earlier siblings, at 10 lb or greater, are at risk for acute lymphatic leukemia.

There is real excitement in watching an infant's growth and development. It is not just a measurement of weight and height and other growth parameters that provides such feelings, but careful attention to the sequence of these measurements and to the child's progressive achievements that is exciting about the care of children.

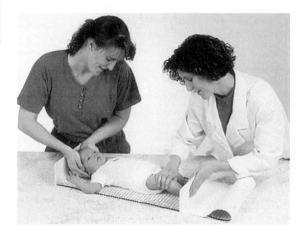

FIGURE 5-10
Measurement of infant length.
Courtesy Seca Corporation.

RECUMBENT LENGTH

Recumbent length is the measurement of choice for infants between birth and 24 to 36 months of age (Figure 5-10). Place the infant supine on the measuring device, and have the parent hold the infant's head against the headboard. Hold the infant's legs straight at the knees, and place the footboard against the bottom of the infant's feet. Read the length measurement to the nearest 0.5 cm or ¼ in. Compare the infant's length to the population standard, using the appropriate growth curve for sex and age, and identify the infant's percentile placement (see Physical Growth Curves for Children, Birth to 36 Months in Appendix E).

At birth, healthy term newborns have length variations between 45 and 55 cm (18 to 22 in). Length increases by 50% in the first year of life.

WEIGHT

Use an infant scale, measuring weight in ounces or grams for infants and small children. Distract the infant and balance the scale as you would for a standing scale. Read the weight to the nearest 10 g or ½ oz when the infant is most still. Plot the infant's weight on the appropriate growth curve for age and sex, comparing the infant's weight to the population standard. Identify the infant's percentile placement (see Appendix E).

Healthy term newborns vary in weight between 2500 and 4000 g (5 lb, 8 oz to 8 lb, 13 oz). In general, they double their birth weight by 4 to 5 months of age and triple their birth weight by 12 months of age. Formula-fed infants are heavier after the first 6 months of life than breast-fed infants. They grow faster in the first 6 months of life with slower growth in the second 6 months of the first year (Binns et al, 1996).

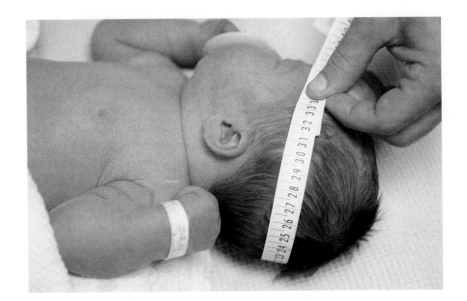

FIGURE 5-11

Appropriate placement of the measuring tape to obtain the head circumference.

HEAD CIRCUMFERENCE

You should measure the infant's head circumference at every health visit until 2 years of age, and then measure the young child's head circumference yearly until 6 years of age. Wrap the measuring tape snugly around the child's head at the occipital protuberance and the supraorbital prominence to find the point of largest circumference, taking care not to cut the skin (Figure 5-11). Make the reading to the nearest 0.5 cm or ⅛ in. (Remember to remeasure the head circumference at least one time to check the accuracy of your measurement.)

Plot the infant's head circumference on the appropriate growth curve, comparing the infant's measurement with expected measurements for the population (Appendix E).

Expected head circumferences for term newborns range between 32.5 and 37.5 cm (12½ to 14½ in) with a mean of 33 to 35 cm (13 to 14 in). At 2 years of age the infant's head circumference is two thirds its adult size. A head circumference increasing rapidly and rising above percentile curves suggests increased intracranial pressure. A head circumference growing slowly enough to fall off percentile curves suggests microcephaly.

CHEST CIRCUMFERENCE

Although the chest circumference is not used universally, it is a useful measurement for comparison with the head circumference when you suspect a problem in either head size or chest size. Wrap the measuring tape around the infant's chest at the nipple line, firmly but not tight enough to cause an indentation of the skin (Figure 5-12). The chest circumference measurement is ideally taken midway between inspiration and expiration and read to the nearest 0.5 cm or ⅛ in.

The newborn's head circumference may equal or exceed the chest circumference by 2 cm (¾ in) for the first 5 months of age. Between the ages of 5 months and 2 years, the infant's chest circumference should closely approximate the head circumference. After 2 years of age the chest circumference should exceed the head circumference, because the chest grows faster than the head (Table 5-5).

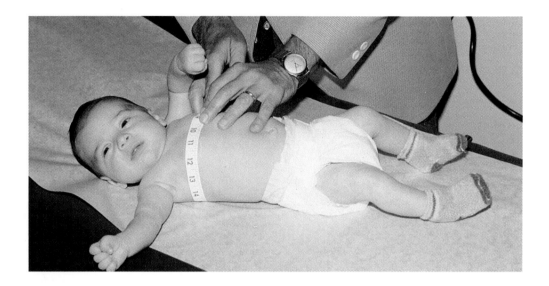

FIGURE 5-12
Measurement of infant chest circumference.

TABLE 5-5	Average Chest and Head Circumference for U.S. Children		
		Head Circumference (cm)	
Age	Chest Circumference (cm)	Males	Females
Birth	35	35.3	34.7
3 months	40	40.9	40.0
6 months	44	43.9	42.8
12 months	47	47.3	45.8
18 months	48	48.7	47.1
2 years	50	49.7	48.1
3 years	52	50.4	49.3

Data from Lowrey, 1986; Waring, Jeansonne, 1982.

GESTATIONAL AGE

Gestational age is an indicator of a newborn's maturity. One method of determining gestational age is calculation of the number of completed weeks since the first day of the mother's last menstrual period to the date of birth. An estimate of gestational age is used for evaluating an infant's developmental progress and for differentiating between preterm newborns who are appropriate size and term newborns who are small for gestational age.

The Dubowitz Clinical Assessment is a standardized tool that uses a newborn's physical and neuromuscular characteristics within 48 hours of birth to establish or confirm the newborn's gestational age. The Dubowitz scoring criteria include 11 physical characteristics and 10 neuromuscular signs. Figure 5-13 provides directions and criteria for scoring each characteristic. The assessment is accurate within 2 weeks of the assigned gestational age.

The gestational ages of 37 through 41 weeks, which are considered *term,* are associated with the best health outcomes. Infants born before 37 weeks' gestation are *preterm,* whereas infants born after 41 completed weeks of gestation are *postterm.*

A

External sign	Score				
	0	**1**	**2**	**3**	**4**
Edema	Obvious edema of hands and feet; pitting over tibia	No obvious edema of hands and feet; pitting over tibia	No edema		
Skin texture	Very thin, gelatinous	Thin and smooth	Smooth; medium thickness. Rash or superficial peeling	Slight thickening. Superficial cracking and peeling, especially of hands and feet	Thick and parchmentlike; superficial or deep cracking
Skin color	Dark red	Uniformly pink	Pale pink; variable over body	Pale; only pink over ears, lips, palms, or soles	
Skin opacity (trunk)	Numerous veins and venules clearly seen, especially over abdomen	Veins and tributaries seen	A few large vessels clearly seen over abdomen	A few large vessels seen indistinctly over abdomen	No blood vessels seen
Lanugo (over back)	No lanugo	Abundant; long and thick over whole back	Hair thinning especially over lower back	Small amount of lanugo and bald areas	At least ¹/₂ of back devoid of lanugo
Plantar creases	No skin creases	Faint red marks over anterior half of sole	Definite red marks over > anterior ¹/₂; indentations over < anterior ¹/₃	Indentations over > anterior ¹/₃	Definite deep indentations over > anterior ¹/₃
Nipple formation	Nipple barely visible; no areola	Nipple well defined; areola smooth and flat, diameter <0.75 cm	Areola stippled, edge not raised, diameter <0.75 cm	Areola stippled, edge raised, diameter >0.75 cm	
Breast size	No breast tissue palpable	Breast tissue on one or both sides, <0.5 cm diameter	Breast tissue both sides; one or both 0.5-1 cm	Breast tissue both sides; one or both >1 cm	
Ear form	Pinna flat and shapeless, little or no incurving of edge	Incurving of part of edge of pinna	Partial incurving whole of upper pinna	Well-defined incurving whole of upper pinna	
Ear firmness	Pinna soft, easily folded, no recoil	Pinna soft, easily folded, slow recoil	Cartilage to edge of pinna, but soft in places, ready recoil	Pinna firm, cartilage to edge; instant recoil	
Genitals Male	Neither testis in scrotum	At least one testis high in scrotum	At least one testis right down		
Female (with hips ¹/₂ abducted)	Labia majora widely separated, labia minora protruding	Labia majora almost cover labia minora	Labia majora completely cover labia minora		

B

Neurologic signs	Score					
	0	**1**	**2**	**3**	**4**	**5**
Posture						
Square window	90°	60°	45°	30°	0°	
Ankle dorsiflexion	90°	75°	45°	20°	0°	
Arm recoil	180°	90°-180°	<90°			
Leg recoil	180°	90°-180°	<90°			
Popliteal angle	180°	160°	130°	110°	90°	<90°
Heel to ear						
Scarf sign						
Head lag						
Ventral suspension						

Posture: Observed with infant quiet and in supine position. Score 0: Arms and legs extended; 1: beginning of flexion of hips and knees, arms extended; 2: stronger flexion of legs, arms extended; 3: arms slightly flexed, legs flexed and abducted; 4: full flexion of arms and legs.

Square window: The hand is flexed on the forearm between the thumb and index finger of the examiner. Enough pressure is applied to get as full a flexion as possible, and the angle between the hypothenar eminence and the ventral aspect of the forearm is measured and graded according to diagram. (Care is taken not to rotate the infant's wrist while doing this maneuver.)

Ankle dorsiflexion: The foot is dorsiflexed onto the anterior aspect of the leg, with the examiner's thumb on the sole of the foot and other fingers behind the leg. Enough pressure is applied to get as full flexion as possible, and the angle between the dorsum of the foot and the anterior aspect of the leg is measured.

Arm recoil: With the infant in the supine position the forearms are first flexed for 5 seconds, then fully extended by pulling on the hands, and then released. The sign is fully positive if the arms return briskly to full flexion (Score 2). If the arms return to incomplete flexion or the response is sluggish it is graded as Score 1. If they remain extended or are only followed by random movements the score is 0.

Leg recoil: With the infant supine, the hips and knees are fully flexed for 5 seconds, then extended by traction on the feet, and released. A maximal response is one of full flexion of the hips and knees (Score 2). A partial flexion scores 1, and minimal or no movement scores 0.

Popliteal angle: With the infant supine and his pelvis flat on the examining couch, the thigh is held in the knee-chest position by the examiner's left index finger and thumb supporting the knee. The leg is then extended by gentle pressure from the examiner's right index finger behind the ankle and the popliteal angle is measured.

Heel to ear maneuver: With the baby supine, draw the baby's foot as near to the head as it will go without forcing it. Observe the distance between the foot and the head as well as the degree of extension at the knee. Grade according to diagram. Note that the knee is left free and may draw down alongside the abdomen.

Scarf sign: With the baby supine, take the infant's hand and try to put it around the neck and as far posteriorly as possible around the opposite shoulder. Assist this maneuver by lifting the elbow across the body. See how far the elbow will go across and grade according to illustrations. Score 0: Elbow reaches opposite axillary line; 1: Elbow between midline and opposite axillary line; 2: Elbow reaches midline; 3: Elbow will not reach midline.

Head lag: With the baby lying supine, grasp the hands (or the arms if a very small infant) and pull him slowly towards the sitting position. Observe the position of the head in relation to the trunk and grade accordingly. In a small infant the head may initially be supported by one hand. Score 0: Complete lag; 1: Partial head control; 2: Able to maintain head in line with body; 3: Brings head anterior to body.

Ventral suspension: The infant is suspended in the prone position, with examiner's hand under the infant's chest (one hand in a small infant, two in a large infant). Observe the degree of extension of the back and the amount of flexion of the arms and legs. Also note the relation of the head to the trunk. Grade according to diagram. If score differs on the two sides, take the mean.

FIGURE 5-13

Assessment of gestational age. **A,** Scoring system of physical signs for assessment of gestational age. Assign a score for each of the 11 external signs based on the descriptions for each. **B,** Scoring system of neurologic signs for assessment of gestational age. Follow directions for assessing each of the 10 neurologic signs and assign a score for each. **C,** Add the scores from the 21 signs and compare the total with this table to determine the neonate's gestational age in weeks. Note the age of the neonate at the time of assessment.

From Dubowitz, Dubowitz, Goldberg, 1970.

Total score	Weeks of gestation	C
0-9	26	
10-12	27	
13-16	28	
17-20	29	
21-24	30	
25-27	31	
28-31	32	
32-35	33	
36-39	34	
40-43	35	
44-46	36	
47-50	37	
51-54	38	
55-58	39	
59-62	40	
63-65	41	
66-69	42	

SIZE FOR GESTATIONAL AGE

A newborn's fetal growth pattern and size for gestational age can be determined once gestational age is assigned. Standardized intrauterine growth curves are used to plot the newborn's birth weight, length, and head circumference (Figure 5-14). The infant is then classified as either small, appropriate, or large for gestational age by percentile curve placement for weeks of gestation (Figure 5-15). The classification system is as follows:

CLASSIFICATION	WEIGHT PERCENTILES
Appropriate for gestational age (AGA)	10th to 90th
Small for gestational age (SGA)	>10th
Large for gestational age (LGA)	<90th

There is an associated risk of morbidity and mortality with infants that are either small or large for gestational age. Risks increase further if the infant is preterm or postterm.

PHYSICAL VARIATIONS

The length of gestation for black infants averages 9 days shorter than that of white infants; black infants are generally more mature than white infants at a similar gestational duration.

Term black infants are also more mature than term white infants, and related to this increased maturity, premature black infants also have a better survival rate than premature white infants.

Data from Papiernik et al, 1986; Zhang, Savitz, 1992; Falkner, Tanner, 1978; Resnick et al, 1989; Collins, David, 1990.

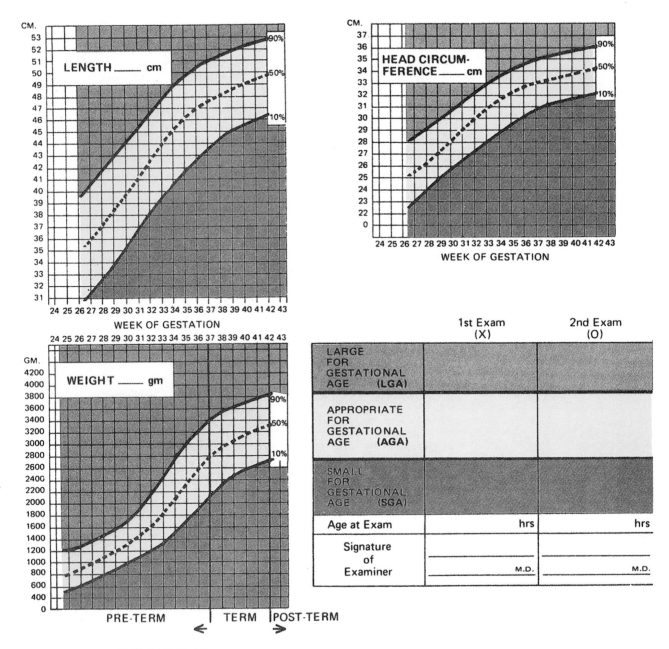

CLASSIFICATION OF NEWBORNS —
BASED ON MATURITY AND INTRAUTERINE GROWTH
Symbols: X - 1st Exam O - 2nd Exam

FIGURE 5-14

Intrauterine growth curves for length, weight, and head circumference by weeks of gestation.

Modified from Lubchenco, 1966 and Battaglia, Lubchenco, 1967.

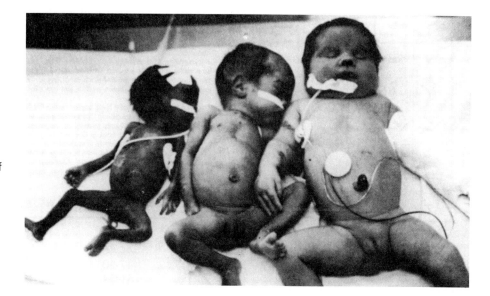

FIGURE 5-15

Three infants, each 32 weeks of gestational age, demonstrating the difference in size between SGA, AGA, and LGA newborns. Birth weights are 600, 1400, and 2750 g, respectively, from left to right.

From Korones, 1986.

CHILDREN

STATURE AND WEIGHT

PHYSICAL VARIATIONS

Children of different races vary in height. Tallest are black and white children, followed by Native American children, who are similar or a little shorter. Next in height are Mexican American children, followed by the shortest group—Oriental children. Black children achieve their growth earlier than white children—white boys catch up with black boys around 9 or 10 years; white girls catch up to black girls around 14 to 15 years.

Within the same racial group, children from families with higher socioeconomic status are taller than those from lower socioeconomic status families. Obese children are taller than lean children; the difference in height can be as much as one standard deviation above their leaner cohorts.

Data from Foster et al, 1977; Strauss, 1993; Dewey et al, 1986; Roche et al, 1990; Lin, 1992; Malina, Hamill, Lemeshow, 1974; Hamill, Johnston, Lemeshow, 1973; Schutte, 1980; Chrzastek-Spruch, Wolanski, Wrebiakowski, 1984; Garn, Clark, Guire, 1974.

Standing height is obtained beginning at 24 to 36 months when the child is walking well. To get the most accurate measurement, use a stature-measuring device (stadiometer) that is mounted on the wall rather than the height-measurement device on a scale. Have the child stand erect with heels, buttocks, and shoulders against the wall or freestanding stadiometer, looking straight ahead (Figure 5-16). The outer canthus of the eye should be on the same horizontal plane as the external auditory canal while you position the headpiece at the crown. The stature reading is made to the nearest 0.5 cm or ¼ in. Table 5-6 lists the expected yearly stature growth, or height velocity, for age and gender.

TABLE 5-6	Expected Height Velocity for Specified Time Intervals During Childhood*	
	Height Velocity (cm)	
Age (yr)	**Males**	**Females**
2-3	8.3	8.6
3-4	7.4	7.6
4-5	6.8	6.8
5-6	6.4	6.4
6-7	6.0	6.1
7-8	5.8	5.9
8-9	5.4	5.7
9-10	5.2	5.8
10-11	5.1	6.7
11-12	5.3	8.3
12-13	6.8	5.9
13-14	9.5	3.0
14-15	6.5	0.9
15-16	3.3	0.1
16-17	1.5	
17-18	0.5	

Modified from Tanner, Davies, 1985.

*Peak height velocity during adolescence is given for average times (13.5 years in males and 11.5 years in females).

FIGURE 5-16
Measuring the stature of a child.

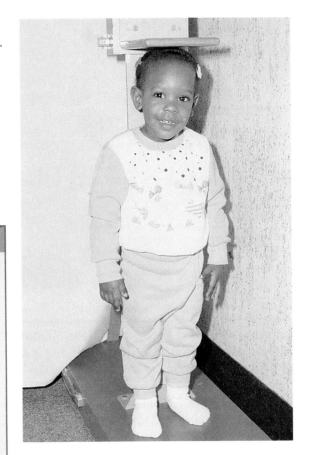

To calculate height velocity, determine the change in height over a time interval, such as a year. Shorter time intervals may reflect seasonal variations in growth. Make height measurements as close to 12 months apart as possible, no fewer than 10 months and no more than 14 months. See Appendix E for the gender-specific height velocity curves.

Weigh the young child over 2 years of age on a standing scale, in standard light garments. Read the weight to the nearest 0.1 kg or ¼ lb. Remember to measure the child's head circumference once a year.

Plot the child's height, weight, and head circumference measurements on the appropriate growth curves for gender and age, comparing the child's growth with the population standards (See Appendix E for physical growth curves for height and weight of children ages 2 through 18). Population standards reflecting various times of the growth spurt for adolescents can be found in the physical growth curves for height and sexual development of children and adolescents ages 2 through 19 in Appendix E. The Nellhaus head circumference curve may be used for children older than age 3 (Figure 5-17).

Over time, interval measurements should demonstrate that the child has established a growth pattern, indicated by consistently following a percentile curve on the growth chart. Children of first generation immigrants may not fit the U.S. population standard, but they should follow a growth pattern consistent with other children, even if it is near or below the fifth percentile. Infants and children who suddenly fall below or rise above their established percentile growth curve should be examined more closely to determine the cause.

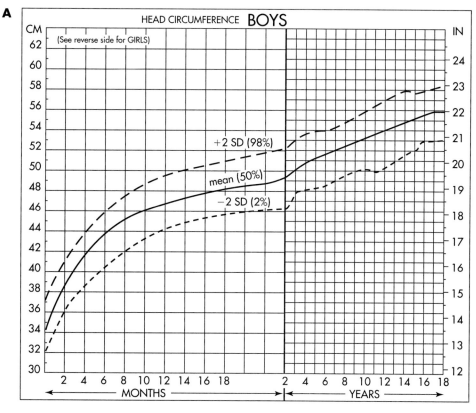

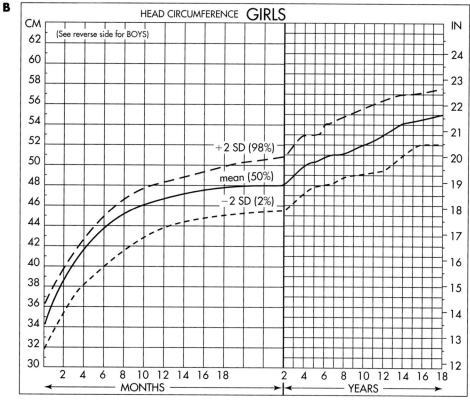

FIGURE 5-17
Head circumference growth curves, birth to 18 years. **A,** Boys. **B,** Girls.
From Nellhaus, 1968.

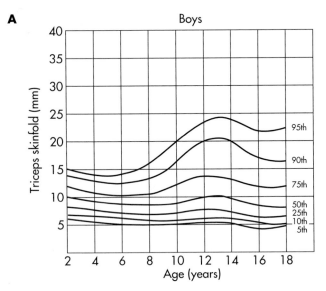
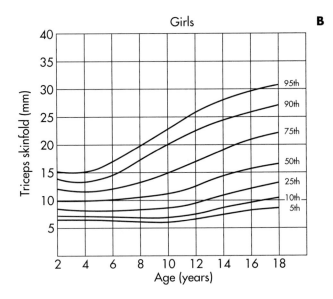

FIGURE 5-18
Skinfold thickness curves for children, ages 2 to 18 years. **A,** Boys. **B,** Girls.
Redrawn from Owen, 1982.

SKINFOLD THICKNESS

Triceps skinfold thickness measurement is not routinely recommended for children, being reserved for those children who have weight for stature greater than the 90th percentile. It is often difficult to differentiate fatfolds from lean muscle tissue in children. This measurement is more commonly used with adolescents for whom no weight-for-stature standard currently exists. Using the technique described for adults, take the triceps skinfold measurement. Plot the reading on the sex-appropriate standardized curves of triceps skinfold thickness for children and adolescents (Figure 5-18).

SITTING HEIGHT

Take the sitting height measurement and compare it with the total height when a child is suspected of having a growth problem or unusual body proportions. Have the child sit erect at the stature-measuring device with buttocks and shoulders against the wall, legs extended and flat against the floor. Position the headpiece at the child's crown while the child looks straight ahead, with the outer eye canthus and external auditory canal on the same plane. The proportion of sitting height to total body height is then calculated. The expected proportion of sitting height to total height by age is as follows (Barness, 1991):

Birth	70%
2 years	60%
10 years	52%
Adult	50%

Infantile stature is a sitting height greater than half the standing height, and *adult stature* is a sitting height approximately half that of the standing height. Adult stature in the young child may indicate precocious sexual development or certain types of dwarfism. Infantile stature in the older child may suggest delayed puberty or hypothyroidism.

PHYSICAL VARIATIONS

Black and white children differ in sitting/standing height ratio. Black children have longer legs in proportion to their height than do white or Mexican-American children; therefore their sitting/standing height ratio at age 10 is 51% in contrast to white and Mexican-American children's ratio of 53%.

Data from Malina, Hamill, Lemeshow, 1974; Hamill, Johnston, Lemeshow, 1973; Malina, Zavaleta, Little, 1987; Najjar, 1987.

ARM SPAN

The arm-span measurement, although not routinely obtained, may be useful when evaluating a child with tall stature. Have the child hold his or her arms fully extended from the sides of the body. Measure the distance from the middle fingertip of one hand to that of the other hand. The arm span should equal the child's height or stature. Arm span that exceeds height is associated with Marfan syndrome.

ADOLESCENTS

The changes of puberty do not occur at exactly the same time in each boy and girl, which can cause great concern when adolescents feel they are growing too fast or too slow. This is a good time to share your knowledge about the various rates of speed in human development, reassuring adolescents that almost all of them get there in good time. The Tanner charts are valuable for explaining to older children, particularly adolescents, where they are in reference to others and where they are going. Show them the pictures and talk about them. All adolescents are curious and will gain from your respectful candor.

Assessing growth and development of the older child and adolescent includes evaluating the patient's sexual maturation. In girls, breast and pubic hair development are evaluated, and genital and pubic hair development are evaluated in boys. The expected stages of pubertal changes for each secondary sexual characteristic are described in Figures 5-19 through 5-22. The duration and tempo of each sequence are quite variable between individuals.

A sexual maturity rating (SMR) may be assigned, or each secondary sexual characteristic may be rated separately, to determine the child's pubertal development. The SMR is calculated by averaging the girl's stages of pubic hair and breast development or the boy's stages of pubic hair and genital development. The stage of each secondary sexual characteristic is then related to the timing of other physiologic events occurring during puberty.

The stage of breast and pubic hair development in the female is related to her chronologic age, age at menarche, and evidence of the height spurt. Breasts begin developing before pubic hair appears in two thirds of girls. The breasts do not always develop at the same rate, so some asymmetry is common. Menarche generally occurs in SMR 4 or breast stage 3 to 4. These physiologic events may be plotted on the growth curve (see Appendix E). The peak height velocity usually occurs before menarche. Development of breast tissue or pubic hair in prepubertal girls younger than 8 years old should be further investigated for cause.

The stage of genital and pubic hair development in the male is related to his age and evidence of the height spurt. External genital changes usually precede pubic hair development. Ejaculation generally occurs at SMR 3, with semen appearing between SMR 3 and 4. The peak height velocity usually occurs later, in SMR 4 or genital development stage 4 to 5. These events may be plotted on a standardized growth curve (see Appendix E). Development of genitals or pubic hair in prepubertal boys younger than 9 years old should be further investigated for cause.

Delayed onset of adolescence, in which the secondary sexual characteristics begin development at a later than average age, is often a normal variant in both boys and girls. It is accompanied by a lag of stature growth. Parents often had a similar adolescent pattern. Once pubertal changes begin, the sequence of development is the same as for other adolescents, but it may occur over a shorter time span. Ultimate height may still be the same.

Early development of sexual hair without signs of sexual maturation may be an indication of premature pubarche. Pubescence usually occurs at the expected time in children with premature pubarche as with healthy children.

Text continued on p. 124

FIGURE 5-19

Five stages of pubic hair development in males.

From Van Wieringen et al, 1971.

P₁—Tanner 1 (preadolescent). No growth of pubic hair; that is, hair in pubic area no different from that on the rest of the abdomen.

P₂—Tanner 2. Slightly pigmented, longer, straight hair, often still downy; usually at base of penis, sometimes on scrotum. Stage is difficult to photograph.

P₃—Tanner 3. Dark, definitely pigmented, curly pubic hair around base of penis. Stage 3 can be photographed.

P₄—Tanner 4. Pubic hair definitely adult in type but not in extent (no further than inguinal fold).

P₅—Tanner 5 (adult distribution). Hair spread to medial surface of thighs, but not upward.

P₆—Hair spread along linea alba (occurs in 80% of men).

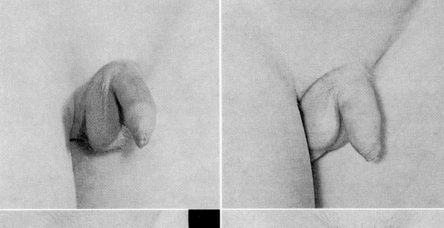
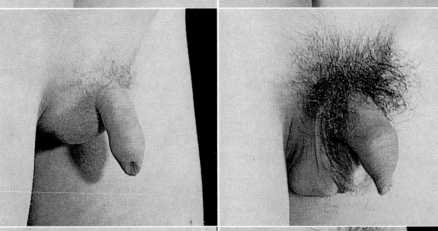
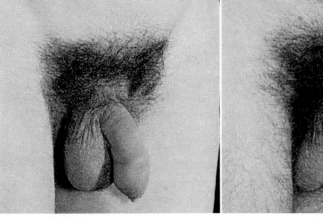

FIGURE 5-20

Five stages of penis and testes/scrotum development in males.

From Van Wieringen et al, 1971.

G_1—Tanner 1. Testes, scrotum, and penis are the same size and shape as in the young child.

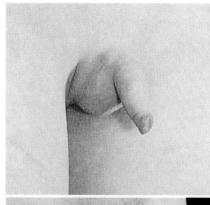

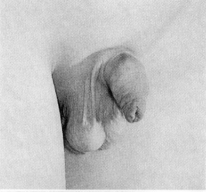

G_2—Tanner 2. Enlargement of scrotum and testes. The skin of the scrotum becomes redder, thinner, and wrinkled. Penis no larger or scarcely so.

G_3—Tanner 3. Enlargement of the penis, especially in length; further enlargement of testes; descent of scrotum.

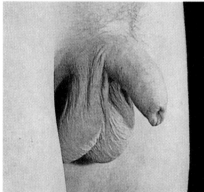

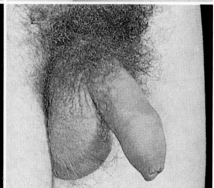

G_4—Tanner 4. Continued enlargement of the penis and sculpturing of the glans; increased pigmentation of scrotum. This stage is sometimes best described as "not quite adult."

G_5—Tanner 5 (adult stage). Scrotum ample, penis reaching nearly to bottom of scrotum.

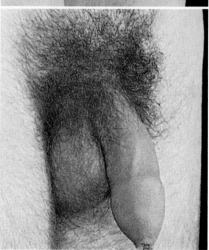

FIGURE 5-21

Five stages of pubic hair development in females.

From Van Wieringen et al, 1971.

P₁—Tanner 1 (preadolescent). No growth of pubic hair.

P₂—Tanner 2. Initial, scarcely pigmented straight hair, especially along medial border of the labia.

P₃—Tanner 3. Sparse, dark, visibly pigmented, curly pubic hair on labia.

P₄—Tanner 4. Hair coarse and curly, abundant but less than adult.

P₅—Tanner 5. Lateral spreading; type and triangle spread of adult hair to medial surface of thighs.

P₆—Tanner 6. Further extension laterally, upward, or dispersed (occurs in only 10% of women).

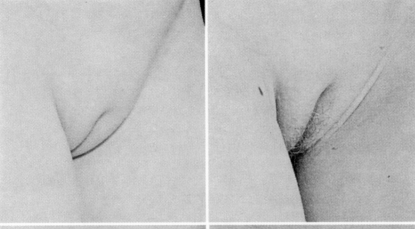
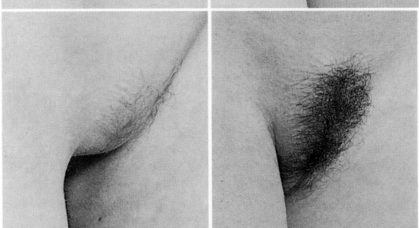
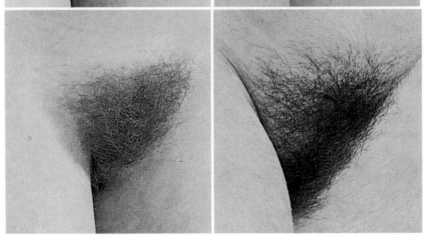

FIGURE 5-22

Five stages of breast development in females.

From Van Wieringen et al, 1971.

M₁—Tanner 1 (preadolescent). Only the nipple is raised above the level of the breast, as in the child.

M₂—Tanner 2. Budding stage: bud-shaped elevation of the areola; areola increased in diameter and surrounding area slightly elevated.

M₃—Tanner 3. Breast and areola enlarged. No contour separation.

M₄—Tanner 4. Increasing fat deposits. The areola forms a secondary elevation above that of the breast. This secondary mound occurs in approximately half of all girls and in some cases persists in adulthood.

M₅—Tanner 5 (adult stage). The areola is (usually) part of general breast contour and is strongly pigmented. Nipple projects.

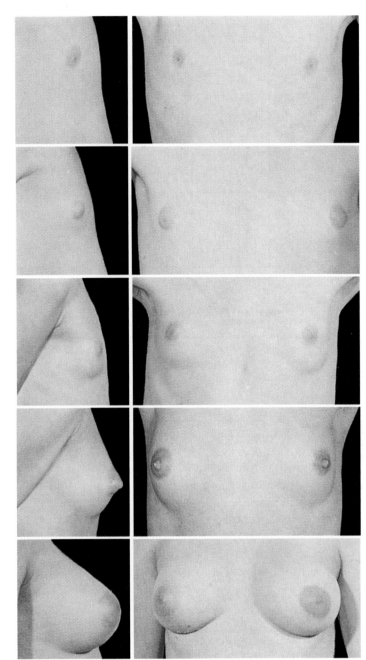

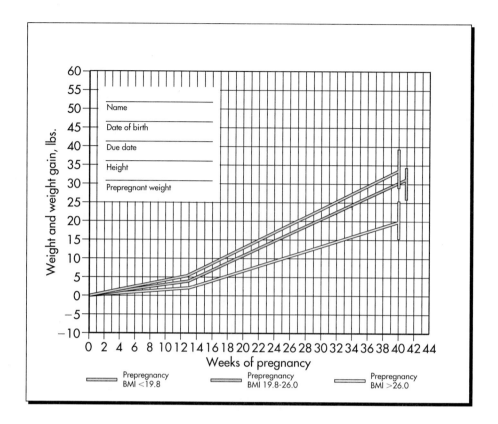

FIGURE 5-23

Prenatal weight gain curve by weeks of gestation.

From Food and Nutrition Board, 1992.

| PREGNANT WOMEN |

Weight gain during pregnancy should be calculated from the woman's prepregnant weight (Figure 5-23). To provide guidance in weight gain during pregnancy, first determine the prepregnancy body mass index (BMI) (see Box 6-4, p. 152). Women with a wide variation in weight gain during pregnancy have good reproductive outcomes. However, inadequate weight gain of less than 20 lb in pregnant adolescents may be associated with low–birth-weight infants and other perinatal complications. Women with an appropriate weight for height or prepregnancy BMI of 19.8 to 26.0 should gain 11.5 to 16 kg (25 to 35 lb) over the entire pregnancy. First trimester gain is variable. In the second trimester, weekly weight gain should range from 0.15 to 0.69 kg (0.3 to 1.5 lb), and in the third trimester it should be between 0.18 to 0.65 kg (0.4 to 1.4 lb).

Calculate the pregnant woman's prepregnancy BMI. Then monitor the woman's weight throughout pregnancy using the BMI weight gain curve guidelines on the prenatal weight gain chart. Note any variation from the expected weight gain. Consider the woman's dietary habits, source of calories, and health status.

| OLDER ADULTS |

Measurement procedures for the older adult are the same as those used for the general population. Compare the individual's triceps skinfold thickness with his or her height in the appropriate gender and frame-size categories to determine the appropriateness of the patient's weight (Tables 5-7 and 5-8).

TABLE 5-7   Selected Percentiles of Weight and Triceps Skinfold Thickness for Height in U.S. Men Ages 55 to 74 Years[*]

Height		Weight (kg)					Triceps (mm)						
In	Cm	5th	15th	50th	85th	95th	5th	10th	15th	50th	85th	90th	95th
Small Frames, Men													
62	157	45	56	61	68	77			6	9	12		
63	160	47	51	62	71	79		5	5	10	16	17	
64	163	47	54	63	72	80	4	4	4	9	20	21	22
65	165	48	59	70	80	90	5	6	7	11	18	19	24
66	168	51	59	68	77	84	5	6	7	11	16	20	20
67	170	55	61	69	79	88	5	6	6	10	15	17	25
68	173	54	58	70	79	86		5	5	10	15	17	
69	175	56	63	75	81	88			8	10	15		
70	178	57	63	76	83	89				11			
71	180	59	65	69	85	91				9			
72	183	60	66	76	86	92							
73	185	62	68	78	88	94							
74	188	63	69	77	89	95							
Medium Frames, Men													
62	157	50	59	68	77	85			5	12	25		
63	160	51	60	70	80	87		7	7	11	20	23	
64	163	55	62	71	82	91	5	6	6	10	17	20	26
65	165	56	64	72	83	89	5	6	7	11	17	19	24
66	168	57	66	74	83	89	6	6	7	12	18	19	22
67	170	59	66	78	87	94	5	6	7	12	18	20	23
68	173	62	68	78	89	101	6	7	8	12	18	21	23
69	175	62	68	77	90	99	5	6	7	12	19	22	25
70	178	62	71	80	90	101	6	7	7	11	18	19	21
71	180	68	72	84	94	101	5	6	6	11	16	17	20
72	183	66	69	81	96	101		6	8	11	19	20	
73	185	68	79	88	93	103			8	13	16		
74	188	69	76	95	98	104				11			
Large Frames, Men													
62	157	54	63	77	91	100							
63	160	55	64	80	92	101				15			
64	163	57	65	77	94	102				21			
65	165	58	73	79	89	103			11	14	22		
66	168	59	73	80	101	105		7	8	13	21	25	
67	170	65	73	85	103	112	6	8	9	16	21	25	27
68	173	67	73	83	95	111	6	7	8	13	20	21	23
69	175	65	74	84	96	105	6	7	8	12	18	20	23
70	178	68	77	87	102	117	5	6	8	14	22	25	31
71	180	65	70	84	102	111		6	6	13	18	22	
72	183	67	81	90	108	112		8	8	13	23	26	
73	185	68	76	88	105	113				11			
74	188	69	78	89	106	114				12			

Modified from Frisancho, 1984.

*Data from National Center for Health Statistics, 1981.

| TABLE 5-8 | Selected Percentiles of Weight and Triceps Skinfold Thickness for Height in U.S. Women Ages 55 to 74 Years[*] |

Height		Weight (kg)					Triceps (mm)						
In	Cm	5th	15th	50th	85th	95th	5th	10th	15th	50th	85th	90th	95th
Small Frames, Women													
58	147	39	48	54	63	71		14	16	21	31	34	
59	150	41	48	55	66	74	11	13	15	21	30	31	33
60	152	43	47	54	67	73	10	11	13	20	29	31	35
61	155	43	45	56	65	71	10	12	14	22	29	29	32
62	157	47	52	58	67	73	11	11	12	21	29	30	32
63	160	42	49	58	67	74		12	13	20	29	30	
64	163	43	49	60	68	75		12	13	21	27	29	
65	165	43	49	60	69	75				18			
66	168	44	50	68	70	76				23			
67	170	45	51	61	71	77							
68	173	45	51	61	71	77							
69	175	46	52	62	72	78							
70	178	47	52	63	73	79							
Medium Frames, Women													
58	147	40	49	57	72	85	5	13	17	28	40	40	41
59	150	47	52	62	74	86	12	15	18	26	34	38	41
60	152	47	52	65	76	86	13	17	18	25	33	34	38
61	155	49	54	64	78	86	13	16	18	25	35	37	42
62	157	49	54	64	78	88	13	15	17	24	33	36	39
63	160	52	55	65	79	89	12	14	16	24	32	35	38
64	163	51	57	66	78	87	12	14	16	25	33	34	37
65	165	54	59	67	78	88	14	16	17	24	33	35	39
66	168	54	57	66	79	88	12	13	16	24	33	33	36
67	170	51	61	72	82	89		17	17	27	35	35	
68	173	52	59	70	83	90				25			
69	175	53	60	72	84	91							
70	178	54	61	73	85	92							
Large Frames, Women													
58	147	53	63	92	95	104				45			
59	150	54	63	78	95	105				36			
60	152	54	69	78	87	105		25	26	35	44	45	
61	155	64	69	79	94	106	18	22	24	33	40	44	46
62	157	59	63	82	93	111	19	24	24	32	40	43	50
63	160	61	67	80	100	118	20	24	25	33	41	43	45
64	163	60	67	77	97	119	18	22	23	29	42	46	50
65	165	60	69	80	98	111	15	17	20	30	43	44	46
66	168	57	63	82	98	109		18	18	27	35	40	
67	170	58	68	80	105	109			22	32	44		
68	173	58	68	79	100	110				26			
69	175	59	69	85	101	110							
70	178	60	69	85	101	111							

Modified from Frisancho, 1984.
[*]Data from National Center for Health Statistics, 1981.

SUMMARY OF EXAMINATION | Growth and Measurement

1. From the history, assess the patient's size (pp. 102-103), including the following:
   * Recent growth, weight gain, or weight loss
   * Chronic illnesses affecting weight gain or loss

2. Obtain the following anthropometric measurements (pp. 104-108), and compare them to those in standardized tables:
   * Standing height
   * Weight
   * Frame size
   * Skinfold thickness

COMMON ABNORMALITIES

METABOLIC DISORDERS

ACROMEGALY

Gradual marked enlargement and elongation of the bones of the face, jaw, and extremities are indicative of acromegaly. This disorder is associated with a pituitary tumor that causes excessive production of growth hormone in middle-age adults. It is characterized by facial feature exaggeration and massive hands and feet but no change in height (Figure 5-24).

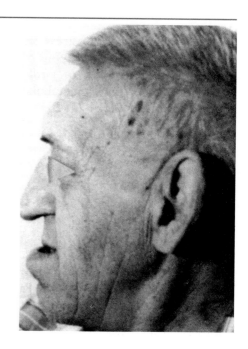

FIGURE 5-24
Acromegaly. Note the coarse facial features, prominent forehead, large nose, and large jaw with prognathism.
From Mazzaferri, 1975.

CUSHING SYNDROME

This disorder results from chronic excessive cortisol production by the adrenal cortex or from the long-term administration of large doses of glucocorticoids. Cushing syndrome is seen most commonly with steroid therapy. However, on rare occasions it is the result of an adrenal malignancy in the very young. It is characterized by muscle weakness, oligomenorrhea or decreased testosterone levels, and abnormally pigmented, fragile skin. There is a redistribution of fat tissue to include a pendulous pad of fat on the chest and abdomen covered with striae, as well as supraclavicular fat pads, moon facies, and thin extremities (Figure 5-25).

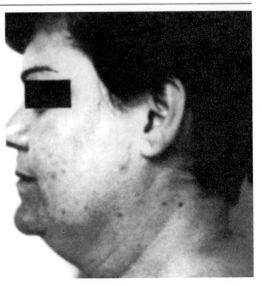

FIGURE 5-25

Cushing syndrome. The characteristic appearance of this syndrome is the round "moon" face with prominent jowls, preauricular fat, and hyperpigmentation and the "buffalo hump" in the low posterior cervical area.

From Mazzaferri, 1975.

OTHER DISORDERS

CHILDREN

HYDROCEPHALUS

This disorder originates when an excessive amount of cerebrospinal fluid accumulates between the brain and the dura mater or within the ventricular system. The resultant increased intracranial pressure leads to head enlargement, widening sutures and fontanels, lethargy, irritability, weakness, and "setting sun" eyes. Without intervention, irreversible neurologic damage results (Figure 5-26).

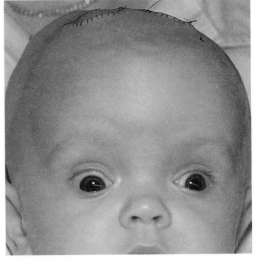

FIGURE 5-26

Infantile hydrocephalus. Paresis of the upward gaze is seen in an infant with hydrocephalus resulting from aqueductal stenosis. It appears more apparent on the right. This phenomenon is often termed the *sunsetting sign.*

From Zitelli, Davis, 1997. Courtesy Dr. Albert Biglan, Children's Hospital of Pittsburgh.

FAILURE TO THRIVE

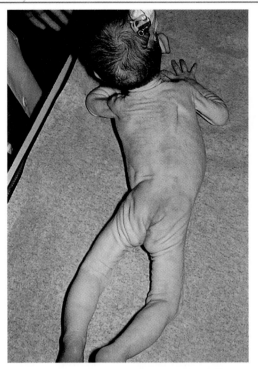

FIGURE 5-27
Psychosocial failure to thrive as the result of neglect. This 4-month-old infant was brought to the emergency department because of congestion, where she was found to be below weight and suffering from severe developmental delay. Note the marked loss of subcutaneous tissue manifested by the wrinkled skin folds over the buttocks, shoulders, and upper arms.
From Zitelli, Davis, 1997.

The failure of an infant to grow at rates considered appropriate for the population often occurs without organic cause. It may be related to chronic disease, inadequate calories and protein in the diet, improper feeding methods, intrauterine growth retardation, or emotional deprivation. The infant who fails to thrive may be the victim of congenital disorders of the brain, heart, or kidney. These are usually easy to discover. It is also possible that there are social and emotional causes. An emotionally deprived infant, one who is hungry for affection, will not grow. Growth hormone will be absent in that child. Once the child is given attention, such as being held, rocked, and provided physical and emotional warmth, the growth hormone will be produced and the child will grow (Figure 5-27).

ACHONDROPLASIA

This genetic disorder causes abnormalities in endochondral ossification. It is characterized by dwarfism with short curved arms and legs, dorsal kyphosis and lumbar lordosis, and a normal-sized head and trunk (Figure 5-28).

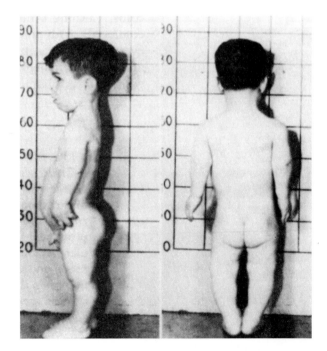

FIGURE 5-28
Achondroplasia.
From McKusick, 1972.

MORQUIO SYNDROME — This genetic mucopolysaccharidosis disorder causes dwarfism with skeletal abnormalities such as pectus carinatum, crouching posture, and prominent joints. The child appears normal at birth, but the defect becomes apparent by 2 years of age (Figure 5-29).

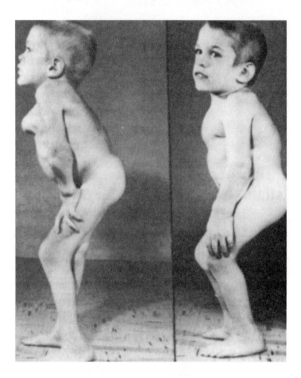

FIGURE 5-29
Morquio syndrome.
From Goodman, Gorlin, 1977.

HYPOPITUITARY DWARFISM

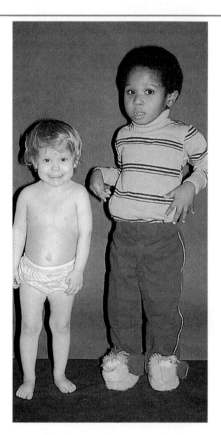

A growth hormone deficiency results in a child with short stature who appears younger than his or her chronologic age. Growth occurs normally for the first 1 or 2 years and then slows markedly, leading to dwarfism unless identified early and treated (Figure 5-30).

FIGURE 5-30
The normal 3-year-old boy is in the fiftieth percentile for height. The short 3-year-old girl exhibits the characteristic "Kewpie doll" appearance, suggesting a diagnosis of growth hormone deficiency.
From Zitelli, Davis, 1997.

PITUITARY GIGANTISM	Excessive stature growth with normal proportions during early childhood is associated with overproduction of growth hor-	mone caused by a pituitary tumor. Headaches and other symptoms of increased intracranial pressure may be present.
PRECOCIOUS PUBERTY	This disorder is characterized by sexual development with all pubertal changes before age 8 in females and age 9 in males.	It is usually idiopathic, but it may be related to organic brain lesions or McCune-Albright syndrome (Figure 5-31).

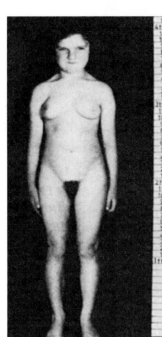
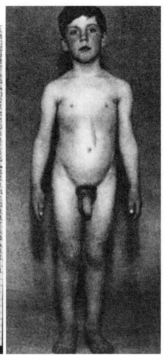

FIGURE 5-31
A, Constitutional sexual precocity in a 5-year-old girl. **B,** Constitutional sexual precocity in a 5-year-old boy.
From Jolly, 1981.

TURNER SYNDROME

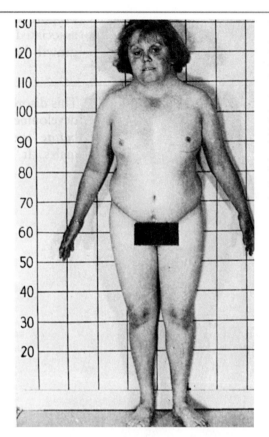

This abnormality of sex chromosomes produces a phenotypic female, usually identified during adolescence because of the absence of sexual development. Some of the following characteristics may be present in any affected child: webbed neck, increased carrying angle of the elbow, shield-shaped chest deformity with hypoplastic nipples, short stature, and congenital anomalies of heart or urinary tract (Figure 5-32).

FIGURE 5-32
Turner syndrome.
From Goodman, Gorlin, 1977.

CHAPTER 6

NUTRITION

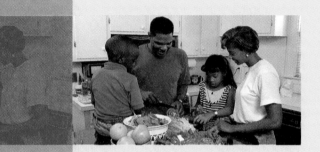

Nutrition may be defined as the science of food as it relates to optimal health and performance. Therefore nutritional intake and status may offer insight into an individual's total health status. In some instances, abnormalities such as anemia and hyperlipidemia may be a direct result of their food intake. A nutritional assessment encompasses analysis of an individual's approximate nutrient intake and relates it to the review of related history, physical examination and findings, and anthropometric and biochemical measures. This chapter reviews the utilization of nutrients for growth, development, and maintenance of health and provides guidelines for assessing an individual's intake. Use of related history, anthropometric (refer to Chapter 5, Growth and Measurement) and biochemical measures, and physical findings to complete a nutrition assessment is discussed in detail for the pediatric and adult populations.

ANATOMY AND PHYSIOLOGY

Food nourishes the body by supplying necessary nutrients and calories to function in one or all of three ways: provide energy for necessary activities, provide for the building and maintenance of body tissues, and regulate body processes. The nutrients necessary to the body are classified as macronutrients, micronutrients, and water. Energy requirements are based on the balance of energy expenditure associated with an individual's body size and composition, and of level of physical activity. An appropriate balance contributes to long-term health and allows for the maintenance of desirable physical activity.

MACRONUTRIENTS

Carbohydrate, protein, and fat are referred to as macronutrients because they are required in large amounts. These three macronutrients provide the calories needed to produce energy in the human body.

Carbohydrate

Carbohydrate, a nutrient found mostly in plants and in milk, is considered the body's main source of energy. Though about 365 g are stored as glycogen in the liver and muscle tissues and is present in circulating blood, this amount provides energy for

133

only about 13 hours of moderate activity. Moderate amounts of carbohydrate must be ingested in frequent intervals to meet the energy demands of the body. Carbohydrate also serves major functions in the liver (sparing the use of protein for energy and participating in specific detoxifying metabolic pathways), heart (as glycogen stored in cardiac muscle), and the central nervous system (as the only energy source to the brain). If more carbohydrate is eaten than is needed for energy, the excess is stored in fatty tissues throughout the body. It is recommended that carbohydrate content of the diet be at least 50% of total calories, with no less than 100 g per day. One gram of carbohydrate supplies 4 calories.

Protein

Protein, which is present in all animal and plant products, is essential to life. It is a part of over half the organic matter in the body, including hair, skin, nails, muscle and glandular organs, connective tissue, and blood plasma and hemoglobin. In all, 20 different amino acids combine in different ways to form proteins. Eight amino acids are considered essential, as they cannot be manufactured by the body, and they are essential for normal growth and development. During the digestion process, protein is broken down into amino acids, the building blocks of the protein molecule. Absorp-

---

TABLE 6-1   **Food and Nutrition Board, National Academy of Sciences— National Research Council Recommended Dietary Allowances*, Revised 1989**
Designed for the maintenance of good nutrition of practically all healthy people in the United States

Category	Age (years) or Condition	Weight† (kg)	Weight† (lb)	Height† (cm)	Height† (in)	Protein (g)	Fat-Soluble Vitamins Vitamin A (μg RE)‡	Vitamin D (μg)§	Vitamin E (mg α-TE)‖	Vitamin K (μg)	Water-Soluble Vitamins Vitamin C (mg)	Thiamin (mg)	Riboflavin (mg)
Infants	0.0-0.5	6	13	60	24	13	375	7.5	3	5	30	0.3	0.4
	0.5-1.0	9	20	71	28	14	375	10	4	10	35	0.4	0.5
Children	1-3	13	29	90	35	16	400	10	6	15	40	0.7	0.8
	4-6	20	44	112	44	24	500	10	7	20	45	0.9	1.1
	7-10	28	62	132	52	28	700	10	7	30	45	1.0	1.2
Males	11-14	45	99	157	62	45	1,000	10	10	45	50	1.3	1.5
	15-18	66	145	176	69	59	1,000	10	10	65	60	1.5	1.8
	19-24	72	160	177	70	58	1,000	10	10	70	60	1.5	1.7
	25-50	79	174	176	70	63	1,000	5	10	80	60	1.5	1.7
	51+	77	170	173	68	63	1,000	5	10	80	60	1.2	1.4
Females	11-14	46	101	157	62	46	800	10	8	45	50	1.1	1.3
	15-18	55	120	163	64	44	800	10	8	55	60	1.1	1.3
	19-24	58	128	164	65	46	800	10	8	60	60	1.1	1.3
	25-50	63	138	163	64	50	800	5	8	65	60	1.1	1.3
	51+	65	143	160	63	50	800	5	8	65	60	1.0	1.2
Pregnant						60	800	10	10	65	70	1.5	1.6
Lactating	1st 6 months					65	1,300	10	12	65	95	1.6	1.8
	2nd 6 months					62	1,200	10	11	65	90	1.6	1.7

From Subcommittee on the Tenth Edition of the RDAs, 1989.

*The allowances, expressed as average daily intakes over time, are intended to provide for individual variations among most normal persons as they live in the United States under usual environmental stresses. Diets should be based on a variety of common foods in order to provide other nutrients for which human requirements have been less well defined.

†Weights and heights of Reference Adults are actual medians for the U.S. population of the designated age, as reported by NHANES II. The median weights and heights of those under 19 years of age were taken from Hamill et al. (1979). The use of these figures does not imply that the height-to-weight ratios are ideal.

‡Retinol equivalents. 1 retinol equivalent = 1 μg retinol or 6 μg β-carotene.

§As cholecalciferol. 10 æg cholecalciferol = 400 iu of vitamin D.

‖α-Tocopherol equivalents. 1 mg d-α tocopherol = 1 α-te.

tion into the bloodstream occurs, and the amino acids are carried to the tissues, with each tissue utilizing a specific amino acid to build its own individual protein. The major functions of protein are building and maintaining tissues, regulating internal water and acid-base balances, and as a precursor for enzymes, antibodies, and several hormones. If more protein is eaten than is needed for these major functions, the extra is used to supply energy or stored as body fat if total calorie intake is in excess of needs. It is recommended that protein content of the diet be between 14% and 20% of total calories, or a minimum of 13 g in infants, 25 g in children, and 45 g in adults each day. Table 6-1 shows the Recommended Dietary Allowances (RDAs) as established by the National Research Council for protein needs, from birth to adult. One gram of protein supplies 4 calories.

Fat

Fat, which is present in animal and some plant products, particularly the seeds of the plant, is necessary as the main source of linoleic acid, a fatty acid essential for normal growth and development. Other major functions of fat include synthesis and regulation of certain hormones, tissue structure, nerve impulse transmission, memory storage, and energy metabolism. Again, if more fat is eaten than is needed for these func-

				Minerals						
Niacin (mg NE)**	Vitamin B$_6$ (mg)	Folate (µg)	Vitamin B$_{12}$ (µg)	Calcium (mg)	Phosphorus (mg)	Magnesium (mg)	Iron (mg)	Zinc (mg)	Iodine (µg)	Selenium (µg)
5	0.3	25	0.3	400	300	40	6	5	40	10
6	0.6	35	0.5	600	500	60	10	5	50	15
9	1.0	50	0.7	800	800	80	10	10	70	20
12	1.1	75	1.0	800	800	120	10	10	90	20
13	1.4	100	1.4	800	800	170	10	10	120	30
17	1.7	150	2.0	1,200	1,200	270	12	15	150	40
20	2.0	200	2.0	1,200	1,200	400	12	15	150	50
19	2.0	200	2.0	1,200	1,200	350	10	15	150	70
19	2.0	200	2.0	800	800	350	10	15	150	70
15	2.0	200	2.0	800	800	350	10	15	150	70
15	1.4	150	2.0	1,200	1,200	280	15	12	150	45
15	1.5	180	2.0	1,200	1,200	300	15	12	150	50
15	1.6	180	2.0	1,200	1,200	280	15	12	150	55
15	1.6	180	2.0	800	800	280	15	12	150	55
13	1.6	180	2.0	800	800	280	10	12	150	55
17	2.2	400	2.2	1,200	1,200	320	30	15	175	65
20	2.1	280	2.6	1,200	1,200	355	15	19	200	75
20	2.1	260	2.6	1,200	1,200	340	15	16	200	75

**1 ne (niacin equivalent) is equal to 1 mg of niacin or 60 mg of dietary tryptophan.

tions, the extra is stored in fatty tissues in the body. Some of these fatty tissues, especially those under the skin and around the abdominal organs, serve a purpose, such as being a reserve store of fuel to be used when calorie intake does not meet needs, to support and protect organs from injury, and to prevent undue loss of heat from the body surface. It is recommended that fat content of the diet be less than 30% of total calories, or at least 20 g per day. One gram of fat supplies 9 calories.

MICRONUTRIENTS

Vitamins and minerals are known as micronutrients because they are required and stored in very small quantities by the body. Even though they are not used as a source of energy, they are essential for growth, development, and hundreds of metabolic processes that occur daily. Vitamins and minerals must be taken in by food or supplement. They cannot be metabolized by the body with the exception of vitamin K and biotin (produced by certain intestinal microorganisms), vitamin D (synthesized from cholesterol), and niacin (synthesized from tryptophan). Tables 6-2, 6-3, and 6-4 provide information on the major vitamins and minerals, their functions, problems occurring from deficiency/excess, and major food sources. Tables 6-1 and 6-5 provide the National Research Council's 1989 RDAs for selected vitamins and minerals.

WATER

Water, although listed last in this section, is the most vital nutrient. An individual can exist without food for several weeks, but without water one would last only a few days. The body of an adult is about 55% to 65% water. The major functions of water include:

- Providing turgor to body tissues;
- Altering the configuration of substances dissolved in it, thus changing their behavior to that necessary for metabolic processes;
- Transporting dissolved nutrients and wastes throughout the body; and
- Maintaining a stable body temperature.

There is a continual loss of water from the body by the kidneys in urine, by the lungs as water vapor in expired air, and by the skin as perspiration. Approximately 2 to 2½ liters of water are lost daily. This loss of water is replaced in the form of fluids taken in, water contained in solid foods eaten, and that produced in the body as a result of oxidative processes. The body is able to maintain a fluid balance except during some acute or chronic illnesses.

ENERGY REQUIREMENTS

Total energy expenditure for a day includes energy used at rest, in physical activity, and as a result of thermogenesis, the metabolic response to food intake. Also affecting these components are age, sex, body size and composition, genetics, physiologic state (growth period, pregnancy, lactation), presence of disease, and body temperature. At all ages, if energy in the form of calories taken in through food exceeds or is deficient to meet an individual's needs, a change in body energy stored as fat occurs.

Resting Energy Expenditure

Resting energy expenditure (REE) contributes the largest proportion of total energy expenditure by the body. REE represents the energy expended by a person at rest under conditions of stable temperature. Although basal metabolic rate (BMR) is defined as the REE measured soon after awakening in the morning (12 hours after the last meal), these two values are often interchangeable (their variability is less than 10%). Table 6-6 presents equations developed by the World Health Organization (WHO), 1985. These equations are meant to serve as a guide, as they are not completely accurate for all individuals, but can assist in determining approximate energy needs. Notice that the tables account for age, weight, and sex, but not height. Height does not appear to affect the accuracy of the calculation.

Physical Activity

Physical activity contributes the second largest proportion of total energy expenditure by the body. The energy expended by numerous activities has been studied thoroughly by a number of researchers. Variations on the energy expended by a given activity can vary greatly among individuals and is most affected by body weight and muscle mass. A heavier person will expend more energy for a given task than a lighter weight individual. This makes calculating exact energy expenditure difficult and often time-consuming. Table 6-7 provides estimates for energy needs, infants through adults, and is based on an activity level of light to moderate. These will need to be adjusted for individuals with higher activity levels and of great or smaller body size. The energy requirements listed for infants and children were derived from estimates of intake associated with normal growth by the WHO. The increase in energy requirements for pregnancy and lactation also come from the WHO and are based on the energy costs estimated during both physiologic states.

Text continued on p. 141

TABLE 6-2 Fat-Soluble Vitamin Summary

Vitamins	Metabolism/Function	Deficiency or Excess	Food Sources
Vitamin A Retinol Retinal Retinoic acid	Bile needed for absorption Mineral oil prevents absorption Stored in liver	Night blindness Keratomalacia Lowered resistance to infection Severe drying and scaling of skin; eye infections; blindness	Liver, kidney
Provitamin A Carotenes	Bone and tooth structure Healthy skin and mucous membranes Vision in dim light	Overdoses are toxic: skin, hair, and bone changes, petechiae	Egg yolk, butter, fortified margarine Milk, cream, cheese, Dark-green leafy and deep-yellow vegetables Deep-yellow fruits

Vitamin D
Precursors:
  Ergosterol in plants
  7-dehydrocholesterol; in skin
	Some storage in liver
	Liver synthesizes calcidiol
	Kidney converts calcidiol to *calcitriol*
	Functions as hormone in absorption of calcium and phosphorus; mobilization and mineralization of bone
		Rickets
		  Soft bones
		  Enlarged joints
		  Enlarged skull
		  Deformed chest
		  Spinal curvature
		  Bowed leg
		Osteomalacia
		Renal osteodystrophy
		Even small excess is toxic
			Fortified milk
			Concentrates: calciferol; viosterol
			Fish-liver oils
			Exposure to ultraviolet rays of sun

Vitamin E Tocopherols	Prevents oxidation of vitamin A in intestine Protects cell membranes against oxidation Protects red blood cells Limited stores in body Polyunsaturated fats increase need	Deficiency not common Red cell hemolysis in malnourished infants Low toxicity	Salad oils, shortenings, margarines Whole grains, legumes, nuts, dark leafy vegetables
Vitamin K	Forms prothrombin for normal blood clotting Synthesized in intestines	Prolonged clotting time Hemorrhage, especially in newborn infants, and biliary tract disease Large amounts toxic	Synthesized by intestinal bacteria Dark-green leafy vegetables

From Robinson, Weigley, Mueller, 1993.

TABLE 6-3   **Water-Soluble Vitamin Summary**

Vitamins	Metabolism/Function	Deficiency	Food Sources

Ascorbic acid
Vitamin C
	Forms collagen
	Teeth firm in gums
	Hormone synthesis
	Resistance to infection
	Improves iron absorption
		Poor wound healing
		Poor bone, tooth development
		Scurvy
		   Bruising and hemorrhage
		   Bleeding gums
		   Loose teeth
			Citrus fruits
			Strawberries, cantaloupe
			Tomatoes, broccoli
			Raw green vegetables

Thiamin
Vitamin B_1
	Coenzyme for breakdown of
	   glucose for energy
	Healthy nerves
	Good digestion
	Normal appetite
	Good mental outlook
		Beriberi
		   Fatigue
		   Poor appetite
		   Constipation
		   Depression
		   Neuropathy
		   Angular stomatitis
		   Polyneuritis
		   Edema
		   Heart failure
			Pork, liver, other meats,
			   poultry
			Dry beans and peas, peanut
			   butter
			Enriched and whole-grain
			   bread
			Milk, eggs

Riboflavin
Vitamin B_2
	Coenzymes for protein and
	   glucose metabolism
	Fatty acid synthesis
	Healthy skin
	Normal vision in bright light
		Cheilosis
		   Scaling skin
		   Burning, itching, sensitive eyes
			Dairy products
			Meat, poultry, fish
			Dark-green leafy vegetables
			Enriched and whole-grain
			   breads, cereals

Niacin
Nicotinic acid
Niacinamide
	Coenzymes for energy metabo-
	   lism
	Normal digestion
	Healthy nervous system
	Healthy skin
	Tryptophan a precusor:
	   60 mg = 1 mg niacin
		Pellagra
		   Dermatitis
		   Angular stomatitis
		   Diarrhea
		   Depression
		   Disorientation
		   Delirium
			Meat, poultry, fish
			Dark-green leafy vegetables
			Whole-grain or enriched
			   breads, cereals

Vitamin B_6
Pyridoxine
Pyridoxal
Pyridoxamine
	Coenzymes for protein
	   metabolism
	Conversion of tryptophan
	   to niacin
	Formation of heme
		Cheliosis
		Gastrointestinal upsets
		Weak gait
		Irritability
		Neuropathy
		Convulsions
			Meat, whole-grain cereals,
			   dark-green leafy vegeta-
			   bles, potatoes

Vitamin B_{12}	Formation of mature red
	   blood cells
	Synthesis of DNA, RNA
	Requires intrinsic factor from
	   stomach for absorption
		Pernicious anemia: lack of intrinsic
		   factor, or after gastrectomy
		Macrocytic anemia: neurologic
		   degeneration, pallor
			Animal foods only: milk,
			   eggs, meat, poultry, fish

Folate
Folacin
Folic acid
	Maturation of red blood cells
	Synthesis of DNA, RNA
		Macrocytic anemia in pregnancy,
		   sprue, pallor
			Dark-green leafy vegetables,
			   meat, fish, poultry, eggs,
			   whole-grain cereals

Biotin	Components of coenzymes
	   in energy metabolism
	Some synthesis in intestine
	Avidin, a protein in raw egg
	   white, interferes with
	   absorption
		Occurs only when large amounts of
		   raw egg whites are eaten
		Dermatitis, loss of hair
			Organ meats, egg yolk,
			   legumes, nuts

Pantothenic acid	Component of coenzyme A
	Synthesis of sterols, fatty acids,
	   heme
		Occurs rarely
		Neuritis of arms, legs; burning
		   sensation of feet
			Meat, poultry, fish,
			   legumes, whole-grain
			   cereals
			Lesser amounts in milk,
			   fruits, and vegetables

From Robinson, Weigley, Mueller, 1993.

TABLE 6-4 Mineral Summary

Element	Function	Utilization/Deficiency	Food Sources
Calcium	99% in bones, teeth Nervous stimulation Muscle contraction Blood clotting Activates enzymes	10% to 40% absorbed Aided by vitamin D and lactose; hindered by oxalic acid Parathyroid hormone regulates blood levels *Deficiency:* fragile bones; osteoporosis	Dairy products Mustard and turnip greens Cabbage, broccoli Clams, oysters, salmon
Phosphorus	80%-90% in bones, teeth Acid-balance Transport of fats Enzymes for energy metabolism; protein synthesis	Vitamin D favors absorption and use by bones Dietary deficiency unlikely	Dairy products Meat, poultry, fish Whole-grain cereals, nuts, legumes
Magnesium	60% in bones, teeth Transmits nerve impulses Muscle contraction Enzymes for energy metabolism	Salts relatively insoluble Acid favors absorption Dietary deficiency unlikely; occurs in alcoholism, renal failure	Milk, meat, green-leafy vegetables, legumes, whole-grain cereals
Sodium	Extracellular fluid Water balance Acid-base balance Nervous stimulation Muscle contraction	Almost completely absorbed Body levels regulated by adrenal; excess excreted in urine and by skin *Deficiency:* rare, occurs with excessive perspiration	Table salt Baking powder, baking soda Milk, meat, poultry, fish, eggs
Potassium	Intracellular fluid Protein and glycogen synthesis Water balance Transmits nerve impulse Muscle contraction	Almost completely absorbed Body levels regulated by adrenal; excess excreted in urine *Deficiency:* starvation, duiretic therapy	Ample amounts in meat, cereals, fruits, fruit juices, vegetables
Iron	Mostly in hemoglobin Muscle myoglobin Oxidizing enzymes for release of energy	5%-20% absorption Acid and vitamin C aid absorption Daily losses in urine and feces Menstrual loss *Deficiency:* anemia, cheilosis, pallor	Organ meats, meat, fish, poultry Whole-grain and enriched cereal Green vegetables, dried fruits
Iodine	Forms thyroxine for energy metabolism	Chiefly in thyroid gland *Deficiency:* endemic goiter	Iodized salt Shellfish, saltwater fish
Fluoride	Prevents tooth decay	Storage in bones and teeth Excess leads to tooth mottling	Flouridated water
Copper	Utilization of iron for hemoglobin formation Pigment formation Myelin sheath of nerves	In form of ceruloplasmin in blood Abnormal storage in Wilson's disease *Deficiency:* rare	Liver, shellfish, meats, nuts, legumes, whole-grain cereals
Zinc	Enzymes for transfer of carbon dioxide Taste, protein synthesis	*Deficiency:* growth retardation; altered taste	Plant and animal proteins

From Robinson, Weigley, Mueller, 1993.

TABLE 6-5 Summary Table: Estimated Safe and Adequate Daily Dietary Intakes of Selected Vitamins and Minerals*

Category	Age (years)	Vitamins	
		Biotin (μg)	Pantothenic Acid (mg)
Infants	0-0.5	10	2
	0.5-1	15	3
Children and adolescents	1-3	20	3
	4-6	25	3-4
	7-10	30	4-5
	11+	30-100	4-7
Adults		30-100	4-7

Trace Elements†

Category	Age (years)	Copper (mg)	Manganese (mg)	Fluoride (mg)	Chromium (μg)	Molybdenun (μg)
Infants	0-0.5	0.4-0.6	0.3-0.6	0.1-0.5	10-40	15-30
	0.5-1	0.6-0.7	0.6-1.0	0.2-1.0	20-60	20-40
Children and adolescents	1-3	0.7-1.0	1.0-1.5	0.5-1.5	20-80	25-50
	4-6	1.0-1.5	1.5-2.0	1.0-2.5	30-120	30-75
	7-10	1.0-2.0	2.0-3.0	1.5-2.5	50-200	50-150
	11+	1.5-2.5	2.0-5.0	1.5-2.5	50-200	75-250
Adults		1.5-3.0	2.0-5.0	1.5-4.0	50-200	75-250

From Subcommittee on the Tenth Edition of the RDAs, 1989.
*Because there is less information on which to base allowances, these figures are not given in the main table of RDA and are provided here in the form of ranges of recommended intakes.
†Because the toxic levels for many trace elements may be only several times usual intakes, the upper levels for the trace elements given in this table should not be habitually exceeded.

TABLE 6-6 Equations for Predicting Resting Energy Expenditure From Body Weight*

Sex and Age Range (years)	Equation to Derive REE in kcal/day
Males	
0-3	$(60.9 \times wt^{\dagger}) - 54$
3-10	$(22.7 \times wt) + 495$
10-18	$(17.5 \times wt) + 651$
18-30	$(15.3 \times wt) + 679$
30-60	$(11.6 \times wt) + 879$
>60	$(13.5 \times wt) + 487$
Females	
0-3	$(61.0 \times wt) - 51$
3-10	$(22.5 \times wt) + 499$
10-18	$(12.2 \times wt) + 746$
18-30	$(14.7 \times wt) + 496$
30-60	$(8.7 \times wt) + 829$
>60	$(10.5 \times wt) + 596$

Modified from Subcommittee on the Tenth Edition of the RDAs, 1989.
*From WHO, 1985. These equations were derived from BMR data.
†Weight of person in kilograms.

| TABLE 6-7 | Median Heights and Weights and Recommended Energy Intake |

Category	Age (years) or Condition	Weight (kg)	Weight (lb)	Height (cm)	Height (in)	REE[a] (kcal/day)	Average Energy Allowance (kcal) Multiples of REE	Average Energy Allowance (kcal) Per kg Body Weight	Average Energy Allowance (kcal) Per Day[b]
Infants	0.0-0.5	6	13	60	24	320		108	650
	0.5-1.0	9	20	71	28	500		98	850
Children	1-3	13	29	90	35	740		102	1,300
	4-6	20	44	112	44	950		90	1,800
	7-10	28	62	132	52	1,130		70	2,000
Males	11-14	45	99	157	62	1,440	1.70	55	2,500
	15-18	66	145	176	69	1,760	1.67	45	3,000
	19-24	72	160	177	70	1,780	1.67	40	2,900
	25-50	79	174	176	70	1,800	1.60	37	2,900
	51+	77	170	173	68	1,530	1.50	30	2,300
Females	11-14	46	101	157	62	1,310	1.67	47	2,200
	15-18	55	120	163	64	1,370	1.60	40	2,200
	19-24	58	128	164	65	1,350	1.60	38	2,200
	25-50	63	138	163	64	1,380	1.55	36	2,200
	51+	65	143	160	63	1,280	1.50	30	1,900
Pregnant	1st Trimester								+0
	2nd Trimester								+300
	3rd Trimester								+300
Lactating	1st 6 months								+500
	2nd 6 months								+500

From Wardlaw, Insel, Seyler, 1994.
[a] Resting energy expenditure (REE): calculation based on FAO equations, then rounded. This is the same as resting metabolic rate (RMR).
[b] Figure is rounded.

Thermogenesis

After eating, the metabolic rate increases, depending on the size and composition of the meal. This accounts for about 7% of the total energy expended during a day. The increased rate peaks after about 1 hour and disappears after 4 hours. It has little long-term effect on energy requirements, being lost in the day-to-day variations in energy metabolism.

REVIEW OF RELATED HISTORY

For any of these presenting problems, a nutrient analysis must be completed by using a method of diet history or recall. Three nutrition screening forms have been developed by representatives of the American Academy of Family Physicians, The American Dietetic Association, and The National Council on the Aging, Inc (Appendix G). These are intended for use in obtaining specific information from individuals about their current nutrition status and intake and determining whether problem areas exist. Which screen form is used is depends on how in-depth the assessment will be and the availability of anthropometric and laboratory values. The questions can be modified for infants, children, older adults, or particular circumstances.

The history of an individual's food intake allows estimation of the adequacy of the diet. Histories may be obtained through 24-hour diet recalls or by having the patient keep a food diary for 3 to 4 days, including 1 weekend day. Various methods for measuring nutrient intake are available.

24-HOUR DIET RECALL

The 24-hour recall is the quickest and most simple method for obtaining a food intake history. The patient completes the 24-hour recall form found in Appendix G, listing all foods, beverages, and snacks eaten during the last 24 hours. You may also just ask the patient to recite what he or she had to eat and drink during the last 24 hours. Unfortunately, this method provides a very limited view of an individual's actual intake over time and therefore may be misleading. Most individuals also are unable to accurately remember everything they ate the day before, which causes further inaccuracies in interpreting the information.

FOOD DIARY

The food diary is the most accurate and time-consuming of the methods for both the patient and health professional. It provides a retrospective view of an individual's eating habits and dietary intake, recorded as it happened. It can also collect relevant data that may aid in identifying problem areas. The patient is provided the food diary form found in Appendix G and requested to keep at least 3 days of specific food and beverage intake, with 1 day being a weekend day.

MEASURES OF NUTRIENT ANALYSIS

Computerized nutrient analysis programs offer the quickest and most efficient method of analyzing an individual's nutrient intake. Analysis may be performed for 1 or more days and averages obtained for all or selected nutrients. A nutrition textbook containing food composition tables may also be used; however, it is time-consuming, and the tables found in these books are often not as complete as those in computerized programs. The quickest method of estimating adequacy with reliable accuracy is simply to compare the individual's intake with the recommended servings and portions listed in the Food Guide Pyramid and Vegetarian Food Guide Pyramid (Figures 6-1 and 6-2).

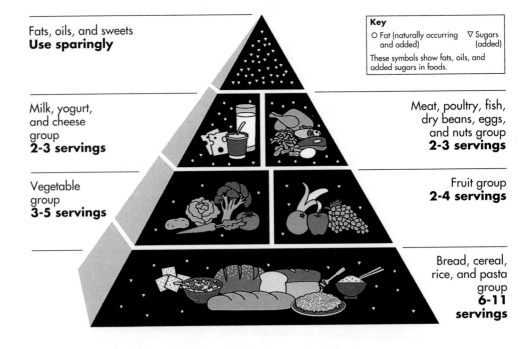

FIGURE 6-1
Food guide pyramid.

Food Guide Pyramid

The Food Guide Pyramid indicates the number of servings and portion sizes to eat from each food group, depending on the person's age. When using the Food Guide Pyramid, remember the following:

- The guide does not deal with infant feeding.
- No one food is absolutely essential to good nutrition. Each food is low in at least one essential nutrient.
- No one food group provides all essential nutrients in adequate amounts. Each food group makes an important, distinct contribution to nutritional intake.
- Variety is the key to the Food Guide Pyramid. Variety is guaranteed by using all the groups. Furthermore, one should consume a variety of foods within each group (Table 6-8).

Vegetarian Food Guide Pyramid

The Vegetarian Food Guide Pyramid indicates the number of servings and portion sizes to eat from each food group, depending on the person's age and energy needs.

When using the Vegetarian Food Guide Pyramid, remember the following:

- The guide does not deal with infant feeding.
- No one food is absolutely essential to good nutrition. Each food is low in at least one essential nutrient.
- No one food group provides all essential nutrients in adequate amounts. Each food group makes an important, distinct contribution to nutritional intake.
- Variety is the key to the Vegetarian Food Guide Pyramid. Variety is guaranteed by using all the groups. Furthermore, one should consume a variety of foods within each group (Table 6-9).
- Five nutrients may be deficient in a vegetarian diet if it is not carefully planned: protein, calcium (lacto-ovo and vegan), iron, vitamin B_{12} (vegan) and vitamin D.

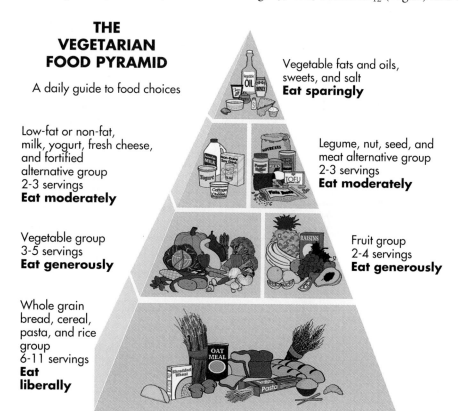

FIGURE 6-2

Vegetarian food guide pyramid.

From The Health Connection, 1994. Illustration by Merle Poirier. The Vegetarian Food Guide Pyramid is available as posters and handouts by calling The Health Connection 1-800-548-8700 or 301-790-9735.

		Major	Foods and
Food Group	Serving	Contributions	Serving Sizes*
Milk, yogurt, and cheese	2 (adult†) 3 (children, teens, young adults, and pregnant or lactating women)	Carbohydrate Calcium Riboflavin Protein Potassium Zinc	1 cup milk 1½ ounces cheese 2 ounces processed cheese 1 cup yogurt 2 cups cottage cheese 1 cup custard/pudding 1½ cups ice cream
Meat, poultry, fish, dry beans, eggs, and nuts	2-3	Protein Niacin Iron Vitamin B_6 Zinc Thiamin Vitamin B_{12}‡	2-3 ounces cooked meat, poultry, or fish 1-1½ cups cooked dry beans 2 tablespoons peanut butter 2 eggs ½-1 cup nuts
Fruits	2-4	Carbohydrate Vitamin C Dietary fiber	¼ cup dried fruit ½ cup cooked fruit ¾ cup juice 1 whole piece of fruit 1 melon wedge
Vegetables	3-5	Carbohydrate Vitamin A Vitamin C Folate Magnesium Dietary fiber	½ cup raw or cooked vegetables 1 cup raw leafy vegetables 3-4 small crackers
Bread, cereals, rice, and pasta	6-11	Carbohydrate Thiamin Riboflavin§ Iron Niacin Folate Magnesium‖ Dietary fiber‖ Zinc‖	1 slice of bread 1 ounce ready-to-eat cereal ½-¾ cup cooked cereal, rice, or pasta
Fats, oils, and sweets		Foods from this group should not replace any from the other groups. Amounts consumed should be determined by individual energy needs.	

TABLE 6-8 The Food Guide Pyramid—A Summary

From Wardlaw, Insel, Seyler, 1994.
*May be reduced for child servings.
† ≥25 years of age.
‡ Only in animal food choices.
§ If enriched.
‖ Whole grains especially.

TABLE 6-9 Vegetarian Food Pyramid—A Summary

Food Group	Daily Serving	Nutrient Contributions	Food and Serving Sizes
Whole grains and legumes	Eat liberally; 6-11	Complex CHO Fiber Protein Vitamin B_1 (Thiamine) Vitamin B_2 (Riboflavin) Vitamin B_6 and niacin Iron Magnesium Calcium Trace minerals	1 slice bread ½ cup hot cereal ¾ cup dry cereal ¼ cup granola ½ cup rice or pasta 1 tortilla 1 chapati ½ bagel or English muffin 3-4 crackers ½ muffin ½ cup cooked beans
Vegetables	Eat generously; 3-5	Fiber Potassium Beta-carotene Folate Vitamin C Calcium Magnesium	1 cup raw, leafy vegetable salad ½ cup cooked vegetables ½ cup chopped raw vegetables ¾ cup vegetable juice
Fruits	Eat generously; 2-4	Vitamin C Beta-carotene Fiber Potassium Folate Magnesium	1 medium, whole fruit ½ cup canned fruit 1 cup berries ¾ cup fruit juice
Legumes, nuts, seeds, meat alternatives	Eat moderately; 2-3	Protein Zinc Iron Fiber Calcium Vitamin B_6 Vitamin E Niacin (B_3) Linoleic acid	½ cup cooked beans or peas ⅓ cup nuts (1 oz) ½ cup tofu 2 Tbsp nut butter (1 oz) ¼ cup meat alternative 2 egg whites
Dairy products and/or fortified alternatives	Eat moderately; 2-3	Calcium Protein Vitamins A and D Riboflavin (B_2) Vitamin B_{12}	1 cup milk, nonfat or lowfat 1 cup soymilk (fortified) ¾ cup lowfat cottage cheese ½ cup soy cheese 1½ oz. fresh cheese 1 cup low-fat or non-fat yogurt
Fats, oils, sugar, salt	Eat sparingly; limit desserts to 2-3/wk; use honey, jams, jelly, corn syrups, molasses, sugar sparingly; use soft drinks and candies very sparingly, if at all; limit foods high in salt.	Low in nutrients; oils contain essential fatty acids; every Tblsp of fat added to 2200 calorie diet increases % of calories as fat × approx 5%; every Tblsp sugar adds 2% calories as sugar	1 tsp salt = 2000 mg sodium 1 T oil = 13.6 g fat 1 tsp oil = 4.5 g fat 1 T marg = 11.4 g fat 1 T mayo = 11 g fat 1 T sour cream = 3 g fat 1 T cream cheese = 5 g fat 1 T sugar = 12 g 1 T honey = 21 g 1 tsp honey = 7 g

Data from General Conference Nutrition Council.

MEASURES OF NUTRIENT ADEQUACY

An individual's diet can be measured for nutritional adequacy based on energy needs and/or a variety of macronutrients or micronutrients.

- Energy: A variety of methods can be used for calculating an individual's energy needs. Refer to Table 6-7 for those patients who are at or within 10% of the listed weight for their height. The "Rule of Thumb" calculations also offer a quick estimate for energy needs for those needing to gain, maintain, or lose weight. Adjustments to the calculations may be made to meet the needs of certain individuals (e.g., those who appear to have a higher metabolic rate and continue to lose weight even when the higher calculation is used). It is important to note that overweight individuals under-report their energy intake by 30% to 55% and lean individuals by only 0% to 20%.
- Fat: For those over 2 years of age, a diet of <30% of the calories consumed in a day should come from fat, with a distribution of <10% saturated fat, <10% polyunsaturated fat and the rest monounsaturated fat. Before age 2, fat intake may reach 35% to 40% of calories. To obtain essential fatty acids, an intake of at least 20 g per day is recommended.
- Protein: For adults, an average of 0.8 g per kilogram body weight is sufficient to meet needs. Refer to Table 6-1 for the recommended daily protein needs for all individuals, including infants, children, and adolescents.
- Vitamins and Minerals: An individual who eats a variety of foods from the food groups will meet his or her needs for most vitamins and minerals. Several that may be of concern if food intake is restricted include vitamins C, E, and A; calcium; iron; and folate.
- Fiber: Although fiber is not classified as a nutrient, it is recommended that an adult obtain 25 to 30 g of fiber per day. In children 3 to 18 years of age the formula "age + 5 g" should be used to determine fiber needs.

PRESENT PROBLEM

Weight Loss

- Total weight lost, compared with usual weight; time period, sudden, gradual, desired or undesired.
- Desired weight loss: eating habits, diet plan used, food preparation, food group avoidance, calorie intake; appetite; exercise pattern; support group participation; weight goal.
- Undesired weight loss: anorexia; vomiting or diarrhea, time period; possibility of diabetes, celiac sprue; change in life-style, activity and stress levels.
- Preoccupation with body weight or body shape: never feeling thin enough, fasting, unusually strict caloric intake, unusual food restrictions or cravings, bulimia, laxative abuse, induced vomiting, amenorrhea, excessive exercise, alcohol intake.
- Medications: chemotherapy, diuretics, insulin, fluoxetine (Prozac); prescription and nonprescription diet pills, laxatives, oral hypoglycemics; herbal supplements.

Weight Gain

- Total weight gained; time period, sudden or gradual, desired or undesired, possibility of pregnancy.
- Change in life-style; change in social aspects of eating; more meals eaten out of the home; meals eaten quickly and on the go; change in meal preparation patterns; exercise patterns, stress level, alcohol intake.
- Medications: steroids, oral contraceptives, antidepressants, insulin.

Increased Metabolic Requirements

- Fever, infection, burns, trauma, pregnancy, infancy, hyperthyroidism.
- External losses (e.g., fistulas, wounds, abscesses, chronic blood loss, chronic dialysis).

PAST MEDICAL HISTORY

- Chronic illness: cystic fibrosis, phenylketonuria (PKU), maple syrup urine disease, inborn errors of carbohydrate metabolism, tyrosinemia, Prader-Willi, Wilson's disease, homocystinuria, diabetes, hypothyroidism, hyperthyroidism, pancreatic insufficiency, celiac disease, surgical resection of GI tract.
- Previous weight loss or gain efforts: weight at 25 years, maximum body weight, minimum weight as an adult.
- Previously diagnosed eating disorder, hypoglycemia.

FAMILY HISTORY

- Obesity.
- Constitutionally short or tall stature.
- Genetic or metabolic disorder: diabetes, see Chronic illness, Past Medical History.

PERSONAL AND SOCIAL HISTORY

- Nutrition: appetite; usual calorie intake, calories adequate or excessive for maintenance of weight; vegetarianism practiced; proportion of fat, protein, carbohydrate in the diet; intake of major vitamins and minerals (A, C, iron, calcium, folate). Refer to Tables 6-1, 6-5, 6-6, and 6-7 in Anatomy and Physiology section.
- Use of vitamin, mineral, and herbal supplements.
- Usual weight and height; current weight and height; goal weight.
- Use of alcohol.
- Use of street drugs.
- Adequate income for food purchases.
- Typical mealtime situations, companions, living environment.
- Use of oral supplements, tube feedings, parenteral nutrition.
- Dentition: dentures, missing teeth, gum disease.
- Refer to "Determine Your Nutritional Health" and "Level I Screen" in Appendix G.

RISK FACTORS   **Eating Disorder**

Weight preoccupation
Poor self-esteem, perfectionist personality
Self-image perceptual disturbances
Chronic medical illness (insulin-dependent diabetes)
Family history of eating disorders, obesity, alcoholism, or affective disorders
Cultural pressure for thinness or outstanding performance
Athlete; drive to excel in sports (particularly females)
Food cravings, restrictions
Compulsive/binge eating
Difficulties with communication, conflict resolution, and separation from families

---

INFANTS AND CHILDREN

- Nutrition: breast-feeding frequency, type and amount of infant formula, time it takes to drink one feeding, intake of protein, calories, vitamins and minerals adequate for growth (refer to Tables 6-1 and 6-5), vegetarianism practiced; food allergies, vitamin and mineral supplements.

- Chronic illness: PKU, maple syrup urine disease, inborn errors of carbohydrate metabolism, tyrosinemia, homocystinuria, Wilson's disease.
- Congenital anomalies: prematurity, cleft palate, malformed palate, tongue thrust, swallowing disorders, neurologic disorders, gastrointestinal reflux.

ADOLESCENTS

- Nutrition: intake of protein, calories, vitamins and minerals adequate for growth (Refer to Tables 6-1 and 6-5); vegetarianism practiced; fast food intake; fad diets; food allergies, vitamin and mineral supplements, herbal supplements.
- Preoccupation with weight (particularly girls)
  - overconcern with developing muscle mass, losing body fat
  - excessive exercise
  - weighs daily, boasts about weight loss
  - omits perceived "fattening" foods and food groups from diet

PREGNANT WOMEN

- Prepregnancy weight, nutrient intake (particularly folate).
- Weight gain during pregnancy, nutrient intake during pregnancy (particularly protein, calories, iron, folate, calcium).
- Lactation, nutrient intake during lactation (particularly protein, calories, calcium, vitamins A and C).
- Pica.

OLDER ADULTS

- Nutrition: weight gain or loss, adequate income for food purchases, medical nutrition therapy needs, participant in elderly feeding programs, social interaction at mealtime, number of daily meals and snacks, transportation to grocery stores. Refer to the Level II Nutrition Screen in Appendix G.
- Chronic illnesses: diabetes, renal disease, cancer, heart disease, and others.
- Food/nutrient/medication interactions (Box 6-1). Also refer to the Medications Use Checklist in Appendix G.

RISK FACTORS | **Possible Medication Effects on Nutritional Intake and Status**

- Alter food intake (taste/smell, drug mouth, gastric irritation, bezoars, appetite increase/decrease, nausea/vomiting)
- Modify nutrient absorption (alter GI pH, bile acid activity, alter GI motility, inhibit enzymes, mucosal cell wall damage, insoluble nutrient-drug complexes)
- Modify nutrient metabolism (vitamin antagonist, vitamin inactivation)
- Modify nutrient excretion (urinary loss, fecal loss)

BOX 6-1 | **Food/Nutrient/Medication Interactions**

Medications can affect nutritional intake and status just as some nutrients can affect absorption, metabolism, and excretion of medications. It is important to assess the medications a patient is taking to determine appropriateness and if there are any possible interactions. The term *medications* should be interpreted to include those by prescription as well as over-the-counter. Often patients are taking vitamin, mineral, herbal, and protein supplements they do not consider to be medications. Thus they do not remember to relate these during the examination unless specifically asked about them.

EXAMINATION AND FINDINGS

EQUIPMENT

- Tape measure with millimeter markings
- Calculator

Nutrition can be assessed through many body systems. Refer to Table 6-10, which summarizes clinical findings often associated with nutrient deficiencies. The section below discusses the specific anthropometric and biochemical measures of nutritional status.

TABLE 6-10	Clinical Signs and Symptoms of Various Nutrient Deficiencies	
Area of Examination	**Sign/Symptom**	**Potential Nutrient Deficiency**
Hair	Alopecia	Zinc, essential fatty acids
	Easy pluckability	Protein, essential fatty acids
	Lackluster	Protein, zinc
	"Corkscrew" hair	Vitamin C, vitamin A
	Decreased pigmentation	Protein, copper
Eyes	Xerosis of conjunctiva	Vitamin A
	Corneal vascularization	Riboflavin
	Keratomalacia	Vitamin A
	Bitot spots	Vitamin A
GI tract	Nausea, vomiting	Pyridoxine
	Diarrhea	Zinc, niacin
	Stomatitis	Pyridoxine, riboflavin, iron
	Cheilosis	Pyridoxine, iron
	Glossitis	Pyridoxine, zinc, niacin, folate, vitamin B_{12}
	Magenta tongue	Riboflavin
	Swollen, bleeding gums	Vitamin C
	Fissured tongue	Niacin
	Hepatomegaly	Protein
Skin	Dry and scaling	Vitamin A, essential fatty acids, zinc
	Petechiae/ecchymoses	Vitamin C, vitamin K
	Follicular hyperkeratosis	Vitamin A, essential fatty acids
	Nasolabial seborrhea	Niacin, pyridoxine, riboflavin
	Bilateral dermatitis	Niacin, zinc
Extremities	Subcutaneous fat loss	Kcalories
	Muscle wastage	Kcalories, protein
	Edema	Protein
	Osteomalacia, bone pain, rickets	Vitamin D
	Arthralgia	Vitamin C
Neurologic	Disorientation	Niacin, thiamin
	Confabulation	Thiamin
	Neuropathy	Thiamin, pyridoxine, chromium
	Paresthesia	Thiamin, pyridoxine, vitamin B_{12}
Cardiovascular	Congestive heart failure, cardiomegaly, tachycardia	Thiamin
	Cardiomyopathy	Selenium

Data from Ross Products Division, Abbot Laboratories Inc.

ANTHROPOMETRICS

Procedures for accurately measuring height, weight, and triceps skin fold and the tables of the norms for the relevant age and gender groups are addressed in Chapter 5, Growth and Measurement. These measures are useful in assessing a patient's nutritional status and possible disease risk.

Assessing Height and Weight

Comparing a patient's height and weight over time is essential in the continuum of patient care (Figure 6-3). This is obvious for pediatrics, but during adulthood patients are weighed at each visit and asked how tall they are, but height is rarely taken. During the aging process, the vertebrae become more compact and height decreases; therefore it is important to obtain an accurate height on middle-aged and elderly patients yearly. Refer to Box 6-2 to perform measures and calculations. See Box 6-3 for adjusting desirable weights for amputations and paraplegia/quadriplegia.

Body Mass Index

The body mass index (BMI) is a formula used to assess nutritional status and total body fat (Box 6-4). It is a measure of kg per (m^2). For adults, a BMI between 20.7 and 27.8 in men and 19.1 and 27.3 in women is expected. A BMI above 27.8 or 27.3, respectively, in men and women, corresponds with being at least 20% overweight.

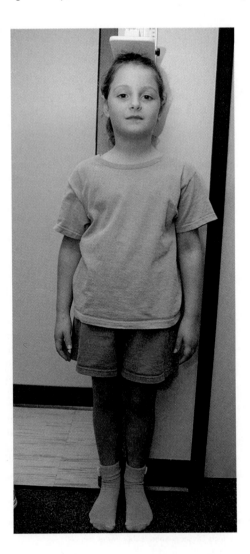

FIGURE 6-3

Measurement of height in a school-age child.

BOX 6-2 **Assessing Height and Weight**

Current Weight _____ Current Height _____
Usual Weight _____
Desirable Body Weight _____ (women: 100 lb for first 5 ft; plus 5 lb for each inch thereafter)
(men: 106 lb for first 5 ft; plus 6 lb for each in thereafter)
This is a quick method for determining desirable weight.
Refer to Chapter 5, Growth and Measurement for
Height/Weight Tables and below for Body Mass Index
measurements.
Add 10% for a large frame; subtract 10% for a small frame.
Refer to Chapter 5, Growth and Measurement for
methods used to determine body frame size.
% Desirable Weight _____ *current weight* $\times$ 100 desirable body weight
% Usual Weight _____ *current weight* $\times$ 100 usual weight
% Weight Change _____ *usual weight − current weight* $\times$ 100 usual weight
A significant weight loss equals or exceeds:
   1% to 2% in 1 week
   5% in 1 month
   7.5% in 3 months
   10% in 6 months
For pediatric patients (birth to age 18) refer to the growth charts in Appendix E.

BOX 6-3 **Desirable Body Weight (DBW) Adjustments**

Adjustment for Amputation

To make adjustments for amputation, subtract the percent weight contributed by the
   amputated body part(s).

Trunk without limbs	42.7%
Entire upper extremity	6.5%
Hand	0.8%
Forearm	2.3%
Forearm and hand	3.1%
Upper arm	3.5%
Entire lower extremity	18.65%
Foot	1.8%
Lower leg	5.3%
Lower leg and foot	7.1%
Thigh	11.6%

Adjustment for Paraplegia/Quadriplegia

To make adjustment for paraplegia: subtract 5% to 10% from calculated DBW
To make adjustment for quadriplegia: subtract 10% to 15% from calculated DBW

Tracking the change of a patient's BMI over time can often quickly signal nutritional problems and/or illness. See Table 6-11 for calculating BMI using pounds and inches. A nomogram for calculating BMI is available on the Level II Nutrition Screen form found in Appendix G.

BMI has not been standardized for use in pediatric and adolescent populations. Measurement of body fat in children and adolescents should be through a combination of measures, including BMI, waist/hip ratio, and skinfold thickness and evaluated with consideration also to maturation stage, race, and gender. Continue to use the growth charts in Appendix E to assess appropriate height and weight relevant to age and gender.

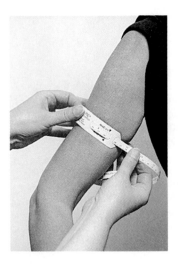

FIGURE 6-4

Measurement of mid upper arm circumference.

Mid Upper Arm Circumference

The mid upper arm circumference, not routinely obtained, provides a rough estimate of muscle mass and available fat and protein stores. A depressed value, however, is usually found only in the most severe forms of protein-calorie malnutrition. The measurement is of more value in the calculation of arm muscle circumference and arm muscle mass, both of which are very sensitive to changes in muscle and/or protein stores. Select the patient's bare right arm for measurement. (Note: The same side of the body should always be used as for other anthropometric measures.) Place the millimeter measuring tape around the patient's upper arm, midway between the tips of the olecranon and acromial processes, the same location where the triceps skinfold thickness measurement is made (see Chapter 5, Growth and Measurement) (Figure 6-4). Hold the measuring tape snugly, but not tight enough to cause an indentation, and make the reading to the nearest 5 mm (0.5 cm). Use the value obtained along with the triceps skinfold measure (Chapter 5, Growth and Measurement) to calculate midarm muscle circumference.

BOX 6-4 **Calculating BMI**

Quick calculation for BMI: wt (lb) $\times$ 705 / height (inches) / height (inches)
Example: a man 6′2 inches weighing 185 lb has a BMI of 25.2

$$185 \text{ lb} \times 705 = 130{,}425$$
$$130425 / 72 = 1811.4583$$
$$1811.4583 / 72 = 25.2$$

TABLE 6-11 Body Weight in Pounds According to Height and Body Mass Index

Height (inches)	Body Mass Index (kg per m²)													
	19.0	20.0	21.0	22.0	23.0	24.0	25.0	26.0	27.0	28.0	29.0	30.0	35.0	40.0
	Body Weight (pounds)													
58.0	90.7	95.5	100.3	105.0	109.8	114.6	119.4	124.1	128.9	133.7	138.5	143.2	167.1	191.0
59.0	93.9	98.8	103.8	108.7	113.6	118.6	123.5	128.5	133.4	138.3	143.3	148.2	172.9	197.6
60.0	97.1	102.2	107.3	112.4	117.5	122.6	127.7	132.9	138.0	143.1	148.2	153.3	178.8	204.4
61.0	100.3	105.6	110.9	116.2	121.5	126.8	132.0	137.3	142.6	147.9	153.2	158.4	184.8	211.3
62.0	103.7	109.1	114.6	120.0	125.5	130.9	136.4	141.9	147.3	152.8	158.2	163.7	191.0	218.2
63.0	107.0	112.7	118.3	123.9	129.6	135.2	140.8	146.5	152.1	157.7	163.4	169.0	197.2	225.3
64.0	110.5	116.3	122.1	127.9	133.7	139.5	145.3	151.2	157.0	162.8	168.6	174.4	203.5	232.5
65.0	113.9	119.9	125.9	131.9	137.9	143.9	149.9	155.9	161.9	167.9	173.9	179.9	209.9	239.9
66.0	117.5	123.7	129.8	136.0	142.2	148.4	154.6	160.8	166.9	173.1	179.3	185.5	216.4	247.3
67.0	121.1	127.4	133.8	140.2	146.5	152.9	159.3	165.7	172.0	178.4	184.8	191.1	223.0	254.9
68.0	124.7	131.3	137.8	144.4	151.0	157.5	164.1	170.6	177.2	183.8	190.3	196.9	229.7	262.5
69.0	128.4	135.2	141.9	148.7	155.4	162.2	168.9	175.7	182.5	189.2	196.0	202.7	236.5	270.3
70.0	132.1	139.1	146.1	153.0	160.0	166.9	173.9	180.8	187.8	194.7	201.7	208.6	243.4	278.2
71.0	135.9	143.1	150.3	157.4	164.6	171.7	178.9	186.0	193.2	200.3	207.5	214.6	250.4	286.2
72.0	139.8	147.2	154.5	161.9	169.2	176.6	183.9	191.3	198.7	206.0	213.4	220.7	257.5	294.3
73.0	143.7	151.3	158.8	166.4	174.0	181.5	189.1	196.7	204.2	211.8	219.3	226.9	264.7	302.5
74.0	147.7	155.4	163.2	171.0	178.8	186.5	194.3	202.1	209.9	217.6	225.4	233.2	272.0	310.9
75.0	151.7	159.7	167.7	175.6	183.6	191.6	199.6	207.6	215.6	223.5	231.5	239.5	279.4	319.4
76.0	155.8	164.0	172.2	180.4	188.6	196.8	205.0	213.2	221.4	229.5	237.7	245.9	286.9	327.9

From U.S. Department of Health and Human Services, 1992.

NOTE: A body mass index (BMI) of 27.8 for men and 27.3 for women is the cutoff point for obesity used in the National Health and Nutrition Examination Survey (NHANES II). The National Academy of Sciences' diet and health report suggests that a BMI of 22 to 27 is normal for persons 45 to 54 years of age, a BMI of 23 to 28 is normal for persons 55 to 65 years of age, and a BMI of 24 to 29 is normal for persons over 65 years old.

Midarm Muscle Circumference/Midarm Muscle Area

Midarm muscle circumference and arm muscle area are estimated from measures of mid upper arm circumference (MAC) and triceps skinfold (TSF). The procedure for obtaining triceps skinfold measures is in Chapter 5, Growth and Measurement. The midarm muscle circumference (MAMC) is well accepted as a sensitive index of body protein reserves. The cross-sectional midarm muscle area (MAMA) can also be estimated. Both measures are commonly decreased in the presence of protein malnutrition. Arm muscle area is useful in children, as the muscle area changes more with age than does arm muscle circumference. Remember, this measure of arm muscle is only an estimate as the thickness of the humerus bone is not taken into account and upper arms are not perfectly round as the formula assumes. Tables 6-12 through 6-15 show the percentiles for both of these measures for men, women, and children ages 1 to 75 years. The Level II Nutrition Screen (Appendix G) provides a summary for the percentiles for these measurements for men and women ages 55 to 75.

Calculations

MAMC: $[MAC(mm) - [3.14 \times TSF(mm)]]$

MAMA: $[MAC(mm) - 3.14 \times TSF(mm)]^2/12.56$

BIOCHEMICAL MEASUREMENT

Relevant Laboratory Measures

This list is intended as a guideline. Not all indicators may be necessary or appropriate for a given patient. Likewise, other laboratory measures not listed here may be useful or necessary in a particular situation. Compare laboratory data to the norms for the relevant age and gender group (Table 6-16). A laboratory may have different reference ranges established based on testing equipment and procedure.

Hemoglobin (g/100 ml)
Hematocrit (%)
Transferrin saturation (%)
Serum albumin (g/100 ml)
Serum cholesterol (CHOL)(mg/100 ml)
Serum triglycerides (TRI) (mg/100 ml)

High density lipoproteins (HDL) (mg/100 ml)
Low density lipoproteins (LDL) (mg/100 ml)
CHOL/HDL ratio
Serum glucose (mg/100 ml)
Serum folate

Text continued on p. 157

TABLE 6-12	Midarm Muscle Circumference Percentiles (mm) for Males						
Age Group	5th	10th	25th	50th	75th	90th	95th
1-2	110	113	119	127	135	144	147
2-3	111	114	122	130	140	146	150
3-4	117	123	131	137	143	148	153
4-5	123	126	133	141	148	156	159
5-6	128	133	140	147	154	162	169
6-7	131	135	142	151	161	170	177
7-8	137	139	151	160	168	177	190
8-9	140	145	154	162	170	182	187
9-10	151	154	161	170	183	196	202
10-11	156	160	166	180	191	209	221
11-12	159	165	173	183	195	205	230
12-13	167	171	182	195	210	223	241
13-14	172	179	196	211	226	238	245
14-15	189	199	212	223	240	260	264
15-16	199	204	218	237	254	266	272
16-17	213	225	234	249	269	287	296
17-18	224	231	245	258	273	294	312
18-19	226	237	252	264	283	298	324
19-25	238	245	257	273	289	309	321
25-35	243	250	264	279	298	314	326
35-45	247	255	269	286	302	318	327
45-55	239	249	265	281	300	315	326
55-65	236	245	260	278	295	310	320
65-75	223	235	251	268	284	298	306

Data from Frisancho, 1981.

TABLE 6-13	Midarm Muscle Circumference Percentiles (mm) for Females						
Age Group	5th	10th	25th	50th	75th	90th	95th
1-2	105	111	117	124	132	139	143
2-3	111	114	119	126	133	142	147
3-4	113	119	124	132	140	146	152
4-5	115	121	128	136	144	152	157
5-6	125	128	134	142	151	159	165
6-7	130	133	138	145	154	166	171
7-8	129	135	142	151	160	171	176
8-9	138	140	151	160	171	183	194
9-10	147	150	158	167	180	194	198
10-11	148	150	159	170	180	190	197
11-12	150	158	171	181	196	217	223
12-13	162	166	180	191	201	214	220
13-14	169	175	183	198	211	226	240
14-15	174	179	190	201	216	232	247
15-16	175	178	189	202	215	228	244
16-17	170	180	190	202	216	234	249
17-18	175	183	194	205	221	239	257
18-19	174	179	191	202	215	237	245
19-25	179	185	195	207	221	236	249
25-35	183	188	199	212	228	246	264
35-45	186	192	205	218	236	257	272
45-55	187	193	206	220	238	260	274
55-65	187	196	209	225	244	266	280
65-75	185	195	208	225	244	264	279

Data from Frisancho, 1981.

TABLE 6-14 Midarm Muscle Area Percentiles (mm²) for Males

Age Group	5th	10th	25th	50th	75th	90th	95th
1-2	956	1014	1133	1278	1447	1644	1720
2-3	973	1040	1190	1345	1557	1690	1787
3-4	1095	1201	1357	1484	1618	1750	1853
4-5	1207	1264	1408	1579	1747	1926	2008
5-6	1298	1411	1550	1720	1884	2089	2285
6-7	1360	1447	1605	1815	2056	2297	2493
7-8	1497	1548	1808	2027	2246	2494	2886
8-9	1550	1664	1895	2089	2296	2628	2788
9-10	1811	1884	2067	2288	2657	3053	3257
10-11	1930	2027	2182	2575	2903	3486	3882
11-12	2016	2156	2382	2670	3022	3359	4226
12-13	2216	2339	2649	3022	3496	3968	4640
13-14	2363	2546	3044	3553	4061	4502	4794
14-15	2830	3147	3586	3963	4575	5368	5530
15-16	3138	3317	3788	4481	5134	5631	5900
16-17	3625	4044	4352	4951	5753	6576	6980
17-18	3998	4252	4777	5286	5950	6886	7726
18-19	4070	4481	5066	5552	6374	7067	8355
19-25	4508	4777	5274	5913	6660	7606	8200
25-35	4694	4963	5541	6214	7067	7847	8436
35-45	4844	5181	5740	6490	7265	8034	8488
45-55	4546	4946	5589	6297	7142	7918	8458
55-65	4422	4783	5381	6144	6919	7670	8149
65-75	3973	4411	5031	5716	6432	7074	7453

Data from Frisancho, 1981.

TABLE 6-15 Midarm Muscle Area Percentiles (mm²) for Females

Age Group	5th	10th	25th	50th	75th	90th	95th
1-2	885	973	1084	1221	1378	1535	1621
2-3	973	1029	1119	1269	1405	1595	1727
3-4	1014	1133	1227	1396	1563	1690	1846
4-5	1058	1171	1313	1475	1644	1832	1958
5-6	1238	1301	1423	1596	1825	2012	2159
6-7	1354	1414	1513	1683	1877	2182	2323
7-8	1330	1441	1602	1815	2045	2332	2469
8-9	1513	1566	1808	2034	2327	2657	2996
9-10	1723	1788	1976	2227	2571	2987	3112
10-11	1740	1784	2019	2296	2583	2873	3093
11-12	1784	1987	2316	2612	3071	3739	3953
12-13	2092	2182	2579	2904	3225	3655	3847
13-14	2269	2426	2657	3130	3529	4061	4568
14-15	2418	2562	2874	3220	3704	4294	4850
15-16	2426	2518	2847	3248	3689	4123	4756
16-17	2306	2567	2865	3248	3718	4353	4946
17-18	2442	2674	2996	3336	3883	4552	5251
18-19	2396	2538	2917	3243	3694	4461	4767
19-25	2538	2728	3026	3406	3877	4439	4940
25-35	2661	2826	3148	3573	4138	4806	5541
35-45	2750	2948	3359	3783	4428	5240	5877
45-55	2784	2956	3378	3858	4520	5375	5964
55-65	2784	3063	3477	4045	4750	5632	6247
65-75	2737	3018	3444	4019	4739	5566	6214

Data from Frisancho 1981.

TABLE 6-16	Biochemical Indicators of Good Nutrition Status			
Nutrient or Measurement	Test	Age Group	Average or Acceptable Levels	
			Male	Female
Iron	Hemoglobin (g/100 ml)	Adults	≥14.0	≥12.0
		Infants (under 2 years)	≥10.0	≥10.0
		Children (2-5 years)	≥11.0	≥11.0
		Children (6-12 years)	≥11.5	≥11.5
		Adolescents (13-16 years)	≥13.5	≥11.5
		Pregnancy		
		(2nd trimester)		≥11.0
		(3rd trimester)		≥10.5
	Hematocrit (%)	Adults	≥40.0	≥37.0
		Infants (under 2 years)	≥31.0	≥31.0
		Children (2-5 years)	≥34.0	≥34.0
		Children (6-12 years)	≥36.0	≥36.0
		Adolescents (13-16 years)	≥40.0	≥36.0
		Adolescents (16 + years)	≥44.0	≥38.0
		Pregnancy (>6 months)		≥33.0
	Transferrin saturation (%)	Adults	≥20.0	≥20.0
		Infants (under 2 years)	≥15.0	≥15.0
		Children (2-12 years)	≥20.0	≥20.0
		Adolescents (12 + years)	≥20.0	≥15.0
Protein	Serum albumin (g/100 ml)		≥3.5	≥3.5
Normal lipid metabolism	Serum cholesterol (mg/100 ml)	Adults	<200	<200
		Children and Adolescents	<170	<170
	Serum triglyceride (mg/100 ml)		<200	<200
	High density lipoprotein (mg/100 ml)		>35	>35
	Low density lipoprotein (mg/100 ml)	Adults	<130	<130
		Children and Adolescents	<110	<110
	Cholesterol/high density lipoprotein ratio		<4.5	<4.5
Normal carbohydrate metabolism	Serum glucose (mg/100 ml)		75-110	75-110
Folate	Serum folate (ng/ml)		>6.0	>6.0

SAMPLE DOCUMENTATION

Male, age 45
Height: 173 cm (68 inches)
Weight: 90.9 kg (200 lb)
123% of desirable body weight;
BMI 30.5; triceps skinfold thickness 20 mm, 90th percentile, mid arm circumference 327.8 mm; mid arm muscle circumference 265 mm, 25th percentile, 2200 calories daily, estimated for appropriate weight loss 73 g protein (0.8 × 90.9)

For additional sample documentation see Chapter 24, Recording Information.

SUMMARY OF EXAMINATION **Nutrition Assessment**

1. From the history and physical examination, assess the patient's nutritional status, including the following:
   - Nutrition screen
   - Assessment of nutrient intake
   - Recent growth, weight loss, or weight gain
   - Chronic illnesses affecting nutritional status or intake
   - Laboratory values
   - Clinical signs or symptoms of nutrient or energy deficiency
   - Medication and supplement use
2. Obtain the following anthropometric measurements and compare them to those in standardized tables:
   - Standing height
   - Weight
   - Calculate body mass index
   - Triceps skin fold thickness and mid upper arm circumference measurements; calculate midarm muscle circumference (MAMC) and midarm muscle area (MAMA)

COMMON ABNORMALITIES

OBESITY

Two types of obesity are defined based on the characteristics of the adipose tissue and the area of fat distribution. In exogenous obesity, there is an increase in the number of fat cells, hyperplasia, as much as three to five times normal. The cells may or may not be enlarged. This is the type most often found in children and women. Excess fat tissue is generally located in the breasts, buttocks, and thighs and is associated with excessive caloric intake, thick skin, pale striae, preservation of muscle strength, and no evidence of osteoporosis. Exogenous obesity is associated with a higher risk of breast cancer (Figure 6-5, *A*).

In endogenous obesity, the fat cells are greatly enlarged or hypertrophied. The actual number of cells may be normal or increased. Excess fat tissue is distributed to certain regions of the body, such as the trunk or abdominal area. Men are more likely to present with this type of obesity, although it is often seen in women as well. This type of obesity is associated with a higher risk of diabetes, heart disease, high blood pressure, and stroke. (Figure 6-5, *B*).

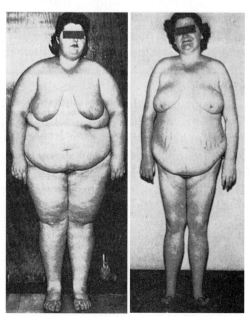

A B

FIGURE 6-5
A, Fat distribution associated with exogenous obesity (female pattern). **B,** Fat distribution associated with endogenous obesity (Cushing syndrome).
From Prior et al, 1981.

ANOREXIA NERVOSA

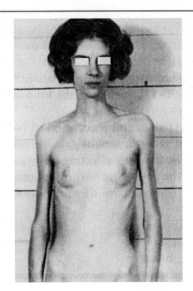

FIGURE 6-6

Wasting associated with anorexia nervosa.

From Ezrein, Godden, Volpe, 1979.

Anorexia nervosa is a psychological disorder in which the patient has a perceptual distortion of body shape, with a relentless drive for thinness through self-imposed starvation, bizarre food habits, obsessive exercise, and self-induced vomiting or laxative abuse. Adolescent and young adult women, usually from middle and upper class families, are most commonly involved. In young adults, the individual usually has a history of being overweight as a child. Anorexia nervosa is characterized by weight loss to 85% or less of expected weight, or failure to attain expected weight. Common signs and symptoms include those of starvation: dry skin, lanugo hair, brittle nails, bloating, constipation, slow heart rate, orthostatic hypotension, stunted growth, amenorrhea, intolerance to cold, carotene (orange) pigmentation, food preoccupation, depression or irritability decreased libido, and interrupted sleep. Visceral protein levels are adequate. Anemia is not common as serum iron and folate levels are normal (Figure 6-6).

BULIMIA

This eating disorder is characterized by binge eating, the rapid intake of a large amount of food, usually consisting of high-calorie sweets or high-carbohydrate foods. Laxative or diuretic abuse often follows the bingeing episode. If binge eating is followed by self-induced vomiting, it is termed bulimarexia. Bulimic individuals, male or female, are usually in their late teens or early twenties and may have a history of substance (alcohol or drug) abuse. Generally the bingeing occurs during a time when they are trying to lose weight, but the repeated episodes become habitual. Bulimic individuals do not usually become malnourished unless their body weight continues to drop to less than 85% of their expected weight.

ANEMIAS

Several types of anemias exist, each dependent on which nutrient is deficient, but all associated with a lowering of serum hemoglobin and hematocrit levels and a change in the size, appearance, and production of red blood cells. Symptoms of severe anemias include skin pallor, weakness, easy fatiguability, headaches, dizziness, sensitivity to cold, paresthesia, cheilosis, glossitis, loss of appetite, and concave fingernails with longitudinal ridging. With increasing severity, tachycardia, palpitations, and shortness of breath may occur. Refer to Table 6-17 to determine type of anemia based on laboratory testing.

TABLE 6-17	Comparison of Laboratory Test Results for Anemias			
Test	Normal Value	Iron Deficiency Anemia	Folic Acid Deficiency Anemia	Vitamin B$_{12}$ Deficiency Anemia
Hemoglobin, g/100 ml	Men: 14-16 Women: 12-14	Decreased	Decreased	Decreased
Hematocrit, %	Men: 40-54 Women: 37-47	Decreased	Decreased	Decreased
MCV, μm^3	82-92	↓ (<80)	↑ (>92)	↑ (>92)
MCH, μg	27-31	↓ (<27)	↑ (>35)	↑ (>35)
MCHC, %	32-36	↓ (<32)	Normal	Normal
Serum iron, μg/100 ml	60-180	Decreased	Increased	Increased
TIBC, μg/100 ml	250-450	↑ (>350)	Normal	Normal
Transferrin saturation, %	20-55	↓ (<20)	Normal	Normal

HYPERLIPIDEMIA

The point that defines high blood cholesterol (240 g/100 ml) is a value above which risk for coronary heart disease rises more steeply and corresponds approximately to the 80th percentile of the adult U.S. population (NHANES III). For patients with blood cholesterol values between 200 and 239, the presence or absence of other risk factors for coronary heart disease (CHD) (see the Risk Factors Box) and the blood levels of HDL and LDL cholesterol determine whether further lipoprotein assessment is necessary. Refer to Table 6-18 for diagnosing hyperlipidemia based on LDL cholesterol and the presence of other risk factors, which include an HDL cholesterol <35 mg/100 ml.

In children, the aim is to identify and treat children and adolescents who are at the greatest risk of having high blood cholesterol as adults and an increased risk of CHD. This would include selective screening of those with a family history of premature cardiovascular disease or at least one parent with high blood cholesterol. Universal screening of all children is not recommended. Refer to Table 6-19 for the diagnosis of hyperlipidemia in children and adolescents.

RISK FACTORS   Coronary Heart Disease

Positive
- Age: Male ≥ 45 years
    Female ≥ 55 years or premature menopause without estrogen replacement therapy
- Family history of premature coronary heart disease
- Smoking
- Hypertension
- HDL-cholesterol <35 mg/100 ml
- Diabetes

Negative
- HDL-cholesterol ≥ 60

Data from National Institutes of Health, 1993.

TABLE 6-18 DIFFERENTIAL DIAGNOSIS	Diagnosis of Hyperlipidemia Based on LDL-Cholesterol Risk Factors Present	
	LDL-Cholesterol Risk Factors	**LDL level**
	Without CHD and with fewer than two risk factors	>160 mg/100 ml
	Without CHD and with two or more risk factors	>130 mg/100 ml
	With CHD	>100 mg/100 ml

Data from National Institutes of Health, September 1993.

TABLE 6-19 DIFFERENTIAL DIAGNOSIS	Classification of Total and LDL-Cholesterol Levels in Children and Adolescents from Families with Hypercholesterolemia or Premature Cardiovascular Disease		
	Category	**Total Cholesterol**	**LDL-Cholesterol**
	Acceptable	<170 mg/100 ml	<110 mg/100 ml
	Borderline	170-199 mg/100 ml	110-129 mg/100 ml
	High	≥200 mg/100 ml	≥130 mg/100 ml

From National Cholesterol Education Program Coordinating Committee, 1991.

Remember to check   *http://www1.mosby.com/physexam_seidel*

CHAPTER 7

Skin, Hair, and Nails

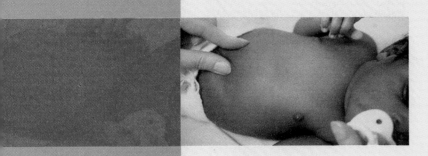

ANATOMY AND PHYSIOLOGY

Skin provides an elastic, rugged, self-regenerating, protective covering for the body. However, it has another important function: the skin and its appendages are our primary physical presentation to the world.

The skin is a stratified structure composed of several functionally related layers. Figure 7-1 shows the main structural components and their approximate spatial relationships. The anatomy of the skin varies somewhat from one part of the body to another.

Skin structure and physiologic processes allow several integral functions:

- Protect against microbial and foreign substance invasion and minor physical trauma
- Retard body fluid loss by providing a mechanical barrier
- Regulate body temperature through radiation, conduction, convection, and evaporation
- Provide sensory perception via free nerve endings and specialized receptors
- Produce vitamin D from precursors in the skin
- Contribute to blood pressure regulation through constriction of skin blood vessels
- Repair surface wounds by exaggerating the normal process of cell replacement
- Excrete sweat, urea, and lactic acid
- Express emotions

EPIDERMIS

The epidermis, the outermost portion of the skin, consists of two major layers: the stratum corneum, which protects the body against harmful environmental substances and restricts water loss, and the cellular stratum in which the keratin cells are synthesized. The basement membrane lies beneath the cellular stratum and connects the epidermis to the dermis. The epidermis is avascular and depends on the underlying dermis for its nutrition.

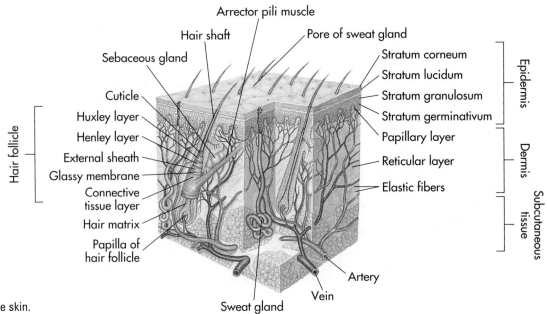

FIGURE 7-1
Anatomic structures of the skin.

The stratum corneum consists of closely packed dead squamous cells that contain the waterproofing protein keratin and form the protective barrier of the skin. These keratin cells are formed in the deepest sublayer of the cellular stratum, the stratum germinativum. The keratinocytes mature as they make their way to the surface through the stratum spinosum and stratum granulosum to replace the cells in the stratum corneum. This basal cell layer also contains melanocytes, the cells that synthesize melanin, which gives the skin its color. An additional sublayer of the cellular stratum, the stratum lucidum, is present only in the thicker skin of the palms and soles and lies just below the stratum corneum.

DERMIS

The dermis is the richly vascular connective tissue layer of the skin that supports and separates the epidermis from the cutaneous adipose tissue. Upward projecting papillae penetrate the epidermis and provide nourishment for the living epidermal cells. Elastin, collagen, and reticulin fibers provide resilience, strength, and stability. Sensory nerve fibers located in the dermis form a complex network to provide sensations of pain, touch, and temperature. The dermis also contains autonomic motor nerves that innervate blood vessels, glands, and the arrectores pilorum muscles.

HYPODERMIS

The dermis is connected to underlying organs by the hypodermis, a subcutaneous layer that consists of loose connective tissue filled with fatty cells. This adipose layer generates heat and provides insulation, shock absorption, and a reserve of calories.

APPENDAGES

The epidermis invaginates into the dermis at myriad points and forms the following appendages: eccrine sweat glands, apocrine sweat glands, sebaceous glands, hair, and nails.

The eccrine sweat glands open directly onto the surface of the skin and regulate body temperature through water secretion. The glands are distributed throughout the body except for the lip margins, eardrums, nail beds, inner surface of the prepuce, and glans penis.

The apocrine glands are specialized structures found only in the axillae, nipples, areolae, anogenital area, eyelids, and external ears. These glands are larger and located more deeply than the eccrine glands. In response to emotional stimuli, the glands secrete a white fluid containing protein, carbohydrate, and other substances. Secretions from these glands are odorless. Bacterial decomposition of apocrine sweat produces a characteristic adult body odor in Blacks and Whites.

The sebaceous glands secrete sebum, a lipid-rich substance that keeps the skin and hair from drying out. Secretory activity, which is stimulated by sex hormones (primarily testosterone), varies according to hormonal levels throughout the life span.

Hair is formed by epidermal cells that invaginate into the dermal layers. Hair consists of a root, a shaft, and a follicle (the root and its covering). The papilla, a loop of capillaries at the base of the follicle, supplies nourishment for growth. Melanocytes in the shaft provide its color. Adults have two kinds of hair: vellus and terminal. Vellus hair is short, fine, soft, and nonpigmented. Terminal hair is coarser, longer, thicker, and usually pigmented. Each hair goes through cyclic changes: anagen (growth), catagen (atrophy), and telogen (rest), after which the hair is shed. Males and females have about the same number of hair follicles that are stimulated to differential growth by hormones.

The nails are epidermal cells converted to hard plates of keratin. The highly vascular nail bed lies beneath the plate, giving the nail its pink color. The white crescent-shaped area extending beyond the proximal nail fold marks the end of the nail matrix, the site of nail growth. The stratum corneum layer of skin covering the nail root is the cuticle, or eponychium, which pushes up and over the lower part of the nail body. The paronychium is the soft tissue surrounding the nail border. Figure 7-2 shows the structures of the nail.

FIGURE 7-2

Anatomic structures of the nail.

From Thompson et al, 1997.

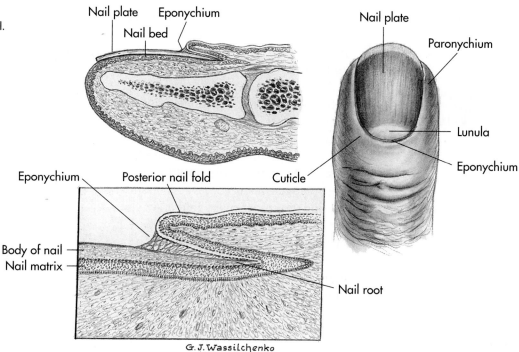

G. J. Wassilchenko

INFANTS AND CHILDREN

The skin of infants and children appears smoother than that of adults, partly because of the relative absence of coarse terminal hair and partly because the skin has not been subjected to years of exposure to the elements. Desquamation of the stratum corneum may be present at birth or very shortly after. The degree of desquamation varies from mild flakiness to shedding of large sheets of cornified epidermis. Vernix caseosa, a mixture of sebum and cornified epidermis, covers the infant's body at birth. The subcutaneous fat layer is poorly developed in newborns, predisposing them to hypothermia. The newborn's body, particularly the shoulders and back, is also covered with fine, silky hair called lanugo. This hair is shed within 10 to 14 days. Some newborns are bald, whereas others have an inordinate amount of head hair. Either way, most of the hair is shed by about 2 to 3 months of age, to be replaced by more permanent hair with a new texture and often a different color.

The eccrine sweat glands begin to function after the first month of life. Apocrine function has not yet begun, giving the skin a less oily texture and resulting in characteristic inoffensive perspiration.

ADOLESCENTS

During adolescence the apocrine glands enlarge and become active, causing increased axillary sweating and sometimes body odor. Sebaceous glands increase sebum production in response to increased hormone levels, primarily androgen, giving the skin an oily appearance and predisposing the individual to acne.

Coarse terminal hair appears in the axillae and pubic areas of both female and male adolescents and on the face of males. Hair production is one response to changing androgen levels. Refer to Chapter 5 (Growth and Measurement) for a more thorough discussion of maturational changes during adolescence.

PREGNANT WOMEN

Increased blood flow to the skin, especially that of the hands and feet, results from peripheral vasodilation and increased numbers of capillaries. Acceleration of sweat and sebaceous gland activity occurs. Both processes assist in dissipating the excess heat caused by the increased metabolism during pregnancy. Vascular spiders and hemangiomas that are present may increase in size.

The skin thickens, and fat is deposited in the subdermal layers. Because of increased fragility of connective tissues, separation may occur with stretching. Hormonal changes also cause increased pigmentation of the face, nipples, areolae, axillae, and vulva.

OLDER ADULTS

Sebaceous and sweat gland activity decreases in older adults, and as a result the skin becomes drier and less perspiration is produced. The epidermis begins to thin and flatten, taking on the look of parchment as the vascularity of the dermis decreases. Epidermal permeability is increased, thus reducing the efficiency of the barrier function of the stratum corneum.

The dermis becomes less elastic, loses collagen and elastic fibers, and shrinks, causing the epidermis to fold and assume a wrinkled appearance. A lifetime of exposure to the sun also predisposes the skin to wrinkling. Wrinkling is less marked in individuals with black and yellow skins and in those who are obese.

Subcutaneous tissue decreases, particularly in the extremities, giving joints and bony prominences a sharp, angular appearance. There is a deepening of the hollows in the thoracic, axillary, and supraclavicular regions.

Gray hair results from a decrease in the number of functioning melanocytes. The hair of Whites turns gray before the hair of Blacks and Orientals does. Axillary and pubic hair production declines because of reduced hormonal functioning. The density and rate of scalp hair growth (anagen phase) decline with age. The size of hair follicles also changes, and there is a progressive transition of terminal hair into vellus hair on the scalp, causing age-associated baldness in both men and women. The opposite transition, from vellus to terminal, occurs in the hair of the nares and on the tragus of men's ears. Women produce increased coarse facial hair because of higher androgen/estrogen ratios. Both genders experience overall loss of hair from the trunk and extremities. Peripheral extremity hair loss may also occur when peripheral vascular disease is present. The loss of axillary and pubic hair results from diminished androgen production.

Nail growth slows because of decreased peripheral circulation. The nails, particularly the toenails, become thicker, brittle, hard, and yellowish. They develop longitudinal ridges and are prone to splitting into layers.

REVIEW OF RELATED HISTORY

PRESENT PROBLEM

Skin

- Changes in skin: dryness, pruritus, sores, rashes, lumps, color, texture, odor, amount of perspiration; changes in wart or mole; lesion that does not heal or is chronically irritated
- Temporal sequence: date of initial onset; time sequence of occurrence and development; sudden or gradual onset; date of recurrence, if any
- Symptoms: itching, pain, exudate, bleeding, color changes, seasonal or climate variations
- Location: skin folds, extensor or flexor surfaces, localized or generalized
- Associated symptoms: presence of systemic disease or high fever, relationship to stress or leisure activities
- Recent exposure to drugs, environmental or occupational toxins or chemicals; to persons with similar skin condition
- Apparent cause, patient's perception of cause
- Travel history: where, when, length of stay, exposure to diseases, contact with travelers
- What the patient has been doing for the problem, response to treatment, what makes the condition worse or better
- How the patient is adjusting to the problem
- Medications: topical or systemic; nonprescription or prescription

---

RISK FACTORS   **Skin Cancer**

- Age (over 50)
- Male
- Fair, freckled, ruddy complexion
- Light-colored hair or eyes
- Tendency to burn easily
- Overexposure to frost, wind, or ultraviolet B radiation from sun (recreation or occupation)
- Geographic location: near equator or at high altitudes
- Exposure to arsenic, creosote, coal tar, and/or petroleum products
- Family history of skin cancer
- Overexposure to radium, radioisotopes, x-rays
- Repeated trauma or irritation to skin
- Precancerous dermatoses

Hair
- Changes in hair: loss or growth, distribution, texture, color
- Occurrence: sudden or gradual onset, symmetric or asymmetric pattern, recurrence
- Associated symptoms: pain, itching, lesions, presence of systemic disease or high fever, recent psychologic or physical stress
- Exposure to drugs, environmental or occupational toxins or chemicals, commercial hair care chemicals
- Nutrition: dietary changes, dieting, malnutrition
- What the patient has been doing for the problem, response to treatment, what makes the problem worse or better
- How the patient is adjusting to the problem
- Medications: nonprescription or prescription; minoxidil

Nails
- Changes in nails: splitting, breaking, discoloration, ridging, thickening, markings, separation from nail bed
- Associated symptoms: pain, swelling, exudate, presence of systemic disease or high fever, recent psychologic or physical stress
- Temporal sequence: sudden or gradual onset, relationship to injury of nail or finger
- Recent exposure to drugs, environmental or occupational toxins or chemicals; frequent immersion in water
- What the patient has been doing for the problem, response to treatment, what makes the problem worse or better
- Medications: nonprescription or prescription

PAST MEDICAL HISTORY

Skin
- Previous skin problems: sensitivities, allergic skin reactions, allergic skin disorders (such as infantile eczema), lesions, treatment
- Tolerance to sunlight
- Diminished or heightened sensitivity to sensory stimuli
- Cardiac, respiratory, liver, endocrine, or other systemic diseases

Hair
- Previous hair problems: loss, thinning, unusual growth or distribution, brittleness, breakage, treatment
- Systemic problems: thyroid or liver disorder, any severe illness, malnutrition, associated skin disorder

Nails
- Previous nail problems: injury; bacterial, fungal, or viral infection
- Systemic problems: associated skin disorder; congenital anomalies; respiratory, cardiac, endocrine, hematologic, or other systemic disease

FAMILY HISTORY

- Current or past dermatologic diseases or disorders in family members: skin cancer, psoriasis, allergic skin disorders, infestations, bacterial, fungal, or viral infections
- Allergic hereditary diseases such as asthma or hay fever
- Familial hair loss or coloration patterns

PERSONAL AND SOCIAL HISTORY

- Skin care habits: cleansing routine, soaps, oils, lotions, or local applications used, cosmetics, home remedies or preparations used, sun exposure patterns, use of sunscreen agents, recent changes in skin care habits
- Skin self-examination (Box 7-1)

| BOX 7-1 | Patient Instructions for Skin Self-Examination |

Always use a good light, positioned to minimize distracting glare.

Be aware of the locations and appearance of moles and birthmarks.

Examine your back and other hard-to-see areas of the body using full-length and hand-held mirrors. Ask a friend or relative to help inspect those areas that are difficult to see, such as the scalp and back.

Begin with your face and scalp and proceed downward, examining your head, neck, shoulders, back, chest, arms, legs, and so on. Concentrate especially on areas where dysplastic nevi (those with unexpected changes) are most common—the shoulders and back—and areas where ordinary moles are rarely found—the scalp, breast, and buttocks. Check the soles of your feet and between the toes.

See rather than feel any early signs of a mole change. Compare photographs of your moles (if you have them) with the appearance of those same moles on self-examination. Monitor change in size by measuring. It can be simply done with a small ruler or even relative to the size of your thumb or fingernail, a measure that is ever present.

Consult your physician promptly if any pigmented skin spots look like melanoma, if new moles have appeared, or any existing moles have changed.

- Hair care habits: cleansing routine, shampoos and rinses used, coloring preparations used, permanents, recent changes in hair care habits
- Nail care habits: any difficulty in clipping or trimming nails, instruments used; biting nails
- Exposure to environmental or occupational hazards: dyes, chemicals, plants, toxic substances, frequent immersion of hands in water, frequent sun exposure
- Recent psychologic or physiologic stress
- Use of alcohol
- Use of street drugs

INFANTS

- Feeding history: breast or formula, type of formula, what foods introduced and when
- Diaper history: type of diapers used, skin cleansing routines, use of rubber pants, method of cleaning washable diapers
- Types of clothing and washing practices, soaps and detergents used, new blanket or clothing
- Bath practices, types of soap, oils, or lotions used
- Dress habits: amount and type of clothing in relation to environmental temperature
- Temperature and humidity of the home environment: air conditioning, heating system (drying or humidified)
- Rubbing head against mattress, rug, furniture, wall

CHILDREN

- Eating habits and types of food, including chocolate, candy, soft drinks, bubble gum
- Exposure to communicable diseases
- Allergic disorders: eczema, urticaria, pruritus, hayfever, asthma, other chronic respiratory disorders
- Pets or animal exposure
- Outdoor exposures such as play areas, hiking, camping, picnics
- Skin injury history: frequency of falls, cuts, abrasions; repeated history of unexplained injuries
- Chronic manipulation of hair
- Nail biting

PREGNANT WOMEN	■ Weeks of gestation or postpartum ■ Hygiene practices ■ Presence of skin problems before pregnancy ■ Effects of pregnancy on preexisting conditions (e.g., psoriasis may remit; condylomata acuminata frequently become larger and more numerous)

OLDER ADULTS	■ Increased or decreased sensation to touch or the environment ■ Generalized chronic itching: exposure to skin irritants, detergents, lotions with high alcohol content, woolen clothing, humidity of environment ■ Susceptibility to skin infections ■ Healing response: delayed or interrupted ■ Frequent falls resulting in multiple cuts or bruises ■ History of diabetes mellitus or peripheral vascular disease ■ Hair loss history: gradual versus sudden onset, loss pattern (symmetric or asymmetric)

EXAMINATION AND FINDINGS

EQUIPMENT

- ■ Centimeter ruler (flexible, clear)
- ■ Wood's lamp (to view fluorescing lesions)
- ■ Flashlight with transilluminator
- ■ Magnifying glass (optional)
- ■ Episcope (optional)

SKIN

Examination of the skin is performed by inspection and palpation. The most important tools are your own eyes and powers of observation. Sometimes when gross inspection leaves you uncertain, a hand-held magnifying glass or episcope may help.

Inspection

Adequate lighting is essential; daylight provides the best illumination for determining color variations, particularly jaundice. If daylight is unavailable or insufficient, it should be supplemented with overhead fluorescent lighting. Tangential lighting is helpful in assessing contour, but inadequate lighting can result in inadequate assessment.

Although the skin is commonly observed as each part of the body is examined, it is important to make a brief but careful overall visual sweep of the entire body. This "bird's-eye view" gives a good idea of the distribution and extent of any lesions. It also allows you to observe skin symmetry, detect differences between body areas, and compare sun-exposed to non-sun-exposed areas. You can also be alert for special conditions that require attention as the examination progresses (Box 7-2).

> **BOX 7-2   Cutaneous Manifestation of Traditional Health Practices**
>
> The use of certain traditional health practices by various cultural groups can produce cutaneous manifestations that could be wrongly confused with disease or physical abuse. One such practice is that of "coining" as used by some Asian subcultures. The placement of a heated coin on the skin to treat certain conditions can produce a burn in the shape of the coin, thus confounding the clinician who is unaware of such practices. The lesson: in your history ask about home remedies or practices. Be aware of and open to traditional modalities that may conflict with your own experience.

PHYSICAL VARIATIONS

Individuals with dark skin often show pigmentary demarcation lines. These lines, a normal variation, mark the border between the darker skin of outward facing surfaces and the lighter skin of inward facing surfaces. They are seen on the arms, legs, chest, and back. About 70% of Black adults have such lines compared with 11% of Whites. Statistics for Orientals and Native Americans fall in between these two figures.

Data from Rampen, 1988; James et al, 1987.

PHYSICAL VARIATIONS

Nevi occur more often in lighter-skinned than in darker-skinned individuals. Blacks have the fewest nevi, Whites the most, with Orientals and Native Americans intermediate. Nevi are thought to result from chronic sun exposure. They are more common in persons who burn rather than tan, and their numbers increase with age.

Data from Rampen, de Wit, 1989; Gallagher et al, 1991.

Adequate exposure of the skin is necessary. It is essential to remove encumbering clothing and to fully remove drapes or coverings as each section of the body is examined. Make sure that the room temperature is comfortable. Look carefully at areas not usually exposed, such as the axillae, buttocks, perineum, backs of thighs, and inner upper thighs. Remove shoes and socks to look at the feet. Pay careful attention to intertriginous surfaces, especially in elderly and bedridden patients. As the examination is completed for each area, the patient should be redraped or covered. Begin by inspecting the skin and mucous membranes (especially oral) for color and uniform appearance, thickness, symmetry, hygiene, and the presence of any lesions.

Skin thickness varies over the body, with the thinnest skin on the eyelids and the thickest at areas of pressure or rubbing, most notably the soles, palms, and elbows. Note callusing on the hands or feet.

The range of expected skin color varies from dark brown to light tan with pink or yellow overtones. Although color should assume an overall uniformity, there may be sun-darkened areas and darker skin around knees and elbows. Knuckles may be darker in dark skinned patients. Callused areas may appear yellow. Vascular flush areas (cheeks, neck, upper chest, and genital area) may appear pink or red, especially with anxiety or excitement. Be aware that skin color may be masked by cosmetics and tanning agents. Look for localized areas of discoloration.

Nevi (moles) occur in forms that vary in size and degree of pigmentation. Nevi are present on most persons, regardless of skin color, and may occur anywhere on the body. They may be flat, slightly raised, dome shaped, smooth, rough, or hairy. Their color ranges from tan, gray, and shades of brown to black. Table 7-1 describes the features and occurrence of various types of pigmented nevi.

TABLE 7-1	Features and Occurrence of Various Types of Pigmented Nevi		
Type	**Features**	**Occurrence**	**Comments**
Halo Nevus	Sharp, oval, or circular; depigmented halo around mole; may undergo many morphologic changes; usually disappears and halo repigments (may take years)	Usually on back in young adult	Usually benign; biopsy indicated because same process can occur around melanoma
Intradermal Nevus	Dome shaped; raised; flesh to black color; may be pedunculated or hair bearing	Cells limited to dermis	No indication for removal other than cosmetic
Junction Nevus	Flat or slightly elevated; dark brown	Nevus cells lining dermoepidermal junction	Should be removed if exposed to repeated trauma
Compound Nevus	Slightly elevated brownish papule: indistinct border	Nevus cells in dermis and lining dermoepidermal junction	Should be removed if exposed to repeated trauma
Hairy Nevus	May be present at birth; may cover large area; hair growth may occur after several years		Should be removed if changes occur

From Thompson et al, 1997.

While most nevi are harmless, some may be dysplastic, precancerous, or cancerous. Table 7-2 describes differences in the features of normal and dysplastic moles. Dysplastic nevi tend to occur on the upper back in men and on the legs in women. See pp. 204-205 for malignant abnormalities.

Several variations in skin color occur in almost all healthy adults and children, including nonpigmented striae (silver or pink "stretch marks" that occur during pregnancy or weight gain), freckles in sun-exposed areas, some birth marks, and some nevi (Figure 7-3). Adult women will frequently have chloasma (also called melasma), areas of hyperpigmentation on the face and neck that are associated with pregnancy or the use of hormones. This condition is more noticeable in darker-skinned women. The absence of melanin will produce patches of unpigmented skin or hair (Figure 7-4).

Color hues in dark-skinned persons are best seen in the sclera, conjunctiva, buccal mucosa, tongue, lips, nail beds, and palms. Be aware, however, that heavily callused palms in dark-skinned persons will have an opaque yellow cast. Particular variations in skin color may be the result of physiologic pigment distribution. The palms and soles are lighter in color than the rest of the body. Hyperpigmented macules on the soles of the feet are common. Freckling of the buccal cavity, gums, and tongue is common. The sclera may appear yellowish brown (often described as "muddy") or may contain brownish pigment that looks like petechiae. A bluish hue of the lips and gums can be a normal finding in persons with dark skin. Some dark-skinned persons have very blue lips, giving a false impression of cyanosis.

Systemic disorders can produce generalized or localized color changes, which are described in Table 7-3 on p. 171. Localized redness often results from an inflammatory process. Pale shiny skin of the lower extremities may reflect peripheral changes that occur with such systemic diseases as diabetes mellitus and cardiovascu-

TABLE 7-2	Features of Normal and Dysplastic Moles	
Feature	**Normal Mole**	**Dysplastic Mole**
Color	Uniformly tan or brown; all moles on one person tend to look alike.	Mixture of tan, brown, black, and red/pink; moles on one person often look quite different from one another
Shape	Round or oval with a clearly defined border which separates the mole from surrounding skin.	Irregular borders which may include include notches. May fade into surrounding skin and include a flat portion level with skin.
Surface	Begins as flat, smooth spot on skin; becomes raised; forms a smooth bump.	May be smooth, slightly scaly, or have a rough, irregular "pebbly" appearance.
Size	Usually less than 5 mm (size of a pencil eraser).	Often larger than 5 mm and sometimes larger than 10 mm.
Number	Typical adult has between 10 and 40 moles scattered over the body.	Many persons do not have increased number; however, persons severely affected may have more than 100 moles.
Location	Usually above the waist on sun-exposed surfaces of the body; scalp, breast, and buttocks rarely have normal moles.	May occur anywhere on the body. but most commonly on back; may also appear below the waist and on scalp, breasts, and buttocks.

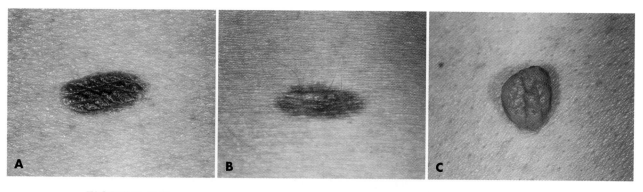

FIGURE 7-3

Commonly occurring nevi. **A,** Junction nevus. Color and shape of this black lesion are uniform. **B,** Compound nevus. Center is elevated and surrounding area is flat, retaining features of a junction nevus. **C,** Dermal nevus. Papillomatous with soft, flabby, wrinkled surface.

From Habif, 1996.

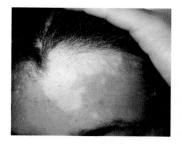

FIGURE 7-4

Vitiligo.

Courtesy Jaime A. Tschen, BD, Baylor College of Medicine, Department of Dermatology; Houston: from Thompson et al, 1993.

TABLE 7-3	**Cutaneous Color Changes**		
Color	**Cause**	**Distribution**	**Select Conditions**
Brown	Darkening of melanin pigment	Generalized	Pituitary, adrenal, liver disease
		Localized	Nevi, neurofibromatosis
White	Absence of melanin	Generalized	Albinism
		Localized	Vitiligo
Red (erythema)	Increased cutaneous blood flow	Localized	Inflammation
		Generalized	Fever, viral exanthems, urticaria
	Increased intravascular red blood cells	Generalized	Polycythemia
Yellow	Increased bile pigmentation (jaundice)	Generalized	Liver disease
	Increased carotene pigmentation	Generalized (except sclera)	Hypothyroidism, increased intake of vegetables containing carotene
	Decreased visibility of oxyhemoglobin	Generalized	Anemia, chronic renal disease
Blue	Increased unsaturated hemoglobin secondary to hypoxia	Lips, mouth, nail beds	Cardiovascular and pulmonary diseases

lar disease. Injury, steroids, vasculitis, and several systemic disorders can cause localized hemorrhage into cutaneous tissues, producing red-purple discolorations. The discolorations produced by injury are called ecchymoses; when produced by other causes they are called petechiae if smaller than 0.5 cm in diameter (Figure 7-5), or purpura if larger than 0.5 cm in diameter (Figure 7-6). Vascular skin lesions are characterized in Figure 7-7. Pale, shiny skin of the lower extremities may reflect peripheral changes that occur with systemic diseases such as diabetes mellitus and cardiovascular disease.

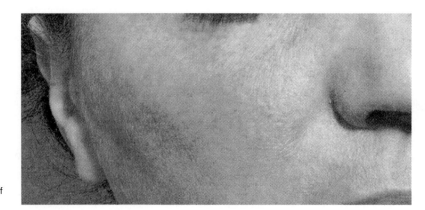

FIGURE 7-5
Petechiae.
Courtesy Antoinette, MD, Department of Dermatology, Indiana University School of Medicine, Indianapolis.

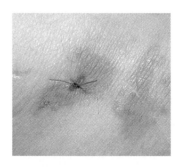

FIGURE 7-6
Purpura.
Courtesy Antoinette Hood, MD, Department of Dermatology, Indiana University School of Medicine, Indianapolis.

Palpation

As you inspect, palpate the skin for moisture, temperature, texture, turgor, and mobility. Palpation may yield additional data for describing lesions, particularly in relation to elevation or depression.

Minimal perspiration or oiliness should be present. Increased perspiration may be associated with activity, warm environment, obesity, anxiety, or excitement and may be especially noticeable on the palms, scalp, and forehead and in the axillae, usually the dampest area. The intertriginous areas should evidence minimal dampness. Pay particular attention to areas that get little or no exposure to circulating air, such as in the folds of large breasts or obese abdomens or in the inguinal area (Figure 7-8, p. 174).

The skin should range from cool to warm to the touch. Use the dorsal surface of your hands or fingers, because these areas are most sensitive to temperature perception. At best, this assessment is a rough estimate of skin temperature; what you are really looking for is bilateral symmetry. Environmental conditions, including the temperature of the examining room, may affect surface temperature.

The texture should feel smooth, soft, and even. Roughness on exposed areas or areas of pressure, particularly the elbows, soles, and palms, may be caused by heavy or woolen clothing, cold weather, or soap. Extensive or widespread roughness may be the result of a keratinization disorder or healing lesions. Hyperkeratoses, especially of the palms and soles, may be the sign of a systemic disorder such as arsenic or other toxic exposure.

To assess turgor and mobility, gently pinch a small section of skin on the forearm or sternal area between the thumb and forefinger and then release the skin (Figure 7-9). Turgor should not be tested on the back of a patient's hand because of the looseness and thinness of the skin in that area. The skin should feel resilient, move easily when pinched, and return to place immediately when released. Turgor will be altered if the patient is substantially dehydrated or if edema is present. For example, turgor is decreased in a dehydrated patient as evidenced by the pinched skin's failing to spring back to place after you release it. Some of the connective tissue diseases, notably the forms of scleroderma, will affect skin mobility.

SKIN LESIONS

As you assess the skin, pay particular attention to any lesions that may be present. "Skin lesion" is a catch-all term that collectively describes any pathologic skin change or occurrence. Lesions may be primary (those that occur as initial spontaneous manifestations of a pathologic process) or secondary (those that result from later evolution of or external trauma to a primary lesion).

Purpura—red-purple nonblanchable discoloration greater than 0.5 cm diameter.
Cause: Intravascular defects, infection

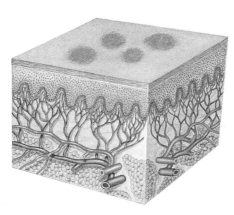

Petechiae—red-purple nonblanchable discoloration less than 0.5 cm diameter
Cause: Intravascular defects, infection

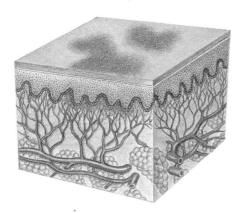

Ecchymoses—red-purple nonblanchable discoloration of variable size
Cause: Vascular wall destruction, trauma, vasculitis

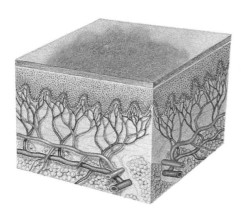

Spider angioma—red central body with radiating spiderlike legs that blanch with pressure to the central body
Cause: Liver disease, vitamin B deficiency, idiopathic

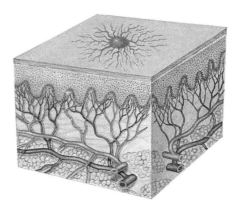

Venous star—bluish spider, linear or irregularly shaped; does not blanch with pressure
Cause: Increased pressure in superficial veins

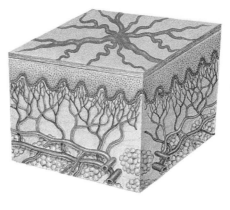

Telangiectasia—fine, irregular red line
Cause: Dilation of capillaries

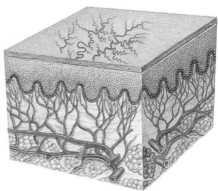

Capillary hemangioma (nevus flammeus)—red irregular macular patches
Cause: Dilation of dermal capillaries

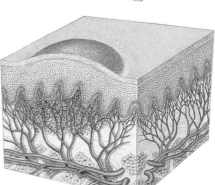

FIGURE 7-7
Characteristics and causes of vascular skin lesions.

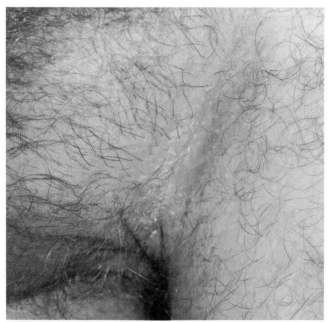

FIGURE 7-8

Examining an intertriginous area. Note fissure and maceration in the crural fold.

From Habif, 1996.

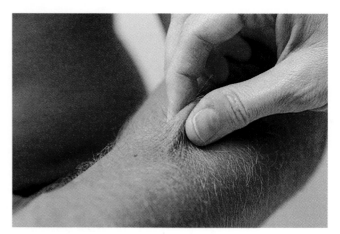

FIGURE 7-9

Testing skin turgor.

Tables 7-4 and 7-5 show the characteristics of primary and secondary lesions. The nomenclature is often used inaccurately; if you are uncertain about a lesion, use the descriptors rather than the name. Be aware that several types of lesions may occur concurrently and that secondary changes may obscure primary characteristics.

Describe lesions according to characteristics (Table 7-6, p. 181), exudates, configuration, and location and distribution:

Characteristics
- Size: measure all dimensions
- Shape
- Color
- Texture
- Elevation or depression
- Pedunculation
- Exudates
  - Color
  - Odor
  - Amount
  - Consistency
- Configuration
  - Annular (rings)
  - Grouped
  - Linear
  - Arciform (bow-shaped)
  - Diffuse
- Location and distribution
  - Generalized or localized
  - Region of the body (Box 7-3)
  - Patterns (Figures 7-10 to 7-12)
  - Discrete or confluent

Text continues on p. 182.

TABLE 7-4   Primary Skin Lesions

Description	Examples		
Macule A flat, circumscribed area that is a change in the color of the skin; less than 1 cm in diameter	Freckles, flat moles (nevi), petechlae, measles, scarlet fever	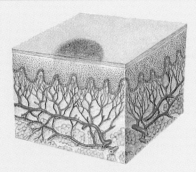	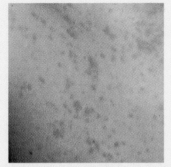 Measles. (From Habif, 1996.)
Papule An elevated, firm, circumscribed area less than 1 cm in diameter	Wart (verruca), elevated moles, lichen planus	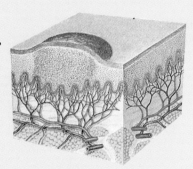	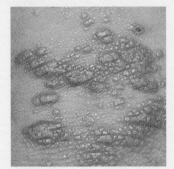 Lichen planus. (From Weston, Lane, Morelli, 1996.)
Patch A flat, nonpalpable, irregular-shaped macule more than 1 cm in diameter	Vitiligo, port-wine stains, mongolian spots, café au lait spot	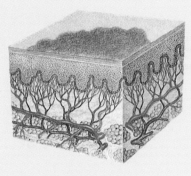	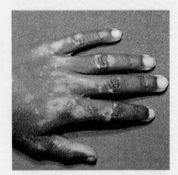 Vitiligo. (From Weston, Lane, Morelli, 1991.)
Plaque Elevated, firm, and rough lesion with flat top surface greater than 1 cm in diameter	Psoriasis, seborrheic and actinic keratoses	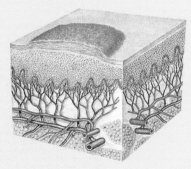	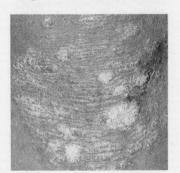 Plaque. (From Habif, 1996.)

Continued

TABLE 7-4	Primary Skin Lesions—cont'd	
Description	**Examples**	

Wheal
Elevated irregular-shaped area of cutaneous edema; solid, transient; variable diameter

Insect bites, urticaria, allergic reaction

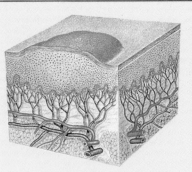
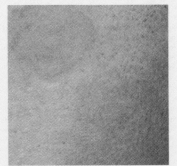

Wheal. (From Farrar et al, 1992.)

Nodule
Elevated, firm, circumscribed lesion; deeper in dermis than a papule; 1 to 2 cm in diameter

Erythema nodosum, lipomas

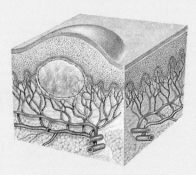
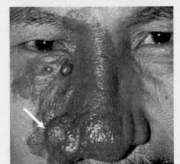

Hypertrophic nodule. (From Goldman and Fitzpatrick, 1994.)

Tumor
Elevated and solid lesion; may or may not be clearly demarcated; deeper in dermis; greater than 2 cm in diameter

Neoplasms, benign tumor, lipoma, hemangioma

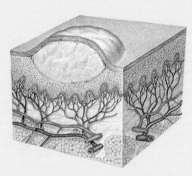
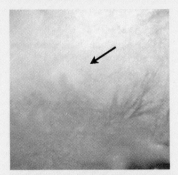

Hemangioma. (From Weston, Lane, Morelli, 1996.)

Vesicle
Elevated, circumscribed, superficial, not into dermis; filled with serous fluid; less than 1 cm in diameter

Varicella (chickenpox), herpes zoster (shingles)

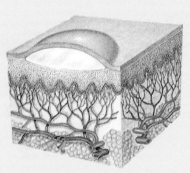
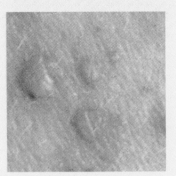

Vesicles caused by varicella. (From Farrar, et al, 1992.)

TABLE 7-4	Primary Skin Lesions—cont'd

Description	Examples		
Bulla Vesicle greater than 1 cm in diameter	Blister, pemphigus vulgaris	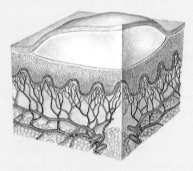	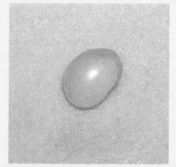Blister. (From White, 1994.)
Pustule Elevated, superficial lesion; similar to a vesicle but filled with purulent fluid	Impetigo, acne	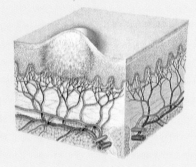	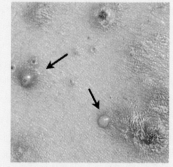Acne. (From Weston, Lane, Morelli, 1996.)
Cyst Elevated, circumscribed, encapsulated lesion; in dermis or subcutaneous layer; filled with liquid or semisolid material	Sebaceous cyst, cystic acne	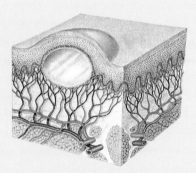	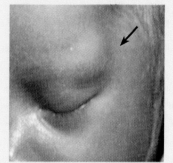Sebaceous cyst. (From Weston, Lane, Morelli, 1996.)
Telangiectasia Fine, irregular red lines produced by capillary dilation	Telangiectasia in rosacea	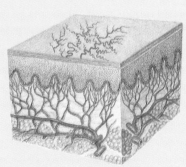	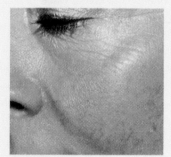Telangiectasia. (From Goldman and Fitzpatrick, 1994.)

Modified from Thompson, Wilson, 1995.

TABLE 7-5 Secondary Skin Lesions

Description	Examples		
Scale Heaped-up keratinized cells; flaky skin; irregular; thick or thin; dry or oily; variation in size	Flaking of skin with seborrheic dermatitis following scarlet fever, or flaking of skin following a drug reaction; dry skin	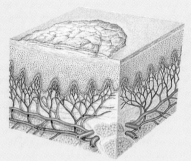	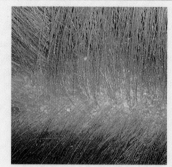 Fine scaling. (From Baran et al, 1991.)
Lichenification Rough, thickened epidermis secondary to persistent rubbing, itching, or skin irritation; often involves flexor surface of extremity	Chronic dermatitis	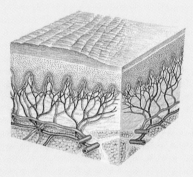	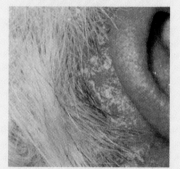 Statis dermatitis in an early stage.
Keloid Irregular-shaped, elevated, progressively enlarging scar; grows beyond the boundaries of the wound; caused by excessive collagen formation during healing	Keloid formation following surgery	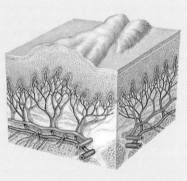	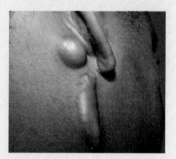 Keloid. (From Weston, Lane, Morelli, 1996.)
Scar Thin to thick fibrous tissue that replaces normal skin following injury or laceration to the dermis	Healed wound or surgical incision	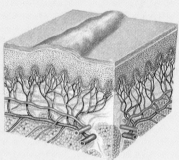	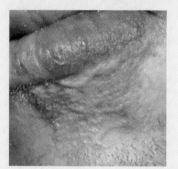 Hypertrophic scar. (From Goldman and Fitzpatrick, 1994.)

TABLE 7-5	Secondary Skin Lesions—cont'd
Description	**Examples**

Excoriation
Loss of the epidermis; linear hollowed-out crusted area

Abrasion or scratch, scabies

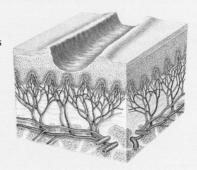
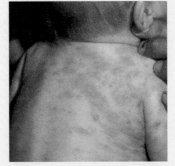

Scabies. (From Weston and Lane, 1991.)

Fissure
Linear crack or break from the epidermis to the dermis; may be moist or dry

Athlete's foot, cracks at the corner of the mouth

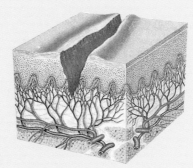
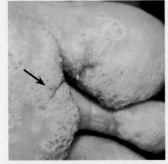

Fissures. (From Goldman and Fitzpatrick, 1994.)

Erosion
Loss of part of the epidermis; depressed, moist, glistening; follows rupture of a vesicle or bulla

Varicella, variola after rupture

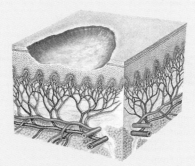
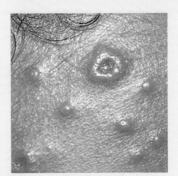

Erosion. (From Cohen, 1993.)

Ulcer
Loss of epidermis and dermis; concave; varies in size

Decubiti, stasis ulcers

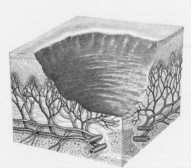
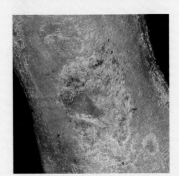

Statis ulcer. (From Habif, 1996.)

Continued

TABLE 7-5	Secondary Skin Lesions—cont'd	
Description	**Examples**	
Crust Dried serum, blood, or purulent exudate; slightly elevated; size varies; brown, red, black, tan, or straw. Scab on abrasion; eczema	Scab on abrasion, eczema	 Scab
Atrophy Thinning of skin surface and loss of skin markings; skin translucent and paperlike	Striae; aged skin	 Striae

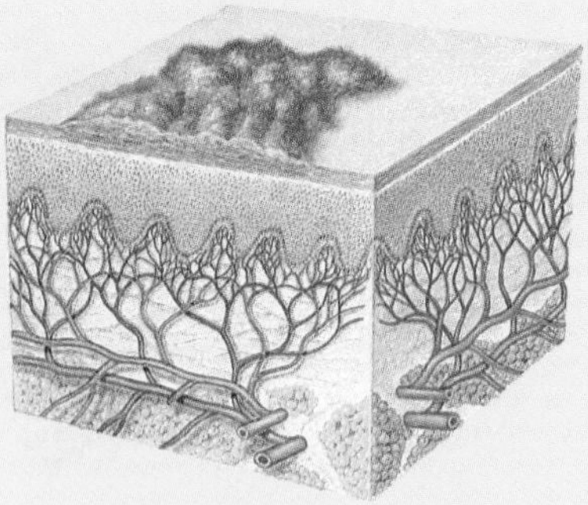

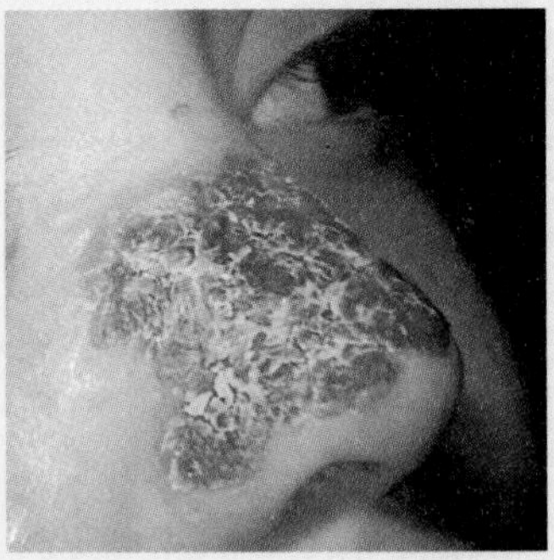

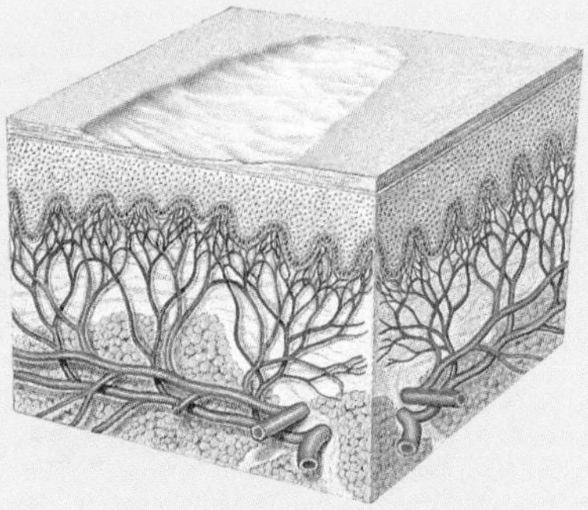

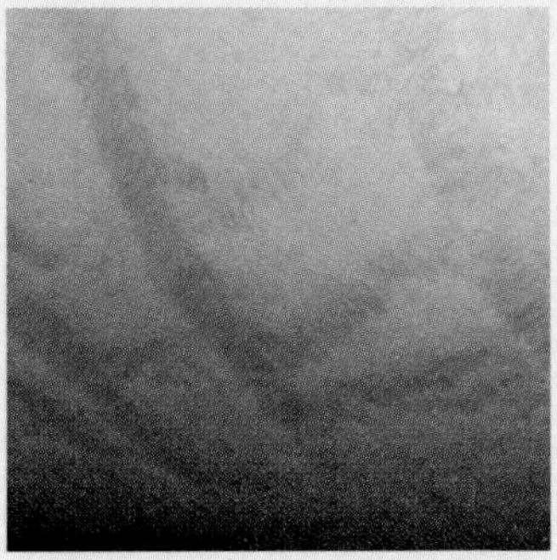

Modified from Thompson, Wilson, 1995.

BOX 7-3   Regional Distribution of Skin Lesions

Sun-Exposed Areas

Sunburn
Lupus erythematosus
Viral exanthem
Porphyria

Clothing Covered Areas

Contact dermatitis
Miliaria

Flexural Aspects of Extremities

Atopic dermatitis
Intertrigo
Candidiasis
Tinea cruris

Extensor Aspects of Extremities

Psoriasis

Stocking and Glove (Acrodermatitis)

Viral exanthem/atopic dermatitis
Tinea pedis with "id" reaction
Post streptococcal infection

Truncal

Pityriasis rosea (Christmas tree pattern)
Atopic dermatitis
Drug reaction

Face, Shoulder, Back

Acne vulgaris
Drug-induced acne
Cushing syndrome

TABLE 7-6   Morphologic Characteristics of Skin Lesions

Characteristic	Description	Examples
Distribution		
localized	lesion appears in one small area	impetigo, herpes simplex (e.g., labialis), tinea corporis ("ringworm")
regional	lesions involve a specific region of the body	acne vulgaris (pilosebaceous gland distribution), herpes zoster (nerve dermatomal distribution), psoriasis (flexural surfaces and skin folds)
generalized	lesions appear widely distributed or in numerous areas simultaneously	urticaria, disseminated drug eruptions
Shape/Arrangement		
round/discoid	coin- or ring-shaped (no central clearing)	nummular eczema
oval	ovoid shape	pityriasis rosea
annular	round, active margins with central clearing	tinea corporia, sarcoidosis
zosteriform (dermatomal)	following a nerve or segment of the body	herpes zoster
polycyclic	interlocking or coalesced circles (formed by enlargement of annular lesions)	psoriases, urticaria
linear	in a line	contact dermatitis
iris/target lesion	pink macules with purple central papules	erythema multiforme
stellate	star-shaped	meningococcal septicemia
serpiginous	snakelike or wavy line track	cutanea larva migrans
reticulate	netlike or lacy	polyarteritis nodosa, lichen planus lesions of erythema infectiosum
morbilliform	measles-like: maculopapular lesions that become confluent on the face and body	measles, roseola
Border/Margin		
discrete	well demarcated or defined, able to draw a line around it with confidence	psoriasis
indistinct	poorly defined, have borders that merge into normal skin or outlying ill defined papules	nummular eczema
active	margin of lesion shows greater actively than center	tinea sp. eruptions
irregular	nonsmooth or notched margin	malignant melanoma
border raised above center	center of lesion is depressed compared to the edge	basal cell carcinoma
advancing	expanding at margins	cellulitis
Associated Changes Within Lesions		
central clearing	an erythematous border surrounds lighter skin	tinea eruptions
desquamation	peeling or sloughing of skin	rash of toxic shock syndrome
keratotic	hypertrophic stratum corneum	callouses, warts
punctation	central umbilication or dimpling	basal cell carcinoma
telangiectasias	dilated blood vessels within lesion blanch completely, may be markers of systemic disease	basal cell carcinoma, actinic keratosis
Pigmentation		
flesh		neurofibroma, some nevi
pink		eczema, pityriasis rosea
erythematous		tinea eruptions, psoriasis
salmon		psoriasis
tan-brown		most nevi, pityriasis versicolor
black		malignant melanoma
pearly		basal cell carcinoma
purple		purpura, Kaposi sarcoma
violaceous		erysipelas
yellow		lipoma
white		lichen planus

From Dains J, Baumann L, Scheibel P, 1998.

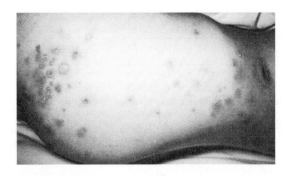

FIGURE 7-10

Clustering of lesions.

Reproduced by permission of the Wellcome Foundation, Ltd.

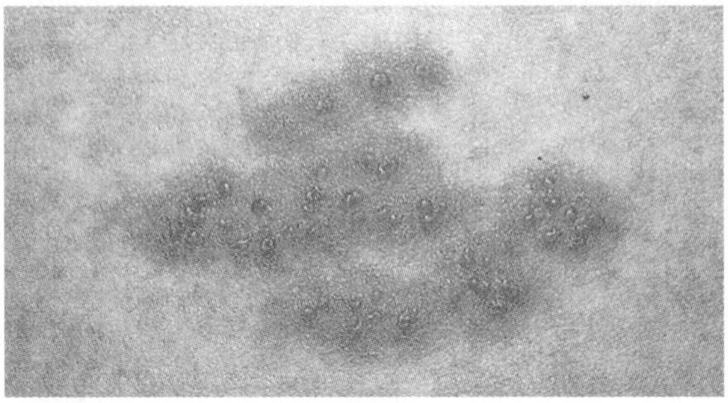

FIGURE 7-11

Linear formation of lesions (herpes zoster).

From White, 1994.

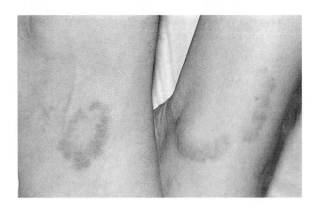

FIGURE 7-12

Annular formation of lesions (granuloma annulare). An annular plaque or plaques may occur on the dorsa of the feet or hands as a manifestation of granuloma annulare.

From White, 1994.

A small, clear, flexible ruler is necessary for measuring the size of lesions. Examiners frequently rely on household measures such as fruit, vegetables, and coins to estimate the size of lesions, nodules, or eruptions; but the resulting descriptions can be as inaccurate as they are interesting. Subjective estimates should not be used as measures of size; instead, use the ruler and report sizes in centimeters (inches may also be used, but centimeters is the preferred unit of measure). Try to measure size in all dimensions (height, width, depth) when possible.

Use a flashlight for closer inspection of a particular lesion to detect its nuances of color, elevation, and borders. Transillumination may be used to determine the presence of fluid in cysts and masses. Darken the room and place the tip of the transilluminator against the side of the cyst or mass. Fluid-filled lesions will transilluminate with a red glow, whereas solid lesions will not.

The Wood's lamp can be used to distinguish fluorescing lesions. Darken the room and shine the light on the area to be examined. Look for the characteristic yellow-green fluorescence that indicates the presence of fungal infection.

HAIR

Inspection and Palpation

Palpate the hair for texture, while at the same time inspecting it for color, distribution, and quantity. The scalp hair may be coarse or fine, curly or straight, and should be shiny, smooth, and resilient. Palpate the scalp hair for dryness and brittleness that could indicate a systemic disorder. Color will vary from very light blond to black to gray and may show alterations with rinses, dyes, or permanents.

The quantity and distribution of hair vary according to individual genetic makeup. Hair is commonly present on scalp, lower face, neck, nares, ears, chest, axillae, back and shoulders, arms, legs and toes, pubic area, and around nipples. Note hair loss, which can be either generalized or localized. Inspect the feet and toes for hair loss that may indicate poor circulation or nutritional deficit. Look for any inflammation or scarring that accompanies hair loss, particularly when it is localized. Diffuse hair loss usually occurs without inflammation and scarring. The presence of scarring is helpful in diagnosis. Note whether the hair shafts are broken off or are completely absent.

Genetically predisposed men often display a gradual symmetric hair loss on the scalp during adulthood as a response to elevated androgen levels. Asymmetric hair loss may indicate a pathologic condition. Women in their twenties and thirties may also develop adrenal androgenic female-pattern alopecia, with a gradual loss of hair from the central scalp.

Fine vellus hair covers the body, whereas coarse terminal hair occurs on the scalp, pubic, and axillary areas, to some extent on the arms and legs, and in the beard of males. The male pubic hair configuration is an upright triangle with the hair extending midline to the umbilicus. The female pubic configuration is an inverted triangle; the hair may extend midline to the umbilicus. Look for hirsutism in women—growth of terminal hair in a male distribution pattern on the face, body, and pubic area. Hirsutism, by itself or associated with other signs of virilization, may be a sign of an endocrine disorder.

NAILS

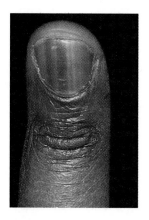

FIGURE 7-13
Pigmented bands in nails are expected in persons with dark skin.
From Habif, 1996.

Inspection

Inspect the nails for color, length, configuration, symmetry, and cleanliness. The condition of the fingernails can provide important insight to the patient's sense of self. Are they bitten down to the quick? Are they clean? Are they kept smooth and neat, or do they look unkempt? There are, of course, physical clues to pathophysiologic problems in the nails, just as in the hair. The condition of the hair and nails gives a clue about the patient's level of self-care and some sense of emotional order and social integration.

The shape and opacity of nails vary considerably among individuals. Nail bed color should be variations of pink. Pigment deposits or bands may be present in the nail beds of persons with dark skin (Figure 7-13). The sudden appearance of such a band in whites may indicate melanoma. Yellow discoloration occurs with several nail diseases including psoriasis and fungal infections and may also occur with chronic respiratory disease. Proximal subungual fungal infection is associated with HIV infection. Diffuse darkening of the nails may arise from antimalarial drug therapy, candidal infection, hyperbilirubinemia, and chronic trauma, such as occurs from tight-fitting shoes. Green-black discoloration, which is associated with *Pseudomonas* infection, may be confused with similar discoloration caused by injury to the nail bed (subungual hematoma). Pain accompanies a subungual hematoma, whereas *Pseudomonas* infection is painless. Splinter hemorrhages, longitudinal red or brown streaks, may occur with severe psoriasis of the nail matrix or as the result of minor injury to

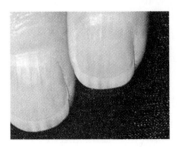

FIGURE 7-14

Aging nails. Longitudinal ridging of the nail is a common expected variation.

From White, 1994.

the proximal nail fold. White spots in the nail plate, a common finding, result from cuticle manipulation or other forms of mild trauma. These spots need to be differentiated from longitudinal white streaks or transverse white bands that are indicative of a systemic disorder. Separation of the nail plate from the bed produces a white, yellow, or green tinge on the nonadherent portion of the nail.

Nail edges should be smooth and rounded. Jagged, broken, or bitten edges or cuticles are indicators of poor care habits and may predispose the patient to localized infection. Peeling nails (from the plate splitting into layers) are usually found in individuals whose hands are subject to repeated water immersion.

The nail plate should appear smooth and flat or slightly convex. Complete absence of the nail (anonychia) may occur as a congenital condition. Look for nail ridging, grooves, depressions, and pitting. Longitudinal ridging and beading are common expected variants (Figure 7-14). Longitudinal ridging and grooving may also occur with lichen planus of the nail. Transverse grooves result from repeated injury to the nail, usually the thumb, as with chronic manipulation to the proximal nail fold. The most common cause is picking at the thumb with the index finger. Chronic inflammation, such as occurs with chronic paronychia or chronic eczema, produces transverse rippling of the nail plate. Transverse depressions that appear at the base of the lunula occur after stress that temporarily interrupts nail formation. Involvement of a single nail usually points to injury to the nail matrix. Assure the patient that the nail will grow out and assume normal appearance in about 6 months. Depressions that occur in all the nails are usually in response to systemic disease, including syphilis, disorders producing high fevers, peripheral vascular disease, and uncontrolled diabetes mellitus. Pitting is seen most commonly with psoriasis. Broadening and flattening of the nail plate may be seen in secondary syphilis (Figure 7-15).

The nail base angle should measure 160 degrees. One way to observe this is to place a ruler or a sheet of paper across the nail and dorsal surface of the finger and examine the angle formed by the proximal nail fold and nail plate. In clubbing, the angle increases and approaches or exceeds 180 degrees. Another method of assessment is the Schamroth technique. Have the patient place together the nail (dorsal) surfaces of the fingertips of corresponding fingers from the right and left hands. When the nails are clubbed, the diamond-shaped window at the base of the nails disappears, and the angle between the distal tips increases (Figure 7-16). Clubbing is associated with a variety of respiratory and cardiovascular diseases, cirrhosis, colitis, and thyroid disease (Figure 7-17).

Examine the proximal and lateral nail folds for redness, swelling, pus, warts, cysts, and tumors. Pain usually accompanies ingrown nails and infections.

Palpation

The nail plates should feel hard and smooth with a uniform thickness. Thickening of the nail may occur from tight-fitting shoes, chronic trauma, and some fungal infections. Thinning of the nail plate may also accompany some nail diseases. Pain in the area of a nail groove may be secondary to ischemia.

Gently squeeze the nail between your thumb and the pad of your finger to test for adherence of the nail to the nail bed. Separation of the nail plate from the bed is common with psoriasis, trauma, candidal or *Pseudomonas* infections, and some medications. The nail base should feel firm (Figure 7-18). A boggy nail base accompanies clubbing.

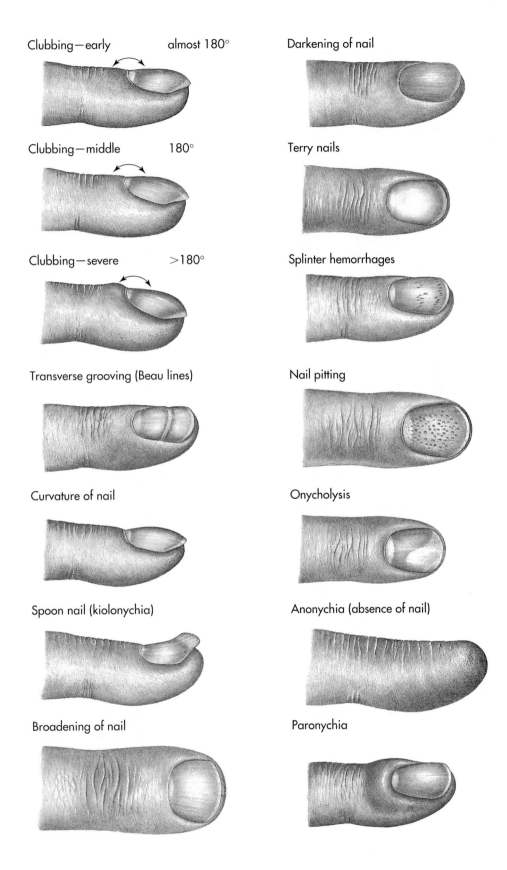

FIGURE 7-15
Nails: unexpected findings and appearance.

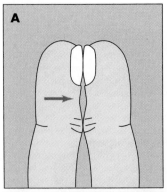

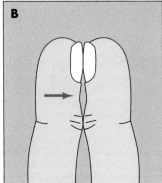

FIGURE 7-16
Schamroth technique. **A,** Patient with healthy nails, illustrating window. **B,** Patient with nail clubbing, illustrating loss of the window and prominent distal angle *(arrows).*

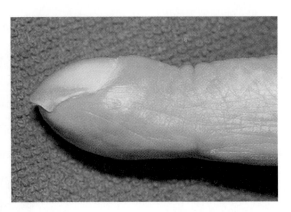

FIGURE 7-17
Finger clubbing. Nail is enlarged and curved.
From Lawrence, Cox, 1993.

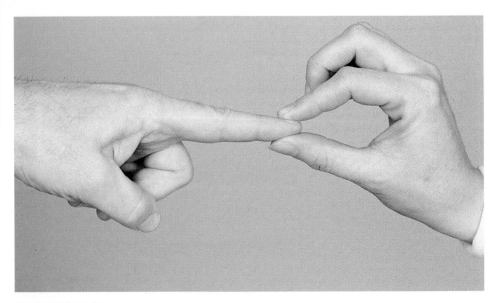

FIGURE 7-18
Testing nail bed adherence.

INFANTS AND CHILDREN

Inspection and Palpation

In the first few hours of life, the infant's skin may look very red (Figure 7-19). The more gentle pink coloring that predominates in infancy usually surfaces in the first day after birth. Skin color is partly determined by chubbiness; the less fat, the redder and more transparent the skin. Dark-skinned newborns do not always manifest the intensity of melanosis that will be readily evident in 2 to 3 months. The exceptions in this regard are the nail beds and skin of the scrotum. The expected color changes in newborns are described in Box 7-4.

Physiologic jaundice may be present to a mild degree in as many as 50% or more of newborn infants. It usually starts after the first day of life and disappears by the eighth to tenth day but may persist for as long as 3 to 4 weeks. Intense and persistent jaundice should suggest liver disease or severe, overwhelming infection. Risk factors for hyperbilirubinemia in the newborn are listed in the Risk Factors box on the next page.

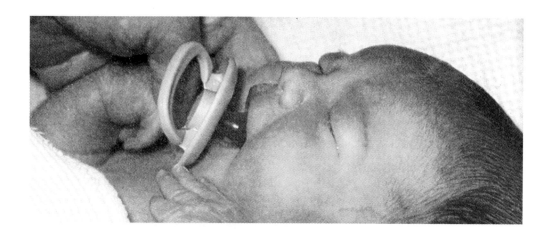

FIGURE 7-19
Ruddy color of newborn.

BOX 7-4 | **Expected Color Changes in the Newborn**

- **Acrocyanosis** Cyanosis of hands and feet
- **Cutis marmorata** Transient mottling when infant is exposed to decreased temperature
- **Erythema toxicum** Pink papular rash with vesicles superimposed on thorax, back, buttocks, and abdomen; may appear in 24 to 48 hours and resolves after several days
- **Harlequin color change** Clearly outlined color change as infant lies on side; dependent lower half of body becomes pink and upper half is pale
- **Mongolian spots** Irregular areas of deep blue pigmentation, usually in the sacral and gluteal regions; seen predominantly in newborns of African, Native American, Asian, or Latin descent
- **Telangiectatic nevi ("stork bites")** Flat, deep pink localized areas usually seen in back of neck

From Whaley, Wong, 1995.

RISK FACTORS | **Hyperbilirubinemia in the Newborn**

- Breast feeding (possibly because of β-glucuronidase in breast milk)
- Cephalhematoma or other cutaneous or subcutaneous bleeds
- Too much extra water
- Hemolytic disease
- Infection

In examining the newborn for hyperbilirubinemia, look at the whole body. Jaundice begins on the face and descends. The bilirubin level is not high if only the face is involved. However, the bilirubin may well be at a worrisome level if the jaundice descends below the nipples. Be sure to examine the oral mucosa and sclera of the eyes, as jaundice can be detected more easily there than in the skin. Examine the baby in natural daylight if possible. Both artificial light and environmental colors such as orange drapes can produce a false color.

The skin of the newborn should be checked carefully for small defects, especially over the entire length of the spine, the midline of the head from the nape of the neck to the bridge of the nose, and the neck extending to the ear. This may offer a clue to sinus tracts, brachial clefts, or cysts. The skin should feel soft and smooth. Also look for skin findings that may signal underlying systemic conditions (Box 7-5).

BOX 7-5   **Skin Lesions: External Clues to Internal Problems**

Many systemic conditions or disorders may present congenital external clues that are apparent on physical examination. The following are but a few examples of cutaneous markers that may signal underlying disease. A thorough evaluation is necessary, although some clues may be isolated findings and may require no intervention, follow-up, or treatment.

Faun tail nevus Tuft of hair overlying the spinal column at birth, usually in the lumbosacral area; may be associated with spina bifida occulta

Epidermal verrucous nevi Warty lesions in a linear or whorled pattern that may be pigmented or skin colored; present at birth or in early childhood; associated most commonly with skeletal, central nervous system, and ocular abnormalities

Café au lait spots Flat, evenly pigmented spots varying in color from light brown to dark brown or black in dark skin; larger than 5 mm in diameter; present at birth or shortly thereafter; may be associated with neurofibromatosis or miscellaneous other conditions including pulmonary stenosis, temporal lobe dysrhythmia, and tuberous sclerosis

Freckling in the axillary or inguinal area Multiple flat pigmented macules associated with neurofibromatosis; may occur in conjunction with café au lait spots

Facial port-wine stain When it involves the ophthalmic division of trigeminal nerve, it may be associated with ocular defects, most notably glaucoma; or it may be accompanied by angiomatous malformation of the meninges (Sturge-Kalischer-Weber syndrome), resulting in atrophy and calcification of the adjacent cerebral cortex

Port-wine stain of limb and/or trunk When accompanied by venous varicosities and hypertrophy of underlying soft tissues and bones, it may be associated with visceral involvement, resulting in bleeding, and/or with limb hypertrophy, resulting in orthopedic problems (Klippel-Trenaunay-Weber syndrome)

Congenital lymphedema with or without transient hemangiomas May be associated with gonadal dysgenesis caused by absence of an X chromosome, producing an XO karyotype (Turner syndrome)

Supernumerary nipples Congenital accessory nipples with or without glandular tissue, located along the mammary ridge (see Chapter 14, Breasts and Axillae); may be associated with renal abnormalities, especially in the presence of other minor anomalies, particularly in Whites

"Hair collar" sign A ring of long, dark coarse hair surrounding the a midline scalp nodule in infants may indicate neural tube closure defects of the scalp

Persistent pruritus Persistent pruritis in the absence of skin disease may indicate chronic renal failure, cholestatic liver disease, Hodgkin disease, or diabetes mellitus

---

Inspect the skin for distortions in contour suggestive of hygromas, fluid-containing masses, subcutaneous angiomas, lymphangiomas, hemangiomas, nodules, and tumors. Transillumination may help if there is a question about the density of the mass or the amount of fluid. With more density and less fluid, there is less tendency to glow on transillumination.

Examine the hands and feet of newborns for skin creases. Flexion results in creases that are readily discernible on the fingers, palms, and soles (Figure 7-20). One indicator of maturity is the number of creases; the older the baby, the more creases. Beyond that, it is appropriate to examine the crease patterns of the fingers and palms, because certain abnormalities are associated with specific derangements of the patterns (the study of which is known as dermatoglyphics). The most commonly recognized crease is the simian line, a single transverse crease in the palm that may be seen in individuals who are otherwise well; however, it is also frequently seen in children with Down syndrome (Figure 7-21).

All newborn infants are covered to some degree by vernix caseosa, a whitish, moist, cheeselike substance. Transient puffiness of the hands, feet, eyelids, legs, pubis, or sacrum occurs in some newborns. It has no discernible cause and should not create concern if it disappears within 2 to 3 days.

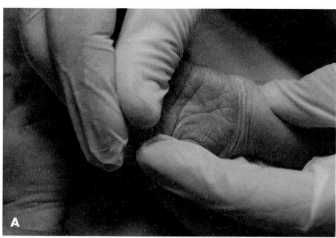
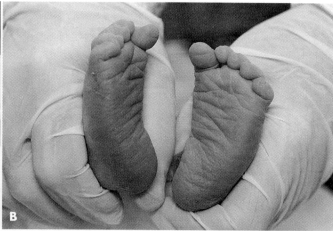

FIGURE 7-20
Expected creases of newborn's hands **(A)** and feet **(B)**.

FIGURE 7-21
Unexpected palmar crease. Simian crease in child with Down syndrome. Compare to Figure 7-20, *A*.
From Zitelli, Davis, 1997.

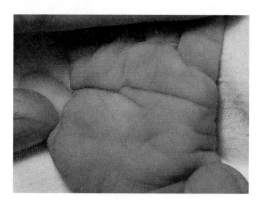

Newborn infants are particularly prone to hypothermia, partly because of their poorly developed subcutaneous fat. In addition, infants have a relatively large body surface area, providing greater area for heat loss. Combined with an inability to shiver, these factors cause term newborns to lose heat at a rate four times that of an adult, per unit of body weight.

Cutis marmorata, a mottled appearance of the body and extremities, is part of the newborn's response to changes in ambient temperature, whether cooling or heating. It is more common in premature infants and children with Down syndrome and hypothyroidism (Figure 7-22). Cyanosis of the hands and feet (acrocyanosis) may be present at birth and may persist for several days or longer if the newborn is kept in cool ambient temperatures. It often recurs when the baby is chilled. Generally, when the cyanosis persists, it is more intense in the feet than in the hands, and an underlying cardiac defect should be suspected (Figure 7-23).

Harlequin color change (dyschromia) often occurs in the normal newborn. One half of the body is more red than the other, with a rather sharp demarcation down the midline. The condition is self-resolving and does not last long.

Bluish black to slate gray spots are sometimes seen on the back, buttocks, shoulders, and legs of well babies. These patches, called mongolian spots, occur most often in babies with dark skin and usually disappear in the preschool years. Mongolian spots are easily mistaken for bruises by the inexperienced examiner (Figure 7-24).

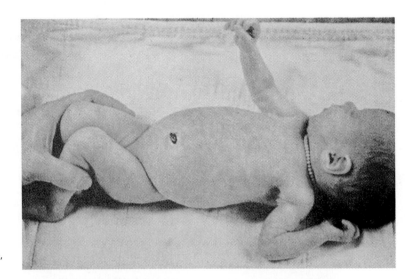

FIGURE 7-22
Mottling (cutis marmorata).
Courtesy Mead Johnson & Co, Evansville, Indiana.

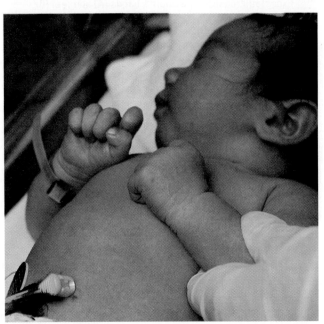

FIGURE 7-23
Acrocyanosis of hands in newborn.

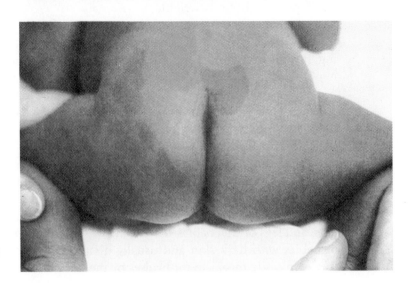

FIGURE 7-24
Mongolian spots are common in babies with dark skin.

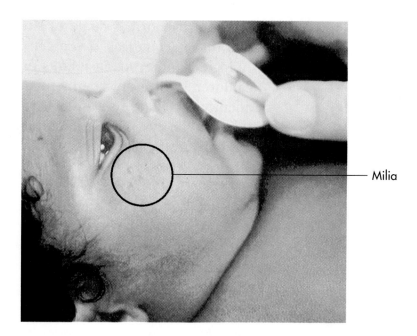

Milia

FIGURE 7-25
Milia in infant.

Milia, small whitish, discrete papules on the face, are commonly found during the first 2 to 3 months of life. The sebaceous glands function in an immature fashion at this age and are easily plugged by sebum (Figure 7-25).

Sebaceous hyperplasia produces numerous tiny yellow macules and papules in the newborn, probably the result of androgen stimulation from the mother. It frequently occurs on the forehead, cheeks, nose, and chin of the full-term infant. Sebaceous hyperplasia disappears quickly within 1 to 2 months of life.

Mothers and fathers sometimes define the excellence of their parenting by the condition of their baby's skin. Diaper rashes are distressing, a false message to the world that parents may not be clean or knowledgeable in baby care. When you notice a skin problem such as diaper rash or impetigo, try to avoid comments or questions that imply that the parent has done something wrong. This, of course, is a guiding principle whenever you are serving children and their parents.

Turgor

The skin and subcutaneous tissues of an infant and young child, more readily than in the older child and adolescent, can give an important indication of the state of hydration and nutrition (Table 7-7). The tissue turgor is best evaluated by gently pinching a fold of the abdominal skin between the index finger and thumb. As with the adult, resiliency will allow it to return to its undisturbed state when released. A child who is seriously dehydrated (more than 3% to 5% of body weight) or very poorly nourished will have skin that retains "tenting" after it is pinched. How quickly the tent disappears provides a clue to the degree of dehydration or malnutrition (Figure 7-26).

Because the normal range of skin moisture is broad, you need to look at other factors that may suggest a problem. Excessive sweating or dryness alone rarely has pathologic significance in infants or children.

Children with atopic dermatitis or chronic skin changes involving the face will frequently rub their eyes, sufficiently sometimes to cause an extra crease or pleat of skin below the eye. This is known as the Dennie-Morgan fold; it is probably secondary to chronic rubbing and inflammation.

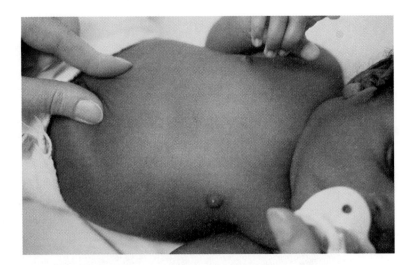

FIGURE 7-26
Testing skin turgor in infant.

TABLE 7-7	Estimating Dehydration	
Return to Normal After the Pinch	**Degree of Dehydration**
<2 seconds	<5% loss of body weight
2-3 seconds	5%-8% loss of body weight
3-4 seconds	9%-10% loss of body weight
>4 seconds	>10% loss of body weight

ADOLESCENTS

The examination of the adolescent's skin is the same as that for the adult. The adolescent's skin may have increased oiliness and perspiration, and hair oiliness may also be increased. Increased sebum production predisposes the adolescent to develop acne. Acne is a matter of deep concern to the adolescent. By all means, mention it, and do not hesitate to say quite candidly that you understand how much of a problem it can be. This is a time when you might refer to your own adolescent experience.

As a reflection of maturing apocrine gland function, increased axillary perspiration occurs, and the characteristic adult body odor develops during adolescence. Hair on the extremities darkens and becomes coarser. Pubic and axillary hair in both males and females develops and assumes adult characteristics. Males develop facial and chest hair that varies in quantity and coarseness. Chapter 5, Growth and Measurement, provides a more thorough discussion of the maturational changes that occur during adolescence.

PREGNANT WOMEN

Striae gravidarum (stretch marks) may appear over the abdomen, thighs, and breasts during the second trimester of pregnancy. They fade after delivery but never disappear (Figure 7-27). Telangiectasias (vascular spiders) may be found on the face, neck, chest, and arms, appearing during the second to fifth month of pregnancy. They usually resolve after delivery. Hemangiomas that were present before pregnancy may increase in size, or new ones may develop. Cutaneous tags (molluscum fibrosum gravidarum) are either pedunculated or sessile skin tags that are most often found on the neck and upper chest. They result from epithelial hyperplasia and are not inflammatory.

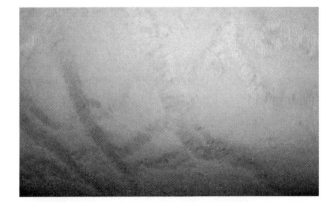

FIGURE 7-27
Striae.

Courtesy Antoinette Hood, MD,
Department of Dermatology, Indiana
University School of Medicine,
Indianapolis.

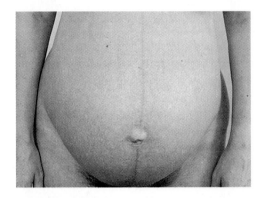

FIGURE 7-28
Linea nigra on abdomen of pregnant woman.

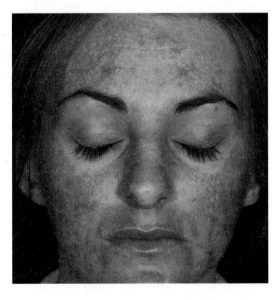

FIGURE 7-29
Facial hyperpigmentation:
chloasma (melasma).

From Habif, 1996.

An increase in pigmentation is common and is found to some extent in all pregnant women. The areas usually affected include the areolae and nipples, vulvar and perianal regions, axillae, and the linea alba. Pigmentation of the linea alba is called the linea nigra. It extends from the symphysis pubis to the top of the fundus in the midline (Figure 7-28). Preexisting pigmented moles (nevi) and freckles may darken, with some nevi increasing in size. New nevi may form. The chloasma or "mask of pregnancy" occurs in approximately 70% of pregnant women and is found on the forehead, cheeks, bridge of the nose, and chin. It is blotchy in appearance and is usually symmetric (Figure 7-29).

PHYSICAL VARIATIONS

Areola pigmentation varies by race, with Blacks having the darkest areolae, Whites the lightest, and Orientals and Native Americans intermediate. Despite common belief, there is no correlation between the color of the areola and nipple damage from breast-feeding.

Data from Pawson, Petrakis, 1975; Gans, 1958; Brown, Hurlock, 1975.

Palmar erythema is a common finding in pregnancy. A diffuse redness covers the entire palmar surface or the thenar and hypothenar eminences. The cause is unknown, and it usually disappears after delivery.

Itching over the abdomen and breasts resulting from stretching is common and not a cause for concern. However, generalized itching that starts in the third trimester and initially affects the palms and soles before spreading is a sign of a more serious condition. Be alert to these more serious manifestations of underlying pathology.

Hair growth is altered in pregnancy by the circulating hormones. The result is a uniform increase in the shedding of hair from 3 to 4 months after delivery, which may continue for 6 to 24 weeks. Acne vulgaris may be aggravated during the first trimester of pregnancy but often improves in the third trimester.

OLDER ADULTS

The skin of the older adult may appear more transparent and paler in light-skinned individuals. Pigment deposits, increased freckling, and hypopigmented patches may develop, causing the skin to take on a less uniform appearance.

Flaking or scaling, associated with the drier skin that comes with aging, occurs most commonly over the extremities. The skin also becomes thinner—especially over bony prominences, the dorsal surface of hands and feet, forearms, and lower legs—and takes on a parchment-like appearance and texture (Figure 7-30).

The skin often appears to hang loosely on the bony frame as a result of a general loss of elasticity, loss of underlying adipose tissue, and years of gravitational pull (Figure 7-31). You may observe tenting of the skin when testing for turgor (Figure 7-32). Thus, in older adults turgor may not be a reliable or valid estimate of hydration status.

The immobility of some older adults, especially when combined with decreased peripheral vascular circulation, places them at risk for the development of decubitus ulcers (pressure sores). In your examination pay particular attention to bony prominences and areas subject to persistent pressure or shearing forces. Heels and the sacrum are common sites in patients who are confined to bed. Don't neglect to examine less obvious areas such as the elbows, scapulae, and back of the head. Assess the diameter and depth of the ulcer and stage it accordingly. The staging criteria are described in Box 7-6.

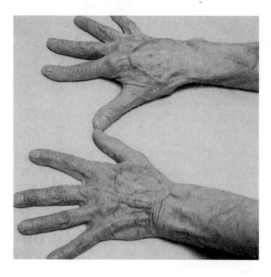

FIGURE 7-30
Hands of older adult. Note prominent veins and thin appearance of skin.

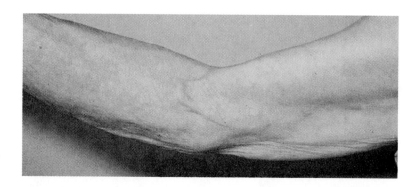

FIGURE 7-31
Skin hanging loosely, especially around bony prominences.

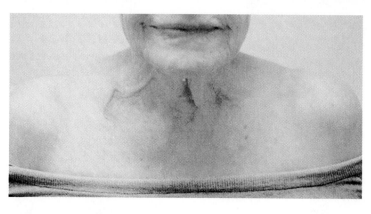

FIGURE 7-32
Skin turgor in older adult. Note tenting.

BOX 7-6	**Staging for Decubitus Ulcers**
STAGE I	Skin red but not broken
STAGE II	Damage through epidermis and dermis
STAGE III	Damage through to subcutaneous tissue
STAGE IV	Muscle and possible bone involvement

PHYSICAL VARIATIONS

Whites wrinkle sooner and their hair turns gray earlier than that of other races; this can cause Whites to underestimate the age of persons from other races. Conversely, persons from other races often overestimate the age of White individuals.

Increased wrinkling is evident, especially in areas exposed to sun and in expressive areas of the face. Sagging or drooping is most obvious under the chin, beneath the eyes, and in the earlobes, breasts, and scrotum.

Several kinds of lesions may occur on the skin of healthy older adults. The following lesions are considered expected findings:

- Cherry angiomas are tiny, bright ruby red, round papules that may become brown with time. They occur in virtually everyone over the age of 30 and increase numerically with age (Figure 7-33).
- Seborrheic keratoses are pigmented, raised, warty lesions, usually appearing on the face or trunk. These must be distinguished from actinic keratoses, which have malignant potential. Since the lesions may look similar, seek the assistance of an experienced practitioner for differential diagnosis (Figure 7-34).
- Sebaceous hyperplasia occurs as yellowish flattened papules with central depressions (Figure 7-35).
- Cutaneous tags (acrochordon) are small, soft tags of skin, usually appearing on the neck and upper chest. They are attached to the body by a narrow stalk (pedunculated) and may or may not be pigmented (Figure 7-36).
- Cutaneous horns are small, hard projections of the epidermis, usually occurring on the forehead and face (Figure 7-37).

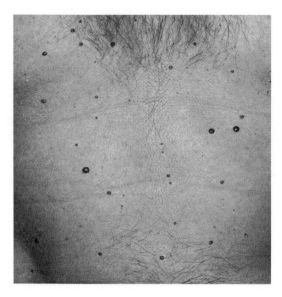

FIGURE 7-33
Cherry angioma in older adult.
From Habif, 1996.

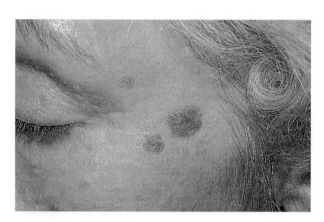

FIGURE 7-34
Seborrheic keratoses in older adult.
From Lawrence, Cox, 1993.

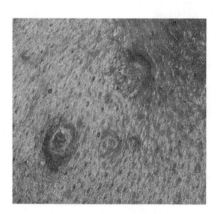

FIGURE 7-35
Sebaceous hyperplasia in older adult.
From Habif, 1996.

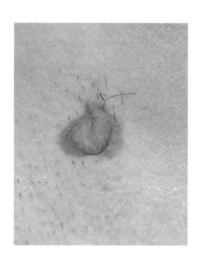

FIGURE 7-36
Cutaneous tag in older adult.
From Habif, 1996.

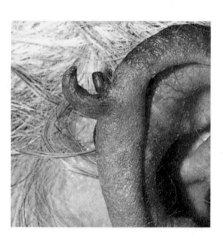

FIGURE 7-37
Cutaneous horn.
From White, 1994.

■ Senile lentigines are irregular, round, gray-brown lesions with a rough surface that occur in sun-exposed areas. These are often referred to as "age spots" or incorrectly as "liver spots" (Figure 7-38).

The hair turns gray or white as melanocytes cease functioning. You will note that the head, body, pubic, and axillary hair thins and becomes sparse and drier. Men may show an increase in coarse aural, nasal, and eyebrow hair; women tend to develop coarse facial hair. Symmetric balding, usually frontal or occipital, often occurs in men.

The nails thicken, become more brittle, and may be deformed, misshapen, striated, distorted, or peeling. They can take on a yellowish color and may lose their transparency. These changes occur most often in the toenails.

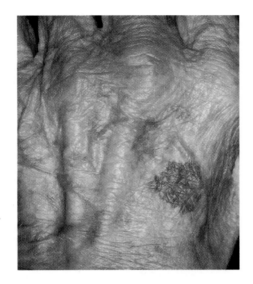

FIGURE 7-38
Lentigo, a brown macule that appears in chronically sun-exposed areas.
From Habif, 1996.

SUMMARY OF EXAMINATION   Skin, Hair, and Nails

Skin

1. Perform overall inspection of entire skin surface (p. 168). During evaluation of each organ system evaluate the overlying skin for the following characteristics:
   - Color
   - Uniformity
   - Thickness
   - Symmetry
   - Hygiene
   - Lesions (record size, shape, location, configuration, color, blanching, texture, elevation or depression, pedunculation, presence of exudates, pattern of distribution, configuration) (p. 172)
   - Odors
2. Palpate skin surfaces for p. 172):
   - Moisture
   - Temperature
   - Texture
   - Turgor
   - Mobility

Hair

1. Inspect hair for the following (p. 183):
   - Color
   - Distribution
   - Quantity
2. Palpate hair for texture (p. 183)

Nails

1. Inspect for the following: (p. 183)
   - Pigmentation of nails and beds
   - Length
   - Symmetry
   - Ridging, beading, pitting, pealing
2. Measure nail base angle (p. 184)
3. Inspect and palpate proximal and lateral nail folds for (p. 184):
   - Redness
   - Swelling
   - Pain
   - Exudate
   - Warts, cysts, tumors
4. Palpate nail plate for the following (p. 184)
   - Texture
   - Firmness
   - Thickness
   - Uniformity
   - Adherence to nail bed

COMMON ABNORMALITIES

SKIN: NONMALIGNANT ABNORMALITIES

CORN (CLAVUS)

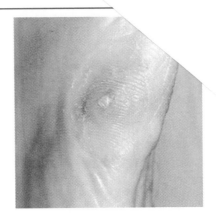

FIGURE 7-39
Corn.

From White, 1994.

...pear ...y between ... "Hard" corn... and have a conical a... ...cur most often over bo... ...ces where pressure is exerted, ... s from shoes pressing on the interphalangeal joints of the toes (Figure 7-39).

CALLUS

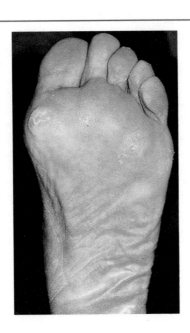

FIGURE 7-40
Calluses are common on both the sole (heels and metatarsal heads) and the dorsum of the foot (especially in women).

From Lawrence, Cox, 1993.

A superficial area of hyperkeratosis is called a callus. Calluses usually occur on the weight-bearing areas of the feet and on the palmar surface of the hands. Calluses are less well demarcated than corns and are usually not tender (Figure 7-40).

ECZEMATOUS DERMATITIS

The most common inflammatory skin disease is eczematous dermatitis. There are several types, including primary contact dermatitis, allergic contact dermatitis, and atopic dermatitis. The common factor of the various forms is epidermal breakdown, usually as a result of intracellular vesiculation. Eczematous dermatitis has three stages: acute, subacute, and chronic. The acute phase is characterized by erythematous, pruritic, weeping vesicles (Figure 7-41). Excoriation from scratching predisposes to infection and causes crust formation. Subacute eczema is characterized by erythema and scaling. Itching may or may not be present. In the chronic stage, thick, lichenified, pruritic plaques are present.

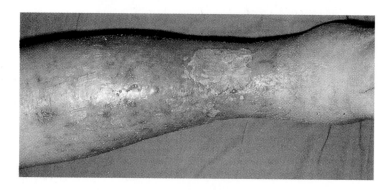

FIGURE 7-41
Contact dermatitis.
From Morison, Moffatt, 1994.

FURUNCLE

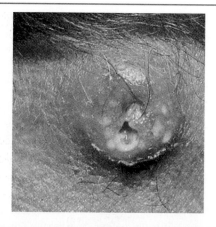

FIGURE 7-42
Furuncle.
Courtesy Jaime A. Tschen, MD, Baylor College of Medicine, Department of Dermatology, Houston; from Thompson et al, 1993.

A furuncle is an acute localized staphylococcal infection. It develops initially as a small perifollicular abscess and spreads to the surrounding dermis and subcutaneous tissue. The initial nodule becomes a pustule surrounded by erythema and edema. The skin is red, hot, and tender. The center of the lesion fills with pus and forms a core that may rupture spontaneously or require surgical incision (Figure 7-42).

FOLLICULITIS

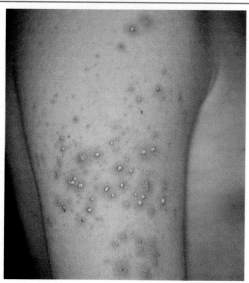

FIGURE 7-43
Staphylococcal folliculitis.
From Habif, 1996.

Staphylococcal infection of the hair follicle and surrounding dermis produces folliculitis. The primary lesion is a small pustule 1 to 2 cm in diameter that is located over a pilosebaceous orifice and may be perforated by a hair. The pustule may be surrounded by inflammation or nodular lesions. After the pustule ruptures, a crust forms (Figure 7-43).

CELLULITIS

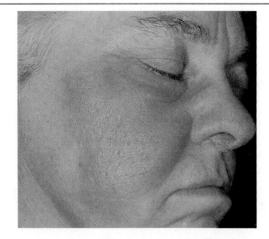

FIGURE 7-44
Streptococcal cellulitis. Acute phase with intense erythema (erysipelas).
From Habif, 1996.

Diffuse, acute, streptococcal, or staphylococcal infection of the skin and subcutaneous tissue is called cellulitis. The skin is red, hot, tender, and indurated. Lymphangitic streaks and regional lymphadenopathy may be present (Figure 7-44).

TINEA (DERMATOPHYTOSIS)

Tinea is a group of noncandidal fungal infections that involve the stratum corneum, nails, or hair. The lesions are usually classified according to anatomic location and can occur on nonhairy parts of the body (tinea corporis), on the groin and inner thigh (tinea cruris), scalp (tinea capitis), feet (tinea pedis), and nails (tinea unguium). The lesions vary in appearance and may be papular, pustular, vesicular, erythematous, or scaling. Secondary bacterial infection may be present (Figure 7-45).

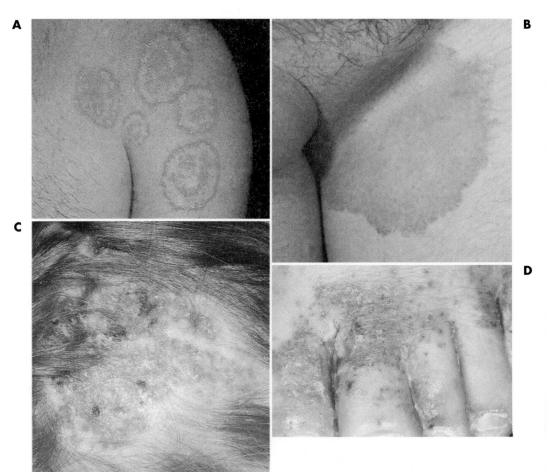

FIGURE 7-45
A, Tinea corporis. **B,** Tinea cruris. **C,** Tinea capitis. **D,** Tinea pedis.
From Habif, 1996.

PITYRIASIS ROSEA

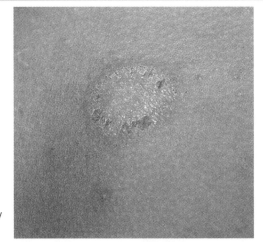

FIGURE 7-46

Pityriasis rosea herald patch.

Courtesy Walter Tunnessen, MD, University of Pennsylvania School of Medicine, Philadelphia.

Pityriasis rosea is a self-limiting inflammation of unknown cause. Onset is sudden with occurrence of a primary (herald) oval or round plaque with fine, superficial scaling (Figure 7-46). A generalized eruption occurs 1 to 3 weeks later and lasts for several weeks. The lesions develop on the extremities and trunk; the palms and soles are not involved, and facial involvement is rare. The trunk lesions are characteristically distributed in parallel alignment following the direction of the ribs in a Christmas tree-like pattern. The lesions are usually pale, erythematous, and macular with fine scaling, but they may be papular or vesicular. Pruritus may be present. The condition is not infectious or contagious.

PSORIASIS

Psoriasis is a chronic and recurrent disease of keratin synthesis that is characterized by well-circumscribed, dry, silvery, scaling papules and plaques. Lesions commonly occur on the back, buttocks, extensor surfaces of the extremities, and the scalp (Figure 7-47).

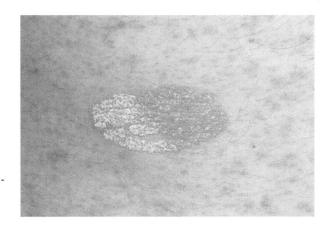

FIGURE 7-47

Psoriasis. Note characteristic silvery scaling.

From Lawrence, Cox, 1993.

ROSACEA

Rosacea is a chronic inflammatory skin disorder that is characterized by telangiectasia, erythema, papules, and pustules that occur particularly in the central area of the face (Figure 7-48). Tissue hypertrophy of the nose, rhinophyma, may occur. Rhinophyma is characterized by sebaceous hyperplasia, redness, prominent vascularity, and swelling of the skin of the nose (Figure 7-49). The cause of rosacea is unknown, but it occurs most often in persons with a fair complexion. Although rosacea resembles acne, comedomes are never present. Antibiotic therapy is usually effective in treating the condition. Rhinophyma may require surgical intervention.

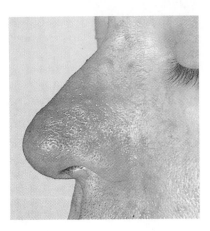

FIGURE 7-48
Rosacea.
From White, 1994

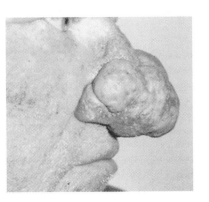

FIGURE 7-49
Rhinophyma.
Courtesy Michael O. Murphy, MD; from White, 1994.

DRUG ERUPTIONS

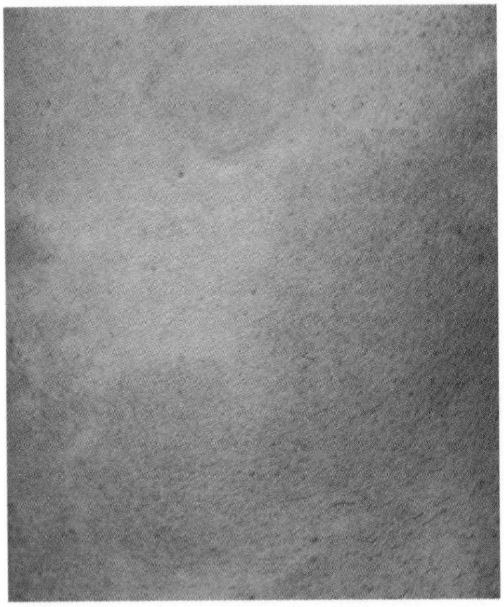

FIGURE 7-50

Drug eruption—hives. The most characteristic presentation is uniformly red edematous plaques surrounded by a faint white halo. These superficial lesions occur from transudation of fluid into the dermis.
From Habif, 1996.

The most common skin reaction to a drug consists of discrete or confluent erythematous maculopapules on the trunk, face, extremities, palms, or soles of the feet. The rash appears from 1 to several days after starting the drug and fades in 1 to 3 weeks. Pruritus is characteristic (Figure 7-50).

HERPES ZOSTER (SHINGLES)

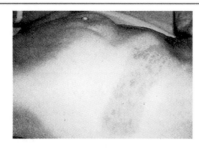

FIGURE 7-51
Herpes zoster lesions confined to one dermatome.
Reproduced by permission of the Wellcome Foundation, Ltd.

Herpes zoster is a viral (varicella-zoster) infection, usually of a single dermatome, that consists of red, swollen plaques or vesicles that become filled with purulent fluid. Pain, itching, or burning of the dermatome area usually precedes eruption by 4 to 5 days (Figure 7-51).

HERPES SIMPLEX

Viral infection by herpes simplex produces tenderness, pain, paresthesia, or mild burning at the infected site before onset of the lesions. Grouped vesicles appear on an erythematous base and then erode, forming a crust. Lesions last 2 to 6 weeks. Two different virus types cause the infection. Type 1 is usually associated with oral infection and type 2 with genital infection; however, crossover infections are becoming increasingly common (Figure 7-52).

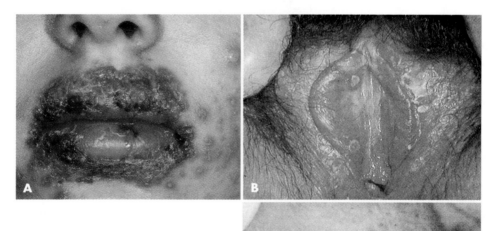

FIGURE 7-52
Herpes simplex. **A,** Oral. **B,** Female genital. **C,** Male genital.
A and **B** from Habif, 1996; **C** from Morse, Moreland, 1996.

SKIN: MALIGNANT ABNORMALITIES

BASAL CELL CARCINOMA

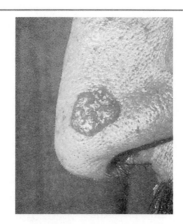

FIGURE 7-53

Basal cell carcinoma, the most commonly occurring skin cancer.

Courtesy Gary Monheit, MD, University of Alabama at Birmingham School of Medicine; from Thompson et al, 1993.

This most common malignant cutaneous neoplasm is commonly found on the face. Fair skin and solar exposure are risk factors. It occurs in various clinical forms including nodular, pigmented, cystic, sclerosing, and superficial (Figure 7-53).

SQUAMOUS CELL CARCINOMA

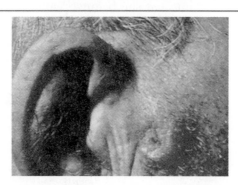

FIGURE 7-54

Squamous cell carcinoma.

Courtesy Gary Monheit, MD, University of Alabama at Birmingham School of Medicine; from Thompson et al, 1993.

This malignant tumor arises in the epithelium. It occurs most commonly in sun-exposed areas, particularly the scalp, back of hands, lower lip, and ear. The lesions are soft, mobile, elevated masses with a surface scale. The base of the lesion may be inflamed (Figure 7-54).

MALIGNANT MELANOMA

MNEMONICS

THE ABCD RULE OF MELANOMA

Here is a simple way to remember the characteristics that should alert you to the possibility of malignant melanoma.

A Asymmetry of lesion

B Borders; irregular

C Color blue/black or variegated

D Diameter > 6 mm

Malignant melanoma (Figure 7-55) is a skin cancer that develops from melanocytes. These cells migrate into the skin, eye, central nervous system, and mucous membrane during fetal development. Less than half of the melanomas develop from nevi; the majority arise de novo from melanocytes. The exact cause of malignancy is not known; heredity, hormonal factors, ultraviolet light exposure,

or an autoimmunologic effect may contribute to causation. Box 7-7 below lists relative risk factors for melanoma. Malignant melanoma is recognizable in its early stages and should be suspected in any patient with a history of change in a preexisting nevus or with a new pigmented lesion that exhibits any of the irregularities described in Box 7-7.

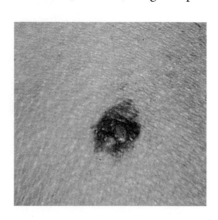

FIGURE 7-55

Malignant melanoma.

Courtesy Walter Tunnessen, MD, University of Pennsylvania, Philadelphia.

RISK FACTORS Melanoma	
Factor	**Increased Risk**
▪ Previous history	▪ 10× risk
▪ Family history	▪ 8× risk
▪ Immune suppression	▪ 4× risk
▪ Blistering sunburn before age 20	▪ 2× risk

BOX 7-7   **Findings Associated with Malignant Changes**

Sores that do not heal
Persistent lump or swelling
New or preexisting nevi that exhibit any of the following:
▪ Various shades of brown and black occurring with red, white, or blue and the half tones of pink or gray
▪ Notching or indentation of the border, with pigment streaming from the edges
▪ Loss of skin markings
▪ Development of a nodule, especially with erosion or ulceration
▪ Bleeding
▪ Changes in color, size, or thickness

KAPOSI SARCOMA

Kaposi sarcoma (KS) is a malignant tumor of the endothelium and epithelial layer of the skin. Lesions are characteristically soft, vascular, bluish-purple, and painless. Lesions may be either macular or papular and may appear as plaques, keloids, or ecchymotic areas (Figure 7-56). Until recently, KS was rare in the United States and was limited to a mild cutaneous form. With the spread of HIV infection, KS has become a common opportunistic infection. The form of the disease is aggressive, with cutaneous lesions, as well as lesions in the GI tract and other organs such as the lungs, liver, viscera, bones, and lymph nodes. Patients have varying degrees of cutaneous and systemic involvement. Diagnosis of KS is made by biopsy of suspect tissue or skin lesions.

A 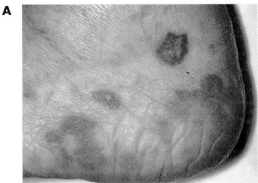 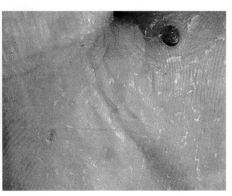 **B**

FIGURE 7-56
A, Violaceous plaques on the heel and lateral foot. **B,** Brown nodule of Kaposi sarcoma.

HAIR

ALOPECIA AREATA

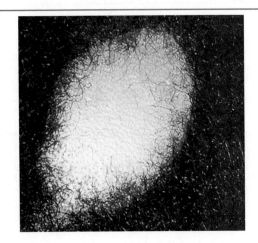

FIGURE 7-57

Alopecia areata.

Courtesy Stephen B. Tucker, MD, Department of Dermatology, University of Texas Health Science Center at Houston; from Thompson et al, 1993.

The sudden, rapid, patchy loss of hair, usually from the scalp or face, is called alopecia areata. The hair shaft is poorly formed and breaks off at the skin surface. Regrowth begins in 1 to 3 months. The prognosis for total regrowth is excellent in cases with limited involvement (Figure 7-57).

SCARRING ALOPECIA

This type of alopecia results from skin diseases of the scalp that cause scarring and destruction of hair follicles.

TRACTION ALOPECIA

Alopecia can result from prolonged tension of the hair. It can occur from wearing certain hairstyles such as braids or using hair rollers and hot combs. The area of loss corresponds directly to the area of stress. The scalp may or may not be inflamed.

HIRSUTISM

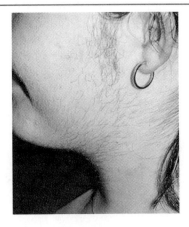

FIGURE 7-58

Facial hirsutism. Terminal hair growth is visible on the chin of this 40-year-old woman with idiopathic hirsutism.

From Lawrence, Cox, 1993.

Hirsutism is the growth of terminal hair in women in the male distribution pattern on the face, body, and pubic areas. Hirsutism may or may not be accompanied by other signs of virilization (Figure 7-58).

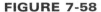

NAILS: INFECTION

PARONYCHIA

Inflammation of the paronychium produces redness, swelling, and tenderness at the lateral and proximal nail folds. Purulent drainage often accumulates under the cuticle. It can occur as an acute or chronic process. Chronic paronychia can produce rippling of the nails (Figure 7-59).

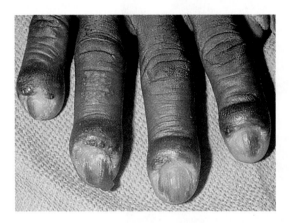

FIGURE 7-59

Chronic paronychia with nail dystrophy.

Courtesy Jaime A. Tschen, MD, Baylor College of Medicine, Department of Dermatology, Houston; from Thompson et al, 1993.

TINEA UNGUIUM

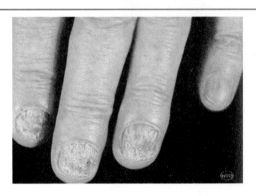

FIGURE 7-60

Tinea unguium.

Courtesy American Academy of Dermatology and Institute for Dermatologic Communication and Education, Evanston, Illinois.

Fungal infection of the nail occurs in four distinct patterns. In the most common form the distal nail plate turns yellow or white as hyperkeratotic debris accumulates, causing the nail to separate from the nail bed (onycholysis). The fungus grows in the nail plate, causing it to crumble (Figure 7-60).

NAILS: INJURY

INGROWN NAILS

Ingrown nails most commonly involve the large toe. The nail pierces the lateral nail fold and grows into the dermis, causing pain and swelling (Figure 7-61).

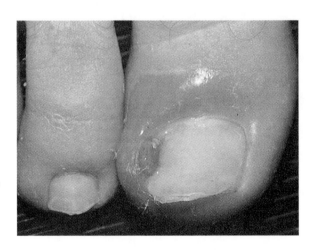

FIGURE 7-61

Ingrown toenail. Swelling and inflammation occur at lateral nail fold.

From White, 1994.

SUBUNGUAL HEMATOMA

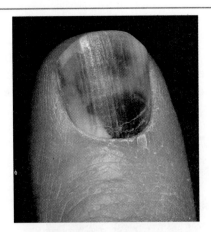

FIGURE 7-62
Subungual hematoma.
From Habif, 1996.

Trauma to the nail plate severe enough to cause immediate bleeding and pain produces a subungual hematoma. The amount of bleeding may be sufficient to cause separation and loss of the nail plate. Trauma to the proximal nail fold may also cause bleeding that is not apparent for several days. In either case, the hematoma remains until the nail grows out (Figure 7-62) or is drilled to release the blood and relieve the pressure.

LEUKONYCHIA PUNCTATA

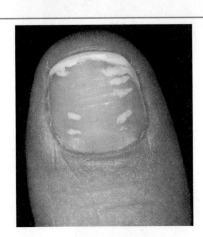

FIGURE 7-63
White spots on nail from injury (leukonychia punctata).
From Habif, 1996.

These white spots appear in the nail plate as a result of minor injury or manipulation of the cuticle. They either resolve spontaneously or grow out (Figure 7-63).

HABIT-TIC DEFORMITY

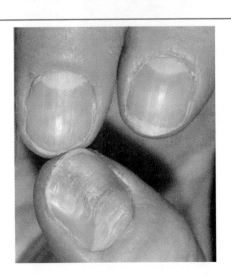

FIGURE 7-64
Habit-tic deformity.
From Habif, 1996.

This abnormality is caused by biting or picking the proximal nail fold of the thumb with the index fingernail. This results in horizontal sharp grooving in a band that extends to the tip of the nail (Figure 7-64).

ONYCHOLYSIS

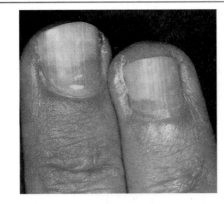

FIGURE 7-65
Onycholysis. Separation of nail plate starts at distal groove.
From Habif, 1996.

Onycholysis is loosening of the nail plate with separation from the nail bed that begins at the distal groove (Figure 7-65). This condition is associated most commonly with minor trauma to long fingernails. Other causes include psoriasis, *Candida* or *Pseudomonas* infections, allergic contact dermatitis, and hyperthyroidism.

CURVATURE

Inward folding of the lateral edges of the nail causes the nail bed to draw up and often become painful. Curvature is most common in the toenails and is thought to be caused by shoe compression (see Figure 7-15).

NAILS: CHANGES ASSOCIATED WITH SYSTEMIC DISEASE

KOILONYCHIA (SPOON NAILS)

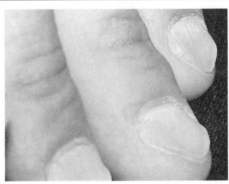

FIGURE 7-66
Koilonychia.
From White, 1994.

Central depression of the nail with lateral elevation of the nail plate produces a concave curvature and spoon appearance. This is associated with iron deficiency anemia, syphilis, fungal dermatoses, and hypothyroidism (Figure 7-66) (see also Figure 7-15).

BEAU LINES

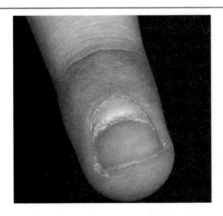

FIGURE 7-67
Beau lines following systemic disease.
From Habif, 1996.

Transverse depressions in all of the nails appear at the base of the lunula weeks after a stress that temporarily interrupts nail formation. Beau lines are associated with coronary occlusion, hypercalcemia, and skin disease. The grooves disappear when the nails grow out (Figure 7-67).

WHITE BANDING (TERRY NAILS)

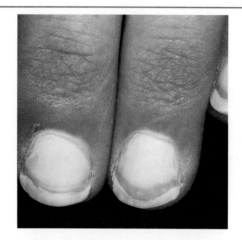

FIGURE 7-68

Terry nails: transverse white bands.

From Habif, 1996.

Transverse white bands cover the nail except for a narrow zone at the distal tip. The changes are associated with cirrhosis and hypoalbuminemia (Figure 7-68).

PSORIASIS

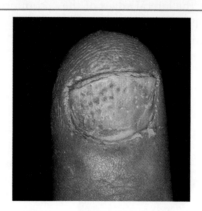

FIGURE 7-69

Nail pitting from psoriasis.

From Habif, 1996.

Psoriasis can produce pitting, onycholysis, discoloration, and subungual thickening. Yellow scaly debris often accumulates, elevating the nail plate. Severe psoriasis of the matrix and nail bed results in grossly malformed nails and splinter hemorrhages (Figure 7-69).

NAILS: PERIUNGUAL GROWTHS

WARTS

Warts are epidermal neoplasms caused by viral infection. They can occur at the nail folds and extend under the nail. A longitudinal nail groove may occur from warts located over the nail matrix (Figure 7-70).

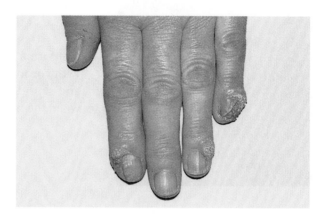

FIGURE 7-70

Periungual warts.

From Lawrence, Cox, 1993.

DIGITAL
MUCOUS CYSTS

These cysts contain a clear jelly-like substance and occur on the dorsal surface of the distal phalanx. A longitudinal nail groove may occur from cysts located at the proximal nail fold (Figure 7-71).

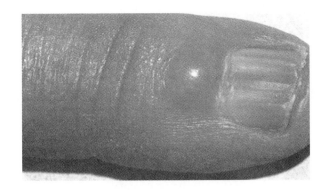

FIGURE 7-71
Digital mucous cyst causing a groove in the nail plate.
From White, 1994.

CHILDREN

CAFÉ AU LAIT PATCHES

FIGURE 7-72
Café au lait patches.

These coffee-colored patches may be either harmless or indicative of underlying disease. The presence of more than five patches with diameters of more than 1 cm in children under age 5 suggests neurofibromatosis (von Recklinghausen disease). Any café au lait patches should be considered suspicious by a beginning practitioner (Figure 7-72).

SEBORRHEIC
DERMATITIS

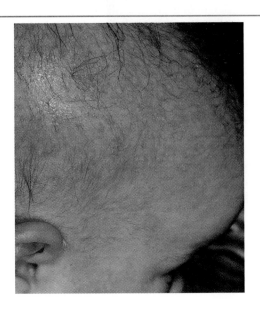

FIGURE 7-73
Seborrheic dermatitis.
From Habif, 1996.

This chronic, recurrent, erythematous scaling eruption is localized in areas where sebaceous glands are concentrated, such as scalp, back, intertriginous, and diaper areas. The scalp lesions are scaling, adherent, thick, yellow, and crusted ("cradle cap") and can spread over the ear and down the nape of the neck. Lesions elsewhere are erythematous, scaling, and fissured (Figure 7-73).

MILIARIA ("PRICKLY HEAT")

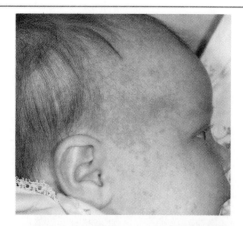

FIGURE 7-74
Miliaria in infant.
From Habif, 1996.

Miliaria is an irregular, red, macular rash caused by occlusion of sweat ducts during periods of heat and high humidity. Overdressed babies are prone to this condition in the summertime (Figure 7-74).

IMPETIGO

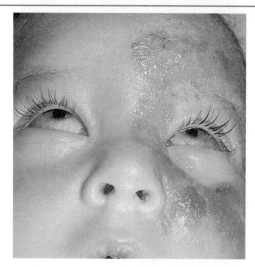

FIGURE 7-75
Impetigo. Note characteristic crusting.
Courtesy Antoinette Hood, MD, Department of Dermatology, Indiana University School of Medicine, Indianapolis.

This highly contagious staphylococcal or streptococcal infection of the epidermis commonly causes pruritus, burning, and regional lymphadenopathy. The initial lesion is a small erythematous macule that changes into a vesicle or bulla with a thin roof. Crusts with a characteristic honey color form from the exudate as the vesicles or bullae rupture (Figure 7-75).

ACNE VULGARIS

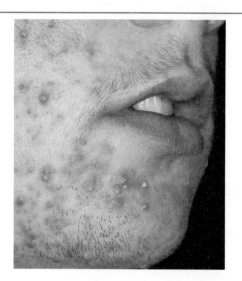

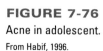

FIGURE 7-76
Acne in adolescent.
From Habif, 1996.

The inflamed lesions of acne involve stagnation of sebum and comedo formation in the pilosebaceous follicle, with bacterial invasion. Acne is seen most commonly in adolescents, though it may occur initially or continue into the adult years (Figure 7-76).

REDDENED PATCHINESS

Irregular reddened areas can occur on the nape of the neck, upper eyelids, forehead, and upper lip that suggest a richer capillary bed. These lesions include capillary hemangioma, nevus flammeus, nevus vasculosus, and telangiectatic nevus. They usually disappear by about 1 year of age, although they may occasionally recur, even in adults (Figure 7-77).

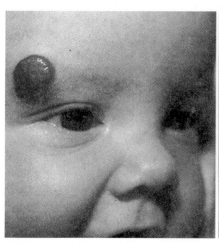
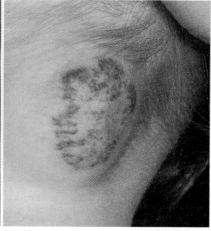

FIGURE 7-77
A, Strawberry hemangioma in infant. **B,** Cavernous hemangioma in infant.
From Habif, 1996.

CHICKENPOX (VARICELLA)

Chickenpox is an acute, highly communicable disease common in children and young adults, caused by the varicella-zoster virus. It is characterized by fever, mild malaise, and a pruritic maculopapular skin eruption that lasts for a few hours and then becomes vesicular. Lesions usually occur in successive outbreaks, with several stages of maturity present at one time. The lesions start on the scalp and trunk and spread centrifugally to the extremities. Lesions may also occur on the buccal mucosa, palate, or conjunctivae. The incubation period is 2 to 3 weeks; the period of communicability lasts from 1 or 2 days before onset of the rash until lesions have crusted over. Complications include conjunctival involvement, secondary bacterial infection, viral pneumonia, encephalitis, aseptic meningitis, myelitis, Guillain-Barré syndrome, and Reye syndrome (Figure 7-78).

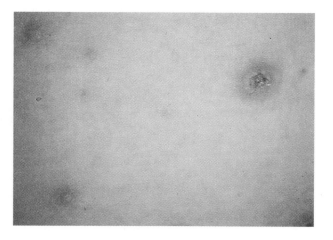

FIGURE 7-78
Chickenpox.
Courtesy Walter Tunnessen, MD, University of Pennsylvania School of Medicine, Philadelphia.

MEASLES (RUBEOLA)

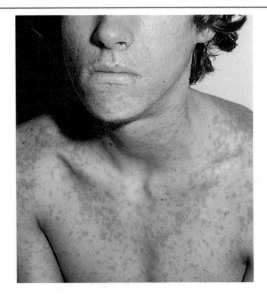

FIGURE 7-79
Rubeola.
From Zitelli, Davis, 1997.

Rubeola, also called hard measles or red measles, is a highly communicable viral disease. A characteristic prodromal fever, conjunctivitis, coryza, and bronchitis followed by a characteristic red blotchy rash occur. Koplik spots appear on the buccal mucosa, and a macular rash develops on the face and neck. The lesions become maculopapular and spread to the trunk and extremities in 24 to 48 hours in irregular confluent patches. The rash lasts 4 to 7 days. The incubation period is commonly 10 days; the period of communicability lasts from a few days before the fever to 4 days after appearance of the rash. Symptoms may be mild or severe. Complications involve infection of the respiratory tract and central nervous system. The disease is preventable by immunization (Figure 7-79).

GERMAN MEASLES (RUBELLA)

Rubella is a mild, febrile, highly communicable viral disease characterized by a generalized light pink to red maculopapular rash. During the prodromal period, low-grade fever, coryza, sore throat, and cough develop, followed by the appearance of a macular rash on the face and trunk that rapidly becomes papular. By the second day, the rash spreads to the upper and lower extremities and fades within 3 days. Reddish spots occur on the soft palate during the prodrome or on the first day of the rash (Forchheimer spots). The incubation period is 14 to 23 days; the period of communicability lasts from 1 week before to 4 days after the appearance of the rash. Infection during the first trimester of pregnancy may lead to infection of the fetus and may produce a variety of congenital anomalies (congenital rubella syndrome). The disease is preventable by immunization (Figure 7-80).

A
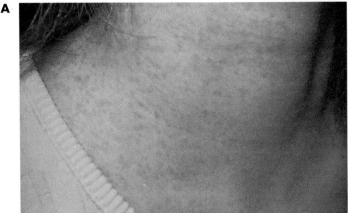

B
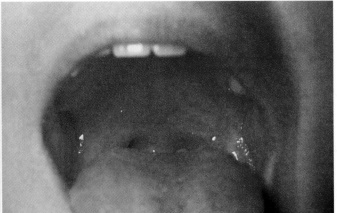

FIGURE 7-80
Rubella/German measles. **A,** The exanthem of rubella usually consists of a fine, pinkish-red, maculopapular eruption that appears first at the hairline and rapidly spreads cephalocaudally. Lesions tend to remain discrete. **B,** The presence of red palatal lesions (Forchheimer spots), seen in some patients on day 1 of the rash, and occipital and posterior cervical adenopathy are findings suggestive of rubella.
Courtesy Dr. Michael Sherlock; from Zitelli, Davis, 1997.

TRICHOTILLOMANIA

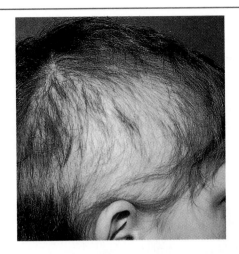

FIGURE 7-81
Trichotillomania in young child.
From Habif, 1996.

Loss of scalp hair can be caused by physical manipulation. Hair is twisted around the finger and pulled or rubbed until it breaks off. The act of manipulation is usually an unconscious habit. The affected area has an irregular border, and hair density is greatly reduced, but the site is not bald (Figure 7-81).

PATTERNS OF INJURY IN PHYSICAL ABUSE

Physical findings in children who are physically abused include bruises, burns, lacerations, scars, bony deformities, alopecia (hair loss), retinal hemorrhages, dental trauma, and head and abdominal injuries. Skin and hair abnormalities may be the most visible clues in detecting this problem. It is important to examine the skin that is usually covered by clothing. Some skin and hair findings commonly associated with physical abuse are described in the following paragraphs.

Bruises: These may be patterned consistent with the implement used such as belt marks (Figure 7-82), looped electric cord, and oval or finger tip grab marks. Bruising associated with abuse occurs over soft tissue; toddlers and older children who bruise themselves accidentally do so over bony prominences. Any bruise in an infant who is not yet developmentally able to be mobile should be cause for concern.

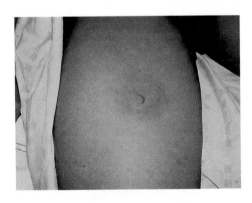

FIGURE 7-82
This contusion in the configuration of a closed horseshoe with a central linear abrasion was inflicted with a belt buckle.
From Zitelli, Davis, 1997.

PATTERNS OF INJURY IN PHYSICAL ABUSE—CONT'D

Lacerations: Lacerations of the frenulum and lips are associated with forced feeding. Human bites can cause breaks in the skin and leave a characteristic bite mark.

Burns: Patterns that are common include scald burns in stocking and glove distribution (hand or feet placed on hot surface or immersed), buttock burns consistent with immersion (Figure 7-83), and cigarette burns (Figure 7-84) (a characteristic small round burn), often on areas hidden by clothing. The absence of splash marks or a pattern consistent with spills of hot liquids may be helpful in differentiating accidental from deliberate burns.

Hair loss: Patchy hair loss or bald spots, in the absence of a scalp disorder (such as ringworm), may indicate repeated hair pulling.

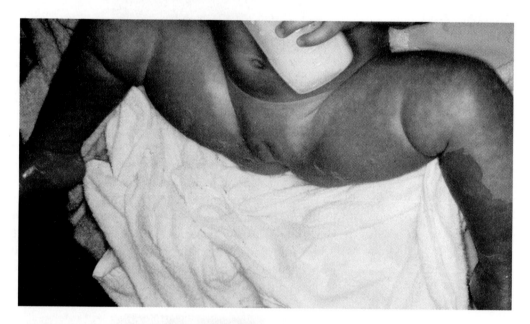

FIGURE 7-83

Burns on the perineum, thighs, legs, and feet.

Courtesy Dr. Thomas Layton, Mercy Hospital, Pittsburgh; from Zitelli, Davis, 1997.

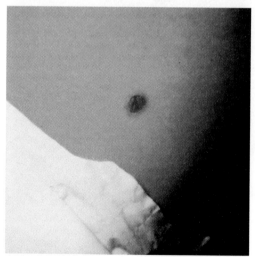

FIGURE 7-84

Cigarette burn. This older burn has begun to granulate.

From Zitelli, Davis, 1997.

OLDER ADULTS

STASIS DERMATITIS

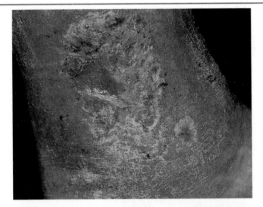

FIGURE 7-85
Stasis dermatitis in older adult with impaired peripheral circulation.
From Habif, 1996.

The lower legs and ankles are affected with erythematous, scaling, weeping patches. Stasis dermatitis is secondary to edema of chronic peripheral vascular disease (Figure 7-85).

SOLAR KERATOSIS (SENILE ACTINIC KERATOSIS)

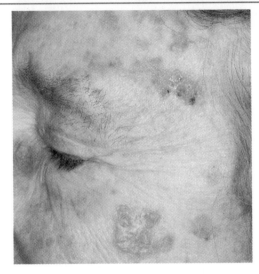

FIGURE 7-86
Actinic keratosis in older adult in area of sun exposure.
From Habif, 1996.

This disorder produces a slightly raised erythematous lesion that is usually less than 1 cm in diameter with an irregular, rough surface. The lesion is most common on the dorsal surface of the hands, arms, neck, and face. Solar keratosis occurs secondary to chronic sun damage and has malignant potential (Figure 7-86).

PHYSICAL ABUSE IN THE ELDERLY

Abuse in older adults can assume the form of physical abuse, neglect, sexual abuse, psychologic abuse, financial abuse, or violation of rights. Physical neglect is probably the most frequent type of abuse encountered by health care professionals. However, be aware that when one form of abuse is present, it is typically accompanied by other forms.

Physical abuse and neglect may present with clues that aid in detection. Assessment of general appearance may indicate poor hygiene, emaciation, healed fractures with deformity, and unexplained trauma. Carefully inspect the skin, particularly on the hidden areas such as the axillae, inner thighs, soles of the feet, palms, and abdomen, looking for bruising, burns, abrasions, or areas of tenderness. Bruising on extensor surfaces is common and usually occurs accidentally; bruising at various stages of resolution located on inner soft surfaces is more likely to indicate abuse.

Careful history taking is essential. When abuse is suspected, it is important to ask direct questions such as, "Is anyone hurting or harming you?" or "Have you been confined against your will?" This should occur in a private setting away from an accompanying family member or caregiver. Determination of mental status is also essential (see Chapter 4), as unintended self-neglect or abuse is also possible. If the patient is cognitively impaired, abuse by another may still be present but needs to be corroborated.

Check it out— 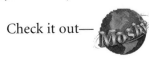 *http:www1.mosby.com/physexam_seidel*

CHAPTER 8

LYMPHATIC SYSTEM

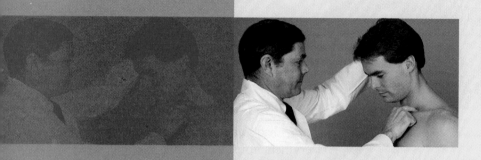

ANATOMY AND PHYSIOLOGY

The lymphatic system consists of lymph fluid, the collecting ducts, and various tissues including the lymph nodes, spleen, thymus, tonsils and adenoids, and Peyer patches. Bits of lymph tissue are found in other parts of the body, including the mucosa of the stomach and appendix, bone marrow, and lungs (Figure 8-1). The entire mass of the system is no more than 3% of the total body weight. An integral part of the immune system, it supports a network of defense against the invasion of microorganisms.

The immune system protects the body from the antigenic substances of invading organisms, removes damaged cells from the circulation, and provides a partial, but often inefficient, barrier to the maturation of malignant cells within the body. When it functions well, the individual is *immunocompetent.* When it fails, for whatever reason, *immunoincompetence* can lead to a variety of illnesses: allergic, immunodeficient (either congenital or acquired [e.g., HIV infection]), or autoimmune (i.e., allergy to oneself such as lupus erythematosus). Tissue rejection of transplanted organs, on the other hand, is an unwanted manifestation of competence.

Every tissue supplied by blood vessels has lymphatic vessels except the placenta and the brain. This wide-ranging presence is essential to the system's role in immunologic and metabolic processes. That role, not yet completely understood, involves the following:

- Movement of lymph fluid in a closed circuit with the cardiovascular system
- Production of lymphocytes within the lymph nodes, tonsils, adenoids, spleen, and bone marrow
- Production of antibodies
- Phagocytosis, the ingestion and digestion by cells of solid substances such as other cells, bacteria, bits of necrosed tissue or foreign particles, a specific function of cells that line the sinuses of lymph nodes
- Absorption of fat and fat-soluble substances from the intestinal tract
- Manufacture of blood when the primary sources are pathophysiologically compromised

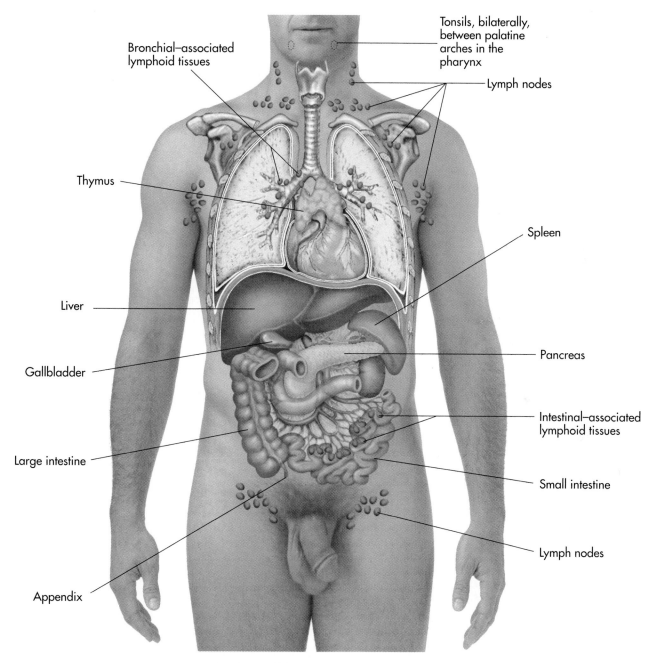

FIGURE 8-1
Lymphatic system (lymphoreticular system).

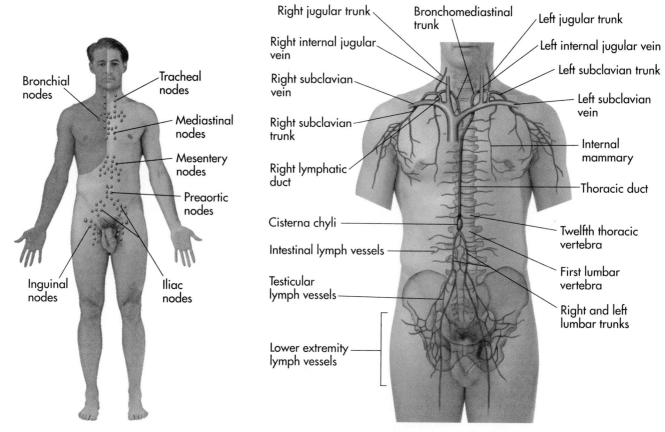

FIGURE 8-2

Lymphatic drainage pathways. Shaded area of the body is drained via the right lymphatic duct, which is formed by the union of three vessels: right jugular trunk, right subclavian trunk, and right bronchomediastinal trunk. Lymph from the remainder of the body enters the venous system by way of the thoracic duct.

In addition, the lymphatic system plays an unwanted role in providing at least one pathway for the spread of malignancy.

Lymph is a clear, sometimes opalescent and sometimes yellow-tinged fluid; it contains a variety of white blood cells (mostly lymphocytes) and occasional red blood cells. The lymphatic and cardiovascular systems are intimately related. The fluids and proteins that constitute lymphatic fluid originally move from the bloodstream into the interstitial spaces. They are then collected throughout the body by a profusion of microscopic tubules (Figure 8-2). These tubules unite, forming larger ducts that collect lymph and carry it to the lymph nodes around the body.

The lymph nodes receive lymph from the collecting ducts in the various regions (Figures 8-3 to 8-11), passing it on through efferent vessels. Ultimately the large ducts merge into the venous system at the subclavian veins.

The drainage point for the right upper body is a lymphatic trunk that empties into the right subclavian vein. The thoracic duct, the major vessel of the lymphatic system, drains lymph from the rest of the body into the left subclavian vein. It returns the various fluids and proteins to the cardiovascular system, forming a closed but porous circle.

Text continues on p. 224.

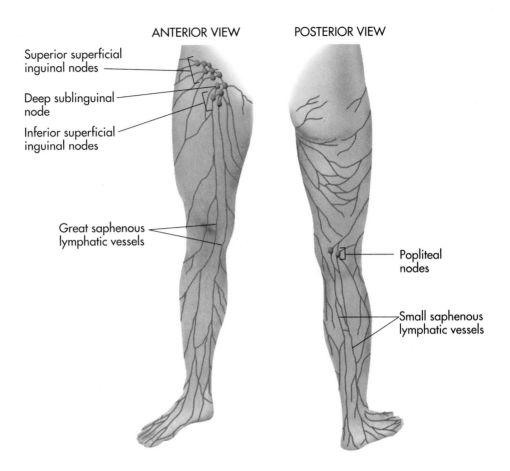

ANTERIOR VIEW   POSTERIOR VIEW

Superior superficial inguinal nodes

Deep sublinguinal node

Inferior superficial inguinal nodes

Great saphenous lymphatic vessels

Popliteal nodes

Small saphenous lymphatic vessels

FIGURE 8-3
Lymphatic drainage of lower extremity.

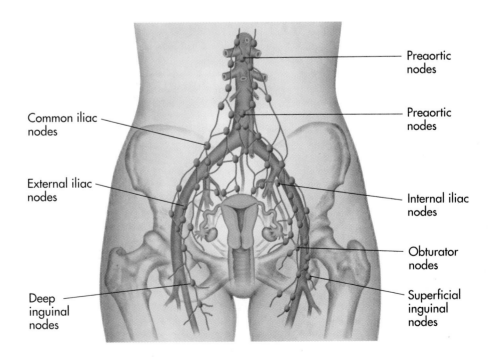

Common iliac nodes

External iliac nodes

Deep inguinal nodes

Preaortic nodes

Preaortic nodes

Internal iliac nodes

Obturator nodes

Superficial inguinal nodes

FIGURE 8-4
Lymphatic drainage of female genital tract.

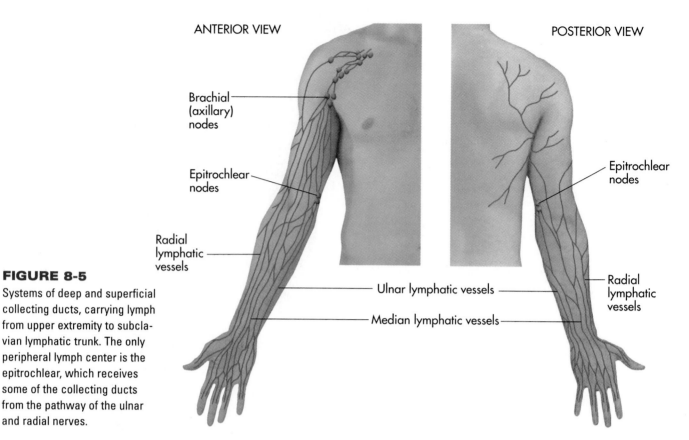

ANTERIOR VIEW

POSTERIOR VIEW

Brachial (axillary) nodes

Epitrochlear nodes

Radial lymphatic vessels

Epitrochlear nodes

Radial lymphatic vessels

Ulnar lymphatic vessels

Median lymphatic vessels

FIGURE 8-5

Systems of deep and superficial collecting ducts, carrying lymph from upper extremity to subclavian lymphatic trunk. The only peripheral lymph center is the epitrochlear, which receives some of the collecting ducts from the pathway of the ulnar and radial nerves.

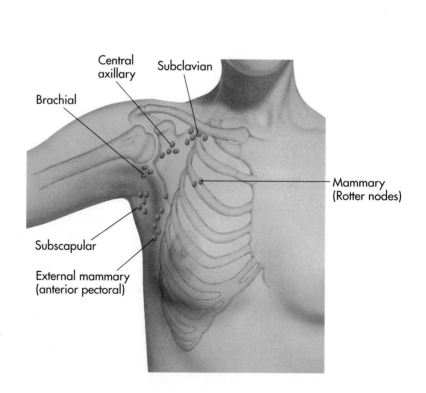

Central axillary

Subclavian

Brachial

Mammary (Rotter nodes)

Subscapular

External mammary (anterior pectoral)

FIGURE 8-6

Six groups of lymph nodes may be distinguished in the axillary fossa.

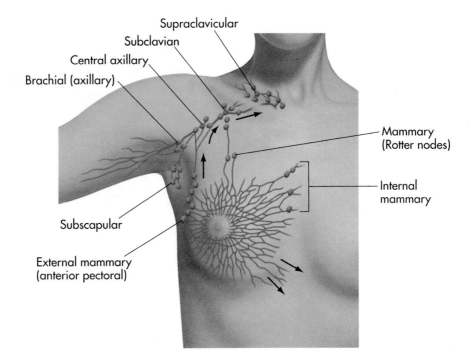

FIGURE 8-7
Lymphatic drainage of breast.

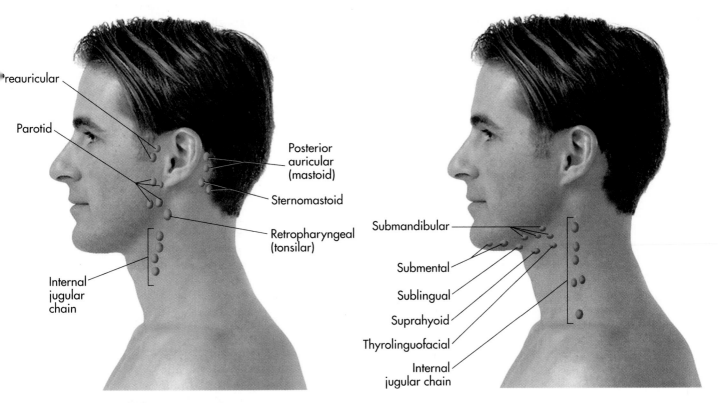

FIGURE 8-8
Lymph nodes involved with the ear.

FIGURE 8-9
Lymph nodes involved with the tongue.

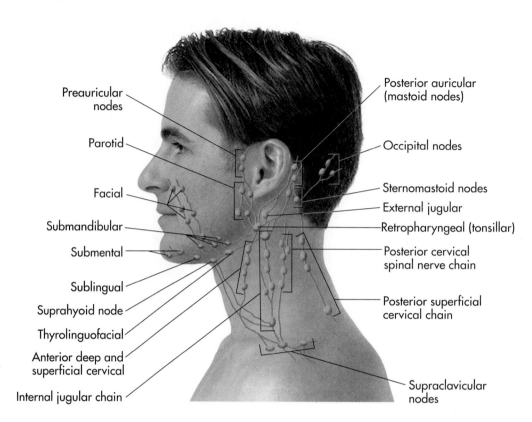

Preauricular nodes

Posterior auricular (mastoid nodes)

Parotid

Occipital nodes

Facial

Sternomastoid nodes

External jugular

Submandibular

Retropharyngeal (tonsillar)

Submental

Posterior cervical spinal nerve chain

Sublingual

Suprahyoid node

Posterior superficial cervical chain

Thyrolinguofacial

Anterior deep and superficial cervical

Internal jugular chain

Supraclavicular nodes

FIGURE 8-10
Lymphatic drainage system of head and neck. If the group of nodes is often referred to by another name, the second name appears in parentheses.

The lymphatic system has no built-in pumping mechanisms of its own. Because it depends on the cardiovascular system for this, the movement of lymph is sluggish compared with that of blood. As lymph fluid volume increases, it flows faster in response to mounting capillary pressure, greater permeability of the capillary walls of the cardiovascular system, increased bodily or metabolic activity, and massage. Conversely, mechanical obstruction will slow or stop the movement of lymph, dilating the system. The permeability of the lymphatic system is protective; if it is obstructed, lymph may diffuse into the vascular system, or collateral connecting channels may develop.

LYMPH NODES

Lymph nodes usually occur in groups. Superficial nodes are located in subcutaneous connective tissues, and deeper nodes lie beneath the fascia of muscles and within the various body cavities. The nodes are numerous and tiny, but some of them may have diameters as large as 0.5 to 1 cm.

The superficial lymph nodes are the gateway to assessing the health of the entire lymphatic system. Readily accessible to inspection and palpation, they provide some of the earliest clues to the presence of infection or malignancy.

LYMPHOCYTES

Lymphocytes are central to the body's response to antigenic substances. They are not identical in size or function. Some are small, approximately 7 to 8 mm in diameter; others range in size to as much as five times that of the small lymphocyte. Some are long-lived, and others short-lived. The maximum life expectancy of lymphocytes is perhaps 200 days. They arise from a number of sites in the body: the lymph nodes, tonsils, adenoids, and spleen, but primarily the bone marrow, where early cells—"stem cells"—capable of developing in a variety of pathways, arise. Lymphocytes derived primarily from bone marrow—B lymphocytes—produce antibodies and are characterized by the various arrangements of immunoglobulins on their surface.

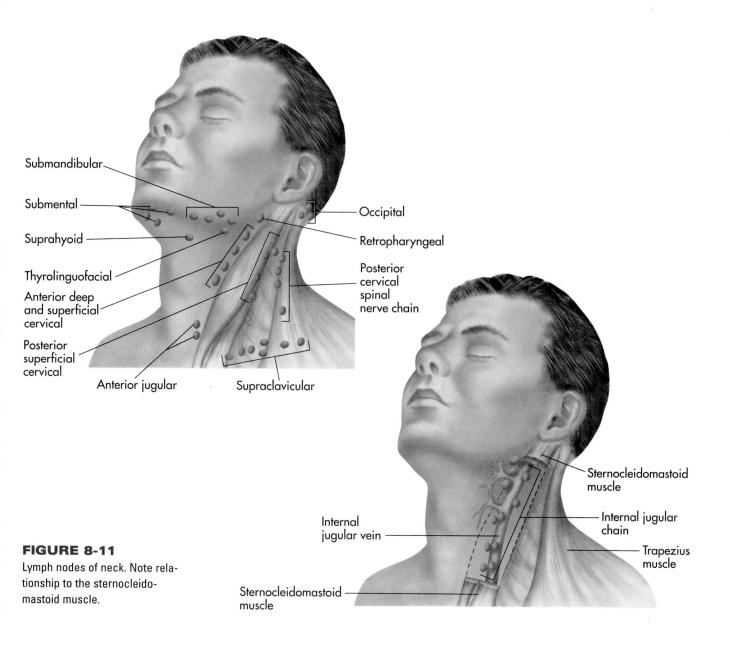

FIGURE 8-11
Lymph nodes of neck. Note relationship to the sternocleidomastoid muscle.

Marrow-derived cells, which flow first to the thymus, can be further differentiated in the thymus as T lymphocytes. They can sense the difference in cells of the body that have been invaded by any foreign substance, for example, a living virus, bacterium, or parasite; some invasive chemical; or even a malignant change. Found in profusion in the centers of lymph nodes, T lymphocytes have an important role in controlling the immune responses brought about by B lymphocytes. There are two types of immunity, humoral (involving the antibodies produced by B cells) and cellular (involving attacks on "invaders" by the cells themselves). Among lymphocytes, B cells have a relatively short life span of 3 to 4 days; T cells, four or five times as numerous as B cells, have a life span of 100 to 200 days. An increased number of lymphocytes in the blood represents a systemic response to most viral infections and to some bacterial infections.

THYMUS

The thymus is located in the superior mediastinum, extending upward into the lower neck. In early life the thymus is essential to the development of the protective immune function (Figure 8-12). It is the site for production of T lymphocytes, the effector cells for cell-mediated immunity reactions and the controlling agent for the humoral immune responses generated by B lymphocytes. In adult life, however, it has little or no demonstrated function.

SPLEEN

The spleen is situated in the left upper quadrant of the abdominal cavity between the stomach and the diaphragm. A highly vascular organ, it is composed of two systems: the white pulp, made up of lymphatic nodules and diffuse lymphatic tissue, and the red pulp, made up of venous sinusoids. The spleen is a blood-forming organ early in life, a site for the storage of red corpuscles, and—with its plethora of blood-filtering macrophages—part of the body's defense system. Its examination therefore is essential to the evaluation of the immune system. (See Chapter 15, Abdomen, for further discussion of the spleen.)

TONSILS AND ADENOIDS

The palatine tonsils are commonly referred to as "the tonsils" without further description. Small and diamond shaped, they are set between the palatine arches on either side of the pharynx, just beyond the base of the tongue. Composed principally of lymphoid tissue, the tonsils are organized as follicles and crypts, covered by mucous membrane. The pharyngeal tonsils, or adenoids, are located at the nasopharyngeal border. When the adenoids are enlarged as a result of frequent bacterial or viral invasion, they can obstruct the nasopharyngeal passageway.

PEYER PATCHES

Peyer patches are small, raised areas of lymph tissue on the mucosa of the small intestine. They consist of many clustered lymphoid nodules, serving the intestinal tract.

INFANTS AND CHILDREN

The immune system and the lymphoid system begin developing at about 20 weeks' gestation. The ability to produce antibodies is still immature at birth, thus increasing an infant's vulnerability to infection during the first few months of life. The mass of lymphoid tissue is relatively plentiful in infants, increases during childhood, especially between 6 and 9 years of age, and then regresses to adult levels by puberty (see Figure 5-3, Chapter 5, Growth and Measurement).

The thymus is at its largest relative to the rest of the body shortly after birth but reaches its greatest absolute weight at puberty. Then it begins to involute, replacing much of its tissue with fat and becoming a rudimentary organ in the adult.

The palatine tonsils, like all lymphoid tissue, are much larger during early childhood than after puberty. An enlargement of the tonsils in children is not necessarily an indication of problems.

The lymph nodes have the same distribution in children as in adults. The finding of small, palpable nodes in the neonate is not unusual. However, they react readily to any mild stimulus and may quickly become larger, particularly in the cervical and postauricular chains. Supraclavicular nodes are not usually found, and their presence, associated with a high incidence of malignancy, is always a cause for concern. Circumcision does not increase the likelihood of the finding of inguinal nodes. It is possible that the infant's relatively large mass of lymphoid tissue is needed to compensate for a rather immature ability to produce antibodies, thus adding to the demand for filtration and phagocytosis.

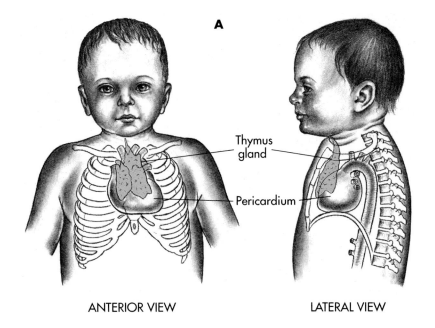

ANTERIOR VIEW   LATERAL VIEW

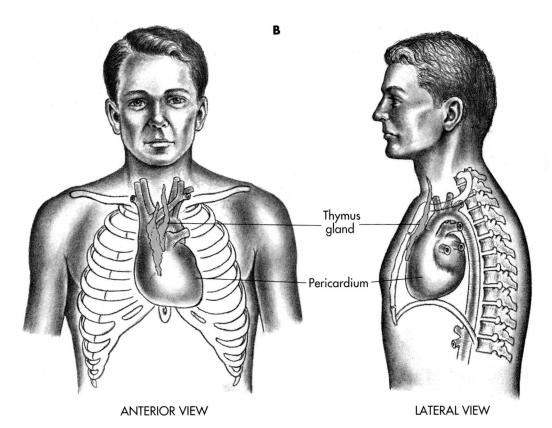

ANTERIOR VIEW   LATERAL VIEW

FIGURE 8-12

Location of thymus gland and its size relative to the rest of the body. **A,** During infancy. **B,** During adult life.

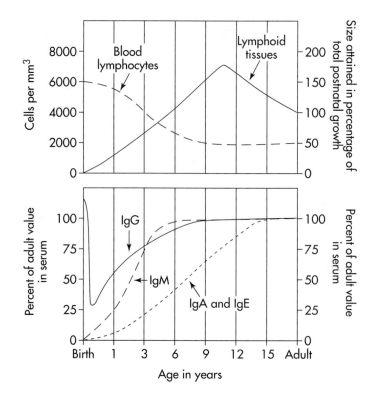

FIGURE 8-13

Relative levels of presence and function of the immune factors.

The lymphatic system gradually reaches adult competency during childhood (Figure 8-13).

PREGNANT WOMEN

For implantation and fetal development to occur, changes occur in the immune system during pregnancy. These changes are not fully understood but seem to reflect a balance between enhancement of certain immune mechanisms and suppression of others. During pregnancy, the leukocyte count increases from a usual level of about 7200 cells/mm³ at 2 months and reaches a plateau during the second and third trimesters at a mean level of 10,350/mm³, with a usual range of 6000 to 12,000/mm³. This increase is due to polymorphonuclear leukocytes, as lymphocytes do not increase in number.

There is impaired immunologic response mediated both by cellular and humoral mechanisms. T-cell function depression occurs (as a result of a change in the helper T cells/suppressor T cells ratio), which increases attack rate, morbidity, and mortality from viral and opportunistic infections. However, immunologic factors may ameliorate certain inflammatory conditions found in autoimmune disorders. Normal T-cell response returns at 1 month postpartum (Gladman and Urowitz, 1995; Priddy, 1997).

OLDER ADULTS

The number of lymph nodes may diminish and size may decrease with advanced age; some of the lymphoid elements are lost. The nodes of older patients are more likely to be fibrotic and fatty than those of the young, a contributing factor in an impaired ability to resist infection.

REVIEW OF RELATED HISTORY

PRESENT PROBLEM

- Bleeding
  - Site: nose, mouth, gums, rectal (blood in stools; black, tarry stools), skin petechiae, easy bruising, blood in vomitus
  - Character: onset, frequency, duration, amount, color (bright red brown, coffee-colored)
  - Associated symptoms: pallor, dizziness, headache, shortness of breath
- Enlarged nodes (bumps, kernels, swollen glands)
  - Character: onset, location, duration, number, tenderness
  - Associated symptoms: pain, fever, redness, warmth, red streaks, itching (some tumors cause pruritus)
  - Predisposing factors: infection, surgery, trauma
- Swelling of extremity
  - Unilateral or bilateral, intermittent or constant, duration
  - Predisposing factors: cardiac or renal disorder, surgery, infection, trauma, venous insufficiency
  - Associated symptoms: warmth, redness or discoloration, ulceration
  - Efforts at treatment and their effect: support stockings, elevation
- Medications: chemotherapy, antibiotics

PAST MEDICAL HISTORY

- Chest x-rays
- Tuberculosis and other skin testing
- Blood transfusions, use of blood products
- Chronic illness: cardiac, renal, malignancy, HIV infection (see the Risk Factors box)
- Surgery: trauma to regional lymph nodes
- Recurrent infections

FAMILY HISTORY

- Malignancy
- Anemia
- Recent infections
- Tuberculosis
- Agammaglobulinemia, severe combined immune deficiency, other immune disorders
- Hemophilia

INFANTS AND CHILDREN

- Recurrent infections: tonsillitis, adenoiditis, bacterial infections, oral candidiasis, chronic diarrhea
- Present or recent infections, trauma distal to nodes
- Poor growth, failure to thrive
- Loss of interest in play or eating
- Immunization history
- Maternal HIV infection
- Hemophilia
- Illness in siblings

PREGNANT WOMEN

- Weeks of gestation, estimated date of delivery
- Exposure to rubella and other infections
- Presence of children and pets in household

OLDER ADULTS

- Present or recent infection or trauma distal to nodes
- Delayed healing

RISK FACTORS   HIV Infection

Adolescents and Adults

Sexual contact with persons infected with HIV
Men with history of homosexual or bisexual activities
Heterosexual contact with homosexual or bisexual men
Multiple and indiscriminate sexual contacts
- Prostitution
- Unprotected sexual activity with persons of known history of risk or unknown history

IV drug use
- Parenteral exposure to HIV–blood-contaminated needles and/or syringes
- Sexual contact with IV drug users

Hemophilia
- Transfusion with infected blood or blood concentrates (Factor VIII, Factor IX) (particularly in the era *before* blood bank screening for HIV)

Blood transfusion
- Transfusion with infected blood or blood concentrates (particularly in the era *before* blood bank screening for HIV)

Work related *(very rare)*
- Rupture of the skin with needles or other sharp objects contaminated with the blood of an HIV-positive patient

Infants and Children

Mother either with or at risk for HIV infection
- During gestation
- At parturition
- During breast-feeding

Hemophilia
- Same as adults

Blood transfusion
- Same as adults

Sexual abuse

EXAMINATION AND FINDINGS

EQUIPMENT

- Centimeter ruler
- Marking (skin) pencil

The lymphatic system is examined by inspection and palpation, region by region as you examine the other body systems, and also by palpating the spleen, an integral part of the system (see Chapter 15, Abdomen, p. 540 for further discussion of the spleen). On occasion you may prefer to examine the entire lymphatic system at once, exploring all the areas in which the nodes are accessible, regardless of their distribution. Individual chapters in this book discuss the lymphatic system in specific body areas. Always during this part of the examination ask the patient if he or she is aware of any "lumps."

INSPECTION AND PALPATION

Inspect each area of the body for apparent lymph nodes, edema, erythema, red streaks, and skin lesions. Using the pads of the second, third, and fourth fingers, gently palpate for superficial lymph nodes (Box 8-1; Figure 8-14). Try to detect any inapparent enlargement, and note the consistency, mobility, tenderness, size, and warmth of the nodes. In areas where the skin is more mobile, move the skin over the area of the nodes. Press lightly at first, increasing pressure gradually. Heavier pressure alone can push nodes out of the way before you have had a chance to recognize their presence. Easily palpable lymph nodes are generally not found in healthy adults. Superficial nodes that are accessible to palpation but not large or firm enough to be felt are common. You may detect small, movable, discrete "shotty" nodes less than a centimeter in diameter that move under your fingers. When the node seems fixed in its setting, there is a greater cause for concern.

MNEMONICS

IF AN ENLARGED LYMPH NODE IS FOUND, EXAMINE: PALS

P   Primary site
A   All associated nodes
L   Liver
S   Spleen

Modified from Shipman, 1984.

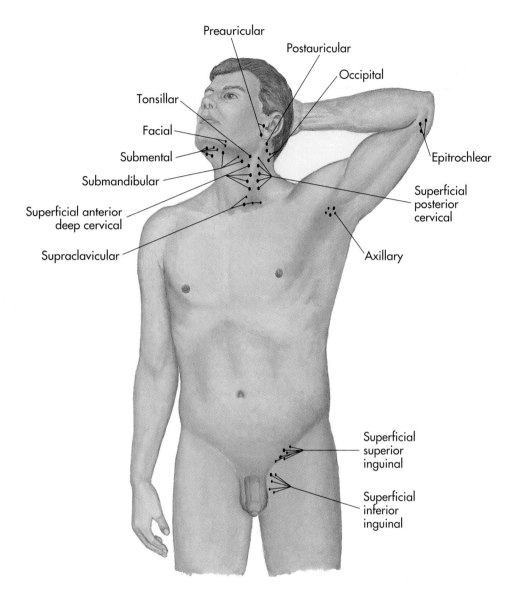

FIGURE 8-14
Some of the accessible lymph nodes.

BOX 8-1	The Lymph Nodes Most Accessible to Inspection and Palpation

Obviously, the more superficial the node, the more accessible.

The "Necklace" of Nodes

Parotid and retropharyngeal (tonsillar)
Submandibular
Submental
Sublingual (facial)
Superficial anterior cervical
Superficial posterior cervical
Preauricular and postauricular
Sternocleidomastoid
Occipital
Supraclavicular

The Arms

Axillary
Epitrochlear (cubital)

The Legs

Superficial superior inguinal
Superficial inferior inguinal
Occasionally, popliteal

When enlarged lymph nodes are encountered, explore the accessible adjacent areas and regions drained by those nodes for signs of possible infection or malignancy. Examine other regions for enlargement. Enlarged lymph nodes in any region should be characterized according to location, size, shape, consistency, tenderness, movability or fixation to surrounding tissues, and discreteness. Lymph nodes that are enlarged and juxtaposed so that they feel like a large mass rather than discrete nodes are described as "matted." Marking the skin with a skin pencil to define the extent of the node at the 12, 3, 6, and 9 o'clock positions is helpful as a guide to the assessment of change.

Note if there is tenderness on touch or on rebound, the degree of discoloration or redness, and any unusual increase in vascularity, heat, or pulsations. (If bruits are audible with the stethoscope, it may be a blood vessel, not a lymph node.) Check to see if any large mass transilluminates when you are uncertain of its nature; as a rule, nodes do not and cysts do. Lymph nodes that are large, fixed or matted, inflamed, or tender indicate a problem. Tenderness is almost always indicative of inflammation; cancerous nodes are not usually tender. With bacterial infection, nodes may become warm or tender to the touch, matted, and much less discrete, particularly if the infection persists. It is possible to infer the site of an infection from the pattern of lymph node enlargement. For example, infections of the ear will usually drain to the preauricular, retropharyngeal, and deep cervical nodes (see Figure 8-8). A child with such an infection is apt to complain of an earache, although the pain originates in a node.

Lymph nodes to which a malignancy has spread are not usually tender. They vary greatly in size, from tiny to many centimeters in diameter. They are sometimes discrete and tend to be harder than expected. Involvement is often asymmetric; contralateral nodes in similar locations may not be palpable.

In tuberculosis the lymph nodes are usually "cold" (actually, body temperature), soft, matted, and often not tender or painful.

Features of a lump are described in the mnemonics box in the margin.

Each of these observations suggests an aspect of the physical examination of a "lump." If you keep them in mind, you can provide an accurate written description for the record by describing each of the observations in sequence. The differentiation of an enlarged lymph node from other masses will depend on many variables, for example, a site incompatible with the distribution of nodes, or a palpable sensation (thrill, consistency) not possible with the basic structure of nodes (Box 8-2).

BOX 8-2   Some Conditions Simulating Lymph Node Enlargement

DIFFERENTIAL DIAGNOSIS

Lymphangioma
Cystic hygroma (thin-walled, contains clear lymph fluid)
Hemangioma (tends to feel spongy; appears reddish-blue, depending on size and extent of angiomatous involvement
Branchial cleft cyst (sometimes accompanied by a tiny orifice in the neck on a line extending to the ear)
Thyroglossal duct cyst
Granular cell tumor
Laryngocele
Esophageal diverticulum
Thyroid goiter
Graves disease
Hashimoto thyroiditis
Parotid swelling (e.g., from mumps or tumor)

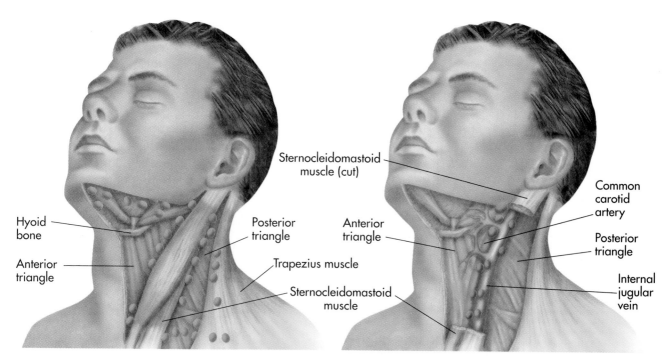

FIGURE 8-15
The triangles of the neck.

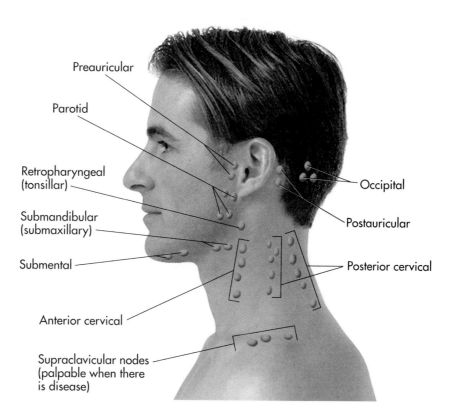

FIGURE 8-16
Palpable lymph nodes of the head and neck.

HEAD AND NECK

Palpate the entire neck lightly for nodes. The anterior border of the sternocleidomastoid muscle is the dividing line for the anterior and posterior triangles of the neck and is a useful landmark for describing location. The muscles and bones of the neck together create these "triangles" (Figure 8-15).

Bending the patient's head slightly forward or to the side will ease taut tissues and allow better accessibility to palpation. Feel for nodes on the head in the following six-step sequence (Figure 8-16):

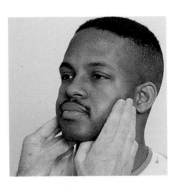

FIGURE 8-17
Palpation of preauricular lymph nodes. Compare the nodes bilaterally.

1. The occipital nodes at the base of the skull
2. The postauricular nodes located superficially over the mastoid process
3. The preauricular nodes just in front of the ear (Figure 8-17)
4. The parotid and retropharyngeal (tonsillar) nodes at the angle of the mandible
5. The submandibular nodes halfway between the angle and the tip of the mandible
6. The submental nodes in the midline behind the tip of the mandible

Then move down to the neck, palpating in the following four-step sequence:

1. The superficial cervical nodes at the sternocleidomastoid muscle
2. The posterior cervical nodes along the anterior border of the trapezius muscle (Figure 8-18)
3. The cervical nodes deep to the sternocleidomastoid (The deep cervical nodes may be difficult to feel if you press too vigorously. Probe gently with your thumb and fingers around the muscle.)
4. The supraclavicular areas, probing deeply in the angle formed by the clavicle and the sternocleidomastoid muscle, the area of Virchow's nodes (Figure 8-19). (Detection of these nodes should always be considered a cause for concern.)

On occasion, postauricular nodes affected by ear infection, particularly external otitis, may be surrounded by some cellulitis. This may cause the ears to protrude.

Supraclavicular nodes are frequently the sites of metastatic disease, because they are located at the end of the thoracic duct and other associated lymphatic ducts. A Virchow node in the left supraclavicular region may be the result of either abdominal or thoracic malignancy. Mediastinal collecting ducts from the lungs go to both sides of the neck, and supraclavicular nodes may be palpated on both sides.

AXILLAE

Think of the axillary examination by imagining a pentagonal structure: the pectoral muscles anteriorly, the back muscles (latissimus dorsi and subscapularis) posteriorly, the rib cage medially, the upper arm laterally, and the axilla at the apex. Let the soft tissues roll between your fingers, the chest wall, and muscles as you palpate. A firm, deliberate, yet gentle touch will feel less ticklish to the patient.

FIGURE 8-18
Palpation of posterior cervical nodes. Dorsal surfaces (pads) of the fingertips are used to palpate along the anterior surface of the trapezius muscle and then moved slowly in a circular motion toward the posterior surface of the sternocleidomastoid muscle.

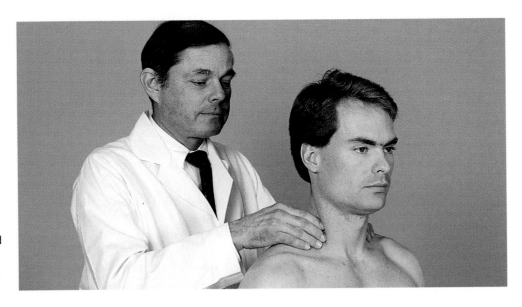

On palpation of the axillary lymph nodes, support the patient's forearm with your contralateral arm and bring the palm of your examining hand flat into the axilla, or alternatively let the patient's forearm rest on that of your examining hand (Figure 8-20). Rotate your fingertips and palm, feeling the nodes; if they are palpable, attempt to glide your fingers beneath the nodes.

A more complete examination of the breast, the axilla, and adjacent areas is described in Chapter 14 (Breasts and Axillae).

OTHER LYMPH NODES

Use a systematic approach when palpating other sites of lymph node clusterings. Move the hand in a circular fashion, probing gently without pressing hard. Relieve tension by flexion of the extremity. To palpate the epitrochlear nodes, support the el-

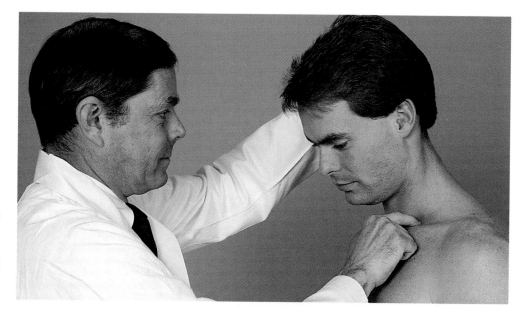

FIGURE 8-19
Palpation for supraclavicular lymph nodes. The patient is encouraged to relax the musculature of the upper extremities so that the clavicles drop. The examiner's free hand is used to flex the patient's head forward to relax the soft tissues of the anterior neck. The fingers are hooked over the clavicle lateral to the sternocleidomastoid muscle.

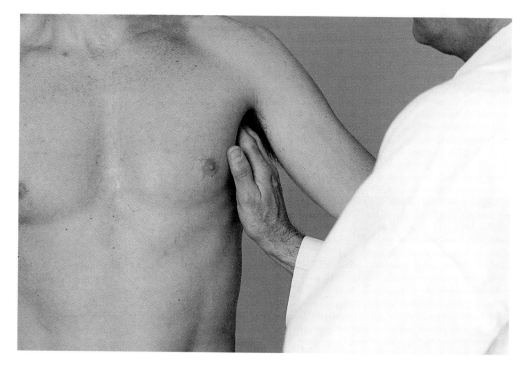

FIGURE 8-20
Soft tissues of axilla are gently rolled against the chest wall and the muscles surrounding the axilla.

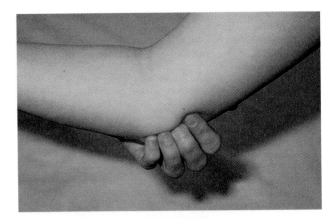

FIGURE 8-21
Palpation for epitrochlear lymph nodes is performed in the depression above and posterior to the medial condyle of the humerus.

A

B

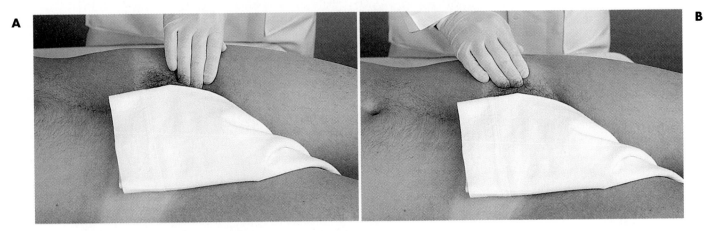

FIGURE 8-22
A, Palpation of inferior superficial inguinal (femoral) lymph nodes. **B,** Palpation of superior inguinal lymph nodes.

bow in one hand as you explore with the other (Figure 8-21). To palpate the inguinal and popliteal area, have the patient lie supine with the knee slightly flexed (Figure 8-22). The superior superficial inguinal (femoral) nodes are close to the surface over the inguinal canals. The inferior superficial inguinal nodes lie deeper in the groin.

The lymphatic drainage of the testes is into the abdomen. Enlarged nodes there are not accessible to inspection and palpation. Nodes in the inguinal area enlarge if there are lesions of the penile and scrotal surfaces.

Similarly, the internal female genitalia drain into the pelvic and paraaortic nodes and are not accessible to inspection and palpation. However, the vulva and lower one third of the vagina drain into the inguinal nodes.

INFANTS AND CHILDREN

The technique of examination is similar for all ages. You will commonly find small, firm, discrete, and movable nodes that are neither warm nor tender located in the occipital, postauricular, cervical, and inguinal chains. The very thin child's inguinal nodes may even be readily visible. In children such nodes are not as worrisome as in the adult. The shape is usually globular or ovoid, sometimes flatter or more cylindrical.

The widespread occurrence of enlarged lymph nodes in children has been frequently documented and demonstrated to be unassociated with serious illness. It is not unusual to find enlarged postauricular and occipital nodes in children younger than 2 years old. Past that age, such enlargement is relatively uncommon and may be significant (Boxes 8-3 and 8-4). Conversely, cervical and submandibular nodal enlargement is relatively less frequent in children less than 1 year old and much more frequent in older children. These age distributions should be considered in your decision to evaluate further lymph node enlargement (Herzog, 1983). The discovery of small lymph nodes in the inguinal, cervical, or axillary chains of neonates may not in itself require further investigation (Box 8-5).

Nodes smaller than 0.5 cm are not generally cause for concern, and nodes with a diameter of 1 cm or less in the cervical and inguinal chains do not always indicate a problem. If nodes have grown rapidly and are suspiciously large (perhaps 2 to 3 cm), even mildly painful, or fixed to contiguous tissues and relatively immovable, investigate further.

The palatine tonsils may be enlarged in children, which is not in itself a problem. Excessive enlargement may obstruct the nasopharynx, increasing the risk of sleep apnea and, on rare occasions, pulmonary hypertension.

DIFFERENTIAL DIAGNOSIS

BOX 8-3 **Mumps Versus Cervical Adenitis**

Mumps, epidemic parotiditis, is characterized by a somewhat painful swelling of the parotid glands unilaterally or bilaterally and, occasionally, by swelling and tenderness of the other salivary glands along the mandible. The swelling can obscure the angle of the jaw and may appear on inspection as a cervical adenitis. On palpation, however, the two are easily distinguished. A cervical adenitis does not ordinarily obscure the angle of the jaw. Your fingers can separate the node from the angle so that you can feel the hard sharpness of the bone, a finding generally not associated with parotid swelling.

DIFFERENTIAL DIAGNOSIS

BOX 8-4 **How to Discover an Immune Deficiency Disease in a Child**

Begin with a thorough history in all regards:
- The family history
- Risk factors for HIV infection
- Illness in siblings
- Previous infections
- Previous hospitalizations
- Most important, serious recurring infections and infections that are uncommon (e.g., *Pneumocystis carinii*); other infections, particularly fungal, that do not yield to therapy

Note unusual findings on the physical examination (e.g., generalized lymphadenopathy and enlargement of the liver and/or spleen).

The child who is not doing well, who has recurrent infection, and in whom unusual findings *persist* could possibly have an immune deficiency. HIV infection in the young can have a very long clinical latency. The least suspicion in a child at risk should lead to testing.

BOX 8-5 **When Physical Examination May Not be Enough**

The number of diseases with which lymphadenopathy is associated is great, and the detection of lymphadenopathy is common. It is infrequently necessary to go beyond physical examination and to resort to biopsy. Still, older patients with localized and persistent lymphadenopathy without evidence of infection or inflammation might be assumed to have cancer unless a biopsy proves otherwise. Young adults and children are more likely to have demonstrable infection, often Epstein-Barr virus mononucleosis. However, the young need biopsy with localized supraclavicular lymphadenopathy as much as the old.

SUMMARY OF EXAMINATION Lymphatic System

The lymphatic system is examined region by region during the examination of the other body systems (head and neck, breast and axillary, genitalia, and extremities).

1. Inspect the visible nodes for the following (p. 230):
   - Edema
   - Erythema
   - Red streaks

2. Palpate the superficial lymph nodes and compare side to side for the following (pp. 230-237):
   - Size
   - Consistency
   - Mobility
   - Discrete borders or matted
   - Tenderness
   - Warmth

COMMON ABNORMALITIES

ACUTE LYMPHANGITIS	Acute lymphangitis is an inflammation of one or more lymphatic vessels. It is characterized by pain, a feeling of malaise and illness, and possibly fever. On inspection you may find a red streak following the course of the lymphatic collecting duct. It appears as a tracing of	rather fine lines streaking up the extremity. The inflammation is sometimes slightly indurated and palpable to gentle touch. Look distal to the inflammation for sites of infection, particularly interdigitally.
ACUTE SUPPURATIVE LYMPHADENITIS	Group A beta-hemolytic streptococci and coagulase-positive staphylococci cause most instances of acute lymphadenitis. The involved node is usually quite firm and tender. The overlying tissue becomes edematous, and the skin appears erythematous, usually within 72 hours. Other pathogens may play a role, for example, actinomycotic adenitis as a result of dental disease; mycobacterial	lymphadenitis in the presence of the tuberculosis organism; organisms both typical and atypical as a result of cat scratch (cat scratch disease), or *Pasteurella multocida* infection at the site of a scratch or bite from a dog or cat. Mycobacterial adenitis is characterized by an inflammation without warmth that may or may not be slightly tender.
NONHODGKIN LYMPHOMA	Malignant neoplasms of the lymphatic system and the reticuloendothelial tissues are usually well defined and solid. Histologically, their cells are often undifferentiated but resemble lymphocytes, histiocytes, or plasma cells. Lymphomas occur most often in lymph nodes, the spleen, and other sites in which lymphoreticular cells are found. The nodes	involved in this and other malignancies may be localized in the posterior cervical triangle or may become matted, crossing into the anterior triangle. It is often not possible or appropriate to attempt to distinguish the findings of these conditions from those in Hodgkin disease through physical examination alone.

HODGKIN DISEASE

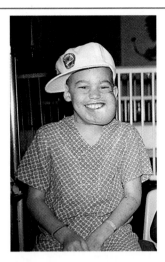

FIGURE 8-23
Hodgkin disease. Note the impressive extent of the enlargement.

Hodgkin disease is a malignant lymphoma that occurs in the young of all races, generally in late adolescence and young adulthood (Figure 8-23), although it also occurs in people over 50. Males are twice as likely to develop Hodgkin disease as are females. Its clinical presentation is variable. Most commonly, there is a painless enlargement of the cervical lymph nodes that is generally asymmetric and inexorably progressive. Occasionally, pressure of the node on surrounding structures will produce symptoms that prompt the patient to seek medical care. The nodes are sometimes matted and generally feel very firm, almost rubbery. Although asymmetry is the rule, nodes are occasionally enlarged in similar patterns on both sides of the body. The nodal size may fluctuate.

EPSTEIN-BARR VIRUS MONONUCLEOSIS

Epstein-Barr virus mononucleosis (infectious mononucleosis) occurs at almost any age but is most common in adolescents and young adults. Initial symptoms include pharyngitis and, usually, fever, fatigue, and malaise. Frequently, splenomegaly and, on occasion, hepatomegaly and/or a rash may be noted. The affected nodes may be generalized but are more commonly felt in the anterior and posterior cervical chains. They vary in firmness and are generally discrete and occasionally a bit tender. Other common viral causes of cervical adenitis include cytomegalovirus, adenovirus, varicella, and enterovirus.

STREPTOCOCCAL PHARYNGITIS

Streptococcal pharyngitis is a fairly common condition. Symptoms usually include a sore throat and often a runny nose. There can be a variety of accompanying symptoms including headache, fatigue, and abdominal pain. On physical examination, anterior cervical nodes are commonly felt. They tend to be somewhat firm, discrete, and quite often tender. It is said that streptococcal pharyngitis may be diagnosed on physical examination when, for example, there are palatal petechiae. The *Streptococcus*, however, presents such a variety of findings in the throat, the tonsillar fossae, and palate that diagnosis is not ensured without a throat culture.

RETROPHARYNGEAL ABSCESS

Retropharyngeal abscess is most common in very young children, because the retropharyngeal lymph nodes, which form chains on either side of the midline in the retropharyngeal area, tend to atrophy by 5 or 6 years of age (Figure 8-24). The condition may result from a puncture wound of the posterior pharyngeal wall. Group A beta-hemolytic streptococcus is the most common causative organism. The child is usually acutely ill, febrile, drooling, anorexic, and restless. Breathing is difficult because of the occluded airway. This is a pediatric emergency, and the child often sits up with arms placed stiffly behind (tripod position) and the head and neck hyperextended to keep the airway open.

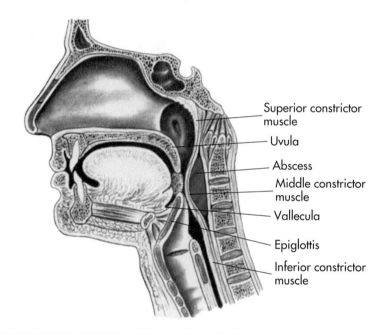

Superior constrictor muscle
Uvula
Abscess
Middle constrictor muscle
Vallecula
Epiglottis
Inferior constrictor muscle

FIGURE 8-24
Retropharyngeal abscess.
Modified from Thompson et al, 1993.

RHEUMATOID ARTHRITIS

Rheumatoid arthritis is a chronic, systemic inflammatory disorder of the joints that is common throughout life (see Chapter 19, Musculoskeletal System). It is frequently associated with localized or generalized lymphadenopathy, which is discovered in more than 25% of such patients. The nodes are not dramatic in presentation. Rather, they tend to be nontender, firm, and freely movable. They do not generally complicate the patient's illness. Splenomegaly, when it occurs in this disorder, is usually accompanied by lymphadenopathy.

HERPES SIMPLEX

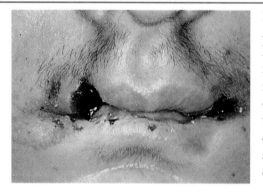

FIGURE 8-25
Herpes simplex.

Herpes simplex can cause discrete labial and gingival ulcers, high fever, and enlargement of the anterior cervical and submandibular nodes (Figure 8-25). These nodes tend to be somewhat firm, quite discrete, movable, and tender. Fever is often high. The relative frequency of this condition and the symptoms are generally sufficient to establish the diagnosis. A viral culture can be obtained if necessary.

CAT SCRATCH DISEASE

Cat scratch disease is among the most common causes of chronic lymphadenopathy in children. The diagnosis can be made in the presence of a nodal enlargement lasting longer than 3 weeks, accompanied by a primary lesion of the skin or eye and following an interaction with a cat, a cat scratch, or cat lick on a break in the skin. Early in the disease, there may be a papule or pustule, which may or may not subside over a short period of time. Tender nodes are most commonly found in the areas of the head, neck, and axillae. The accessible nodal areas in the arms and legs are less frequently involved. The nodes can be very large—up to several centimeters—and they may occasionally suppurate. The lymphadenopathy can last for 2 to 4 months, even longer, making more serious malignant disease a frequent diagnostic concern.

ACQUIRED IMMUNE DEFICIENCY SYNDROME (AIDS)

Acquired immune deficiency syndrome (AIDS) is characterized by the dysfunction of cell-mediated immunity. It is manifested clinically as the development of recurrent, often severe, opportunistic infections. Common life-threatening diseases associated with full-blown AIDS include Kaposi sarcoma, *Pneumocystis carinii* pneumonia, pulmonary tuberculosis, recurrent pneumonia, and invasive cervical cancer. Initial symptoms include lymphadenopathy, fatigue, fever, and weight loss. In children, although there may be a prolonged clinical latent period, neurodevelopmental problems with loss of developmental milestones, a parotid enlargement simulating mumps, anemia and thrombocytopenia, chronic diarrhea, and recurrent infections may be initial signs. AIDS is caused by the human immunodeficiency virus (HIV). A CD4+ T-lymphocyte count of less than 14% is a significant marker for HIV-related immunosuppression.

HIV SEROPOSITIVITY

A person with HIV antibodies who has not yet developed the sequelae of recurrent infections and neoplastic disease is said to be *HIV positive*. Warning signs and symptoms may include severe fatigue, malaise, weakness, persistent unexplained weight loss, persistent lymphadenopathy, fevers, arthralgias, and persistent diarrhea.

SERUM SICKNESS

Serum sickness is an immune complex disease characterized by urticaria, other rashes, lymphadenopathy, joint pain, fever, and at times facial edema. Urticaria usually appears first. Lymphadenopathy, a common finding, is most prominent in the area draining the site of the injection of an antiserum from animal sources or, more often recently, by a variety of drugs. The nodal enlargement can be generalized. Facial edema is not unusual. These findings become apparent about 7 to 10 days following the use of a provoking substance. They subside rather more slowly, recurring at times over several weeks. The patient can react similarly to repeated exposure to the stimuli; subsequent reactions may be even more severe and even fatal.

LYMPHEDEMA

Congenital lymphedema (Milroy disease) is the hypoplasia and maldevelopment of the lymphatic system, resulting in swelling and often grotesque distortion of the extremities (Figure 8-26). The degree varies with the severity and distribution of the abnormality. Acquired lymphedema results from trauma to the ducts of regional lymph nodes (particularly axillary and inguinal) after surgery or metastasis. In each case obstruction and sometimes infection block the lymphatic ducts, producing lymphedema. Lymphedema does not pit, and the overlying skin will eventually thicken and feel tougher than usual. Congenital lymphedema is usually apparent at birth and involves most often the legs, particularly the dorsum of the foot. A later appearance, *praecox* in adolescence and *tarda* in middle age, is possible.

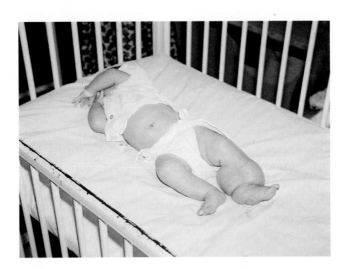

FIGURE 8-26
Lymphedema.

LYMPHANGIOMA AND CYSTIC HYGROMA

Lymphangioma and cystic hygroma are the results of obstruction of developing lymphatic vessels. Most lymphangiomas are present at birth and are apparent early in life, usually in the neck or axilla, less commonly in the chest or extremities. Cystic hygromas can be so large as to distort the face and neck. They feel soft and are fluid-containing. In severe circumstances, they may obstruct the airway or compromise swallowing. These malformations are generally accessible to physical examination.

ELEPHANTIASIS

Elephantiasis is a massive accumulation of lymphedema throughout the body that results from widespread inflammation and obstruction of the lymphatics by the filarial worms, *Wuchereria bancrofti* or *Brugia malayi*. Adequate drainage is prevented, and the patient becomes more susceptible to infection, cellulitis, and fibrosis. The term is often loosely used to describe the result of any obstruction, congenital or acquired (Box 8-6).

DIFFERENTIAL DIAGNOSIS

BOX 8-6 | **When the Body Swells**

Milroy disease and elephantiasis remind us that a significant number of pathologic processes can cause swelling of the extremities and other areas in the body. These can stem from, but are not limited to, the cardiovascular system—for example, congestive heart failure or constrictive pericarditis; diseases of the liver—for example, obstruction of the hepatic vein (Chiari syndrome) and portal vein thrombosis; and kidney malfunction. The most frequent cause, particularly of the feet and the ankles, is stasis, the result of deep venous thrombosis, which may occur in otherwise well men and women who must stand or sit for long periods. The failure to move with some regularity increases orthostatic pressure in the legs. Pregnancy is also a frequent contributor, even in the absence of venous abnormality in the legs. There can also be a significant disruption of lymphatic circulation in the legs with Milroy disease and elephantiasis. When lymphatic disruption is at the root of swelling, the edema does *not* have the characteristic pitting usually seen with other causes of edema. Patients with myxedema, a finding associated with hypothyroidism that is typified by a dry, waxy swelling, share this characteristic. The edema in this circumstance can cause a rather typical facies, with swollen lips and a thick nose. It too does not pit.

CHAPTER 9

HEAD AND NECK

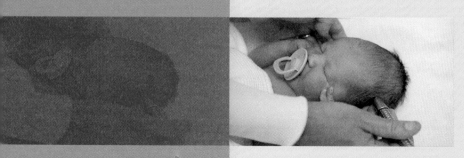

Together the head and neck provide the bony housing and protective cover for the brain, including the special senses of vision, hearing, smell, and taste. Before examining the special senses and the neurologic system, it is important to evaluate carefully the overlying structures.

ANATOMY AND PHYSIOLOGY

The skull is composed of seven bones (two frontal, two parietal, two temporal, and one occipital) that are fused together and covered by the scalp. Bones of the skull are used to identify the location of findings referable to the head (Figure 9-1). The facial skull has several cavities for the eyes, nose, and mouth. The bony structure of the face is formed from the fused frontal, nasal, zygomatic, ethmoid, lacrimal, sphenoid, and maxillary bones and the movable mandible.

Major landmarks of the face are the palpebral fissures and the nasolabial folds (Figure 9-2). Facial muscles are innervated by cranial nerves V and VII. The temporal artery is the major accessible artery of the face, passing just anterior to the ear, over the temporal muscle, and onto the forehead.

The parotid, submandibular, and sublingual salivary glands are paired and produce saliva, which serves to moisten the mouth, inhibit dental caries formation, and initiate digestion of carbohydrates. The parotid gland is located anterior to the ear and above the mandible; the submandibular, medial to the mandible at the angle of the jaw; and the sublingual, anteriorly in the floor of the mouth.

The structure of the neck is formed by the cervical vertebrae, ligaments, and the sternocleidomastoid and trapezius muscles, which give it support and movement (Figure 9-3). Horizontal mobility is greatest at the level of cervical vertebrae 4-5 or 5-6. The sternocleidomastoid muscle extends from the upper sternum and medial third of the clavicle to the mastoid process. The trapezius muscle extends from the scapula, the lateral third of the clavicle, and the vertebrae to the occipital prominence.

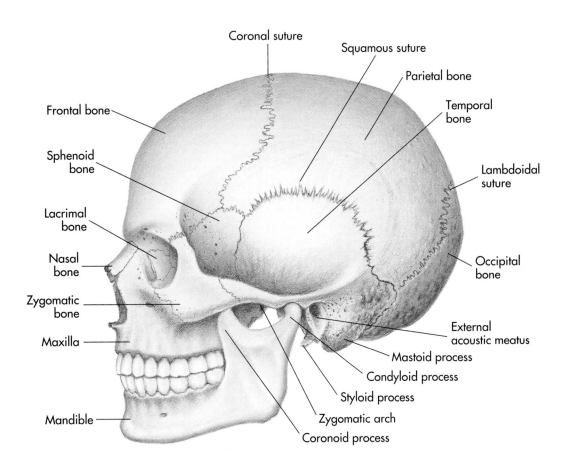

FIGURE 9-1
Bones of the skull.

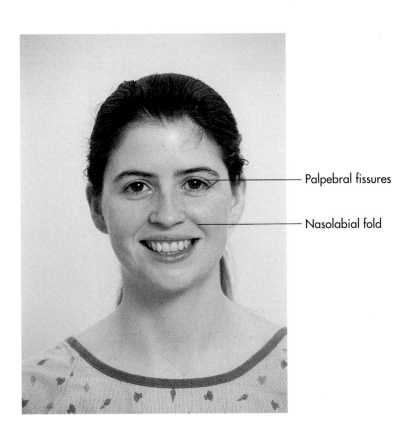

FIGURE 9-2
Landmarks of the face.

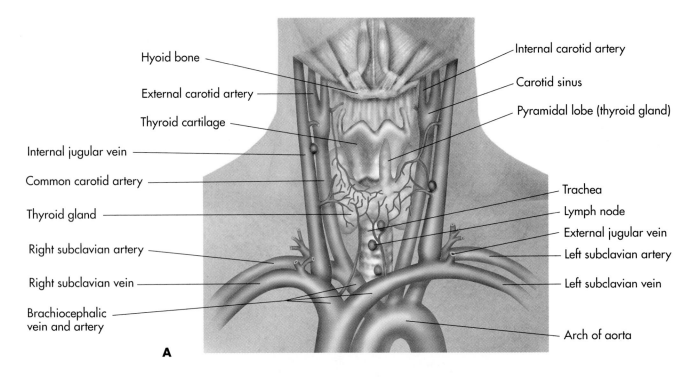

Hyoid bone

External carotid artery

Thyroid cartilage

Internal jugular vein

Common carotid artery

Thyroid gland

Right subclavian artery

Right subclavian vein

Brachiocephalic vein and artery

Internal carotid artery

Carotid sinus

Pyramidal lobe (thyroid gland)

Trachea

Lymph node

External jugular vein

Left subclavian artery

Left subclavian vein

Arch of aorta

A

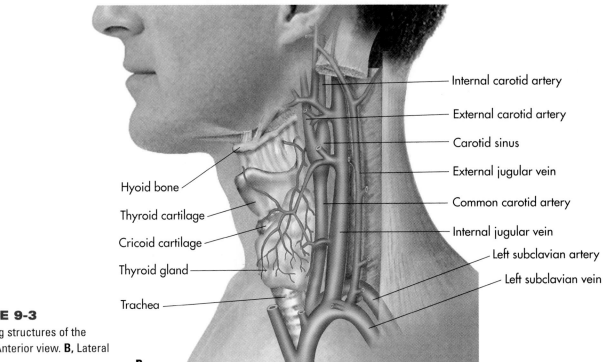

Internal carotid artery

External carotid artery

Carotid sinus

External jugular vein

Common carotid artery

Internal jugular vein

Left subclavian artery

Left subclavian vein

Hyoid bone

Thyroid cartilage

Cricoid cartilage

Thyroid gland

Trachea

FIGURE 9-3
Underlying structures of the neck. **A,** Anterior view. **B,** Lateral view.

B

The relationship of these muscles to each other and to adjacent bones creates triangles used as anatomic landmarks. The posterior triangle is formed by the trapezius and sternocleidomastoid muscles and the clavicle (Figure 9-4) and contains the posterior cervical lymph nodes (Figure 9-5). For a more complete description of the lymph nodes of the head and neck, see Figures 8-8 to 8-11 (pp. 223-225).

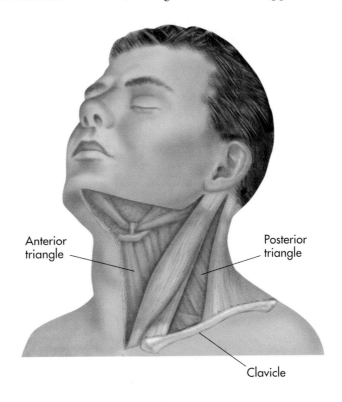

FIGURE 9-4
Anterior and posterior triangles of the neck.

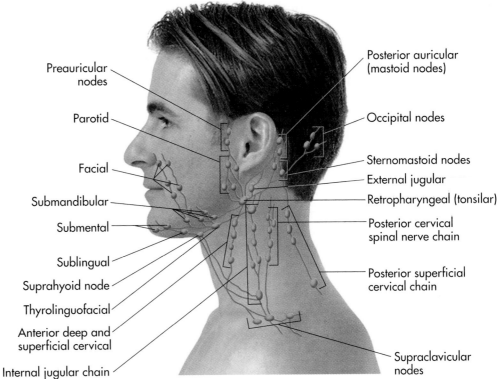

FIGURE 9-5
Lymphatic drainage system of head and neck. (If the group of nodes is often referred to by another name, the second name appears in parentheses.)

The anterior triangle is formed by the medial border of the sternocleidomastoid muscles and the mandible. The hyoid bone, cricoid cartilage, trachea, thyroid, and anterior cervical lymph nodes lie inside this triangle. The carotid artery and internal jugular vein lie deep and run parallel to the sternocleidomastoid muscle along its anterior aspect. The external jugular vein crosses the surface of the sternocleidomastoid muscle diagonally. The hyoid bone lies just below the mandible. The thyroid cartilage is shaped like a shield, its notch on the upper edge marking the level of bifurcation of the common carotid artery. The cricoid cartilage is the uppermost ring of the tracheal cartilages.

The thyroid is the largest endocrine gland in the body, producing two hormones, thyroxine (T_4) and triiodothyronine (T_3). Its two lateral lobes are butterfly shaped and joined by an isthmus at their lower aspect. This isthmus lies across the trachea below the cricoid cartilage. A pyramidal lobe, extending upward from the isthmus slightly to the left of midline, is present in about one third of the population. The lobes curve posteriorly around the cartilages and are in large part covered by the sternocleidomastoid muscles.

INFANTS

The seven cranial bones are soft and separated by the sagittal, coronal, and lambdoidal sutures (Figure 9-6). The anterior and posterior fontanels are the membranous spaces formed where four cranial bones meet and intersect. Spaces between the cranial bones permit the expansion of the skull to accommodate brain growth. Ossification of the sutures begins after completion of brain growth, at about 6 years of age, and is finished by adulthood. The fontanels ossify earlier, with the posterior fontanel usually closing by 2 months of age and the anterior fontanel closing by 24 months of age. The time of closure of the fontanel does not correlate with term or premature delivery, sex, size of the fontanel, or head circumference. Black infants tend to have somewhat larger fontanels than do whites.

The process of birth through the vaginal canal often causes molding of the newborn skull, during which the cranial bones may shift and overlap. Within days the newborn skull resumes its appropriate shape and size.

ADOLESCENTS

Subtle changes in facial appearance occur throughout childhood. In the male adolescent the nose and thyroid cartilage enlarge, and facial hair develops, emerging first on the upper lip, then the cheeks, lower lip, and chin.

PREGNANT WOMEN

There are a number of changes that occur in the thyroid gland and in thyroid hormones during pregnancy. Pregnancy is, however, a euthyroid state. There is an early and sustained rise in the renal clearance of iodine, and the thyroid compensates by enlarging and increasing the plasma clearance of iodine to produce sufficient thyroid hormones (Figure 9-7). Serum bioassayable thyroid-stimulating activity is increased in the first trimester because of human chorionic gonadotropin (hCG). The hCG may cause an increase in the T_4 and T_3 levels. There is also a rise in thyroxine-binding globulin (TBG) concentration.

Some women develop the "mask of pregnancy" (chloasma) characterized by tan or brown pigmentation on the forehead, nose, and the malar prominence (see Figure 7-29). It may be permanent, or it may disappear after delivery.

OLDER ADULTS

With aging the rate of T_4 production and degradation gradually decreases, and the thyroid gland becomes more fibrotic.

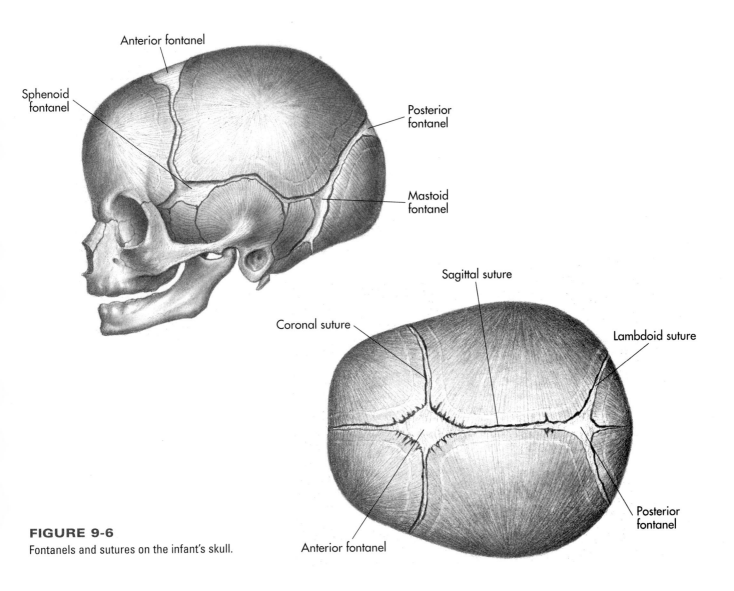

FIGURE 9-6

Fontanels and sutures on the infant's skull.

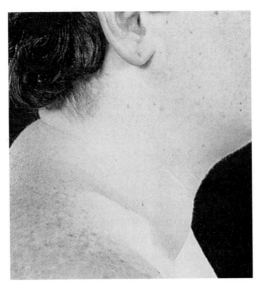

FIGURE 9-7

Thyroid enlargement (in profile) in a normal pregnancy. Some degree of goiter is physiologically normal.

From Symonds, Macpherson, 1994.

REVIEW OF RELATED HISTORY

PRESENT PROBLEM

- Head injury
  - Independent observer's description of event
  - State of consciousness after injury: immediately and 5 minutes later; duration of unconsciousness; combative, confused, alert, or dazed
  - Predisposing factors: seizure disorder, poor vision, light-headedness, blackouts
  - Associated symptoms: head or neck pain, laceration, altered level of consciousness, local tenderness, change in breathing pattern, blurred or double vision, discharge from nose or ears, nausea or vomiting, urinary or fecal incontinence, ability to move all extremities (see Chapter 23, Assessment of the Emergency or Life-Threatening Situation)
  - Medications: prescription or nonprescription
- Headache
  - Onset: early morning, during day, during night; gradual versus abrupt
  - Duration: minutes, hours, days, weeks; relieved by medication, sleep; resolves spontaneously; occurs in clusters, headache-free periods
  - Location: entire head, unilateral, specific site (neck, sinus region, behind eyes, hatband distribution)
  - Character: throbbing, pounding, boring, shocklike, dull, nagging, constant pressure, aggravated with movement
    - Severity: same or different with each event (gradation 1-10)
    - Visual prodromal event: scotoma; hemianopia; distortion of size, shape, or location
  - Pattern: worse in AM or PM, worse or better as day progresses, occurs only during sleep
    - Episodes closer together or worsening, lasting longer
    - Change in level of consciousness as pain increases
  - Associated symptoms: nausea, vomiting, diarrhea, photophobia, visual disturbance, difficulty falling asleep, increased lacrimation, nasal discharge, tinnitus, paresthesias, mobility impairment
  - Precipitating factors: fever, fatigue, stress, food additives, prolonged fasting, alcohol, seasonal allergies, menstrual cycle, intercourse, oral contraceptives
  - Efforts to treat: sleep, pain medication
  - Medications: anticonvulsants; antiarrhythmics; beta blockers, calcium channel blockers; oral contraceptives; serotonin antagonists or agonists, uptake inhibitors; antidepressants; nonsteroidal antiinflammatory drugs (NSAIDs); narcotics; caffeine-containing drugs, nonprescription drugs
- Stiff neck
  - Neck injury or strain, head injury, swelling of neck
  - Fever, bacterial or viral illness
  - Character: limitation of movement; pain with movement, pain relieved by movement; continuous or cramping pain; radiation patterns to arms, shoulders, hands, or down the back
  - Predisposing factors: unilateral vision or hearing loss
  - Efforts to treat: heat, pain medication, physical therapy
  - Medications: prescription or nonprescription
- Thyroid problem
  - Change in temperature preference: more or less clothing, different from patient's family

- Swelling in the neck; interference with swallowing; redness; pain with touch, swallowing, or hyperextension of the neck; difficulty buttoning shirt
- Change in texture of hair, skin, or nails; increased pigmentation of skin at pressure points
- Change in emotional stability: increased energy, irritability, nervousness, or lethargy, complaisance, disinterest
- Increased prominence of eyes, puffiness in periorbital area, blurred or double vision
- Tachycardia, palpitations
- Change in menstrual flow
- Change in bowel habits
- Medications: thyroid preparations, prescription or nonprescription

PAST MEDICAL HISTORY

- Head trauma, subdural hematoma, recent lumbar puncture
- Radon or radium treatment around head and neck
- Headaches: migraine, vascular
- Surgery for tumor
- Seizure disorder
- Thyroid dysfunction, surgery

PERSONAL AND SOCIAL HISTORY

- Employment: risk of head injury, use of helmet, exposure to toxins or chemicals
- Stress; tension; demands at home, work, or school
- Potential risk of injury: participation in sports, handrails available, use of seat belts, unsafe environment
- Nutrition: recent weight gain or loss, food intolerances, eating habits (skipping meals)
- Use of alcohol
- Use of street drugs

FAMILY HISTORY

- Headaches: type, character, similarity to patient's
- Thyroid dysfunction

INFANTS

- Prenatal history: mother's use of drugs or alcohol, treated for hyperthyroidism
- Birth history: vaginal or Caesarean section delivery; presentation, difficulty of delivery, use of forceps (associated with caput succedaneum, cephalhematoma, Bell palsy, molding)
- Unusual head shape: bulging or flattening (congenital anomaly or positioning in utero), preterm infant, head held at angle, preferred position at rest
- Quality of head control
- Acute illness: diarrhea, vomiting, fever, stiff neck, irritability (associated with meningitis)
- Congenital anomalies: meningomyelocele, encephalocele, microcephaly, or hydrocephaly
- Neonatal screening for congenital hypothyroidism

PREGNANT WOMEN

- Weeks' gestation or postpartum
- Presence of preexisting disease (e.g., hypothyroidism, hyperthyroidism)
- History of pregnancy-induced hypertension (PIH)
- Use of street drugs
- Medications: prescription or nonprescription

OLDER ADULTS

- Dizziness with head or neck movement
- Weakness or impaired balance increasing risk of falling and head injury

EXAMINATION AND FINDINGS

EQUIPMENT

- Tape measure
- Stethoscope
- Cup of water (for evaluation of thyroid gland)
- Transilluminator (electronic or flashlight attachment, for infants)

HEAD AND FACE

Inspection

Begin examining the head and neck with inspection of head position and facial features, making observations throughout the history and physical examination. The patient's head should be held upright and still. A horizontal jerking or bobbing motion may be associated with a tremor, whereas a nodding movement may be associated with aortic insufficiency, especially if nodding is synchronized with the pulse. Holding the head tilted to one side to favor a good eye or ear occurs with unilateral hearing or vision loss, but it is also associated with shortening of a sternocleidomastoid muscle (torticollis) (see Figure 9-34).

Facial features (eyelids, eyebrows, palpebral fissures, nasolabial folds, and mouth) should be inspected for shape and symmetry with rest, movement, and expression. The integrity of cranial nerves V and VII (trigeminal and facial) has been partially tested, as detailed in Chapters 4 (Mental Status) and 20 (Neurologic System). Facial characteristics vary according to race, sex, and body build. Some slight asymmetry is common.

When facial asymmetry is present, note whether all features on one side of the face are affected or only a portion of the face, such as the forehead, lower face, or mouth. Suspect facial nerve paralysis when the entire side of the face is affected and facial nerve weakness when the lower face is affected. If only the mouth is involved, suspect a problem with the peripheral trigeminal nerve.

Tics, spasmodic muscular contractions of the face, head, or neck, should be noted. They may be associated with pressure on or degenerative changes of the facial nerves, or they may be psychogenic.

Note any change in the shape of the face or unusual features, such as edema, puffiness, coarsened features, prominent eyes, hirsutism, lack of expression, excessive perspiration, pallor, or pigmentation variations. Certain disorders will cause characteristic changes in facial appearance (see Common Abnormalities, pp. 263-266).

Inspect the skull for size, shape, and symmetry. Examine the scalp by systematically parting the hair from the frontal to occipital region, noting any lesions, scabs, tenderness, parasites, nits, or scaliness. Pay special attention to the areas behind the ears, at the hairline, and at the crown of the head. Note any hair loss pattern. In men it is common to see bitemporal recession of hair or balding over the crown of the head.

Palpation

The skull is palpated in a gentle rotary movement progressing systematically from front to back. The skull should be symmetric and smooth. The bones should be indistinguishable, because the sites of fusion are not generally palpable after 6 months of age. However, the ridge of the sagittal suture may be felt on some individuals. The scalp should move freely over the skull, and no tenderness, swelling, or depressions on palpation are expected. An indentation or depression of the skull may indicate a skull fracture.

Palpate the patient's hair, noting its texture, color, and distribution. Hair should be smooth, symmetrically distributed, and have no splitting or cracked ends. Coarse, dry, and brittle hair is associated with hypothyroidism. Fine, silky hair is associated with hyperthyroidism.

Palpate the temporal arteries and note their course. Any thickening, hardness, or tenderness over the arteries may be associated with temporal arteritis. Palpate the temporomandibular joint space bilaterally, as described in Chapter 19, p. 707.

Inspect for any asymmetry or enlargement of the salivary glands. If noted, palpate for possible discrete enlargement, noting whether it is fixed or movable, soft or hard, tender or nontender. Ask the patient to open the mouth and see if any material can be expressed through the salivary duct as you press on the gland itself. An enlarged, tender gland may suggest infection, either viral or bacterial, or a ductal stone preventing saliva from exiting the gland. A discrete nodule may represent a cyst or tumor, either benign or malignant.

Percussion

Percussion of the head and neck is not routinely performed. If one suspects that a patient has sinusitis, percussion of the sinuses may elicit tenderness, which helps confirm the diagnosis (see Chapter 11, p. 329, Figure 11-25). Some investigators have also described a sign of hyperparathyroidism. They noted that percussion of the skull of individuals with hyperparathyroidism produced a low-pitched note that is far different from the high-pitched crack elicited from the skull of healthy individuals.

Auscultation

Auscultation of the skull is not routinely performed. In individuals who have developed diplopia, a bruit or blowing sound over the orbit may rarely be heard. It suggests that an expanding cerebral aneurysm may be responsible for the diplopia. If you have any reason to suspect a vascular anomaly of the brain, listen for bruits over the skull and eyes. Place the bell of the stethoscope over the temporal region, over the eyes, and below the occiput (Figure 9-8). A bruit over any of these areas indicates a vascular anomaly.

NECK

Inspection

Inspect the neck in the usual anatomic position, in slight hyperextension, and as the patient swallows. Look for bilateral symmetry of the sternocleidomastoid and trapezius muscles, alignment of the trachea, the landmarks of the anterior and posterior triangles, and any subtle fullness at the base of the neck. Note any apparent masses,

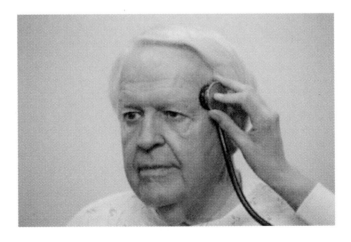

FIGURE 9-8

Auscultation for a temporal bruit.

From Thompson, Wilson, 1996.

webbing, excess skin folds, unusual shortness, or asymmetry. Observe for any distention of the jugular vein or prominence of the carotid arteries. Carotid artery and jugular vein examination is described in Chapter 13 (Heart and Blood Vessels).

Webbing, excessive posterior cervical skin, and an unusually short neck may be associated with chromosomal anomalies. The transverse portion of the omohyoid muscle in the posterior triangle can sometimes be mistaken for a mass. Marked edema of the neck is associated with local infections. A mass filling the base of the neck or visible thyroid tissue that glides upward when the patient swallows may indicate an enlarged thyroid.

Evaluate range of motion by asking the patient to flex, extend, rotate, and laterally turn the head and neck (see Chapter 19, Musculoskeletal System, for details). Movement should be smooth and painless and should not cause dizziness.

Palpation

The ability to palpate and identify structures in the neck varies with the patient's habitus. It is more difficult to examine a short, thick, muscular neck than a long, slender one.

Palpate the trachea for midline position. Place a thumb along each side of the trachea in the lower portion of the neck (Figure 9-9). Compare the space between the trachea and the sternocleidomastoid muscle on each side. An unequal space indicates displacement of the trachea from the midline and may be associated with a mass or pathologic condition in the chest.

Identify the hyoid bone and the thyroid and cricoid cartilages. They should be smooth and nontender, and they should move under your finger when the patient swallows. On palpation, the cartilaginous rings of the trachea in the lower portion of the neck should be distinct and nontender.

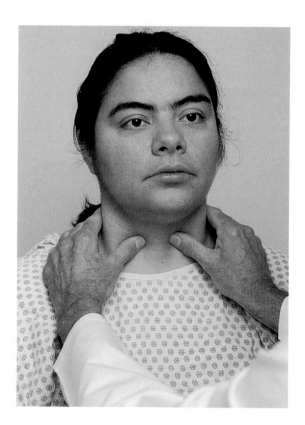

FIGURE 9-9

Position of the thumbs to evaluate the midline position of the trachea.

With the patient's neck extended, position the index finger and thumb of one hand on each side of the trachea below the thyroid isthmus (Figure 9-10). A downward tugging sensation, synchronous with the pulse, is evidence of tracheal tugging, suggesting the presence of an aortic aneurysm.

Lymph Nodes

Inspect and palpate the head and neck for lymph nodes. A description of the sequence is on pp. 234 in Chapter 8 (Lymphatic System).

Thyroid Gland

Examination of the thyroid gland involves inspection, palpation, and auscultation. Begin the evaluation by asking the patient to hyperextend the head so that the neck skin is tightened. Note any asymmetry. After offering the patient a sip of water and positioning again in the hyperextended state, ask the patient to swallow. An enlarged thyroid gland may be visible in the neck with swallowing. Note whether it is symmetric or asymmetric.

Palpation. Palpation of the thyroid gland mandates a gentle touch. Nodules and asymmetric position will be more difficult to detect if you press too hard. Allow your fingers to almost drift over the gland. Palpate the thyroid for size, shape, configuration, consistency, tenderness, and the presence of any nodules. Use one of two approaches, standing either facing or behind the patient, to palpate the isthmus, main body, and lateral lobes of the thyroid gland. Choose one approach to use consistently.

For both approaches the patient should be positioned to relax the sternocleidomastoid, with the neck flexed slightly forward and laterally toward the side being ex-

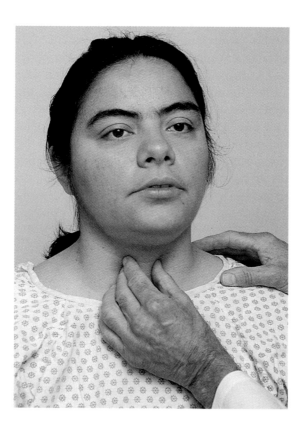

FIGURE 9-10
Position of the thumb and finger to detect tracheal tugging.

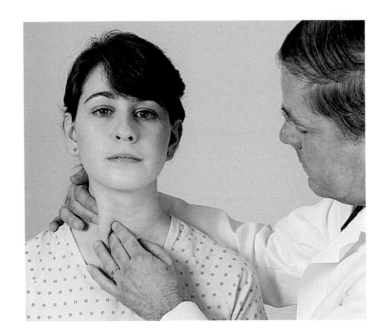

FIGURE 9-11

Palpation of the right thyroid lobe and lateral border from in front of the patient.

amined. To facilitate swallowing, give the patient a cup of water. Ask the patient to hold a sip of water in his or her mouth until you have your hands positioned, then instruct the patient to swallow.

To palpate the thyroid using the frontal approach, have the patient sit on the examining table. Using the pads of the first two fingers, palpate the left lobe with your right hand and the right lobe with your left hand. To increase your access to the lobe, gently move the skin medially over the sternocleidomastoid muscle and reach under its anterior borders with your fingers just beneath the cricoid cartilage. Ask the patient to swallow while you palpate the movement of the thyroid isthmus. Slightly displace the trachea to the left to palpate the main body of the right thyroid lobe (Figure 9-11). The thyroid should move beneath your fingers when the patient swallows. Place your left thumb on the lower left portion of the cricoid cartilage, clasping the right side of the patient's neck, and hook your fingers behind the patient's right sternocleidomastoid muscle. (Make sure your fingernails are well trimmed.) Again ask the patient to swallow. Attempt to palpate the right thyroid lobe between your thumb and fingers, noting its lateral borders. To examine the left lobe, move your hands to the reverse corresponding positions. By palpating above the cricoid cartilage, you may be able to feel the pyramidal lobe of the thyroid, if one is present.

For examining the thyroid from behind, seat the patient on a chair with the neck at a comfortable level. Using both hands, position two fingers of each hand on the sides of the trachea just beneath the cricoid cartilage. Ask the patient to swallow, feeling for movement of the isthmus. Then displace the trachea to the left, ask the patient to swallow, and palpate the main body of the right lobe. To palpate the right lateral border, move the fingers of your left hand between the trachea and the right sternocleidomastoid, placing the fingers of your right hand behind the right sternocleidomastoid muscle. Press your hands together and palpate the right lobe as the patient swallows (Figure 9-12). Repeat the maneuver for the left lobe with your hands in the reverse corresponding positions.

The thyroid lobes, if felt, should be small, smooth, and free of nodules. The gland should rise freely with swallowing. The thyroid at its broadest dimension is ap-

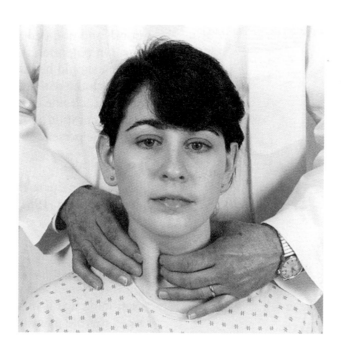

FIGURE 9-12
Palpation of the right thyroid lobe main body from behind the patient.

proximately 4 cm, and the right lobe is often 25% larger than the left. The consistency of the thyroid tissue should be firm yet pliable. Coarse tissue or a gritty sensation implies that an inflammatory process has been present. If nodules are present, they need to be characterized by number, whether they are smooth or irregular, and whether they are soft or hard. An enlarged tender thyroid may indicate thyroiditis.

If the thyroid gland is enlarged, auscultate for vascular sounds with the bell of the stethoscope. In a hypermetabolic state, the blood supply is dramatically increased and a vascular bruit, a soft, rushing sound, may be heard.

INFANTS

Inspection
Measure the infant's head circumference and compare it with expected size for age on a growth chart, as detailed in Chapter 4, Growth and Measurement. Inspect the infant's head from all angles for symmetry of shape, noting any prominent bulges or swellings. Inspect the scalp for scaling and crusting, dilated scalp veins, the presence of excessive hair, or an unusual hairline.

You can always tell a pediatric specialist by the first movement in the examination of an infant. The hand goes almost instinctively to palpate the fontanel. Even in a social situation, you will find the pediatric specialist's fingers saying "hello" by drifting over the soft spot.

Birth trauma may cause swelling of the scalp. Caput succedaneum is subcutaneous edema over the presenting part of the head at delivery (Figure 9-13). It is the most common form of birth trauma of the scalp and usually occurs over the occiput and crosses suture lines. The affected part of the scalp feels soft, and the margins are poorly defined. Generally the edema goes away in a few days.

Cephalhematoma is a subperiosteal collection of blood and is therefore bound by the suture lines. It is commonly found in the parietal region and, unlike caput, may not be immediately obvious at birth. A cephalhematoma is firm, and its edges are well defined; it does not cross suture lines. As it ages, the cephalhematoma may liquefy and become fluctuant on palpation (Figure 9-14).

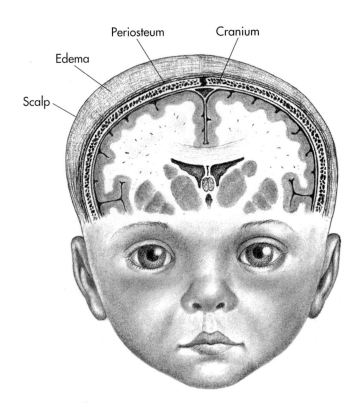

FIGURE 9-13
Caput succedaneum.

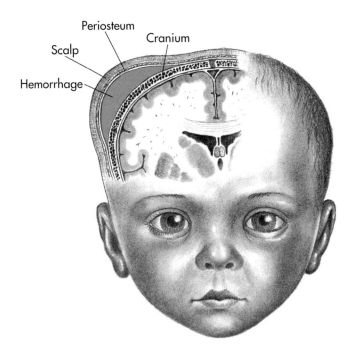

FIGURE 9-14
Cephalhematoma. Note that the swelling does not cross suture lines.

Head shape with an unusual contour may be related to premature or irregular closing of suture lines. Preterm infants often have long, narrow heads because their soft cranial bones become flattened with positioning and the weight of the head. Bossing (bulging of the skull) of the frontal areas is associated with prematurity and rickets. Bulging in other areas of the skull may indicate cranial defects or intracranial masses. Dilated scalp veins and a head circumference increasing faster than expected may indicate increased intracranial pressure.

Inspect the face for spacing of the features, symmetry, paralysis, skin color, and texture. Uterine positioning can cause some facial asymmetry.

Observe the infant's head control, position, and movement. Note any jerking, tremors, or inability to move the head in one direction. Chapters 19 (Musculoskeletal System) and 20 (Neurologic System) provide further details.

Inspect the infant's neck for symmetry, size, and shape. Note the presence of edema, distended neck veins, pulsations, masses, webbing, or excess posterior cervical skin. To observe the newborn's neck, which is usually not easily visible in the supine position, elevate the upper back of the infant and permit the head to fall back into extension. The neck appears short during infancy and lengthens by 3 to 4 years of age. Marked edema may indicate localized infections. A cystic mass high in the neck may be a thyroglossal duct cyst or a branchial cleft cyst. A mass over the clavicle, changing size with crying or respiration, suggests a cystic hygroma. Nuchal rigidity, resistance to flexion of the neck, is associated with meningeal irritation.

Palpation

Palpate the infant's head, identifying suture lines and fontanels. Note any tenderness over the scalp. Suture lines feel ridgelike until about 6 months of age, after which they are usually no longer palpable. Vaginally delivered newborns may have molding with prominent ridges from overriding sutures. Fontanels may be small or not palpable at birth. Molding of the head at delivery can be very distressing for parents. The football shape disappears relatively quickly, but reassurance is necessary. Drawings can help you explain that the infant's cranial bones overlap and that their relative lack of development is a protective device for the brain. Assure the parents that symmetry of the head is usually regained within 1 week of birth, with fontanels and suture line resuming their appropriate shape and size. A third fontanel (the mastoid fontanel), located between the anterior and posterior fontanels, may be an expected variant but is common in infants with Down syndrome. Any palpable ridges in addition to the expected suture lines may indicate fractures.

Measure the size of the anterior and posterior fontanels using two dimensions (anteroposterior and lateral). The anterior fontanel diameter in infants under 6 months of age should not exceed 4 to 5 cm. It should get progressively smaller beyond that age, closing completely by 18 to 24 months of age.

With the infant in a sitting position, palpate the anterior fontanel for bulging or depression. It should feel slightly depressed, and some pulsation is expected. A bulging fontanel feels tense, similar to the fontanel of an infant during the expiratory phase of crying. A bulging fontanel with marked pulsations may indicate increased intracranial pressure. The infant fontanel gives important clues to what is going on inside the body. If there is infection or increased intracranial pressure, the fontanel will bulge. Interestingly, in the early months of life the fontanel may not be the sensitive indicator it becomes later in the first year. You cannot assume that an infant of 3 months whose fontanel is not bulging is free of meningitis. Indeed, an infant who is symptomatic should be evaluated for meningitis even in the absence of a bulging fontanel.

Palpate the scalp firmly above and behind the ears to detect craniotabes, any softening of the outer table of the skull. A snapping sensation, similar to the bounce of a Ping-Pong ball, indicates craniotabes, which may be associated with rickets and hydrocephalus.

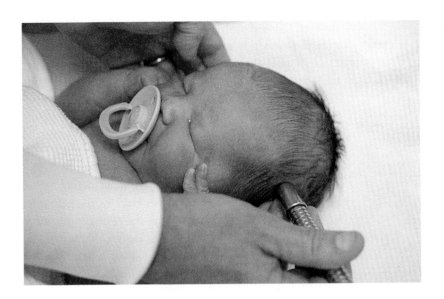

FIGURE 9-15
Transillumination of the infant's scalp.

Palpate the sternocleidomastoid muscle, noting its tone and the presence of any masses. A mass in the lower third of the muscle may indicate a hematoma. Palpate the trachea. A palpatory thud felt over the trachea suggests the presence of a foreign body. The thyroid is difficult to palpate in an infant unless it is enlarged. The presence of a goiter, which may cause respiratory distress, results from intrauterine deprivation of thyroid hormone.

Transillumination

Transilluminate the skull of every newborn and of older infants who have a suspected intracranial lesion or rapidly increasing head circumference. Perform the procedure in a completely darkened room, allowing a few minutes to elapse for your eyes to adjust. The transilluminator is placed firmly against the infant's scalp so that no light escapes (Figure 9-15). Begin at the midline frontal region and inch the transilluminator over the entire head. Observe the ring of illumination through the scalp and skull around the light, noting any asymmetry. A ring of 2 cm or less beyond the rim of the transilluminator is expected on all regions of the head except the occiput, where the ring should be 1 cm or less. Illumination beyond these parameters suggests excess fluid or decreased brain tissue in the skull. Transillumination, performed less often than in the past because examiners now place greater reliance on the computed tomography (CT) scan, is much cheaper and still quite helpful.

CHILDREN

Direct percussion of the skull with one finger is useful to detect the Macewen sign, a cracked-pot sound. The sound, which is physiologic when the fontanels are open, may indicate increased intracranial pressure after fontanel closure.

Bruits are common in children up to 5 years of age or in children with anemia. After age 5 their presence may suggest vascular anomalies or increased intracranial pressure.

The thyroid of the young child may be palpable. Using techniques described for adults, note the size, shape, position, mobility, and any tenderness. No tenderness should be present. An enlarged tender thyroid may indicate thyroiditis.

PREGNANT WOMEN	Beginning after 16 weeks of gestation, many pregnant women develop blotchy, brownish hyperpigmentation of the face, particularly over the malar prominences and the forehead (see Figure 7-29). This chloasma, also called "mask of pregnancy," may further darken with sun exposure, but it generally fades after delivery. The thyroid gland hypertrophies and may become palpable. Because of increased vascularity, a thyroid bruit may be heard.
OLDER ADULTS	The facies of older adults vary with their nutritional status. The eyes may appear sunken with soft bulges underneath, and the eyelids may appear wrinkled and hang loose. Use caution when evaluating range of motion in the older adult's neck. Rather than have the patient perform an entire rotational maneuver, go slowly and evaluate each movement separately. Note any pain, crepitus, dizziness, jerkiness, or limitation of movement. With aging the thyroid becomes more fibrotic, feeling more nodular or irregular to palpation.

SAMPLE DOCUMENTATION

HEAD AND NECK

Head: held erect and midline. Skull normocephalic, symmetrical and smooth without deformities. Facial features symmetrical. No frontal or maxillary sinus tenderness elicited with palpation or percussion. Salivary glands not tender. Temporal artery pulsations visible bilaterally, soft and nontender to palpation. No bruits.

Neck: Trachea midline. No jugular venous distention (JVD) or carotid artery prominence. Thyroid palpable, firm, smooth, not enlarged. Thyroid and cartilages move with swallowing. No nodules, tenderness, or bruits. Full range of motion (ROM) of the neck without discomfort.

For additional sample documentation, see Chapter 24, Recording Information.

SUMMARY OF EXAMINATION   Head and Neck

Head

1. Observe head position (p. 252).
2. Inspect skull and scalp for the following (p. 252):
   - Size
   - Shape
   - Symmetry
   - Lesions
3. Inspect facial features, including the following (p. 252):
   - Symmetry
   - Shape
   - Unusual features
   - Tics
   - Characteristic facies
4. Palpate head and scalp, noting the following (p. 252):
   - Symmetry
   - Tenderness (particularly over areas of frontal and maxillary sinuses)
   - Scalp movement
5. Palpate the temporal arteries, noting the following (p. 253):
   - Thickening
   - Hardness
   - Tenderness
6. Auscultate the temporal arteries for bruits (p. 253).
7. Inspect and palpate the salivary glands (p. 253).

Neck

1. Inspect the neck for the following (p. 253):
   - Symmetry
   - Alignment of trachea
   - Fullness
   - Masses, webbing, and skin folds
   - Jugular vein distention
   - Carotid artery prominence
2. Palpate the neck, noting the following (pp. 253-254):
   - Tracheal position
   - Tracheal tug
   - Movement of hyoid bone and cartilages with swallowing
3. Palpate the thyroid gland for the following (p. 255):
   - Size
   - Shape
   - Configuration
   - Consistency
   - Tenderness
   - Nodules
   (If gland is enlarged, auscultate for bruits.)
4. Evaluate range of motion of the neck (p. 254).

COMMON ABNORMALITIES

HEAD

HEADACHES

Headaches are one of the common complaints and probably one of the most self-medicated. They are not always benign. A history of insistent headache, severe and recurrent, must always be given attention. Sometimes the underlying cause is life threatening, such as a brain tumor. Sometimes it is life intimidating, such as migraines. At other times it is easily confronted, such as when it is the result of drinking wine. The patient's history is fully as important as the physical examination in getting at the root of a headache. Various kinds of headaches are compared in Table 9-1.

DIFFERENTIAL DIAGNOSIS

| TABLE 9-1 | Comparison of Various Kinds of Headaches |

Characteristic	Classic Migraine	Common Migraine	Cluster	Hypertensive	Muscular Tension	Temporal Artertis
Age at onset	Childhood	Childhood	Adulthood	Adulthood	Adulthood	Older adulthood
Location	Unilateral	Generalized	Unilateral	Bilateral or occipital	Unilateral or bilateral	Unilateral or bilateral
Duration	Hours to days	Hours to days	½ to 2 hours	Hours	Hours to days	Hours to days
Time of onset	Morning or night	Morning or night	Night	Morning	Anytime, commonly in afternoon or evening	Anytime
Quality of pain	Pulsating or throbbing	Pulsating or throbbing	Intense burning, boring, searing, knifelike	Throbbing	Bandlike, constricting	Throbbing
Prodromal event	Well-defined neurologic event, scotoma, aphasia, hemianopsia, aura	Vague neurologic changes, personality change, fluid retention, appetite loss	Personality changes, sleep disturbances	None	None	None
Precipitating event	Menstrual period, missing meals, birth control pills, letdown after stress	Menstrual period, missing meals, birth control pills, letdown after stress	Alcohol consumption	None	Stress, anger, bruxism	None
Frequency	Twice a week	Twice a week	Several times nightly for several nights, then none	Daily	Daily	Daily
Gender predilection	Females	Females	Males	Equal	Equal	Equal
Other symptoms	Nausea, vomiting	Nausea, vomiting	Increased lacrimation, nasal discharge	Generally remits as day progresses	None	None

Modified from Sapar, 1983.

FACIES

Facies is defined as an expression or appearance of the face and features of the head and neck that, when considered together, are characteristic of a clinical condition or syndrome. Once a facies is recognized, the examiner may be able to diagnose the condition or syndrome even before completing the examination of the patient. Facies develop slowly and should therefore not be considered a subtle diagnostic clue. As biochemical testing permits diagnosis before gross changes occur, the examiner should be more alert to early changes suggesting a developing facies. As an example, a patient with early changes of acromegaly is included. Figures 9-16 through 9-31 demonstrate some facies and their associated disorders.

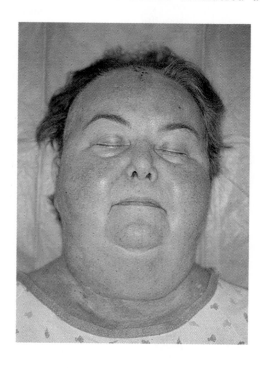

FIGURE 9-16
Cushing syndrome. Facies include a rounded or "moon-shaped" face with thin, erythematous skin. Hirsutism may also be present.

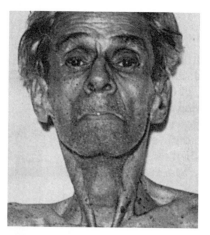

FIGURE 9-17
Hippocratic facies. Note sunken appearance of the eyes, cheeks, and temporal areas; sharp nose; and dry rough skin, seen in the terminal stages of illness.
From Prior et al, 1981.

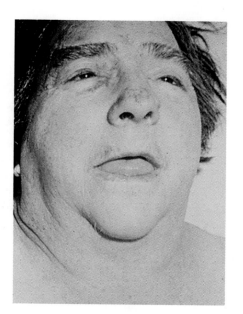

FIGURE 9-18
Myxedema facies. Note dull, puffy, yellowed skin; coarse, sparse hair; temporal loss of eyebrows; periorbital edema; prominent tongue.

Courtesy Paul W. Ladenson, MD, The Johns Hopkins University and Hospital, Baltimore.

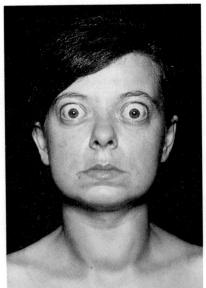

FIGURE 9-19

Hyperthyroid facies. Note fine, moist skin with fine hair, prominent eyes and lid retraction, and staring or startled expression.

FIGURE 9-20

Butterfly rash of systemic lupus erythematosus. Note butterfly-shaped rash over malar surfaces and bridge of nose. Either a blush with swelling or scaly, red, maculopapular lesions may be present.

Courtesy Walter Tunnessen, MD, Chapel Hill, NC.

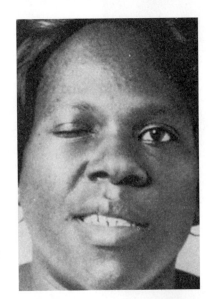

FIGURE 9-21

Left facial palsy. Facies include asymmetry of one side of the face, eyelid not closing completely, drooping lower eyelid and corner of mouth, and loss of nasolabial fold.

From Dyken, Miller, 1980.

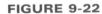

FIGURE 9-22

Acromegaly. **A,** Note large head, forward projection of jaw, and protrusion of frontal bone.
B, Early acromegaly. Note the coarsening of features with broadening of the nasal alae and prominence of the zygomatic arches.

A, From *400 More Self Assessment Picture Tests in Clinical Medicine,* 1988, by permission of Mosby International;
B, Courtesy Gary Wand, MD, The Johns Hopkins University and Hospital, Baltimore.

A

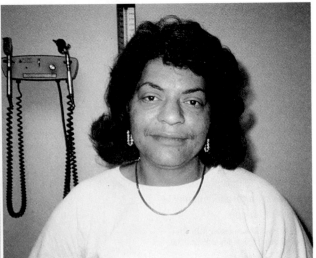

B

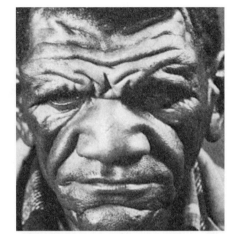

FIGURE 9-23
Pachydermoperiostosis. Coarsening of facial features and thickening and furrowing of face and scalp are seen.
From Goodman, Gorlin, 1977.

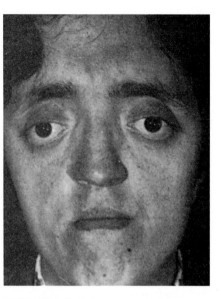

FIGURE 9-24
Craniofacial dysostosis, with characteristic mandibular prognathism, drooping lower lip and short upper lip, parrot beak nose, and proptotic eyes.
From Goodman, Gorlin, 1977.

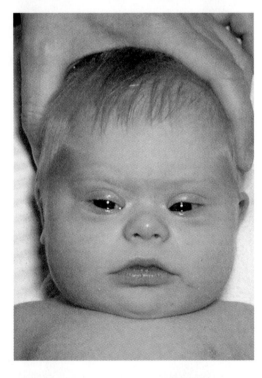

FIGURE 9-25
Down syndrome. Note depressed nasal bridge, epicanthal folds, mongoloid slant of eyes, low set ears, and large tongue.
From Zitelli, Davis, 1997.

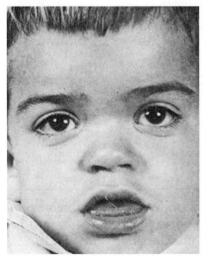

FIGURE 9-26
Hurler syndrome. Facies includes enlarged skull with low forehead, corneal clouding, and short neck.
From Goodman, Gorlin, 1977.

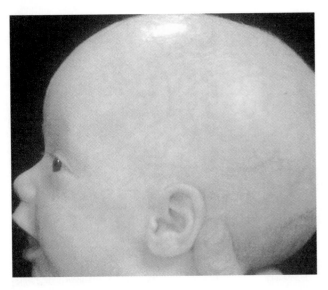

FIGURE 9-27
Hydrocephalus, with characteristic enlarged head, bulging fontanel, dilated scalp veins, bossing of the skull, and sclerae visible above the iris.
From Zitelli, Davis, 1997.

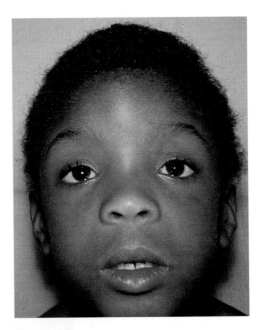

FIGURE 9-28
Fetal alcohol syndrome. Note the poorly formed philtrum; widespread eyes, with inner epicanthal folds and mild ptosis; hirsute forehead; short nose; and relatively thin upper lip.
From Zitelli, Davis, 1997.

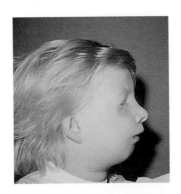

FIGURE 9-29
Treacher-Collins syndrome. Note the maxillary hypoplasia, micrognathia, and auricular deformity.
From Zitelli, Davis, 1997.

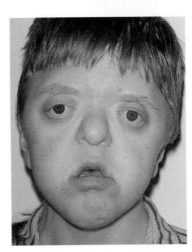

FIGURE 9-30
Apert syndrome. Note the severe maxillary and midfacial hypoplasia.
From Zitelli, Davis, 1997.

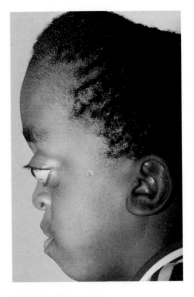

FIGURE 9-31
Crouzon syndrome. Observe the severe maxillary and midfacial hypoplasia with low-set ears.
From Zitelli, Davis, 1997.

NECK

THYROGLOSSAL DUCT CYST

This freely movable cystic mass lies high in the neck at the midline with the duct at the base of the tongue. It is a remnant of fetal development (Figure 9-32).

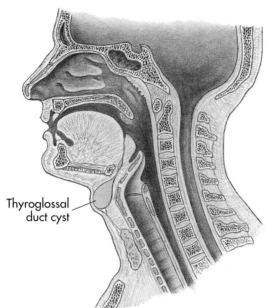

FIGURE 9-32
Thyroglossal duct cyst location.

BRANCHIAL CLEFT CYST

An oval, moderately movable cystic mass appears near the upper third of the sternocleidomastoid muscle and is a remnant of embryologic development. It may be associated with a fistula (Figure 9-33).

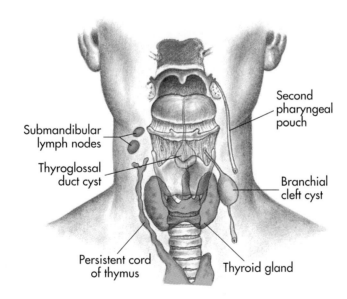

FIGURE 9-33
Branchial cleft cyst location in relation to other neck masses.

TORTICOLLIS

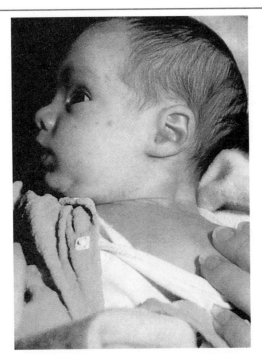

FIGURE 9-34
Torticollis, or wry neck.
From Zitelli, Davis, 1997.

Torticollis, or wry neck, is often the result of injury during the birth process. The head is tilted and twisted toward the sternocleidomastoid muscle. A hematoma may be palpated shortly after birth, and within 2 to 3 weeks a firm, fibrous mass may be felt in the muscle (Figure 9-34). Torticollis can also occur in older children and adults as a result of trauma, muscle spasms, viral infection, or drug ingestion.

SALIVARY GLAND TUMOR

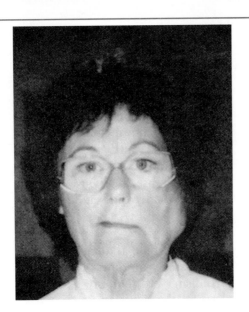

Salivary gland tumors may arise in any of the salivary glands, most commonly the parotid (Figure 9-35).

FIGURE 9-35
Parotid gland tumor. This individual has a tumor of the left parotid gland, characterized by enlargement of the gland and asymmetry of the left jaw. There appear to be additional lesions present on the left mandible and below the left zygomatic arch. The patient also has paresis of the left facial nerve with drooping of the mouth. That finding raises the concern that the tumor has invaded the facial nerve as it passes through the parotid gland.
Courtesy John P. Saunders, Jr., MD, Department of Surgery, The Johns Hopkins University and Hospital, Baltimore.

THYROID

HYPOTHYROIDISM AND HYPERTHYROIDISM	The thyroid hormone influences the metabolism of most cells in the body. An overabundance or a paucity of the hormone can therefore cause symptoms affecting many body systems. Table 9-2 contrasts the signs and symptoms produced by hyperthyroidism and hypothyroidism.	

TABLE 9-2   Hyperthyroidism Versus Hypothyroidism

System or Structure Affected	Hyperthyroidism	Hypothyroidism
Constitutional		
Temperature preference	Cool climate	Warm climate
Weight	Loss	Gain
Emotional state	Nervous, easily irritated, highly energetic	Lethargic, complacent, disinterested
Hair	Fine, with hair loss; failure to hold a permanent wave	Coarse, with tendency to break
Skin	Warm, fine, hyperpigmentation at pressure points	Coarse, scaling, dry
Fingernails	Thin, with tendency to break; may show onycholysis	Thick
Eyes	Bilateral or unilateral proptosis, lid retraction, double vision	Puffiness in periorbital region
Neck	Goiter, change in shirt neck size, pain over the thyroid	No goiter
Cardiac	Tachycardia, dysrhythmia, palpitations	No change noted
Gastrointestinal	Increased frequency of bowel movements; diarrhea rare	Constipation
Menstrual	Scant flow, amenorrhea	Menorrhagia
Neuromuscular	Increasing weakness, especially of proximal muscles	Lethargic, but good muscular strength

MYXEDEMA	Adult-onset hypothyroidism associated with a decreased metabolic rate produces myxedema. The deposition of glycosaminoglycan in all organ systems leads to the characteristic mucinous edema of facial features (see Figure 9-18). Signs and symptoms of hyperthyroidism and hypothyroidism are compared in Table 9-2.	
GRAVES DISEASE	This thyroid disorder is thought to be autoimmune in origin. It is more common in women during the third and fourth decades of life. Multiple systems are affected, and the disease is often characterized by diffuse thyroid enlargement, hyperthyroidism, and ophthalmologic, dermatologic, and musculoskeletal pathologic conditions (see Figure 9-19 and signs and symptoms in Table 9-2).	Pregnancy can make the diagnosis of hyperthyroidism more difficult. The presence of goiter may not be specific. The presence of weight loss, marked tachycardia, eye signs, and bruit over the thyroid are suggestive. Confirmation of the diagnosis is made by measuring free T_4 and T_3 levels in the blood.
HASHIMOTO DISEASE	Hashimoto disease is a chronic autoimmune disorder that causes symptoms of either hyperthyroidism or hypothyroidism, depending on the duration of the disease. It is common in children and in women between 30 and 50 years of age.	

ENCEPHALOCELE

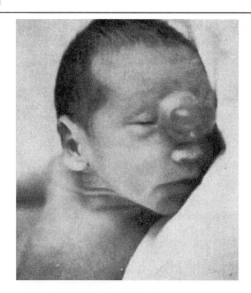

A protrusion of nervous tissue through a defect in the skull may occur any place on the scalp (Figure 9-36).

FIGURE 9-36

Newborn with frontal, nasal, interocular encephalocele.

Courtesy Charles Linder, MD, Medical College of Georgia; from Dyken, Miller, 1980.

MICROCEPHALY

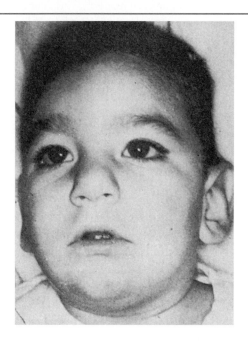

Microcephaly is evident by a congenitally small skull caused by cerebral dysgenesis or craniostenosis and is usually associated with mental retardation and failure of the brain to develop normally (Figure 9-37).

FIGURE 9-37

Primary familial microcephaly.

From Dyken, Miller, 1980.

CRANIOSYNOSTOSIS

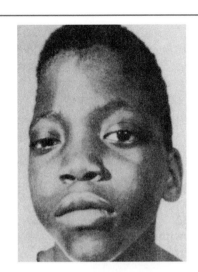

FIGURE 9-38

Fourteen-year-old with dolichoscaphocephaly, one of the less threatening of the craniosynostoses.

From Dyken, Miller, 1980.

Premature union of cranial sutures leads to a misshapen skull, usually not accompanied by mental retardation. The sutures involved determine the shape of the head (Figure 9-38).

 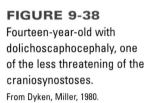

EYES

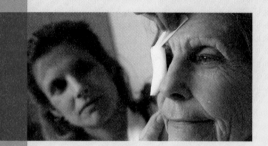

ANATOMY AND PHYSIOLOGY

The eye is the sensory organ that transmits visual stimuli to the brain for interpretation (Figure 10-1). It occupies the orbital cavity with only its anterior aspect exposed. The four rectus and two oblique muscles attached to the eye are innervated by cranial nerves III (oculomotor), IV (trochlear), and VI (abducens) (Figure 10-2). The eye itself is a direct embryologic extension of the brain and is connected to the brain by cranial nerve II, the optic nerve.

EXTERNAL EYE

The external eye is composed of the eyelid, conjunctiva, lacrimal gland, eye muscles, and the bony skull orbit (Figure 10-3).

Eyelids
The eyelids are composed of skin, conjunctiva, and both striated and smooth muscle. Their function is to distribute tears over the surface of the eye, to limit the amount of light entering it, and to protect the eye from foreign bodies. Eyelashes extend from the border of each lid.

Conjunctiva
The conjunctiva is a thin membrane covering most of the anterior surface of the eye and the surface of the eyelid in contact with the globe. The conjunctiva protects the eye from foreign bodies and desiccation.

Lacrimal Gland
The lacrimal gland is located in the temporal region of the superior eyelid and produces tears that moisten the eye (Figure 10-3). Tears flow over the cornea and drain via the lacrimal sac into the nasal meatus.

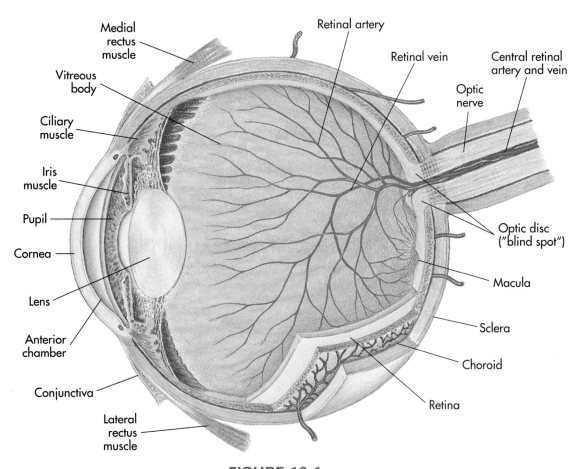

FIGURE 10-1
Anatomy of the human eye.

INTERNAL EYE

The internal structures of the eye are composed of three separate coats, or tunics. The outer fibrous layer is composed of the sclera posteriorly and the cornea anteriorly. The middle tunic, or choroid coat, consists of the choroid posteriorly and the ciliary body and iris anteriorly. The inner nervous tunic is the retina.

Sclera

The sclera is the dense, avascular structure that appears anteriorly as the white of the eye. It physically supports the internal structure of the eye.

Cornea

The cornea constitutes the anterior sixth of the globe and is continuous with the sclera. It has sensory innervation primarily for pain. The cornea separates the watery fluid of the anterior chamber (aqueous humor) from the external environment and permits the transmission of light through the lens to the retina.

Iris

The iris is a circular, contractile muscular disc containing pigment cells that produce the color of the eye. The central aperture of the iris is the pupil, through which light travels to the retina. By dilating and contracting, the iris controls the amount of light reaching the retina.

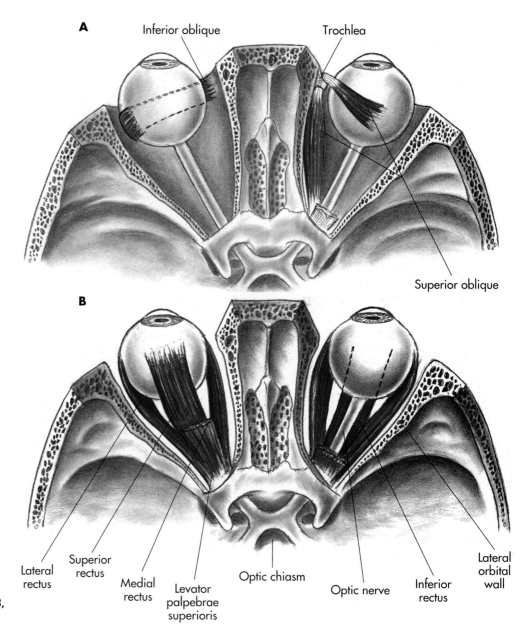

FIGURE 10-2

Extraocular muscles of the eye as viewed from above. In **A,** the oblique muscles are shown. In **B,** the recti are shown.

Lens

The lens is a cellular structure containing crystalline matter that is located immediately behind the iris. It is biconvex and transparent. It is supported circumferentially by fibers arising from the ciliary body of the iris. The lens is highly elastic, and contraction or relaxation of the ciliary body changes its thickness, thereby permitting images from varied distances to be focused on the retina.

Retina

The retina is the sensory network of the eye. It transforms light impulses into electrical impulses, which are transmitted through the optic nerve, optic tract, and optic radiation to consciousness in the cerebral cortex. The optic nerve communicates with the brain, passing through the optic foramen along with the ophthalmic artery and vein, and the autonomic nervous system innervation of the eye. Accurate vision is achieved

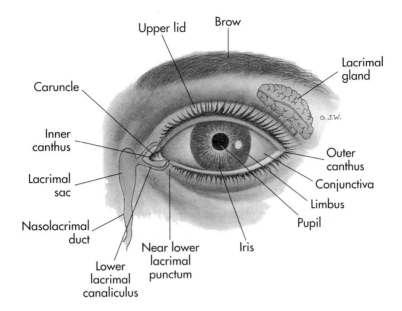

FIGURE 10-3
Important landmarks of the external eye.
From Thompson et al, 1997.

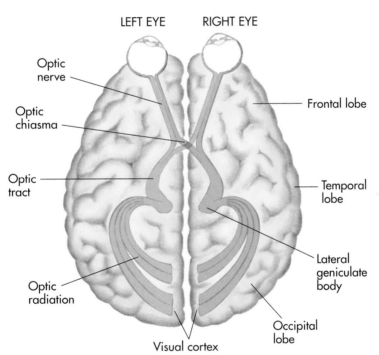

FIGURE 10-4
The visual pathway.
Modified from Thompson et al, 1997.

by focusing an image on the retina through accommodation of the lens. The neural impulses so generated are transmitted along the optic nerve and optic tract, reaching the optic cortex for interpretation. An object may be perceived in each optic cortex, even when one eye is covered, if the light impulse is cast on both the temporal and the nasal retina. Fibers located on the nasal retina decussate in the optic chiasm (Figure 10-4). Accurate vision also requires the synchronous functioning of the extraocular muscles.

Major landmarks of the retina include the optic disc, from which the optic nerve originates, together with the central retinal artery and vein. The macula, or fovea, is the site of central vision and color perception. The direct ophthalmoscope is used primarily to examine these structures in the posterior pole of the eye.

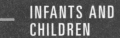
INFANTS AND CHILDREN

The eye forms during the first 8 weeks of gestation and may become malformed from the insult of maternal drug ingestion or infection during this time. The development of vision, which is dependent on maturation of the nervous system, occurs over a longer period (Table 10-1). Term infants are hyperopic, with a visual acuity of 20/200. Although peripheral vision is fully developed at birth, central vision develops later. By 2 to 3 months of age the lacrimal ducts begin carrying tears into the nasal meatus, and the infant gains voluntary control of the eye muscles. By 8 months, vision has developed sufficiently so that the infant can differentiate colors. The eye muscles begin to coordinate, allowing a single image to be perceived by 9 months of age.

Young children have myopic acuity, primarily because the shape of their eyeball is less spherical than that of adults. The globe of the eye grows as the child's head and brain grow, and adult visual acuity is achieved at about 6 years of age.

TABLE 10-1	Chronology of Visual Development
Age	**Level of Development**
Birth	Awareness of light and dark. Infant closes eyelids in bright light.
Neonatal	Rudimentary fixation on near objects (3-30 inches).
2 weeks	Transitory fixation, usually monocular at a distance of roughly 3 feet.
4 weeks	Follows large conspicuously moving objects.
6 weeks	Moving objects evoke binocular fixation briefly.
8 weeks	Follows moving objects with jerky eye movements. Convergence beginning to appear.
12 weeks	Visual following now a combination of head and eye movements. Convergence improving. Enjoys light objects and bright colors.
16 weeks	Inspects own hands. Fixates immediately on a 1-inch cube brought within 1-2 feet of eye. Vision 20/300-20/200 (6/100-6/70).
20 weeks	Accommodative convergence reflexes all organizing. Visually pursues lost rattle. Shows interest in stimuli more than 3 feet away.
24 weeks	Retrieves a dropped 1-inch cube. Can maintain voluntary fixation of stationary object even in the presence of competing moving stimulus. Hand-eye coordination appearing.
26 weeks	Will fixate on a string.
28 weeks	Binocular fixation clearly established.
36 weeks	Beginning of depth perception.
40 weeks	Marked interest in tiny objects. Tilts head backward to gaze up. Vision 20/200 (6/70).
52 weeks	Fusion beginning to appear. Discriminates simple geometric forms (squares and circles). Vision 20/180 (6/60).
12-18 months	Looks at pictures with interest.
18 months	Convergence well established. Localization in distance crude—runs into large objects.
2 years	Accommodation well developed. Vision 20/40 (6/12).
3 years	Convergence smooth. Fusion improving. Vision 20/30 (6/9).
4 years	Vision 20/20 (6/6).

From Kemp, 1987.

| PREGNANT WOMEN | The eyes undergo several changes throughout pregnancy because of physiologic and hormonal adaptations. Mild corneal edema occurs, especially in the third trimester. Corneal thickening may also occur. These changes can result in hypersensitivity and can change the refractory power of the eye. Diabetic retinopathy may worsen significantly. An increase in corneal epithelial pigmentation (Krukenberg spindles) may also occur. Tears contain an increased level of lysozyme, resulting in a "greasy" sensation for contact lens wearers, which may result in blurred vision. Therefore the patient who wears contact lenses may decide to discontinue their use during pregnancy. Because of the various changes in the eye, new lens prescriptions should not be obtained until several weeks after delivery.

Intraocular pressure falls most notably during the latter half of pregnancy. Ptosis may develop for unknown reasons. Subconjunctival hemorrhages may occur spontaneously in pregnancy or during labor; these resolve spontaneously. |
|---|---|
| **OLDER ADULTS** | The major physiologic change that occurs with aging is a progressive change in the near point of accommodation. Generally by age 45, the lens becomes more rigid and the ciliary muscle of the iris becomes weaker. This combination results in presbyopia. The lens also continues to form fibers throughout life. Old fibers are compressed centrally, forming a more dense central region that may cause loss of clarity of the lens and cataract formation. |

REVIEW OF RELATED HISTORY

PRESENT PROBLEM

- Eyelids: recurrent hordeola; ptosis of the lids so that they interfere with vision (unilateral or bilateral)
- Difficulty with vision: one or both eyes, corrected by lenses, involving near or distant vision, primarily central or peripheral, transient or sustained; cataracts (bilateral or unilateral, types [senile, diabetic, secondary to hyperparathyroidism, or central], surgical treatment); adequacy of color vision; presence of halos around lights, floaters, or diplopia (when one eye is covered or when both eyes are open)
- Pain: in or around the eye, superficial or deep, insidious or abrupt in onset; burning, itching, or nonspecific uncomfortable sensation
- Secretions: color (clear or yellow), consistency (watery or foamy), duration, tears that run down the face, decreased tear formation with sensation of gritty eyes; presence of conjunctival redness
- Medications: use of any eyedrops or ointments, antibiotics, artificial tears, mydriatics, myotics; prescription or nonprescription

PAST MEDICAL HISTORY

- Trauma: to the eye as a whole or a specific structure (e.g., cornea) or supporting structures (e.g., the floor of the orbit); events surrounding the trauma; efforts at correction and degree of success
- Eye surgery: condition requiring surgery, date surgery performed, outcome
- Chronic illness that may affect vision: hypertension, diabetes, glaucoma

FAMILY HISTORY

- Retinoblastoma or cancer of the retina (often an autosomal dominant disorder)
- Conditions similar to the patient's
- Color blindness, cataract formation, diabetes, glaucoma, retinitis pigmentosa, macular degeneration, or allergies affecting the eye
- Nearsightedness, farsightedness, or strabismus

PERSONAL AND SOCIAL HISTORY

- Employment: exposure to irritating gases, foreign bodies, or high-speed machinery
- Activities: participation in sporting activities that might endanger the eye (e.g., squash, racquetball, fencing, motorcycle riding)
- Allergies: type, seasonal, associated symptoms
- Lenses: when last changed, how long worn, type (glasses or contact), adequacy of corrected vision; methods of cleaning and storage, insertion and removal procedures of contact lenses; date of last eye examination
- Use of protective devices during work or activities that might endanger the eye

INFANTS AND CHILDREN

- Preterm: resuscitated, ventilator or oxygen used, given diagnosis of retinopathy of prematurity (retrolental fibroplasia)
- Failure of infant to gaze at mother's face or other objects, uncertainty of mother that infant looks at her; failure of infant to blink when bright lights or threatening movements are directed at the face
- White area in the pupil on a photograph; inability of one eye to reflect light properly (may indicate retinoblastoma)
- Excessive tearing over the lower eyelid
- Strabismus some or all of the time
- Young children: excessive rubbing of the eyes, frequent hordeola, inability to reach for and pick up small objects, necessity of bringing objects close to examine them
- School-age children: necessity of sitting near the front of the classroom to see the board; poor progress in school not explained by intellectual ability

PREGNANT WOMEN

- Weeks gestation or postpartum
- History of diabetes or disorders of the eye
- Presence of disorders that can cause ocular complications such as pregnancy-induced hypertension or diabetes
- Use of topical eye medications (they may cross the placental barrier)

OLDER ADULTS

- Visual acuity: decrease in central vision, distortion of central vision, use of dim light to increase visual acuity, complaints of glare
- Production of excess tearing or complaints of blurred vision (caused by loss of contact of the lacrimal duct with the nasal lacrimal lake)
- Dry eyes
- Development of scleral brown spots
- Difficulty in performing near work without lenses
- Nocturnal eye pain

EXAMINATION AND FINDINGS

EQUIPMENT

- Snellen chart or E chart
- Rosenbaum or Jaeger near vision card
- Penlight
- Cotton wisp
- Ophthalmoscope
- Eye cover, gauze, or opaque card

VISUAL TESTING

Measurement of visual acuity—the discrimination of small details—tests cranial nerve II (optic nerve) and is essentially a measurement of central vision. Position the patient 20 ft (6.1 m) away from the Snellen chart (see Figure 3-16), making sure it is well lighted. Test each eye individually by covering one eye with an opaque card or a gauze, being careful to avoid applying pressure to the eye. Ask the patient to identify all of the letters beginning at any line. Determine the smallest line in which the patient can identify all of the letters and record the visual acuity designated by that line. (If a more precise determination is needed, see p. 66.) When testing the second eye, you may want to ask the patient to read the line from right to left. If you test the patient with and without corrective lenses, record the readings separately. Always test vision without glasses first. The test should be done rapidly enough to prevent the patient from memorizing the chart. However, one of the problems patients confront during the examination of the vision is that the examiner sometimes goes too fast, asking that lines on the chart be read or that other judgments be made more quickly than feels comfortable to the patient. The patient's quick judgment may be helpful. However, it is wise to pace it a bit more slowly to let the patient be comfortable and to allow time to puzzle out a response. The patient should not have to leave the examination feeling that something had been said too quickly or was not understood fully.

Visual acuity is recorded as a fraction in which the numerator indicates the distance of the patient from the chart (20 ft or 6.1 m), and the denominator indicates the distance at which the average eye can read the line. Thus 20/200 (6.1/61.0) means that the patient can read at 20 ft (6.1 m) what the average person can read at 200 ft (61.0 m). The smaller the fraction, the worse the myopia. Vision not correctable to better than 20/200 is considered legal blindness.

If the visual acuity is recorded at a fraction less than 20/20 (or 6.1/6.1 m), you can perform a pinhole test to see if the observed decrease in acuity was caused by a refractive error. Ask the patient to hold a piece of paper with a small hole in it over the uncovered eye. This maneuver permits light to enter only the central portion of the lens. It should result in an improvement in visual acuity by at least one line on the chart if refractive error is responsible for the diminished acuity.

Measurement of near vision should also be tested in each eye separately, with a handheld card such as the Rosenbaum Pocket Vision Screener (Figure 3-17). Have the patient hold the card a comfortable distance (about 35 cm, or 14 in) from the eyes and read the smallest line possible.

Peripheral vision can be accurately measured with sophisticated instruments, but it is generally estimated by means of the confrontation test. Sit or stand opposite the patient at eye level at a distance of about 1 m. Ask the patient to cover the right eye while you cover your left eye, so the open eyes are directly opposite each other (Figure 10-5). Both you and the patient should be looking at each other's eye. Fully extend your arm midway between the patient and yourself and then move it centrally with fingers moving. Have the patient tell you when the moving fingers are first seen. Compare the patient's response to the time you first noted the fingers. Test the nasal, temporal, superior, and inferior fields. Remember that the nasal portion of the visual field is interfered with by the nose itself. Unless you are aware of a problem with your vision, you can feel comfortable that the fields are full if they correspond with yours. Actually one anticipates that the fields describe an angle of 60 degrees nasally, 90 degrees temporally, 50 degrees superiorly, and 70 degrees inferiorly. The confrontation test is imprecise, however, and can be considered significant only when it is abnormal.

Color vision is rarely tested in the routine physical examination. Color plates are available in which numerals are produced in primary colors and surrounded by confusing colors. The tests vary in degree of difficulty. For routine testing check the patient's ability to appreciate primary colors.

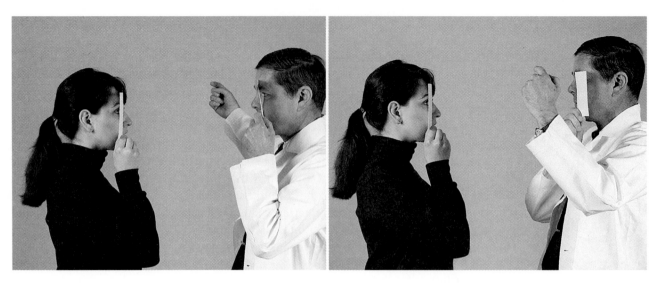

FIGURE 10-5
Estimation of peripheral fields of vision.

Remember that testing of visual acuity involves many complex factors not necessarily related to the ability to see the test object. Motivation and interest, as well as intelligence and attention span, can modify the results of all sensory testing.

EXTERNAL EXAMINATION

Examination of the eyes is carried out in a systematic manner, beginning with the appendages, that is, the eyebrows and surrounding tissues, and moving inward.

Surrounding Structure

Inspect the eyebrows for size, extension, and texture of the hair. Note whether the eyebrows extend beyond the eye itself or end short of it. The coarseness of the hair is also important. If the patient's eyebrows are coarse or do not extend beyond the temporal canthus, the patient may have hypothyroidism. If the brows appear unusually thin, ask if the patient waxes or plucks them.

Inspect the orbital area for edema, puffiness, or sagging tissue below the orbit. Although puffiness may represent the loss of elastic tissue that occurs with aging, periorbital edema is always abnormal; the significance varies directly with the amount. It may represent the presence of thyroid hypoactivity, allergies, or (especially in youth) the presence of renal disease. You may see flat, slightly raised, irregularly shaped, yellow-tinted lesions on the periorbital tissues that represent depositions of lipids and *may* suggest that the patient has an abnormality of lipid metabolism. These lesions are called xanthelasma (Figure 10-6), an elevated plaque of cholesterol deposited most commonly in the nasal portion of either the upper or lower lid.

Eyelid

Examine the patient's lightly closed eyes for fasciculations or tremors of the lids, a sign of hyperthyroidism. Inspect the eyelids for their ability to close completely and open widely. Observe for flakiness, redness, or swelling on the eyelid margin. Eyelashes should be present on both lids and should turn outward.

When the eye is open, the superior eyelid should cover a portion of the iris but not the pupil itself. If one superior eyelid covers more of the iris than the other or extends over the pupil, then ptosis of that lid may be present, indicating a congenital or

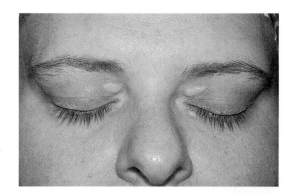

FIGURE 10-6
Xanthelasma.

Courtesy John W. Payne, MD, The Wilmer
Ophthalmological Institute, The Johns
Hopkins University and Hospital,
Baltimore.

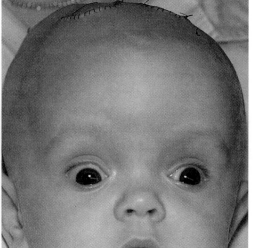

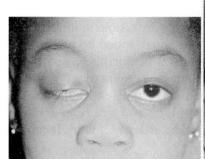

FIGURE 10-7
A, Ptosis, a drooping of the upper eyelid. **B,** Paresis of the upward gaze is seen in an infant
with hydrocephalus resulting
from aqueductal stenosis.

A from Stein, Slatt, Stein, 1994; **B** from
Zitelli, Davis, 1996.

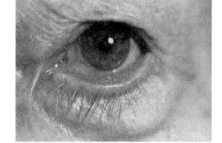

FIGURE 10-8
Ectropion.

From Stein, Slatt, Stein, 1988.

acquired weakness of the levator muscle or a paresis of a branch of the third cranial
nerve (Figure 10-7). Record the difference between the two lids in millimeters.

You should also note whether the lids evert or invert. When the lower lid is
turned away from the eye, ectropion is present and may result in excessive tearing
(Figure 10-8). The inferior punctum, which serves as the tear-collecting system, is
pulled outward and cannot collect the secretions of the lacrimal gland.

When the lid is turned inward toward the globe, a condition known as entropion (Figure 10-9), the lid's eyelashes may cause corneal and conjunctival irritation,
increasing the risk of a secondary infection.

An acute suppurative inflammation of the follicle of an eyelash can cause an
erythematous or yellow lump. This hordeolum or sty is generally caused by staphylococcal organisms (Figure 10-10).

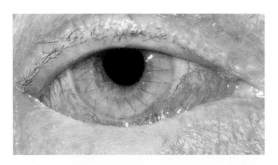

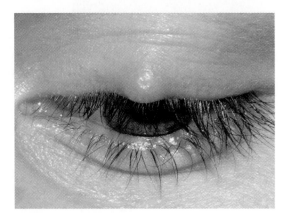

FIGURE 10-9

Involutional entropion. Note that this patient has undergone corneal transplantation.

From Palay, Krachmer, 1997.

FIGURE 10-10

Acute hordeolum of upper eyelid.

From Palay, Krachmer, 1997.

Palpation

Palpate the eyelids for nodules. Ask the patient to close the eyes, and note whether the eyelids meet completely. When the closed lids do not completely cover the globe, a condition called lagophthalmos, the cornea may become dried and be at increased risk of infection.

Next palpate the eye itself. Determine whether it feels hard or can be gently pushed into the orbit without causing discomfort. An eye that feels very firm and resists palpation may indicate glaucoma, hyperthyroidism, or the presence of a retroorbital tumor.

Conjunctivae

The conjunctivae are usually inapparent, clear, and free of erythema. Inspection of the conjunctival covering of the lower lid is easily performed by having the patient look upward while you draw the lower lid downward (Figure 10-11).

Inspect the upper tarsal conjunctiva only when there is a suggestion that a foreign body may be present. Ask the patient to look down while you pull the eyelashes gently downward and forward to break the suction between the lid and globe (Figure 10-12). Next evert the lid on a small cotton-covered applicator. After you inspect and remove any foreign body that may be present, return the eyelid to its regular position by asking the patient to look up while you apply forward pressure against the eyelid.

Observe the conjunctiva for increased erythema or exudate. An erythematous or cobblestone appearance may indicate an allergic or infectious conjunctivitis (Figure 10-13). Bright red blood in a sharply defined area surrounded by healthy appearing conjunctiva indicates subconjunctival hemorrhage (Figure 10-14). The blood stays red because of direct diffusion of oxygen through the conjunctiva.

A pterygium is an abnormal growth of conjunctiva that extends over the cornea from the limbus. It occurs more commonly on the nasal side (Figure 10-15). A pterygium is more common in people heavily exposed to ultraviolet light. It can interfere with vision if it advances over the pupil.

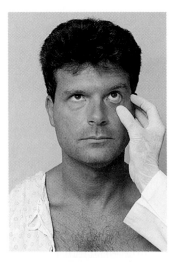

FIGURE 10-11

Pulling lower eyelid down to inspect the conjunctiva.

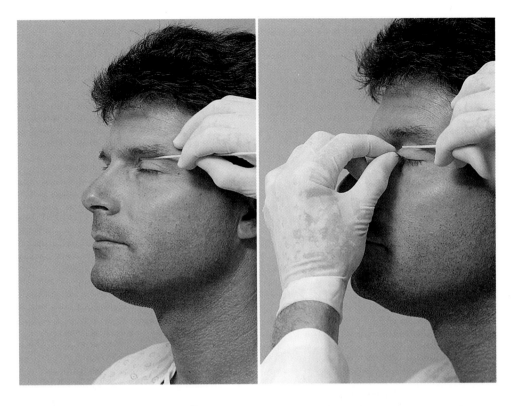

FIGURE 10-12
Everting upper eyelid.

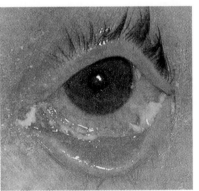

FIGURE 10-13
Acute purulent conjunctivitis.
From Newell, 1996.

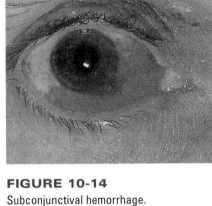

FIGURE 10-14
Subconjunctival hemorrhage.
From Newell, 1996.

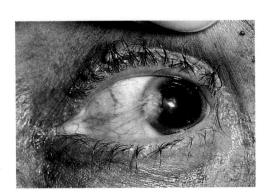

FIGURE 10-15
Pterygium.

Courtesy John W. Payne, MD, The Wilmer
Ophthalmological Institute, The Johns
Hopkins University and Hospital,
Baltimore.

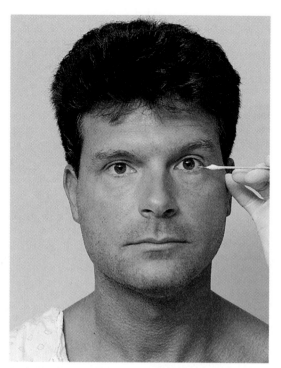

FIGURE 10-16
Testing corneal sensitivity.

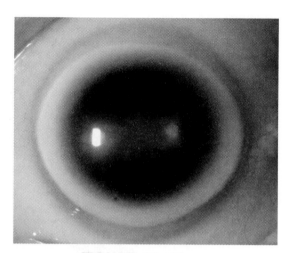

FIGURE 10-17
Corneal circus senilis.
From Palay, Krachmer, 1997.

Cornea

Examine the cornea for clarity by shining a light tangentially on it. Since the cornea is avascular, blood vessels should not be present. Corneal sensitivity, controlled by cranial nerve V (trigeminal nerve), is tested by touching a wisp of cotton to the cornea (Figure 10-16). The expected response is a blink, which requires intact sensory fibers of cranial nerve V and motor fibers of cranial nerve VII (facial nerve).

You may note a corneal arcus (arcus senilis), which is composed of lipids deposited in the periphery of the cornea. It may in time form a complete circle (circus senilis) (Figure 10-17). An arcus is seen in the majority of individuals over age 60. If present before age 40, arcus senilis may indicate a lipid disorder, most commonly type II hyperlipidemia.

Iris and Pupil

The iris pattern should be clearly visible. Generally the irides are the same color. Note any irregularity in the shape of the pupils. They should be round, regular, and equal in size. Pupil abnormalities are described on p. 300.

Test the pupils for response to light both directly and consensually. Dim the lights in the room so that the pupils dilate. Shine a penlight directly into one eye and note whether the pupil constricts. Note the consensual response of the opposite pupil constricting simultaneously with the tested pupil. Repeat the test by shining the light in the other eye.

Test the pupils for constriction to accommodation as well. Ask the patient to look at a distant object and then at a test object (either a pencil or your finger) held

10 cm from the bridge of the nose. The pupils should constrict when the eyes focus on the near object. With some patients, especially those with dark irides, it may be easier to observe pupillary dilation when the patient looks from near to far. Testing for pupillary response to accommodation is of diagnostic importance only if there is a defect in the pupillary response to light. A failure to respond to direct light but retaining constriction during accommodation is sometimes seen in patients with diabetes or syphilis.

Estimate the pupillary sizes and compare them for equality. Pupils may show size variation in a number of ways. Miosis is pupillary constriction to less than 2 mm. The miotic pupil fails to dilate in the dark. It is commonly caused by ingestion of drugs such as morphine, but drugs that control glaucoma may cause miosis as well. Mydriasis is characterized by pupillary dilation of more than 6 mm and failure of the pupils to constrict with light. Mydriasis is an accompaniment of coma, whether caused by diabetes, alcohol, uremia, epilepsy, or head trauma. Anisocoria, the inequality of pupillary size, is a common variation but may also occur in a large variety of disease states.

Lens

Inspect the lens, which should be transparent. Shining a light on the lens may cause it to appear gray or yellow, but its ability to transmit light may still be great. Later examination of the lens with the ophthalmoscope will help judge the clarity.

Sclera

The sclera should be examined primarily to ensure that it is white. The sclera should be visible above the iris only when the eyelids are wide open. If liver disease is present, the sclerae may become pigmented and appear either yellow or green. Senile hyaline plaque appears as a dark, rust-colored pigment just anterior to the insertion of the medial rectus muscle (Figure 10-18). Its presence does not imply disease but should be noted.

Lacrimal Apparatus

Inspect the region of the lacrimal gland, and palpate the lower orbital rim near the inner canthus. The puncta should be seen as slight elevations with a central depression on both the upper and lower lid margins. If the temporal aspect of the upper lid feels full, evert the lid and inspect the gland. The lacrimal glands are rarely enlarged but may become so in some conditions, such as sarcoid disease and Sjögren syndrome. Despite the enlargement, the patient may complain of dry eyes because the glands produce inadequate tears.

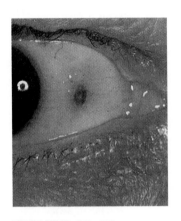

FIGURE 10-18
Senile hyaline plaque.
From Newell, 1996.

EXTRAOCULAR EYE MUSCLES

Full movement of the eyes is controlled by the integrated function of the cranial nerves III (oculomotor), IV (trochlear), and VI (abducens) and the six extraocular muscles. Hold the patient's chin to prevent movement of the head and ask him or her to watch your finger as it moves through the six cardinal fields of gaze (Figure 10-19). Then ask the patient to look to the extreme lateral (temporal) positions. Do not be surprised to observe a few horizontal nystagmic beats.

Occasionally you may note sustained nystagmus, the involuntary rhythmic movements of the eyes that can occur in a horizontal, vertical, rotary, or mixed pattern. Jerking nystagmus, characterized by faster movements in one direction, is defined by its rapid phase. If the eye moves rapidly to the right and then slowly drifts leftward, the patient is said to have nystagmus to the right.

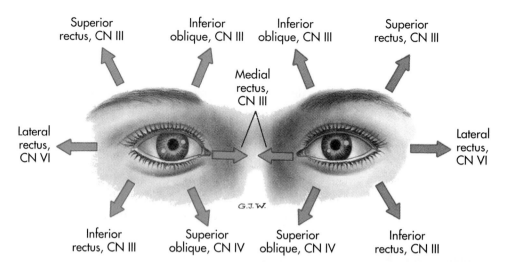

FIGURE 10-19
Cranial nerves and extraocular muscles associated with the six cardinal fields of gaze.

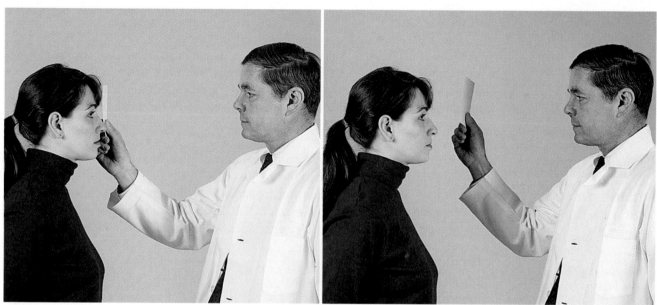

FIGURE 10-20
Evaluating eye fixation by the cover-uncover test.

Finally, have the patient follow your finger in the vertical plane, going from ceiling to floor. Observe the coordinated movement of the globes and the superior lid. The movement should be accomplished smoothly and without exposure of the sclera. Full movements indicate integrity of muscle strength and cranial nerve action. Lid lag, the exposure of the sclera above the iris when the patient is asked to follow your finger as you direct the eye in a smooth movement from ceiling to floor, may indicate hyperthyroidism.

Use the corneal light reflex to test the balance of the extraocular muscles. Direct a light source at the nasal bridge from a distance of about 30 cm. Ask the patient to look at a nearby object (but not the light source). This will encourage the effort to converge. The light should be reflected symmetrically from both eyes. When there is an imbalance found with the corneal light reflex test, then perform the cover-uncover test (Figure 10-20).

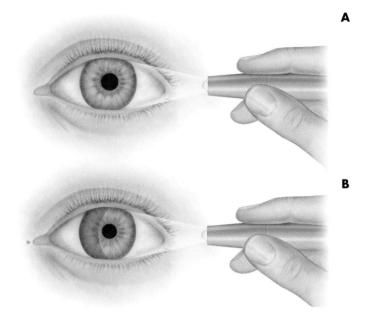

A

B

FIGURE 10-21

Evaluation of depth of anterior chambers. **A,** Normal anterior chamber. **B,** Shallow anterior chamber.

To perform the cover-uncover test, ask the patient to stare straight ahead at a near fixed point. Cover one eye and observe the uncovered eye for movement as it focuses on the designated point. Remove the cover and watch for movement of the newly uncovered eye as it fixes on the object. Repeat the process, covering the other eye. Movement of the covered or uncovered eye may indicate either esotropia or exotropia.

OPHTHALMOSCOPIC EXAMINATION

TEST FOR APPLYING MYDRIATRICS

Before instillation of a mydriatic, inspect the patient's anterior chamber by shining a focused light tangentially at the limbus (the union of the conjunctiva and the sclera). Note the illumination of the iris nasally (Figure 10-21). This portion of the iris is not lighted when the patient has a shallow anterior chamber, indicating a risk of acute angle glaucoma. Mydriatics should be avoided in these patients.

The ophthalmoscopic examination of the eyes is a tiring process. Avoid prolonging it while still giving the patient at least brief intervals for rest from the bright light, a respectful consideration that reduces fatigue and improves comfort.

Inspection of the interior of the eye permits visualization of the optic disc, arteries, veins, and retina. Adequate pupillary dilation is necessary and can often be achieved by dimming the lights in the examining room. Instillation of medications that cause mydriasis is used in some cases.

Examine the patient's right eye with your right eye and the patient's left eye with your left. Hold the ophthalmoscope in the hand that corresponds to the examining eye. (A photograph of the ophthalmoscope appears in Figure 3-13, p. 64.) Change the lens of the ophthalmoscope with your index finger. Start with the lens on the 0 setting, and stabilize yourself and the patient by placing your other hand on the patient's shoulder or head (Figure 10-22).

With the patient looking at a distant fixation point, direct the light of the ophthalmoscope at the pupil from about 30 cm (12 in) away. First visualize a red reflex, caused by the light illuminating the retina. Any opacities in the path of the light will stand out as black densities. Absence of the red reflex is often the result of an improperly positioned ophthalmoscope, but it may also indicate total opacity of the pupil by a cataract or by hemorrhage into the vitreous humor. If you locate the red reflex and then lose it as you approach the patient, simply move back and start again.

The fundus, or retina, appears as a yellow or pink background, depending on the amount of melanin in the pigment epithelium. The pigment generally varies with the complexion of the patient (Figure 10-23). No discrete areas of pigmentation should be seen in the fundus except for crescents or dots at the disc margin, most commonly along the temporal edge.

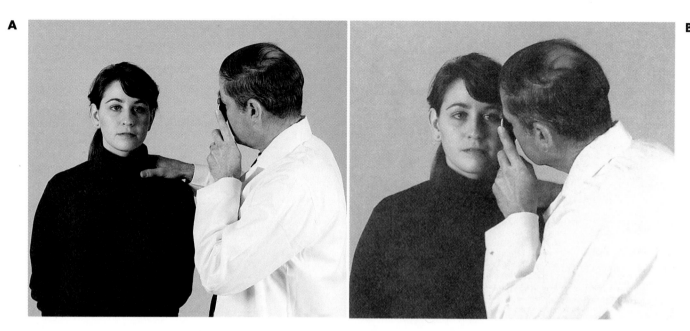

FIGURE 10-22
A, Visualization of the red reflex. **B,** Examination of the optic fundus.

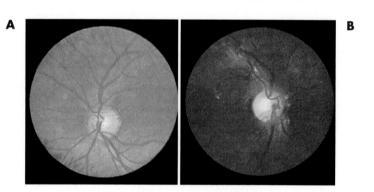

FIGURE 10-23
Fundus of **A,** white patient, and
B, black patient.
From MEDCOM, 1983.

As you approach the eye gradually, the retinal details should become apparent (Figure 10-24). Recall that at any one time, you will see only a small portion of the retina. A blood vessel will probably be the first structure seen when you are about 3 to 5 cm from the patient. You may have to adjust the ophthalmoscope lens to be able to see the retinal details. If your patient is myopic, you will need to use a minus (red) lens, and if the patient is hyperopic or lacks a lens (aphakic), you will need a plus (black) lens (see Chapter 3, p. 64). When fundus details come into focus, you will note the branching of blood vessels. Since they always branch away from the optic disc, you can use these landmarks to find the optic disc.

Next look at the vascular supply of the retina. The blood vessels divide into superior and inferior branches and then into nasal and temporal ones. Venous pulsations may be seen on the disc and should be noted. Arterioles are smaller than venules, generally at a ratio of 3:5 to 2:3. The light reflected from arterioles is brighter than that from venules, and the oxygenated blood is a brighter red. Follow the blood vessels distally as far as you can see them in each of the four quadrants. Note especially the sites of crossing of the arterioles and venules, because their characteristics may change when hypertension is present.

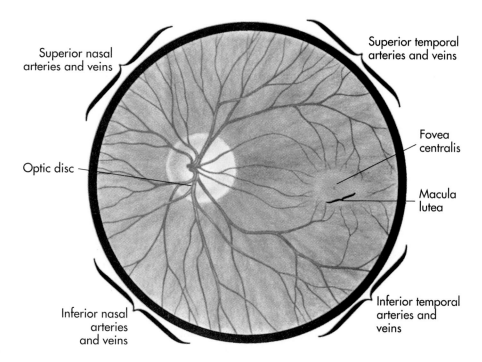

FIGURE 10-24
Retinal structures of the left eye.

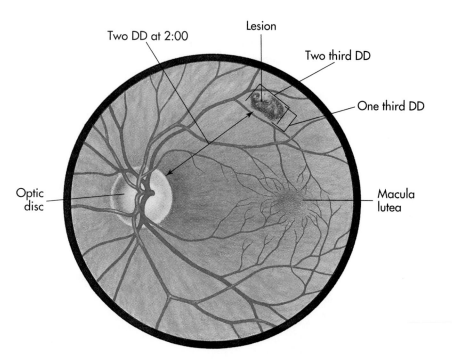

FIGURE 10-25
Method of describing the position and dimension of a lesion in terms of disc diameter. The lesion is this illustration is described as being 2 disc diameters (DD) from the optic disc at the 2 o'clock position. The lesion is two-thirds DD long and one-third DD wide.

The disc margin should be sharp and well defined, especially in the temporal region. The disc is generally yellow to creamy pink in color, but the color varies with race, being darker in individuals whose skin is dark. It is about 1.5 mm in diameter and is the unit of measurement in describing lesion size and location on the fundus. For example, an abnormality of a blood vessel may occur 2 disc diameters from the optic nerve at the 2 o'clock position (Figure 10-25).

Next examine the macula, also called the fovea centralis or macula lutea. The site of central vision, it is located approximately two disc diameters temporal to the optic disc. It may be impossible to examine when the pupil is not dilated, because shining light on it induces strong pupillary constriction. To bring it into your field of vision, ask the patient to look directly at the light of the ophthalmoscope. No blood vessels enter the fovea, and it appears as a yellow dot surrounded by a deep pink periphery.

Unexpected Findings

Occasionally you may see such unexpected findings as myelinated nerve fibers, papilledema, glaucomatous cupping, drusen bodies, or hemorrhages.

Myelinated nerve fibers appear as a white area with soft, ill-defined peripheral margins (Figure 10-26). The area is continuous with the optic disc. The nerve fiber layer is on the innermost surface of the retina. Note how the myelinated nerve fibers obscure areas of the retinal blood vessels, particularly inferiorly. This finding is due to the fact that the vessels lie deeper in the retina. The absence of pigment, feathery margins, and full visual fields help distinguish this benign condition from chorioretinitis.

Papilledema is characterized by loss of definition of the optic disc that initially occurs superiorly and inferiorly and then nasally and temporally. It is caused by increased intracranial pressure transmitted along the optic nerve. The central vessels are pushed forward, and the veins are markedly dilated. Venous pulsations are not visible and cannot be induced by pressure applied to the globe. Venous hemorrhages may occur. Initially vision is not altered (Figure 10-27).

Glaucomatous cupping is a result of increased intraocular pressure and the consequent interruption of the vascular supply to the optic nerve (Figure 10-28). Blood vessels may disappear over the edge of the physiologic disc and be seen again deep within the disc. Blood vessels may also be displaced nasally. Impairment of the blood supply may lead to optic atrophy, causing the disc to appear much whiter than usual. Peripheral visual fields are constricted.

Drusen bodies can appear as small, discrete spots that are slightly pinker than the retina. With time the spots enlarge and become more yellow. They may occur in many conditions that affect the pigment layers of the retina, but most commonly they are a consequence of the aging process and may be the precursor of senile macular degeneration (Figure 10-29).

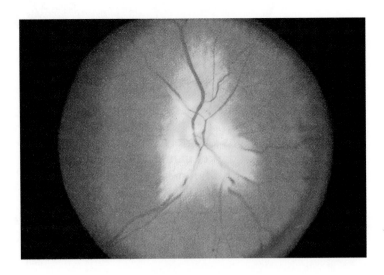

FIGURE 10-26

Myelinated retinal nerve fibers.

Courtesy Andrew P. Schachat, MD, The Wilmer Ophthalmological Institute, The Johns Hopkins University and Hospital, Baltimore.

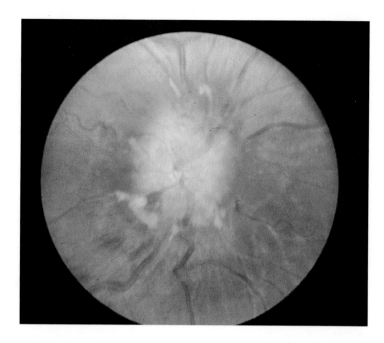

FIGURE 10-27

Severe papilledema.

Courtesy John W. Payne, MD, The Wilmer Ophthalmological Institute, The Johns Hopkins University and Hospital, Baltimore.

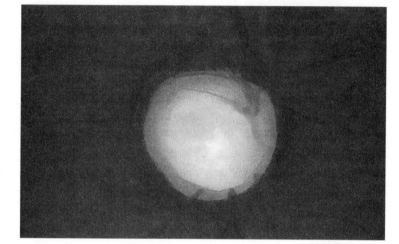

FIGURE 10-28

Marked glaucomatous optic nerve head cupping. Compare the disappearance of blood vessels here with the blood vessels of the optic disc in Figure 10-23.

Courtesy Andrew P. Schachat, MD, The Wilmer Ophthalmological Institute, The Johns Hopkins University and Hospital, Baltimore.

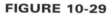

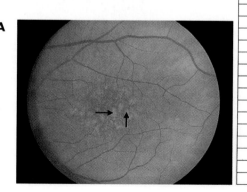

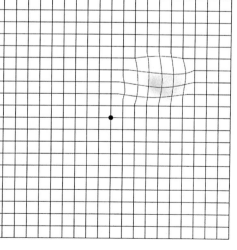

FIGURE 10-29

A, Drusen bodies. **B,** Amsler grid showing visual changes seen with central serous retinopathy.

A, Courtesy Robert P. Murphy, MD, Glaser Murphy Retina Treatment Center, Baltimore. **B,** Courtesy Brent A. Bauer, MFA, The Wilmer Ophthalmological Institute, The Johns Hopkins University and Hospital, Baltimore.

When Drusen bodies are noted to be increasing in number or in intensity of color, the individual should be given an Amsler grid. The grid is used to evaluate central vision. The patient is instructed to observe the grid with each eye and note any distortion of the grid pattern. Figure 10-29, *B* shows the grid of an individual with Drusen bodies who has developed leakage in the area of the macula (central serous retinopathy).

Hemorrhages in the retina vary in color and shape, depending on the cause and location (Figure 10-30, *A*). A hemorrhage at the disc margin often indicates poorly controlled glaucoma or undiagnosed glaucoma. Flame-shaped hemorrhages occur in the nerve fiber layers, and the blood spreads parallel to the nerve fibers (Figure 10-30, *B*). Round hemorrhages tend to occur in the deeper layers and may appear as a dark color instead of the bright red that is characteristic of flame hemorrhages. Dot hemorrhages may actually represent microaneurysms, which are common in diabetic retinopathy. The direct ophthalmoscope does not permit the distinction between dot hemorrhages and microaneurysms. Vascular changes that suggest systemic hypertension may be observed in the retina and are described in Box 10-1.

BOX 10-1   **Hypertensive Retinopathy**

Retinal changes associated with hypertension are generally classified according to the Keith-Wagner-Barker (KWB) system (Keith, Wagner, and Barker, 1939), which evaluates changes in the vascular supply, the retina itself, and the optic disc. For accurate rating the changes should be present bilaterally.

The arterial-venous size ratio is usually 3:5. As arterioles become smaller because of smooth muscle contraction, hyperplasia, or fibrosis, that ratio decreases. Venules do not have a smooth muscle coat but share the adventitia of the arteriole where the arteriole and venule cross. Thickening of the arteriolar coat results in apparent nicking of the venule where the venule passes beneath the arteriole, or the venule may appear elevated when it passes over the arteriole.

Group I of the KWB classification is characterized by increased light reflex from the arterioles. There are moderate arteriolar attenuation and focal constriction. No arterial-venous changes at crossing are noted.

Group II is marked by the appearance of arterial-venous crossing changes. Arterioles are reduced to about one half usual size, and areas of localized constriction may be observed.

Group III is characterized by a shiny retina and by the appearance of cotton wool spots, which represent ischemic infarcts of the retina. These are yellow areas with poorly defined margins. Hemorrhages may also be present.

Group IV is characterized by the appearance of papilledema.

A 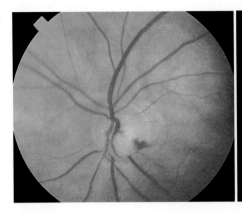 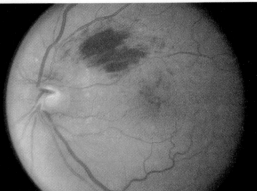 B

FIGURE 10-30

A, Hemorrhage at the disc margin. **B,** Flame hemorrhages.

A, Courtesy John W. Payne, MD, The Wilmer Ophthalmological Institute, The Johns Hopkins University and Hospital, Baltimore. **B,** Courtesy Robert P. Murphy, MD, Glaser Murphy Retina Treatment Center, Baltimore.

INFANTS

Infants often shut their eyes tightly when eye examination is attempted. It is difficult to separate the eyelids, and often the lids will evert when too much effort is exerted. Examining the newborn's eyes in a dimly lit room often encourages the baby to open the eyes. Holding the infant upright, suspended under its arms, also encourages the eyes to open. If a parent is present, have him or her hold the infant over a shoulder, and position yourself behind the parent. Even when the infant is crying, there will often be a moment when the eyes open. This gives you an opportunity to learn something about the eyes, their symmetry and extraocular muscular balance, and whether there is a red reflex. The child may then start crying again, but progress has been made.

Begin by inspecting the infant's external eye structures. Note the size of the eyes, paying particular attention to small or different sized eyes. Inspect the eyelids for swelling, epicanthal folds, and position. To detect epicanthal folds, look for a vertical fold of skin nasally that covers the lacrimal caruncle (Figure 10-31). Prominent epicanthal folds are common in Asian infants, but they may be suggestive of Down syndrome in children of other ethnic groups. Observe the alignment and slant of the palpebral fissures of the infant's eyes. Draw an imaginary line through the medial canthi and extend the line past the outer canthi of the eyes. The medial and lateral canthi should be horizontal. When the outer canthi are above the line, an upward, or mongolian, slant is present. When the outer canthi are below the line, a downward, or antimongolian, slant is present (Figure 10-32).

Inspect the level of the eyelid covering the eye. To detect the setting sun sign, rapidly lower the infant from upright to supine position. Look for sclera above the iris. This sign may be an expected variant in newborns; however, it also may be observed in infants with hydrocephalus and brainstem lesions.

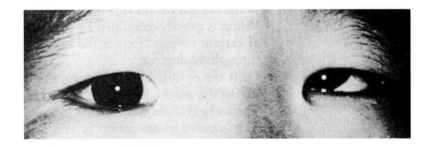

FIGURE 10-31

Epicanthal folds.

From Stein, Slatt, Stein, 1994.

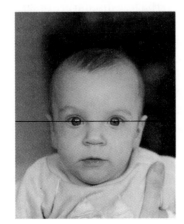

FIGURE 10-32

Drawing a line between medial and lateral canthi to determine if a Mongolian or antimongolian slant is present.

Courstesy Matthew Watson.

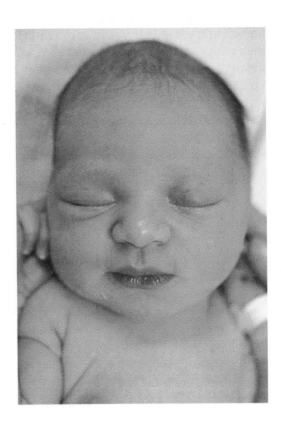

FIGURE 10-33
Swollen eyelids in a newborn.

Observe the distance between the eyes, looking for widely spaced eyes, or hypertelorism, which may be associated with mental retardation. Asian and Native American infants often have pseudostrabismus, the false appearance of strabismus because of a flattened nasal bridge or epicanthal fold. Pseudostrabismus generally disappears by about 1 year of age. Use the corneal light reflex to distinguish pseudostrabismus from strabismus. An asymmetric light reflex may indicate a real strabismus or hypertelorism.

Inspect the sclera, conjunctiva, pupil, and iris of each eye. The newborn's eyelids may be swollen or edematous, accompanied by conjunctival inflammation and drainage (Figure 10-33). This may be a consequence of routinely administered antibiotics. Any redness, hemorrhages, discharge, or granular appearance beyond the newborn period may indicate infection, allergy, or trauma. Inspect each iris and pupil for any irregularity in shape. A coloboma, or keyhole pupil, is often associated with other congenital anomalies. White specks scattered in a linear pattern around the entire circumference of the iris, called Brushfield spots, strongly suggest Down syndrome or mental retardation.

Test the cranial nerves II, III, IV, and VI in the following manner:

- Vision is grossly examined by observing the infant's preference for looking at certain objects. Expect the infant to focus on and track a light or face through 60 degrees.
- Elicit the optical blink reflex by shining a bright light at the infant's eyes, noting the quick closure of the eyes and dorsiflexion of the head.
- The corneal reflex is performed as in adults.

TABLE 10-2	Eye and Vision Examination Recommendations for Primary Care Physicians	
Age	**Screening Method**	**Indicators Requiring Further Evaluation**
Newborn to 3 months old	Red reflex	Abnormal or asymmetric
	Corneal light reflex	Asymmetric
	Inspection	Structural abnormality
6 months to 1 year old	Red reflex	Abnormal or asymmetric
	Corneal light reflex	Asymmetric
	Differential occlusion	Failure to object equally to covering each eye
	Fix and follow with each eye	Failure to fix and follow
	Inspection	Structural abnormality
3 years old (approximately)	Visual acuity*	20/50 or worse or two lines of difference between the eyes
	Red reflex	Abnormal or asymmetric
	Corneal light reflex/cover-uncover	Asymmetric/ocular refixation movements
	Stereoacuity†	Failure to appreciate random dot or Titmus Stereogram
	Inspection	Structural abnormality
5 years old (approximately)	Visual acuity*	20/30 or worse
	Red reflex	Abnormal or asymmetric
	Corneal light reflex/cover-uncover	Asymmetric/ocular refixation movements
	Stereoacuity†	Failure to appreciate random dot or Titmus Sterogram
	Inspection	Structural abnormality

From American Academy of Ophthalmology, 1992.
*Allen figures, HOTV, Tumbling E, or Snellen.
†Optional, sometimes advocated in lieu of visual acuity; Random Dot E Game (RDE), Titmus Stereograms, Randot Stereograms.

A funduscopic examination is very difficult to conduct on a newborn or young infant and is generally deferred until the infant is 2 to 6 months of age, unless, as with the visual problems of prematurity, there is a compelling need. Dilation of the eyes for effective visualization of the fundi can be safely achieved in the nursery by using solutions of weak mydriatics. If an infant's irides are blue, very little of a weak solution is necessary; one drop in each eye is generally enough. With darker colored eyes, a second drop a few seconds later is indicated. Cyclopentolate hydrochloride 0.5% is a popular mydriatic.

The red reflex should be elicited bilaterally in every newborn. Observe for any opacities, dark spots, or white spots within the circle of red glow. Opacities or interruption of the red reflex may indicate congenital cataracts or retinoblastoma (Table 10-2).

CHILDREN

Perform the inspection of the young child's external eye structures as described for the infant.

Visual acuity is tested (when the child is cooperative with the Snellen E game) usually at about 3 years of age (Figure 3-16, *B*). Have one examiner point to the line on the chart and another assist the child with covering one eye. As with adults, have the child stand 20 ft (6.1 m) away. Allow the child to practice following the instructions before you administer the test. Instruct the child to point his or her arm or finger in the direction of the legs of the E. If the child has difficulty following these directions, a card with a large E on it can be given the child with instructions to turn the E to match the letter indicated on the chart. Test each eye separately. If the child wears glasses, vision should be tested both with and without corrective lenses.

Examine visual acuity of younger children by observing their activities. Provide an opportunity for the child to play with toys in the examining room. Watch the child stacking, building, or placing objects inside of others. Children should have no visual difficulties if these tasks are performed well. The anticipated visual acuity of young children is as follows (Sprague, 1983):

AGE	VISUAL ACUITY
3 years	20/50
4 years	20/40
5 years	20/30
6 years	20/20

When you are testing visual acuity in the child, any difference in the scores between the eyes should be detected. A two-line difference (for example, 20/50 and 20/30) may indicate amblyopia.

Examination of extraocular movements and cranial nerves III, IV, and VI is performed as with adults. You may, however, need to hold the child's head still and use an appealing object such as a teddy bear for the child to follow through the six cardinal fields of gaze. Peripheral vision can be tested in cooperative children; the young child may prefer to sit on the parent's lap while these tests are performed.

Patience is very often needed to gain the child's cooperation for the funduscopic examination. The young child is often unable to keep the eyes still and focused on a distant object. Position the young child supine on the examining table, with the head near one end. Stand at the end of the table and use your right eye to examine the child's left eye and vice versa. Do not hold the child's eyelids open forcibly, because that effort will only lead to some resistance. Remember all retinal findings will appear upside down. Rather than move the ophthalmoscope to visualize all retinal fields, inspect the optic disc, the fovea, and the vessels as they pass by. Often the results are better when the child sits on the parent's lap. If this position is used, examine as is done with an adult.

PREGNANT WOMEN

Retinal examination in the pregnant woman can help differentiate between chronic hypertension and pregnancy-induced hypertension (PIH). Vascular tortuosity, angiosclerosis, hemorrhage, and exudates may be seen in patients with a long-standing history of hypertension. In the patient with PIH, however, there is segmental arteriolar narrowing with a wet, glistening appearance indicative of edema. Hemorrhages and exudates are rare. Detachment of the retina may occur with spontaneous reattachment after successful control of hypertension is achieved.

Because of systemic absorption, cycloplegic and mydriatic agents should be avoided unless there is a need to evaluate for retinal disease. Use of nasolacrimal occlusion after instillation of topical eye medications may reduce systemic absorption.

Eyes: near vision 20/40 in each eye uncorrected, corrected to 20/20 with glasses. Distant vision 20/20 Snellen. Visual fields full by confrontation.
Extraocular movements intact and full, no nystagmus.
Corneal light reflex equal.
Lids and globes are symmetrical. No ptosis. Eyebrows full, no edema or lesions evident. Conjunctiva pink, sclerae clear. No discharge evident. Cornea clear, corneal reflex intact. Irides brown, pupils equal, round and reactive to light and accommodation. Ophthalmoscopic examination reveals a red reflex. Discs cream colored, borders well defined with temporal pigmentation in both eyes (OU). No venous pulsations evident at the disc. Arteriole-venule ratio is 3:5, no nicking or crossing changes, hemorrhages or exudates noted.
Maculae are yellow OU.

For additional sample documentation, see Chapter 24, Recording Information.

SUMMARY OF EXAMINATION Eyes

1. Measure visual acuity, noting the following (pp. 278-279):
   - Near vision
   - Distant vision
   - Peripheral vision
2. Inspect the eyebrows for the following (p. 280):
   - Hair texture
   - Size
   - Extension
3. Inspect the orbital area for the following (p. 280):
   - Edema
   - Sagging tissues or puffiness
   - Lesions
4. Inspect the eyelids for the following (pp. 280-282):
   - Ability to open wide and close completely
   - Eyelash position
   - Ptosis
   - Fasciculations or tremors
   - Flakiness
   - Redness
   - Swelling
5. Palpate the eyelids for nodules.
6. Palpate the eye for firmness.
7. Inspect the orbits.
8. Pull down the lower lids and inspect the conjunctivae and sclerae for the following (pp. 282-283):
   - Color
   - Discharge
   - Lacrimal gland punctate
   - Pterygium
9. Inspect the external eyes for the following (pp. 284-285):
   - Corneal clarity
   - Corneal sensitivity
   - Corneal arcus
   - Color of irides
   - Pupillary size and shape
   - Pupillary response to light and accommodation
   - Depth of anterior chamber
10. Palpate the lacrimal gland in the superior temporal orbital rim (p. 285).
11. Evaluate muscle balance and movement of eyes with the following (pp. 285-287):
    - Corneal light reflex
    - Cover-uncover test
    - Six cardinal fields of gaze
    - Nystagumus
12. Ophthalmoscopic examination (pp. 287-290):
    - Lens clarity
    - Red reflex
    - Retinal color and lesions
    - Characteristics of blood vessels
    - Disc characteristics
    - Macula characteristics

COMMON ABNORMALITIES

EXTERNAL EYE

EXOPHTHALMOS

The mean protrusion of the eye for black males exceeds that of white males by 2 mm. The same measurement in black females exceeds that of white females by 2.4 mm.

From Migliori ME, Gladstone GJ, 1984.

Exophthalmos is an increase in the volume of the orbital content, causing a protrusion of the globes forward (Figure 10-34). It may be bilateral or unilateral. The most common cause is Graves disease, but when the exophthalmos is unilateral, a retroorbital tumor must be considered. The exophthalmos may be exaggerated by retraction of the upper lid and exposure of the sclera above the iris. Examination for exophthalmos is best conducted with the patient seated and the examiner standing above and looking down over the forehead. Precise quantification of the exophthalmos requires the use of an exophthalmometer. Blacks and individuals of Mediterranean descent may have prominent eyes as an expected variant.

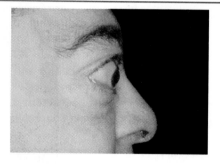

FIGURE 10-34
Thyroid exophthalmos.
From Stein, Slatt, Stein, 1994.

EPISCLERITIS

Episcleritis is an inflammation of the superficial layers of the sclera anterior to the insertion of the rectus muscles (Figure 10-35). It is generally localized, with a purplish elevation of a few millimeters. Often the cause of the inflammation is unknown, but it is a common manifestation of Crohn disease, rheumatoid arthritis, and other autoimmune disorders.

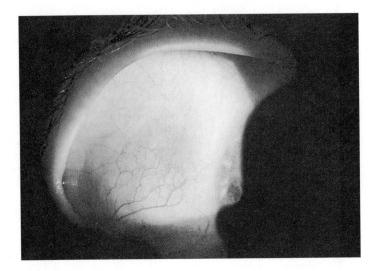

FIGURE 10-35

Episcleritis.

Courtesy Andrew P. Schachat, MD, The Wilmer Ophthalmological Institute, The Johns Hopkins University and Hospital, Baltimore.

BAND KERATOPATHY

Band keratopathy is produced by the deposition of calcium in the cornea (Figure 10-36). It appears as horizontal grayish bands interspersed with dark areas that look like holes. Band keratopathy appears as a line where the eyelids close just below the pupil and passes over the cornea rather than around the iris as arcus senilis does. This finding is most commonly seen in patients with hyperparathyroidism, but it occasionally occurs in individuals with renal failure or syphilis.

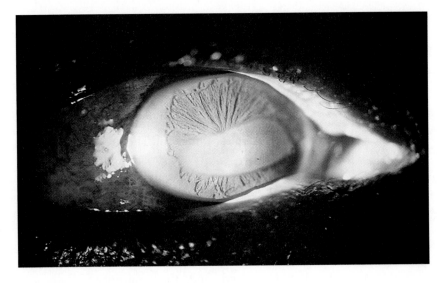

FIGURE 10-36

Band keratopathy.

Courtesy John W. Payne, MD, The Wilmer Ophthalmological Institute, The Johns Hopkins University and Hospital, Baltimore.

CORNEAL ULCER

Corneal ulcers are a disruption of the corneal epithelium and stroma caused by viral or bacterial infection, or desiccation because of incomplete lid closure or poor lacrimal gland function. Wearing contact lenses increases the risk of developing bacterial ulceration in the otherwise healthy eye. Figure 10-37 shows an ulcer in the lower temporal quadrant of the left cornea stained with rose Bengal.

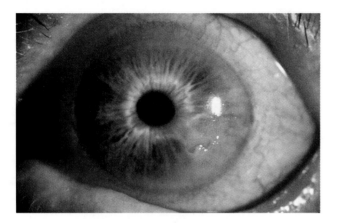

FIGURE 10-37
Corneal ulcer.

Courtesy John W. Payne, MD, The Wilmer Ophthalmological Institute, The Johns Hopkins University and Hospital, Baltimore.

EXTRAOCULAR MUSCLES

STRABISMUS (PARALYTIC AND NONPARALYTIC)

Strabismus is a condition in which both eyes do not focus on an object simultaneously. The condition may be paralytic, caused by impairment of one or more extraocular muscles or their nerve supply.

If a nerve supplying an extraocular muscle has been interrupted or the muscle itself has become weakened, the eye will fail to move in the direction controlled by that muscle. For example, if the right sixth nerve is damaged, the right eye does not move temporally.

Nonparalytic strabismus has no primary muscle weakness. The patient can focus with either eye but not with both simultaneously (Figure 10-38). It is detected by having the patient observe a near object. When one eye is covered, the other one will move to focus on the object if the covered eye was the dominant one. (Review cover-uncover testing in Figure 10-20.)

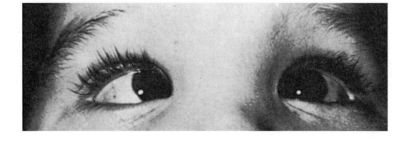

FIGURE 10-38
Right convergent strabismus.
From Stein, Slatt, Stein, 1994.

INTERNAL EYE   Pupil Abnormalities

TABLE 10-3   Descriptions of Various Pupil Abnormalities

Abnormality	Contributing Factors	Appearance
Bilateral		
Miosis (pupillary constriction; usually less than 2 mm in diameter)	Iridocyclitis; miotic eye drops (such as pilocarpine given for glaucoma)	
Mydriasis (pupillary dilation; usually more than 6 mm in diameter)	Iridocyclitis; mydriatic or cycloplegic drops (such as atropine); midbrain (reflex arc) lesions or hypoxia; oculomotor (CN III) damage; acute-angle glaucoma (slight dilation)	
Failure to respond (constrict) with increased light stimulus	Iridocyclitis; corneal or lens opacity (light does not reach retina); retinal degeneration; optic nerve (CN II) destruction; midbrain synapses involving afferent pupillary fibers or oculomotor nerve (CN III) (consensual response is also lost); impairment of efferent fibers (parasympathetic) that innervate sphincter pupillae muscle	
Argyll Robertson pupil	Bilateral, miotic, irregularly shaped pupils that fail to constrict with light but retain constriction with convergence; pupils may or may not be equal in size; commonly caused by neurosyphilis or lesions in midbrain where afferent pupillary fibers synapse	
Unilateral		
Anisocoria (unequal size of pupils)	Congenital (approximately 20% of healthy people have minor or noticeable differences in pupil size, but reflexes are normal) or caused by local eye medications (constrictors or dilators), amblyopia, or unilateral sympathetic or parasympathetic pupillary pathway destruction (see also Figure 3-39) (NOTE: Examiner should test whether pupils react equally to light; if response is unequal, examiner should note whether larger or smaller eye reacts more slowly [or not at all], since either pupil could represent the abnormal size)	Normal eye Affected eye
Iritis constrictive response	Acute uveitis is frequently unilateral; constriction of pupil accompanied by pain and circumcorneal flush (redness)	Normal eye Affected eye
Oculomotor nerve (CN III) damage	Pupil dilated and fixed; eye deviated laterally and downward; ptosis	Normal eye Affected eye
Adie pupil (tonic pupil)	Affected pupil dilated and reacts slowly or fails to react to light; responds to convergence; caused by impairment of postganglionic parasympathetic innervation to sphincter pupillae muscle or ciliary malfunction; often accompanied by diminished tendon reflexes (as with diabetic neuropathy or alcoholism)	

Modified from Thompson et al, 1997.

HORNER SYNDROME

Horner syndrome is caused by the interruption of the sympathetic nerve supply to the eye and results in ipsilateral miosis and mild ptosis. It is often caused by interruption of the cervical sympathetic trunk by mediastinal tumors, bronchogenic carcinoma, metastatic tumors, or operative trauma. Congenital Horner syndrome has also been described (Figure 10-39).

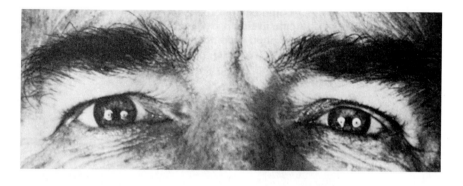

FIGURE 10-39
Horner syndrome, left eye.
From Trevor-Roper, Curran, 1984.

CATARACTS

The only common abnormality of the lens is cataract formation. A cataract is an opacity occurring in the lens, most commonly from denaturation of lens protein caused by aging. Almost everyone over the age of 65 has some evidence of lens opacification. With aging the lesion is generally central, but peripheral cataracts occur in conditions such as hypoparathyroidism. Congenital cataracts can result from maternal rubella or other fetal insults during the first trimester of pregnancy (Figure 10-40).

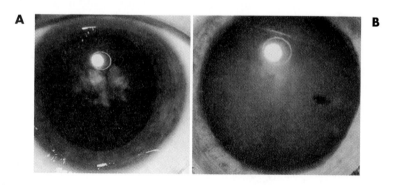

FIGURE 10-40
A, Snowflake cataract of diabetes. **B,** Senile cataract.
From Donaldson, 1976.

OPTIC ATROPHY

Optic atrophy is the result of death of nerve fibers and myelin sheaths. The primary symptom of optic atrophy is loss of central or peripheral vision or both. The disc or a portion of it loses its yellowish hue and becomes stark white. It is often helpful to compare the disc color in each eye when assessing for optic atrophy (Figure 10-41).

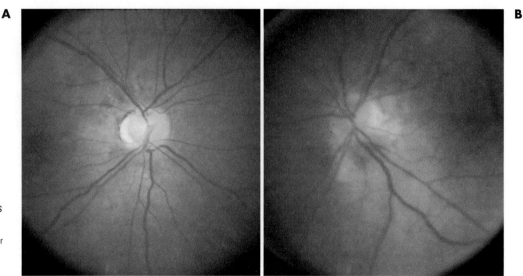

A   **B**

FIGURE 10-41

Optic atrophy. **A,** Patient's right eye shows atrophy. **B,** Left eye is unaffected.

Courtesy John W. Payne, MD, The Wilmer Ophthalmological Institute, The Johns Hopkins University and Hospital, Baltimore.

DIABETIC RETINOPATHY (BACKGROUND)

Diabetic retinopathy is generally divided into background and proliferative retinopathy. Background retinopathy is marked by dot hemorrhages or microaneurysms and the presence of hard and soft exudates. Hard exudates, thought to be the result of lipid transudation through incompetent capillaries, have sharply defined borders and tend to be bright yellow. Soft exudates are caused by infarction of the nerve layer and appear as dull yellow spots with poorly defined margins (Figure 10-42).

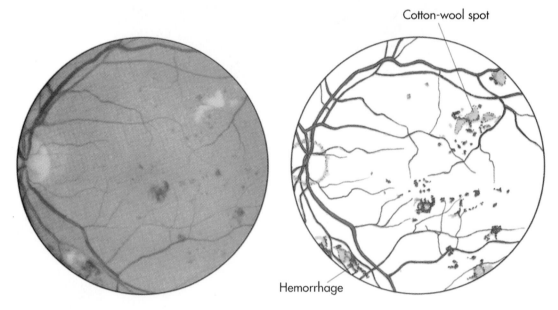

Cotton-wool spot

Hemorrhage

FIGURE 10-42

Background diabetic retinopathy. Note flame-shaped and dot-blot hemorrhages, cotton-wool spots, and microaneurysms.

From Barkauskas et al, 1998.

DIABETIC RETINOPATHY (PROLIFERATIVE)

Proliferative retinopathy is the development of new vessels as the result of anoxic stimulation (Figure 10-43). It may occur in the peripheral retina or on the optic nerve itself. The new vessels lack the supporting structure of healthy vessels and are likely to hemorrhage. These vessels grow out of the retina toward the vitreous humor, and visualization may require change in the lens setting of the ophthalmoscope. Bleeding from these vessels is a major cause of blindness in patients with diabetes. The same lesion may be seen in the infant born prematurely who has retinopathy of prematurity associated with oxygen therapy. Laser therapy for diabetic retinopathy can often control this neovascularization and prevent blindness from occurring. Laser therapy in the premature infant is still experimental.

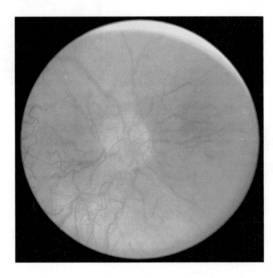

FIGURE 10-43
Proliferative diabetic retinopathy.

Courtesy John W. Payne, MD, The Wilmer Ophthalmological Institute, The Johns Hopkins University and Hospital, Baltimore.

LIPEMIA RETINALIS

Lipemia retinalis is a dramatic condition that occurs when the serum triglyceride level exceeds 2000 mg/dl (Figure 10-44). The blood vessels become progressively pink and then white as the triglyceride level rises. This condition may be seen in diabetic ketoacidosis and in some of the hyperlipidemic states.

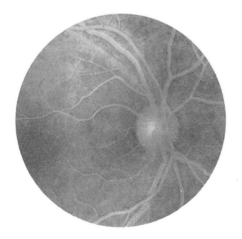

FIGURE 10-44
Lipemia retinalis.

From Newell, 1996.

RETINITIS PIGMENTOSA

Retinitis pigmentosa is an inherited condition characterized by the development of night blindness and loss of peripheral vision. Optic atrophy, narrowing of the arterioles, and peripheral "bone spicule" pigmentation are hallmarks of the disease (Figure 10-45).

A 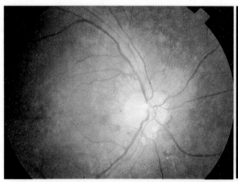 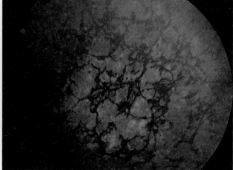 **B**

FIGURE 10-45

Retinitis pigmentosa. **A,** Optic atrophy and narrowing of the arterioles. **B,** Classic "bone spicule" pigmentation in the retinal periphery.

Courtesy John W. Payne, MD, The Wilmer Ophthalmological Institute, The Johns Hopkins University and Hospital, Baltimore.

CYTOMEGALOVIRUS INFECTION

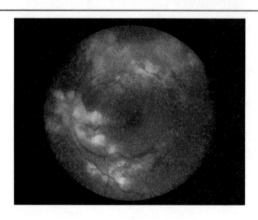

FIGURE 10-46

Cytomegalovirus retinitis.

Courtesy Douglas A. Jabs, MD, The Wilmer Ophthalmological Institute, The Johns Hopkins University and Hospital, Baltimore.

Cytomegalovirus (CMV) infection is an increasingly common cause of blindness as the human immunodeficiency virus (HIV) epidemic spreads. It is characterized by hemorrhage, exudates, and necrosis of the retina following the vascular pattern. CMV infection is said to create a "pizza pie" appearance in the retina (Figure 10-46).

GLAUCOMA

Glaucoma is an abnormal condition of elevated pressure within an eye caused by obstruction of the outflow of aqueous humor. It may occur acutely because the pupil dilates widely and the thickened iris blocks the exit of aqueous humor from the anterior chamber. Acute glaucoma is accompanied by intense ocular pain, blurred vision, a red eye, and a dilated pupil. Glaucoma may also occur chronically in which symptoms are absent except for gradual loss of peripheral vision over a period of years (Figure 10-28).

CHORIORETINAL INFLAMMATION

Chorioretinal inflammation (Figure 10-47) is an inflammatory process that involves both the choroid and the retina. It results in a sharply defined lesion that is generally whitish yellow and stippled with dark pigment. The most common cause of these lesions today is laser therapy for diabetic retinopathy, but it may also be seen as a consequence of infectious agents such as cytomegalovirus or toxoplasmosis during fetal life.

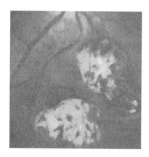

FIGURE 10-47

Patches of chorioretinitis adjacent to the optic disc.

From Stein, Slatt, Stein, 1994.

CHOROIDAL NEVUS

Choroidal nevi are pigmented lesions of the choroid (Figure 10-48). They appear as darkened, well-defined areas of varying size beneath the retina. They should be carefully observed to detect any enlargement or elevation that would suggest malignant change, for example, melanoma.

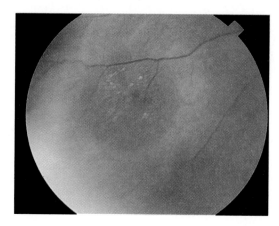

FIGURE 10-48

Choroidal nevus.

Courtesy John W. Payne, MD, The Wilmer Ophthalmological Institute, The Johns Hopkins University and Hospital, Baltimore.

VISUAL FIELDS

HEMIANOPIA

Defective vision or blindness in half the visual field may be a consequence of degenerative changes within the eye itself, such as a cataract, or it may stem from a lesion of the optic nerve anterior to its decussation (Figure 10-49).

Homonymous hemianopia can be caused by a lesion arising in either of two areas of the optic nerve radiation in the brain. The lesion may occur after the op-

tic chiasma and therefore involve nerve fibers arising from the same side of each eye. This disorder is also caused by the complete interruption of the nerve fibers as they progress to the optic cortex (Figure 10-50, *A*).

Bitemporal hemianopia (Figure 10-50, *B*) is caused by a lesion interrupting the optic chiasma, most commonly a pituitary tumor.

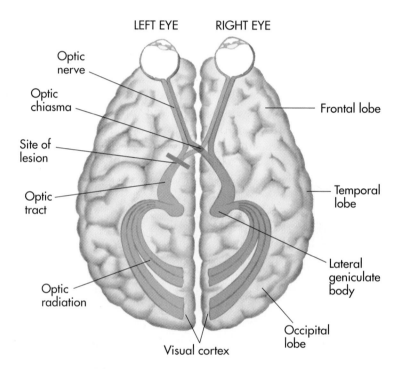

FIGURE 10-49
Site of lesion causing homonymous hemianopia.

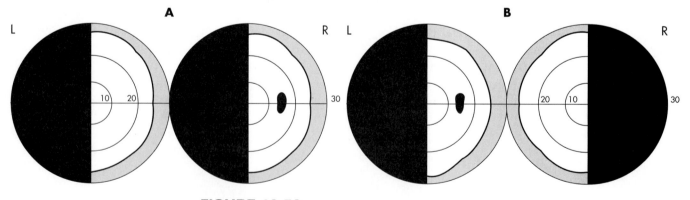

FIGURE 10-50
A, Left homonymous hemianopia. **B,** Bitemporal hemianopia.
From Stein, Slatt, Stein 1994.

CHILDREN

RETINOBLASTOMA

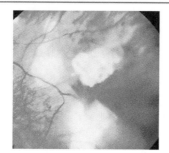

FIGURE 10-51

Retinoblastoma, the most common retinal tumor in children.

From Stein, Slatt, Stein 1994.

Retinoblastoma is a congenital malignant tumor arising from the retina, often during the first 2 years of life. The retinoblastoma may be transmitted either by an autosomal dominant trait or by a chromosomal mutation. Initial signs are a white reflex, also called a cat's eye reflex, rather than the usual red reflex. Funduscopic examination reveals an ill-defined mass arising from the retina. Often chalky-white areas of calcification can be seen (Figure 10-51).

RETINOPATHY OF PREMATURITY (RETROLENTAL FIBROPLASIA)

Figure 10-52 shows the changes found in the posterior pole of the left eye in the cicatricial (late) stage of the disease. Note that the blood vessels are straightened and diverted temporally. There is temporal traction on the retina in the posterior pole. Cicatricial changes may be much more severe and lead to retinal detachment, glaucoma, and blindness. Peripheral changes are seen only with the indirect ophthalmoscope.

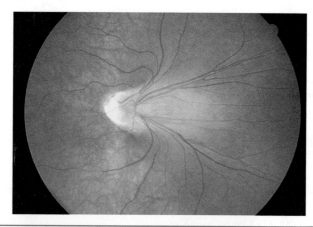

FIGURE 10-52

Retinopathy of prematurity.

Courtesy John W. Payne, MD, The Wilmer Ophthalmological Institute, The Johns Hopkins University and Hospital, Baltimore.

RETINAL HEMORRHAGES IN INFANCY

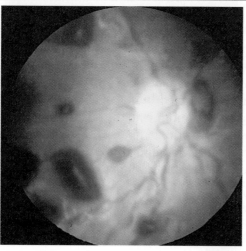

FIGURE 10-53

Multiple retinal hemorrhages are seen on funduscopic examination of this infant who was a victim of the shaken-baby syndrome.

From Zitelli, Davis, 1996; courtesy Stephen Ludwig, MD, Children's Hospital of Philadelphia.

Figure 10-53 shows multiple hemorrhages in the optic fundus of an infant who was a victim of the shaken-baby syndrome. Whenever retinal hemorrhages are seen, one must suspect infant abuse and investigate carefully.

Remember to check 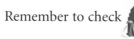 *http://www1.mosby.com/physexam_seidel*

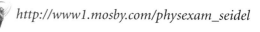

CHAPTER 11

Ears, Nose, and Throat

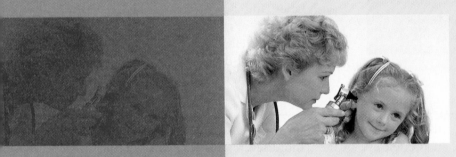

Much information about the function of the respiratory and digestive tracts can be gleaned from their accessible orifices—the ears, nose, mouth, and throat. The special senses of smell, hearing, equilibrium, and taste are also located in the ears, nose, and mouth.

ANATOMY AND PHYSIOLOGY

EARS

The ear is a sensory organ that functions in the identification, localization, and interpretation of sound, as well as in the maintenance of equilibrium. Anatomically, it is divided into the external, middle, and inner ear (Figures 11-1 and 11-2).

The *external ear,* including the auricle (or pinna) and external auditory canal, is composed of cartilage covered with skin. The auricle, extending slightly outward from the skull, is positioned on a nearly vertical plane. Note its structural landmarks in Figure 11-3.

The external auditory canal, an S-shaped pathway leading to the middle ear, is approximately 2.5 cm long in adults. Its skeleton of bone and cartilage is covered with very thin, sensitive skin. This canal lining is protected and lubricated with cerumen, secreted by the sebaceous glands in the distal third of the canal.

The *middle ear* is an air-filled cavity in the temporal bone. It contains the ossicles, three small connected bones (malleus, incus, and stapes) that transmit sound from the tympanic membrane to the oval window of the inner ear. The air-filled cells of the mastoid area of the temporal bone are continuous with the middle ear. The tympanic membrane, surrounded by a dense fibrous ring (annulus), separates the external ear from the middle ear. It is concave, being pulled in at the center (umbo) by the malleus. The tympanic membrane is translucent, permitting visualization of the middle ear cavity, including the malleus. Its oblique position to the auditory canal and conical shape account for the triangular light reflex. Most of the tympanic membrane is tense (the pars tensa), but the superior portion (pars flaccida) is more flaccid (Figure 11-4).

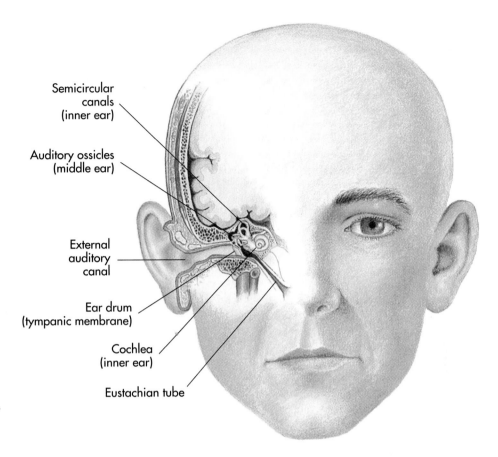

FIGURE 11-1
Cross section of the external, middle, and inner ear in relationship to other structures of the head and face.

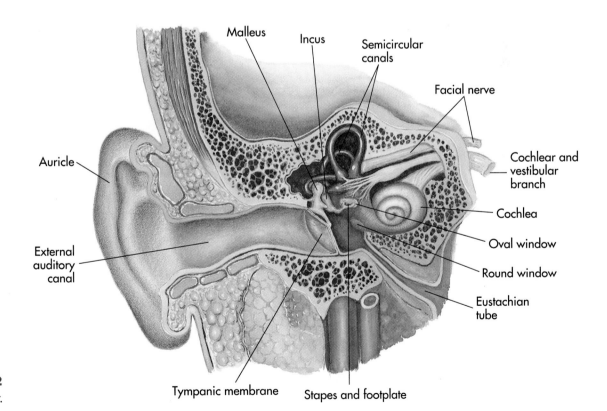

FIGURE 11-2
Anatomy of the ear.

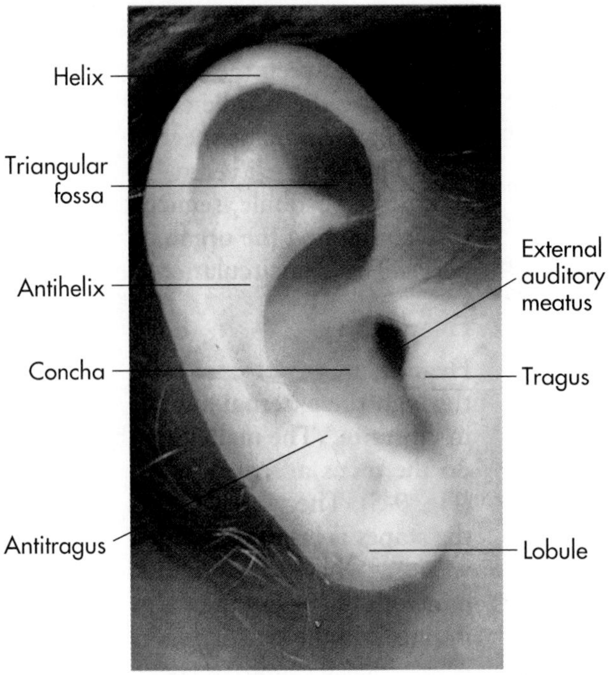

FIGURE 11-3

Anatomic structures of the auricle. The helix is the prominent outer rim, whereas the antihelix is the area parallel and anterior to the helix. The concha is the deep cavity containing the auditory canal meatus. The tragus is the protuberance lying anterior to the auditory canal meatus, and the antitragus is the protuberance on the antihelix opposite the tragus. The lobule is the soft lobe on the bottom of the auricle.

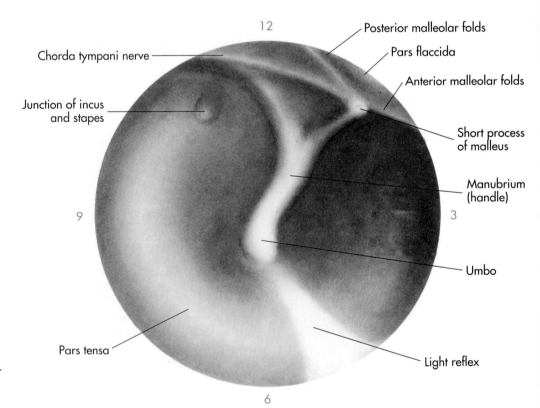

FIGURE 11-4

Structural landmarks of the tympanic membrane.

From Barkauskas et al, 1998.

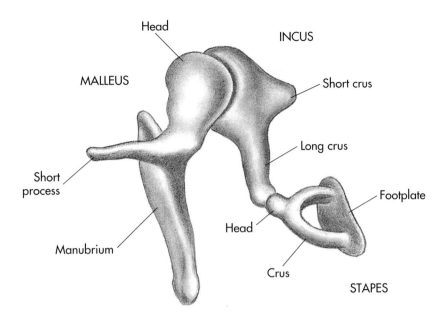

FIGURE 11-5

Ossicles of the right middle ear.

From Thompson et al, 1997.

The middle ear mucosa produces a small amount of mucus, which is rapidly cleared by the ciliary action of the eustachian tube, a cartilaginous and bony passageway between the nasopharynx and the middle ear. This passage opens briefly to equalize the middle ear pressure with that of atmospheric pressure when swallowing, yawning, or sneezing.

The *inner ear* is a membranous curved cavity inside a bony labyrinth consisting of the vestibule, semicircular canals, and cochlea. The cochlea, a coiled structure containing the organ of Corti, transmits sound impulses to the eighth cranial nerve. The semicircular canals contain the end organs for vestibular function.

Hearing

Hearing is an interpretation of sound waves by the brain. Sound waves travel through the external auditory canal and strike the tympanic membrane, setting it in vibration. The malleus, attached to the tympanic membrane, begins vibrating as do the incus and stapes, which are attached to the malleus on its medial surface (Figure 11-5). The vibrations are passed to the oval window of the inner ear in which the stapes is inserted. From here they travel via the fluid of the cochlea to the round window where they are dissipated. Vibrations in the membrane cause the delicate hair cells of the organ of Corti to strike against the membrane of Corti, stimulating impulses in the sensory endings of the auditory division of the eighth cranial nerve. These impulses are transmitted to the temporal lobe of the brain for interpretation. Sound vibrations may also be transmitted by bone directly to the inner ear.

NOSE AND NASOPHARYNX

The nose and nasopharynx have several functions:
- Identification of odors
- Passageway for inspired and expired air
- Humidification, filtration, and warmth of inspired air
- Resonance of laryngeal sound

The external nose is formed by bone and cartilage and covered with skin. The nares, which are the anterior openings of the nose, are surrounded by the cartilaginous ala nasi and columella. The frontal and maxillary bones form the nasal bridge (Figure 11-6).

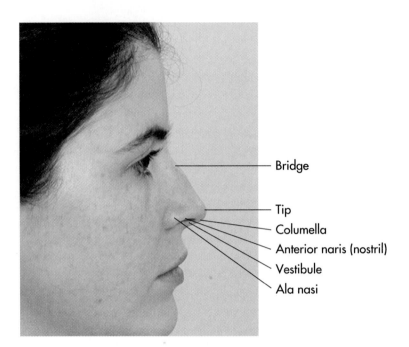

FIGURE 11-6
Anatomic structures of the external nose.

Bridge

Tip

Columella

Anterior naris (nostril)

Vestibule

Ala nasi

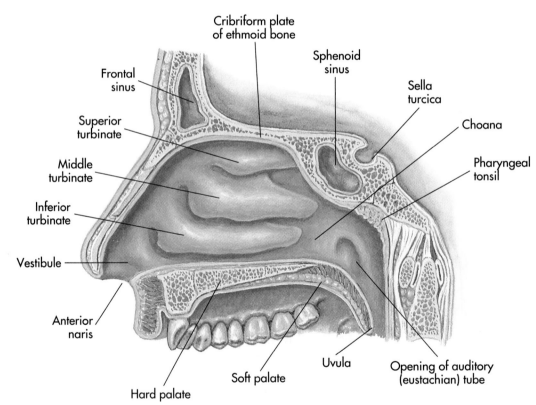

FIGURE 11-7
Cross-sectional view of the anatomic structures of the nose and nasopharynx.

Cribriform plate of ethmoid bone

Sphenoid sinus

Sella turcica

Choana

Pharyngeal tonsil

Frontal sinus

Superior turbinate

Middle turbinate

Inferior turbinate

Vestibule

Anterior naris

Hard palate

Soft palate

Uvula

Opening of auditory (eustachian) tube

The floor of the nose is formed by the hard and soft palate, whereas the roof is formed by the frontal and sphenoid bone. The internal nose is covered by a vascular mucous membrane thickly lined with small hairs and mucous secretions. This membrane collects and carries debris and bacteria from the inspired air to the nasopharynx for swallowing or expectoration.

The internal nose is divided by the septum into two anterior cavities, the vestibules. Inspired air enters the nose through the nares and passes through the vestibules to the choanae, which are posterior openings leading to the nasopharynx. The cribriform plate, housing the sensory endings of the olfactory nerve, lies on the roof of the nose. The Kiesselbach plexus is a convergence of small fragile arteries and veins located superficially on the anterior superior portion of the septum. The adenoids lie on the posterior wall of the nasopharynx (Figure 11-7).

The lateral walls of the nose are formed by turbinates, curved bony structures covered by vascular mucous membrane, that run horizontally and protrude into the nasal cavity. The inferior, medial, and superior turbinates increase the surface area of the nose to warm, humidify, and filter inspired air. A meatus in the area below each turbinate is named for the turbinate above it. The nasolacrimal duct drains into the inferior meatus, while the paranasal sinuses drain into the medial meatus.

Sinuses

The paranasal sinuses are air-filled, paired extensions of the nasal cavities within the bones of the skull. They are lined with mucous membranes and cilia that move secretions along excretory pathways. Their openings into the medial meatus of the nasal cavity are easily obstructed.

The maxillary sinuses lie along the lateral wall of the nasal cavity in the maxillary bone. The frontal sinuses are in the frontal bone superior to the nasal cavities. Only the maxillary and frontal sinuses are accessible for physical examination. The ethmoid sinuses lie behind the frontal sinuses and near the superior portion of the nasal cavity. The sphenoid sinuses are deep in the skull behind the ethmoid sinuses (Figures 11-8 and 11-9).

MOUTH AND OROPHARYNX

The mouth and oropharynx have the following functions:

- Emission of air for vocalization and non-nasal expiration
- Passageway for food, liquid, and saliva, either swallowed or vomited
- Initiation of digestion by masticating solid foods and by salivary secretion
- Identification of taste

The oral cavity is divided into the mouth and the vestibule. The vestibule is the space between the buccal mucosa and the outer surface of the teeth and gums. The mouth, housing the tongue, teeth, and gums, is the anterior opening of the oropharynx. The roof of the mouth is formed by the bony arch of the hard palate and fibrous soft palate. The uvula hangs from the posterior margin of the soft palate (Figure 11-10).

The floor of the mouth is formed by loose, mobile tissue covering the mandibular bone. The tongue is anchored to the back of the oral cavity at its base and to the floor of the mouth by the frenulum. The dorsal surface of the tongue is covered with thick mucous membrane, supporting the filiform papillae. The ventral surface of the tongue has visible veins and fimbriated folds, a thin mucous membrane with ridges (Figure 11-11).

The parotid, submandibular, and sublingual salivary glands are located in tissues surrounding the oral cavity. The secreted saliva initiates digestion and moistens the mucosa. Stensen ducts are outlets of the parotid gland that open on the buccal mucosa opposite the second molar on each side of the upper jaw. Wharton ducts, outlets of the submandibular glands, open on each side of the frenulum under the tongue. The sublingual glands have many ducts opening along the sublingual fold.

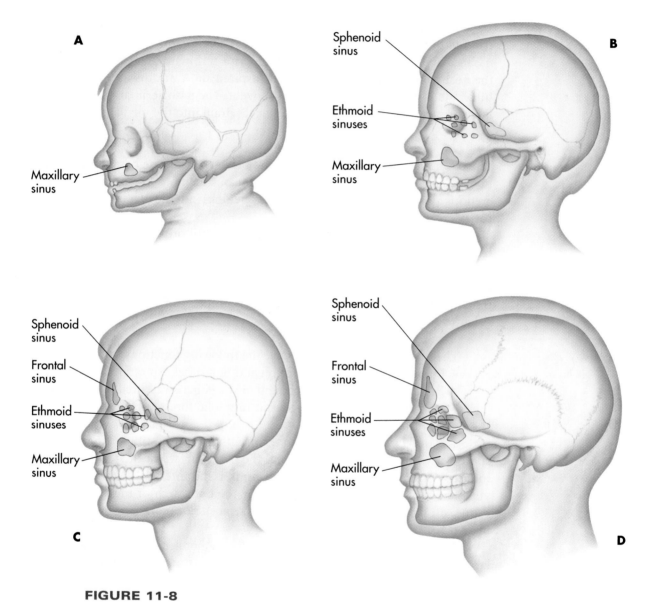

FIGURE 11-8
Location of the paranasal sinuses and comparison of their size by age. **A,** Infant, 1 year. **B,** Young child, 6 years. **C,** School-age child, 10 years. **D,** Adult, 21 years.

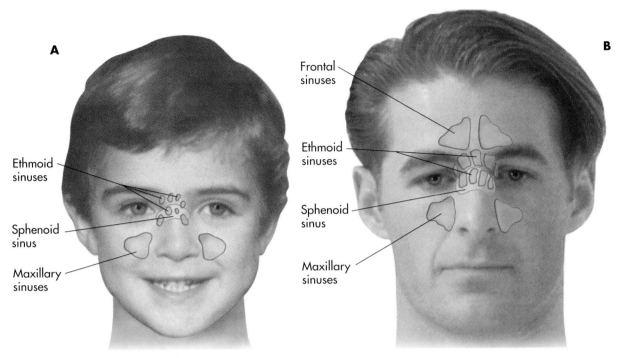

FIGURE 11-9
Anterior view of the cranial sinuses. **A,** Six-year-old child. **B,** Adult.

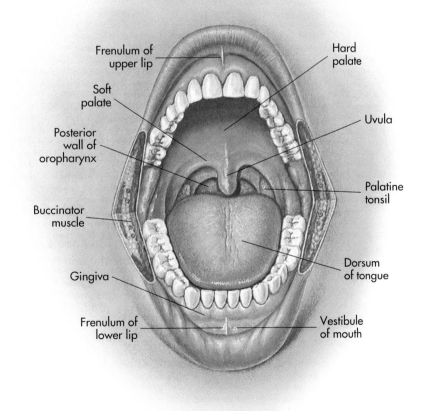

FIGURE 11-10
Anatomic structures of the oral cavity.

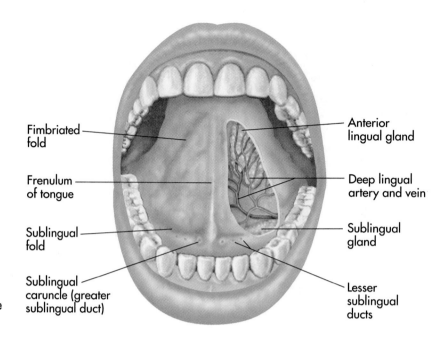

Fimbriated fold

Frenulum of tongue

Sublingual fold

Sublingual caruncle (greater sublingual duct)

Anterior lingual gland

Deep lingual artery and vein

Sublingual gland

Lesser sublingual ducts

FIGURE 11-11

Landmark of the ventral surface of the tongue.

The gingivae, fibrous tissue covered by mucous membrane, are attached directly to the alveolar surface. The roots of the teeth are anchored to the alveolar ridges, and the gingivae cover the neck and roots of each tooth. Adults generally have 32 permanent teeth consisting of 4 incisors, 2 canines, 4 premolars, and 6 molars, including wisdom teeth, in each jaw (Figure 11-12).

The oropharynx, continuous with but inferior to the nasopharynx, is separated from the mouth by the anterior and posterior tonsillar pillars on each side. The tonsils, lying in the cavity between these pillars, have crypts that collect cell debris and food particles.

INFANTS AND CHILDREN

Because development of the inner ear occurs during the first trimester of pregnancy, an insult to the fetus during that time may impair hearing. The infant's external auditory canal is shorter than the adult's and has an upward curve. The infant's eustachian tube is relatively wider, shorter, and more horizontal than the adult's, which allows easier reflux of nasopharyngeal secretions. As the child grows, the eustachian tube lengthens and its pharyngeal orifice moves inferiorly. With the growth of lymphatic tissue, specifically the adenoids, the eustachian tube may become occluded, interfering with aeration of the middle ear.

Although the maxillary and ethmoid sinuses are present at birth, they are very small. The sphenoid sinus is a tiny cavity at birth that is not fully developed until puberty. The frontal sinus develops by 7 to 8 years of age.

Salivation increases by the time the infant is 3 months old, and the infant drools until swallowing is learned. Deciduous teeth begin to calcify in the third month of fetal life, each tooth erupting when it has sufficient calcification to withstand chewing. The 20 deciduous teeth usually appear between 6 and 24 months of age. The permanent teeth begin forming in the jaw by 6 months of age. Pressure from these teeth leads to the resorption of the roots of the deciduous teeth until the crown is shed. Eruption of the permanent teeth begins about 6 years of age and is completed around 14 or 15 years of age in most races. White children's third molars erupt around 18 years of age.

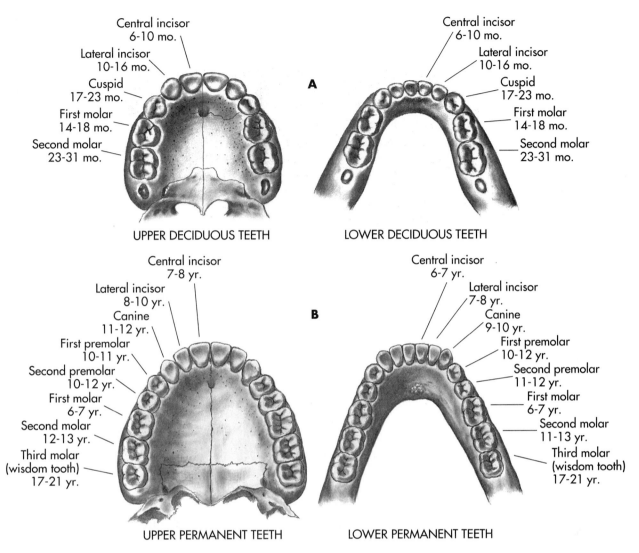

FIGURE 11-12

A, Dentition of deciduous teeth and their sequence of eruption. **B,** Dentition of permanent teeth and their sequence of eruption.

PREGNANT WOMEN	Elevated levels of estrogen cause increased vascularity of the upper respiratory tract. The capillaries of the nose, pharynx, and eustachian tubes become engorged, leading to symptoms of nasal stuffiness, decreased sense of smell, epistaxis, a sense of fullness in the ears, and impaired hearing. Increased vascularity and proliferation of connective tissue of the gums also occur. Laryngeal changes are also hormonally induced so that hoarseness, deepening or cracking of the voice, vocal changes, or persistent cough may occur.

OLDER ADULTS	Hearing tends to deteriorate with degeneration of hair cells in the organ of Corti, usually after age 50. The stria vascularis, a network of capillaries that secrete endolymph and promote the sensitization of hair cells in the cochlea, may atrophy, contributing to hearing loss. Sensorineural hearing loss first occurs with high-frequency sounds and then progresses to lower frequency tones.

Hearing deterioration may also result from an excess deposition of bone cells along the ossicle chain, causing fixation of the stapes in the oval window. Fewer sebaceous glands are active, and consequently the cerumen may become very dry. Cerumen may totally obstruct the external auditory canal, interfering with sound transmission. The tympanic membrane becomes more translucent and sclerotic. Conductive hearing loss occurs in each case.

Cartilage formation continues in the ears and nose, making the auricle and nose larger and more prominent. The soft tissues of the mouth change as the granular lining on the lips and cheeks becomes more prominent. The gingival tissue is less elastic and more vulnerable to trauma. The tongue becomes more fissured. The older adult may have altered motor function of the tongue, leading to problems with swallowing.

Saliva production may decrease as a result of disease or medications taken. Lost teeth may contribute to diet changes or difficulty chewing. Sensitivity to odors and taste declines.

REVIEW OF RELATED HISTORY

PRESENT PROBLEM

- Dizziness or vertigo
  - Time of onset, duration of attacks
  - Description (to and fro movement or rotary motion—room moving around patient or patient rotating), change of sensation with position change, associated with head and neck movement
  - Associated symptoms: nausea, vomiting, presence or absence of tinnitus and hearing loss, visual changes
  - Unsteadiness, loss of balance, falling
  - Medications: prescription or nonprescription
- Earache
  - Onset, duration, pain, fever, discharge (waxy, serous, mucoid, purulent, sanguinous)
  - Concurrent upper respiratory infection, frequent swimming, trauma to the head; related complaints in the mouth, teeth, sinuses, or throat
  - Associated symptoms: reduced hearing, ringing in ear, vertigo
  - Method of ear canal cleaning
  - Medications: antibiotics, ear drops (acetic acid, Auralgan, topical steroids)
- Hearing loss: one or both ears (see the Risk Factors box for hearing loss)
  - Onset: instant (may indicate vascular disruption), over a few hours or days (may indicate viral infection), slow or gradual
  - Repeated history of cerumen impaction
  - Hears best: on telephone, in quiet or noisy environment; all sounds reduced or some sounds garbled; inability to discriminate words
  - Speech: soft or loud, articulation of speech sounds
  - Management: hearing aid, when worn, battery change frequency; lip reading, sign language used
  - Medications: ototoxic (aminoglycosides, salicylates, furosemide, streptomycin, quinine, ethacrynic acid, cisplatin)
- Nasal discharge
  - Character (watery, mucoid, purulent, crusty, bloody), odor, amount, duration, unilateral or bilateral
  - Associated symptoms: sneezing, nasal congestion, itching nasal mucosa, habitual sniffling, nasal obstruction, mouth breathing, malodorous breath, conjunctival burning or itching
  - Seasonality of symptoms; allergies or concurrent upper respiratory infection; frequency of occurrence
  - Tenderness over sinuses, postnasal drip, daytime cough, face pain, headache
  - Medications: nose drops or sprays, antihistamines, decongestants

---

RISK FACTORS   **Hearing Loss**

Adults
- Exposure to industrial or recreational noise
- Genetic disease: Ménière disease
- Neurodegenerative disorder

Infants and Children
- Prenatal factors: maternal infection, irradiation, drug abuse, syphilis
- Birth weight less than 1500 g
- Excessively high bilirubin level
- Infection: bacterial meningitis, recurrent otitis media
- Cleft palate, craniofacial abnormalities
- Ototoxic antibiotic use
- Head trauma
- Hypoxic episode

- Snoring
  - Change in snoring pattern, complaints of snoring loudness by partner
  - Daytime sleepiness (associated with obstructive apnea)
  - Medications: prescription or nonprescription
- Nosebleed
  - Frequency, amount of bleeding, nasal obstruction, treatment, difficulty stopping the bleeding
  - Predisposing factors: concurrent upper respiratory infection, dry heat, nose picking, forceful nose blowing, trauma, allergies
  - Site of bleeding: unilateral or bilateral, alternating sides
  - Medications: prescription or nonprescription
- Dental problems
  - Pain: with chewing, localized to tooth or entire jaw, severity, interference with eating, foods no longer eaten; tooth grinding; associated with temporomandibular joint problems
  - Swollen or bleeding gums, mouth ulcers, tooth loss
  - Dentures or dental appliances: snugness of fit, areas of irritation, length of time dentures or appliances worn daily
  - Malocclusion: difficulty chewing, tooth extractions, previous orthodontic work
  - Medications: phenytoin, cyclosporine, calcium channel blockers, mouth rinses
- Mouth lesions
  - Intermittent or constantly present, duration, pain; excessive dryness of mouth; halitosis
  - Associated with stress, foods, seasons, fatigue, tobacco use, alcohol use, dentures (see the Risk Factors box for oral cancer)
  - Variations in tongue character: swelling, size change, color, coating ulceration, difficulty moving tongue
  - Medications: mouth rinses

RISK FACTORS   **Oral Cancer**

- >40 years of age
- Gender: men have twice the rate of women
- African American
- Excessive alcohol use
- Tobacco use: cigarettes, cigars, pipes, chewing tobacco, snuff
- Occupation: textile industry, leather manufacturing

- Sore throat
  - Pain with swallowing: associated with upper respiratory infection symptoms; exposure to streptococcus or gonorrhea; postnasal drip; or mouth breathing
  - Exposure to dry heat, smoke, or fumes
  - Hoarseness: voice overuse, infection, gastroesophageal reflux, need to clear throat frequently
  - Medications: antibiotics, nonprescription lozenges or sprays
- Difficulty swallowing
  - Solids, liquids, or both
  - Tightness, "catching," substernal fullness, vomiting
  - Drooling
  - Aspiration when swallowing
  - Swallowed liquids coming out of nose

PAST MEDICAL HISTORY

- Systemic disease: hypertension, cardiovascular disease, diabetes mellitus, nephritis, bleeding disorder, gastrointestinal disease, reflux esophagitis
- Ear: frequent ear problems during childhood; surgery; labyrinthitis; antibiotic use, dosage, and duration
- Nose: trauma, surgery, chronic nosebleeds
- Sinuses: chronic postnasal drip, repeated sinusitis, allergies
- Throat: frequent documented streptococcal infections, tonsillectomy, adenoidectomy

FAMILY HISTORY

- Hearing problems or hearing loss, Ménière disease
- Allergies
- Hereditary renal disease

PERSONAL AND SOCIAL HISTORY

- Environmental hazards: exposure to loud, continuous noises (factory, airport, playing in rock band); types of protective hearing devices used (associated with hearing loss)
- Nutrition: excessive sugar intake, foods eaten (associated with caries)
- Oral care patterns: tooth brushing and flossing; last visit to dentist; current condition of teeth; braces, dentures, bridges, crowns
- Tobacco use: pipe, cigarettes, cigars, smokeless; amount, number of years (associated with oral cancer)
- Use of alcohol
- Intranasal use of cocaine

INFANTS AND CHILDREN

- Prenatal: maternal infection, irradiation, alcohol and drug abuse, hypertension, Rh incompatibility, diabetes
- Prematurity: birth weight less than 1500 g, anoxia, ototoxic antibiotic use
- Erythroblastosis fetalis, bilirubin greater than 20 mg/100 ml serum
- Infection: meningitis, encephalitis, recurrent or chronic otitis media, unilateral mumps, congenital syphilis
- Breast-feeding, secondary tobacco smoke exposure, day care (associated with occurrence of otitis media)
- Congenital defect: cleft palate, craniofacial abnormality
- Playing with small objects (could place in nose or ears)
- Behaviors indicating hearing loss: no reaction to loud or strange noises, no babbling after 6 months of age, no communicative speech and reliance on gestures after 15 months of age, inattention to children of the same age
- Dental care: fluoride supplementation or fluoridated water; goes to sleep with bottle of milk or juice; when first tooth erupted; number of teeth present; thumb-sucking, pacifier use

PREGNANT WOMEN	■ Weeks' gestation or postpartum
	■ Presence of symptoms before pregnancy
	■ Accompanying symptoms suggestive of pathology
	■ Pattern of dental care

OLDER ADULTS	■ Hearing loss causing any interference with daily life
	■ Any physical disability: interference with oral care or denture care, problems operating hearing aid
	■ Deterioration of teeth, extractions, difficulty chewing
	■ Dry mouth (xerostomia)
	■ Medications decreasing salivation: anticholinergics, diuretics, antihypertensives, antihistamines, antispasmodics, antidepressants, tranquilizers; ototoxic drugs

EXAMINATION AND FINDINGS

EQUIPMENT

- Otoscope with pneumatic attachment
- Nasal speculum
- Tongue blades
- Tuning fork (500 to 1000 Hz, approximates vocal frequencies)
- Gauze
- Gloves
- Penlight, sinus transilluminator, or light from otoscope
- Vials with different odors such as mint, banana, coffee

EARS

External Ear

Inspect the auricles for size, shape, symmetry, landmarks, color, and position on the head. Examine the lateral and medial surfaces and surrounding tissue, noting color, presence of deformities, lesions, and nodules. (Figure 11-13 depicts the three earlobe shapes.) The auricle should have the same color as the facial skin, without moles, cysts or other lesions, deformities, or nodules. No openings or discharge should be present in the preauricular area. Darwin tubercle, a thickening along the upper ridge of the helix, is an expected variation, as are preauricular pits, which are found in front of the ear where the upper auricle originates.

FIGURE 11-13
The three earlobe shapes.
A, Soldered. **B,** Attached.
C, Free.

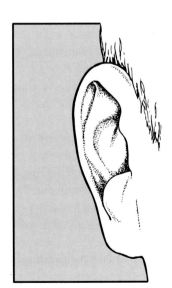
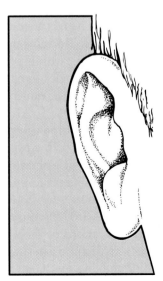
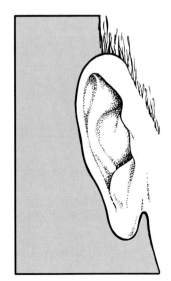

A   B   C

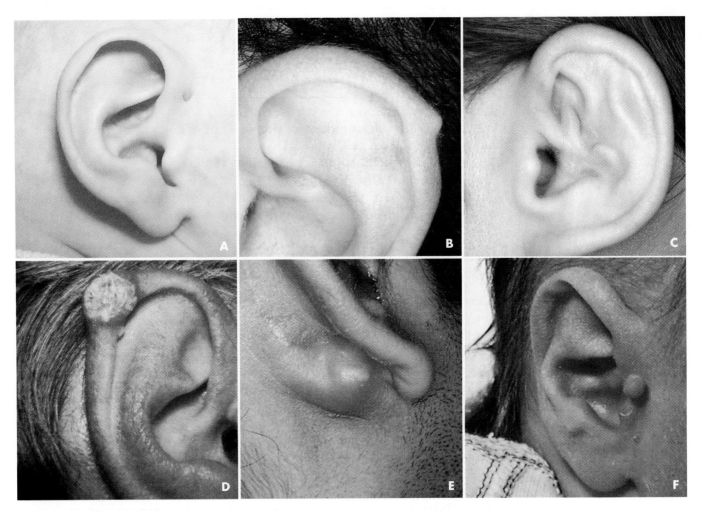

FIGURE 11-14
A, Auricular sinus. **B,** Darwin tubercle. **C,** Cauliflower ear. **D,** Tophi. **E,** Sebaceous cysts. **F,** Preauricular skin tag.

A and **F** from Zitelli, Davis, 1997; **B, C,** and **E** from Bingham, Hawke, and Kwok, 1992; **D** from Sigler and Schuring, 1993.

The color of the auricles may vary with certain conditions. Blueness may indicate some degree of cyanosis. Pallor or excessive redness may be the result of vasomotor instability. Frostbite can cause extreme pallor.

An unusual size or shape of the auricle may be a familial trait or indicate abnormality. A cauliflower ear is the result of blunt trauma and necrosis of the underlying cartilage. Tophi—small, whitish uric acid crystals along the peripheral margins of the auricles—may indicate gout. Sebaceous cysts, which are elevations in the skin with a punctum indicating a blocked sebaceous gland, are common (Figure 11-14).

To determine the position of the auricle, draw an imaginary line between the outer canthus of the eye and the most prominent protuberance of the occiput. The top of the auricle should touch or be above this line. Then draw another imaginary line perpendicular to the previous line just anterior to the auricle. The auricle's position should be almost vertical, with no more than a 10-degree lateral posterior angle (Figure 11-15). An auricle with a low-set or unusual angle may indicate chromosomal aberrations or renal disorders.

Inspect the external auditory canal for discharge and note any odor. A purulent, foul-smelling discharge is associated with an otitis or foreign body. In cases of head trauma, a bloody or serous discharge is suggestive of a skull fracture.

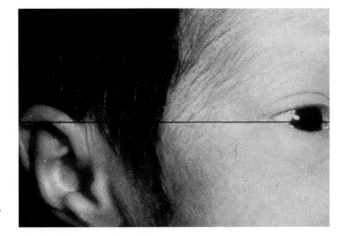

FIGURE 11-15
Assessment of auricle alignment, showing expected position.

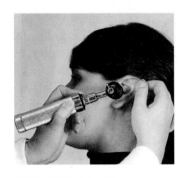

FIGURE 11-16
Straighten the external auditory canal by pulling the auricle up and back to examine the ear with the otoscope.

Palpate the auricles and mastoid area for tenderness, swelling, or nodules. The consistency of the auricle should be firm, mobile, and without nodules. If folded forward it should readily recoil to its usual position. Pulling gently on the lobule should cause no pain. If pain is present, inflammation of the external auditory canal may be present. Tenderness or swelling in the mastoid area may indicate mastoiditis.

Otoscopic Examination

The otoscope is used to inspect the external auditory canal and middle ear. (See Figure 3-19, p. 69, for a photograph of the otoscope.) Select the largest size speculum that will fit comfortably in the patient's ear. Hold the handle of the otoscope between your thumb and index finger, supported on the middle finger (right hand for the right ear and left hand for the left ear). This leaves the ulnar side of your hand to rest against the patient's head, stabilizing the otoscope as it is inserted into the canal. The handle of the otoscope can be held facing either up or down, whichever is most comfortable for you. Tilt the patient's head toward the opposite shoulder and simultaneously pull the patient's auricle upward and back as the speculum is inserted, thereby straightening the auditory canal to give the best view (Figure 11-16).

Examination of the tympanic membrane with the otoscope requires that you manipulate the auricle. This is one of innumerable times when the admonition to be gentle is underscored. A viselike grip is not necessary; a firm, gentle grasp is. The entire procedure need not be at all uncomfortable for the patient.

Slowly insert the speculum to a depth of 1.0 or 1.5 cm (0.5 in), and inspect the auditory canal from the meatus to the tympanic membrane, noting discharge, scaling, excessive redness, lesions, foreign bodies, and cerumen. Avoid touching the bony walls of the auditory canal (the inner two thirds) with the speculum, as this will be painful for the patient. Expect to see minimal cerumen, a uniformly pink color, and hairs in the outer third of the canal. Cerumen may vary in color and texture but should have no odor. No lesions, discharge, or foreign body should be present. See Box 11-1 for suggestions to clean an obstructed auditory canal.

BOX 11-1   Cleaning an Obstructed Auditory Canal

If the tympanic membrane is obscured by cerumen, the canal can be cleaned by warm water irrigation or by a cerumen spoon. Although a cerumen spoon is an acceptable tool for clearing out ear wax, you must remember that the auditory canal is easily abraded and bleeds readily, and when this happens, you cause pain. Water irrigation with body temperature water is the preferable approach, particularly with the young. Water irrigation should never be performed in the presence of otitis externa, a perforated tympanic membrane, myringotomy tubes, or a mastoid cavity.

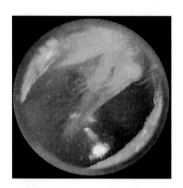

FIGURE 11-17

Healthy tympanic membrane.

From Barkauskas et al, 1998; courtesy Richard A. Buckingham, Clinical Professor, Otolaryngology, Abraham Lincoln School of Medicine, University of Illinois, Chicago.

Inspect the tympanic membrane for landmarks, color, contour, and perforations. Vary the direction of the light to see the entire tympanic membrane and the annulus. The landmarks (umbo, handle of malleus, and light reflex) should be visible (Figure 11-17). The tympanic membrane should have no perforations and be a translucent pearly gray color. Its contour should be slightly conical with a concavity at the umbo. A bulging tympanic membrane is more conical, usually with a loss of bony landmarks and a distorted light reflex. A retracted tympanic membrane is more concave, usually with accentuated bony landmarks and a distorted light reflex (Figure 11-18).

The pneumatic attachment of the otoscope is used to evaluate the mobility or compliance of the tympanic membrane. Make sure the speculum inserted into the canal seals it from the outside air. If a soft-tipped speculum is not available, a piece of rubber tubing around the end of the speculum tip may help achieve a seal with the canal. *Gently* apply positive (squeeze) and negative (release) pressure into the canal by using the pneumatic bulb attachment. Observe the membrane moving in and out, indicated by a change in the appearance of the cone of light. The tympanic membrane does not move when a tympanostomy tube is properly in place. Pathologic conditions in the middle ear may be suggested by characteristics of the tympanic membrane (Table 11-1).

Although pneumatic otoscopy has made it easier to assess the mobility of the tympanic membrane and the pressures within the middle ear, improper technique may produce misleading results. Dilation of the vessels overlying the malleus can result from applying negative pressure too slowly. The consequent redness, described as a mallear blush, may be the result of the otoscopy and can occur in the absence of infection (Bluestone and Shurin, 1974).

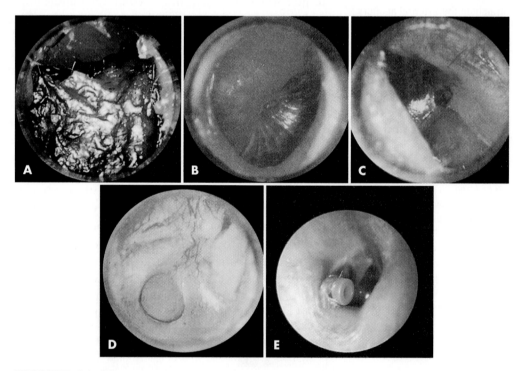

FIGURE 11-18

A, Tympanic membrane partially obscured by cerumen. **B,** Bulging tympanic membrane with loss of bony landmarks. **C,** Perforated tympanic membrane. **D,** Perforated tympanic membrane that has healed. **E,** Tympanostomy tube protruding from the right tympanic membrane.

A to **D** from Barkauskas et al, 1998; courtesy Richard A. Buckingham, Clinical Professor, Otolaryngology, Abraham Lincoln School of Medicine, University of Illinois, Chicago; **E** from Bingham, Hawke, Kwok, 1992.

TABLE 11-1	Tympanic Membrane Signs and Associated Conditions
Signs	**Associated Conditions**
Mobility	
Bulging with no mobility	Pus or fluid in middle ear
Retracted with no mobility	Obstruction of eustachian tube with or without effusion
Mobility with negative pressure only	Obstruction of eustachian tube with or without effusion
Excess mobility in small areas	Healed perforation, atrophic tympanic membrane
Color	
Amber or yellow	Serous fluid in middle ear
Blue or deep red	Blood in middle ear
Chalky white	Infection in middle ear
Redness	Infection in middle ear, prolonged crying
Dullness	Fibrosis
White flecks, dense white plaques	Healed inflammation
Air Bubbles	Serous fluid in middle ear

Hearing Evaluation

Cranial nerve VIII is tested by evaluating hearing. Screening of auditory function begins when the patient responds to your questions and directions. The patient should respond without excessive requests for repetition. Speech with a monotonous tone and erratic volume may indicate hearing loss.

Whispered voice. Check the patient's response to your whispered voice, one ear at a time. Mask the hearing in the other ear by having the patient place a finger in the ear canal and gently move it rapidly up and down. Stand to the side of the patient at a consistent distance best for you, about 30 to 60 cm (1 to 2 ft) away from the ear being tested. Whisper one- and two-syllable words very softly and ask the patient to repeat the words heard. If the patient has difficulty, increase the loudness of the whisper gradually until the patient responds appropriately. Repeat the procedure with the other ear. The patient should hear softly whispered words in each ear at a distance of 30 to 60 cm (1 to 2 ft), responding correctly at least 50% of the time.

Ticking watch test. Use a nonelectric ticking watch to test high-frequency hearing. Because of the variable loudness of ticking between watches, determine the average distance from the ear at which the ticking of your watch is heard by several people. Use this distance as the criterion to judge the patient's hearing. Mask the hearing in one ear, as described previously, and position the watch about 12.7 cm (5 in) from the other ear, slowly moving it toward the ear. Ask the patient to tell you when the ticking is heard. Repeat the procedure with the other ear.

Weber, Rinne, and Schwabach tests. The tuning fork is used to compare hearing by bone conduction with that by air conduction. Hold the base of the tuning fork with one hand without touching the tines, and stroke or tap the tines gently with your other hand, setting the tuning fork in vibration.

Perform the Weber test by placing the base of the vibrating tuning fork on the midline vertex of the patient's head (Figure 11-19). Ask the patient if the sound is heard equally in both ears or is better in one ear (lateralization of sound). Avoid giving the patient a cue as to the best response. The patient should hear the sound equally in both ears. If the sound is lateralized, have the patient identify which ear hears the sound better. To test the reliability of the patient's response, repeat the procedure while occluding one ear, asking the patient in which ear the sound is best heard. It should be heard best in the occluded ear.

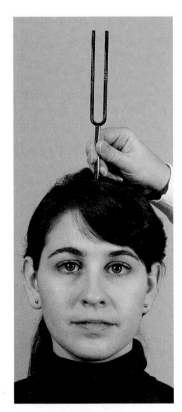

FIGURE 11-19
Weber test. Place the tuning fork on the midline of the skull.

A 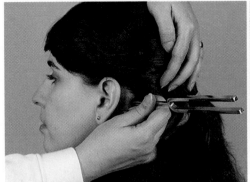 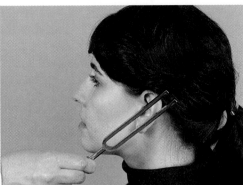 B

FIGURE 11-20
Rinne test. **A,** Place the tuning fork on the mastoid bone for bone conduction. **B,** Place the tuning fork on front of the ear for air conduction.

The Rinne test is performed by placing the base of the vibrating tuning fork against the patient's mastoid bone. Begin counting or timing the interval with your watch. Ask the patient to tell you when the sound is no longer heard, noting the number of seconds. Quickly position the still vibrating tines 1 to 2 cm (0.5 to 1 in) from the auditory canal, and ask the patient to tell you when the sound is no longer heard. Continue counting or timing the interval to determine the length of time the sound is heard by air conduction (Figure 11-20). Compare the number of seconds sound is heard by bone conduction versus air conduction. Air-conducted sound should be heard twice as long as bone-conducted sound after bone conduction stops. For example, if bone conduction is heard for 15 seconds, air conduction should be heard for an additional 30 seconds.

The Schwabach test is a comparison of the patient's and examiner's hearing by bone conduction. Alternately place the vibrating tuning fork against the patient's mastoid bone and your mastoid bone, until one of you no longer hears the sound. You should both hear the sound an equal length of time.

Unexpected findings from the three tuning fork tests must be integrated to differentiate between conductive and sensorineural hearing loss (Table 11-2). *Conductive hearing loss* results when sound transmission is impaired through the external or middle ear. *Sensorineural hearing loss* results from a defect in the inner ear that leads to distortion of sound and misinterpretation of speech. Any patient with unexpected findings should be referred for a thorough auditory evaluation.

TABLE 11-2	Interpretation of Tuning Fork Tests		
Test	**Expected Findings**	**Conductive Hearing Loss**	**Sensorineural Hearing Loss**
Weber	No lateralization, but will lateralize to ear occluded by patient	Lateralization of deaf ear unless sensorineural loss	Lateralization to better ear unless conductive loss
Rinne	Air conduction heard longer than bone conduction by 2:1 ratio (*Rinne positive*)	Bone conduction heard longer than air conduction in affected ear (*Rinne negative*)	Air conduction heard longer than bone conduction in affected ear, but less than 2:1 ratio
Schwabach	Examiner hears equally as long as the patient	Patient hears longer than the examiner	Examiner hears longer than the patient

NOSE AND NASOPHARYNX

External Nose

The nose is inspected for deviations in shape, size, and color. Observe the nares for discharge and for flaring or narrowing. The skin should be smooth without swelling and conform to the color of the face. The columella should be directly midline, and its width should not exceed the diameter of a naris. The nares are usually oval in shape and symmetrically positioned.

If discharge is present, describe its character (watery, mucoid, purulent, crusty, or bloody), amount, and color and whether it is unilateral or bilateral. The characteristics of nasal discharge are associated with various conditions. A bilateral watery discharge, associated with sneezing and nasal congestion, is indicative of an allergy. A unilateral watery discharge occurring after head trauma may indicate a fracture of the cribriform plate. The discharge may be spinal fluid. Bloody discharge usually results from epistaxis or trauma. Mucoid discharge is typical of rhinitis, and bilateral purulent discharge can occur with an upper respiratory infection. Unilateral, purulent, thick, greenish, and extremely malodorous discharge may indicate a foreign body.

A depression of the nasal bridge can result from a fractured nasal bone. Nasal flaring is associated with respiratory distress, whereas narrowing of the nares on inspiration may be indicative of chronic nasal obstruction and mouth breathing. A transverse crease at the junction between the cartilage and bone of the nose may indicate chronic nasal itching and allergies (Figure 11-21).

Palpate the ridge and soft tissues of the nose. Note any displacement of bone and cartilage, tenderness, or masses. Place one finger on each side of the nasal arch and gently palpate, moving the fingers from the nasal bridge to the tip. The nasal structures should feel firm and stable to palpation. No tenderness or masses should be present.

Evaluate the patency of the nares. Occlude one naris by placing a finger on the side of the nose, and ask the patient to breathe in and out with mouth closed. Repeat the procedure with the other naris. Nasal breathing should be noiseless and easy through the open naris.

Nasal Cavity

Use a nasal speculum and good light source to inspect the nasal cavity. Hold the speculum in the palm of the hand and use the index finger for stabilization. Use your other hand to change the patient's head position. The speculum should be inserted slowly and cautiously. Make sure you do not overdilate the naris or touch the nasal septum, which causes pain (Figure 11-22). Inspect the nasal mucosa for color, discharge, masses, lesions, and swelling of the turbinates. Inspect the nasal septum for alignment, perforation, bleeding, and crusting.

Only the inferior and middle turbinates will be visible. Keep the patient's head erect to examine the vestibule and inferior nasal turbinate. Tilt the patient's head back to visualize the middle meatus and middle turbinate. Then cautiously move the speculum tip toward the midline to examine the septum. Repeat the procedure in the other naris (Figure 11-23).

The nasal mucosa should appear deep pink (pinker than the buccal mucosa) and glistening. A film of clear discharge is often apparent on the nasal septum. Hairs may be present in the vestibule. Increased redness of the mucosa may occur with an infection, whereas localized redness and swelling in the vestibule may indicate a furuncle.

The turbinates should be the same color as the surrounding area and have a firm consistency. Turbinates that appear bluish gray or pale pink with a swollen, boggy consistency may indicate allergies. A rounded, elongated mass projecting into the nasal cavity from boggy mucosa may be a polyp.

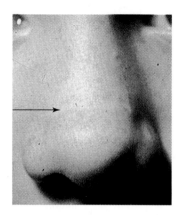

FIGURE 11-21
Transverse nasal crease.

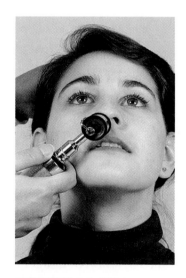

FIGURE 11-22
Use of the nasal speculum. Avoid touching the nasal septum.

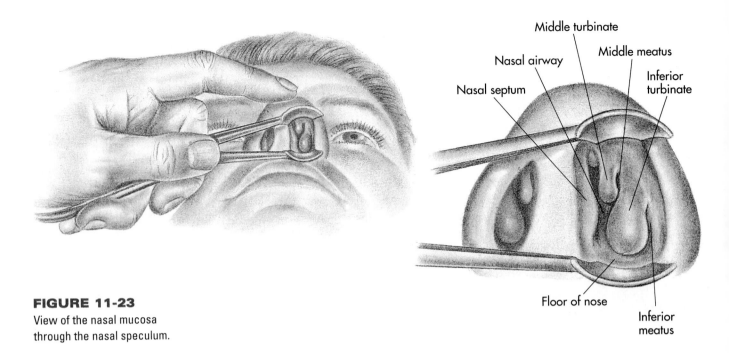

FIGURE 11-23
View of the nasal mucosa through the nasal speculum.

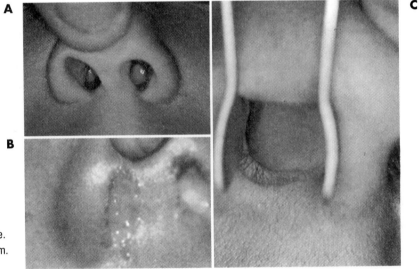

FIGURE 11-24
Unexpected findings on nasal examination. **A,** Nasal polyp (allergic). **B,** Purulent discharge. **C,** Deviation of the nasal septum.
C from Bull, 1974.

The nasal septum should be close to midline and fairly straight, appearing thicker anteriorly than posteriorly. Asymmetric size of the posterior nasal cavities may indicate deviation of the nasal septum. No perforations, bleeding, or crusting should be apparent. Crusting over the anterior portion of the nasal septum may occur at the site of epistaxis (Figure 11-24).

The sense of smell *(cranial nerve I)* is often tested with recognition of different odors. This procedure is described in Chapter 20 (Neurologic System) in the examination of cranial nerves.

A 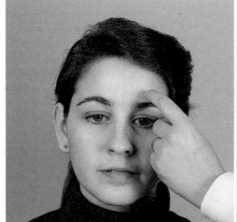 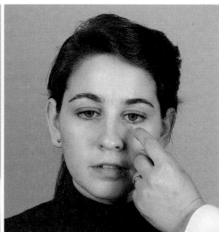 B

FIGURE 11-25
Percussion of **A**, frontal, and
B, maxillary sinuses.

Sinuses

Inspect the frontal and maxillary sinus areas for swelling. To palpate the frontal sinuses, use your thumbs to press up under the bony brow on each side of the nose. Then press up under the zygomatic processes, using either your thumbs or index and middle fingers to palpate the maxillary sinuses. No tenderness or swelling over the soft tissue should be present.

Percuss the sinus areas to detect tenderness. Lightly tap directly over each sinus area with your index finger, using your wrist to produce the force behind the finger (Figure 11-25). Swelling, tenderness, and pain over the sinuses may indicate infection or obstruction.

MOUTH AND OROPHARYNX

Lips

With the patient's mouth closed, inspect and palpate the lips for symmetry, color, edema, and surface abnormalities. Make sure the female patient removes her lipstick. The lips should be pink and have vertical and horizontal symmetry, both at rest and with movement. The distinct border between the lips and the facial skin should not be interrupted by lesions. The surface characteristics of the lips should be smooth and free of lesions.

Dry, cracked lips (cheilitis) may be caused by dehydration from wind chapping, dentures, braces, or excessive lip licking. Deep fissures at the corners of the mouth (cheilosis) may indicate riboflavin deficiency or overclosure of the mouth, allowing saliva to macerate the tissue. Swelling of the lips may be caused by infection, whereas angioedema may indicate allergy. Lesions, plaques, vesicles, nodules, and ulcerations may be signs of infections, irritations, or skin cancer (Figure 11-26).

The color of the lips is influenced by various conditions. Pallor of the lips is associated with anemia, whereas circumoral pallor is associated with scarlet fever. Cyanosis from a respiratory or cardiovascular problem produces bluish purple lips. A cherry red color is associated with acidosis and carbon monoxide poisoning. Round, oval, or irregular bluish gray macules of various intensity on the lips and buccal mucosa are associated with Peutz-Jeghers syndrome (Figure 11-27).

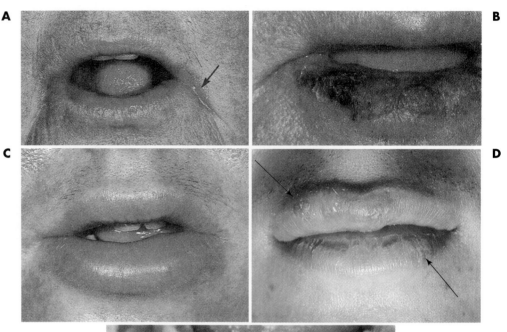

FIGURE 11-26
Unexpected findings on the lips.
A, Angular cheilitis. **B,** Actinic cheilitis. **C,** Angioedema. **D,** Herpes labialis. **E,** Squamous cell carcinoma of the lip.

A to C from Habif, 1996; D courtesy Antoinette Hood, MD, University of Indiana, School of Medicine, Indianapolis; E from Stewart et al, 1978.

Buccal Mucosa, Teeth, and Gums

Ask the patient to clench his or her teeth and smile so you can observe the occlusion of the teeth. The facial nerve *(cranial nerve VII)* is also tested with this maneuver. Proper tooth occlusion is apparent when the upper molars rest directly on lower molars and the upper incisors slightly override the lower incisors (Figure 11-28). Protrusion of the upper or lower incisors, failure of the upper incisors to overlap with the lower incisors, and back teeth that do not meet are indications of malocclusion (Figure 11-29). Three classes of malocclusion are listed in Table 11-3.

Have the patient remove any dental appliances and open the mouth partially. Using a tongue blade and bright light, inspect the buccal mucosa, gums, and teeth. The mucous membrane should be pinkish red, smooth, and moist. The Stensen duct should appear as a whitish yellow or whitish pink protrusion in approximate alignment with the second upper molar.

Fordyce spots are ectopic sebaceous glands that appear on the buccal mucosa and lips as numerous small, yellow-white raised lesions and are an expected variant. Deeply pigmented buccal mucosa may indicate an endocrine pathologic condition. Whitish or pinkish scars are a common result of trauma from poor tooth alignment. A red spot on the buccal mucosa at the opening of the Stensen duct is associated with parotitis (mumps). Aphthous ulcers on the buccal mucosa appear as white, round, or oval ulcerative lesions with a red halo (Figure 11-30).

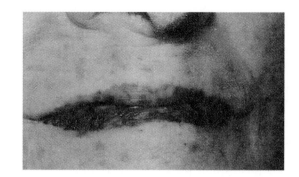

FIGURE 11-27

Peutz-Jeghers syndrome.

From *Diagnostic picture tests in clinical medicine,* 1984.

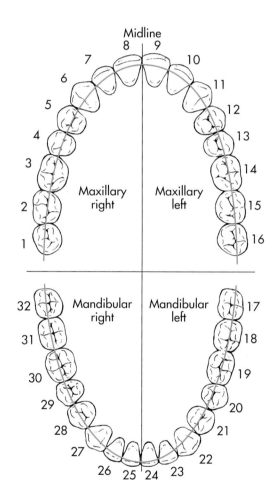

FIGURE 11-28

The line of occlusion and American Dental Association sequential tooth numbering system.

Modified from Miyasaki-Ching, 1996.

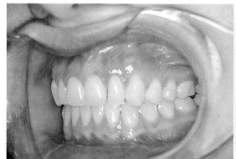

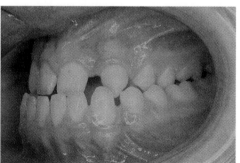

FIGURE 11-29

A, Class I malocclusion. **B,** Class III malocclusion.

Courtesy Drs. Abelson and Cameron, Lutherville, Maryland.

TABLE 11-3	Classes of Malocclusion
Class I	Molars have customary relationship, but the line of occlusion is incorrect because of malpositioned teeth from rotations or other causes.
Class II	Lower molars are distally positioned in relation to the upper molars; the line of occlusion may or may not be correct.
Class III	Lower molars are medially positioned in relation to the upper molars; the line of occlusion may or may not be correct.

The gingiva should have a slightly stippled, pink appearance with a clearly defined, tight margin at each tooth. The gum surface beneath dentures should be free of inflammation, swelling, or bleeding.

Using gloves, palpate the gums for any lesions, induration, thickening, or masses. No tenderness on palpation should be elicited. Epulis, a localized gingival enlargement or granuloma, is usually an inflammatory rather than neoplastic change. Enlargement of the gums occurs with pregnancy, puberty, phenytoin (Dilantin) therapy, and leukemia. A blue-black line about 1 mm from the gum margin may indicate chronic lead or bismuth poisoning. Easily bleeding, swollen gums that have enlarged crevices between the teeth and gum margins, or pockets containing debris at tooth margins are associated with gingivitis or periodontal disease (Figure 11-31).

Inspect and count the teeth, noting wear, notches, caries, and missing teeth. Make sure teeth are firmly anchored, probing each with a tongue blade. The teeth generally have an ivory color but may be stained yellow from tobacco or brown from coffee or tea. Loose teeth can be the result of periodontal disease or trauma. Discolorations on the crown of a tooth should raise the suspicion of caries.

Oral Cavity

Inspect the dorsum of the tongue, noting any swelling, variation in size or color, coating, or ulcerations. Ask the patient to extend the tongue while you inspect for deviation, tremor, and limitation of movement. The procedure also tests the hypoglossal nerve *(cranial nerve XII)*. The protruded tongue should not be atrophied and should be maintained at the midline without fasciculations. Deviation to one side indicates tongue atrophy and hypoglossal nerve impairment (Figure 11-32).

The tongue should appear dull red, moist, and glistening. Its anterior portion should have a smooth, yet roughened surface with papillae and small fissures. The posterior portion should have a smooth, slightly uneven or rugated surface with a thinner mucosa than the anterior portion. The geographic tongue, an expected variant, has superficial denuded circles or irregular areas exposing the tips of papillae. A smooth red tongue with a slick appearance may indicate niacin or vitamin B_{12} deficiency. The hairy tongue with yellow-brown to black elongated papillae on the dorsum sometimes follows antibiotic therapy (Figure 11-33).

A

B

FIGURE 11-30

Findings on the buccal mucosa. **A,** Fordyce spots. **B,** Aphthous ulcer.

A from Wood, Goaz, 1991; **B** courtesy Antoinette Hood, MD, Indiana University School of Medicine, Indianapolis.

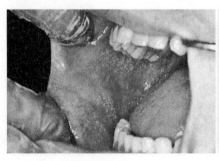
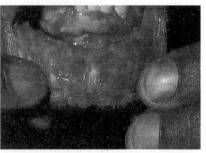

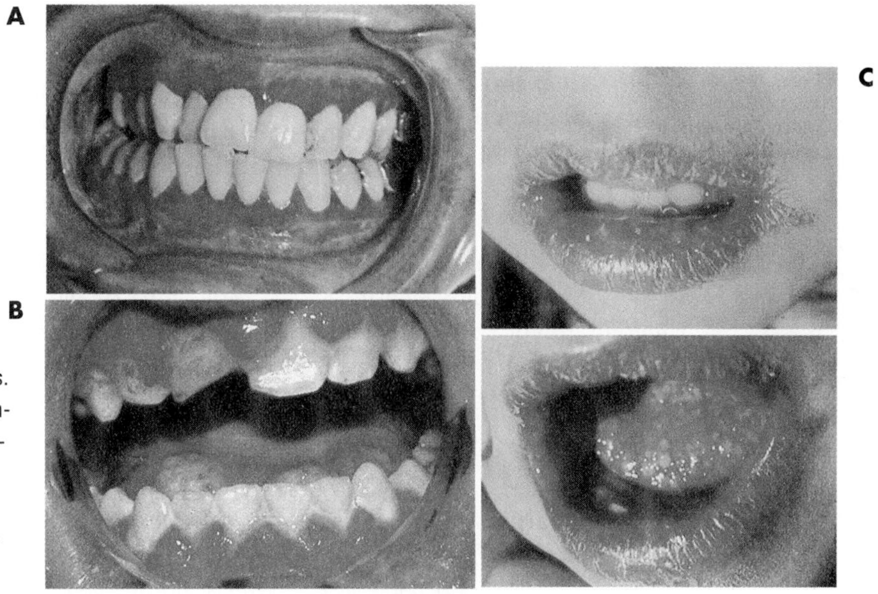

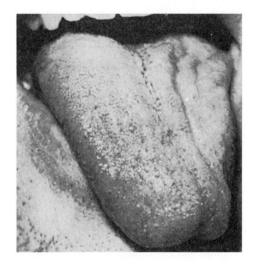

FIGURE 11-31

Unexpected findings of the gingiva. **A,** Plasma cell gingivitis. **B,** Primary herpetic gingivostomatitis. **C,** Primary gingivostomatitis showing lesions on the lips, tongue, and gums.

A and **B** from Wood, Goaz, 1991; **C** reproduced with permission of the Wellcome Foundation Ltd.

FIGURE 11-32

Left hypoglossal paralysis. The tongue deviates toward the weak side. Note atrophy on the left side of the tongue.

From Saunders et al, 1979.

FIGURE 11-33

Findings on the tongue. **A,** Geographic tongue. **B,** Smooth tongue resulting from vitamin deficiency. **C,** Glossitis. **D,** Black hairy tongue. **E,** Dome-shaped varicosity resembling a ranula.

A and **C** courtesy Antoinette Hood, MD, Indiana University School of Medicine, Indianapolis; **D** from Wood, Goaz, 1991; **E** from Bull, 1974.

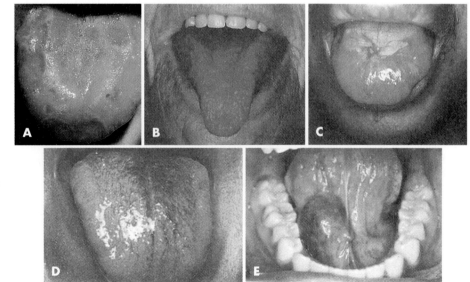

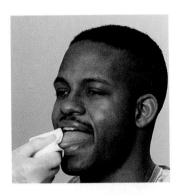

FIGURE 11-34
Inspection of lateral borders of the tongue.

Ask the patient to touch the tongue tip to the palate area directly behind the upper incisors. Inspect the floor of the mouth and the ventral surface of the tongue for swelling and varicosities, also observing the frenulum, sublingual ridge, and Wharton ducts. The tip of the tongue should have no difficulty touching the hard palate behind the upper central incisors. The ventral surface of the tongue should be pink and smooth with large veins between the frenulum and fimbriated folds. Wharton ducts should be apparent on each side of the frenulum.

Wrapping the tongue with a piece of gauze, pull the tongue to each side, inspecting its lateral borders (Figure 11-34). Any white or red margins should be scraped to differentiate food particles from leukoplakia or another fixed abnormality. Then palpate the tongue and the floor of the mouth for lumps, nodules, or ulceration.

The tongue should have a smooth, even texture without nodules, ulcerations, or areas of induration. Any ulcer, nodule, or thickened white patch on the lateral or ventral surface of the tongue may be suggestive of malignancy. Table 11-4 presents the oral manifestations of HIV infection.

Ask the patient to tilt his or her head back for you to inspect the palate and uvula. The whitish hard palate should be dome shaped with transverse rugae. The pinker soft palate should be contiguous with the hard palate. The uvula, a midline continuation of the soft palate, varies in length and thickness. The hard palate may have a bony protuberance at the midline, called torus palatinus, which has no clinical consequence (Figure 11-35). A nodule on the palate that is not at the midline may indicate a tumor. Figure 11-36 shows oral Kaposi sarcoma, moderately advanced and advanced lesions.

Movement of the soft palate is evaluated by asking the patient to say "ah." Depressing the tongue may be necessary for this maneuver. As the patient vocalizes, observe the soft palate rise symmetrically with the uvula remaining in the midline. This maneuver also tests the glossopharyngeal and vagus nerves *(cranial nerves IX and X)*. Failure of the soft palate to rise bilaterally with vocalization may result from paralysis of the vagus nerve. The uvula will deviate to the unaffected side.

TABLE 11-4	Oral Manifestations of HIV Infection
Lesion	**Characteristics**
Oral hairy leukoplakia	White, irregular lesions on lateral side of tongue or buccal mucosa; may have prominent folds or "hairy" projections
Angular cheilitis	Red, unilateral or bilateral fissures at corners of mouth
Candidiasis	Creamy white plaques on oral mucosa that bleed when scraped
Herpes simplex	Recurrent vesicular, crusting lesions on the vermilion border of the lip
Herpes zoster	Vesicular and ulcerative oral lesions in the distribution of the trigeminal nerve; may also be on gingiva
Human papillomavirus	Single or multiple, sessile or pedunculated nodules in the oral cavity
Aphthous ulcers	Recurrent circumscribed ulcers with an erythematous margin
Periodontal disease	In a mouth with little plaque or calculus, gingivitis with rapid bone and soft tissue degeneration accompanied by severe pain
Kaposi sarcoma	In the mouth, incompletely formed blood vessels proliferate, forming lesions of various shades and size as blood extravasates in response to the malignant tumor of the epithelium

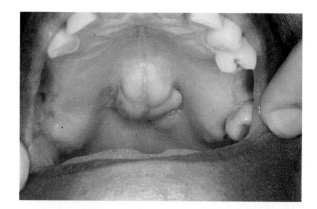

FIGURE 11-35

Torus palatinus.

Courtesy Drs. Abelson and Cameron, Lutherville, Maryland.

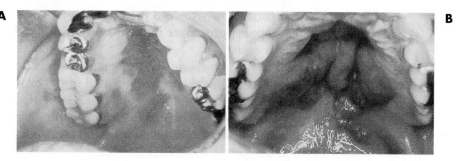

A

B

FIGURE 11-36

Oral Kaposi sarcoma. **A,** Moderately advanced. **B,** Advanced lesion.

From Grimes, 1991; courtesy Sol Silverman, Jr., DDS, University of California, San Francisco.

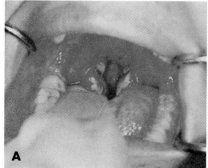
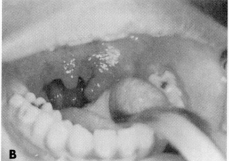
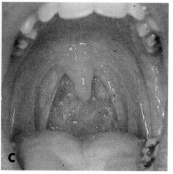

A

B

C

FIGURE 11-37

Findings of the oropharynx. **A,** Tonsillitis and pharyngitis. **B,** Acute viral pharyngitis. **C,** Postnasal drip.

A and **B** from Barkauskas et al, 1998; courtesy Edward L. Applebaum, MD, Head, Department of Otolaryngology, University of Illinois Medical Center, Chicago.

Oropharynx

Inspect the oropharynx using a tongue blade to depress the tongue. A patient of any age will possibly anticipate the use of the tongue blade with some degree of anxiety. If the patient is an easy gagger, there probably is little you can do to avoid setting off this reflex. Moistening the tongue blade with warm water helps, because a warm, wet blade will not trigger the gag as frequently as a dry one. Observe the tonsillar pillars, noting the size of tonsils, if present, and the integrity of the retropharyngeal wall. The tonsils usually blend into the pink color of the pharynx and should not project beyond the limits of the tonsillar pillars. Tonsils may have crypts where cellular debris and food particles collect. If the tonsils are reddened, hypertrophied, and covered with exudate, an infection may be present (Figure 11-37).

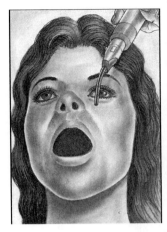
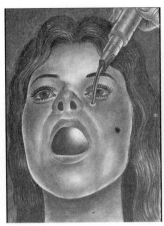
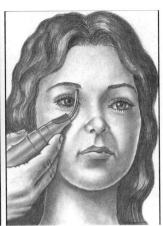
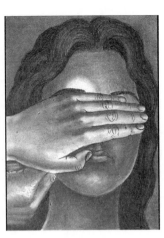

A   B

FIGURE 11-38
Transillumination of the sinuses: placement of the light source and expected area of transillumination.
A, For the maxillary sinus. **B,** For the frontal sinus.

The posterior wall of the pharynx should be smooth, glistening pink mucosa with some small irregular spots of lymphatic tissue and small blood vessels. A red bulge adjacent to the tonsil and extending beyond the midline may indicate a peritonsillar abscess. A yellowish mucoid film in the pharynx is typical of postnasal drip. A grayish adherent membrane is associated with diphtheria.

After preparing the patient for a gag response, touch the posterior wall of the pharynx on each side. Elicitation of the gag reflex tests the glossopharyngeal and vagus nerves *(cranial nerves IX and X)*. Expect a bilateral response.

ADDITIONAL PROCEDURES

Equilibrium

The Romberg test, described in Chapter 20 (Neurologic System), is used to screen for equilibrium in most patients. When a vestibular function disorder is suspected, as indicated by a loss of balance by the Romberg test, further evaluation of the vestibular branch of the auditory nerve *(cranial nerve VIII)* is indicated. In most cases, the patient is referred to a specialist for the cold caloric test or Nylen-Bárány test.

For the cold caloric test, have the patient sit and hyperextend the head to 60 degrees. Irrigate one auditory canal with cold water (32 to 50° F) for 20 seconds. (*Caution!* Do not perform this test if the patient has an acute middle ear infection or a perforated tympanic membrane.) The patient should feel nausea and dizziness and demonstrate nystagmus. All should appear in about 30 seconds and last about 90 seconds. Normal response is horizontal nystagmus, with conjugate eye movement, turning slowly toward the ear being irrigated and then quickly to the other side. Repeat the procedure in the other auditory canal. The response should be bilaterally equal.

For the Nylen-Bárány test, the patient should be supine with the head hyperextended about 45 degrees over the end of the examining table. When the patient turns his or her head to one side, observe for nystagmus. Repeat the procedure with the patient's head turned to the other side. Nystagmus is an unexpected finding, and if it is present, note the duration and direction of eye movement (horizontal or vertical).

Transillumination

Transillumination of the frontal and maxillary sinuses is performed if sinus tenderness is present or infection is suspected (Figure 11-38). The examination must be performed in a completely darkened room. A sinus transilluminator or small bright light is used.

To transilluminate the maxillary sinuses, place the light source lateral to the nose, just beneath the medial aspect of the eye. Look through the patient's open mouth for illumination of the hard palate. To transilluminate the frontal sinuses, place the light source against the medial aspect of each supraorbital rim. Look for a dim red glow as light is transmitted just above the eyebrow. The sinuses will usually show differing degrees of illumination. The absence of a glow indicates that either the sinus is filled with secretions or it never developed.

INFANTS

Because the ears, nose, mouth, and throat are frequent sites of congenital malformations in the newborn, thorough examination is important.

EARS

The auricle should be well formed, with all landmarks present on inspection. The tip of the auricle should cross the imaginary line between the outer canthus of the eye and the prominent portion of the occiput, varying no more than 10 degrees from vertical. Auricles either poorly shaped or positioned below the imaginary line are associated with renal disorders and congenital anomalies.

The newborn's auricle is very flexible but should have instant recoil after bending. The premature infant's auricles may appear flattened with limited incurving of the upper auricle, and ear recoil is slower.

No skin tags should be present. A small preauricular skin tag or pit is sometimes found just anterior to the tragus, indicating a remnant of the first branchial cleft.

The newborn's auditory canals are often obstructed with vernix, but they should be examined within the first few weeks of life. The tympanic membrane is usually in an extremely oblique position until the infant is 1 month old. The infant is placed in either supine or prone position so the head can be turned side to side. Hold the otoscope so that the ulnar surface of your hand rests against the infant's head, alternating the hand used (right hand for the right ear and left hand for the left ear). As the infant's head moves, the otoscope moves, preventing trauma to the auditory canal. Use your other hand to stabilize the infant's head as the thumb and index finger pull the auricle down to straighten the upward curvature of the canal. Because the tympanic membrane does not become conical for several months, the light reflex may appear diffuse. Limited mobility, dullness, and opacity of a pink or red tympanic membrane may be noted in neonates. As the middle ear matures during the infant's first months of life, the tympanic membrane takes on the expected appearance.

Knowledge of the sequence of hearing development is necessary to evaluate the infant's hearing (Table 11-5). Use a bell or your voice, or clap your hands as a sound stimulus, taking care that the infant does not respond to the air movement generated by any of these maneuvers. Remember that responses to repeated sound stimuli will diminish as the infant tunes out the stimulus.

TABLE 11-5	The Sequence of Expected Hearing Response
Age	**Response**
Birth to 3 months	Startle reflex, crying, cessation of breathing or movement in response to sudden noise; quiets to parent's voice
4 to 6 months	Turns head toward source of sound but may not always recognize location of sound; responds to parent's voice; enjoys sound-producing toys
6 to 10 months	Responds to own name, telephone ringing, and person's voice, even if not loud; begins localizing sounds above and below, turns head 45 degrees toward sound
10 to 12 months	Recognizes and localizes source of sound; imitates simple words and sounds

Adapted from Caufield, 1978.

NOSE AND SINUSES

The external nose should have a symmetric appearance and be positioned in the vertical midline of the face. Only minimal movement of the nares with breathing should be apparent. A deviation of the nose may be related to fetal position. A saddle-shaped nose with a low bridge and broad base, a short small nose, or a large nose may suggest a congenital anomaly.

Inspect the internal nose by shining a light inside after gently tilting the nose tip upward with your thumb. Small amounts of clear fluid discharged with crying may be seen in infants.

Newborns are obligatory nose breathers, so nasal patency must be determined at the time of birth. With the infant's mouth closed, occlude one naris and then the other, observing the respiratory pattern. With total obstruction, the infant will not be able to inspire or expire through the noncompressed naris. With any breathing difficulty, pass a small catheter through each naris to the choana, the posterior nasal opening. An obstruction may indicate choanal atresia or septal deviation from delivery trauma.

Because the maxillary and ethmoid sinuses are small during infancy, few problems arise in these areas, and examination is generally unnecessary.

MOUTH

The lips should be well formed with no cleft. The newborn may have sucking calluses on the upper lips appearing as plaques or crusts for the first few weeks of life. Healthy newborns may have circumoral cyanosis at birth and for a short while afterward.

The crying infant provides the opportune time to examine the mouth. Avoid depressing the tongue, because this stimulates a strong reflex protrusion, making visualization of the mouth difficult.

The buccal mucosa should be pink and moist with sucking pads but have no other lesions. Scrape any white patches on the tongue or buccal mucosa with a tongue blade. Nonadherent patches are usually milk deposits, whereas adherent patches may indicate candidiasis (thrush) (Figure 11-39, *A*). Secretions that accumulate in the newborn's mouth requiring frequent suctioning may indicate esophageal atresia.

Drooling is common in infants between 6 weeks and 6 months of age; however, it may be indicative of a neurologic disorder in infants over 12 months of age.

The newborn's gums should be edentulous, smooth with a serrated edge of tissue along the buccal margins. Occasionally you will find a tooth or tooth buds in a newborn (Figure 11-39, *B*). Determine if natal teeth are loose and their potential for aspiration. The question is whether to leave them there or remove them. Such teeth are not usually firmly fixed, and it is probably wisest, in most instances, to remove them. Never do this without consulting the parents first, however. In older infants, count the deciduous teeth, noting any unusual sequence of eruption. Pearl-like retention cysts that sometimes appear along the buccal margin disappear in 1 to 2 months.

The tongue should fit well in the floor of the mouth. The frenulum of the tongue usually attaches at a point midway between the ventral surface of the tongue and its tip (Figure 11-39, *C*). If the tongue protrudes beyond the alveolar ridge, no feeding difficulties should occur. Macroglossia is associated with congenital anomalies—another reminder that external clues to pathophysiologically severe problems abound (Figure 11-39, *D*). A large tongue protruding from the mouth so that it does not close should make you think of congenital hypothyroidism, for example.

The palatal arch should be dome shaped with no clefts in either the hard or soft palate. A narrow, flat palate roof or a high, arched palate (associated with congenital anomalies) will affect the tongue's placement, leading to feeding and speech problems. The soft palate should rise symmetrically when the infant cries. Petechiae are often seen on the newborn's soft palate. Epstein pearls, small, whitish-yellow masses at

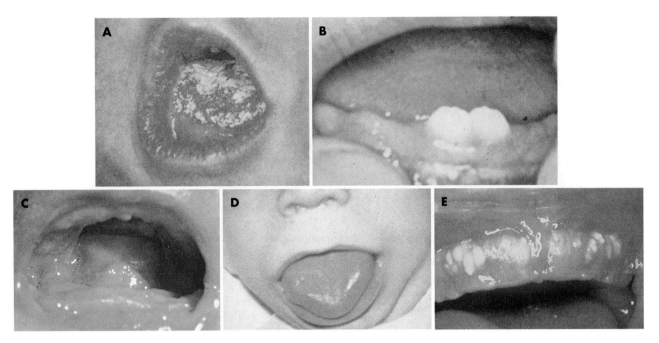

FIGURE 11-39
Findings in the infant's mouth. **A,** Thrush. **B,** Natal teeth. **C,** Short frenulum. **D,** Macroglossia. **E,** Epstein pearls.
Courtesy Mead Johnson & Co., Evansville, Indiana.

the juncture between the hard and soft palate, are common and disappear within a few weeks after birth (Figure 11-39, *E*).

Insert your index finger into the infant's mouth, with the fingerpad to the roof of the mouth. Simultaneously evaluate the infant's suck and palpate the hard and soft palates. (This maneuver may be performed when quieting the infant to auscultate the heart and lungs.) The infant should have a strong suck, the tongue pushing vigorously upward against the finger. Neither the hard nor soft palate should have palpable clefts. Stimulate the gag reflex by touching the tonsillar pillars. A bilateral gag reflex should be present.

CHILDREN

Because the young child often resists otoscopic and oral examination, it may be wise to postpone these procedures until the end. Be prepared to use restraint if encouraging the child to cooperate fails. Another person, usually the parent, may be needed to effectively restrain the child.

Children of any age who are not too big to sit on their parent's lap are better examined there than in a prone or supine position on the examining table. If the baby or toddler is comfortably seated in the parent's lap, back to the parent and legs between the adult's legs, the parent can then reach comfortably around to restrain the child's arms with one arm and control the child's head with the other. This can usually be accomplished without forcing, which avoids extra grief for the child, the parent, and you (Figure 11-40, *A*).

For the otoscopic examination, face the child sideways with one arm placed around the parent's waist. The parent holds the child firmly against his or her trunk, using one arm to restrain the child's head and the other arm to restrain the child's body. You further stabilize the child's head as you insert the otoscope. For the oral examination, face the child forward.

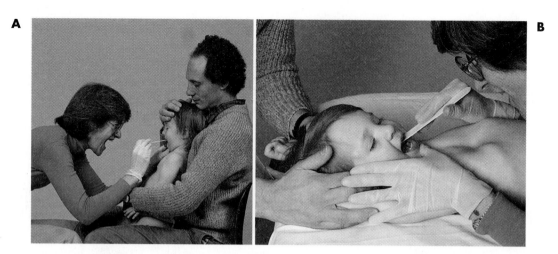

FIGURE 11-40
Positioning of toddler for oral examination. **A,** Sitting position. **B,** Supine position.

When the child actively resists your efforts to examine the ears and mouth, place him or her in supine position on the examining table. The parent holds the child's arms extended above the head and assists in restraining the head. You lie across the child's trunk and stabilize the child's head with your hands as you insert the otoscope or tongue blade. A third person may hold the child's legs, if necessary (Figure 11-40, *B*).

EARS

When performing the otoscopic examination, pull the auricle either downward and back or upward and back to gain the best view of the tympanic membrane. As the child grows, the shape of the auditory canal changes to the S-shaped curve of the adult. If the child is crying or has recently cried vigorously, dilation of blood vessels in the tympanic membrane can cause redness. Thus you cannot assume that redness of the membrane alone is a hallmark of middle ear infection. The pneumatic otoscope is especially important to differentiate a red tympanic membrane caused by crying (the membrane is mobile) from that resulting from disease (no mobility). Tympanometry provides an accurate way to identify middle ear effusion. (Figure 11-41). Make sure the ear piece is sealed in the canal.

Evaluate the toddler's hearing by observing the response to a whispered voice and various noisemakers (for example, rattle, bell, tissue paper). Position yourself behind the child while the parent distracts the child. Whisper or use noisemakers outside of the child's field of vision. The child should turn toward the sound consistently. Development of speech provides another indication of hearing acuity. When whispering, particularly to children, use words that will have more meaning for them, such as the name of a popular television personality or a comic strip character—Big Bird, Mickey Mouse, or Barney, for example.

In addition to these procedures, evaluate the young child's hearing by asking the child to perform tasks, using a soft voice. Avoid giving visual cues. The Weber, Rinne, and Schwabach tests are used when the child understands directions and can cooperate with the examiner, usually between 3 and 4 years of age. Audiometric evaluation should be performed in all young children.

NOSE AND SINUSES

As with infants, when inspecting the internal nose, it is usually adequate to tilt the nose tip upward with your thumb. However, if visualization of a larger area is needed, the largest otoscopic speculum may be used.

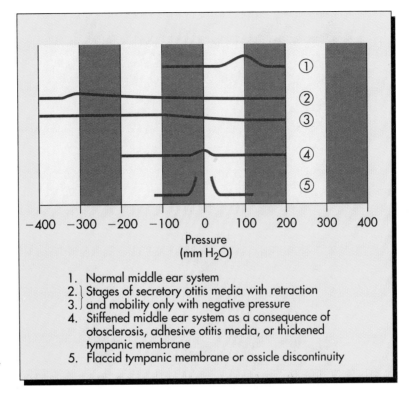

FIGURE 11-41
Tympanometric configuration for middle ear conditions.

The transverse crease at the juncture between the cartilage and the bone of the nose is often the result of the "adenoidal" or "allergic salute." Children are particularly prone to wipe their noses with an upward sweep of the palm of the hand, which if repeated often enough causes the crease.

The maxillary sinuses may be palpated, but few sinus problems occur in this age group, since the sinuses develop during childhood. However, there is a wide variation in the development of sinuses; do not assume that young children will not have sinusitis simply on the basis of age.

MOUTH

Encourage the child to cooperate with the oral examination. Letting the child hold and manipulate the tongue blade and light may reduce the fear of the procedure. Begin by asking the child to show you his or her teeth, usually not a threatening request. Flattened edges on the teeth may indicate bruxism, unconscious grinding of the teeth. Multiple brown areas or caries on the upper and lower incisors may be the result of a bedtime bottle of juice or milk, commonly called baby bottle syndrome (Figure 11-42). Teeth with a black or gray color may indicate pulp decay or oral iron therapy. Mottled or pitted teeth are often the result of tetracycline treatment during tooth development or enamel dysplasia.

If the child will protrude the tongue and say "ah," the tongue blade is often unnecessary for the oral examination. Ask the child to pant "like a puppy" to raise the palate. When the child refuses to open the mouth, insert a tongue blade through the lips to the back molars. Gently but firmly insert the tongue blade between the back molars and press the tongue blade to the tongue. This maneuver should stimulate the gag reflex and give you a brief view of the mouth and oropharynx.

Koplik spots, white specks with a red base on the buccal mucosa opposite the first and second molars, occur with rubeola in a child with fever, coryza, and cough. A highly arched palate may be observed in children who are chronic mouth breathers.

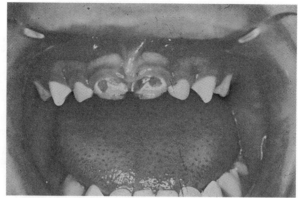

FIGURE 11-42

Baby bottle syndrome.

Courtesy Drs. Abelson and Cameron, Lutherville, Maryland.

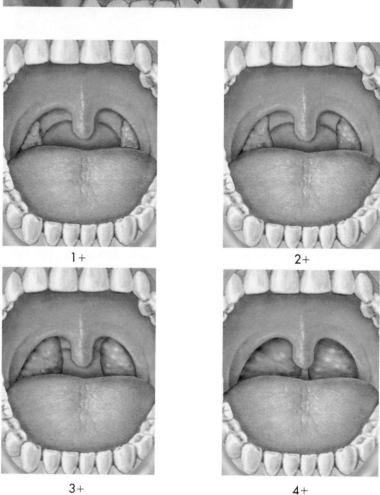

FIGURE 11-43

Enlarged tonsils are graded to describe their size: 1+, visible; 2+, halfway between tonsillar pillars and the uvula; 3+, nearly touching the uvula; 4+, touching each other.

The tonsils, lying deep in the oral cavity, should blend with the color of the pharynx. They gradually enlarge to their peak size between 2 and 6 years of age, but the oropharynx should retain an unobstructed passage. Enlarged tonsils are graded to describe their size (Figure 11-43).

If the tonsils appear pushed backward or forward, possibly displacing the uvula, consider a peritonsillar abscess.

When the tongue is depressed, the epiglottis is visible as a glistening pink structure behind the base of the tongue.

> ### BOX 11-2 Caution: Special Procedure if Epiglottitis Is Suspected
>
> Even though it is becoming rare, you should suspect epiglottitis when a child's symptoms include a sudden high fever, croupy cough, sore throat, drooling, apprehension, and a focus on breathing, as evidenced by the child's sitting in tripod position with the neck extended to keep the airway as open as possible. These are all indications of an impending airway obstruction resulting from acute inflammation of the epiglottis. Treat this as a *medical emergency.* No one should examine the child's mouth until an anesthesiologist or other skilled physician is present with intubation equipment. Examination is often performed in the operating room, followed by immediate intubation because the examination may result in a complete airway obstruction. A markedly swollen, cherry-red epiglottis is diagnostic of epiglottitis.

PREGNANT WOMEN

Edema and erythema in the nose and pharynx of the pregnant woman result from the increased vascularization of the respiratory tract. Tympanic membranes may have increased vascularity and be retracted or bulging with serous fluid. The gums will appear reddened, swollen, and spongy, with the hypertrophy resolving within 2 months of delivery. Frequently there is an increased incidence of nasal congestion and sinusitis.

OLDER ADULTS

EARS AND HEARING

Inspect the auditory canal of the patient who wears a hearing aid for areas of irritation from the ear mold. Coarse, wirelike hairs are often present along the periphery of the auricle. On otoscopic examination, the tympanic membrane landmarks may appear slightly more pronounced from sclerotic changes.

Some degree of sensorineural hearing deterioration with advancing age (presbycusis) may be noted. This is marked by greater difficulty understanding speech rather than a reduction in all sounds heard. Problems will be most prominent when the patient is in a room with considerable background noise. Conductive hearing loss from otosclerosis and cerumen impaction may also occur.

NOSE

The nasal mucosa may appear dryer, less glistening. An increased number of bristly hairs in the vestibule are common, especially in men.

MOUTH

The lips will have increased vertical markings and appear dryer when salivary flow is reduced. The buccal mucosa is thinner, less vascular, and less shiny than that of the younger adult. The tongue may appear more fissured, and veins on its ventral surface may appear varicose (Figure 11-44).

Many adults over 65 years of age are edentulous. Natural teeth may be worn down, and dental restorations may have deteriorated. The teeth often appear longer as resorption of the gum and bone progresses. Dental malocclusion is commonly caused by the migration of remaining teeth after extractions. The lower jaw may protrude in patients with a stooping and head-thrusting posture.

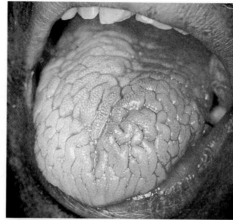

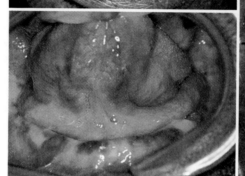

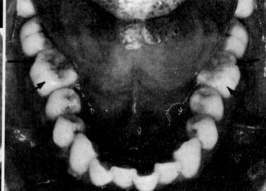

FIGURE 11-44

Common findings in the older adult's mouth. **A,** Fissured tongue. **B,** Varicose veins on tongue. **C,** Attrition of teeth.

A and **B** courtesy Drs. Abelson and Cameron, Lutherville, Maryland; **C** from Halstead et al, 1982.

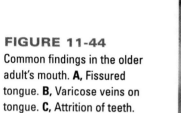

FUNCTIONAL ASSESSMENT

Ears, Nose, and Throat

The ability to perform activities of daily living is often dependent on the person's ability to hear, speak, chew food, and swallow. Hearing and speech are important for the personal social components of the functional assessment. The ability to chew and swallow food is important for adequate nutrition. When the patient has dentures, a hearing aid, or other assistive device, evaluate how effectively the patient uses these devices and is able to care for them.

Ears: Auricles in alignment, lobes are pierced without masses, lesions, or tenderness. Canals unobstructed and coated with minimal amount of brown cerumen. Tympanic membranes are pearly gray, noninjected, intact, with bony landmarks and light reflex visualized bilaterally. No evidence of fluid or retraction. Conversational hearing appropriate. Able to hear whispered voice. Weber—lateralizes equally to both ears; Rinne—air conduction greater than bone conduction bilaterally.

Nose: No discharge or polyps, mucosa pink and moist, septum midline, patent bilaterally. No edema over frontal or maxillary sinuses. No sinus tenderness to palpation. Correctly identifies mint, banana, and ammonia odors.

Mouth: Buccal mucosa pink and moist without lesions. Twenty-six teeth present in various states of repair. Lower second molars (18, 30) absent bilaterally. Gingiva pink and firm. Tongue midline with no tremors or fasciculation.

Pharynx: Clear without erythema, tonsils 1+ without exudates. Uvula rises evenly and gag reflex is intact. No hoarseness. Patient identifies tastes of salt and sugar.

For additional sample documentation see Chapter 24, Recording Information.

SUMMARY OF EXAMINATION   **Ears, Nose, and Throat**

The following steps should be performed with the patient sitting.

Ears

1. Inspect the auricles and mastoid area for the following (pp. 321-322):
   - Size
   - Shape
   - Symmetry
   - Landmarks
   - Color
   - Position
   - Deformities or lesions
2. Palpate the auricles and mastoid area for the following (p. 323):
   - Tenderness
   - Swelling
   - Nodules
3. Inspect the auditory canal with an otoscope, noting the following (p. 323):
   - Cerumen
   - Color
   - Lesions
   - Discharge, or foreign bodies
4. Inspect the tympanic membrane for the following (p. 324):
   - Landmarks
   - Color
   - Contour
   - Perforations
   - Mobility
5. Assess hearing through the following (pp. 325-326):
   - Response to questions during history
   - Response to a whispered voice
   - Response to tuning fork for air and bone conduction

Nose and Sinuses

1. Inspect the external nose for the following (p. 327):
   - Shape
   - Size
   - Color
   - Nares
2. Palpate the ridge and soft tissues of the nose for the following (p. 327):
   - Tenderness
   - Displacement of cartilage and bone
   - Masses
3. Evaluate the patency of the nares (p. 327):
4. Inspect the nasal mucosa and nasal septum for the following (pp. 327-328):
   - Color
   - Alignment
   - Discharge
   - Swelling of turbinates
   - Perforation
5. Inspect the frontal and maxillary sinus area for swelling (p. 329).
6. Palpate and percuss the frontal and maxillary sinuses for the following (p. 329):
   - Tenderness or pain
   - Swelling

Mouth

1. Inspect and palpate the lips for the following (p. 329):
   - Symmetry
   - Color
   - Edema
   - Surface abnormalities
2. Inspect and palpate the gingivae for the following (p. 332):
   - Color
   - Lesions
   - Tenderness
3. Inspect the teeth for the following (p. 332):
   - Occlusion
   - Caries
   - Loose or missing teeth
4. Inspect the tongue and buccal mucosa for the following (pp. 330-334):
   - Color
   - Symmetry
   - Swelling
   - Ulcerations
   - Cranial nerve XII (hypoglossal)
5. Palpate the tongue (p. 334).
6. Inspect the palate and uvula (p. 334).
7. Inspect the following oropharyngeal characteristics (pp. 335-336):
   - Tonsils
   - Posterior wall of pharynx
8. Elicit gag reflex (cranial nerves IX and X) (p. 336).

COMMON ABNORMALITIES

EAR

| OTITIS EXTERNA (SWIMMER'S EAR) | Otitis externa is an infection of the auditory canal resulting when trauma or a | moist environment favors bacterial or fungal growth (Table 11-6). |

BACTERIAL OTITIS MEDIA

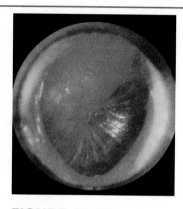

FIGURE 11-45
Acute otitis media.
From Barkauskas et al, 1998; courtesy Richard A. Buckingham, MD, Clinical Professor, Otolaryngology, Abraham Lincoln School of Medicine, University of Illinois, Chicago.

This infection of the middle ear often follows or accompanies an upper respiratory infection (Figure 11-45; Table 11-6). This is the most common infection of childhood, with a lower incidence in adults.

TABLE 11-6 Differentiating Between Otitis Externa, Bacterial Otitis Media, and Otitis Media with Effusion

Signs and Symptoms	Otitis Externa	Bacterial Otitis Media	Otitis Media with Effusion
Initial symptoms	Itching in ear canal	Fever, feeling of blockage, tugging earlobe, anorexia, irritability, dizziness, vomiting and diarrhea	Sticking or cracking sound on yawning or swallowing; no signs of acute infection
Pain	Intense with movement of pinna, chewing	Deep-seated earache	Uncommon; feeling of fullness
Discharge	Watery, then purulent and thick, mixed with pus and epithelial cells; musty, foul-smelling	Only if tympanic membrane ruptures or through tympanostomy tubes; foul-smelling	Uncommon
Hearing	Conductive loss caused by exudate and swelling of ear canal	Conductive loss as middle ear fills with pus	Conductive loss as middle ear fills with fluid
Inspection	Canal is red, edematous; tympanic membrane obscured	Tympanic membrane may be red, thickened, bulging; full, limited, or no movement to +/− pressure	Tympanic membrane is retracted, impaired mobility, yellowish; air fluid level and/or bubbles

OTITIS MEDIA WITH EFFUSION

This is an inflammation of the middle ear resulting in the collection of liquid (effusion) in the middle ear when the tympanic membrane is intact. The effusion may be serous, mucoid, or purulent. Causes of this disorder include an obstructed or dysfunctional eustachian tube, allergies, and enlarged lymphoid tissue in the nasopharynx. Once the obstruction occurs, the middle ear absorbs the air, creating a vacuum, and the mucosa secretes a transudate into the middle ear. The average duration of a persistent effusion is 23 days (Figure 11-46; Table 11-6).

A

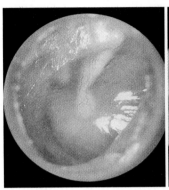 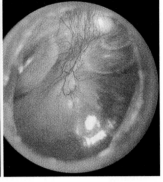

B

FIGURE 11-46
Otitis media with effusion. **A,** Middle ear filled with serous fluid. **B,** Air fluid levels in upper middle ear.

From Barkauskas et al, 1998; courtesy Richard A. Buckingham, MD, Clinical Professor, Otolaryngology, Abraham Lincoln School of Medicine, University of Illinois, Chicago.

CHOLESTEATOMA

An epithelial growth that migrates through a perforation in the tympanic membrane often results in a cholesteatoma. White, shiny, greasy flacks of debris are visualized in the posterior superior section of the middle ear through the tympanic membrane or through a perforation. A foul-smelling discharge may be found when a perforation is present. Symptoms include progressive hearing loss, fullness in the ear, tinnitus, and mild vertigo. If untreated, the cholesteatoma can lead to intracranial complications by eroding the temporal bone (Figure 11-47).

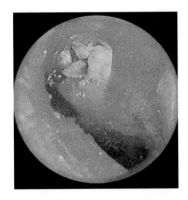

FIGURE 11-47
Cholesteatoma.

From Barkauskas et al, 1998; courtesy Richard A. Buckingham, MD, Clinical Professor, Otolaryngology, Abraham Lincoln School of Medicine, University of Illinois, Chicago.

OTOSCLEROSIS

Otosclerosis is a hereditary condition that is more common in women. Irregular ossification occurs within the bony labyrinth or otic capsule, resulting in fixation of the stapes. Symptoms include tinnitus and slowly progressive low- to medium-pitch conductive hearing loss, usually noticed between late teens and 30 years of age. Sensorineural hearing loss may also develop, causing a mixed hearing loss.

MÉNIÈRE DISEASE	Ménière disease affects the vestibular labyrinth, leading to profound sensorineural hearing loss. Symptoms include attacks of severe vertigo, tinnitus, and	progressive hearing loss of low tones initially. The disorder may be unilateral at first and then may involve other ear.
LABYRINTHITIS	Inflammation of the labyrinthine canal of the inner ear occurs as a complication of an acute upper respiratory infection. Symptoms of severe vertigo, associated	with nystagmus, increase in severity with head movement. Total sensorineural hearing loss occurs on the affected side.

NOSE AND SINUSES

SINUSITIS	An infection of one or more of the paranasal sinuses may be a complication of a viral upper respiratory infection, dental infection, allergies, or a structural defect of the nose. A blockage of the sinus meatus prevents secretions from draining out of the sinus cavity. Symptoms include fever, headache, local tenderness, and pain. There may be swelling	of the skin overlying the involved sinus and copious purulent nasal discharge (Figure 11-48). Children may alternately suffer from upper respiratory symptoms, nasal discharge, low-grade fever, daytime cough, malodorous breath, cervical adenopathy, and intermittent painless morning eye swelling with no facial pain or headache.

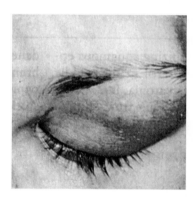

FIGURE 11-48
Acute frontal sinusitis with orbital edema.
From Saunders et al, 1979.

COCAINE ABUSE	Nasal insufflation (snorting) of cocaine, a currently favored substance for abuse, must be considered when examining all adolescents and adults. Commonly, patients complain of such chronic nasal symptoms as sniffling, nasal congestion, recurrent nosebleeds, and sinus problems. Signs of very recent insufflation include hyperemia and edema of the nasal	mucosa and rhinorrhea. White powder may still be present on the nasal hairs and mustache. Signs of chronic cocaine insufflation include scabs on the nasal mucosa, decreased perception of taste and smell, and perforation of the nasal septum due to ischemic necrosis of the septal cartilage resulting from chronic irritation.

MOUTH AND OROPHARYNX

TONSILLITIS

Inflammation or infection of the tonsils is frequently caused by streptococci. Symptoms include sore throat, referred pain to the ears, dysphagia, fever, fetid breath, and malaise. The tonsils appear red and swollen, and tonsillar crypts are filled with purulent exudate (Figure 11-49). Tonsils studded with yellow follicles are associated with streptococcal infections. Anterior cervical lymph nodes are enlarged.

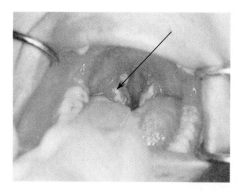

FIGURE 11-49
Tonsillitis and pharyngitis.
From Barkauskas et al, 1998; courtesy Edward L. Applebaum, MD, Head, Department of Otolaryngology, University of Illinois Medical Center, Chicago.

PERITONSILLAR ABSCESS

Infection of the tissue between the tonsil and pharynx occurs as a complication of tonsillitis. Symptoms include dysphagia, drooling, severe sore throat with pain radiating to the ear, muffled voice, and fever. The tonsil, tonsillar pillar, and adjacent soft palate become red and swollen (Figure 11-50). The tonsil may appear pushed forward or backward, possibly displacing the uvula.

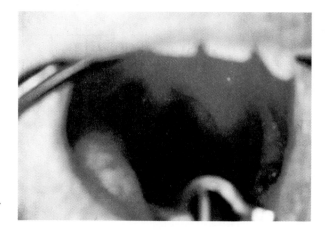

FIGURE 11-50
Swelling of peritonsillar abscess.
From Sigler, Schuring, 1993.

SLEEP APNEA

Sleep apnea is a periodic cessation of breathing during sleep that is associated with either an obstruction to airflow or failure of the central nervous system to stimulate the respiratory effort to breathe. In obstructive sleep apnea, muscles in the nasopharynx, hypopharynx, and pharynx relax during sleep, resulting in loud snoring, restless sleep, and a pause in nasal and oral airflow with respiratory effort. This can result in progressive hypercapnia, hypoxemia, increased pulmonary arterial pressures, and possibly life-threatening cardiac arrhythmias. Patients are typically overweight, middle-aged men who complain of excessive daytime sleepiness and morning headaches.

CHOANAL ATRESIA

Choanal atresia is a congenital nasal obstruction of the posterior nares at the junction between the nasal cavity and nasopharynx. Without prompt intervention, newborns who have this anomaly experience respiratory distress because they are obligatory nose breathers. The infant will breathe when crying because the mouth is open (Figure 11-51).

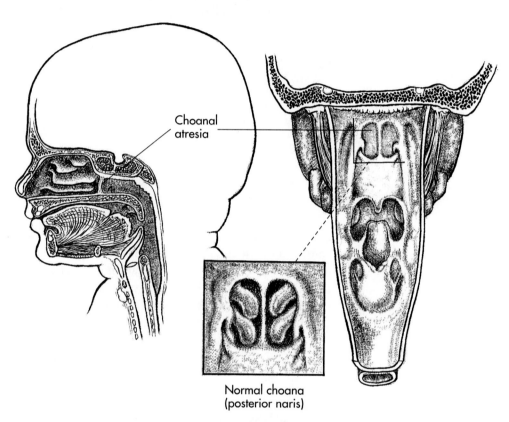

Choanal atresia

Normal choana (posterior naris)

FIGURE 11-51
Choanal atresia.

CLEFT LIP AND PALATE

PHYSICAL VARIATIONS

The incidence is higher in whites and Japanese, lower in blacks.

Bluestone, 1995.

This congenital malformation of the face appears as a fissure of the upper lip or palate. Each may occur without the other; however, they often occur together. There may be a complete cleft extending through the lip and hard and soft palates to the nasal cavity, or there may be a partial cleft in any of these tissues. Long-term problems for the affected child include hearing loss, chronic otitis media, speech difficulties, feeding problems, and improper tooth development and alignment (Figure 11-52).

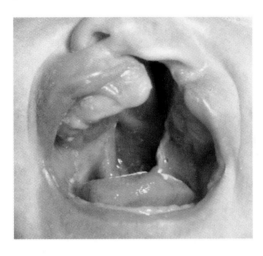

FIGURE 11-52
Unilateral cleft lip and palate.
From Zitelli, Davis, 1997.

OLDER ADULTS

PRESBYCUSIS

Presbycusis is a common auditory disorder in which there is bilateral sensorineural hearing loss associated with aging. It is caused by degenerative changes in the inner ear or auditory nerve. There is a loss in the perception of auditory stimuli, initially of high-frequency sounds and tinnitus. Speech may be poorly understood when spoken quickly or when background noise is present.

XEROSTOMIA

Xerostomia is a dry mouth caused by the ingestion of anticholinergic or antidepressant drugs that interfere with the production of saliva. Xerostomia is also caused by systemic diseases such as rheumatoid arthritis, scleroderma, polymyositis, and Sjögren syndrome. The condition is also found in patients who are heavy smokers or who have received radiation to the head and neck.

Check it out— *Mosby* *http://www1.mosby.com/physexam_seidel*

CHAPTER 12

CHEST AND LUNGS

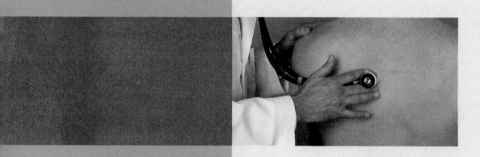

ANATOMY AND PHYSIOLOGY

The chest, or thorax, is a cage of bone, cartilage, and muscle capable of movement as the lungs expand. It consists anteriorly of the sternum, manubrium, xiphoid process, and costal cartilages; laterally, of the 12 pairs of ribs; and posteriorly, of the 12 thoracic vertebrae (Figures 12-1 and 12-2). All the ribs are connected to the thoracic vertebrae; the upper 7 are attached anteriorly to the sternum by the costal cartilages. The transverse diameter of the chest generally exceeds the anteroposterior diameter in adults.

The primary muscles of respiration are the diaphragm and the intercostal muscles. The diaphragm contracts and moves downward during inspiration, lowering the abdominal contents to increase the intrathoracic space. The external intercostal muscles increase the anteroposterior chest diameter during inspiration, and the internal intercostals decrease the transverse diameter during expiration. The sternocleidomastoid and trapezius muscles may also contribute to respiratory movements (Figure 12-3).

The interior of the chest is divided into three major spaces: the right and left pleural cavities and the mediastinum. The mediastinum, situated between the lungs, contains all of the thoracic viscera except the lungs. The pleural cavities are lined with the parietal and visceral plurae, serous membranes that enclose the lungs. The spongy and highly elastic lungs are paired but not symmetric, the right having three lobes and the left two (Figure 12-4). The left upper lobe has an inferior tonguelike projection, the lingula, which is a counterpart of the right middle lobe. Each lung has a major fissure—the oblique—which divides the upper and lower portions. In addition, a lesser horizontal fissure divides the upper portion of the right lung into the upper and middle lobes at the level of the fifth rib in the axilla and the fourth rib anteriorly. Each lobe consists of blood vessels, lymphatics, nerves, and an alveolar duct connecting with the alveoli (as many as 300 million in an adult). The entire lung parenchyma is shaped by an elastic subpleural tissue that limits its expansion. Each lung is conical; the apex is rounded and extends anteriorly about 4 cm above the first rib into the base of the neck in adults. Posteriorly, the apices of the lungs rise to about the level of T1. The lower borders descend on deep inspiration to about T12 and rise on forced expiration to about T9. The base of each lung is broad and concave, resting on the convex

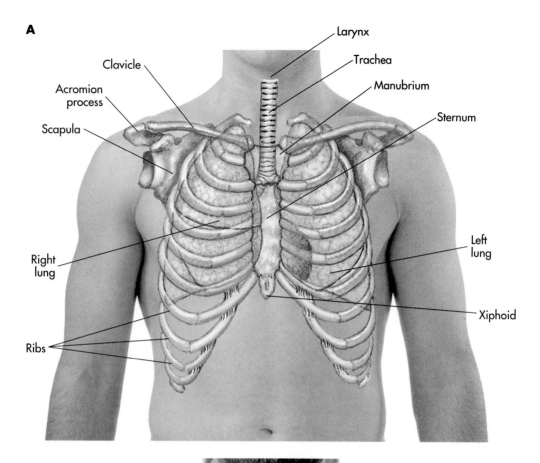

A

Larynx

Clavicle

Trachea

Acromion process

Manubrium

Scapula

Sternum

Right lung

Left lung

Xiphoid

Ribs

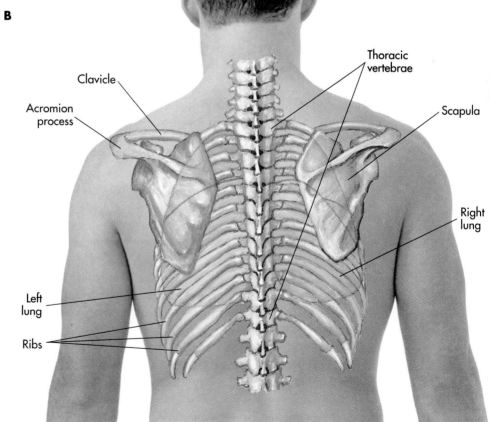

B

Clavicle

Thoracic vertebrae

Acromion process

Scapula

Right lung

Left lung

Ribs

FIGURE 12-1

The bony structures of the chest form a protective expandable cage around the lungs and heart. **A,** Anterior view. **B,** Posterior view.

From Thompson, Wilson, 1996.

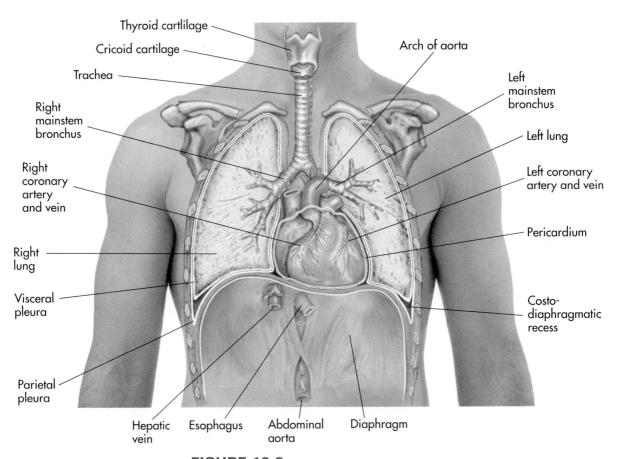

FIGURE 12-2
Chest cavity and related anatomic structures.

surface of the diaphragm. The medial surfaces of the lung are to some extent concave, providing a cradle for the heart.

The tracheobronchial tree is a tubular system that provides a pathway for air to move from the upper airway to the farthest alveolar reaches. The trachea is 10 to 11 cm long and about 2 cm in diameter. It lies anterior to the esophagus and posterior to the isthmus of the thyroid. The trachea divides into the right and left main bronchi at about the level of T4 or T5 and just below the manubriosternal joint.

The right bronchus is wider, shorter, and more vertically placed than the left bronchus (and therefore more susceptible to aspiration of foreign bodies). The main bronchi are divided into three branches on the right and two on the left, each branch supplying one lobe of the lungs. The branches then begin to subdivide into terminal bronchioles and ultimately into respiratory bronchioles so small that each is associated with one acinus, or terminal respiratory unit. The acini consist of the respiratory bronchioles, alveolar ducts, alveolar sacs, and alveoli. The bronchi transport air and, to some extent, trap noxious foreign particles in the mucus of their cavities and sweep them toward the pharynx with their cilia.

The bronchial arteries branch from the anterior thoracic aorta and the intercostal arteries, supplying blood to the lung parenchyma and stroma. The bronchial vein is formed at the hilum of the lung, but most of the blood supplied by the bronchial arteries is returned by the pulmonary veins (Figure 12-5 and Box 12-1).

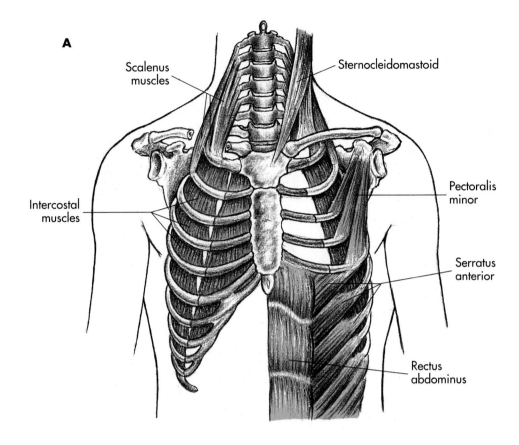

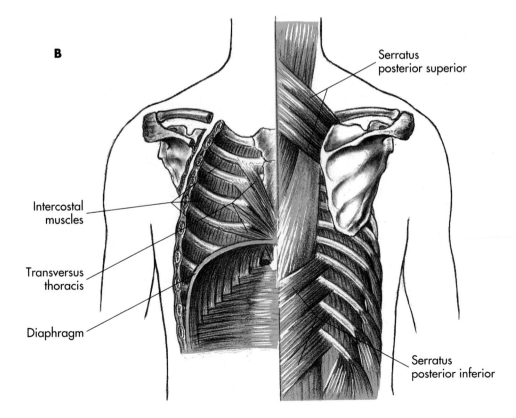

FIGURE 12-3
Muscles of ventilation. **A,** Anterior view. **B,** Posterior view.

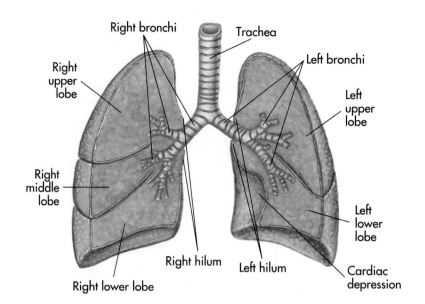

Right bronchi

Trachea

Right upper lobe

Left bronchi

Left upper lobe

Right middle lobe

Left lower lobe

Right hilum   Left hilum

Cardiac depression

Right lower lobe

FIGURE 12-4
The lobes of the lungs.
From Wilson, Thompson, 1990.

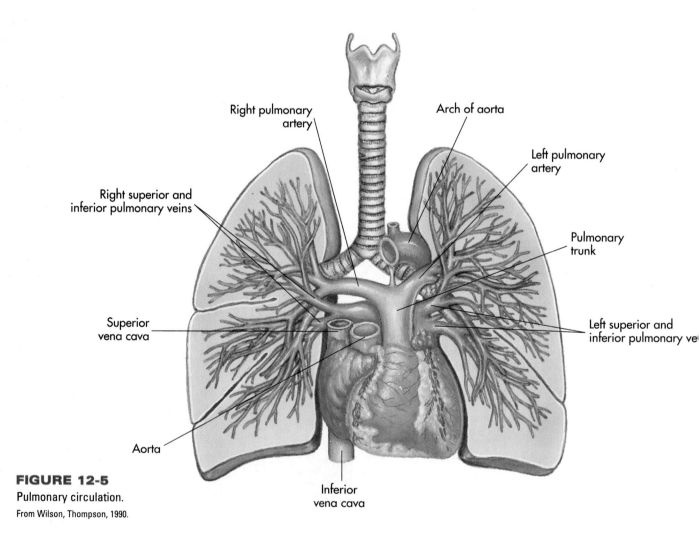

Right pulmonary artery

Arch of aorta

Left pulmonary artery

Right superior and inferior pulmonary veins

Pulmonary trunk

Superior vena cava

Left superior and inferior pulmonary ve

Aorta

Inferior vena cava

FIGURE 12-5
Pulmonary circulation.
From Wilson, Thompson, 1990.

BOX 12-1 ## Visualizing the Lungs from the Surface

Anteriorly

The right lung may ride higher because of the fullness of the dome of the liver. Except for an inferior lateral triangle, the anterior view on the right is primarily the upper and middle lobes, separated by the horizontal fissure at about the fifth rib in the midaxilla to about the fourth at the sternum; on the left as on the right, the lower lobe is set off by a diagonal fissure stretching from the fifth rib at the axilla to the sixth at the midclavicular line.

Posteriorly

Except for the apices, the posterior view is primarily the lower lobe, which extends from about T3 to T10 or T12 during the respiratory cycle.

Right Lateral

Lung underlies the area extending from the peak of the axilla to the seventh or eighth rib. The upper lobe is demarcated at about the level of the fifth rib in the midaxillary line and the sixth rib more anteriorly.

Left Lateral

Lung underlies the area extending from the peak of the axilla to the seventh or eighth rib. The entire expanse is virtually bisected by the oblique fissure from about the level of the third rib medially to the sixth rib anteriorly.

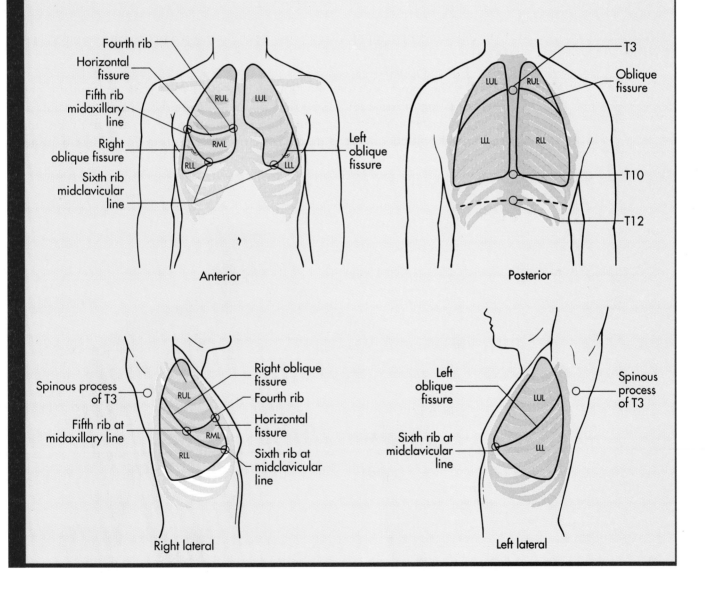

CHEMICAL AND NEUROLOGIC CONTROL OF RESPIRATION

The purpose of respiration is to keep the body adequately supplied with oxygen and protected from excess accumulation of carbon dioxide. It involves the movement of air back and forth from the deepest reaches of the alveoli to the outside (ventilation); gas exchange across the alveolar-pulmonary capillary membranes (diffusion and perfusion); and circulatory system transport of oxygen to, and carbon dioxide from, the peripheral tissues. Control of this complex process is not yet fully understood. Chemoreceptors in the medulla oblongata are exquisitely sensitive and respond quickly to changes in hydrogen ion concentration in the blood and spinal fluid. Peripherally, chemoreceptors in the carotid body at the bifurcation of the common carotid arteries also respond to changes in arterial oxygen and carbon dioxide levels. Both types of chemoreceptors respond by sending signals to the respiratory center in the medulla oblongata. Nerve impulses from here are transmitted to two subcenters in the pons, which regulate the respiratory muscles. Excess levels of carbon dioxide stimulate the rate and depth of respiration.

ANATOMIC LANDMARKS

The following topographic markers on the chest are used to describe findings (Figure 12-6):
1. The nipples
2. The manubriosternal junction (angle of Louis): a visible and palpable angulation of the sternum and the point at which the second rib articulates with the sternum. One can count the ribs and intercostal spaces from this point. The number of each intercostal space corresponds to that of the rib immediately above it.

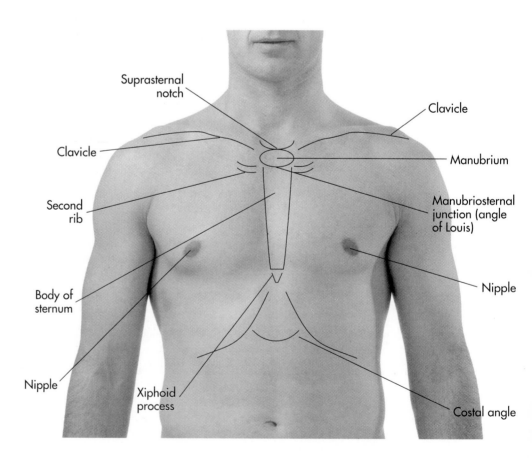

FIGURE 12-6
Topographic landmarks of the chest.

From Thompson, Wilson, 1996.

3. The suprasternal notch: a depression, easily palpable and most often visible at the base of the ventral aspect of the neck, just superior to the manubriosternal junction.
4. Costal angle: the angle formed by the blending together of the costal margins at the sternum. It is usually no more than 90 degrees, with the ribs inserted at approximately 45-degree angles.
5. Vertebra prominens: the spinous process of C7. It can be more readily seen and felt with the patient's head bent forward. If two prominences are felt, the upper is that of the spinous process of C7, and the lower is that of T1. It is difficult to use this as a guide to counting ribs posteriorly, because the spinous processes from T4 down project obliquely, thus overlying the rib *below* the number of its vertebra.
6. The clavicles.

INFANTS AND CHILDREN

At about 4 weeks' gestation, the lung is a groove on the ventral wall of the gut. It evolves ultimately from a simple sac to an involuted structure of tubules and spaces. The lungs contain no air, and the alveoli are collapsed. Relatively passive respiratory movements occur throughout much of gestation; they do not open the alveoli or move the lung fields. Rather, they prepare the term infant to respond to postnatal chemical and neurologic respiratory stimuli. Fetal gas exchange is mediated by the placenta.

At birth the change in respiratory function is rapid and intense. After the cord is cut, the lungs fill with air for the first time; this first respiratory effort is great. No longer coursing through the placenta, blood flows through the lungs more vigorously. The pulmonary arteries expand and relax, offering much less resistance than the systemic circulation. This relative decrease in pulmonary pressure leads to closure of the foramen ovale within minutes after birth, and the increased oxygen tension in the arterial blood stimulates contraction and closure of the ductus arteriosus. The pulmonary and systemic circulations adopt their mature configurations, and the lungs are fully integrated for postnatal function.

The chest of the newborn is generally round, the anteroposterior diameter approximating the transverse, and the circumference is roughly equal to that of the head until the child is about 2 years old (Figure 12-7). With growth, the chest assumes adult proportions, with the lateral diameter exceeding the anteroposterior diameter (see Table 5-5).

FIRST BREATH

The first breath an infant takes provides a moment of drama as intense as any in later life—and is far more often accompanied by joy.

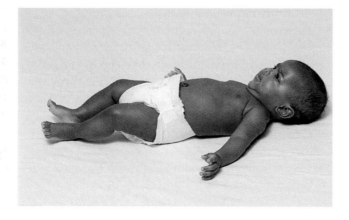
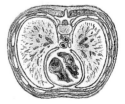

FIGURE 12-7
Chest of healthy infant. Note that anteroposterior diameter is approximately the same as transverse diameter.

The relatively thin chest wall of the infant and young child makes the bony structure more prominent than in the adult. It is more cartilaginous and yielding, and the xiphoid process is often more prominent and a bit more movable.

PREGNANT WOMEN	Mechanical and biochemical factors, including the enlarged uterus and an increased level of circulating progesterone, interact to create changes in the respiratory function of the pregnant woman. Anatomic changes that occur in the chest as the lower ribs flare include an increase in the transverse diameter of about 2 cm, and an increase in the circumference of 5 to 7 cm. In addition, the diaphragm at rest rises as much as 4 cm above its usual resting position, yet diaphragmatic movement increases so that the major work of breathing is done by the diaphragm. The increased level of progesterone acts as a respiratory stimulant that causes an increased tidal volume without changing respiratory frequency.
OLDER ADULTS	The barrel chest that is characteristic of many older adults results from loss of muscle strength in the thorax and diaphragm (Figure 12-9, p. 364), coupled with the loss of lung resiliency. In addition, skeletal changes of aging tend to emphasize the dorsal curve of the thoracic spine, resulting in an increased anteroposterior chest diameter. There may also be stiffening and decreased expansion of the chest wall.

The alveoli become less elastic and relatively more fibrous. The associated loss of some of the interalveolar folds decreases the alveolar surface available for gas exchange. This and the loss of some tensile strength in the muscles of respiration result in underventilation of the alveoli in the lower lung fields and a decreased tolerance for exertion. The net result of these changes is a decrease in vital capacity and an increase in residual volume. Dyspnea can occur when older persons exceed their customary light or moderate exertional demands.

Aging mucous membranes tend to become drier and less able to rid themselves of mucus. Retained mucus encourages bacterial growth and predisposes the older adult to respiratory infection.

REVIEW OF RELATED HISTORY

PRESENT PROBLEM

- Coughing
  - Onset: sudden, gradual; duration
  - Nature of cough: dry, moist, wet, hacking, hoarse, barking, whooping, bubbling, productive, nonproductive
    - Sputum production: duration, frequency, with activity, at certain times of day
    - Sputum characteristics: amount, color (clear, mucoid, purulent, blood-tinged, mostly blood), foul odor
  - Pattern: occasional, regular, paroxysmal; related to time of day, weather, activities, (e.g., exercise), talking, deep breaths; change over time
  - Severity: tires patient, disrupts sleep or conversation, causes chest pain
  - Associated symptoms: shortness of breath, chest pain or tightness with breathing, fever, coryza, stuffy nose, noisy respirations, hoarseness, gagging, choking, stress
  - Efforts to treat: prescription or nonprescription drugs, vaporizers; effectiveness
  - Other medications: prescription or nonprescription
- Shortness of breath
  - Onset: sudden or gradual; duration; gagging or choking event few days before onset

PAIN FROM COCAINE

If an adult, especially a young adult, or an adolescent complains of severe, acute chest pain, ask about drug use, particularly cocaine. This situation will not occur often, but the possibility of drug use causing the pain exists. Cocaine can cause tachycardia, hypertension, coronary arterial spasm (with infarction), and pneumothorax with severe acute chest pain the frequent result.

- Pattern
  - Position most comfortable, number of pillows used
  - Related to extent of exercise, certain activities, time of day, eating
  - Harder to inhale or exhale
- Severity: extent of activity limitation, fatigue with breathing, anxiety about getting air
- Associated symptoms: pain or discomfort (relationship to specific point in respiratory exertion, location), cough, diaphoresis, ankle edema
- Chest pain
  - Onset and duration; associated with trauma, coughing, lower respiratory infection
  - Associated symptoms: shallow breathing, fever, uneven chest expansion, coughing, anxiety about getting air, radiation of pain to neck or arms
  - Efforts to treat: heat, splinting, pain medication
  - Other medications: prescription or nonprescription

PAST MEDICAL HISTORY

- Thoracic trauma or surgery, hospitalizations for pulmonary disorders, dates
- Use of oxygen or ventilation-assisting devices
- Chronic pulmonary diseases: tuberculosis (date, treatment, compliance), bronchitis, emphysema, bronchiectasis, asthma, cystic fibrosis
- Other chronic disorders: cardiac, cancer
- Testing: allergy, pulmonary function tests, tuberculin and fungal skin tests, chest x-ray examinations

FAMILY HISTORY

- Tuberculosis
- Cystic fibrosis
- Emphysema
- Allergy, asthma, atopic dermatitis
- Malignancy

PERSONAL AND SOCIAL HISTORY

- Employment: nature of work, extent of physical and emotional effort and stress, environmental hazards, exposure to chemicals, animals, vapors, dust, pulmonary irritants (e.g., asbestos), allergens, use of protective devices
- Home environment: location, possible allergens, type of heating, use of air conditioning, humidifier, ventilation
- Tobacco use: type of tobacco (cigarettes, cigars, pipe, smokeless), duration and amount (pack years = number of years of smoking × number of packs smoked per day), age started, efforts to quit smoking with factors influencing success or failure, the extent of smoking by others at home or at work (passive smoking)
- Exposure to respiratory infections, influenza, tuberculosis
- Nutritional status: weight loss or obesity
- Regional or travel exposures (e.g., human immunodeficiency virus [HIV] infection in central Africa, the Caribbean; histoplasmosis in southeastern and midwestern United States; schistosomiasis in the Orient, Africa, Caribbean, Southwest Asia)
- Hobbies: owning pigeons or parrots, woodworking, welding; other possibilities of noxious exposure (e.g., with employment)
- Use of alcohol
- Use of illegal drugs
- Exercise tolerance: diminished ability to perform up to expectations

INFANTS AND CHILDREN

- Low birth weight: premature, duration of ventilation assistance if any, respiratory distress syndrome, bronchopulmonary dysplasia, transient tachypnea of the newborn.
- Coughing or difficulty breathing of sudden onset
- Possible aspiration of small object, toy, or food
- Possible ingestion of kerosene or other hydrocarbon
- Difficulty feeding: increased perspiration, cyanosis, tiring quickly, disinterest in feeding, inadequate weight gain (good indication of exercise intolerance)
- Apneic episodes: use of apnea monitor, sudden infant death in sibling
- Recurrent spitting up and choking, recurrent pneumonia (possible gastroesophageal reflux)

PREGNANT WOMEN

- Weeks of gestation or estimated date of conception (EDC)
- Presence of multiple fetuses, polyhydramnios, or other conditions in which a larger uterus displaces the diaphragm upward
- Exercise type and energy expenditure (although energy expenditure effects on pregnancy outcomes is not great [Magann, Evans, Newnham, 1996])
- Exposure to and frequency of respiratory infections, history of annual influenza immunization, history of pneumococcal vaccination

OLDER ADULTS

- Exposure to and frequency of respiratory infections, history of pneumococcal vaccination and annual influenza immunization
- Effects of weather on respiratory efforts and occurrence of infections
- Immobilization or marked sedentary habits
- Difficulty swallowing
- Alteration in daily living habits or activities as a result of respiratory symptoms
- Because older adults are at risk for chronic respiratory diseases (lung cancer, chronic bronchitis, emphysema, and tuberculosis), reemphasize the following:
  - Smoking history
  - Cough, dyspnea on exertion, or breathlessness
  - Fatigue
  - Significant weight changes
  - Fever, night sweats

RISK FACTORS   **Respiratory Disability: Barriers to Competent Function**

- Gender: Greater in men, but the difference between the sexes diminishes with advancing age
- Age: Increases inexorably with advancing age
- Family history of asthma, cystic fibrosis, tuberculosis and other contagious disease, neurofibromatosis
- Smoking
- Sedentary life-style or forced immobilization
- Occupational exposure to asbestos, dust, or other pulmonary irritants and toxic inhalants
- Extreme obesity
- Difficulty swallowing for any reason
- Weakened chest muscles for any reason
- History of frequent respiratory infections

EXAMINATION AND FINDINGS

EQUIPMENT

- Marking pencil or eyeliner (silver is good for dark skin)
- Centimeter ruler and tape measure
- Stethoscope with bell and diaphragm (for children, the diaphragm may, but does not necessarily have to, have a smaller diameter)
- Drapes

The sequence of steps in examination of the chest and lungs is traditional—inspection, palpation, percussion, and auscultation. None of these techniques alone will provide adequate information for the accurate definition of a pathologic process. The integration of all four, together with the history, often will. Listening to the lungs without also inspecting and palpating the chest will deny you the chance to interpret your findings in the most accurate way. Dullness on percussion, for example, is present in both pleural effusion and lobar pneumonia. Breath sounds are absent in the former and may be tubular in the latter. On palpation you will often find that tactile fremitus is absent when an effusion exists and is increased with lobar pneumonia. The differentiation of these conditions may well be established on a complete physical examination.

INSPECTION

Have the patient sit upright, if possible without support, naked to the waist. Clothing of any kind is a real barrier. A drape should be available to cover the patient when full exposure is not necessary. The room and stethoscope should be comfortably warm, and a bright tangential light is needed to highlight chest movement. Positioning the patient so that the light source comes at different angles may accentuate findings that are more subtle and otherwise difficult to detect, such as minimal pulsations or retractions or the presence of deformity (e.g., minimal pectus excavatum). If the patient is in bed and mobility is limited, you should have access to both sides of the bed. Do not hesitate to raise and lower the bed as needed.

Note the shape and symmetry of the chest from both the back and front. The bony framework is obvious, the clavicles prominent superiorly, the sternum usually rather flat and free of an abundance of overlying tissue. (See Box 12-2 for thoracic landmarks to use as you record findings.) The chest will not be absolutely symmetric, but one side can be used as a comparison for the other. The anteroposterior (AP) diameter of the chest is ordinarily less than the transverse diameter, often by as much as half (Figure 12-8).

BOX 12-2 **Thoracic Landmarks**

In conjunction with the anatomic landmarks of the chest, the following imaginary lines on the surface will help localize the findings on physical examination (see Figure 12-10):
1. Midsternal line: vertically down the midline of the sternum
2. Right and left midclavicular lines: parallel to the midsternal line, beginning at midclavicle; the inferior borders of the lungs generally cross the sixth rib at the midclavicular line
3. Right and left anterior axillary lines: parallel to the midsternal line, beginning at the anterior axillary folds
4. Right and left midaxillary lines: parallel to the midsternal line, beginning at the midaxilla
5. Right and left posterior axillary lines: parallel to the midsternal line, beginning at the posterior axillary folds
6. Vertebral line: vertically down the spinal processes
7. Right and left scapular lines: parallel to the vertebral line, through the inferior angle of the scapula when the patient is erect

The spinous process of the seventh cervical vertebra is readily palpated. The thoracic vertebrae can then be counted down from that point (Figure 12-11). Although the head of each rib articulates with its corresponding vertebra, remember that the spinous process of that vertebra is the palpable portion. It extends caudally and is dorsal to the next vertebral body. Thus the rib you feel in apparent association with the spinous process is really the number of that process plus one.

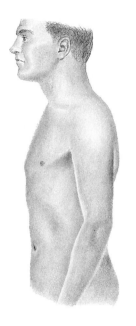

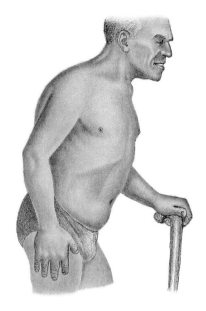

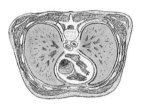

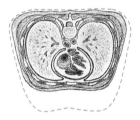

FIGURE 12-8
Thorax of healthy adult male. Note that anteroposterior diameter is less than transverse diameter.

FIGURE 12-9
Barrel chest. Note increase in anteroposterior diameter.

Barrel chest (Figure 12-9) results from compromised respiration as in, for example, chronic asthma, emphysema, or cystic fibrosis. The ribs are more horizontal, the spine at least somewhat kyphotic, and the sternal angle more prominent. The trachea may be posteriorly displaced.

Other changes in chest wall contour may be the result of structural problems in the spine, rib cage, or sternum. The spine may be deviated either posteriorly (kyphosis) or laterally (scoliosis) (see Figures 19-20, *B* and 19-76 in Chapter 19, Musculoskeletal System). Two common structural problems are pigeon chest (pectus carinatum), which is a prominent sternal protrusion, and funnel chest (pectus excavatum), which is an indentation of the lower sternum above the xiphoid process (Figure 12-12).

Inspect the skin, nails, lips, and nipples, noting whether cyanosis or pallor is present. These may be clues to respiratory or cardiac disorder. Smell the breath; intrathoracic infection may make it malodorous. Note whether there are supernumerary nipples, frequently a clue to other congenital abnormalities, particularly in white patients. Look for any superficial venous patterns over the chest, which may be a sign of heart disorders or vascular obstruction or disease. The underlying fat and relative prominence of the ribs give some clue to general nutrition.

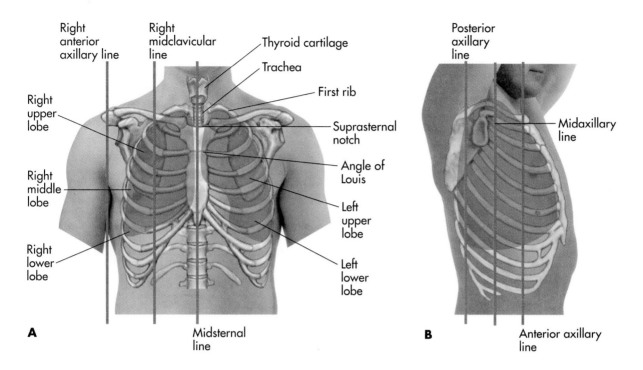

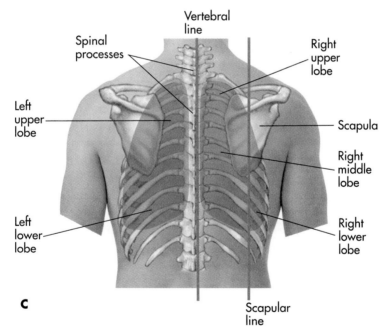

FIGURE 12-10

Thoracic landmarks. **A,** Anterior thorax. **B,** Right lateral thorax. **C,** Posterior thorax.

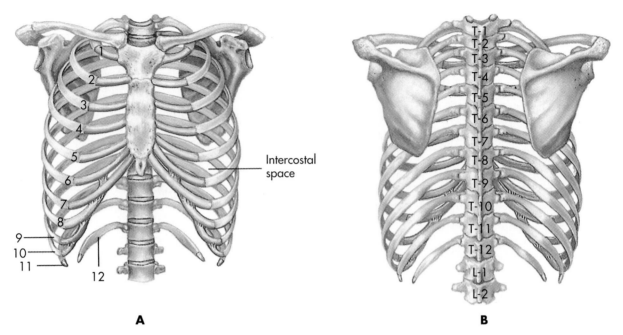

FIGURE 12-11
Rib cage. **A,** Anterior view. **B,** Posterior view.

RESPIRATION

Determine the respiratory rate. The rate should be 12 to 20 respirations per minute; the ratio of respirations to heartbeats is approximately 1:4. You need not tell the patient that you are counting respirations. Frequently the patient will have a self-conscious response that may be misleading; therefore make your count while you are palpating the pulse. Check each of the rates in sequence without the patient being precisely aware of what you are doing. Respiratory rates can vary in the variety of waking and sleep states. Noting the behavior of the patient relative to the rate is often helpful.

Note the pattern (or rhythm) of respiration and the way in which the chest moves (Figure 12-13). Expansion of the chest should be bilaterally symmetric. Expect the patient to breathe easily, regularly, and without apparent distress. The pattern of breathing should be even, neither too shallow nor too deep. Note any variations in respiratory rate.

DESCRIPTORS OF RESPIRATION

Dyspnea, difficult and labored breathing with shortness of breath, is commonly observed with pulmonary or cardiac compromise. A sedentary life-style and obesity can cause it in an otherwise well person. In general, dyspnea increases with the severity of the underlying condition. It is important to establish the amount and kind of effort that produces dyspnea.

- Is it present even when the patient is resting?
- How much walking? On a level surface? Up stairs?
- Is it necessary to stop and rest when climbing stairs?
- With what other activities of daily life does dyspnea begin? With what level of physical demand?

Other manifestations of respiratory difficulty include the following:

- *Orthopnea*—shortness of breath that begins or increases when the patient lies down; ask whether the patient needs to sleep on more than one pillow and whether that helps.

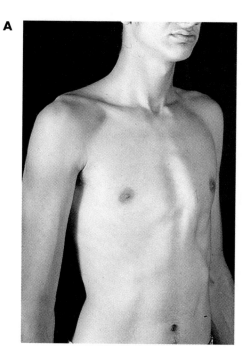

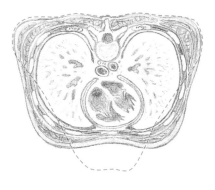

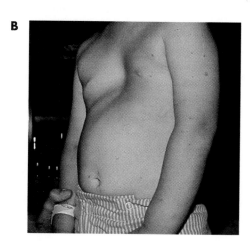

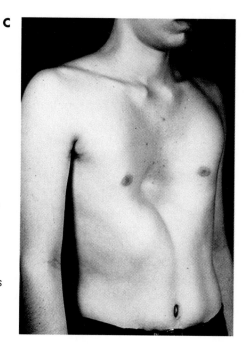

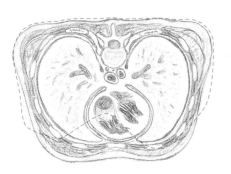

FIGURE 12-12

A, Unilateral pectus carinatum (pigeon chest) in an 18-year-old. **B,** Pectus excavatum (funnel chest) in a 4-year-old. Note the child's poor posture, pot belly, and sunken chest. **C,** The same patient with pectus excavatum is shown 14 years later. (Dotted lines indicate structural deviations.)

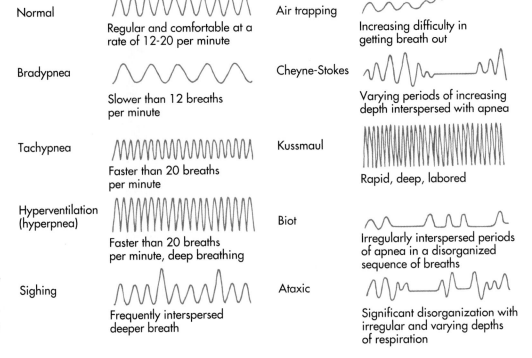

FIGURE 12-13

Patterns of respiration. The horizontal axis indicates the relative rates of these patterns. The vertical swings of the lines indicate the relative depth of respiration.

■ *Paroxysmal nocturnal dyspnea*—a sudden onset of shortness of breath after a period of sleep; sitting upright is helpful.

■ *Platypnea*—dyspnea increases in the upright posture.

Tachypnea is a persistent respiratory rate approaching 25 respirations per minute. Double check to be sure that the respiratory rate is persistent. Rapid, shallow breathing may occur during hyperventilation or simply as a self-conscious response to your observation. It is often a symptom of protective splinting from pain of a broken rib or pleurisy. Massive liver enlargement or abdominal ascites may prevent descent of the diaphragm and produce a similar pattern. *Bradypnea,* a rate slower than 12 respirations per minute, may indicate neurologic or electrolyte disturbance, infection, or a sensible response to protect against the pain of pleurisy or other irritative phenomena. It may also indicate a splendid level of cardiorespiratory fitness.

Note any variations in respiratory rhythm. It may be difficult to discern abnormalities unless they are quite obvious (Box 12-3). If the patient is breathing laboriously, rapidly, and deeply *(hyperpnea),* hyperventilation results. Exercise and anxiety can cause hyperpnea, but so can central nervous system and metabolic disease. *Kussmaul breathing,* always deep and most often rapid, is the eponymic description applied to respiratory effort associated with metabolic acidosis. *Hypopnea,* on the other hand, refers to abnormally shallow respirations, for example, when pleuritic pain limits excursion.

A regular periodic pattern of breathing, with intervals of apnea followed by a crescendo/decrescendo sequence of respiration, is called *periodic breathing* or *Cheyne-Stokes* respiration. Children and older adults may breathe in this pattern during sleep, but otherwise it occurs in patients who are seriously ill, particularly those with brain damage at the cerebral level or with drug-caused respiratory compromise (Box 12-4).

BOX 12-3   **Some Influences on the Rate and Depth of Breathing**

The Rate and Depth of Breathing Will

Increase with
Acidosis (metabolic)
Central nervous system lesions (pons)
Anxiety
Aspirin poisoning
Oxygen need (hypoxemia)
Pain

Decrease with
Alkalosis (matabolic)
Central nervous system lesions (cerebrum)
Myasthenia gravis
Narcotic overdoses
Obesity (extreme)

BOX 12-4   **Apnea**

Apnea, the absence of spontaneous respiration, may have its origin in the respiratory system and, as well, in a variety of central nervous system and cardiac abnormalities. Commonly, seizures, central nervous system trauma or hypoperfusion, a variety of infections of the respiratory passageway, drug ingestions, and obstructive sleep disorders may contribute. Cheyne-Stokes respiration has characteristic moments of apnea. There is the universal expectation of the absence of breathing when one is swallowing *(deglutition apnea)*. *Primary apnea* is a self-limited condition, which is not uncommon after a blow to the head. It is especially noted immediately after the birth of a newborn who will breath spontaneously when sufficient carbon dioxide accumulates in the circulation. If irritating and nausea-provoking vapors or gases are inhaled, there can be an involuntary, obviously temporary halt to respiration *(reflex apnea)*. *Secondary apnea* is grave. The breathing stops and it will not begin spontaneously unless resuscitative measures are immediately instituted. Any event that severely limits the absorption of oxygen into the bloodstream will lead to secondary apnea. *Sleep apnea,* characterized by periods of an absence of breathing effort during sleep, can be very disturbing; the respiratory muscles do not function and air flow is not maintained through the nose and mouth. *Selective apnea* affects only a part of the breathing cycle. *Apneustic breathing* is characterized by a long inspiration and what amounts to expiration apnea. The neural center for control is in the pons. When it is affected, breathing can become gasping, as inspirations are prolonged and expiration constrained. The *apnea of prematurity* is a more intense version of *periodic apnea of the newborn,* a normal condition characterized by an irregular pattern of rapid breathing interspersed with brief periods of apnea usually associated with rapid eye movement sleep.

An occasional deep, audible *sigh* that punctuates an otherwise regular respiratory pattern is associated with emotional distress or an incipient episode of more severe hyperventilation. Sighs are significant only if they exceed the infrequent and relatively inconsequential sighs of daily life.

If the pulmonary tree is seriously obstructed for any reason, inspired air has difficulty overcoming the resistance and getting out. *Air trapping* is the result of a prolonged but inefficient expiratory effort. The rate of respiration increases in order to compensate; as this happens, the effort becomes more shallow, the amount of trapped air increases, and the lungs inflate.

Biot respiration consists of somewhat irregular respirations varying in depth and interrupted by intervals of apnea, but lacking the repetitive pattern of periodic respiration. On occasion, the respirations may be regular, but the apneic periods may occur in an irregular pattern. Biot respiration usually is associated with severe and persistent increased intracranial pressure, respiratory compromise resulting from drug poisoning, or brain damage at the level of the medulla. It may be referred to as *ataxic* in its more extreme expression. Changes in breathing pattern are usually significant. When breathing is labored or respirations are deeper than usual, the accessory muscles of respiration, the sternocleidomastoid and trapezius muscles, may be used.

BOX 12-5   **Is the Airway Patent or Obstructed?**

Determining the patency of the upper airway is essential to a complete evaluation of pulmonary status. When is the upper airway obstructed?

- When there is
  - Inspiratory stridor (with a ratio with expiration of more than 2:1)
  - A hoarse cough or cry
  - Flaring of the alae nasi
  - Retraction at the suprasternal notch
- Severely so, when
  - Stridor is inspiratory and expiratory
  - Cough is barking
  - Retractions also involve the subcostal and intercostal spaces
  - Cyanosis is obvious even with blow-by oxygen
- When the obstruction is above the glottis
  - Stridor tends to be quieter
  - The voice is muffled, as if there is a "hot potato" in the mouth
  - Swallowing is more difficult
  - Cough is not a factor
  - The head and neck may be awkwardly positioned to preserve the airway (extended with retropharyngeal abscess; head to the affected side with peritonsillar abscess)
- When the obstruction is below the glottis
  - Stridor tends to be louder, more rasping
  - The voice is hoarse
  - Swallowing is not affected
  - Cough is harsh, barking
  - Positioning of the head is not a factor

MODES OF RESPIRATION

Respiration may be defined as the act of breathing with the lungs so that the necessary exchange of carbon dioxide for oxygen can take place. *Thoracic (costal) respiration* is primarily the result of the use of intercostal muscles. *Diaphragmatic respiration,* on the other hand, is primarily the result of the movement of the diaphragm responding to intrathoracic pressure. *Abdominal respiration* involves contraction of the diaphragm and the interplay of the abdominal muscles, resulting in the expansion and recoil of the abdominal walls. It is not unusual to see abdominal respiration, particularly in very young infants. Thoracic respiration, however, is the rule at most ages unless the intercostal and other thoracic muscles are compromised or the person has a pathophysiologic need to use every respiratory resource. Men are more likely to use diaphragmatic respiration and women, particularly when they are pregnant, thoracic. *Paradoxic breathing* occurs when a negative intrathoracic pressure is transmitted to the abdomen by a weakened, poorly functioning diaphragm, obstructive airway disease, or during sleep, in the event of upper airway obstruction. Thus on inspiration, the lower thorax is drawn in and the abdomen protrudes, and on expiration, the opposite occurs.

Inspect the chest wall movement during respiration. Again, different angles of illumination will aid inspection and help delineate chest wall deformities. Expansion should be symmetric, without apparent use of accessory muscles. Chest asymmetry can be associated with unequal expansion and respiratory compromise caused by a collapsed lung or limitation of expansion by extrapleural air, fluid, or a mass. Unilateral or bilateral bulging can be a reaction of the ribs and interspaces to respiratory obstruction. A prolonged expiration and bulging on expiration are probably caused by outflow obstruction or the valvelike action of compression by a tumor, aneurysm, or enlarged heart. The costal angle widens beyond 90 degrees.

Retractions suggest an obstruction to inspiration at any point in the respiratory tract. As intrapleural pressure becomes increasingly negative, the musculature "pulls back" in an effort to overcome blockage. Any significant obstruction makes the retraction observable with each inspiratory effort. The degree and level of retraction depend on the extent and level of obstruction (Box 12-5). When the obstruction is high in the respiratory tree (e.g., with tracheal or laryngeal involvement), breathing is characterized by stridor, and the chest wall seems to cave in at the sternum, between the ribs, at the suprasternal notch, above the clavicles, and at the lowest costal margins.

A foreign body in one or the other of the bronchi (usually the right because of its broader bore and more vertical placement) causes unilateral retraction, but the suprasternal notch is not involved. Retraction of the lower chest occurs with asthma and bronchiolitis.

Observe the lips and nails for cyanosis, the lips for pursing, the fingers for clubbing, and the alae nasi for flaring. Any of these peripheral clues suggests pulmonary or cardiac difficulty. Pursing of the lips is an accompaniment of increased expiratory effort. Clubbing of the fingers is associated with chronic fibrotic changes within the lung, the chronic cyanosis of congenital heart disease, or cystic fibrosis. (Note that other chronic problems involving the lungs, for example, asthma and emphysema, are not associated with clubbing.) Flaring of the alae nasi during inspiration is a common sign of air hunger, particularly when the alveoli are considerably involved.

PALPATION

Palpate the thoracic muscles and skeleton, feeling for pulsations, areas of tenderness, bulges, depressions, unusual movement, and unusual positions. There should be bilateral symmetry and some elasticity of the rib cage, but the sternum and xiphoid should be relatively inflexible and the thoracic spine rigid.

Crepitus, a crackly or crinkly sensation, can be both palpated and heard—a gentle, bubbly feeling. It indicates air in the subcutaneous tissue from a rupture somewhere in the respiratory system or by infection with a gas-producing organism. It may be localized (e.g., over the suprasternal notch and base of the neck) or cover a wider area of the thorax, usually anteriorly and toward the axilla. Crepitus is always a sign requiring attention.

A palpable, coarse, grating vibration, usually on inspiration, suggests a *pleural friction rub* caused by inflammation of the pleural surfaces. Think of it as the feel of leather rubbing on leather.

To evaluate thoracic expansion during respiration, stand behind the patient and place your thumbs along the spinal processes at the level of the tenth rib, with your palms lightly in contact with the posterolateral surfaces (Figure 12-14). Watch your thumbs diverge during quiet and deep breathing. A loss of symmetry in the movement of the thumbs suggests a problem on one or both sides. Then face the patient and place your thumbs along the costal margin and the xiphoid process, with your palms touching the anterolateral chest. Again, watch your thumbs diverge as the patient breathes.

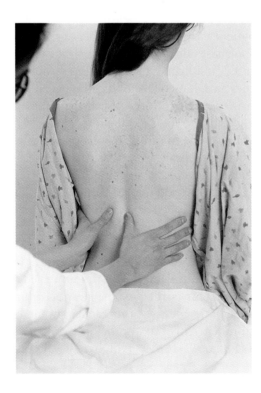

FIGURE 12-14
Palpating thoracic expansion. The thumbs are at the level of the tenth rib.

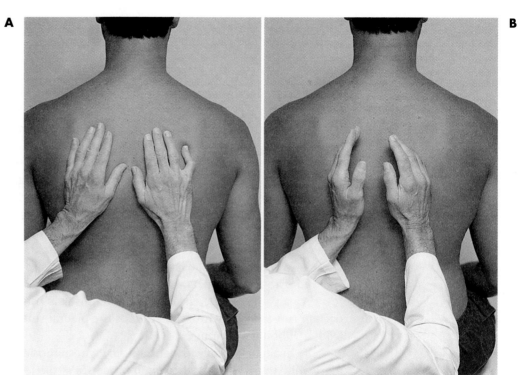

FIGURE 12-15
Two methods for evaluating tactile fremitus. **A,** With palmar surface of both hands. **B,** With ulnar aspect.

Note the quality of the *tactile fremitus,* the palpable vibration of the chest wall that results from speech or other verbalizations. Fremitus is best felt parasternally at the second intercostal space, at the level of the bifurcation of the bronchi. There is great variability depending on the intensity and pitch of the voice and the structure and thickness of the chest wall. In addition, the scapulae obscure fremitus.

Ask the patient to recite a few numbers or say a few words while you systematically palpate the chest with the palmar surfaces of the fingers or with the ulnar aspects of the hand. Use a firm, light touch, establishing even contact. For comparison, palpate both sides simultaneously and symmetrically, or use one hand, quickly alternating between the two sides. Move about the patient, palpating each area carefully: front to back, right side to left side, the lung apices (Figure 12-15).

Decreased or absent fremitus may be caused by excess air in the lungs or may indicate emphysema, pleural thickening or effusion, massive pulmonary edema, or bronchial obstruction. Increased fremitus, often coarser or rougher in feel, occurs in the presence of fluids or a solid mass within the lungs and may be caused by lung consolidation, heavy but nonobstructive bronchial secretions, compressed lung, or tumor. Gentle, more tremulous fremitus than expected occurs with some lung consolidations and inflammatory and infectious processes.

Note the position of the trachea. Place an index finger in the suprasternal notch and move it gently, side to side, along the upper edges of each clavicle and in the spaces above to the inner borders of the sternocleidomastoid muscles. These spaces should be equal on both sides, and the trachea should be in the midline directly above the suprasternal notch. This can also be determined by palpating with both thumbs simultaneously (Figure 12-16). A slight, barely noticeable deviation to the right is not unusual.

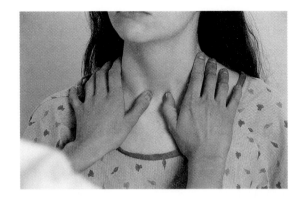

FIGURE 12-16
Palpating to evaluate midline position of the trachea.

The trachea may be deviated because of problems within the chest and may, on occasion, seem to pulsate. It may be displaced by atelectasis, thyroid enlargement, significant parenchymal and/or pleural fibrosis, or pleural effusion, and may be pushed to one side by tension pneumothorax, a tumor, or nodal enlargements on the contralateral side, or pulled by a tumor on the side to which it deviates. Anterior mediastinal tumors may push it posteriorly; with mediastinitis, the trachea may be pushed forward. A palpable pull out of midline with respiration is called a *tug*.

The examination of a woman's chest may be obscured by the breasts. It is permissible, when necessary, to move the breast gently or to ask the patient to do this for you. For example, when percussing, you may shift the breast slightly with the pleximeter hand and, keeping it in place, strike the finger of that hand with the plexor of your free hand.

PERCUSSION

Percussion tones heard over the chest, as elsewhere, are described in Chapter 3 (Examination Techniques and Equipment) and summarized in Table 12-1. You can percuss directly or indirectly, as described in Chapter 3 (Figure 12-17).

Compare all areas bilaterally, using one side as a control for the other. The following sequence serves as one model. First, examine the back with the patient sitting with head bent forward and arms folded in front. This moves the scapulae laterally, exposing more of the lung. Then ask the patient to raise the arms overhead while you percuss the lateral and anterior chest. For all positions percuss at 4- to 5-cm intervals over the intercostal spaces, moving systematically from superior to inferior and medial to lateral (Figures 12-18 and 12-19). This sequence is one of many that you may follow. Adopt the one most comfortable for you, and use it consistently. Resonance can usually be heard over all areas of the lungs. Hyperresonance associated with hyperinflation may indicate emphysema, pneumothorax, or asthma. Dullness or flatness suggests atelectasis, pleural effusion, pneumothorax, or asthma.

TABLE 12-1	Percussion Tones Heard over the Chest			
Type of Tone	**Intensity**	**Pitch**	**Duration**	**Quality**
Resonant	Loud	Low	Long	Hollow
Flat	Soft	High	Short	Extremely dull
Dull	Medium	Medium-high	Medium	Thudlike
Tympanic	Loud	High	Medium	Drumlike
Hyperresonant*	Very loud	Very low	Longer	Booming

From Thompson et al, 1997.
See Chapter 3 for definitions and a more complete discussion of these tones.
*Hyperresonance is an abnormal sound in adults. It represents air trapping such as occurs in obstructive lung diseases.

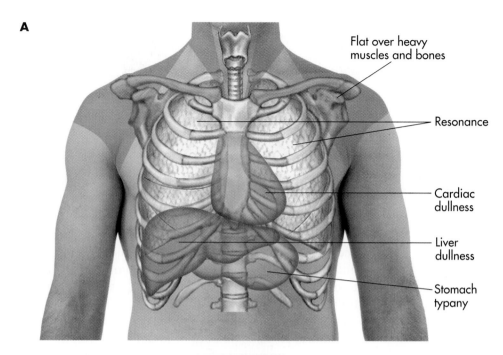

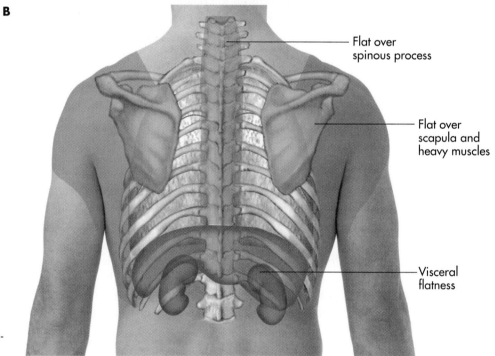

FIGURE 12-17
Percussion tones throughout chest. **A,** Anterior view. **B,** Posterior view

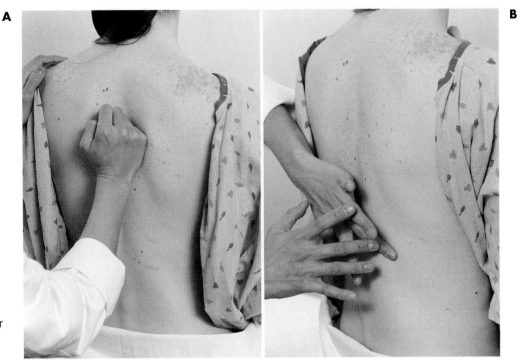

FIGURE 12-18
A, Direct percussion using ulnar aspect of fist. **B,** Indirect percussion.

Diaphragmatic Excursion

Measure the diaphragmatic excursion. Its descent may be limited by several types of lesions—pulmonary (e.g., as a result of emphysema), abdominal (e.g., massive ascites, tumor), or superficial painful (e.g., fractured rib). Remember that the diaphragm is usually higher on the right than on the left because it sits over the bulk of the liver.

The following steps suggest one approach to measuring the diaphragmatic excursion:

- Ask the patient to inhale deeply and hold.
- Percuss along the scapular line until you locate the lower border, the point marked by a change in note from resonance to dullness.
- Mark the point with a skin pencil at the scapular line. Allow the patient to breathe, and then repeat the procedure on the other side.
- Ask the patient to take several breaths and then to exhale as much as possible and hold (Box 12-6).
- Percuss up from the marked point and make a mark at the change from dullness to resonance. Remind the patient to start breathing. Repeat on the other side.
- Measure and record the distance in centimeters between the marks on each side. The excursion distance is usually 3 to 5 cm (Figure 12-20).

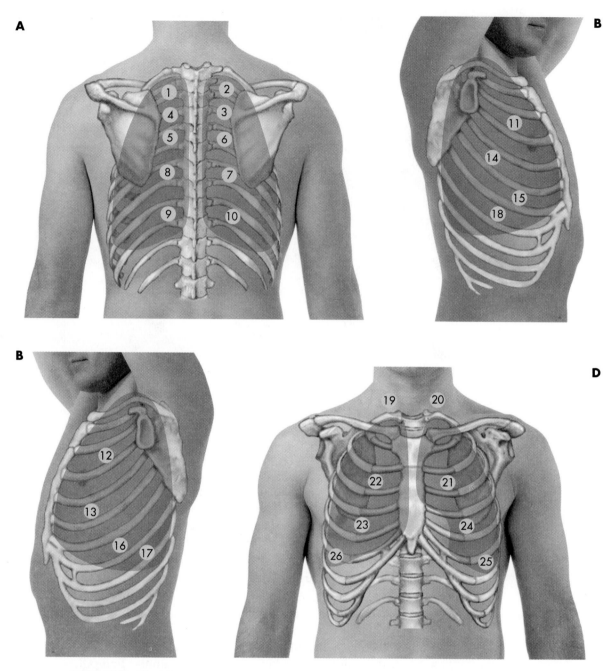

FIGURE 12-19

Suggested sequence for systematic percussion and auscultation of the thorax. **A,** Posterior thorax. **B,** Right lateral thorax. **C,** Left lateral thorax. **D,** Anterior thorax. The pleximeter finger or the stethoscope is moved in the numeric sequence suggested; however, other sequences are possible. It is beneficial to be systematic.

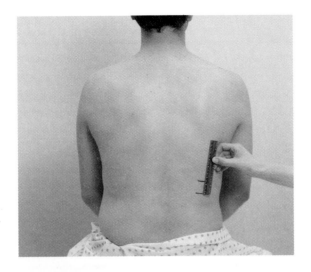

FIGURE 12-20
Measuring diaphragmatic excursion. Excursion distance is usually 3 to 5 cm.

| BOX 12-6 | **Smell the Breath** |

Auscultation of the lungs makes it possible (occasionally uncomfortably so) to become aware of a patient's breath odor. Your nose may provide a significant clue:

- Sweet, fruity — Diabetic ketoacidosis; starvation ketosis
- Fishy, stale — Uremia (trimethylamines)
- Ammonia-like — Uremia (ammonia)
- Musty fish, clover — *Fetor hepaticus*: hepatic failure, portal vein thrombosis, portacaval shunts
- Foul, feculent — Intestinal obstruction/diverticulum
- Foul, putrid — Nasal/sinus pathology: infection, foreign body, cancer; respiratory infections: empyema, lung abscess, bronchiectasis
- Halitosis — Tonsillitis, gingivitis, respiratory infections, Vincent's angina, gastroesophageal reflux
- Cinnamon — Pulmonary tuberculosis

Modified from Wilson, 1997 and McMillan, Stockman, Oski, 1982.

AUSCULTATION

Auscultation with a stethoscope provides important clues to the condition of the lungs and pleura. (On relatively rare occasions, a sound is apparent to the ear directly that might be lost via the stethoscope, for example, the click of an aspirated foreign body.) All sounds can be characterized in the same manner as the percussion notes: intensity, pitch, quality, and duration (Table 12-2).

Have the patient sit upright, if possible, and breathe slowly and deeply through the mouth, exaggerating normal respiration. Demonstrate it yourself. Caution the patient to keep a pace consistent with comfort; hyperventilation, which occurs more easily than one might think, may cause faintness and exaggerated breathing can be tiring, especially for the elderly or the ill. Since most pulmonary pathologic conditions in the elderly occur at the lung bases, it is a good idea to examine these first before fatigue sets in.

The diaphragm of the stethoscope is usually preferable to the bell for listening to the lungs, because it transmits the ordinarily high-pitched sounds better, and it provides a broader area of sound. Place the stethoscope firmly on the skin. When the individual breath sound is being evaluated, there should be *no* movement of patient or stethoscope except for the respiratory excursion.

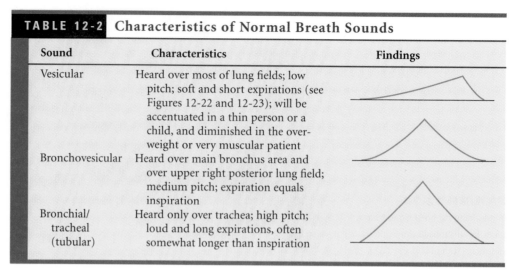

TABLE 12-2	Characteristics of Normal Breath Sounds	
Sound	**Characteristics**	**Findings**
Vesicular	Heard over most of lung fields; low pitch; soft and short expirations (see Figures 12-22 and 12-23); will be accentuated in a thin person or a child, and diminished in the overweight or very muscular patient	
Bronchovesicular	Heard over main bronchus area and over upper right posterior lung field; medium pitch; expiration equals inspiration	
Bronchial/ tracheal (tubular)	Heard only over trachea; high pitch; loud and long expirations, often somewhat longer than inspiration	

Modified from Thompson et al, 1993.

To auscultate the back, ask the patient to sit as for percussion, with head bent forward and arms folded in front to enlarge the listening area (Figure 12-21). Then have the patient sit more erect with arms overhead for auscultating the lateral chest. Finally, ask the patient to sit erect with the shoulders back for auscultation of the anterior chest. As with so much else, the exact sequence you adopt is not as important as using the same sequence each time to ensure that the examination is thorough.

Listen systematically at each position throughout inspiration and expiration, taking advantage of a side-to-side comparison as you move downward from apex to base at intervals of several centimeters. The sounds of the middle lobe of the right lung and the lingula on the left are best heard in the respective axillae.

Breath Sounds

Breath sounds are made by the flow of air through the respiratory tree. They are characterized by pitch, intensity, and quality and relative duration of their inspiratory and expiratory phases, and are classified as vesicular, bronchovesicular, and bronchial (tubular) (Table 12-2 and Figure 12-22).

CONGESTIVE HEART FAILURE

If the patient may have congestive heart failure, you should begin auscultation at the base of the lungs to detect crackles that may disappear with continued exaggerated respiration.

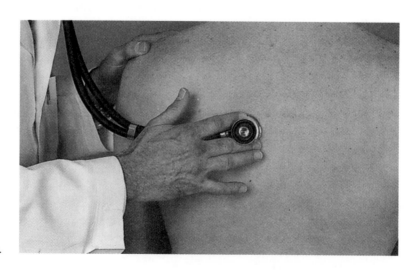

FIGURE 12-21
Auscultation with a stethoscope.

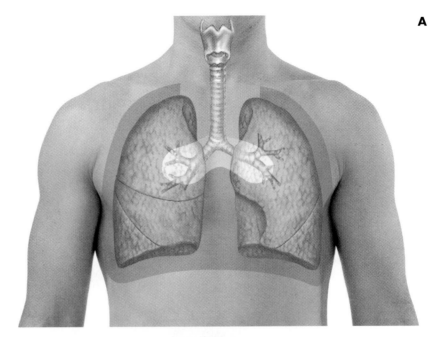

A

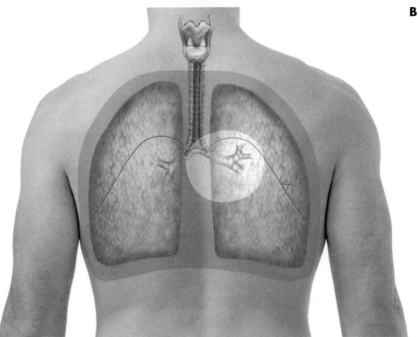

B

KEY:

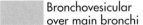
Bronchovesicular
over main bronchi

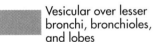
Vesicular over lesser
bronchi, bronchioles,
and lobes

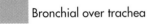
Bronchial over trachea

FIGURE 12-22
Expected auscultatory sounds.
A, Anterior view. **B**, Posterior
view.

Vesicular breath sounds are low-pitched, low-intensity sounds heard over healthy lung tissue. *Bronchovesicular* sounds are heard over the major bronchi and are typically moderate in pitch and intensity. The sounds highest in pitch and intensity are the *bronchial* breath sounds, which are ordinarily heard only over the trachea. Both bronchovesicular and bronchial breath sounds are abnormal if they are heard over the peripheral lung tissue.

Breathing that resembles the noise made by blowing across the mouth of a bottle is defined as *amphoric* and is most often heard with a large, relatively stiff-walled pulmonary cavity or a tension pneumothorax with bronchopleural fistula. *Cavernous breathing,* sounding as if it were coming from a cavern, is commonly heard over a pulmonary cavity in which the wall is rigid.

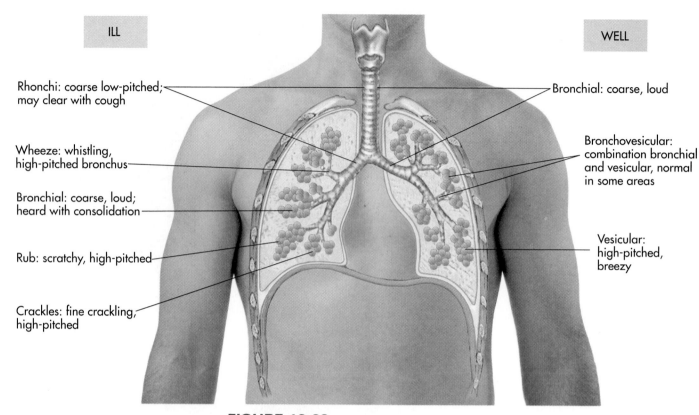

ILL

Rhonchi: coarse low-pitched;
may clear with cough

Wheeze: whistling,
high-pitched bronchus

Bronchial: coarse, loud;
heard with consolidation

Rub: scratchy, high-pitched

Crackles: fine crackling,
high-pitched

WELL

Bronchial: coarse, loud

Bronchovesicular:
combination bronchial
and vesicular, normal
in some areas

Vesicular:
high-pitched,
breezy

FIGURE 12-23
Schema of breath sounds in the ill and well patient.

Breath sounds are relatively more difficult to hear or are absent if fluid or pus has accumulated in the pleural space, secretions or a foreign body obstructs the bronchi, the lungs are hyperinflated, or breathing is shallow from splinting for pain. Breath sounds are easier to hear when the lungs are consolidated; the mass surrounding the tube of the respiratory tree promotes sound transmission better than do air-filled alveoli.

Most of the unexpected sounds heard during lung auscultation are superimposed on the breath sounds. Extraneous sounds such as the crinkling of chest or back hair must be carefully distinguished from far more significant adventitious sounds. Sometimes it helps to moisten chest hair to minimize this problem. The common terms used to describe adventitious sounds are *crackles* (formerly called *rales*), *rhonchi, wheezes,* and *friction rub* (Figure 12-23) (Box 12-7). Crackles are discontinuous; rhonchi and wheezes are continuous. See Box 12-8 for a more detailed description of adventitious breath sounds.

BOX 12-7 **The Terminology of Breath Sounds**

Lung sounds are easier to recognize than to describe. Perhaps that is why the traditional use of the word *rales* has yielded to *crackles*. The terminology we use follows the suggestion of the American Thoracic Society. It is reflected in Table 12-3 (in several languages). However, the terms cannot be rigid, since the airway is continuous and there may be overlapping noises which, while obvious to the ear, may not lend themselves to precise description. The terminology, however, attempts to allow a common understanding in the sometimes frustrated effort to be exact.

TABLE 12-3	Lung Sound Nomenclature				
Lung Sound	**English**	**French**	**German**	**Portuguese**	**Spanish**
Discontinuous					
Fine (high pitched, low amplitude, short duration)	Fine crackles	Râles crepitants	Feines Rassein	Estertores finos	Esterfores finos
Coarse (low pitched, high amplitude, long duration)	Coarse crackles	Râles bulleux ou Sous-crepitants	Grobes Rassein	Estertores grossos	Estertores gruesos
Continuous					
High pitched	Wheezes	Râles sibilants	Pfeifen	Sibilos	Sibilancias
Low pitched	Rhonchus	Râles ronflants	Brummen	Roncos	Roncus

From Cugell, 1987.

BOX 12-8	Adventitious Breath Sounds

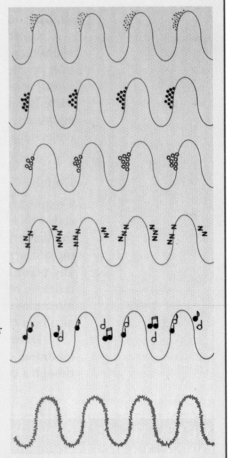

Fine crackles: high-pitched, discrete, discontinuous crackling sounds heard during the end of inspiration; not cleared by a cough

Medium crackles: lower, more moist sound heard during the midstage of inspiration; not cleared by a cough

Coarse crackles: loud, bubbly noise heard during inspiration; not cleared by a cough

Rhonchi (sonorous wheeze): loud, low, coarse sounds like a snore most often heard continuously during inspiration or expiration; coughing may clear sound (usually means mucus accumulation in trachea or large bronchi)

Wheeze (sibilant wheeze): musical noise sounding like a squeak; most often heard continuously during inspiration or expiration; usually louder during expiration

Pleural friction rub: dry, rubbing, or grating sound, usually caused by inflammation of pleural surfaces; heard during inspiration or expiration; loudest over lower lateral anterior surface

Modified from Thompson et al, 1997.

Crackles

A crackle is an abnormal respiratory sound heard more often during inspiration and characterized by discrete discontinuous sounds, each lasting just a few milliseconds. The individual noise tends to be brief and the interval to the next one similarly brief.

Crackles may be fine, high pitched, and relatively short in duration, or coarse, low pitched, and relatively longer in duration. They are caused by the disruptive passage of air through the small airways in the respiratory tree. High-pitched crackles are described as *sibilant;* the more low pitched are termed *sonorous.* Crackles with a dry quality, more crisp than gurgling, are apt to occur higher in the respiratory tree. You might listen for crackles at the open mouth. If their origin is in the upper airways, they will be easily heard; if in the lower, not so easily.

Rhonchi

Rhonchi (sonorous wheezes) are deeper, more rumbling, more pronounced during expiration, more likely to be prolonged and continuous, and less discrete than crackles. They are caused by the passage of air through an airway obstructed by thick secretions, muscular spasm, new growth, or external pressure. The more sibilant, higher-pitched rhonchi arise from the smaller bronchi, as in asthma; the more sonorous, lower-pitched rhonchi arise from larger bronchi, as in tracheobronchitis. They may at times be palpable.

It may be difficult to distinguish between crackles and rhonchi. In general, rhonchi tend to disappear after coughing, whereas crackles do not. If such sounds are present, listen to several respiratory excursions, a few with the patient's accustomed effort, a few with deeper breathing, a few before coughing, and a few after.

Wheezes

A *wheeze (sibilant wheeze)* is sometimes thought of as a form of rhonchus. It is a continuous, high-pitched, musical sound, almost a whistle, heard during inspiration or expiration. It is caused by a relatively high-velocity air flow through a narrowed airway. Wheezes may be composed of complex combinations of a variety of pitches or of a single pitch, and they may vary from area to area and minute to minute. If a wheeze is heard bilaterally, it may be caused by the bronchospasm of asthma (reactive airway disease) or acute or chronic bronchitis. Unilateral or more sharply localized wheezing or stridor may occur with a foreign body. A tumor compressing a part of the bronchial tree can create a consistent wheeze or whistle of single pitch at the site of compression. If infection is the source of wheezing, the organism is usually a virus, not a bacterium. See Box 12-9 for other possible causes of wheezing.

Other Sounds

A *friction rub* occurs outside the respiratory tree. It has a dry, crackly, grating, low-pitched sound and is heard in both expiration and inspiration. It may have a machinelike quality. It may have no significance if heard over the liver or spleen. However, a friction rub heard over the heart or lungs is caused by inflamed, roughened surfaces rubbing together. Over the pericardium, this sound suggests pericarditis; over the lungs, pleurisy. The respiratory rub will disappear when the breath is held; the cardiac rub will not.

Mediastinal crunch (Hamman sign) is found with mediastinal emphysema. There is a great variety of noise—loud crackles and clicking and gurgling sounds. These are synchronous with the heartbeat and not particularly so with respiration, but the sounds can be more pronounced toward the end of expiration. They are easiest to hear when the patient leans to the left or lies down on the left side.

SICKLE CELL DISEASE

Persons with sickle cell disease may have frequent pulmonary complaints. The ever-present concern about pulmonary infarction and a pulmonary crisis, the "chest syndrome," may be suggested by a variety of findings on inspection, palpation, percussion, and auscultation, and also by an arching of the back as the patient attempts to breathe more comfortably.

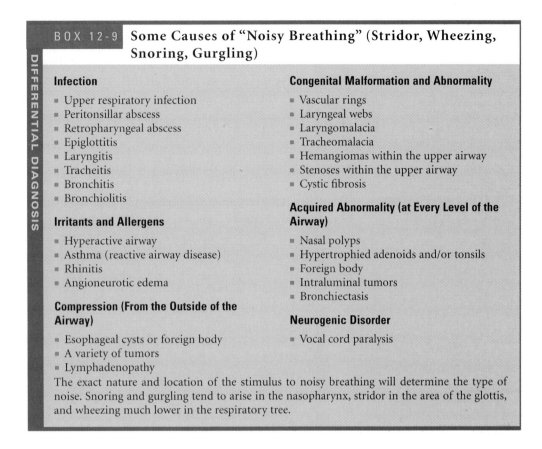

BOX 12-9 **Some Causes of "Noisy Breathing" (Stridor, Wheezing, Snoring, Gurgling)**

DIFFERENTIAL DIAGNOSIS

Infection

- Upper respiratory infection
- Peritonsillar abscess
- Retropharyngeal abscess
- Epiglottitis
- Laryngitis
- Tracheitis
- Bronchitis
- Bronchiolitis

Irritants and Allergens

- Hyperactive airway
- Asthma (reactive airway disease)
- Rhinitis
- Angioneurotic edema

Compression (From the Outside of the Airway)

- Esophageal cysts or foreign body
- A variety of tumors
- Lymphadenopathy

Congenital Malformation and Abnormality

- Vascular rings
- Laryngeal webs
- Laryngomalacia
- Tracheomalacia
- Hemangiomas within the upper airway
- Stenoses within the upper airway
- Cystic fibrosis

Acquired Abnormality (at Every Level of the Airway)

- Nasal polyps
- Hypertrophied adenoids and/or tonsils
- Foreign body
- Intraluminal tumors
- Bronchiectasis

Neurogenic Disorder

- Vocal cord paralysis

The exact nature and location of the stimulus to noisy breathing will determine the type of noise. Snoring and gurgling tend to arise in the nasopharynx, stridor in the area of the glottis, and wheezing much lower in the respiratory tree.

Air and fluid in the pleural cavity simultaneously or in large cavities within the lungs are suspected if one listens over the possibly involved area and gently shakes the patient from side to side. This can be achieved with the patient sitting. First, place a hand on the patient's shoulder and then with your hand, move the patient from side to side, not brusquely but with a bit of vigor. The fluid will splash, and in the presence of air, a *succussion splash* will be heard.

Vocal Resonance

The spoken voice vibrates and transmits sounds through the lung fields that may be judged with reasonable ease. Ask the patient to recite numbers, names, or other words. These transmitted sounds are usually muffled and indistinct and best heard medially. Pay particular attention to vocal resonance if there are other unexpected findings during any part of the examination of the lungs, such as dullness on percussion or changes in tactile fremitus. The factors that influence tactile fremitus similarly influence vocal resonance.

Greater clarity and increased loudness of spoken sounds are defined as *bronchophony*. If bronchophony is extreme in the presence, for example, of consolidation of the lungs, even a whisper can be heard clearly through the stethoscope (*whispered pectoriloquy*). When the intensity of the spoken voice is increased and there is a nasal quality (*e*'s become stuffy broad *a*'s), the auditory quality is called *egophony*. These auditory changes may be present in any condition that consolidates lung tissue. Conversely, vocal resonance diminishes and loses intensity when there is blockage of the respiratory tree for any reason, such as with emphysema.

Cough

Coughs are a common symptom of a respiratory problem. They are usually preceded by a deep inspiration; this is followed by closure of the glottis and contraction of the chest, abdominal, and even the pelvic muscles, and then a sudden, spasmodic expiration, forcing a sudden opening of the glottis. Air and secretions are exhaled. The causes may be related to localized or more general insults at any point in the respiratory tract. Coughs may be voluntary, but they are usually reflexive responses to an irritant such as a foreign body (microscopic or larger), an infectious agent, or a mass of any sort compressing the respiratory tree. They may also be a clue to an anxiety state.

Describe a cough according to its moisture, frequency, regularity, pitch and loudness, and quality. The type of cough may offer some clue to the cause. Although a cough may not have a serious cause, do not ignore it.

Dry or moist. A moist cough may be caused by infection and can be accompanied by sputum production. A dry cough can have a variety of causes (e.g., cardiac problems, allergies, HIV infection), which may be indicated by the quality of its sound.

Onset. An acute onset, particularly with fever, suggests infection; in the absence of fever, a foreign body or inhaled irritants are additional possible causes.

Frequency of occurrence. Note whether the cough is seldom or often present. An infrequent cough may result from allergens or environmental insults.

Regularity. A regular, paroxysmal cough is heard in pertussis. An irregularly occurring cough may have a variety of causes, such as smoking, early congestive heart failure, an inspired foreign body or irritant, or a tumor within or compressing the bronchial tree.

Pitch and loudness. A cough may be loud and high-pitched or quiet and relatively low-pitched.

Postural influences. A cough may occur soon after a person has reclined or assumed an erect position (e.g., with a nasal drip or pooling of secretions in the upper airway).

Quality. A dry cough may sound brassy if it is caused by compression of the respiratory tree (as by a tumor) or hoarse if it is caused by croup. Pertussis produces an inspiratory whoop at the end of a paroxysm of coughing.

BOX 12-10 **Summary of Expected Findings of Chest and Lungs**

When the lungs are healthy, the respiratory tree clear, the pleurae unaffected by disease, and the chest wall symmetrically and appropriately structured and mobile, the following characteristics will be found:

On inspection
- Symmetry of movement on expansion
- Absence of retractions

On palpation
- Midline trachea without a tug
- Symmetric, unaccentuated tactile fremitus

On percussion
- Range of 3 to 5 cm in the descent of diaphragm
- Resonant and symmetric percussion notes

On auscultation
- Absence of adventitious sounds
- Vesicular breath sounds, except for bronchovesicular sounds beside the sternum and the more prominent bronchial components in the area of the larger bronchi

Sputum

The production of sputum is generally associated with cough. Sputum in more than small amounts with any degree of consistency always suggests the presence of disease. If the onset is acute, infection is most probable. Once there is some chronicity, the possibility of a significant anatomic change, for example, tumor, cavitation, or bronchiectasis, becomes apparent. The following list* delineates possible pathologic conditions and their accompanying sputum findings.

CAUSE	POSSIBLE SPUTUM CHARACTERISTICS
Bacterial infection	Yellow, green, rust (blood mixed with yellow sputum), clear, or transparent; purulent; blood streaked; mucoid, viscid
Viral infection	Mucoid, viscid; blood streaked (not common)
Chronic infectious disease	All of the above; particularly abundant in the early morning; slight, intermittent blood streaking; occasionally, large amounts of blood
Carcinoma	Slight, persistent blood streaking
Infarction	Blood clotted; large amounts of blood
Tuberculous cavity	Large amounts of blood

Remember always to ascertain that the blood is not swallowed from a nosebleed.

INFANTS

The approach to examination of the chest and lungs of the newborn follows a sequence similar to that for adults. Inspecting without disturbing the baby is key. Percussion, however, is usually unreliable. The examiner's fingers may be too large for the baby's chest, particularly the premature infant.

A newborn's Apgar scores at 1 and 5 minutes after birth tell you a great deal about the infant's respiratory efforts. An infant whose respirations are inadequate but who is otherwise normal may initially score 1 or even 0 on heart rate, muscle tone, response to a catheter, or color. Depressed respiration often has its origins in the maternal environment during labor, such as sedatives or compromised blood supply to the child, or it may result from mechanical obstruction by mucus. Table 12-4 explains the Apgar scoring system. Remember that this score requires some subjective judgment and cannot be considered absolute.

* Modified from Harvey et al, 1988.

TABLE 12-4	Infant Evaluation at Birth—Apgar Scoring System		
	0	**1**	**2**
Heart rate	Absent	Slow (below 100 beats/min)	Over 100 beats/min
Respiratory effort	Absent	Slow or irregular	Good crying
Muscle tone	Limp	Some flexion of extremities	Active motion
Response to catheter in nostril (tested after oropharynx is clear)	No response	Grimace	Cough or sneeze
Color	Blue or pale	Body pink, extremities blue	Completely pink

Add the scores of the five individual observations to get the full Apgar score. The lower the total, the more likely a problem.

A DIAPHRAGMATIC HERNIA

A diaphragmatic hernia, the result of an imperfectly structured diaphragm, occurs once in slightly more than 2,000 live births. It is on the left side at least 90% of the time; the liver is not there to get in the way. The degree of respiratory distress can be slight or very severe and accompanied by intense cyanosis, dependent really on the extent to which bowel has invaded the chest through the defect. Although prenatal ultrasonography can identify as many as 75% of the cases, physical examination remains essential for the rest. Bowel sounds heard in the chest and a flat or scaphoid abdomen are significant clues. The heart is usually displaced to the right. This abnormal development of the diaphragm can be associated with significant defects in one or both lungs.

Inspect the thoracic cage, noting its size and shape; measure the chest circumference, which in the healthy full-term infant is usually in the range of 30 to 36 cm, sometimes 2 to 3 cm smaller than the head circumference. Such a difference between the two increases with prematurity. An infant with intrauterine growth retardation will have a relatively smaller chest circumference compared to the head, while the infant of a poorly controlled diabetic mother will have a relatively larger chest circumference. As a rough measure, the distance between the nipples is about one-fourth the circumference of the chest.

Observe the nipples for symmetry in size and for the presence of swelling and discharge, as detailed in Chapter 14 (Breasts and Axillae). On occasion you will see supernumerary nipples, ordinarily not fully developed, along a line drawn caudad from the primary nipple. In white children, but not as often in blacks, they may be associated with a variety of congenital abnormalities.

The newborn's lung function is particularly susceptible to a number of environmental factors. The pattern of respirations will vary with room temperature, feeding, and sleep. In the first few hours after birth, the respiratory effort can be depressed by the passive transfer of drugs given to the mother before delivery.

Cyanosis of the hands and feet (acrocyanosis) is common in the newborn and can persist for several days in a cool environment without causing concern.

Count the respiratory rate for 1 minute. The expected rate varies from 40 to 60, although 80 respirations per minute is not uncommon. Babies delivered by cesarean section generally have a more rapid rate than babies delivered vaginally. If the room temperature is very warm or cool, a noticeable variation in the rate occurs, most often tachypnea but sometimes bradypnea.

Note the regularity of respiration. Babies are obligate nose breathers. It sometimes seems that they would prefer respiratory distress to opening their mouths to breathe. The more premature an infant at birth, the more likely some irregularity in the respiratory pattern will be present. *Periodic breathing*, a sequence of relatively vigorous respiratory efforts followed by apnea of as long as 10 to 15 seconds, is common. It is cause for concern if the apneic episodes tend to be prolonged and the baby becomes centrally cyanotic (i.e., cyanotic about the mouth, face, and torso). The persistence of periodic breathing episodes in preterm infants is relative to the gestational age of the baby, with the apneic period diminishing in frequency as the baby approaches term status. In the term infant, periodic breathing should wane a few hours after birth.

Coughing is rare in the newborn and should be considered a problem. Sneezing, on the other hand, is frequent and expected—it clears the nose.

Newborns rely primarily on the diaphragm for their respiratory effort, only gradually adding the intercostal muscles. Infants quite commonly also use the abdominal muscles.

If the chest expansion is asymmetric, suspect some compromise of the baby's ability to fill one of the lungs (e.g., with pneumothorax or diaphragmatic hernia) (Figure 12-24).

Palpate the rib cage and sternum, noting loss of symmetry, unusual masses, or crepitus. Crepitus around a fractured clavicle (with no evidence of pain) is common after a difficult forceps delivery. The newborn's xiphoid process is more mobile and prominent than that of the older child or adult. It has a sharp inferior tip that moves slightly back and forth under your finger.

Listen to the chest. If the baby is crying and restless, it pays to wait for a more quiet moment. Localization of breath sounds is difficult, particularly in the very small

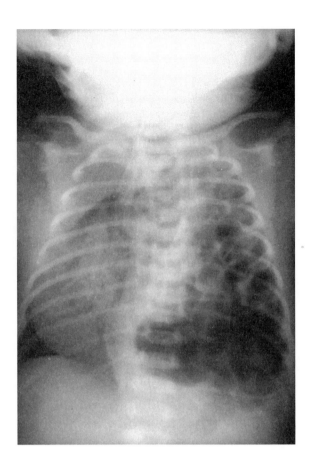

FIGURE 12-24
X-ray film showing diaphragmatic hernia.

chest of the preterm infant. Breath sounds are easily transmitted from one segment of the auscultatory area to another; therefore the absence of sounds in any given area may be difficult to detect. Sometimes it helps to listen to both sides of the chest simultaneously. Some neonatologists use a double-belled stethoscope for this purpose (Box 12-11).

It is not uncommon to hear crackles and rhonchi immediately after birth, since fetal fluid has not been completely cleared. Whenever auscultatory findings are asymmetric, a problem should be suspected as, for example, with the aspiration of meconium. Gurgling from the intestinal tract, slight movement, and mucus in the upper airway may all contribute to adventitious sounds, making evaluation difficult. If gastrointestinal gurgling sounds are persistently heard in the chest, one must suspect diaphragmatic hernia, but wide transmission of these sounds can sometimes be deceptive.

Stridor is a high-pitched, piercing sound, most often heard during inspiration. It is the result of an obstruction high in the respiratory tree. A compelling sound at any age, it cannot be dismissed as inconsequential, particularly when inspiration (I) may be three to four times longer than expiration (E), an I/E ratio of 3:1 or 4:1. If it is accompanied by a cough, hoarseness, and retraction, it signifies a serious problem in the trachea or larynx: a floppy epiglottis, congenital defects, croup, or an edematous response to an infection, allergen, smoke, chemicals, or aspirated foreign body. Infants who have a narrow tracheal lumen readily respond with stridor to its compression by a tumor, abscess, or double aortic arch. Retraction at the supraclavicular notch and contraction of the sternocleidomastoid muscles should be considered significant. Vigorous contraction, when the infant is supine and the head given suboccipital support, might make the head bob.

BOX 12-11 | Comparing Ventilation Regionally

It is sometimes helpful to compare two areas in the lungs fields simultaneously. This is accomplished with a stethoscope that is double-belled or double-diaphragmed and modified so that the chest pieces are connected as illustrated. This procedure is useful in emergent or other stressful situations, particularly with preterm infants. Atelectasis and pneumothorax, for example, can be differentiated and their sites localized.

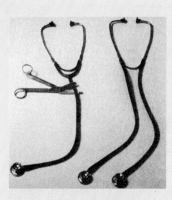

Two conventional single-tube stethoscopes are cut and reassembled into a double-headed stethoscope.

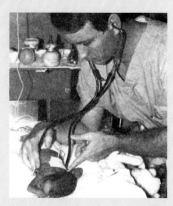

Lateral placement of the stethoscope heads allows the best appreciation of differences in breath sounds.

Courtesy Biomedical Photography, Division of Audiovisual Programs, The Johns Hopkins University School of Medicine.

Respiratory grunting is a mechanism by which the infant tries to expel trapped air or fetal lung fluid while trying to retain air and increase oxygen levels. When persistent, it is cause for concern. *Flaring of the alae nasi* is another indicator of respiratory distress at this, or any, age.

CHILDREN

Children use the thoracic (intercostal) musculature for respiration by the age of 6 or 7 years. In young children, obvious intercostal exertion (retractions) on breathing suggests some pulmonary or airway problem. Usual respiratory rates for children are suggested below (Figure 12-25). Sustained rates that exceed the indicated limits should suggest difficulty (Box 12-12):

AGE	RATE PER MINUTE
Newborn	30-80
1 year	20-40
3 years	20-30
6 years	16-22
10 years	16-20
17 years	12-20

If the "roundness" of the young child's chest persists past the second year of life, be concerned about the possibility of a chronic obstructive pulmonary problem such as cystic fibrosis. The persistence of a barrel chest at the age of 5 or 6 years can be ominous.

FIGURE 12-25

Mean values *(solid line)* ± 2 SD *(dashed lines)* of the usual respiratory rate at rest. There is no significant difference between the sexes, and the regression line represents data from both boys and girls. The respiratory rate decreases with age and shows a greater potential for variation during the first 2 years of life.

Data from Iliff, Lee, 1952. Redrawn from Chernick, 1990.

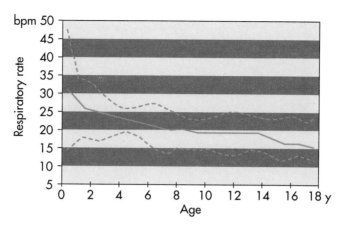

BOX 12-12   Assessment of Respiratory Distress

Important observations to be made of the respiratory effort include the following:

- Does a loss of synchrony between left and right occur during the respiratory effort? Is there a lag in movement of the chest on one side? Atelectasis? Diaphragmatic hernia?
- Is there stridor? Croup? Epiglottitis?
- Is there retraction at the suprasternal notch, intercostally, or at the xiphoid process?
- Do the nares dilate and flare with respiratory effort? Is pneumonia present?
- Is there an audible expiratory grunt? Is it audible with the stethoscope only or without the stethoscope? Is there lower airway obstruction? Focal atelectasis?
- Is there paradoxic breathing?

Seize the opportunity a crying child presents. A sob is frequently followed by a deep breath. The sob itself allows the evaluation of vocal resonance and the feel for tactile fremitus; use the whole hand, palm and fingers, gently. The crying child may pause occasionally, and the heart sounds may be heard. These pauses may be a bit prolonged as the breath is held, giving the chance to distinguish a murmur from a breath sound. In any event, your ear can suppress ambient noise to some extent, much as at a noisy restaurant, allowing you to concentrate on the matter at hand.

Children younger than 5 or 6 years may not be able to give enough of an expiration to satisfy you, particularly when you suspect subtle wheezing. Asking them to "blow out" your flashlight or to blow away a bit of tissue in your hand may help to bring out otherwise difficult to hear end expiratory sounds. It is also easier to hear the breath sounds when the child breathes more deeply after running up and down the hallway.

Children's chests are thinner and ordinarily more resonant than adults' chests; the intrathoracic sounds are easier to hear, and hyperresonance is common in young children. With either direct or indirect percussion, it is easy to miss the dullness of an underlying consolidation. If you sense some loss of resonance, give it as much importance as you would give frank dullness in the adolescent or adult.

Because of the thin chest wall, the breath sounds of the young may sound louder, harsher, and more bronchial than those of the adult. Bronchovesicular breath sounds may be heard throughout the chest.

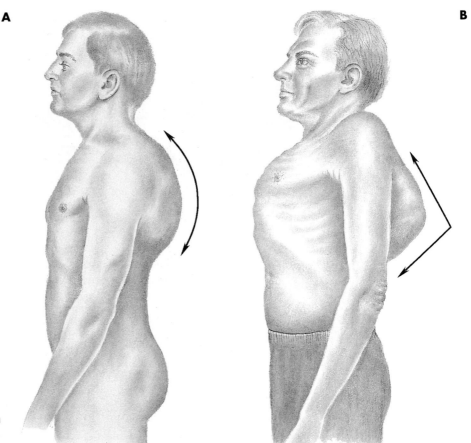

FIGURE 12-26
Pronounced dorsal curvature in older adult. **A**, Kyphosis. **B**, Gibbus (extreme kyphosis).

PREGNANT WOMEN	Pregnant women experience both structural and ventilatory changes. The costal angle of approximately 68 degrees before pregnancy increases to about 103 degrees in the third trimester. Dyspnea is common in pregnancy and is usually a result of normal physiologic changes. There is an increase of 100 to 200 ml in vital capacity, the amount of air that can be expelled at the normal rate of exhalation after a maximum inspiration. The tidal volume, the amount of air inhaled and exhaled during normal breathing, increases 40% along with minute ventilation. Overall, the pregnant woman increases her ventilation by breathing more deeply, not more frequently.
OLDER ADULTS	The examination procedure for older adults is the same as that for younger adults, although there may be variations in some expected findings. Chest expansion is often decreased. The patient may be less able to use the respiratory muscles because of muscle weakness, general physical disability, or a sedentary life-style. Calcification of rib articulations may also interfere with chest expansion, requiring use of accessory muscles. Bony prominences are marked, and there is loss of subcutaneous tissue. The dorsal curve of the thoracic spine is pronounced (kyphosis) with flattening of the lumbar curve (Figure 12-26). The anteroposterior diameter of the chest is increased in relation to the lateral diameter.

Older patients may have more difficulty breathing deeply and holding their breath than younger patients, and they may tire more quickly even when well. The pace and demands of examination should therefore be adapted to individual need.

Some older patients may display hyperresonance as a result of increased distensibility of the lungs. This finding must be evaluated in the context of the presence or absence of other symptoms.

SAMPLE DOCUMENTATION

Minimal increase in the AP diameter of chest, without kyphosis or other distortion. Thoracic expansion symmetric. Respirations rapid and somewhat labored, not accompanied by retractions or stridor. On palpation, trachea in midline without tug; no friction rubs or tenderness over the ribs or other bony prominences. Over the left base posteriorly tactile fremitus diminished; percussion note dull; on auscultation, crackles were heard which did not clear with cough; breath sounds diminished. Remainder of lung fields clear and free of adventitious sounds, with resonant percussion tones. Diaphragmatic excursion 3 cm bilaterally.

For additional sample documentation see Chapter 24, Recording Information.

SUMMARY OF EXAMINATION   **Chest and Lungs**

The following steps are performed with the patient sitting.

1. Inspect the chest, front and back, noting thoracic landmarks, for the following (pp. 363-365):
   - Size and shape (anteroposterior diameter compared with transverse diameter)
   - Symmetry
   - Color
   - Superficial venous patterns
   - Prominence of ribs
2. Evaluate respirations for the following (pp. 366-369):
   - Rate
   - Rhythm or pattern
3. Inspect chest movement with breathing for the following (p. 370):
   - Symmetry
   - Bulging
   - Use of accessory muscles
4. Note any audible sounds with respiration (i.e., stridor or wheezes) (p. 370).
5. Palpate the chest for the following (pp. 371-373):
   - Symmetry
   - Thoracic expansion
   - Pulsations
   - Sensations such as crepitus, grating vibrations
   - Tactile fremitus
6. Perform direct or indirect percussion on the chest, comparing sides, for the following (pp. 373-377):
   - Diaphragmatic excursion
   - Percussion tone intensity, pitch, duration, and quality
7. Auscultate the chest with the stethoscope diaphragm, from apex to base, comparing sides for the following (pp. 377-383):
   - Intensity, pitch, duration, and quality of expected breath sounds
   - Unexpected breath sounds (crackles, rhonchi, wheezes, friction rubs)
   - Vocal resonance

COMMON ABNORMALITIES

Physical findings associated with many common conditions are listed in Table 12-5.

TABLE 12-5 | **Physical Findings Associated with Common Respiratory Conditions**

Condition	Inspection	Palpation	Percussion	Auscultation
Asthma	Tachypnea Dyspnea	Tachycardia Diminished fremitus	Occasional hyper-resonance Occasional limited diaphragmatic descent; diaphragmatic level lower	Prolonged expiration Wheezes Diminished lung sounds
Atelectasis	Delayed and/or diminished chest wall movement, (respiratory lag), narrowed intercostal spaces on affected side Tachypnea	Diminished fremitus Apical cardiac impulse deviated ipsilaterally Trachea deviated ipsilaterally	Dullness over affected lung	In upper lobe, bronchial breathing, egophony, whispered pectoriloquy In lower lobe, diminished or absent breath sounds Wheezes, rhonchi, and crackles in varying amounts depending on extent of collapse
Bronchiectasis	Tachypnea Respiratory distress Hyperinflation	Few, if any, consistent findings	No unusual findings if there are no accompanying pulmonary disorders	A variety of crackles, usually coarse, and rhonchi, sometimes disappearing after cough
Bronchitis	Occasional tachypnea Occasional shallow breathing Often no deviation from expected findings	Tactile fremitus undiminished	Resonance	Breath sounds may be prolonged Occasional crackles Occasional expiratory wheezes
Chronic obstructive pulmonary disease	Respiratory distress Audible wheezing Cyanosis Distention of neck veins, peripheral edema, and—rarely—finger clubbing (in presence of right-sided heart failure)	Somewhat limited mobility of diaphragm Somewhat diminished vocal fremitus	Occasional hyper-resonance	Postpertussive rhonchi (sonorous wheezes) and sibilant wheezing Inspirational crackles (best heard with stethoscope held over open mouth) Breath sounds somewhat diminished
Emphysema	Tachypnea Deep breathing Pursed lips Barrel chest Thin, underweight	Apical impulse may not be felt Liver edge displaced downward Diminished fremitus	Hyperresonance Limited descent of diaphragm on inspiration Upper border of liver dullness pushed downward	Diminished breath and voice sounds with occasional prolonged expiration Diminished audibility of heart sounds Only occasional adventitious sounds
Pleural effusion and/or thickening	Diminished and delayed respiratory movement (lag) on affected side	Diminished and delayed respiratory movement on affected side Cardiac apical impulse shifted contralaterally Trachea shifted contralaterally Diminished fremitus Tachycardia	Dullness to flatness Hyperresonant note in area superior to effusion	Diminished to absent breath sounds Bronchophony, whispered pectoriloquy Egophony in area superior to effusion Occasional friction rub

TABLE 12-5	Physical Findings Associated with Common Respiratory Conditions—cont'd			
Condition	Inspection	Palpation	Percussion	Auscultation
Pneumonia with lobar consolidation	Tachypnea Shallow breathing Flaring of alae nasi Occasional cyanosis Limited movement at times on involved side; splinting	Increased fremitus in presence of consolidation Decreased fremitus in presence of a concomitant empyema or pleural effusion Tachycardia	Dullness if consolidation is great	A variety of crackles and occasional rhonchi Bronchial breath sounds Egophony, bronchophony, whispered pectoriloquy
Pneumothorax	Tachypnea Cyanosis Respiratory distress Bulging intercostal spaces Respiratory lag on affected side Tracheal deviation	Diminished to absent fremitus Cardiac apical impulse, trachea, and mediastinum shifted contralaterally Diminished to absent tactile fremitus Tachycardia	Hyperresonance	Diminished to absent breath sounds Succussion splash audible if air and fluid mix Sternal and precordial clicks and crackling (Hamman sign) if air underlies that area Diminished to absent whispered voice sounds

Physical findings will vary in intensity depending on the severity of the underlying problem and on occasion may not be present in the early stages.

ASTHMA (REACTIVE AIRWAY DISEASE)

Asthma is a chronic obstructive pulmonary disease (COPD) characterized by airway inflammation, generally resulting from airway hyperreactivity triggered by allergens, anxiety, upper respiratory infections, cigarette smoke or other environmental "poisons," or exercise. You might say that the patient's airway is "twitchy." The reaction may be aggravated by cold air and is less likely to be triggered in warm, humid air. The result is mucosal edema, increased secretions, and bronchoconstriction. Airway resistance increases and respiratory flow is impeded.

The episodes are characterized by paroxysmal dyspnea, tachypnea, cough, wheezing on expiration and inspiration, and, as airway resistance increases, more prolonged expiration. Chest pain is not infrequent and, with it, a feeling of chest tightening. The episodes may last for just minutes or hours, or they may be prolonged over days. Unlike other forms of COPD in older adults, the obstruction of asthma is reversible either spontaneously or in response to therapy. Between episodes, the patient may be asymptomatic.

Certainly, asthma can vary in intensity, even from moment to moment and often from one area of the lungs to another, but it is always acutely anxiety provoking. It is an increasingly common disorder that often begins in childhood and can be life-threatening if it is not treated promptly and adequately. A wheezing patient with generalized pulmonary findings may have asthma or a viral infection, but rarely, if ever, a bacterial infection.

ATELECTASIS

Atelectasis is the incomplete expansion of the lung at birth or the collapse of the lung at any age (Figure 12-27). Collapse can be caused by compression from outside (exudates, tumors) or resorption of gas from the alveoli in the presence of complete internal obstruction (loss of elastic recoil of the lung for any reason—thoracic or abdominal surgery, plugging, exudates, foreign body). The affected area of the lung is airless. The overall effect is to dampen or mute the sounds in the involved area.

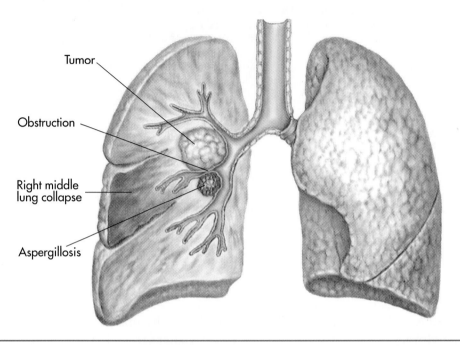

FIGURE 12-27
Atelectasis.
Modified from Wilson, Thompson, 1990.

BRONCHITIS

Bronchitis is an inflammation of the mucous membranes of the bronchial tubes. Acute bronchitis may be more or less severe than chronic bronchitis, and it may be accompanied by fever and chest pain (Figure 12-28). Chronic bronchitis has a wide variety of causes and physical manifestations, including excessive secretion of mucus in the bronchial tree. In either type, the initial stimulus is irritation by an internal or external noxious influence. Either an acute or chronic condition can show varying degrees of involvement, with the possibility of obstructive phenomena and even atelectasis, but bronchitis is most often quite mild.

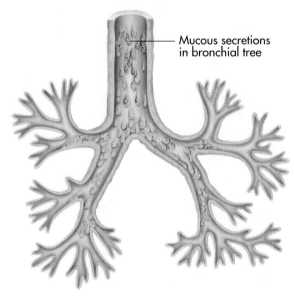

FIGURE 12-28
Acute bronchitis.
From Wilson, Thompson, 1990.

PLEURISY

Pleurisy is an inflammatory process involving the visceral and parietal pleura, often the result of pulmonary infections, bacterial or viral, and sometimes associated with neoplasm or asbestosis. The onset is usually sudden and the typical pleuritic pain is acute. The pleura becomes "dry," actually edematous and fibrinous, making breathing difficult (Figure 12-29). The resultant "rubbing" can be felt and heard. The respirations are rapid and shallow, with diminished breath sounds. The area involved can vary considerably. If it is close to the diaphragm, the pain can be referred to the ipsilateral shoulder. As the process continues, and if pleural effusion results, the pain and rub may disappear; but the fever, tachypnea, and malaise will not.

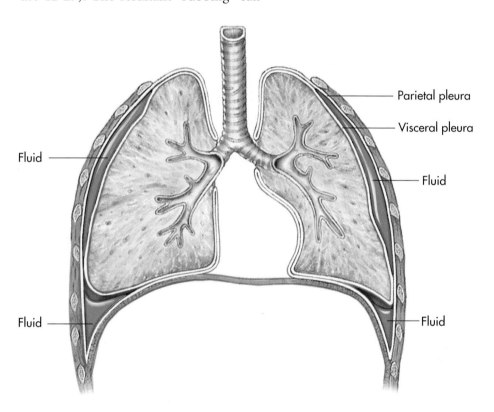

Parietal pleura

Visceral pleura

Fluid

Fluid

Fluid

Fluid

FIGURE 12-29
Pleurisy.
Modified from Wilson, Thompson, 1990.

PLEURAL EFFUSION

Excessive nonpurulent fluid in the pleural space can result in permanent fibrotic thickening. The sources of fluid vary; infection, neoplasm, and trauma are all possible causes. The extent of embarrassment varies with the amount of fluid, and the degree of fibrosis varies with the chronicity of the condition. The findings vary with severity and also with the position of the patient. Fluid is mobile; it will gravitate to the most dependent position. In the affected areas the breath sounds are muted (Figure 12-30).

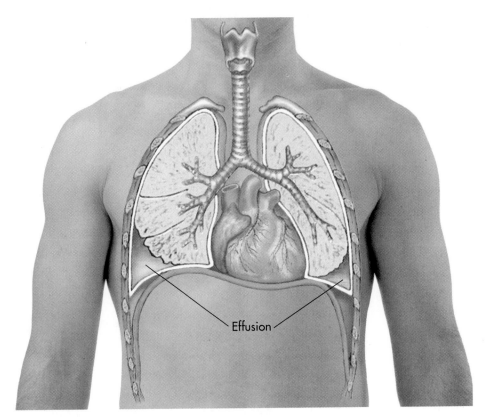

FIGURE 12-30
Pleural effusion.
Modified from Wilson, Thompson, 1990.

EMPYEMA

Empyema is said to occur when fluid collected in the pleural spaces is a purulent exudate, arising most commonly from adjacent infected, sometimes traumatized, tissues (Figure 12-31). It may be complicated by pneumonia, a penetrating injury, simultaneous pneumothorax, or bronchopleural fistulae. Breath sounds are distant or absent in the affected area, the percussion note is dull, vocal fremitus is absent, and the patient is often febrile and tachypneic and appears ill.

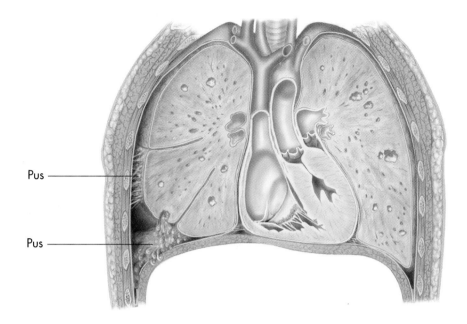

Pus

Pus

FIGURE 12-31
Empyema.
Modified from Wilson, Thompson, 1990.

LUNG ABSCESS

A lung abscess is a well-defined, circumscribed mass defined by inflammation, suppuration, and subsequent central necrosis (Figure 12-32). It may at first appear to be a localized pneumonia, and it may elude diagnosis for a long time unless it invades a bronchus so that resulting drainage will allow detection of an air-fluid level. The causes are many. Aspiration of food or infected material from upper respiratory or dental sources of infection are perhaps most common, given an inoculum of sufficient size in a patient whose immunologic defenses may be down for any reason. The percussion note is dull and the breath sounds distant or absent over the affected area. There may be a pleural friction rub, and cough may produce a purulent, foul-smelling sputum. The patient is usually obviously ill and febrile, sometimes tachypneic. The breath commonly has a foul odor.

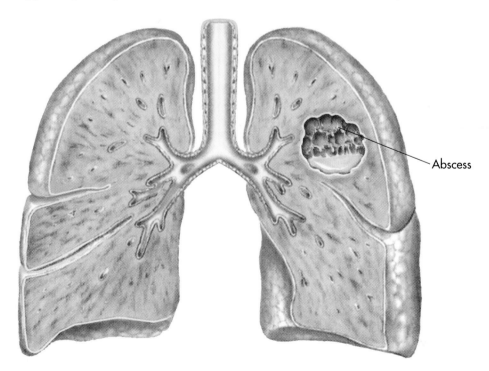

Abscess

FIGURE 12-32
Lung abscess.
Modified from Wilson, Thompson, 1990.

PNEUMONIA

Pneumonia is an inflammatory response of the bronchioles and alveolar spaces to an infective agent (bacterial, fungal, or viral) (Figure 12-33). Exudates lead to lung consolidation, resulting in dyspnea, tachypnea, and crackles. Diminished breath sounds and dullness to percussion occur over the area of consolidation.

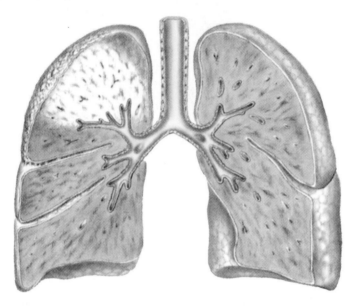

FIGURE 12-33

Lobar pneumonia (right upper lobe).

Modified from Wilson, Thompson, 1990.

PNEUMOCYSTIS CARINII PNEUMONIA (PCP)

Pneumocystis carinii pneumonia is an otherwise rare disease that occurs with disturbing frequency in persons with any acquired or congenital immunodeficiency, not only those with the HIV. When PCP is suspected, the pneumocysts may be seen with special stains of sputum or respiratory tissue. There are no findings on physical examination to distinguish this condition from a variety of other pneumonic conditions.

INFLUENZA

A host of viruses, many frequently mutating, some as yet undiscovered or uncharacterized, cause this acute, generalized, febrile illness. In varying degree, it is characterized by cough, fever, malaise, headache, and the coryza and mild sore throat typical of the common cold. When it is mild, it may seem to be just a cold. However, the aged, the very young, and the chronically ill are particularly susceptible; in these persons it may prove fatal, although yearly immunization is often preventive if it is given. The entire respiratory tract may be overwhelmed by interstitial inflammation and necrosis extending throughout the bronchiolar and alveolar tissue (Figure 12-34). There may be a variety of respiratory findings: crackles, rhonchi, and tachypnea, as well as cough (generally nonproductive) and substernal pain.

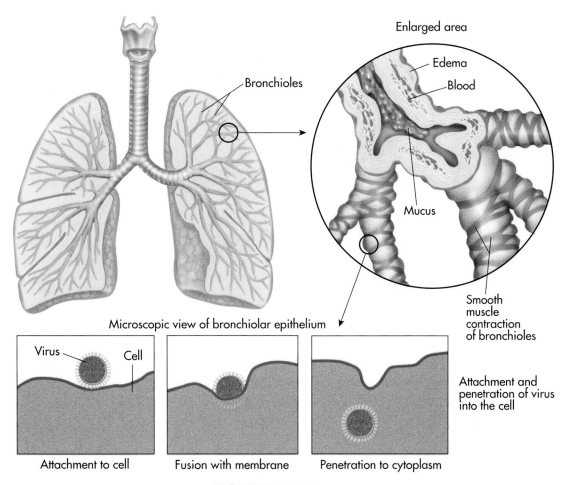

FIGURE 12-34
Influenza.
Modified from Wilson, Thompson, 1990.

TUBERCULOSIS

Tuberculosis is a chronic infectious disease that most often begins in the lung but may then have widespread manifestations in many organs and systems. Most often, at the start, the tubercle bacillus (usually, *Mycobacterium tuberculosis;* occasionally, *M. bovis* or an atypical mycobacterium) is inhaled from the airborne moisture of the coughs and sneezes of infected persons and given the opportunity to settle in the furthest reaches of the lung (Figure 12-35). There is then a latent period as the organism entrenches itself. The patient may not be ill, and only a bit of lung and some regional lymph nodes may be involved. There is always the potential for a post-primary spread locally or throughout the body. While treatment for tuberculosis has been effective in recent decades, the compromise caused by the HIV and the increasing incidence of HIV infection have been paralleled by an increasing incidence of tuberculosis and of mycobacteria that are resistant to treatment, in part because of frequent failure to comply with drug regimens.

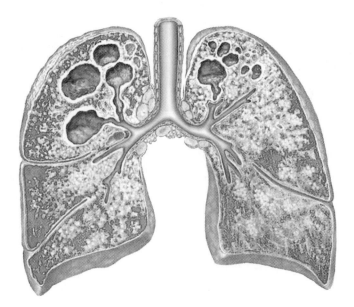

FIGURE 12-35
Tuberculosis.
Modified from Wilson, Thompson, 1990.

PNEUMOTHORAX

The presence of air or gas in the pleural cavity may be the result of trauma or may occur spontaneously, perhaps because of rupture of a congenital bleb. The air in the pleural space may not communicate with that in the lung, but in tension pneumothorax, air leaks continually into the pleural space, becoming trapped on expiration, resulting in increasing pressure in the pleural space (Figure 12-36). Minimal collections of air without the presence of associated inflammatory lesions may easily escape detection at first. Larger collections cause varying degrees of the possible findings. Overall, the breath sounds are distant but the percussion note may boom.

A positive "coin click" can help. Place a coin over the suspicious area in the chest (e.g., posteriorly) and, while listening to the opposite side (anteriorly), have someone strike the coin with the edge of another. A clear click will be heard only in the event of a pronounced pneumothorax.

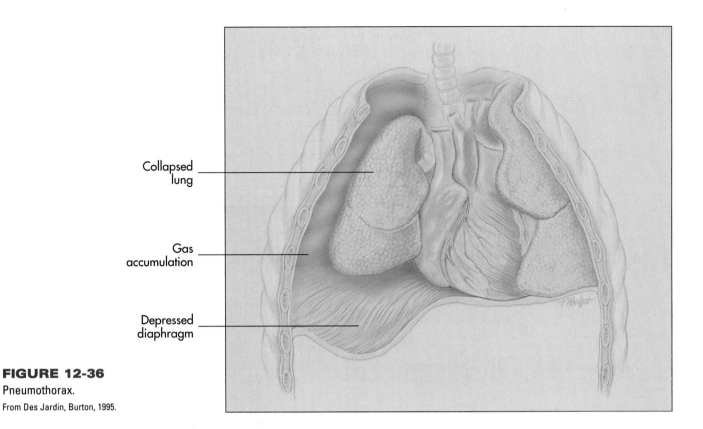

FIGURE 12-36
Pneumothorax.
From Des Jardin, Burton, 1995.

Collapsed lung

Gas accumulation

Depressed diaphragm

HEMOTHORAX

The presence of blood in the pleural cavity, *hemothorax* (Figure 12-37), may be the result, for example, of trauma or invasive medical procedures (thoracentesis, pleural biopsy). Sometimes air may be present with the blood; this is called a *hemopneumothorax.* If there is no air, or if blood predominates, the breath sounds will be distant or absent, the percussion note will be dull, and the "coin click" will be absent.

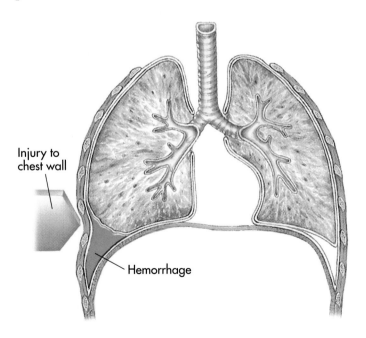

Injury to chest wall

Hemorrhage

FIGURE 12-37
Hemothorax.
Modified from Wilson, Thompson, 1990.

LUNG CANCER

Lung cancer generally refers to broncho-genic carcinoma, a malignant tumor that evolves from bronchial epithelial structures. Etiologic agents include tobacco smoke, asbestos, ionizing radiation, and other inhaled chemicals and noxious agents. It may cause cough, wheezing, a variety of patterns of emphysema and at-electasis, pneumonitis, and hemoptysis. The extent of the tumor and the patterns of its invasion and metastasis are often determined by its histologic nature (Figure 12-38). There are many other less frequent examples of uncontrolled growth primary in the lung, and numerous examples of metastasis from distant sites.

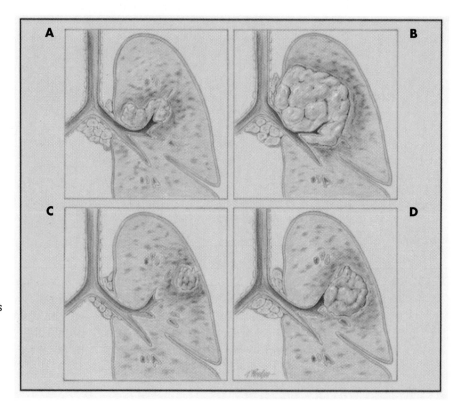

FIGURE 12-38
Cancer of the lung. **A,** Squamous (epidermoid) cell carcinoma. **B,** Small cell (oat cell) carcinoma. **C,** Adenocarcinoma. **D,** Large cell carcinoma.

From Des Jardin, Burton, 1995.

COR PULMONALE

Cor pulmonale is an acute or chronic condition involving right-sided heart failure. In the acute phase, the right side of the heart is dilated and fails, most often as a direct result of pulmonary embolism. In chronic cor pulmonale a chronic, massive disease of the lungs causes gradual obstruction that produces a more gradual hypertrophy of the right ventricle, increasing stress, and ultimate heart failure (Figure 12-39). An isolated failure of the right side of the heart is rare except in the circumstance of pulmonary obstruction caused by emboli, primary pulmonary hypertension, or extensive infection and noxious involvement of the lung.

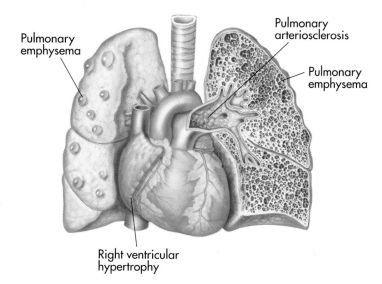

FIGURE 12-39
Cor pulmonale. Notice extensive pulmonary emphysema, pulmonary arteriosclerosis, and right ventricular hypertrophy.
Modified from Wilson, Thompson, 1990.

PULMONARY HYPERTENSION

Pulmonary hypertension is defined as a pulmonary artery pressure greater than 30/15 mm Hg. Elevation must always be recognized as indicative of a disease process, such as pulmonary artery embolism or thrombosis, failure of the left side of the heart, or extensive parenchymal disease of the lung. When pulmonary hypertension is chronic, it clearly adds to the stress imposed on the heart and the coronary vasculature, compounding the initial problem. The patient with pulmonary hypertension may have only vague complaints of weakness, dyspnea, or fatigue. However, severe disease produces intense fatigue, precordial pain, and occasionally, fainting.

CYSTIC FIBROSIS

Cystic fibrosis is an autosomal recessive disorder of exocrine glands involving the lungs, pancreas, and sweat glands. The Scottish and English are particularly at risk. Salt loss in sweat is distinctive. A parent may have noticed that the child's skin tastes unusually salty. Heavy secretions of abnormally thick mucus cause progressive clogging of the bronchi and bronchioles, leading to frequent and progressive pulmonary infections (Figure 12-40). Initially, areas of hyperinflation and atelectasis are evident. As pulmonary dysfunction progresses, the tolerance for exercise diminishes and pulmonary hypertension and cor pulmonale often occur. Recent advances in treatment have extended life expectancy into adulthood.

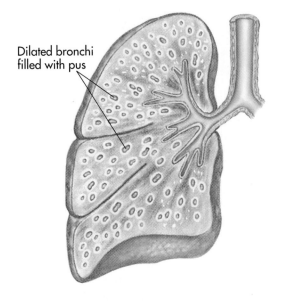

Dilated bronchi filled with pus

FIGURE 12-40
Cystic fibrosis.
Modified from Wilson, Thompson, 1990.

EPIGLOTTITIS

Epiglottitis is an acute, life-threatening disease almost always caused by *Haemophilus influenzae* type B. It begins suddenly and progresses rapidly, often to full obstruction of the airway (Figure 12-41, *A*) resulting in death. It may occur at any age but occurs most often in children between the ages of 3 and 7. The child sits straight up with neck extended and head held forward, appears very anxious and ill, is unable to swallow, and is drooling from an open mouth; cough is not common. The fever may be high. The epiglottis appears beefy red. It is vital to note that *no attempt* should be made to visualize the epiglottis and that any suspicion of epiglottitis should be treated as a medical emergency. Immediate attention is required with the help of an anesthesiologist and/or otolaryngologist and radiologist in an emergency department. The tentative diagnosis should be based on the history and clinical appearance of the child before physical examination. Any attempt to visualize the epiglottis without skilled assistance and appropriate equipment for establishing an artificial airway is not justified. Direct examination of the throat, with or without a tongue blade, is to be avoided. Recently, appropriate immunization has reduced the incidence of this disease significantly but not entirely.

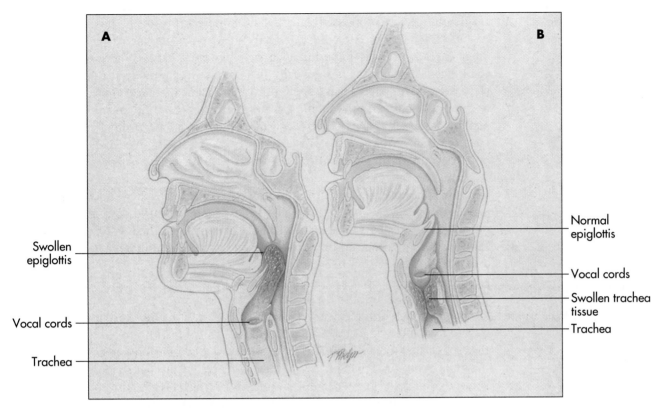

FIGURE 12-41
Croup syndrome. **A,** Acute epiglottitis. **B,** Laryngotracheobronchitis.
From Des Jardins, Burton, 1995.

CROUP

Croup is a syndrome that generally results from infection with a variety of viral agents, particularly the parainfluenza viruses. It occurs most often in very young children, generally from about 1½ to 3 years of age. Boys are more frequently affected than girls, and for reasons unknown, some children are prone to recurrent episodes. It is not unusual to have an episode begin in the evening, often after the child has gone to sleep. The child awakens suddenly, often very frightened, with a harsh stridorous cough, somewhat like the bark of a seal. Labored breathing, retraction, and inspiratory stridor are characteristic. Fever does not always accompany croup. The inflammation is subglottic and may involve areas beyond the larynx (laryngotracheobronchitis) (Figure 12-41, *B*). Children with croup may be frightened, but they do not have the toxic, drooling facies of persons with epiglottitis. An aspirated foreign body may mimic croup on occasion.

TRACHEOMALACIA

"Noisy breathing" in infancy, sometimes described as wheezing, is often inspiratory stridor. It can frequently be attributed to a floppiness of the trachea or airway, a lack of rigidity termed tracheomalacia, which causes the trachea to change in response to the varying pressures of inspiration and expiration. Although tracheomalacia tends to be benign and self-limited with increasing age, it is necessary to eliminate the possibility of fixed lesions, such as a vascular lesion, tracheal stenosis, or even a foreign body. At times, the larynx may also have the same "yielding" characteristic (*laryngomalacia;* if the entire large airway is involved, the condition is called *laryngotracheomalacia*).

| BRONCHIOLITIS | Bronchiolitis occurs most frequently in infants less than 6 months old. The principal characteristic is hyperinflation of the lungs. The cause is viral, usually the respiratory syncytial virus. Expiration becomes difficult, and the infant appears anxious and tachypneic. Generalized retraction and perioral cyanosis are common. Because of lung hyperinflation, the | anteroposterior diameter of the thoracic cage may be increased and percussion hyperresonant. Wheezing may or may not be apparent. In the presence of severe tachypnea, air exchange is poor and the breaths are rapid and short, with the expiratory phase prolonged. Crackles may or may not be heard. The abdomen appears distended from swallowed air. |
| SLIPPING RIB SYNDROME | Slipping rib syndrome is the result of injury to the costal cartilages of the eighth, ninth, and tenth ribs. The associated pain can be sharp at times and continuously dull. Eating, exercise, and deep breathing | can aggravate the pain. The diagnosis is suggested by the demonstration of tenderness over the involved cartilages. Cartilage excision may be necessary. |

OLDER ADULTS

The ability of the lungs to do their work can be quantified. Essentially, the need is to know how much of the air they exchange is of functional use and how easily it can be moved to and fro. The vital capacity (VC) is a valuable indicator of the amount of air that is expelled after the patient takes a maximal inspiration and follows that with a maximal expiration. The physical dimensions of the chest cage, posture, gender (the volume of males is greater than that of females), age, height, and the degree of physical fitness are among the variables that influence VC. When VC is impaired, a wide variety of disease processes can be suspect (e.g., loss of lung tissue, airway obstruction, loss of muscle strength, chest deformity, pneumothorax). The vital capacity cannot differentiate among these. The peak expiratory flow rate (PEFR), a measure of the maximum flow of air that can be achieved during a forced expiratory maneuver, is a useful surrogate for the VC in children as well as adults. It provides an easily reproducible number obtained by using inexpensive, hand-held peak flow meters. The reliability of the PEFR is limited by the patient's ability to cooperate and is useful as a measure only for large airway function; however, it does suggest the extent of impairment and it can be used as a guide to measure the success (or lack of it) of treatment. It is best to compare a patient's PEFR to a previous "personal best," if possible, rather than to an expected predicted value attainable from a nomogram geared to the patient's height and based on the generalization that lung volume parallels height.

| CHRONIC OBSTRUCTIVE PULMONARY DISEASE (COPD) | COPD is a nonspecific designation that includes a group of respiratory problems in which coughs, chronic and frequently excessive sputum production, and dyspnea are prominent features. Ultimately, an irreversible expiratory airflow obstruction occurs. Chronic bronchitis, emphysema (Figure 12-42), asthmatic bronchitis, bronchiectasis, and even cystic fibrosis may be included in that group. One need not be elderly, of course, to have one of these problems. Most patients, however, are certainly not young, and most patients have been smokers. A careful his- | tory will reveal a legacy of episodes of coughs and sputum and limited tolerance for exercise. The chest may be barrel shaped, and scattered crackles or wheezes may be heard. Airway obstruction can be evaluated during forced maximal expiration. Listen over the trachea with the diaphragm of your stethoscope as the patient inhales to the limit and then breathes out as quickly as possible through an open mouth. If this forced expiration time is longer than 4 to 5 seconds, you should suspect airway obstruction. |

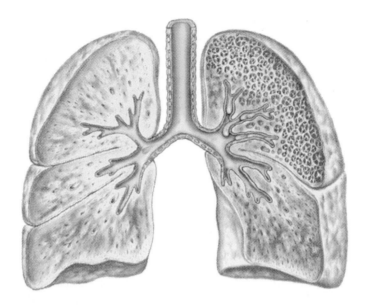

FIGURE 12-42

Chronic obstructive pulmonary disease with lobar emphysema.

Modified from Wilson, Thompson, 1990.

EMPHYSEMA

Emphysema, perhaps the most severe chronic obstructive pulmonary disorder, is a condition in which air may take over and dominate a space in a way that disrupts function. The air spaces beyond the terminal bronchioles dilate, rupturing alveolar walls, permanently destroying them, reducing their number, and permanently hyperinflating the lung. Alveolar gas is trapped, essentially in expiration, and gas exchange is seriously compromised. Chronic bronchitis is the frequent precursor. Involutionary changes as the lungs lose elasticity because of aging, smoking, or impairment of the defenses mediated by a-antitrypsin are also contributors. The overinflated lungs tend to be hyperresonant on percussion. Further expansion on inspiration is limited; occasionally there is a prolonged expiratory effort, longer than 4 or 5 seconds, to expel air. Dyspnea is common even at rest. Cough is infrequent without much production of sputum. The patient is often thin and barrel-chested.

BRONCHIECTASIS

Chronic dilation of the bronchi or bronchioles is caused by repeated pulmonary infections and bronchial obstruction (Figure 12-43). The dilations may involve the tube uniformly (cylindric) or irregularly (saccular); at the terminal ends, the enlargement may be bulbous. Bronchiectasis may lead to malfunction of bronchial muscle tone and loss of elasticity. The extent of findings on physical examination is governed by the degree of "wetness." The cough and expectoration are most often the major clues. Kartagener syndrome, an autosomal recessive condition, is characterized by bronchiectasis, sinusitis, dextrocardia, and male infertility.

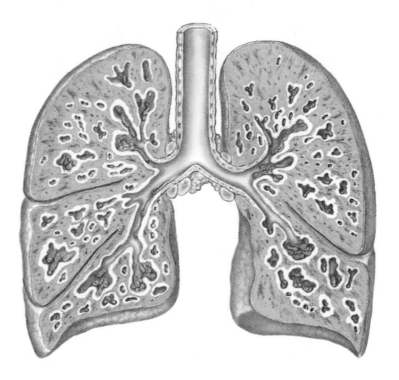

FIGURE 12-43
Bronchiectasis.
Modified from Wilson, Thompson, 1990.

CHRONIC BRONCHITIS

This condition, characterized by excessive mucus and cough, may occur at any age but is primarily a problem of older and elderly patients. The mucus of the bronchi is chronically inflamed, recurrent bacterial infections are common, dyspnea may be present although not severe, and cough and sputum are impressive. Smoking is prominent in the history; many of these patients are emphysematous. These conditions are all clearly correlated.

http://www1.mosby.com/physexam_seidel

CHAPTER 13

HEART AND BLOOD VESSELS

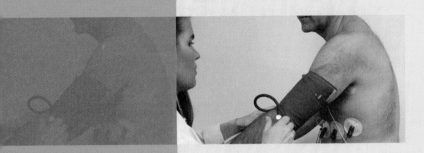

ANATOMY AND PHYSIOLOGY

HEART

The heart lies in the mediastinum, to the left of the midline, just above the diaphragm, and is cradled between the medial and lower borders of the lungs. It is positioned behind the sternum and the contiguous parts of the third to the sixth costal cartilages. The area of the chest overlying the heart is the precordium. Because of the heart's conelike shape, the broader upper portion is called the base, and the narrower lower tip of the heart is the apex (Figure 13-1).

The position of the heart can vary considerably, depending on body build, configuration of the chest, and level of the diaphragm. In a tall, slender person, the heart tends to hang more vertically and to be positioned more centrally. With increasing stockiness and shortness, it tends to lie more to the left and more horizontally. On occasion, the heart may be positioned to the right, either rotated or displaced, or as a complete mirror image of the expected; such a circumstance is called *dextrocardia*. If the heart and stomach are placed to the right and the liver to the left, the situation is termed *situs inversus*.

Structure

The pericardium is a tough, double-walled, fibrous sac encasing and protecting the heart. Several cubic centimeters of fluid are present between the inner and outer layers of the pericardium, providing for easy, low-friction movement (Figure 13-2).

The epicardium, the thin outermost muscle layer, covers the surface of the heart and extends to the great vessels. The myocardium, the thick muscular middle layer, is responsible for the pumping action of the heart. The endocardium, the innermost layer, lines the inner chambers of the heart and covers the heart valves and the small muscles associated with the opening and closing of these valves (Figure 13-3).

The heart is divided into four chambers. The two top chambers are the right and left atria (or auricles, because of their earlike shape), and the bottom chambers are the right and left ventricles. The left atrium and left ventricle together are referred to as the left heart; the right atrium and right ventricle together are referred to as the right heart. The left heart and right heart are divided by a blood-tight partition called the cardiac septum.

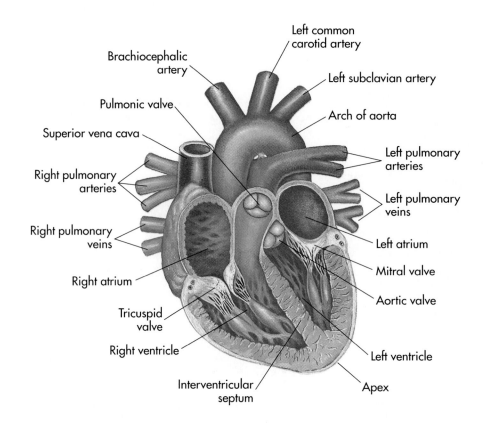

FIGURE 13-1

Frontal section of the heart.

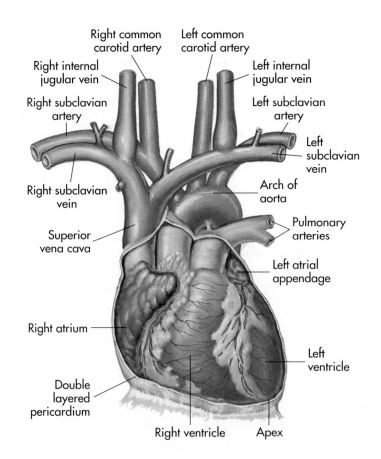

FIGURE 13-2

Heart within the pericardium.

Modified from Canobbio, 1990.

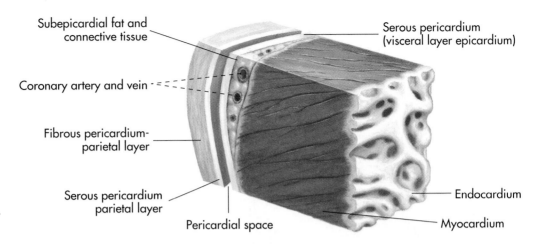

Subepicardial fat and connective tissue

Serous pericardium (visceral layer epicardium)

Coronary artery and vein

Fibrous pericardium-parietal layer

Serous pericardium parietal layer

Pericardial space

Endocardium

Myocardium

FIGURE 13-3
Cross section of cardiac muscle.
From Canobbio, 1990.

The atria are small, thin-walled structures that act primarily as a reservoir for the blood returning to the heart from the veins throughout the body. The ventricles are large, thick-walled chambers that pump blood to the lungs and throughout the body. The right and left ventricles together form the primary muscle mass of the heart.

Most of the anterior surface of the heart is formed by the right ventricle. The left ventricle is positioned behind the right but extends anteriorly, forming the left border of the heart. Its contraction and thrust are responsible for the apical impulse usually felt in the fifth left intercostal space at the midclavicular line. The right atrium lies above and slightly to the right of the right ventricle, participating in the formation of the right border of the heart. The left atrium is above the left ventricle, forming the more posterior aspect of the heart. The heart is, in effect, turned ventrally on its axis, putting its right side more forward. The adult heart is about 12 cm long, 8 cm wide at the widest point, and 6 cm in its anteroposterior diameter (Figure 13-4).

The four chambers of the heart are connected by two sets of valves: the atrioventricular and semilunar valves. In the fully formed heart that is free of defect, these are the only intracardiac pathways. They permit the flow of blood in only one direction (Figure 13-5).

The atrioventricular valves, situated between the atria and the ventricles, include the tricuspid and mitral valves. The tricuspid valve, which has three cusps or leaflets, separates the right atrium from the right ventricle. The mitral valve, which has two cusps, separates the left atrium from the left ventricle. When the atria contract, the atrioventricular valves open, allowing blood to flow into the ventricles. When the ventricles contract, these valves snap shut, preventing blood from flowing back into the atria.

The two semilunar valves each have three cusps. The pulmonic valve separates the right ventricle from the pulmonary artery. The aortic valve lies between the left ventricle and the aorta. Contraction of the ventricles opens the semilunar valves, causing blood to rush into the pulmonary artery and aorta. When the ventricles relax, the valves close, shutting off any backward flow into the ventricles.

The arteries and veins leading from and to the heart are called the *great vessels*. They circulate blood to and from the body and the lungs. The great vessels, located in a cluster at the base of the heart, include the aorta, superior and inferior venae cavae, pulmonary arteries, and pulmonary veins (Figure 13-6). The aorta carries oxygenated blood out of the left ventricle to the body. The superior and inferior venae cavae carry blood from the upper and lower body, respectively, to the right atrium. The pulmonary artery, which leaves the right ventricle and bifurcates almost immediately into its right and left branches, carries blood to the lungs. The pulmonary veins return oxygenated blood from the lungs to the left atrium.

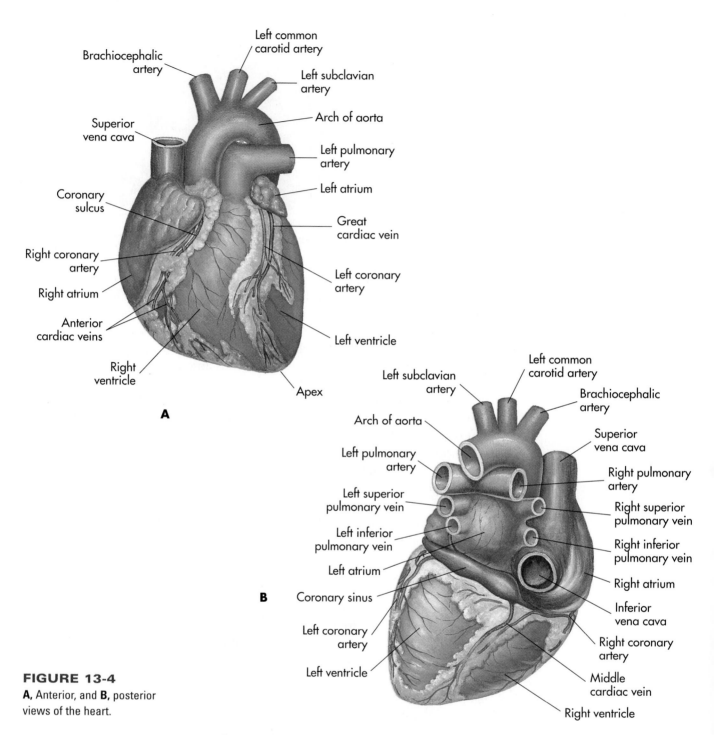

FIGURE 13-4
A, Anterior, and **B,** posterior views of the heart.

Cardiac Cycle

The muscular heart contracts and relaxes rhythmically to ensure proper circulation, a process that creates two phases in the cardiac cycle. During systole the ventricles contract, ejecting blood from the left ventricle into the aorta and from the right ventricle into the pulmonary artery. During diastole the ventricles relax and the atria contract, moving blood from the atria to the ventricles (Figure 13-7). The volume of blood and the pressure under which it is returned to the heart vary with the degree of body activity, for example, with exercise or fever. As the ventricles fill, each must respond to the force under which filling takes place.

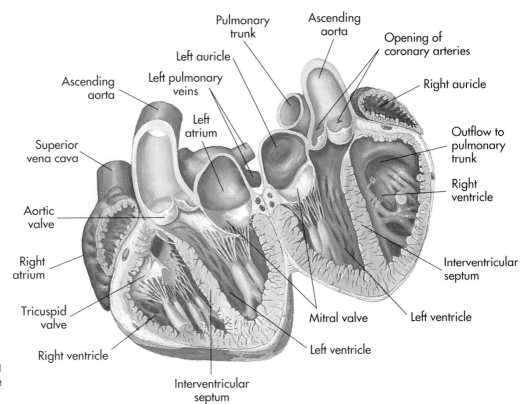

FIGURE 13-5
Anterior cross section showing the valves and chambers of the heart.

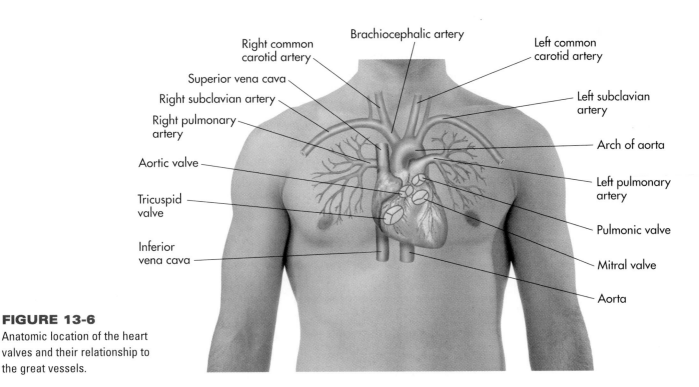

FIGURE 13-6
Anatomic location of the heart valves and their relationship to the great vessels.

A
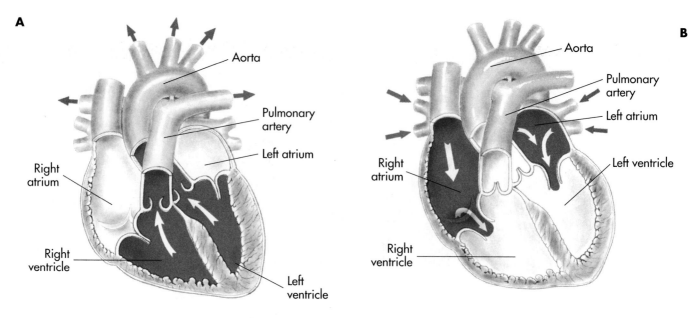
B

FIGURE 13-7
Blood flow. **A,** During systole. **B,** During diastole.
From Canobbio, 1990.

As systole begins, ventricular contraction raises the pressure in the ventricles and forces the mitral and tricuspid valves closed, preventing backflow. This valve closure produces the first heart sound (S_1), the characteristic "lubb." The intraventricular pressure rises until it exceeds that in the aorta and pulmonary artery. Then the aortic and pulmonic valves are forced open, and ejection of blood into the arteries begins. Valve opening is usually a silent event (Figure 13-8).

When the ventricles are almost empty, the pressure in the ventricles falls below that in the aorta and pulmonary artery, allowing the aortic and pulmonic valves to close. Closure of these valves causes the second heart sound (S_2), "dubb," which has two components: A_2 is produced by aortic valve closure, and P_2 is produced by pulmonic valve closure. As ventricular pressure falls below atrial pressure, the mitral and tricuspid valves open to allow the blood collected in the atria to refill the relaxed ventricles. Diastole is a relatively passive interval until ventricular filling is almost complete. This filling sometimes produces a third heart sound (S_3). Then the atria contract to ensure the ejection of any remaining blood. This can sometimes be heard as a fourth heart sound (S_4). The cycle begins anew, with ventricular contraction and atrial refilling occurring at about the same time. The heart fulfills this impressive demand without resting and while adjusting constantly to the variable demands of work, rest, illness, and digestion.

This discussion describes the events of the cardiac cycle as virtually simultaneous on both sides of the heart. Actually, however, the pressures in the right ventricle, right atrium, and pulmonary artery are lower than those on the left side of the heart; and the same events occur slightly later on the right side than on the left. The effect is that heart sounds sometimes have two distinct components, the first produced by the left side and the second by the right side. For example, the aortic valve closes slightly before the pulmonic, so that S_2 is often heard as two distinct components, referred to as "split S_2."

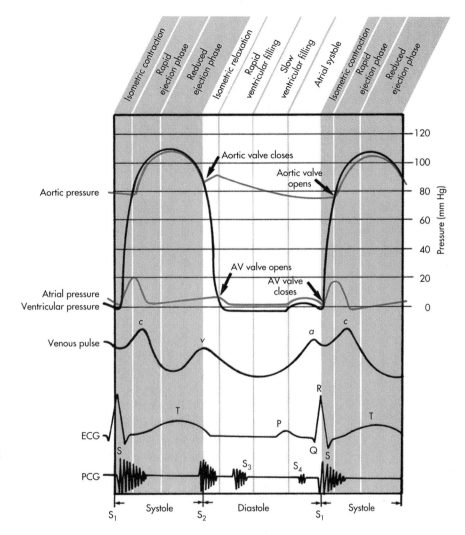

FIGURE 13-8

Events of cardiac cycle, showing venous pressure waves, ECG, and heart sounds in systole and diastole.

Modified from Guzzetta, Dossey, 1992.

Closure of the heart valves during the cardiac cycle produces heart sounds in rapid succession. The simultaneous muscular tension and flow of blood give "body" to the sounds. Although the valves are anatomically close to each other, their sounds are best heard in an area away from the anatomic site (in the direction of blood flow) (see Figure 13-21, p. 434).

Electrical Activity

The heart is, in a sense, autonomous. An intrinsic electrical conduction system enables it to contract within itself, free of any stimulus from elsewhere in the body. The electrical system coordinates the sequence of muscular contractions that take place during the cardiac cycle. An electrical current or impulse stimulates each myocardial contraction. The impulse originates in and is paced by the sinoatrial node (SA node), located in the wall of the right atrium. The impulse then travels through both atria to the atrioventricular node (AV node), located in the atrial septum. In the AV node the impulse is slightly delayed but then passes down the bundle of His to the Purkinje fibers in the ventricular myocardium. Ventricular contraction is initiated at the apex and proceeds toward the base of the heart (Figure 13-9).

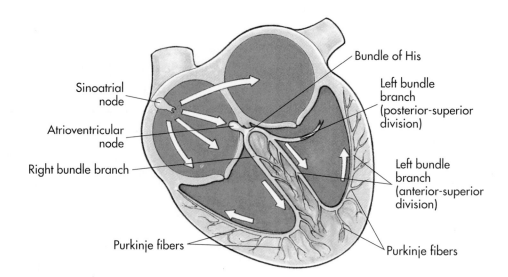

FIGURE 13-9

Cardiac conduction.

From Canobbio, 1990.

An electrocardiogram (ECG) is a graphic recording of electrical activity during the cardiac cycle. The ECG records electrical current generated by movement of ions in and out of the myocardial cell membrane. The ECG records two basic events: depolarization, which is the spread of a stimulus through the heart muscle, and repolarization, which is the return of the stimulated heart muscle to a resting state. The ECG records electrical activity as specific waves (Figure 13-10):

- P wave—the spread of a stimulus through the atria (atrial depolarization)
- PR interval—the time from initial stimulation of the atria to initial stimulation of the ventricles
- QRS complex—the spread of a stimulus through the ventricles (ventricular depolarization)
- ST segment and T wave—the return of stimulated ventricular muscle to a resting state (ventricular repolarization)
- U wave—a small deflection sometimes seen just after the T wave, representing the final phase of ventricular repolarization

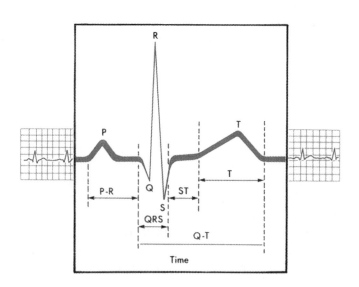

FIGURE 13-10

Usual ECG waveform.

From Berne, Levy, 1997.

Because the electrical stimulus starts the cycle, it must precede the mechanical response by a brief moment; the sequence of myocardial depolarization is a cause of events on the left side of the heart occurring slightly before those on the right. When the heart is beating at a rate of 68 to 72 beats per minute, ventricular systole is shorter than diastole; however, as the rate increases to about 120 because of stress or pathologic factors, the two phases of the cardiac cycle tend to approximate each other in length.

BLOOD CIRCULATION

Once it leaves the heart, the blood flows through two circulatory systems: the pulmonary and the systemic. The heart and these two systems create a closed system that distributes oxygen to all parts of the body (Figure 13-11).

The pulmonary circulation routes blood through the lungs, where it is reoxygenated before being dispatched to the rest of the body. Venous blood arrives at the right atrium via the superior and inferior venae cavae and moves through the tricuspid valve to the right ventricle. During systole, unoxygenated blood is ejected through the pulmonic valve into the pulmonary artery; it travels through increasingly smaller and more numerous arteries, arterioles, and capillaries of the lungs until it reaches the alveoli, where gas exchange occurs.

Oxygenated blood returns to the heart through the pulmonary veins into the left atrium, then through the mitral valve into the left ventricle. The left ventricle contracts, forcing a volume of blood (stroke volume) through the aortic valve into the aorta, through the arterial system and capillaries. In the capilary bed, oxygen is provided to the tissues of the body and the deoxygenated blood passes into the venous system and returns to the heart (Figure 13-12). The stroke volume (SV) multiplied by the heart rate per minute (R) gives the cardiac output (CO), a measure of the heart's ability to adapt to the changing demands of the body.

The structure of the arteries and veins reflects their function. The arteries are tougher, more tensile, and less distensible. They are subjected to much more pressure than are the veins. The veins are less sturdy and more passive than the arteries (Figure 13-13). Because venous return is less forceful than blood flow through the arteries, veins contain valves to keep blood flowing in one direction. If blood volume increases significantly, the veins can expand and act as a repository for extra blood. This compensatory mechanism helps to diminish stress on the heart.

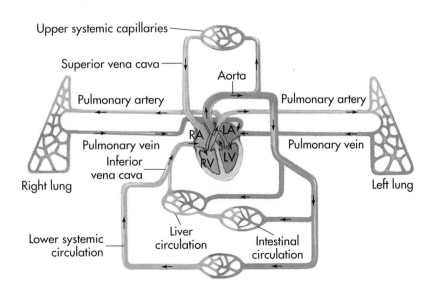

FIGURE 13-11
Circulatory system.
From Canobbio, 1990.

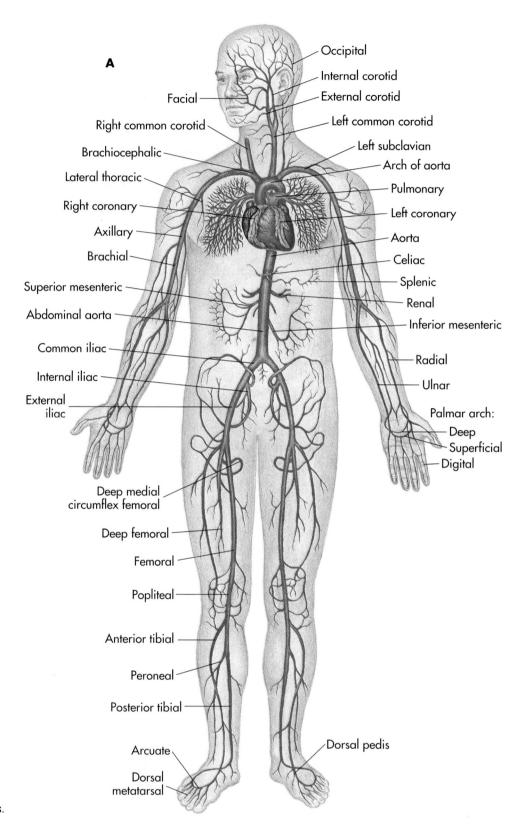

A

Occipital
Internal corotid
External corotid
Facial
Left common corotid
Right common corotid
Left subclavian
Brachiocephalic
Arch of aorta
Lateral thoracic
Pulmonary
Right coronary
Left coronary
Axillary
Aorta
Brachial
Celiac
Superior mesenteric
Splenic
Abdominal aorta
Renal
Inferior mesenteric
Common iliac
Radial
Internal iliac
Ulnar
External iliac
Palmar arch:
Deep
Superficial
Digital
Deep medial circumflex femoral
Deep femoral
Femoral
Popliteal
Anterior tibial
Peroneal
Posterior tibial
Dorsal pedis
Arcuate
Dorsal metatarsal

FIGURE 13-12
Systemic circulation. **A,** Arteries.

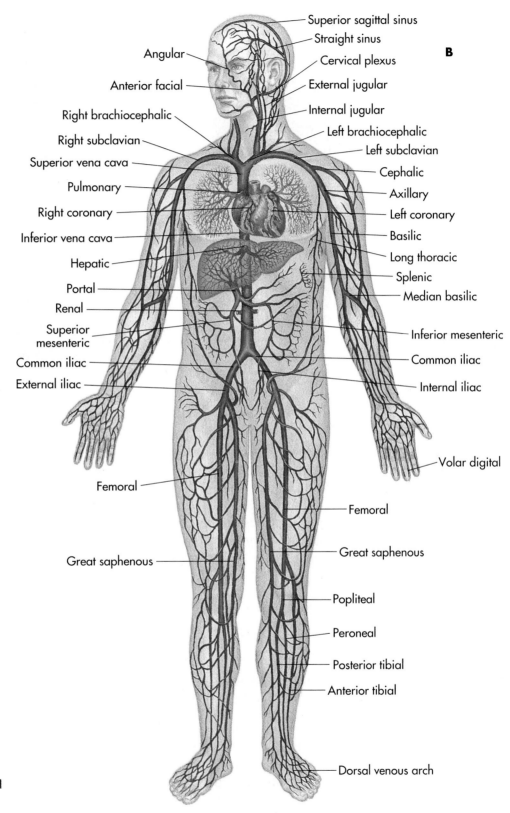

FIGURE 13-12, cont'd
B, Veins.

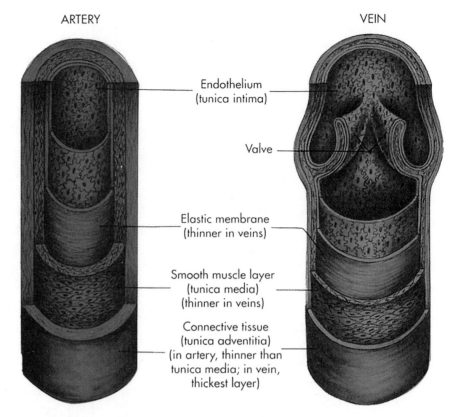

ARTERY   VEIN

Endothelium
(tunica intima)

Valve

Elastic membrane
(thinner in veins)

Smooth muscle layer
(tunica media)
(thinner in veins)

Connective tissue
(tunica adventitia)
(in artery, thinner than
tunica media; in vein,
thickest layer)

FIGURE 13-13
Structure of arteries and veins.
Note the relative thickness of ar-
terial walls.
From Thompson et al, 1997.

Arterial Pulse and Pressure

The palpable and sometimes visible arterial pulses are the result of ventricular systole, which produces a pressure wave throughout the arterial system (arterial pulse). It takes barely 0.2 second for the impact of this wave to be felt in the dorsalis pedis artery and considerably more than 2 seconds for a red blood cell to travel the same distance. The arterial blood pressure is the force exerted by the blood against the wall of an artery as the ventricles of the heart contract and relax.

The pulse usually is felt as a forceful wave that is smooth and more rapid on the ascending part of the wave, becoming domed, less steep, and slower on the descending part. Since the carotid arteries are the most accessible arteries closest to the heart, they have the most suitable pulse for evaluation of cardiac function (Figure 13-14).

Arterial blood pressure has both systolic and diastolic components. Systolic pressure is the force exerted against the wall of the artery when the ventricles contract and is largely the result of cardiac output and blood volume. Blood pressure is highest in systole. Diastolic pressure is the force exerted against the wall of the artery when the heart is in the filling or relaxed state and is primarily the function of peripheral vascular resistance. During diastole, pressure falls to its lowest point. Pulse pressure is the difference between systolic and diastolic pressures (see p. 453). The following variables contribute to the characteristics of the pulses:

- Volume of the blood ejected (stroke volume)
- Distensibility of the aorta and large arteries
- Viscosity of the blood
- Rate of cardiac emptying
- Peripheral arteriolar resistance

FIGURE 13-14
Diagram of usual pulse.
From Barkauskas et al, 1994.

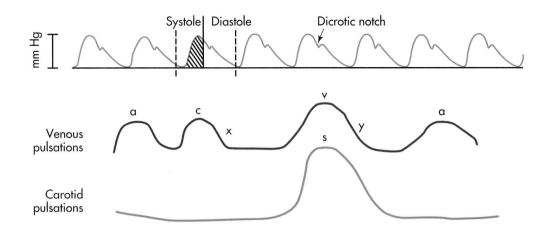

FIGURE 13-15
Expected venous pulsations.

Jugular Venous Pulse and Pressure

The jugular veins, which empty directly into the superior vena cava, reflect the activity of the right side of the heart and offer clues to its competency. The level at which the jugular venous pulse is visible gives an indication of right atrial pressure.

The external jugulars are more superficial and are more visible bilaterally above the clavicle, close to the insertion of the sternocleidomastoid muscles. The larger internal jugulars run deep to the sternocleidomastoids, near the carotid arteries, and are less accessible to inspection (see Figure 13-31, p. 455).

The activity of the right side of the heart is transmitted back through the jugular veins as a pulse* that has five identifiable components—three peaks and two descending slopes (Figure 13-15):

a wave	The a wave, the first and highest component, is the result of a brief backflow of blood to the vena cava during right atrial contraction.
c wave	The c wave is a transmitted impulse from the vigorous backward push produced by closure of the tricuspid valve during ventricular systole.
v wave	The v wave is caused by the increasing volume and concomitant increasing pressure in the right atrium. It occurs a split moment after the c wave, late in ventricular systole.
x slope	The downward x slope is caused by passive atrial filling.
y slope	The y slope following the v wave reflects the open tricuspid valve and the rapid filling of the ventricle.

INFANTS AND CHILDREN

The heart becomes very much like the adult heart early in fetal life. The fetal circulation, including the umbilical vessels, compensates for the nonfunctional fetal lung. The right ventricle pumps blood through the patent ductus arteriosus rather than into the lungs. The right and left ventricles are equal in weight and muscle mass because they both pump blood into the systemic circulation (Figures 13-16 and 13-17).

The changes at birth include closure of the ductus arteriosus, usually within 24 to 48 hours, and the functional closure of the interatrial foramen ovale as the pressure in the left atrium rises. The changing demand on the right ventricle as the pulmonary circulation is established and on the left ventricle as it assumes total responsibility for the

*Although often referred to as a pulse, this is not the same as an arterial pulse, since it is reflected back from the right heart rather than pushed forward by the left heart. Unlike arterial pulses, it cannot be palpated, only visualized.

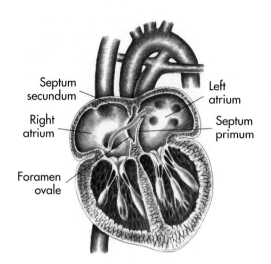

FIGURE 13-16

Anatomy of the fetal heart.

From Thompson et al, 1997.

systemic circulation results in a relative increase in the mass of the left ventricle. By 1 year of age, the relative sizes of the left and right ventricles approximate the adult ratio of 2:1.

In infants and young children, the heart lies more horizontally in the chest than in the adult, and as a result the apex of the heart rides higher, sometimes well out into the fourth left intercostal space. In most cases, the adult heart position is reached by the age of 7 years.

PREGNANT WOMEN

The maternal blood volume increases 40% over prepregnancy volume. The rise is mainly due to an increase in plasma volume, which begins in the first trimester and reaches a maximum after the thirtieth week. On the average, plasma volume increases 50% with a single pregnancy and as much as 70% with a twin pregnancy. The heart works harder to accommodate the increased heart rate and stroke volume required for the expanded blood volume. The left ventricle increases in both wall thickness and mass. In addition, the aorta, pulmonary artery, and mitral orifice increase in size by 12 weeks of pregnancy. Between 32 and 38 weeks, they reach maximum values of 12% to 14% over those in the nonpregnant state. The blood volume returns to prepregnancy levels within 3 to 4 weeks after delivery (Table 13-1).

The cardiac output increases approximately 40% to 50% over that of the nonpregnant state and reaches its highest level by 24 weeks of gestation. This level is maintained until term. Cardiac output returns to prepregnancy levels about 2 weeks after delivery. Both at rest and during strenuous exercise ECG changes are more frequent in pregnancy, but the changes appear to be of questionable significance (Veille, Kitzman, and Bacevice, 1996).

As the uterus enlarges and the diaphragm moves upward in pregnancy, the position of the heart is shifted toward a horizontal position, and there is slight axis rotation.

Systemically, vascular resistance decreases and peripheral vasodilation occurs, often resulting in palmar erythema and spider telangiectases. Blood pressure decreases during the second trimester and may rise thereafter to the prepregnancy level. In general, a blood pressure greater than 140 systolic or 90 mm Hg diastolic is considered hypertension.

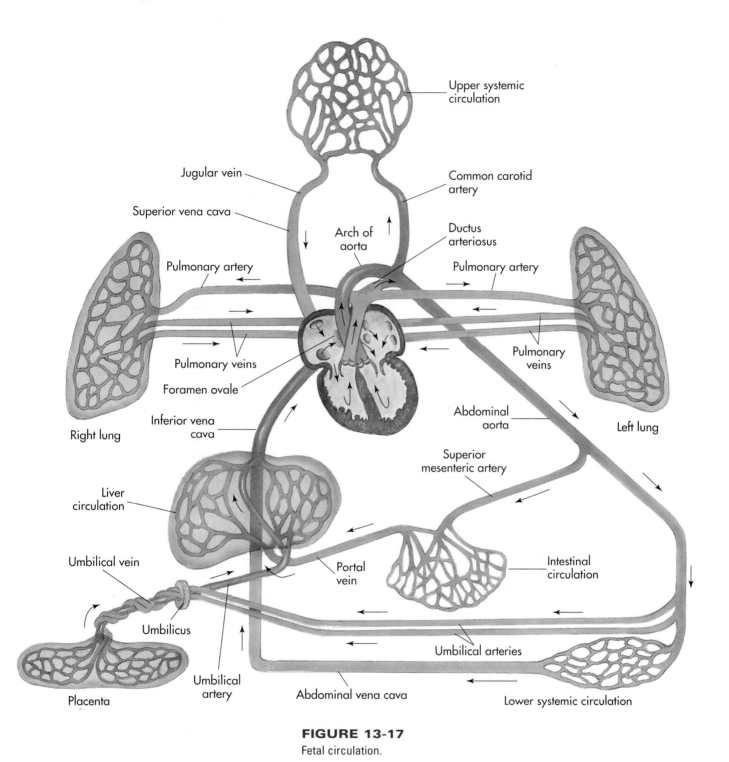

FIGURE 13-17
Fetal circulation.

Blood in the lower extremities tends to stagnate in later pregnancy—except when the woman is in the lateral recumbent position—as a result of occlusion of the pelvic veins and inferior vena cava from pressure created by the enlarged uterus. The occasional result is an increase in dependent edema, varicosities of the legs and vulva, and hemorrhoids.

TABLE 13-1	**Hemodynamic Changes During Pregnancy**				
	Stage				
Hemodynamic Variable	**First Trimester**	**Second Trimester**	**Third Trimester**	**Labor and Delivery**	**Postpartum Period**
HR	Increased	Peaks at 28th week	Slightly decreased	Increased; brady-cardia at delivery	Prepregnancy level within 2-6 weeks
BP	Prepregnancy level	Slightly decreased	Prepregnancy level	Prepregnancy level	Prepregnancy level
BV	Increased	Peaks at 20th week	Gradually decreased	Rises sharply	Prepregnancy level within 2-6 weeks
SV	Increased	Peaks at 28th week	Gradually decreased	Decreased	Prepregnancy level within 2-6 weeks
CO	Increased	Peaks at 20th week	Slightly decreased	Increased	Prepregnancy level within 2-6 weeks
LVEDP	Prepregnancy level	Prepregnancy level	Prepregnancy level	Prepregnancy level	Prepregnancy level
SVR	Decreased	Decreased	Decreased	Sharply decreased at delivery	Prepregnancy level within 2-6 weeks
PVR	Decreased	Decreased	Decreased	Decreased	Prepregnancy level within 2-6 weeks

From Walsh, 1988.

HR, Heart rate; *BP*, blood pressure; *BV*, blood volume; *SV*, stroke volume; *CO*, cardiac output; *LVEDP*, left ventricular end-diastolic pressure; *SVR*, systemic vascular resistance; *PVR*, pulmonary vascular resistance.

OLDER ADULTS

Heart size may decrease with age unless there is enlargement associated with hypertension or heart disease. The left ventricular wall thickens and the valves tend to fibrose and calcify. The heart rate slows (although resting heart rate may not be significantly influenced by age), stroke volume decreases, and cardiac output declines by 30% to 40% during exercise. The endocardium thickens. The myocardium becomes less elastic and more rigid so that recovery of myocardial contractility and irritability is delayed. Thus the response to stress and increased oxygen demand is less efficient, tachycardia is poorly tolerated, and after any type of stress, the return to an expected heart rate takes longer. Thus while the net result of the age-associated changes in heart architecture and contractile properties permits the aged heart to function reasonably well at rest, it is probably long-standing hypertensive disease, infarcts, and/or other insults and physical deconditioning that lead to even more severe compromise of the heart and to increasingly significant decline in cardiac output.

Calcification and other histologic changes in the walls of the arteries, at first proximally and then throughout, cause dilation and tortuosity of the aorta, aortic branches, and the carotid arteries. The superficial vessels of the forehead, neck, and extremities also become tortuous and more prominent. The arterial walls lose elasticity and vasomotor tone, thus diminishing the ability of the artery to comply with changing body needs. Increased peripheral vascular resistance usually elevates blood pressure. Increased vasopressor lability tends to increase both systolic and diastolic pressures progressively. Cardiac function is further compromised by fibrosis and sclerosis in the region of the SA node and in the heart valves (particularly the mitral valve and aortic cusps), by increased vagal tone, and by decreased baroreceptor sensitivity.

Electrocardiographic changes occur secondary to cellular alteration, fibrosis within the conduction system, and neurogenic changes. Common ECG changes in older patients include first-degree atrioventricular block, bundle branch block, ST-T wave abnormalities, premature systole (atrial and ventricular), left anterior hemiblock, left ventricular hypertrophy, and atrial fibrillation.

REVIEW OF RELATED HISTORY

PRESENT PROBLEM

EXERCISE INTENSITY

Light: walking 10-15 steps, preparing simple meal for one, retrieving newspaper from just outside door, pulling down bedspread, brushing teeth

Moderate: making bed, dusting and sweeping, walking a level short block, office filing

Moderately heavy: climbing 1-2 flights of stairs, lifting full cartons, long walks, sexual intercourse

Heavy: jogging, vigorous athletics of any kind, cleaning entire house in less than a day, raking large number of leaves, mowing large lawn, shoveling deep snow

- Chest pain (Boxes 13-1 and 13-2 and Table 13-2)
  - Onset and duration: sudden or gradual, time episode lasted; cyclic nature; related to physical exertion, rest, emotional experience, eating, coughing, cold temperatures
  - Character: aching, sharp, tingling, burning, pressure, stabbing, crushing, or clenched fist sign
  - Location: radiation down arms, to neck, jaws, teeth, scapula; relief with rest or position change
  - Severity: interference with activity, need to stop all activity until subsides, disrupts sleep, how severe on a scale of 0 to 10
  - Associated symptoms: anxiety, dyspnea, diaphoresis, dizziness, nausea and vomiting, faintness, cold clammy skin, cyanosis, pallor, swelling or edema (noted anywhere, constant or certain times during day)

BOX 13-1 **Chest Pain**

The presence of chest pain suggests heart disease in the minds of both the professional health care worker and the layperson. The variety of causes of chest pain, however, is great. *Angina pectoris* is traditionally described as a pressure or choking sensation substernally, or up into the neck. The discomfort, which can be intense, may radiate as high as the jaw and down the left (and sometimes the right) arm. It often begins during strenuous physical activity or eating and frequently during exposure to intense cold, windy weather. Relief may occur in minutes if the activity can be stopped.

There are, however, myriad variations on this theme, sometimes quite similar, sometimes varying in location, intensity, and radiation—and often arising from sources other than the heart. "The precordial catch," for example, is a sudden, sharp, relatively brief pain that does not radiate, occurs most often at rest, and is unrelated to exertion and may not have a discoverable cause. It will, however, cause concern.

Some Possible Causes of Chest Pain

Cardiac
Typical angina pectoris
Atypical angina pectoris, angina equivalent
Prinzmetal variant angina
Unstable angina
Coronary insufficiency
Myocardial infarction
Nonobstructive, nonspastic angina
Mitral valve prolapse
Aortic
Dissection of the aorta
Musculoskeletal
Cervical radiculopathy
Shoulder disorder or dysfunction (arthritis, bursitis, rotator cuff injury, biceps tendinitis)
Costochondral disorder
Xiphodynia

Pleuropericardial pain
Pericarditis
Pleurisy
Pneumothorax
Mediastinal emphysema
Gastrointestinal disease
Hiatus hernia
Reflux esophagitis
Esophageal spasm
Cholecystitis with or without gall stones
Peptic ulcer disease
Pancreatitis
Pulmonary disease
Pulmonary hypertension
Pneumonia
Pulmonary embolus
Bronchial hyperreactivity
Psychoneurotic
Illicit drug use (e.g., cocaine)

Unlike in adults, chest pain in children and adolescents is seldom due to a cardiac problem. It is very often difficult to find a cause, but trauma and exercise-induced asthma and, even in a somewhat younger child as in the adolescent and adult, the use of cocaine should be among the considerations.

Data from Samiy, Douglas, Barondess, 1987; Harvey, 1988.

BOX 13-2 **Characteristics of Chest Pain**

Type	Characteristics
Anginal	Substernal; provoked by effort, emotion, eating; relieved by rest and/or nitroglycerin; often accompanied by diaphoresis, occasionally by nausea.
Pleural	Precipitated by breathing or coughing; usually described as sharp. Present during respiration; absent when breath held.
Esophageal	Burning, substernal, occasional radiation to the shoulder; nocturnal occurrence, usually when lying flat; relief with food, antacids, sometimes nitroglycerin
From a peptic ulcer	Almost always infradiaphragmatic and epigastric; nocturnal occurrence and daytime attacks relieved by food; unrelated to activity
Biliary	Usually under right scapula, prolonged in duration; will trigger angina more often than mimic it
Arthritis/bursitis	Usually of hours' long duration; local tenderness and/or pain with movement
Cervical	Associated with injury; provoked by activity, persists after activity; painful on palpation and/or movement
Musculoskeletal (chest)	Intensified or provoked by movement, particularly twisting or costochondral bending; long lasting; often associated with local tenderness
Psychoneurotic	Associated with/after anxiety; poorly described; located in intramammary region

Data from Samiy, 1987; Harvey, 1988.

- Treatment: rest, position change, exercise, nitroglycerin, digoxin, diuretics, beta blockers, antihypertensives
- Other medications: prescription and nonprescription, prophylactic penicillin, aspirin
- Fatigue
  - Unusual or persistent, inability to keep up with contemporaries, inability to maintain usual activities, bedtime earlier
  - Associated symptoms: dyspnea on exertion, chest pain, palpitations, orthopnea, anorexia, nausea, vomiting
  - Medications: prescription and nonprescription
- Cough
  - Onset and duration
  - Character: dry, wet, nighttime, aggravated by lying down
- Difficult breathing (dyspnea, orthopnea)
  - Aggravated by exertion, lying down (eased by resting on pillows, how many)
- Leg pain or cramps
  - Onset and duration: with activity or rest, with elevation of legs, recent injury or immobilization
  - Character
    - Continuous burning in toes, pain when pointing toes, pain in thighs or buttocks, charley horses, aching, pain over specific location, induced by activity, amount of activity
    - Skin changes: cold skin, pallor, hair loss, sores, redness or warmth over vein, visible veins
    - Fatigue or limping: occurs with walking, improves with walking
    - Wake up at night

TABLE 13-2	**Comparison of Some Types of Chest Pain**		
DIFFERENTIAL DIAGNOSIS	**Angina Pectoris**	**Musculoskeletal**	**Gastrointestinal**
	Presence of cardiac risk factors	History of trauma	History of indigestion
	Specifically noted time of onset	Vague onset	Vague onset
	Related to physical, emotional, or psychosocial effort	Related to physical effort	Related to food consumption
	Disappears if stimulating effort can be terminated	Continues after cessation of effort	May go on for several hours; unrelated to effort
	Frequently forces patients to stop effort	Patients can very often continue activity	Patients can very often continue activity
	Patient may awaken from sleep	Delays falling asleep	Patient may awaken from sleep, particularly during early morning
	Relief at times with nitroglycerin	Relief at times with heat, aspirin, or rest	Relief at times with antacids
	Pain frequently in early morning or after washing and eating	Worse in evening after a day of physical effort	No particular relationship to time of day; related to food, tension
	Greater likelihood in cold weather	Greater likelihood in cold, damp weather	Anytime

Data from Samiy, 1987; Harvey, 1988.

- Loss of consciousness (transient syncope)
  - Associated with: palpitation, arrhythmia, unusual exertion, sudden turning of neck (carotid sinus effect), looking upward (vertebral artery occlusion), change in posture

PAST MEDICAL HISTORY

- Cardiac surgery or hospitalization for cardiac evaluation or disorder
- Acute rheumatic fever, unexplained fever, swollen joints, inflammatory rheumatism, St. Vitus dance (Sydenham chorea)
- Chronic illness: hypertension, bleeding disorder, hyperlipidemia, diabetes, thyroid dysfunction, coronary artery disease, congenital heart defect

FAMILY HISTORY

- Diabetes
- Heart disease
- Hyperlipidemia
- Hypertension
- Congenital heart defects, ventricular septal defects (About 1 in 100 persons has a congenital heart problem; once it occurs in a family the likelihood of it occurring increases to 3 to 5 times the incidence in the general population, particularly with a left-sided lesion.)
- Sudden death, particularly in young and middle-aged relatives
- Family members with risk factors, morbidity, mortality related to cardiovascular system; ages at time of illness or death

PERSONAL AND SOCIAL HISTORY

- Employment: physical demands, environmental hazards such as heat, chemicals, dust, sources of emotional stress

- Tobacco: type (cigarettes, cigars, pipe, chewing tobacco, snuff), duration of use, amount, age started and, perhaps, stopped; pack years (number of years smoking × number of packs per day)
- Nutritional status
  - Usual diet: proportion of fat, food preferences, history of dieting
  - Weight: loss or gain, amount and rate
  - Alcohol consumption: amount, frequency, duration of current intake
  - Known hypercholesterolemia and/or elevated triglyceridemia
- Personality assessment: intensity, hostile attitudes, inability to relax, compulsive behavior
- Relaxation
  - Hobbies
  - Exercise: type, amount, frequency, intensity (see the margin note on p. 425)
  - Sexual activity: frequency of intercourse, sexual practices, number of partners
- Use of alcohol
- Use of illegal drugs: amyl nitrate ("poppers"); cocaine

INFANTS

- Tiring easily during feeding
- Breathing changes: more heavily or more rapidly than expected during feeding or defecation
- Cyanosis: perioral during eating, more widespread and more persistent, related to crying
- Weight gain as expected
- Knee-chest position or other position favored for rest
- Mother's health during pregnancy: rubella in first trimester, unexplained fever, drug use (prescription, nonprescription, and illicit)

CHILDREN

- Tiring during play: amount of time before tiring, activities that are tiring, inability to keep up with other children, reluctance to go out to play
- Naps: longer than expected, usual length
- Positions: squatting instead of sitting when at play or watching television
- Leg pains during exercise
- Headaches
- Nosebleeds
- Unexplained joint pain
- Unexplained fever
- Expected height and weight gain (and any substantiating records)
- Expected physical and cognitive development (and any substantiating records)

PREGNANT WOMEN

- Blood pressure: prepregnancy levels, elevation during pregnancy; associated symptoms and signs, such as headaches, visual changes, nausea and vomiting, epigastric pain, right upper quadrant pain, oliguria, rapid onset of edema (facial, abdominal, or peripheral), hyperreflexia, proteinuria
- Legs: edema, varicosities, pain or discomfort (see the Risk Factors box for varicose veins)
- Dizziness or faintness on standing
- Indications of heart disease during pregnancy include severe or progressive dyspnea, progressive orthopnea, paroxysmal nocturnal dyspnea, hemoptysis, syncope with exertion, chest pain related to effort or emotion, cyanosis, clubbing, persistent neck vein distention, a systolic murmur greater than grade II/VI in intensity, diastolic murmur, and cardiomegaly, general or localized

RISK FACTORS   **Cardiac Disability**

- Gender (men more at risk than women; women's risk is increased in the postmenopausal years and with oral contraceptive use)
- Hyperlipidemia*
- Hypertension (treated or untreated)*
- Smoking*
- Family history of cardiovascular disease, diabetes, hyperlipidemia, hypertension, or sudden death in young adults
- Diabetes mellitus
- Obesity: dietary habits and an excessively fatty diet
- Sedentary life-style without exercise
- Personality type: intense, compulsive behavior with feelings of hostility

*If all factors marked with an asterisk are present, the risk is approximately eight times greater than if none is present.

RISK FACTORS   **Varicose Veins**

- Gender (women more often than men; in fact, four times more often. During pregnancy in particular, increased hormonal levels weaken the walls of the vein and result in failure of the valves.)
- Genetic predisposition: persons of Irish or German descent, daughters of women with varicosities, and genetically predisposed women taking birth control pills.
- Sedentary life-style (habitual inactivity allows blood to pool in the veins, resulting in edema; thus the valves are compromised.)
- Age (the veins of older adults are less elastic and, as a result, more apt to succumb to varicosity.)
- Race: blacks have a lower incidence of varicosities than whites, probably because they have more venous valves in the lower leg than whites.

OLDER ADULTS

- Common symptoms of cardiovascular disorders
  - Confusion, dizziness, blackouts, syncope
  - Palpitations
  - Coughs and wheezes
  - Hemoptysis
  - Shortness of breath
  - Chest pains or chest tightness
  - Incontinence, constipation, impotence, heat intolerance (all associated with many other indications of orthostatic hypotension)
  - Fatigue
  - Leg edema: pattern, frequency, time of day most pronounced
- If heart disease has been diagnosed
  - Drug reactions: potassium excess (weakness, bradycardia, hypotension, confusion); potassium depletion (weakness, fatigue, muscle cramps, dysrhythmias); digitalis toxicity (anorexia, nausea, vomiting, diarrhea, headache, confusion, dysrhythmias, halo, yellow vision)
  - Interference with activities of daily living
  - Ability of the patient and family to cope with the condition, perceived and actual
  - Claudication
  - Orthostatic hypotension

EXAMINATION AND FINDINGS

- Marking pencil
- Centimeter rule
- Stethoscope, with bell and diaphragm (for children, the diaphragm and bell may, but do not need to, have a smaller diameter)
- Sphygmomanometer with appropriately sized cuff (see Figure 3-2)

The examination of the cardiovascular system includes the following: (1) observing and palpating the pulses, comparing each with the contralateral pulse and comparing pulses of the upper extremity with those of the lower; (2) inspecting the veins, particularly the jugular veins; (3) measuring blood pressure in both upper extremities with the patient sitting, standing, and supine, when there is clinical indication, and measuring the blood pressure in both lower extremities again when there is a clinical indication; and (4) inspecting, palpating, percussing, and auscultating the heart.

The parts of the physical examination should be performed in a sequence that is comfortable for you. Findings from examinations of other systems besides the cardiovascular, such as signs of heart failure (crackles in the lungs and engorgement of the liver), have a significant impact on judgments that will be made about the cardiovascular system. Other influencing factors may include the effect of a barrel chest or pectus deformity; the erythema marginatum of rheumatic fever; the Osler nodes or Janeway lesions of bacterial endocarditis; xanthelasma; the funduscopic changes of hypertension; the crackles, wheezes, and rubs in and over the lungs; ascites; and the bruits of aortic aneurysms. No system can be appropriately evaluated outside the context of the entire examination, and performing a successful examination requires both a mastery of the mechanics of each procedure and an ability to integrate and interpret findings in relation to the cardiac events they reflect.

HEART

In assessing cardiac function, it is a common error to listen to the heart first. Rather, it is important to follow the proper sequence, beginning with inspection, palpation, percussion, and then auscultation. Attempt to ensure that lighting includes a tangential source to allow shadows to accent the surface flicker of underlying cardiac movement. The room should be quiet because subtle, low-pitched sounds are hard to hear. Stand to the patient's right, at least at the start. A thorough examination of the heart requires the patient to assume a variety of positions: sitting erect and leaning forward, lying supine, and being in the left lateral recumbent position. These necessary changes in position mandate a comfortable examining table on which movement is easy. Large breasts can make examination difficult. Either you or the patient can move the left breast up or to the left. You must also learn to appreciate the differences in findings when the chest is thin and nonmuscular (sounds are louder, closer) or muscular or obese (sounds are dimmer, distant).

In most adults the apical impulse should be visible at about the midclavicular line in the fifth left intercostal space, but it is easily obscured by obesity, large breasts, and great muscularity. In some it may be visible in the fourth left intercostal space; in any event it should not be seen in more than one space if the heart is healthy. However, the apical impulse may become visible only when the patient sits up and the heart is brought closer to the anterior wall. This is an expected finding.

Readily visible and palpable findings when the patient is supine suggest an intensity that may be the result of a problem. The absence of an apical impulse in addition to faint heart sounds, particularly when the patient is in the left lateral recumbent position, suggests some intervening extracardiac problem, such as pleural or pericardial fluid. In any event, findings are affected by the shape and thickness of the chest wall and the amount of tissue, air, and fluid through which the impulses are transmitted.

Inspection of other organs may reflect important information about the cardiac status. For example, inspecting the skin for cyanosis or venous distention and inspecting the nail bed for cyanosis and capillary refill time provide valuable clues to the cardiac evaluation.

Palpation

Making sure that your hands are warm, and with the patient supine, feel the precordium. Use the proximal halves of the four fingers held gently together or the whole hand. Touch gently and let the movements rise to your hand, because sensation will decrease as you increase pressure.

As always, be methodical. One suggested sequence is to begin at the apex, move to the left sternal border and then to the base, going down to the right sternal border and into the epigastrium or axillae if the circumstance dictates (Figure 13-18).

Feel for the apical impulse and identify its location by the intercostal space and the distance from the midsternal line. Determine the width of the arc in which it is felt. Usually it is palpable within a small radius—no more than 1 cm. The impulse is usually gentle and brief, not lasting as long as systole. If it is more vigorous than expected, characterize it as a *heave* or *lift*. In many adults, you may not be able to feel the apical impulse because of the thickness of the chest wall (Figure 13-19).

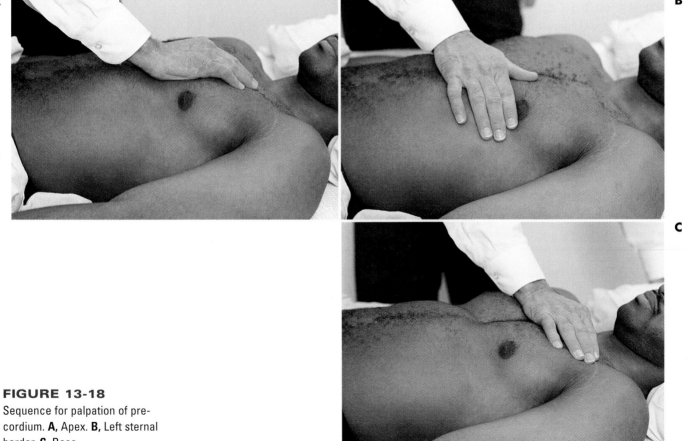

FIGURE 13-18
Sequence for palpation of precordium. **A,** Apex. **B,** Left sternal border. **C,** Base.

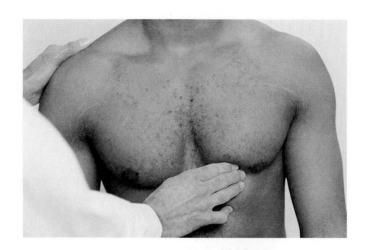

FIGURE 13-19
Palpation of the apical pulse.

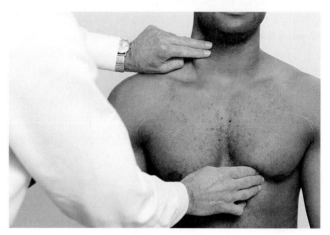

FIGURE 13-20
Palpation of carotid artery to
time events felt over precordium.

An apical impulse that is more forceful and widely distributed, fills systole, or is displaced laterally and downward may indicate increased cardiac output or left ventricular hypertrophy. A lift along the left sternal border may be caused by right ventricular hypertrophy. A loss of thrust may be related to overlying fluid or air or to displacement beneath the sternum. Displacement to the right without a loss or gain in thrust suggests dextrocardia, diaphragmatic hernia, distended stomach, or pulmonary abnormality. The point at which the apical impulse is most readily seen or felt may be described as the *point of maximal impulse* (PMI).

Feel for a *thrill*—a fine, palpable, rushing vibration, a palpable murmur, often, but not always, over the base of the heart in the area of the right or left second intercostal space. It generally indicates a disruption of the expected blood flow related to some defect in the closure of one of the semilunar valves (generally aortic or pulmonic stenosis), pulmonary hypertension, or atrial septal defect (Box 13-3). Locate each sensation in terms of its intercostal space and relationship to the midsternal, midclavicular, and axillary lines. Chapter 12 (Chest and Lungs) describes the method for counting ribs and intercostal spaces.

While palpating the precordium, use your other hand to palpate the carotid artery so that you can describe the carotid pulse in relation to the cardiac cycle. The carotid pulse and S_1 are practically synchronous. The carotid pulse is located just medial to and below the angle of the jaw (Figure 13-20).

BOX 13-3	The Thrill of Heart Examination

A murmur at the grade IV level or more can be felt (see Table 13-5 on p. 441). The sensation delivered to your probing fingers is called a *thrill*. It may be discovered in systole or diastole. The following are among the more common:

Timing	Location	Probable Cause
Systole	Suprasternal notch and/or second and third right intercostal spaces	Aortic stenosis
	Suprasternal notch and/or second and third left intercostal spaces	Pulmonic stenosis
	Fourth left intercostal space	Ventricular septal defect
	Apex	Mitral regurgitation
	Left lower sternal border	Tetralogy of Fallot
	Left upper sternal border, often with extensive radiation	Patent ductus arteriosus
Diastole	Right sternal border	Aortic regurgitation Aneurysm of ascending aorta
	Apex	Mitral stenosis

Percussion

Percussion is of limited value in defining the borders of the heart or determining its size, because the shape of the chest is relatively rigid and can to some extent make the more malleable heart conform. Left ventricular size is better judged by the location of the apical impulse. The right ventricle tends to enlarge in the anteroposterior diameter rather than laterally, thus diminishing the value of percussion of the right heart border. A chest roentgenogram may be far more useful for defining the heart borders.

Should you wish to estimate the size of the heart by percussion, begin tapping at the anterior axillary line, moving medially along the intercostal spaces toward the sternal border. The change from a resonant to a dull note marks the cardiac border. These points can be noted with a marking pencil and the outline of the heart thus visually defined. On the left, the loss of resonance will generally be close to the point of maximal impulse at the apex of the heart. Measure this point from the midsternal line at each intercostal space. When percussing the right cardiac border, one does not note a change in resonance until the right sternal border is encountered. Obesity, unusual muscular development, and some pathologic conditions (such as presence of air or fluids) can easily distort the findings.

Auscultation

Because all heart sounds are of relatively low frequency, in a range somewhat difficult for the human ear to detect, you must be compulsive about ensuring ambient quiet. Because shivering and movement increase adventitious sound and because comfort is important, make certain the patient is warm and relaxed before beginning. Nevertheless, a comfortably warm stethoscope should be placed on the naked chest.

It is a common error to try to hear *all* of the sounds in the cardiac cycle at one time. Take the time to isolate each sound and each pause in the cycle, listening separately and selectively for as many beats as necessary to evaluate the sounds. It takes time to tune in, so you must not rush. Avoid "jumping" the stethoscope from one site to another; instead, "inch" the endpiece along the route. This maneuver helps prevent missing important sounds, particularly more widely transmitted abnormal sounds, and it allows "tracking" of a sound from its loudest point to its farthest reach (e.g., into the axillae or the back).

Because sound is transmitted in the direction of blood flow, specific heart sounds are best heard over areas where the blood flows after it passes through a valve. Approach each of the precordial areas systematically in a sequence that is comfortable for you, working your way from base to apex or apex to base (Box 13-4).

Auscultation should be performed in, but not limited to, each of the five cardiac areas, using first the diaphragm and then the bell of the stethoscope. Use firm pressure with the diaphragm and light pressure with the bell.

There are five traditionally designated auscultatory areas, located as follows (Figure 13-21):

- Aortic valve area: second right intercostal space at the right sternal border
- Pulmonic valve area: second left intercostal space at the left sternal border
- Second pulmonic area: third left intercostal space at the left sternal border
- Tricuspid area: fourth left intercostal space along the lower left sternal border
- Mitral (or apical) area: at the apex of the heart in the fifth left intercostal space at the midclavicular line

---

BOX 13-4   **Procedure for Auscultating the Heart**

Adopt a routine for the various positions the patient is asked to assume, although you should be prepared to alter the sequence if the patient's condition requires it. Instruct the patient when to breathe comfortably and when to hold the breath in expiration and inspiration. Listen carefully for each heart sound, isolating each component of the cardiac cycle, especially while the respirations are momentarily suspended. The following sequence is suggested:

- Patient sitting up and leaning slightly forward and, preferably, in expiration: listen in all five areas (Figure 13-22, *A*). This is the best position to hear relatively high-pitched murmurs with the stethoscope diaphragm.
- Patient supine: listen in all five areas (Figure 13-22, *B*.)
- Patient left lateral recumbent: listen in all five areas. This is the best position to hear the low-pitched filling sounds in diastole with the stethoscope bell (Figure 13-22, *C*).
- Other positions depend on your findings. Patient right lateral recumbent: this is best position for evaluating right rotated heart or dextrocardia. Listen in all five areas.
- Inch, don't jump, your way from area to area.

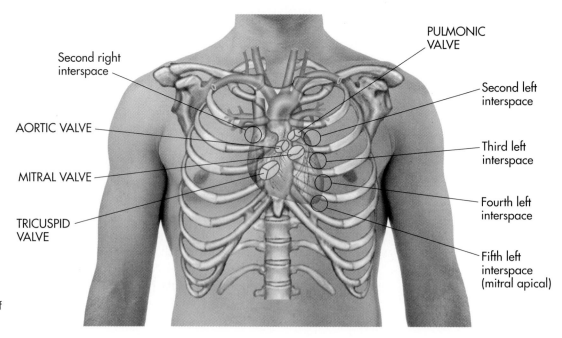

FIGURE 13-21

Areas for auscultation of the heart.

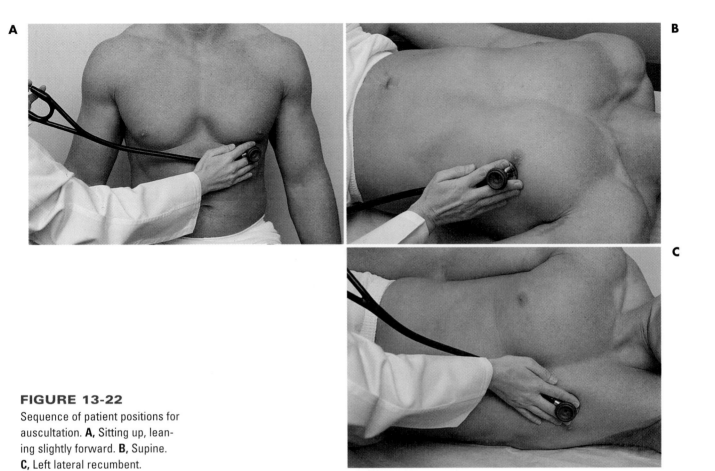

FIGURE 13-22
Sequence of patient positions for auscultation. **A,** Sitting up, leaning slightly forward. **B,** Supine. **C,** Left lateral recumbent.

As you examine each of the five auscultatory areas, remember to inch along. A full hearing cannot be obtained by jumping from one isolated area to the next. At each site pause and listen selectively for each component of the cardiac cycle. Let your stethoscope follow the sounds wherever they lead.

- Assess the overall rate and rhythm of the heart, noting the auscultatory area in which you are listening each time.
- Instruct the patient to breathe normally and then hold the breath in expiration. Listen for S_1 while you palpate the carotid pulse. S_1 coincides with the rise (upswing) of the carotid pulse. Note the intensity, any variations, the effect of respirations, and any splitting of S_1.
- Concentrate on systole, listening for any extra sounds or murmurs. S_1 marks the beginning of systole.
- Concentrate on diastole, which is a longer interval than systole, listening for any extra sounds or murmurs. (Note, however, that systole and diastole are equal in duration when the heart rate is rapid.) S_1 immediately follows diastole.
- Instruct the patient to breathe comfortably, listening closely for S_2 to become two components (split S_2) during inspiration.

Areas for inspection, palpation, and auscultation change if the heart is not located in its expected place in the left mediastinum. In situs inversus, the heart and stomach are placed on the right and the liver on the left. In dextrocardia, the heart alone is rotated. In such a circumstance, adjust to the anatomic alteration by thinking of the examination sites as they would be in a mirror image of the expected.

TABLE 13-3	Heart Sounds According to Auscultatory Area				
	Aortic	**Pulmonic**	**Second Pulmonic**	**Mitral**	**Tricuspid**
Pitch	$S_1 < S_2$	$S_1 < S_2$	$S_1 < S_2$	$S_1 < S_2$	$S_1 < S_2$
Loudness	$S_1 < S_2$	$S_1 < S_2$	$S_1 < S_2$*	$S_1 > S_2$†	$S_1 > S_2$
Duration	$S_1 > S_2$	$S_1 > S_2$	$S_1 > S_2$	$S_1 > S_2$	$S_1 > S_2$
S_2 split	>inhale	>inhale	>inhale	>inhale ‡	>inhale
	<exhale	<exhale	<exhale	<exhale	<exhale
A_2	Loudest	Loud	Decreased		
P_2	Decreased	Louder	Loudest		

*S_1 is relatively louder in second pulmonic area than in aortic area.
†S_1 may be louder in mitral area than in tricuspid area.
‡S_2 split may not be audible in mitral area if P_2 is inaudible.

Basic heart sounds. Heart sounds are characterized in much the same way as respiratory and other body sounds: by frequency (pitch), intensity (loudness), duration, and timing in the cardiac cycle. Heart sounds are relatively low in pitch, except in the presence of significant pathologic events. Table 13-3 summarizes their relative differences according to auscultatory area. (Also see Figure 13-25, p. 442.)

There are four basic heart sounds: S_1, S_2, S_3, and S_4. S_1 and S_2 are the most distinct heart sounds and should be characterized separately, since variations can offer important clues to cardiac function. S_3 and S_4 may or may not be present; their absence is not an unusual finding, but their presence does not necessarily indicate a pathologic condition. Thus S_3 and S_4 must be evaluated in relation to other sounds and events in the cardiac cycle.

S_1 and S_2. S_1, the result of closure of the AV values, indicates the beginning of systole and is best heard toward the apex where it is usually louder than S_2 (Box 13-5). At the base, S_1 is louder on the left than on the right but softer than S_2 in both areas. It is lower in pitch and a bit longer than S_2, and it occurs immediately after diastole (Figure 13-23).

BOX 13-5	S_1 Intensity: Diagnostic Clues

When systole begins with the mitral valve open, the valve snaps shut more vigorously, producing a louder S_1. This occurs in the following situations:
- Blood velocity is increased, such as occurs in anemia, fever, hyperthyroidism, anxiety, and during exercise.
- The mitral valve is stenotic.

If the mitral valve is not completely open, ventricular contraction forces it shut. The loudness produced by valve closure depends on the degree of opening, so the intensity of S_1 varies in the following situations:
- Complete heart block is present.
- Gross disruption of rhythm occurs, such as during fibrillation.

The intensity of S_1 is decreased in the following situations:
- Increased overlying tissue, fat, or fluid (such as occurs in emphysema, obesity, or pericardial fluid) obscures sounds.
- Systemic or pulmonary hypertension is present, which contributes to more forceful atrial contraction. If the ventricle is noncompliant, the contraction may be delayed or diminished, especially if the valve is partially closed when contraction begins.
- Fibrosis and calcification of a diseased mitral valve can result from rheumatic heart disease. Calcification diminishes valve flexibility so that it closes with less force.

Heart sounds   **Site at which
                                        best heard**

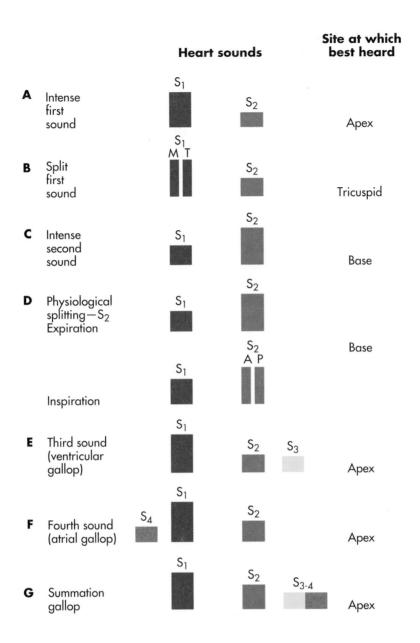

FIGURE 13-23
Heart sounds.

Although there is some asynchrony between closure of the mitral and tricuspid valves, S_1 is usually heard as one sound. If the asynchrony is more marked than usual, the sound may be split and is then best heard in the tricuspid area. Other variations in S_1 depend on the competency of the pulmonary and systemic circulations, the structure of the heart valves, their position when ventricular contraction begins, and the force of the contraction.

S_2, the result of closure of the semilunar valves, indicates the end of systole and is best heard in the aortic and pulmonic areas. It is of higher pitch and shorter duration than S_1 and occurs at the end of systole. S_2 is louder than S_1 at the base of the heart; still it is usually softer than S_1 at the apex (Box 13-6).

S_2 is actually two sounds that merge during expiration. The closure of the aortic valve (A_2) contributes to most of the sound of S_2 when it is heard in the aortic and pulmonic areas. A_2 tends to mask the sound of pulmonic valve closure (P_2). During inspiration P_2 occurs slightly later, giving S_2 two distinct components—this is a split S_2. Splitting is more often heard and easier to detect in the young; it is not well heard

---

BOX 13-6 | **S₂ Intensity: Diagnostic Clues**

The intensity of S_2 increases in the following conditions:
- Systemic hypertension (S_2 may ring or boom), syphilis of the aortic valve, exercise, or excitement accentuates A_2.
- Pulmonary hypertension, mitral stenosis, and congestive heart failure accentuate P_2.
- The valves are diseased but still fully mobile; the component of S_2 affected depends on which valve is compromised.

The intensity of S_2 decreases in the following conditions:
- A shocklike state with arterial hypotension causes loss of valvular vigor.
- The valves are immobile, thickened, or calcified; the component of S_2 affected depends on which valve is compromised.
- Aortic stenosis affects A_2.
- Pulmonic stenosis affects P_2.
- Overlying tissue, fat, or fluid mutes S_2.

---

in the elderly. This may be because of the tendency of the anteroposterior diameter of the chest to increase with age.

Splitting. Splitting of S_1 is not usually heard because the sound of the tricuspid valve closing is too faint to hear. On occasion, however, it may be audible in the tricuspid area, particularly on deep inspiration.

Splitting of S_2 is an expected event, because pressures are higher and depolarization occurs earlier on the left side of the heart. Ejection times on the right are longer, and the pulmonic valve closes a bit later than the aortic valve. As a consequence, the usual S_2 often has two audible components. If P_2 is heard outside the pulmonary area, it is generally unusually loud or delayed. It may also be a different sound with a different source.

Splitting is greatest at the peak of inspiration (Figure 13-23, *D*). During expiration the disparity in ejection times tends to diminish, and the split may disappear. Ejection times tend to equalize when the breath is held in inspiration, so this maneuver also tends to eliminate the split. Thus the degree of S_2 splitting is most evident during inspiration. It may vary widely from easily heard to nondetectable, from inspiration to expiration. The respiratory cycle is not always the dominant factor; the interval between the components may remain easily discernible throughout the respiratory cycle (Box 13-7).

S_3 and S_4. During diastole the ventricles fill in two steps: an early, passive flow of blood from the atria is followed by a more vigorous, atrial ejection. The passive phase occurs quickly relatively early in diastole, distending the ventricular walls and causing vibration. The resultant sound, S_3, is quiet and somewhat difficult to hear (Figure 13-23, *E*).

In the second phase of ventricular filling, vibration in the valves, papillae, and ventricular walls produces S_4 (Figure 13-23, *F*). Because it occurs so late in diastole (presystole), S_4 may be confused with a split S_1.

S_3 and S_4 should be quiet and therefore somewhat difficult to hear. Increasing venous return (by asking the patient to raise a leg) or arterial pressure (by asking the patient to grip your hand vigorously and repeatedly) may make these sounds easier to hear. S_2 and S_4 are commonly heard in pediatric patients. Increased intensity of either sound is suspect.

When S_3 becomes intense and easy to hear, the resultant sequence of sounds simulates a gallop—the protodiastolic gallop rhythm. S_4 may also become more intense, producing a readily discernible presystolic gallop rhythm. This is most frequent in older patients, but it may happen at any age when there is increased resistance to filling because of loss of compliance of the ventricular walls (such as in hypertensive

BOX 13-7 **Unexpected Splitting of Heart Sounds**

Wide Splitting

The split becomes wider when there is delayed activation of contraction or emptying of the right ventricle resulting in delay in pulmonic closure. This occurs, for example, in right bundle branch block, which splits both S_1 and S_2. Wide splitting of S_2 also occurs when stenosis delays closure of the pulmonic valve, when pulmonary hypertension delays ventricular emptying, or when mitral regurgitation induces early closure of the aortic valve. The split becomes narrower and is even eliminated or paradoxic when closure of the aortic valve is delayed, such as in left bundle branch block.

Fixed Splitting

Splitting is said to be fixed when it is unaffected by respiration. This occurs with delayed closure of the pulmonic valve when output of the right ventricle is greater than that of the left (such as occurs in large atrial septal defects, a ventricular septal defect with left to right shunting, or right ventricular failure).

Paradoxic (Reversed) Splitting

Paradoxic splitting occurs when closure of the aortic valve is delayed (such as in left bundle branch block) so that P_2 occurs first, followed by A_2. In this case, the interval between P_2 and A_2 is heard during expiration and disappears during inspiration.

See Figure 13-24 for visual depiction of (variations in splitting of S_2) variations in split heart sounds.

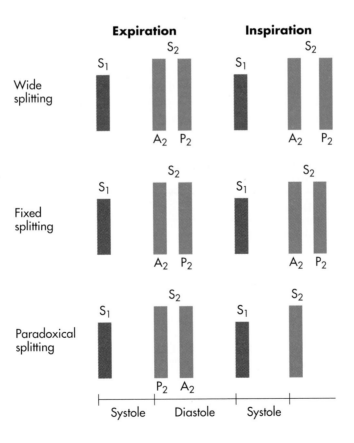

FIGURE 13-24

Variations in splitting of S_2.

From Barkauskus et al, 1998.

disease and coronary artery disease) or the increased stroke volume of high-output states (such as in profound anemia, pregnancy, and thyrotoxicosis). The rhythm of the heart sound when an S_3 is heard resembles the rhythm of Tenn - es - see. When an S_4 is heard, it resembles the rhythm of Ken - tuc - ky. A loud S_4 always suggests pathology and deserves additional evaluation.

Extra heart sounds. The cardiac valves generally open noiselessly unless thickened, roughened, or otherwise altered as a result of disease. Valvular stenosis may produce an opening snap (mitral valve), ejection clicks (semilunar valves), or mid-to-late nonejection systolic clicks (mitral prolapse). The pulmonary ejection click is best heard on expiration, seldom on inspiration; aortic ejection clicks are less sharp, are less involved with S_1, and may be heard as distant as the anterior axillary line. Extra heart sounds often accompany murmurs and should always be considered indicative of a pathologic process.

Pericardial friction rub can be easily mistaken for cardiac-generated sounds. Inflammation of the pericardial sac causes a roughening of the parietal and visceral surfaces, which produces a rubbing sound audible through the stethoscope. It occupies both systole and diastole and overlies the intracardiac sounds. Pericardial friction rub may have three components that are associated in sequence with the atrial component of systole, ventricular systole, and ventricular diastole. It is usually heard widely but is more distinct toward the apex. A three-component friction rub is a grating sound that may be intense enough to obscure the heart sounds. However, if there are only one or two components, the sound may not be particularly intense or machinelike and may then be more difficult to distinguish from an intracardiac murmur. The detection of extra heart sounds is detailed in Table 13-4, along with associated disorders (Figure 13-25).

You should always be aware, based on the history and inspection of the chest, if a patient has had a cardiac surgical procedure. If this involves the placement of a prosthetic mitral valve, listen for a distinct click early in diastole, loudest at the apex and transmitted precordially. A prosthetic aortic valve will cause a sound in early systole. The intensity of these sounds will depend on the type of material used for the prosthesis. Animal tissue is the most quiet, even silent. Pacemakers no longer tend to cause

TABLE 13-4	Extra Heart Sounds	
Sound	**Detection**	**Description**
Increased S_3	Bell at apex; patient left lateral recumbent	Early diastole, low pitch
Increased S_4	Bell at apex; patient supine or part way between lateral and supine	Late diastole or early systole, low pitch
Gallops	Bell at apex; patient supine or left lateral recumbent	Presystole, intense, easily heard
Mitral valve opening snap	Diaphragm medial to apex, may radiate to base; any position, second left intercostal space	Early diastole briefly, before S_3; high pitch, sharp snap or click; not affected by respiration; easily confused with S_2
Ejection clicks	Diaphragm; patient sitting or supine	
Aortic valve	Apex, base in second right intercostal space	Early systole, intense, high pitch; radiates; not affected by respirations
Pulmonary valve	Second left intercostal space at sternal border	Early systole, less intense than aortic click; intensifies on expiration, decreases on inspiration
Pericardial friction rub	Widely heard, sound clearest toward apex	May occupy all of systole and diastole; intense, grating, machinelike; may have 3 components and obliterate heart sounds; if only 1 or 2 components, may sound like murmur

a sound. Earlier models made a high-pitched, clicklike, presystolic "noise" that was extracardiac in origin as skeletal muscle contracted.

Heart murmurs. Heart murmurs are relatively prolonged extra sounds heard during systole or diastole; they frequently indicate a problem. Murmurs are caused by some disruption in the flow of blood into, through, or out of the heart. The characteristics of a murmur depend on the adequacy of valve function, the size of the opening, the rate of blood flow, the vigor of the myocardium, and the thickness and consistency of the overlying tissues through which the murmur must be heard.

Diseased valves, a common cause of murmurs, either do not open or do not close well. When the leaflets are thickened and the passage narrowed, forward blood flow is restricted (stenosis). When valve leaflets, which are intended to fit together snugly, lose competency, the slack openings allow backward flow of blood (regurgitation). Table 13-5 summarizes the characteristics of the heart murmurs. You will find that murmurs have been described in many ways (e.g., harsh, blowing, seagull). Such descriptions may or may not be consistent with the way you hear the sounds. Don't hesitate to use words that best suit your interpretation.

TABLE 13-5	Characterization of Heart Murmurs	
	Classification	**Description**
Timing and duration*	Early systolic	Begins with S_1, decrescendoes, ends well before S_2
	Midsystolic (ejection)	Begins after S_1, ends before S_2; crescendo-decrescendo quality sometimes difficult to discern
	Late systolic	Begins mid to late systole, crescendoes, ends at S_2; often introduced by mid to late systolic clicks
	Early diastolic	Begins with S_2
	Middiastolic	Begins at clear interval after S_2
	Late diastolic (presystolic)	Begins immediately before S_1
	Holosystolic (pansystolic)	Begins with S_1, occupies all of systole, ends at S_2
	Holodiastolic (pandiastolic)	Begins with S_2, occupies all of diastole, ends at S_1
	Continuous	Starts in systole, continues without interruption through S_2 into all or part of diastole; does not necessarily persist throughout entire cardiac cycle
Pitch	High, medium, low	Depends on pressure and rate of blood flow; low pitch is heard best with the bell
Intensity†	Grade I	Barely audible in quiet room
	Grade II	Quiet but clearly audible
	Grade III	Moderately loud
	Grade IV	Loud, associated with thrill
	Grade V	Very loud, thrill easily palpable
	Grade VI	Very loud, audible with stethoscope not in contact with chest, thrill palpable and visible
Pattern	Crescendo	Increasing intensity caused by increased blood velocity
	Decrescendo	Decreasing intensity caused by decreased blood velocity
	Square or plateau	Constant intensity
Quality	Harsh, raspy, machinelike, vibratory, musical, blowing	Quality depends on several factors, including degree of valve compromise, force of contractions, blood volume
Location	Anatomic landmarks (e.g., second left intercostal space on sternal border)	Area of greatest intensity, usually area to which valve sounds are normally transmitted
Radiation	Anatomic landmarks (e.g., to axilla or carotid arteries)	Site farthest from location of greatest intensity at which sound is still heard; sound usually transmitted in direction of blood flow
Respiratory phase variations	Intensity, quality, and timing may vary	Venous return increases on inspiration and decreases on expiration

*Systolic murmurs are best described according to time of onset and termination; diastolic murmurs are best classified according to time of onset only.
†Discrimination among the six grades is more difficult for the diastolic murmur than for the systolic.

Heart sounds	First heart sound $[S_1(M_1T_1)]$	Second heart sound $[S_2(A_2P_2)]$	Third heart sound $(S_3,$ ventricular gallop)	Fourth heart sound $(S_4,$ atrial gallop)
Anatomic reference	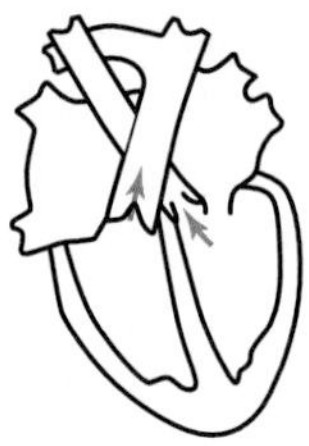	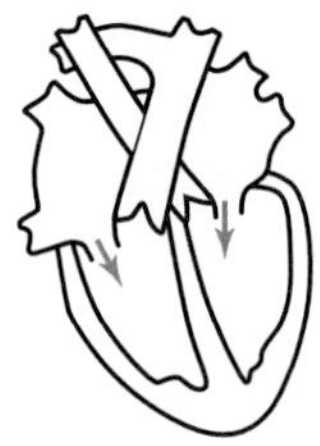	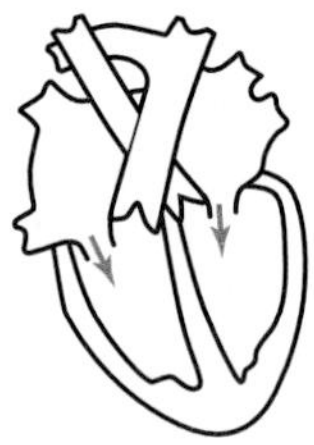	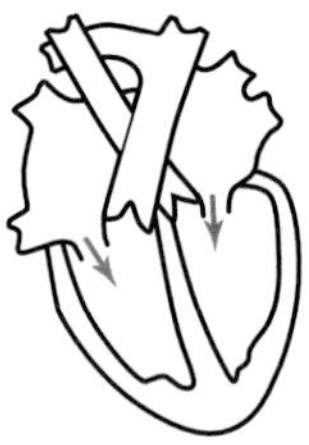
Preferable position of patient	Any position	Sitting or supine	Supine or left lateral	Supine or left semilateral
Area for auscultation	Entire precordium (apex)	A_2 at 2nd RICS* P_2 at 2nd LICS	Apex	Apex
Endpiece	Diaphragm	Diaphragm	Bell	Bell
FINDINGS Pitch	High	High	Low	Low
Effects of respiration	Softer on inspiration	Fusion of A_2P_2 on expiration; physiologic split on inspiration	Increased on inspiration	Increased on forced inspiration
External influences	Increased with excitement, exercise, amyl nitrate, epinephrine, and atropine	Increased with thin chest walls and with exercise	Increased with exercise, fast heart rate, elevation of legs and increased venous return	Same as for S_3
Contributing event	Closure of tricuspid and mitral valves	Closure of pulmonic and aortic valves	Rapid ventricular filling	Forceful atrial ejection into distended ventricle

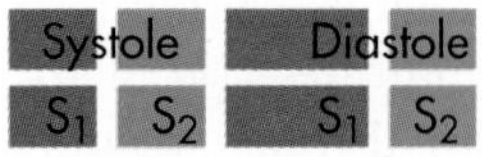

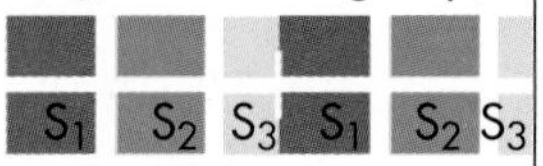

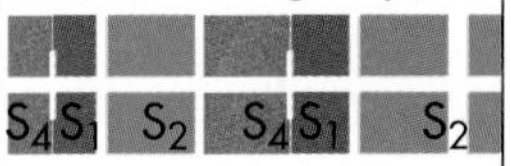

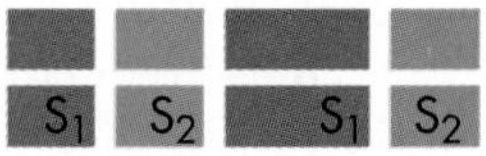

*RICS, right intercostal space; LICS, left intercostal space.

FIGURE 13-25

Assessment of heart sounds.

Modified from Guzetta, Dossey, 1992.

Quadruple rhythm	Summation gallop (triple gallop)	Ejection sounds	Systolic click	Opening snap
$S_4 S_1$ S_2 S_3 $S_4 S_1$ S_2	S_{3-4} S_1 S_2 S_{3-4} S_1 S_2	S_1 S_2 S_1 ¹ S_2	S_1 ¹ S_2 S_1 ¹ S_2	S_1 S_2 ¹ S_1 S_2 ¹
Supine or left lateral	Supine or left lateral	Sitting or supine	Sitting or supine	Any position
Apex	Apex	2nd RICS, 2nd LICS, or apex	Apex	Apex
Bell	Bell	Diaphragm	Diaphragm	Diaphragm
Low	Low	High	High	High
Increased on inspiration	Increased on inspiration	Increased on inspiration with pulmonary stenosis	Increased on inspiration	Uninfluenced by inspiration
Same as for S_3	Same as for S_3	Aortic ejection sound same as S_1 and S_2; pulmonary ejection sound increased on expiration	Occurs later in systole with increased venous return (e.g., with elevated legs or supine position)	May be confused with S_3
S_1, S_2, S_3, and S_4, all heard separately	S_3 and S_4 fuse with fast heart rates	Opening of deformed semi-lunar valves	Prolapse of mitral valve leaflet	Abrupt recoil of stenotic mitral or tricuspid valve

The discovery of a heart murmur requires careful assessment and diagnosis. Although some murmurs are benign (Box 13-8), others represent a noxious process at work. Therefore solid evidence from additional testing is often mandatory before a murmur is dismissed as "functional."

Not all murmurs, however, are the result of valvular defects. Other causes include:

- High output demands that increase speed of blood flow (such as thyrotoxicosis, anemia, pregnancy)
- Structural defects, either congenital or acquired, that allow blood to flow through inappropriate pathways (such as the myocardial septa)
- Diminished strength of myocardial contraction
- Altered blood flow in the major vessels near the heart

It is not always possible on physical examination to identify with consistency the cause of a systolic murmur. However, a number of maneuvers can narrow the choices before diagnostic laboratory studies are performed (Table 13-6).

PERIPHERAL ARTERIES

CAUTION: CAROTID SINUS MASSAGE

When palpating the carotid arteries, *never palpate both sides simultaneously.* Excessive carotid sinus massage can cause slowing of the pulse or a drop in blood pressure and compromise of blood flow to the brain. The resultant effect could be possible circulatory embarrassment, particularly in older adults who may already have compromised cardiovascular function. If you have difficulty feeling the pulse, rotate the patient's head to the side being examined to relax the sternocleidomastoid muscle.

Palpation

The pulses are best palpated over arteries that are close to the surface of the body and lie over bones. These include the carotid, brachial, radial, femoral, popliteal, dorsalis pedis, and posterior tibial (Table 13-7 and Figure 13-26).

An arterial pulsation is essentially a bounding wave of blood with varying vigor that diminishes with increasing distance from the heart. Of all the arterial pulses, the carotids are easily accessible and closest to the cardiac source and thus most useful in evaluating heart activity. The arterial pulses in the extremities are examined to determine the sufficiency of the entire arterial circulation. At least one pulse point is palpated in each extremity, usually at the most distal point.

Examine the arterial pulses with the distal pads of the second and third fingers. Despite traditional advice to the contrary, the thumb may also be used; it is particularly useful in "fixing" the brachial and even the femoral pulses, because these have a tendency to move when probed by the fingers. Palpate firmly but not so hard as to occlude the artery.

If you have difficulty finding a pulse, try varying your pressure, feeling carefully throughout the area. Make sure when you locate it that you are not feeling your own pulse. A pulse is most readily felt over a bony prominence; therefore in some areas, particularly the ankle, fat or edema may make it difficult to feel.

DIFFERENTIAL DIAGNOSIS

TABLE 13-6   **Comparison of Systolic Murmurs**

Origin	Maneuver	Effect on Intensity
Right-sided chambers	Inspiration	Increase
	Expiration	Decrease
Hypertrophic cardio-myopathy	Valsalva	Increase
	Squatting to standing (rapidly for 30 seconds)	Increase
	Standing to squatting (rapidly)	Decrease
	Passive leg elevation to 45 degrees, patient supine	Decrease
	Handgrip (after 1 minute of patient's strongest possible grip)	Decrease
Mitral regurgitation*	Handgrip	Increase
Ventricular septal defect*	Transient arterial occlusion (sphygmo-manometer placed on each of patient's upper arms and simultaneously inflated to 20-40 mm Hg above patient's previously recorded blood pressures; intensity noted after 20 seconds	Increase
	Inhalation of amyl nitrate (3 rapid breaths from a broken ampule) *(Not routinely recommended)*	Decrease
Aortic stenosis	No maneuver distinguishes this murmur; the diagnosis can be made by exclusion	

*The combination of handgrip, transient arterial occlusion, and inhalation of amyl nitrate will distinguish mitral regurgitation and ventricular septal defect from other causes of systolic murmurs; more than just auscultation is needed to make further distinction.
Adapted from Lembo, 1988.

TABLE 13-7   **Locations of Palpable Pulses**

Pulse	Location
Carotid	In the neck, just medial to and below angle of the jaw (do not palpate both sides simultaneously)
Brachial	Just medial to biceps tendon
Radial	Medial and ventral side of wrist (gentle pressure)
Femoral	Inferior and medial to inguinal ligament; if patient is obese, midway between anterior superior iliac spine and pubic tubercle (press harder here than in most areas)
Popliteal	Popliteal fossae (press firmly); the patient should be prone with the knee flexed
Dorsalis pedis	Medial side of dorsum of foot with foot slightly dorsiflexed (pulse may be hard to feel and may not be palpable in some well persons)
Posterior tibial	Behind and slightly inferior to medial malleolus of ankle (pulse may be hard to feel and may not be palpable in some well persons)

PEDAL PULSES

Either the dorsalis pedis or posterior tibial pulses may be bilaterally absent in many persons. Unilateral absences of one pulse or absence of all pulses is a significant finding and should be given attention.

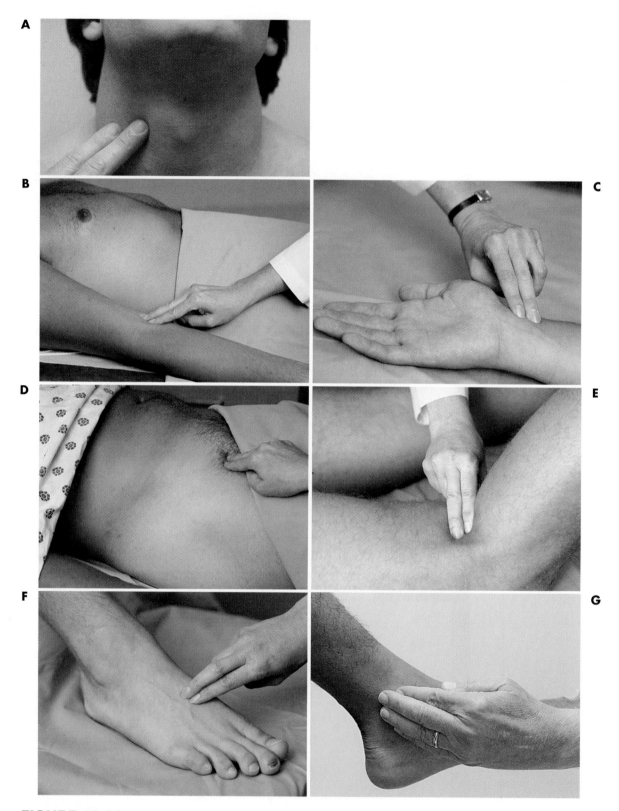

FIGURE 13-26

Palpation of arterial pulses. **A**, Carotid. **B**, Brachial. **C**, Radial. **D**, Femoral. **E**, Popliteal. **F**, Dorsalis pedis. **G**, Posterial tibial.

TABLE 13-8	Arterial Pulse Abnormalities	
Type	**Description**	**Associated Conditions**
Alternating pulse (pulsus alternans)	Regular rate; amplitude varies from beat to beat with weak and strong beats	Left ventricular failure (Figure 13-27, *A*)
Pulsus bisferiens	Two strong systolic peaks separated by a midsystolic dip	Aortic regurgitation alone or with stenosis (Figure 13-27, *B*)
Bigeminal pulse (pulsus bigeminus)	Two beats in rapid succession followed by longer interval; easily confused with alternating pulse	Regularly occurring ventricular premature beats (Figure 13-27, *C*)
Bounding pulse	Increased pulse pressure; contour may have rapid rise, brief peak, rapid fall	Atherosclerosis, aortic rigidity, patent ductus arteriosus, fever, anemia, hyperthyroidism, anxiety, exercise (Figure 13-27, *D*)
Bradycardia	Rate less than 60	Hypothermia, hypothyroidism, drug intoxication, impaired cardiac conduction, excellent physical conditioning
Labile pulse	Normal when patient is resting but increases on standing or sitting	Not necessarily associated with disease; not a specific indicator of a problem
Paradoxic pulse (pulsus paradoxus)	Amplitude decreases on inspiration	Chronic obstructive pulmonary disease, constrictive pericarditis, pericardial effusion (Figure 13-27, *E*)
Pulsus differens	Unequal pulses between left and right extremities	Impaired circulation, usually from unilateral local obstruction
Tachycardia	Rate over 100	Fever, hyperthyroidism, anemia, shock, heart disease, anxiety, exercise
Trigeminal pulse (pulsus trigeminus)	Three beats followed by a pause	Often benign, such as after exercise; but may occur with cardiomyopathy, severe ventricular hypertrophy, severe aortic stenosis, dysfunctional right ventricle
Water-hammer pulse (Corrigan pulse)	Jerky pulse with full expansion followed by sudden collapse	Aortic regurgitation (Figure 13-27, *F*)

Characteristics. Palpation of arterial pulses (most often the radial) can indicate heart rate and rhythm, pulse contour (wave form), amplitude (strength), symmetry, and sometimes obstructions to blood flow. Variations from the expected findings are described in Table 13-8 and Figure 13-27.

The pulse rate (heart rate) is determined by counting the pulsations for 60 seconds (or counting for 30 seconds and doubling the count). The resting pulse rate should range between 60 and 90 per minute.

Determine the steadiness of the heart rhythm, which should be regular. If it is irregular, determine whether there is a consistent pattern. A heart rate that is irregular but occurs in a repeated pattern may indicate *sinus arrhythmia,* a cyclic variation of the heart rate that is characterized by an increasing rate on inspiration and decreasing rate on expiration. A patternless, unpredictable irregular rate may indicate heart disease or conduction system impairment.

The contour of the pulse wave in pliable, healthy arteries has a smooth, rounded, or domed shape. Attention should be paid to the ascending portion, the peak, and the descending portion. Each wave crest should be compared with the next to detect cyclic differences.

PULSE   **POSSIBLE CAUSE**

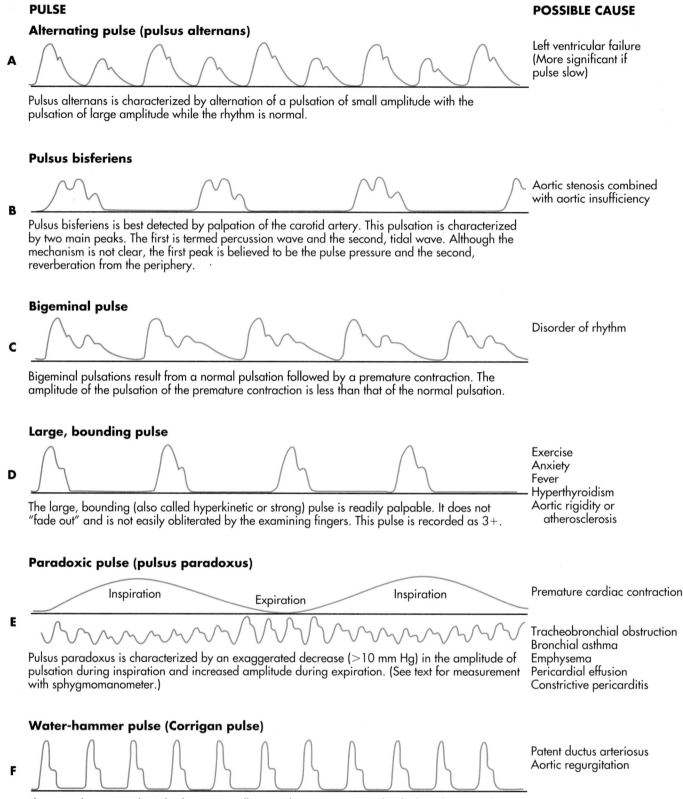

Alternating pulse (pulsus alternans)

A

Left ventricular failure (More significant if pulse slow)

Pulsus alternans is characterized by alternation of a pulsation of small amplitude with the pulsation of large amplitude while the rhythm is normal.

Pulsus bisferiens

B

Aortic stenosis combined with aortic insufficiency

Pulsus bisferiens is best detected by palpation of the carotid artery. This pulsation is characterized by two main peaks. The first is termed percussion wave and the second, tidal wave. Although the mechanism is not clear, the first peak is believed to be the pulse pressure and the second, reverberation from the periphery.

Bigeminal pulse

C

Disorder of rhythm

Bigeminal pulsations result from a normal pulsation followed by a premature contraction. The amplitude of the pulsation of the premature contraction is less than that of the normal pulsation.

Large, bounding pulse

D

Exercise
Anxiety
Fever
Hyperthyroidism
Aortic rigidity or atherosclerosis

The large, bounding (also called hyperkinetic or strong) pulse is readily palpable. It does not "fade out" and is not easily obliterated by the examining fingers. This pulse is recorded as 3+.

Paradoxic pulse (pulsus paradoxus)

Inspiration   Expiration   Inspiration

E

Premature cardiac contraction

Tracheobronchial obstruction
Bronchial asthma
Emphysema
Pericardial effusion
Constrictive pericarditis

Pulsus paradoxus is characterized by an exaggerated decrease (>10 mm Hg) in the amplitude of pulsation during inspiration and increased amplitude during expiration. (See text for measurement with sphygmomanometer.)

Water-hammer pulse (Corrigan pulse)

F

Patent ductus arteriosus
Aortic regurgitation

The water-hammer pulse (also known as collapsing) has a greater amplitude than the normal pulse, a rapid rise to a narrow summit, and a sudden descent.

FIGURE 13-27

Pulse abnormalities.

Modified from Barkauskas, 1998.

The amplitude of the pulse is described on a scale of 0 to 4:

4 = bounding
3 = full, increased
2 = expected
1 = diminished, barely palpable
0 = absent, not palpable

Lack of symmetry between the left and right extremities suggests impaired circulation. Compare the strength of the upper extremity pulses with those of the lower extremities and the left with the right. Ordinarily, the femoral is as strong as or stronger than the radial pulse. If this is reversed or if the femoral pulsation is absent, coarctation of the aorta must be suspected.

Auscultation

Auscultation over an artery for a bruit (murmur or unexpected sound) is indicated when you are following the radiation of murmurs or looking for evidence of local obstruction. These sounds are usually low pitched and relatively hard to hear. Using the bell of the stethoscope and asking the patient to hold a breath for a few heartbeats will help. Sites at which to auscultate for a bruit are the temporal, carotid, subclavian, abdominal aorta, renal, iliac, and femoral arteries (Figure 13-28).

BOX 13-9 | **Determination of a Paradoxic Pulse* by Sphygmomanometer**

Determination of a paradoxic pulse may be an important diagnostic finding. The difference in systolic pressure between expiration and inspiration should be 5 mm Hg. If it is greater than 10 mm Hg, the paradoxic pulse is *exaggerated*. This may be associated with a serious constraint on the heart's action caused by cardiac tamponade or constrictive pericarditis or great respiratory effort as occurs with emphysema. Associated findings include low blood pressure and weak and rapid pulse.

- Ask the patient to breathe as easily and comfortably as possible; remember that this is a difficult assignment when one is being observed.
- Apply the sphygmomanometer and inflate it until no sounds are audible.
- Deflate the cuff *gradually* until sounds are audible *only* during expiration.
- Note the pressure.
- Deflate the cuff further until sounds are also audible during inspiration.
- Note the pressure.

*Paradoxic pulse is the usual fall in systolic pressure during inspiration.

A 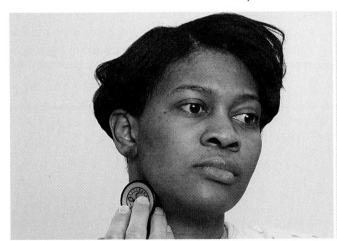   **B**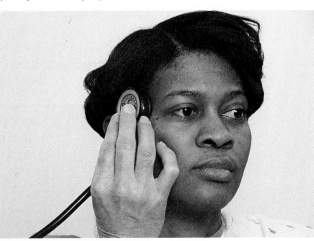

FIGURE 13-28
Auscultation for bruits. **A,** Carotid artery. **B,** Temporal artery.

Carotid artery bruits are best heard at the anterior margin of the sternocleido-mastoid muscle. These may include the following types:

- Transmitted murmurs resulting from valvular aortic stenosis, ruptured chordae tendineae of the mitral valve, or severe aortic regurgitation
- Vigorous left ventricular ejection (more common in children than in adults)
- Obstructive disease in cervical arteries, such as atherosclerotic carotid arteries, fibromuscular hyperplasia, or arteritis.

Mild obstruction produces a short, but not particularly intense, localized bruit; greater obstruction lengthens the duration and heightens the pitch. Complete obstruction eliminates the bruit.

Assessment for Arterial Occlusion and Insufficiency

Arteries in any location can become occluded or in some manner traumatized, making them insufficient to their task. The resultant diminution in circulation to the tissues will lead to signs and symptoms that are related to the following:

- Site
- Degree of occlusion
- Ability of collateral channels to compensate
- Rapidity with which the problem develops

The first symptom is pain that results from muscle ischemia, referred to as "claudication" (Box 13-10). This pain can be characterized as a dull ache with accompanying muscle fatigue and often crampiness. It usually appears during sustained exercise, such as walking a distance or climbing several flights of stairs. Just a few minutes of rest will ordinarily relieve it. It recurs again with the same amount of activity.

The site of pain is distal to the occlusion. After determining the distinguishing characteristics of the pain, you should note the following:

- Pulses (weak and thready, or possibly absent)
- Possible systolic bruits over the arteries that may extend through diastole
- Loss of expected body warmth in the affected area
- Localized pallor and cyanosis
- Collapsed superficial veins, with delay in venous filling
- Thin, atrophied skin; muscle atrophy; and loss of hair (particularly in the case of long-term insufficiency, which accentuates skin mottling and increases the likelihood of ulceration, localized anesthesia, and tenderness)

Three *p*'s therefore characterize occlusion—*pain, pallor,* and *pulselessness*—and, in the presence of an acute occlusion of a major artery, a fourth *p* occurs—*paresthesias,* and occasionally, a fifth—*paralysis,* completing the *compartment syndrome.*

To judge the degree of occlusion and the potential severity of the arterial occlusion, perform the following steps:

BOX 13-10   **Comparison of Pain from Vascular Insufficiencies and Musculoskeletal Disorders**

Arterial	Venous and Musculoskeletal
Comes on during exercise	Comes on during or often several hours after exercise
Quickly relieved by rest	Relieved by rest but sometimes only after several hours or even days; pain tends to be constant
Intensity increases with the intensity and duration of exercise	Greater variability than arterial pain in response to intensity and duration of exercise

- Have the patient lie supine.
- Elevate the extremity.
- Note the degree of blanching.
- Have the patient sit on the edge of the bed or examining table to lower the extremity.
- Note the time for maximal return of color after the extremity is elevated. Slight pallor on elevation and a return to full color as soon as the leg becomes dependent is the expected finding. If there is a delay of many seconds or even minutes before the extremity regains full color, arterial occlusion is present. When return to full color takes as long as 2 minutes, the problem is severe.

A measurement of the *capillary refill time* provides another method of assessing severity (Box 13-11).

The following list provides a general guideline for pain assessment:

LOCATION	PROBABLE OBSTRUCTED ARTERY
Calf muscles	Superficial femoral artery
Thigh	Common femoral artery or external iliac artery
Buttock	Common iliac artery or distal aorta (impotence may accompany occlusion of distal aorta)

If the pain is constant, the occlusion was probably acute, and if it is excruciating, a major artery has probably been severely compromised.

Blood Pressure

Blood pressure is usually measured in the patient's arm and should be measured in both arms at least once (Box 13-12). The patient's arm should be slightly flexed and comfortably supported on a table, pillow, or your hand. Be sure that the arm is free of clothing. Center the deflated bladder over the brachial artery, just medial to the biceps tendon, with the lower edge 2 to 3 cm above the antecubital crease. Apply an appropriately sized cuff (see Chapter 3, Examination Techniques and Equipment) snugly and securely because a loose cuff will give an inaccurate diastolic measurement.

BOX 13-11 Capillary Refill Time

The capillary bed joins the arterial and venous systems. It is the bodywide structure that allows fluid exchange between the vascular and interstitial spaces, as a result of the competitive and complementary interaction of the hydrostatic pressures of the blood and interstitial tissues and the colloid osmotic pressures of plasma and interstitial fluids. This interplay in the healthy person allows dominance of hydrostatic pressure at the arterial end of the capillary bed (pushing fluid out) and of the colloid osmotic pressure at the venous end (pulling fluid in), helping them to maintain the balance of fluids in the intravascular and extravascular spaces.

The time it takes the capillary bed to fill after it is occluded by pressure gives some indication of the health of the system. This is referred to as the *capillary refill time*. To gauge the capillary refill time, perform the following:
- Blanch the nail bed with a sustained pressure of several seconds on a toenail or fingernail.
- Release the pressure.
- Observe the time elapsed before the nail regains its full color.

If the system is intact, this should occur almost instantly—in *less than 2 seconds*. If, however, the system is compromised (e.g., during arterial occlusion, hypovolemic shock, or hypothermia), the refill time will be *more than 2 seconds*, and much longer if circulatory compromise is severe.

CAUTION: Environmental influences, such as even moderately decreased ambient temperature, may influence capillary time by prolonging it, thus suggesting a problem that may not exist. In addition, there is variability among examiners in defining the time. Therefore the capillary refill time should not be considered an observation with exquisite sensitivity and specificity and should be used only cautiously in making clinical judgments.

Checking the palpable systolic blood pressure first will help you avoid being misled by an auscultatory gap when you listen with the stethoscope. Place the fingers of one hand over the brachial or radial artery. Rapidly inflate the cuff with the hand bulb 20 to 30 mm Hg above the point at which you no longer feel the brachial pulse. Deflate the cuff slowly at a rate of 2 to 3 mm Hg per second until you again feel at least two beats of the brachial pulse. This point is the palpable systolic blood pressure. Immediately deflate the cuff completely (Figure 13-29, *A*).

A 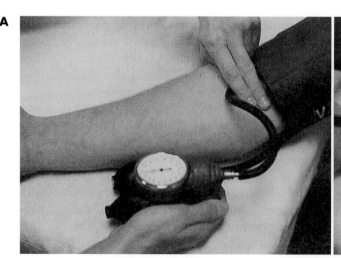 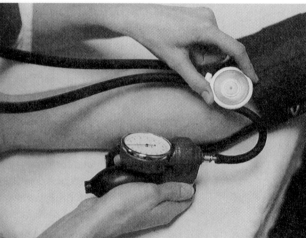 B

FIGURE 13-29
Blood pressure measurement. **A,** Checking palpable systolic pressure. **B,** Using bell of stethoscope.

Now place the bell of the stethoscope over the brachial artery and, pausing for 30 seconds, again inflate the cuff until it is 20 to 30 mm Hg above the palpable systolic blood pressure (Figure 13-29, *B*). The bell of the stethoscope is more effective than the diaphragm in transmitting the low-pitched sound produced by the turbulence of blood flow in the artery (Korotkoff sounds). Deflate the cuff slowly as previously described, listening for the following sounds (Figure 13-30):

- Two consecutive beats indicate the systolic pressure and also the beginning of phase 1 of the Korotkoff sounds.
- Occasionally, the Korotkoff sounds will be heard, disappear, and reappear 10 to 15 mm Hg later (phase 2). The period of silence is the auscultatory gap. You should be aware of the possibility of this gap, or you may underestimate the systolic pressure or overestimate the diastolic pressure. The auscultatory gap widens in the instance of systolic hypertension in elderly persons (with loss of arterial pliability) or a drop in diastolic pressure (with chronic severe aortic regurgitation). It narrows in the event of pulsus paradoxus with cardiac tamponade or other constrictive cardiac events.
- Note the point at which the sounds, which are first crisp (phase 3), become muffled (phase 4). This is the first diastolic sound, which is considered to be the closest approximation of direct diastolic arterial pressure. It signals imminent disappearance of the Korotkoff sounds.
- Note the point at which the sounds disappear (phase 5). This is the second diastolic sound. Now deflate the cuff completely.

The American Heart Association recommends recording three values for the blood pressure: the systolic and both diastolic measures (for example, 110/76/68). If only two values are recorded, they are the systolic and the second diastolic pressures (for example, 100/68). The difference between the systolic and diastolic pressures is the pulse pressure. The expected range is approximately 100 to 140 mm Hg for the systolic pressure and 60 to 90 mm Hg for the (second) diastolic. The pulse pressure should range from 30 to 40 mm Hg, even to as much as 50 mm Hg.

Repeat the process in the other arm. Readings between the arms may vary by as much as 10 mm Hg and tend to be higher in the right arm; the higher reading should be accepted as closest to the patient's blood pressure. Record both sets of measurements.

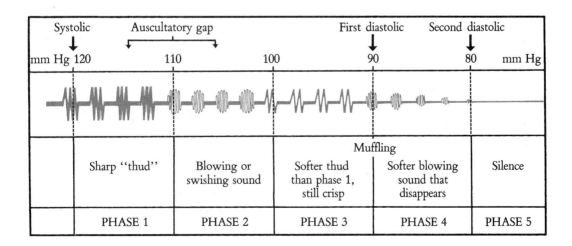

FIGURE 13-30

Phases of Korotkoff sounds, including an example of auscultatory gap.

TABLE 13-9	**Classification of Blood Pressure for Adults Age 18 and Older***		
Category	**Systolic (mm Hg)**		**Diastolic (mm Hg)**
Optimal[†]	<120	and	<80
Normal	<130	and	<85
High-normal	130-139	or	85-89
Hypertension[‡]			
Stage 1	140-159	or	90-99
Stage 2	160-179	or	100-109
Stage 3	≥180	or	≥110

*Not taking antihypertensive drugs and not acutely ill. When systolic and diastolic blood pressures fall into different categories, the higher category should be selected to classify the individual's blood pressure status. For example, 160/92 mm Hg should be classified as stage 2 hypertension, and 174/120 mm Hg should be classified as stage 3 hypertension. Isolated systolic hypertension is defined as systolic blood pressure of 140 mm Hg or greater and diastolic blood pressure below 90 mm Hg and staged appropriately (e.g., 170/82 mm Hg is defined as stage 2 isolated systolic hypertension). In addition to classifying stages of hypertension on the basis of average blood pressure levels, clinicians should specify presence or absence of target organ disease and additional risk factors. This specificity is important for risk classification and treatment.
†Optimal blood pressure with respect to cardiovascular risk is below 120/80 mm Hg. However, unusually low readings should be evaluated for clinical significance.
‡Based on the average of two or more readings taken at each of two or more visits after an initial screening.
From NIH Publication No. 98-4080, November, 1997.

Since the systolic pressure is more labile and more readily responsive to a wide range of physical and emotional stimuli, hypertension is usually defined on the basis of several measurements taken over a period of time. The Joint National Committee on prevention, detection, evaluation, and treatment of high blood pressure has classified blood pressure for adults (Table 13-9). Most cases of hypertension in adults have no discoverable cause and are referred to as "essential hypertension." Since the elevation of blood pressure may, for a time, be the only significant clinical finding, persons with hypertension are often asymptomatic. Individuals who complain of frequent epistaxis or recurrent morning headaches that disappear as the day progresses certainly deserve careful monitoring of their blood pressure.

If the diastolic pressure in the arms is above 90 mm Hg or you suspect coarctation of the aorta or aortic insufficiency, measure the blood pressure in the legs. The patient should be prone, if possible; if supine, the leg should be flexed as little as possible. Center the thigh cuff bladder over the posterior surface and wrap the cuff securely on the distal third of the femur. Measure the pressure over the popliteal artery using the same procedure as for the brachial artery. A Doppler measurement may be helpful in this regard. Leg pressures, which are usually higher than arm pressures, will be lower with coarctation of the aorta or aortic stenosis.

If the patient is taking antihypertensive medications, has a depleted blood volume, or complains of fainting or postural dizziness, blood pressure in the arm should also be measured with the patient standing. Ordinarily, as a patient changes position from supine to standing, there is a slight or no drop in systolic pressure and a slight rise in diastolic pressure. However, if postural hypotension is present, expect to see a significant drop in systolic pressure (greater than 15 mm Hg) and a drop in diastolic pressure. Even a mild blood loss (such as from blood donation), drugs, autonomic nervous system disease, or prolonged stay in a recumbent position can contribute to postural hypotension. Patients at risk in this regard should have the blood pressure taken at first when supine, then standing.

With even impeccable technique, the accuracy of the blood pressure reading may be undermined by some conditions:

- Cardiac arrhythmias: An infrequent odd beat may be ignored, but if the irregularity is sustained, it is a good idea to take the average of several pressures and to write a note about the uncertainty.
- Aortic regurgitation: The sounds of aortic regurgitation do not disappear, thus obscuring the diastolic pressure.
- Venous congestion: Sluggish venous flow from a pathologic event can cause the systolic pressure to be heard lower than it actually is and the diastolic pressure higher. Repeated, slow inflations of the cuff can also cause venous congestion.
- Valve replacement: The sounds may be heard all the way down to a zero gauge reading; listen carefully for the first muffling of the sound (Korotkoff phase 4) to determine the diastolic pressure.

PERIPHERAL VEINS

Jugular Venous Pressure

Careful measurement of the jugular venous pressure (JVP) is an important and, in some instances, critical portion of the physical examination. Several techniques may be utilized. The simplest, most reproducible and reliable method requires a ruler at least 15 cm long. Folding rulers with guides for ECG analysis are widely available and useful for this purpose. In the most convenient mode of examination, a bed or examining table is used whose angle of back support can be adjusted. Ideally, a pen light is also used to supply tangential light across the neck to accentuate the appearance of the jugular venous pulsations. Review Figure 13-15.

The patient is placed in the supine position initially. This position results in engorgement of the jugular veins. The head of the bed is gradually raised until the jugular venous pulsations become evident between the angle of the jaw and the clavicle (Figure 13-31). Palpating the contralateral carotid pulse will help identify the venous pulsations and distinguish them from the carotid pulsations. Table 13-10 provides instructions on differentiating between jugular and carotid pulses.

Several conditions may make the examination more difficult: (1) Severe right heart failure, tricuspid insufficiency, constrictive pericarditis, and cardiac tamponade may all cause extreme elevation of the JVP so that it is not apparent until the patient is sitting upright; 2) severe volume depletion makes it difficult to detect the JVP even when the patient is supine; and 3) extreme obesity obscures the jugular venous pulsations by overlying adipose tissue.

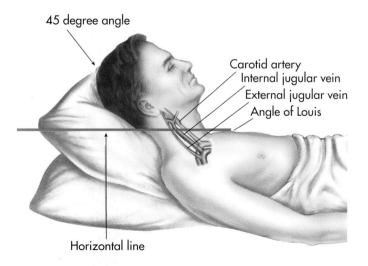

FIGURE 13-31

Inspection of jugular venous pressure.

From Thompson et al, 1997.

	Jugular	Carotid
Quality and Character Palpate the carotid artery on one side of the neck and look at the jugular vein on the other to tell the difference	Three positive waves in normal sinus rhythm More undulating	One wave More brisk
Effect of Respiration	Level of pulse wave decreased on inspiration and increased on expiration	No effect
Effect of Changing Position	More prominent when recumbent; less prominent when sitting	No effect
Venous Compression Apply gentle pressure over vein at base of neck above clavicle	Easily eliminates pulse wave	No effect
Abdominal Pressure Place the palm moderately firmly over the right upper quadrant of the abdomen for half a minute	May cause some increased prominence even in well persons; with right- sided failure, jugular vein may be more visible	No effect

TABLE 13-10 Comparison of the Jugular and Carotid Pulse Waves

A ruler is placed with its origin at the mid-axillary line at the level of the nipple (the position of the heart within the chest) and extended vertically. The level of the meniscus of the JVP is extended horizontally until it intersects the vertical ruler, and the vertical distance above the level of the heart is noted as the mean jugular venous pressure in centimeters water (Figure 13-32). A value of less than 9 cm H_2O is the expected value. The number can be divided by 1.3 to calculate its value in millimeters of mercury.

Maneuvers useful for confirming the jugular venous pressure measurement include hepatojugular reflux and evaluation of the venous engorgement of the hands at various levels of elevation above the heart.

Hepatojugular Reflux

Some have erroneously suggested that the hepatojugular reflux is a sign of right heart failure. All patients will have elevation of the JVP with this maneuver depending on the elevation of their head with respect to the heart and their underlying venous pressure. The hepatojugular reflux is exaggerated when right heart failure is present.

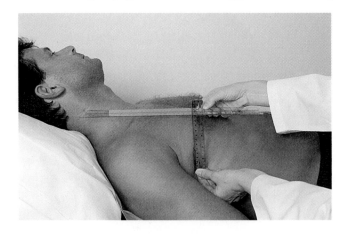

FIGURE 13-32

Measuring jugular venous pressure.

The hepatojugular reflux maneuver entails applying firm and sustained pressure to the abdomen in the mid-epigastric region with the examiner's hand while the patient is instructed to breathe regularly. The neck is then observed for a simultaneous elevation in jugular venous pressure followed by an abrupt fall in JVP as the hand pressure is released. The JVP quickly equilibrates to its true level between the positions it achieved with and immediately after removal of the abdominal hand pressure.

This maneuver is analogous to focusing a camera by turning the focus ring one way and then the other until the picture is the sharpest. If the jugular venous pressure is not obvious with this maneuver, the pressure is either much higher or much lower than the patient's current neck position with relation to the heart. The maneuver should then be repeated with the patient more supine if you suspect the pressure to be lower or with the patient more upright if you suspect the JVP to be higher.

Evaluation of Hand Veins

The veins of the hand can be used as an auxiliary "manometer" of the right heart pressure in the absence of thrombosis of the hand or subclavian vein, the absence of an AV fistula in that arm, and in the absence of the superior vena cava syndrome. With the patient semirecumbent, place the hand on the exam table or mattress. Palpate the hand veins, which should be engorged to make sure they are compressible and not thrombosed. Slowly raise the hand until the hand veins collapse (Figure 13-33). Note the vertical distance between the mid-axillary line at the nipple level (level of the heart) and the level of collapse of the hand veins. Confirm this level by lowering the hand slowly until the veins distend again and raise it back until they once again collapse. This distance should be identical to the mean jugular venous pressure.

The hand vein measurement is particularly helpful at the extremes of jugular venous pressure: severe right heart failure where the pressure may be 20 to 30 cm H_2O (i.e., not evident with the patient sitting upright) or volume depletion (i.e., not visible with the patient supine).

Assessment for Venous Obstruction and Insufficiency

Obstruction of the venous system and a consequent insufficiency will result in signs and symptoms that vary depending on the rapidity with which the occlusion develops and on the degree of localization. An acute process may result from injury, external compression, or thrombophlebitis. Pain—a constant pain—is one of the first symptoms (see Box 13-10). In the affected area, pain occurs simultaneously with the following:

- Swelling and tenderness over the muscles
- Engorgement of superficial veins
- Erythema and/or cyanosis

A 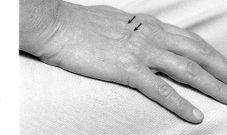 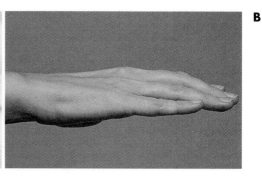 B

FIGURE 13-33
Evaluation of hand veins. **A,** Engorged veins in dependent hand. **B,** Collapsed veins in elevated hand.

The extremities should be inspected for signs of venous insufficiency (thrombosis, varicose veins, or edema). The patient should be examined in both the standing and supine positions, particularly in the case of a suspected chronic venous occlusion.

Thrombosis. Note any redness, thickening, and tenderness along a superficial vein; these findings together suggest thrombophlebitis of a superficial vein. A deep vein thrombosis cannot be confirmed on physical exam alone, but it is suspected if swelling, pain, and tenderness occur over a vein. (An occluded artery does not result in swelling.) Flex the patient's knee slightly with one hand and, with the other, dorsiflex the foot to test for *Homans sign. The complaint of calf pain with this procedure is a positive sign and usually indicates thrombosis.*

Be certain that you do not confuse calf pain with Achilles tendon pain, a common finding in athletes who frequently stress the Achilles tendon and in women who wear high-heeled shoes. Avoid this confusion by keeping the knee slightly flexed when you dorsiflex the foot.

Edema. Inspect the extremities for edema, manifested as a change in the usual contour of the leg. Press your index finger over the bony prominence of the tibia or medial malleolus for several seconds. A depression that does not rapidly refill and resume its original contour indicates orthostatic (pitting) edema, which is not usually accompanied by thickening or pigmentation of the overlying skin. Right-sided heart failure leads to an increased fluid volume, which in turn elevates the hydrostatic pressure in the vascular space, causing edema in dependent parts of the body.

Edema accompanied by some thickening and ulceration of the skin is associated with deep venous obstruction or valvular incompetence. Edema related to valvular incompetence or an obstruction of a deep vein (usually in the legs) is caused by the mechanical-pressure of increased blood volume in the area served by the affected vein. Circulatory disorders that cause edema so tense that it does not pit must be distinguished from lymphedema (see Chapter 8, Lymphatic System).

The severity of edema may be characterized by grading 1+ through 4+ (Figure 13-34). Any concomitant pitting can be mild or severe, as evidenced by the following:

1+: slight pitting, no visible distortion, disappears rapidly

2+: a somewhat deeper pit than in 1+, but again no readily detectable distortion, and it disappears in 10-15 sec

3+: the pit is noticeably deep and may last more than a minute; the dependent extremity looks fuller and swollen

4+: the pit is very deep, lasts as long as 2-5 min, and the dependent extremity is grossly distorted

REMINDER: If edema is unilateral, suspect the occlusion of a major vein. If edema occurs without pitting, suspect arterial disease and occlusion.

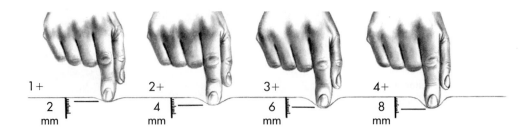

FIGURE 13-34
Assessing for pitting edema.
From Canobbio, 1990.

1+   2 mm

2+   4 mm

3+   6 mm

4+   8 mm

Varicose Veins. Varicose veins are dilated and swollen, with a diminished rate of blood flow and an increased intravenous pressure. These characteristics may be the result of incompetence of the vessel wall or venous valves or an obstruction in a more proximal vein.

Superficial varicosities are easy to detect on inspection, particularly when the patient is standing. The veins appear dilated and often tortuous when the extremities are dependent. If varicose veins are suspected, have the patient stand on the toes 10 times in succession. This will build a palpable pressure in the veins. If the venous system is competent, the pressure in the veins will disappear in just a few seconds. If not, the feeling of pressure in the veins will be sustained for a longer time, and the return to the pretest state will be quite sluggish.

When varicosities are present, the *Trendelenburg test* is used to evaluate venous incompetence. With the patient supine, lift the leg above the level of the heart until the veins empty. Then lower the leg quickly. An incompetent system will allow rapid filling of the veins.

The *Perthes test* is used to evaluate the patency of deep veins. With the patient supine and the extremity elevated, occlude the subcutaneous veins with a tourniquet just above the knee to prevent filling of superficial varicosities from above. As the patient walks, muscular tension will act on the deep veins and empty the dilated superficial varicosities. When these superficial veins fail to empty, suspect that the deep veins are also somewhat incompetent.

To evaluate the direction of blood flow and the competency of the valves in the venous system, distend visible veins by putting the limb in a dependent position. Compress the vein with the finger or thumb of one hand and strip the vein of blood by compressing it with fingers of the second hand. If the compressed vessel fills before either compressing finger is released, there is collateral circulation. If the compressing finger nearest the heart is released, the vessel should fill backward to the first valve only. If the entire venous column fills, the valves in that vessel are incompetent.

INFANTS

The newborn presents a challenge because of the immediate change from fetal to systemic and pulmonary circulation. Examine the heart within the first 24 hours and again at about 2 to 3 days of age.

Complete evaluation of heart function includes examination of the skin, lungs, and liver. Infants with right-sided congestive heart failure have large, firm livers with the inferior edge as much as 5 to 6 cm below the right costal margin. Unlike adults, this finding may precede that of pulmonary crackles.

Inspect the color of the skin and mucous membranes. The well newborn should be reassuringly pink. A purplish plethora is associated with polycythemia, an ashy white color indicates shock, and central cyanosis (cyanosis of the skin and mucous membranes of the head and body) suggests congenital heart disease. Note the distribution and intensity of discoloration, as well as the extent of change after vigorous exertion. Acrocyanosis, cyanosis of the hands and feet without central cyanosis, is of little concern; it usually disappears within a very few days, or even a few hours, after birth.

Cyanosis distinguishes the problems that lead to admixture of arterial and venous blood or prevent the expected oxygenation of blood. Severe cyanosis evident at birth or shortly thereafter suggests transposition of the great vessels, tetralogy of Fallot, tricuspid atresia, a severe septal defect, or severe pulmonic stenosis. Cyanosis that does not appear until after the neonatal period suggests a pure pulmonic stenosis, Eisenmenger complex, tetralogy of Fallot, or large septal defects.

The apical impulse in the newborn is usually seen and felt at the fourth to fifth left intercostal space just medial to the midclavicular line. The smaller the baby or the thinner the chest, the more obvious it will be. It may be somewhat farther to the right in the first few hours of life, sometimes even substernal.

Note any enlargement of the heart. It is especially important to note the position of the heart if a baby is having trouble breathing. A pneumothorax shifts the apical impulse away from the area of the pneumothorax. A diaphragmatic hernia, more commonly found on the left, shifts the heart to the right. Dextrocardia results in an apical impulse on the right.

The right ventricle is relatively more vigorous than the left in a well, full-term newborn. If the baby is thin, you might even be able to feel the closure of the pulmonary valve in the second left intercostal space.

S_2 in infants is somewhat higher in pitch and more discrete than S_1. The vigor and quality of the heart sounds of the newborn (and throughout infancy and early childhood) are major indicators of the function of the heart. Diminished vigor may be the only apparent change when an infant is already in heart failure. Splitting of the heart sounds is common. S_2 is usually heard without a split at birth, then often splits within a few hours.

Murmurs are relatively frequent in the newborn until about 48 hours of age. Most are innocent, caused by the transition from fetal to pulmonic circulation rather than a significant congenital abnormality. These murmurs are usually of grade I or II intensity, systolic, and unaccompanied by other signs and symptoms; they usually disappear within 2 to 3 days. Paradoxically, a significant congenital abnormality may be unaccompanied by a murmur.

If you cannot tell a murmur from respiration, pinch the nares briefly, listen while the baby is feeding, or time the sound with the carotid pulsation. Because of the rapid heart rate in infants, the heart sounds are more difficult to evaluate. A murmur heard immediately at birth is apt to be less significant than one detected after the first few hours of life. If a murmur persists beyond the second or third day of life, is intense, fills systole, occupies diastole to any extent, or radiates widely, it must be investigated. If you push up on the liver, thereby increasing right atrial pressure, the murmur of a left-to-right shunt through a septal opening or patent ductus will disappear briefly, whereas the murmur of a right-to-left shunt will intensify.

Murmurs that extend beyond S_2 and occupy diastole are said to have a machinelike quality; they may be associated with a patent ductus arteriosus. The murmur should disappear when the patent ductus closes in the first 2 or 3 days of life. Diastolic murmurs, almost always significant, may nevertheless be transient and possibly related to an early closing ductus arteriosus or a mild, brief pulmonary insufficiency.

In the newborn suspected of having cardiovascular difficulty, auscultate the head and the abdomen for bruits to detect arteriovenous malformations.

Infants' heart rates are more variable than those of older children. Eating, sleeping, and waking can change the rate considerably. The variation is greatest at birth or shortly after and is even more marked in premature infants. Rates close to 200 per minute are not uncommon, but they may also indicate paroxysmal atrial tachycardia. Ordinarily, the decrease in rate is relatively rapid, and at a few hours of age the rate may be much closer to 120. A relatively fixed tachycardia is a clue to some difficulty.

The brachial, radial, and femoral pulses of the newborn are easily palpable. When the pulse is weaker or thinner than expected, the cardiac output may be diminished, or peripheral vasoconstriction may be present. A bounding pulse is associated with a large left-to-right shunt produced by a patent ductus arteriosus. Differ-

THE INFANT LIVER AND THE HEART

If heart failure is suspected, note that the infant's liver may enlarge before there is any suggestion of moisture in the lungs, and that the left lobe of the liver may be more distinctly enlarged than the right.

ence in pulse amplitude between the upper extremities or between the femoral and radial pulses suggests a coarctation of the aorta, as does absence of the femoral pulses.

The usual blood pressure measurement techniques may be difficult to implement in infants and very young children. A small arm and the problem of obtaining cooperation suggest the alternative of the "flush technique":

- Place the cuff on the upper arm (or leg).
- Elevate and wrap the arm firmly with an elastic bandage from fingers to antecubital space, thus emptying the veins and capillaries.
- Inflate the cuff to a pressure above the systolic reading you expect.
- Lower the arm and remove the bandage. (The arm will be pale.)
- Diminish the pressure gradually until you see a sudden "flush" and a return to usual color in the forearm and hand, a quite definitive endpoint.

The resultant value is generally both lower than the systolic pressure and higher than the diastolic pressure obtained through auscultation and palpation.

Electronic sphygmomanometers with a Doppler or other oscillometric technique work by sensing vibrations, converting them to electrical impulses, and transmitting them to a device that produces a digital readout. They are relatively sensitive and can also simultaneously measure the pulse rate. If the readout and clinical impression are not consistent, you may validate the readout by taking the pressure with a manual cuff. However, Doppler devices are more sensitive than stethoscopes to the first Korotkoff sound. The usual newborn blood pressure ranges from 60 to 96 mm Hg systolic and 30 to 62 mm Hg diastolic. A *sustained* increase in blood pressure is almost always significant.

Hypertension in the newborn may be the result of thrombosis after the use of an umbilical catheter, stenosis of the renal artery, coarctation of the aorta, cystic disease of the kidney, neuroblastoma, Wilms tumor, hydronephrosis, adrenal hyperplasia, or central nervous system disease. Capillary refill times in infants and children younger than 2 years of age are very rapid, less than 1 second. A prolonged capillary refill time, longer than 2 seconds, indicates a significant degree of dehydration or hypovolemic shock.

CHILDREN

The precordium of a child tends to bulge over an enlarged heart if the enlargement is of long standing. A child's thoracic cage, being more cartilaginous and yielding than that of an adult, responds more to the thrust of cardiac enlargement.

Sinus arrhythmia is a physiologic event during childhood. The heart rate varies in a cyclic pattern, usually faster on inspiration and slower on expiration. Most often, other arrhythmias in children are ectopic in origin, for example, supraventricular and ventricular ectopic beats. These and a variety of other seeming "irregularities" require *extensive* investigation only occasionally.

The heart rates of children are more variable than those of adults, reacting with wider swings to stress of any sort (exercise, fever, tension). It is not uncommon to discover an increase of 10 to 20 beats in the heart rate for each degree of temperature elevation. The expected heart rates in children vary with age:

AGE	RATE (BEATS PER MINUTE)
Newborn	120-170
1 year	80-160
3 years	80-120
6 years	75-115
10 years	70-110

A *venous hum,* common in children, usually has no pathologic significance (Box 13-13). It is caused by the turbulence of blood flow in the internal jugular veins. To detect a venous hum, ask the child to sit with the head turned to the left and tilted slightly upward (to the right if you are listening on the left). Auscultate over the right supraclavicular space at the medial end of the clavicle and along the anterior border of the sternocleidomastoid muscle (Figure 13-35). The intensity of the hum is increased when the patient is sitting with the head turned away from the area of auscultation, and it is diminished with a Valsalva maneuver. When present, the hum is a continuous low-pitched sound that is louder during diastole. It may be interrupted by gentle pressure over the vein in the space between the trachea and the sternocleidomastoid muscle at about the level of the thyroid cartilage. Although this hum is heard less often in adults, particularly younger adults, it can be elicited in some by firm pressure with the stethoscope, particularly in those with high cardiac output states (for example, as occur during thyrotoxicoses, pregnancy, or anemia). The venous hum can be confused with patent ductus arteriosus, aortic regurgitation, and the murmur of valvular aortic stenosis transmitted into the carotid arteries.

BOX 13-13 **Listening to the Neck**

Venous Hum

- Heard at medial end of clavicle and anterior border of sternocleidomastoid muscle
- Usually or no clinical significance.
- Confused with carotid bruit, patent ductus arteriosus, and aortic regurgitation
- When in adults, usually occurs with anemia, pregnancy, thyrotoxicosis, and intracranial arteriovenous malformation

Carotid Artery Bruits

- Heard at medial end of clavicle and anterior margin of sternocleidomastoid muscle
- Transmitted murmurs: valvular aortic stenosis, ruptured chordae tendineae of mitral valve, and severe aortic regurgitation
- Can be heard with vigorous left ventricular ejection (more commonly heard in children than in adults)
- Occur with obstructive disease in cervical arteries (e.g., atherosclerotic carotid arteries, fibromuscular hyperplasia, and arteritis.)

Mild obstruction produces a short, not particularly intense, localized bruit; greater obstruction lengthens the duration and increases the pitch. Virtual or complete obstruction will eliminate the bruit.

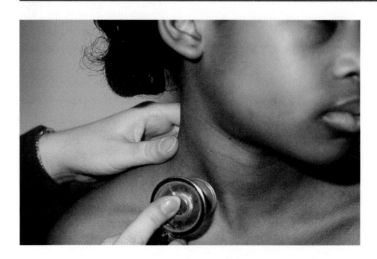

FIGURE 13-35
Auscultation for venous hum.

Most organic murmurs in infants and children are the result of congenital heart disease. However, acute rheumatic fever still accounts for most acquired murmurs, and its occurrence has been on the rise in recent years.

When examining a child with known heart disease, take careful note of weight gain (or loss), developmental delay, cyanosis, and clubbing of fingers and toes. Cyanosis is a major key to congenital heart defects that impede oxygenation of blood.

Regardless of what you may have heard, blood pressure is easy to measure in children past the age of 2 or 3 years. The correct cuff size is mandatory (see Figure 3-2, p. 56). Korotkoff phase 4 sound should be considered the appropriate diastolic reading, until adolescence when Korotkoff phase 5 is used. Children like to explore the sphygmomanometer, and full explanation of the process and a moment of playing with the instrument can facilitate examination. If your ability to hear is compromised by the child's crying or a deeply placed brachial artery, palpate the radial artery if a digital sphygmomanometer is not available. This will yield a systolic pressure about 10 mm Hg less than that at the brachial artery.

Do not make the diagnosis of hypertension on the basis of one reading. Many readings should be taken over time. If the systolic pressure is elevated and the diastolic is not, transient anxiety may be responsible. Take time to reassure the child to alleviate the anxiety. Studies suggest that in children the blood pressure varies with sex and height at any age. Values for significant (90th percentile) and severe (95th percentile) hypertension have been compiled by the Task Force on High Blood Pressure in Children. See Tables 13-11 and 13-12. Children with pressures consistently above the 95th percentile must be carefully studied and followed. It is unlikely for a child to have unexplained hypertension (the possibility is greater in the adolescent). Most often hypertension in children is caused by kidney disease, renal arterial disease, coarctation of the aorta, or pheochromocytoma.

Hypertension occurs in approximately 1% to 3% of all children. Those who have hypertension are by and large not severely afflicted at the start. Perhaps 10% will have serious, even life-threatening, problems. Of these, 80% to 90% will have underlying renal disease. If hypertension is severe and sustained, there is a possibility of great morbidity and mortality. Clearly, early detection and treatment are essential. In childhood as in adult life, blood pressures should always be checked during physical exam. Blood pressures consistently above the expected range, some 10 to 20 mm Hg above the 95th percentile, should be considered carefully. The physical examination is the source of early discovery (Dillon, 1987).

FACIAL PALSY

Severe hypertension in children may be accompanied by a facial palsy that disappears when the hypertension is treated. When there is such a palsy, always be sure to check the blood pressure.

From Siegler, 1991.

PREGNANT WOMEN

The heart rate gradually increases throughout pregnancy until it is 10 to 15 beats per minute higher by the end of the third trimester. Blood pressure readings gradually fall until they reach a nadir at 16 to 20 weeks and then gradually rise to prepregnant levels at term. A sustained systolic blood pressure of 140 mm Hg or greater or a diastolic pressure of 90 mm Hg or more should alert you to the probability of pregnancy-induced hypertension (PIH).

The heart position is shifted during pregnancy, but the position varies with the size and position of the uterus. The apical impulse is upward and more lateral by 1 to 1.5 cm. Some changes in auscultated heart sounds are expected because of the increased blood volume and extra effort of the heart. There is more audible splitting of S_1 and S_2, and S_3 may be readily heard after 20 weeks of gestation. In addition, grade II systolic ejection murmurs may be heard over the pulmonic area in 90% of pregnant women. The murmur is intensified during inspiration or expiration.

| TABLE 13-11 | Blood Pressure Levels for the 90th and 95th Percentiles of Blood Pressure for Boys Aged 1 to 17 Years by Percentiles of Height |

Age, y	Blood Pressure Percentile*	Systolic Blood Pressure by Percentile of Height, mm Hg†							Diastolic Blood Pressure by Percentile of Height, mm Hg†						
		5%	10%	25%	50%	75%	90%	95%	5%	10%	25%	50%	75%	90%	95%
1	90th	94	95	97	98	100	102	102	50	51	52	53	54	54	55
	95th	98	99	101	102	104	106	106	55	55	56	57	58	59	59
2	90th	98	99	100	102	104	105	106	55	55	56	57	58	59	59
	95th	101	102	104	106	108	109	110	59	59	60	61	62	63	63
3	90th	100	101	103	105	107	108	109	59	59	60	61	62	63	63
	95th	104	105	107	109	111	112	113	63	63	64	65	66	67	67
4	90th	102	103	105	107	109	110	111	62	62	63	64	65	66	66
	95th	106	107	109	111	113	114	115	66	67	67	68	69	70	71
5	90th	104	105	106	108	110	112	112	65	65	66	67	68	69	69
	95th	108	109	110	112	114	115	116	69	70	70	71	72	73	74
6	90th	105	106	108	110	111	113	114	67	68	69	70	70	71	72
	95th	109	110	112	114	115	117	117	72	72	73	74	75	76	76
7	90th	106	107	109	111	113	114	115	69	70	71	72	72	73	74
	95th	110	111	113	115	116	118	119	74	74	75	76	77	78	78
8	90th	107	108	110	112	114	115	116	71	71	72	73	74	75	75
	95th	111	112	114	116	118	119	120	75	76	76	77	78	79	80
9	90th	109	110	112	113	115	117	117	72	73	73	74	75	76	77
	95th	113	114	116	117	119	121	121	76	77	78	79	80	80	81
10	90th	110	112	113	115	117	118	119	73	74	74	75	76	77	78
	95th	114	115	117	119	121	122	123	77	78	79	80	80	81	82
11	90th	112	113	115	117	119	120	121	74	74	75	76	77	78	78
	95th	116	117	119	121	123	124	125	78	79	79	80	81	82	83
12	90th	115	116	117	119	121	123	123	75	75	76	77	78	78	79
	95th	119	120	121	123	125	126	127	79	79	80	81	82	83	83
13	90th	117	118	120	122	124	125	126	75	76	76	77	78	79	80
	95th	121	122	124	126	128	129	130	79	80	81	82	83	83	84
14	90th	120	121	123	125	126	128	128	76	76	77	78	79	80	80
	95th	124	125	127	128	130	132	132	80	81	81	82	83	84	85
15	90th	123	124	125	127	129	131	131	77	77	78	79	80	81	81
	95th	127	128	129	131	133	134	135	81	82	83	83	84	85	86
16	90th	125	126	128	130	132	133	134	79	79	80	81	82	82	83
	95th	129	130	132	134	136	137	138	83	83	84	85	86	87	87
17	90th	128	129	131	133	134	136	136	81	81	82	83	84	85	85
	95th	132	133	135	136	138	140	140	85	85	86	87	88	89	89

*Blood pressure percentile was determined by a single measurement.
†Height percentile was determined by standard growth curves.
Data from Update on the Task Force Report (1987) on High Blood Pressure in Children and Adolescents: A working group report from National High Blood Pressure Education Program, NIH 96-3790. Printed in Update on Task Force Report on High Blood Pressure in Children, *Pediatrics* 98:649-658, 1996.

OLDER ADULTS

You may need to slow the pace of your examination when asking some older patients to assume positions that may be uncomfortable or perhaps too difficult. Some may not be able to lie flat for an extended time, and some may not be able to control their breathing pattern at your request. Since the cardiac response to even minimal demand may be slowed or insufficient, even a moderately abrupt position change may cause a transient syncope, as may the drop in arterial pressure after a moderate meal.

The heart rate may be slower because of increased vagal tone, or more rapid, with a wide range from the low 40s to more than 100. Occasional ectopic beats are fairly common and may or may not be significant.

TABLE 13-12 Blood Pressure Levels for the 90th and 95th Percentiles of Blood Pressure for Girls Aged 1 to 17 Years by Percentiles of Height

Age, y	Blood Pressure Percentile*	Systolic Blood Pressure by Percentile of Height, mm Hg†							Diastolic Blood Pressure by Percentile of Height, mm Hg†						
		5%	10%	25%	50%	75%	90%	95%	5%	10%	25%	50%	75%	90%	95%
1	90th	97	98	99	100	102	103	104	53	53	53	54	55	56	56
	95th	101	102	103	104	105	107	107	57	57	57	58	59	60	60
2	90th	99	99	100	102	103	104	105	57	57	58	58	59	60	61
	95th	102	103	104	105	107	108	109	61	61	62	62	63	64	65
3	90th	100	100	102	103	104	105	106	61	61	61	62	63	63	64
	95th	104	104	105	107	108	109	110	65	65	65	66	67	67	68
4	90th	101	102	103	104	106	107	108	63	63	64	65	65	66	67
	95th	105	106	107	108	109	111	111	67	67	68	69	69	70	71
5	90th	103	103	104	106	107	108	109	65	66	66	67	68	68	69
	95th	107	107	108	110	111	112	113	69	70	70	71	72	72	73
6	90th	104	105	106	107	109	110	111	67	67	68	69	69	70	71
	95th	108	109	110	111	112	114	114	71	71	72	73	73	74	75
7	90th	106	107	108	109	110	112	112	69	69	69	70	71	72	72
	95th	110	110	112	113	114	115	116	73	73	73	74	75	76	76
8	90th	108	109	110	111	112	113	114	70	70	71	71	72	73	74
	95th	112	112	113	115	116	117	118	74	74	75	75	76	77	78
9	90th	110	110	112	113	114	115	116	71	72	72	73	74	74	75
	95th	114	114	115	117	118	119	120	75	76	76	77	78	78	79
10	90th	112	112	114	115	116	117	118	73	73	73	74	75	76	76
	95th	116	116	117	119	120	121	122	77	77	77	78	79	80	80
11	90th	114	114	116	117	118	119	120	74	74	75	75	76	77	77
	95th	118	118	119	121	122	123	124	78	78	79	79	80	81	81
12	90th	116	116	118	119	120	121	122	75	75	76	76	77	78	78
	95th	120	120	121	123	124	125	126	79	79	80	80	81	82	82
13	90th	118	118	119	121	122	123	124	76	76	77	78	78	79	80
	95th	121	122	123	125	126	127	128	80	80	81	82	82	83	84
14	90th	119	120	121	122	124	125	126	77	77	78	79	79	80	81
	95th	123	124	125	126	128	129	130	81	81	82	83	83	84	85
15	90th	121	121	122	124	125	126	127	78	78	79	79	80	81	82
	95th	124	125	126	128	129	130	131	82	82	83	83	84	85	86
16	90th	122	122	123	125	126	127	128	79	79	79	80	81	82	82
	95th	125	126	127	128	130	131	132	83	83	83	84	85	86	86
17	90th	122	123	124	125	126	128	128	79	79	79	80	81	82	82
	95th	126	126	127	129	130	131	132	83	83	83	84	85	86	86

*Blood pressure percentile was determined by a single reading.
†Height percentile was determined by standard growth curves.
Data from Update on the Task Force Report (1987) on High Blood Pressure in Children and Adolescents: A working group report from National High Blood Pressure Education Program, NIH 96-3790. Printed in Update on Task Force Report on High Blood Pressure in Children, *Pediatrics* 98:649-658, 1996.

The apical impulse may be harder to find in many persons because of the increased anteroposterior diameter of the chest. In obese older adults, the diaphragm is raised and the heart is more transverse.

The elderly who exercise regularly may reverse or defer some of the age-associated changes.

S_4 is more common in older adults and may indicate decreased left ventricular compliance. Early, soft, physiologic murmurs may be heard, caused by aortic lengthening, tortuosity, and sclerotic changes.

The dorsalis pedis and posterior tibial pulses may be more difficult to find, and the superficial vessels are more apt to appear tortuous and distended.

Because of loss of elasticity of the vessels in the process of aging, the systolic blood pressure may increase. Hypertension in the elderly is defined as a pressure greater than 140/90. The suggestion that the systolic blood pressure should be less than 120 + the patient's age is no longer acceptable. Many practitioners do consider other factors, in addition to the blood pressure itself, when deciding to undertake therapy.

SAMPLE DOCUMENTATION

Heart: No visible pulsations over precordium. The point of maximal impulse (PMI) palpable at the 5th ICS in the MCL, 1 cm in diameter. No lifts, heaves, or thrills felt on palpation. S_1 is crisp. Split S_2 increases with inspiration. No audible S_3, S_4, murmur, click, or rub.

Vessels: Neck veins not distended. Both A and V waves are visualized. The JVP is 4 cm H_2O at 45 degrees. Arterial pulses equal and symmetrical, testing on a scale of x/4.

	C	B	R	F	P	PT	DP
L	2+	2+	2+	2+	2+	2+	2+
R	2+	2+	2+	2+	2+	2+	2+

Vessels soft. No bruits are audible.

Extremities: No edema, skin, or nail changes. Superficial varicosities noted in both lower extremities. No areas of tenderness to palpation.

For additional sample documentation, see Chapter 24, Recording Information.

SUMMARY OF EXAMINATION   Heart and Blood Vessels

Heart

The following steps are performed with the patient sitting and leaning forward, supine, and in the left lateral recumbent positions; these positions are all used to compare findings or enhance the assessment.

1. Inspect the precordium for the following (p. 430):
   - Apical impulse
   - Pulsations
   - Heaves or lifts
2. Palpate the precordium to detect the following (p. 431):
   - Apical impulse
   - Thrills, heaves, or lifts
3. Percussion to estimate the heart size (optional) (p. 433).
4. Systematically auscultate in each of the five areas while the patient is breathing regularly and holding breath for the following (pp. 433-441):
   - Rate
   - Rhythm
   - S_1
   - S_2
   - Splitting
   - S_3 and/or S_4
   - Extra heart sounds (snaps, clicks, friction rubs, and murmurs)
5. Assess the following characteristics of murmurs (pp. 441-444):
   - Timing and duration
   - Pitch
   - Intensity
   - Pattern
   - Quality
   - Location
   - Radiation
   - Variation with respiratory phase

Blood Vessels

1. Palpate the arterial pulses in distal extremities, comparing characteristics bilaterally for the following (p. 444):
   - Rate
   - Rhythm
   - Contour
   - Amplitude
2. Auscultate the carotid, temporal, abdominal aorta, renal, iliac, and femoral arteries for bruits (p. 449).
3. Measure the blood pressure in both arms, first supine and then, in patients at risk for orthostatic hypotension, standing (pp. 451-455).
4. With the patient reclining at a 45-degree angle elevation, inspect for jugular venous pulsations and distention; differentiate jugular and carotid pulse waves, and measure jugular venous pressure (pp. 455-457).
5. Inspect the extremities for sufficiency of arteries and veins through the following (pp. 457-459):
   - Color, skin texture, and nail changes
   - Presence of hair
   - Muscular atrophy
   - Edema or swelling
   - Varicose veins
6. Palpate the extremities for the following (pp. 449, 458):
   - Warmth
   - Pulse quality
   - Tenderness along a superficial vein
   - Pitting edema

COMMON ABNORMALITIES

CARDIAC DISORDERS

HEART MURMURS

The most common source of significant murmurs is anatomic disorder of the valves of the heart (Figure 13-36 and Table 13-13.).

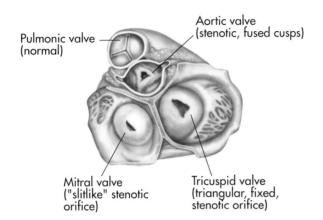

FIGURE 13-36
Valvular heart disease.
Modified from Canobbio, 1990.

TABLE 13-13	Heart Murmurs		
Type and Detection	**Findings on Examination**	**Description**	
Mitral Stenosis			
Heard with bell at apex, patient in left lateral decubitus	Low-frequency diastolic rumble, more intense in early and late diastole, does not radiate; systole usually quiet; palpable thrill at apex in late diastole common; S_1 increased and often palpable at left sternal border; S_2 split often with accented P_2; opening snap follows P_2 closely Visible lift in right parasternal area if right ventricle hypertrophied Arterial pulse amplitude decreased	Narrowed valve restricts forward flow; forceful ejection into ventricle Often occurs with mitral regurgitation Caused by rheumatic fever or cardiac infection	Mitral valve Mitral valve stenosis

Continued

TABLE 13-13   Heart Murmurs—cont'd

Type and Detection	Findings on Examination	Description	
Aortic Stenosis			
Heard over aortic area; ejection sound at second right inter-costal border	Midsystolic (ejection) murmur, medium pitch, coarse, diamond shaped,* crescendo-decrescendo; radiates down left sternal border (sometimes to apex) and to carotid with palpable thrill; S_1 often heard best at apex, disappearing when stenosis is severe, often followed by ejection click; S_2 soft or absent and may not be split; S_4 palpable; ejection sound muted in calcified valves; the more severe the stenosis, the later the peak of the murmur in systole Apical thrust shifts down and left and is prolonged if left ventricular hypertrophy is also present.	Calcification of valve cusps restricts forward flow; forceful ejection from ventricle into systemic circulation Caused by congenital bicuspid (rather than the expected tricuspid) valves, rheumatic heart disease, atherosclerosis May be the cause of sudden death, particularly in children and adolescents, either at rest or during exercise; risk apparently related to degree of stenosis	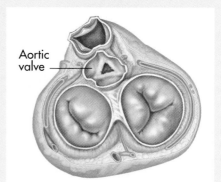 Aortic valve Aortic valve stenosis
Subaortic Stenosis			
Heard at apex and along left sternal border	Murmur fills systole, diamond shaped, medium pitch, coarse; thrill often palpable during systole at apex and right sternal border; multiple waves in apical impulses; S_2 usually split; S_3 and S_4 often present Arterial pulse brisk, double wave in carotid common; jugular venous pulse prominent	Fibrous ring, usually 1 to 4 mm below aortic valve; most pronounced on ventricular septal side; may become progressively severe with time; difficult to distinguish from aortic stenosis on clinical grounds alone	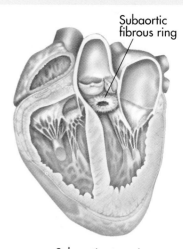 Subaortic fibrous ring Subaortic stenosis

*Diamond-shaped murmur is named for its recorded shape on photocardiogram (a crescendo-decrescendo sound).

TABLE 13-13   Heart Murmurs—cont'd

Type and Detection	Findings on Examination	Description	
Pulmonic Stenosis			
Heard over pulmonic area radiating to left and into neck; thrill in second and third left intercostal space	Systolic (ejection) murmur, diamond shaped, medium pitch, coarse; usually with thrill; S_1 often followed quickly by ejection click; S_2 often diminished, usually wide split; P_2 soft or absent; S_4 common in right ventricular hypertrophy; murmur may be prolonged and confused with that of a ventricular septal defect	Valve restricts forward flow; forceful ejection from ventricle into pulmonary circulation Cause is almost always congenital	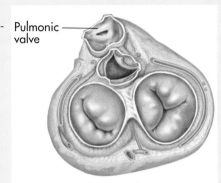 Pulmonic valve stenosis
Tricuspid Stenosis			
Heard with bell over tricuspid area	Diastolic rumble accentuated early and late in diastole, resembling mitral stenosis but louder on inspiration; diastolic thrill palpable over right ventricle; S_2 may be split during inspiration Arterial pulse amplitude decreased; jugular venous pulse prominent, especially a wave; slow fall of v wave	Calcification of valve cusps restricts forward flow; forceful ejection into ventricles Usually seen with mitral stenosis, rarely occurs alone Caused by rheumatic heart disease, congenital defect, endocardial fibroelastosis, right atrial myxoma	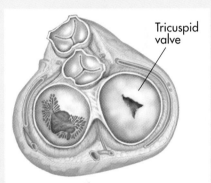 Tricuspid valve stenosis
Mitral Regurgitation			
Heard best at apex; loudest there, transmitted into left axilla	Holosystolic, plateau-shaped intensity, high pitch, harsh blowing quality, often quite loud and may obliterate S_2; radiates from apex to base or to left axilla; thrill may be palpable at apex during systole; S_1 intensity diminished; S_2 more intense with P_2 often accented; S_3 often present; S_3-S_4 gallop common in late disease If mild, late systolic murmur crescendos; if severe, early systolic intensity decrescendos; apical thrust more to left and down in ventricular hypertrophy	Valve incompetence allows backflow from ventricle to atrium Caused by rheumatic fever, myocardial infarction, myxoma, rupture of chordae	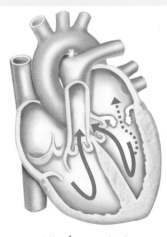 Mitral regurgitation (heart in systole)

Continued

TABLE 13-13 | Heart Murmurs—cont'd

Type and Detection	Findings on Examination	Description	
Mitral Valve Prolapse			
Heard at apex and left lower sternal border; easily missed in supine position; also listen with patient upright	Typically late systolic murmur preceded by midsystolic clicks, but both murmur and clicks highly variable in intensity and timing	Valve is competent early in systole but prolapses into atrium later in systole; may become progressively severe, resulting in a holosystolic murmur; frequently concurrent with pectus excavatum	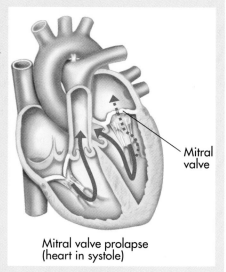 Mitral valve Mitral valve prolapse (heart in systole)
Aortic Regurgitation			
Heard with diaphragm, patient sitting and leaning forward; Austin-Flint murmur heard with bell; ejection click heard in second intercostal space	Early diastolic, high pitch, blowing, often with diamond-shaped midsystolic murmur, sounds often not prominent; duration varies with blood pressure; low-pitched, rumbling murmur at apex common (Austin-Flint); early ejection click sometimes present; S_1 soft; S_2 split may have tambourlike quality; M_1 and A_2 often intensified, S_3-S_4 gallop common In left ventricular hypertrophy, prominent prolonged apical impulse down and to left Pulse pressure wide; water-hammer or bisferiens pulse common in carotid, brachial, and femoral arteries	Valve incompetence allows backflow from aorta to ventricle Caused by rheumatic heart disease, endocarditis, aortic diseases (Marfan syndrome, medial necrosis), syphilis, ankylosing spondylitis, dissection, cardiac trauma	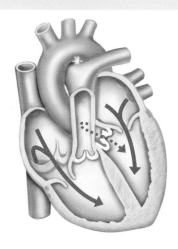 Aortic regurgitation (heart in diastole)

TABLE 13-13 Heart Murmurs—cont'd

Type and Detection	Findings on Examination	Description	
Pulmonic Regurgitation	Difficult to distinguish from aortic regurgitation on physical examination	Valve incompetence allows backflow from pulmonary artery to ventricle Secondary to pulmonary hypertension or bacterial endocarditis	Pulmonic regurgitation (heart in diastole)
Tricuspid Regurgitation Heard at left lower sternum, occasionally radiating a few centimeters to left	Holosystolic murmur over right ventricle, blowing, increased on inspiration; S_3 and thrill over tricuspid area frequent In pulmonary hypertension, pulmonary artery impulse palpable over second left intercostal space and P_2 accented; in right ventricular hypertrophy, visible lift to right of sternum Jugular venous pulse has large v waves	Valve incompetence allows backflow from ventricle to atrium Caused by congenital defects, bacterial endocarditis (especially in IV drug abusers), pulmonary hypertension, cardiac trauma	Tricuspid regurgitation (heart in systole)

LEFT VENTRICULAR HYPERTROPHY

The left ventricle works harder and longer with each beat when it meets increased resistance to the emptying of blood into the systemic circulation, as with aortic stenosis, volume overload, and systemic hypertension. It hypertrophies because of the extra exercise and, sometimes, becomes displaced laterally. A vigorous sustained lift is palpable during ventricular systole, sometimes over a broader area than usual, as much as 2 cm or more. The displacement of the apical impulse can be most impressive, well lateral to the midclavicular line and downward.

RIGHT VENTRICULAR HYPERTROPHY	The right ventricle works harder and enlarges with defects of the pulmonary vascular bed and pulmonary hypertension. This is less common than left ventricular hypertrophy. It can cause a lift along the left sternal border in the third and fourth	left intercostal spaces accompanied by occasional systolic retraction at the apex. The left ventricle is not itself particularly affected, but it is displaced and turned posteriorly by the enlarged right ventricle.

SICK SINUS SYNDROME	In sick sinus syndrome, sinoatrial dysfunction occurs secondary to hypertension, arteriosclerotic heart disease, or rheumatic heart disease; it may also occur idiopathi-	cally. The condition causes fainting, transient dizzy spells, light-headedness, seizures, palpitations, and symptoms of angina and congestive heart failure.

BACTERIAL ENDOCARDITIS

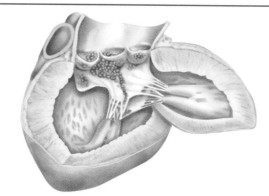

FIGURE 13-37
Bacterial endocarditis.
Modified from Canobbio, 1990.

A bacterial infection of the endothelial layer of the heart and valves should be suspected with prolonged fever, signs of neurologic dysfunctions, and sudden onset of congestive heart failure. A murmur may or may not be present. Individuals with valvular defects, congenital or acquired, and those who use intravenous drugs are particularly susceptible (Figure 13-37). Janeway lesions and Osler nodes are characteristic.

CONGESTIVE HEART FAILURE	Congestive heart failure is a syndrome in which the heart fails to propel blood forward normally, resulting in congestion in the pulmonary or systemic circulation. Decreased cardiac output causes decreased blood flow to the tissues. Congestive heart	failure may be predominantly left- or right-sided. It can develop gradually or suddenly with acute pulmonary edema. The prevalence increases more markedly with age, particularly after 50 years, more rapidly among women than among men.

PERICARDITIS

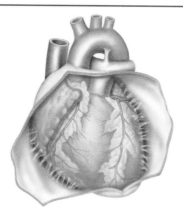

FIGURE 13-38
Pericarditis.
Modified from Canobbio, 1990.

Pericardial disease, which is relatively infrequent, may be confused with more common and occasionally life-threatening cardiac conditions. Chest pain is the usual initial symptom in acute pericarditis, inflammation of the pericardium. The key physical finding is the triphasic friction rub, which comprises ventricular systole, early diastolic ventricular filling, and late diastolic atrial systole. It occurs in well over nine of ten patients with the disease. It is best heard just to the left of the sternum in the third and fourth intercostal spaces and is characteristically scratchy, grating, and very easily heard even in the presence of considerable pericardial effusion. As an acute pericarditis persists and becomes subacute or chronic, the effusion may increase and result in cardiac tamponade (Figure 13-38).

CARDIAC TAMPONADE

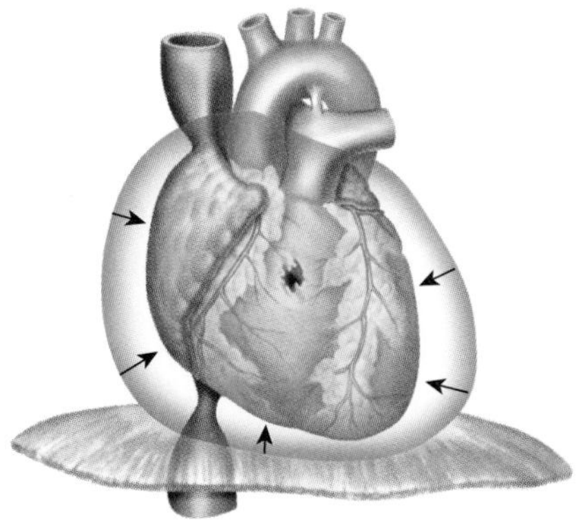

FIGURE 13-39
Hemopericardium and cardiac tamponade.
Modified from Canobbio, 1990.

Hemopericardium and tamponade

An excessive accumulation of effused fluids or blood between the pericardium and heart results in cardiac tamponade (Figure 13-39). *Excessive* is difficult to define because as much as 300 ml of fluid may not constrain cardiac function in the adult. In any event, a sufficient amount seriously constrains cardiac relaxation, impairing access of blood to the right heart and ultimately causing the signs and symptoms of systemic venous congestion—edema, ascites, and dyspnea. A chronically and severely involved pericardium may also scar and constrict, forming in a sense a "shell" around the heart that limits cardiac filling. In this circumstance, heart sounds are muffled, blood pressure drops, the pulse becomes weakened and rapid, and the paradoxic pulse becomes exaggerated. Pericarditis and trauma are frequent causes of tamponade.

COR PULMONALE

Cor pulmonale is the enlargement of the right ventricle secondary to pulmonary malfunction. Usually chronic but occasionally acute, cor pulmonale results from chronic obstructive pulmonary disease. Alterations in the pulmonary circulation lead to pulmonary arterial hypertension, which imposes a mechanical load on right ventricular emptying. Signs include left parasternal systolic lift and a loud S_2 exaggerated in the pulmonic region.

MYOCARDIAL INFARCTION

Ischemic myocardial necrosis is caused by an abrupt decrease in coronary blood flow to a segment of the myocardium. It most commonly affects the left ventricle, but damage may extend into the right ventricle or atria. Symptoms commonly include deep substernal or visceral pain that often radiates to the jaw, neck, and left arm, although discomfort may be mild, especially in older adults or patients with diabetes mellitus. Dysrhythmias are common, and S_4 is usually present. Heart sounds are typically distant, with a soft systolic blowing apical murmur. Pulse may be thready, and blood pressure varies, although hypertension is usual in the early phases. Atherosclerosis and thrombosis are the common underlying causes.

MYOCARDITIS

Focal or diffuse inflammation of the myocardium can result from infectious agents or toxins. Initial symptoms are typically vague and include fatigue, dyspnea, fever, and palpitations. As the disease process advances, cardiac enlargement, murmurs, gallop rhythms, tachycardia, arrhythmias, and pulsus alternans develop.

ABNORMALITIES IN HEART RATES AND RHYTHMS

CONDUCTION DISTURBANCES

Conduction disturbances occur either proximal to the bundle of His or diffusely throughout the conduction system. They produce symptoms of transient weakness, fainting spells, or strokelike episodes. Heart block may result from a variety of disturbances—ischemic, infiltrative, or more rarely, neoplastic. Unusual dysrhythmias—whether fast or slow, with or without block—may result in fainting, particularly in elderly persons. Antidepressant drugs, digitalis, or quinidine can be a precipitating factor. With these attacks, cardiac syncope may occur acutely and without particular warning; sometimes a diminished sensibility, a "gray-out" instead of a "black-out," may precede the event. Heart rates are often labile and disturbances in rhythm not at all unusual (Table 13-14).

TABLE 13-14	**Abnormalities in Rates and Rhythms**	
Type and Detection	**Findings on Examination**	**Description**
Atrial (Auricular) Flutter	Atrial rate far in excess of ventricular rate; heart sounds not necessarily weak	Regular uniform atrial contractions occur in excess of 200/min, but the ventricular response is limited as a result of heart block. The conduction system cannot respond to the rapidity of the atrial rate, causing variance from the ventricular rate. The ECG may look like a saw-tooth cog.
Atrial flutter with a constant 4:1 conduction ratio. From Guzzetta, Dossey, 1984.		
Sinus Bradycardia	Slow rate, sometimes below 50 or 60/min	There is no disruption in conduction; not necessarily suggestive of a problem.
Sinus bradycardia. From Guzzetta, Dossey, 1984.		

TABLE 13-14	Abnormalities in Rates and Rhythms—cont'd		
Type and Detection	**Findings on Examination**	**Description**
Atrial Fibrillation Atrial fibrillation with rapid ventricular response. From Guzzetta, Dossey, 1992.	Dysrhythmic contraction of the atria gives way to rapid series of irregular spasms of the muscle wall; no discernible regularity in rhythm or pattern	The conduction system is malfunctioning and is in an anarchic state. Any contraction of the atria that gets through to the ventricle is irregular. The sounds are best described as irregularly irregular.
Heart Block Sinus rhythm with first-degree AV block. From Guzzetta, Dossey, 1992.	Heart rate slower than expected, often 25-45/min at rest	Conduction from atria to ventricles partially or completely disrupted. If conduction is completely disrupted, the ventricle may be left to beat on its own and the heart rate slows considerably. ECG is necessary to determine the extent and nature of heart block in conduction.
Atrial Tachycardia Paroxysmal atrial tachycardia (PAT). From Guzzetta, Dossey, 1992.	Rapid, regular heart rate (≈200/min) without disruption of the rhythm; may be heard only on occasion (in paroxysms) and without loss of vigor in heart sounds	This is the result of electrical stimulus originating in a focus in the atrium separate from the SA node. Conduction through to the ventricle is usually complete. Often there is no other evidence of disease, and the patient is usually a young adult. The rate will occasionally respond to vagal stimulation, holding a deep breath, or gentle massage of a carotid sinus. (Remember that massage always must be done with care.)

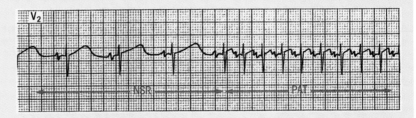

Continued

TABLE 13-14	Abnormalities in Rates and Rhythms—cont'd	
Type and Detection	**Findings on Examination**	**Description**
Ventricular Tachycardia Ventricular tachycardia. From Guzzetta, Dossey, 1992.	Rapid, relatively regular heartbeat (often nearly 200/min) without loss in apparent strength	The electrical source of the beat is in an unusual focus somewhere in the ventricles. This usually arises in serious heart disease and is a grave prognostic sign.
Ventricular Fibrillation Ventricular fibrillation. From Guzzetta, Dossey, 1992.	Complete loss of regular heart rhythm with expected conduction pattern absent; if weakened and rapid, ventricular contraction is irregular	The ventricle has lost the rhythm of its expected response, and all evidence of vigorous contraction is gone. It calls for immediate action and may immediately precede sudden death.

CONGENITAL DEFECTS

TETRALOGY OF FALLOT

Four cardiac defects make up the tetralogy of Fallot: ventricular septal defect, pulmonic stenosis, dextroposition of the aorta, and right ventricular hypertrophy. Infants with tetralogy of Fallot often have paroxysmal dyspnea with loss of consciousness and central cyanosis; older children develop clubbing of fingers and toes. There is a parasternal heave and precordial prominence. A systolic ejection murmur is heard over the third intercostal space, sometimes radiating to the left side of the neck. A single S_2 is heard (Figure 13-40). Surgical correction, currently initiated after the first "spell" in infancy, may allow the tolerance of effort to approach the expected for ordinary day-to-day living.

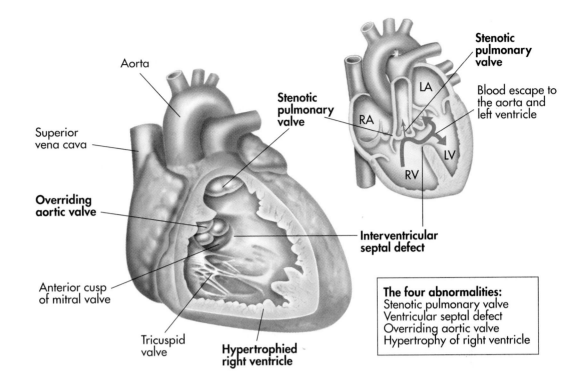

FIGURE 13-40
Tetralogy of Fallot.
Modified from Canobbio, 1990.

The four abnormalities:
Stenotic pulmonary valve
Ventricular septal defect
Overriding aortic valve
Hypertrophy of right ventricle

VENTRICULAR SEPTAL DEFECT

Ventricular septal defect is an opening between the left and right ventricles. The arterial pulse is small, and the jugular venous pulse is unaffected. Regurgitation occurs through the septal defect; as a result, the murmur tends to be holosystolic. It is frequently loud, coarse, high-pitched, and best heard along the left sternal border in the third to fifth intercostal spaces. A distinct lift is often discernible along the left sternal border and the apical area. A smaller defect causes a louder murmur and a more easily felt thrill than a large one (Figure 13-41). This murmur does not radiate to the neck, whereas a similar murmur—the result of subaortic stenosis—does.

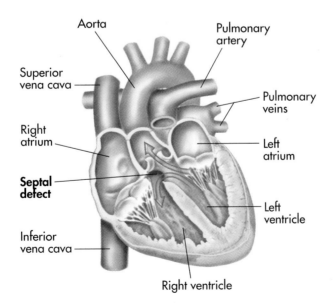

FIGURE 13-41
Ventricular septal defect.
Modified from Canobbio, 1990.

COARCTATION OF THE AORTA

Coarctation of the aorta is a congenital stenosis or narrowing most commonly in the descending aortic arch near the origin of the left subclavian artery and ligamentum arteriosum (Figure 13-42). If present, it will be detected most often during infancy and should be routinely sought. When the radial and femoral pulses are palpated simultaneously, they will ordinarily be perceived to peak at the same time, the femoral slightly earlier perhaps than the radial. If there is a delay and/or a palpable diminution in amplitude (not necessarily an absence) of the femoral pulse, coarctation must be suspected. The findings will be the same on both the right and left sides of the body. Blood pressure readings taken in the arms and legs should confirm the suspicion. They will be distinctly, even severely, higher in the arms than in the legs. (Blood pressure in the legs will ordinarily be the same as or even slightly higher than that in the arms.) A systolic murmur may be audible over the precordium and, at times, over the back relative to the area of the coarctation. In adults, x-ray film may show notching of the ribs and a "3" sign in the contour of the left upper border of the heart, caused by dilation of the aorta distal to the area of the coarctation, which is then adjacent to the shadow of the descending thoracic aorta. If coarctation remains undetected, the aorta may dissect or rupture, and endocarditis and congestive heart failure are possible. The results of surgery are usually excellent.

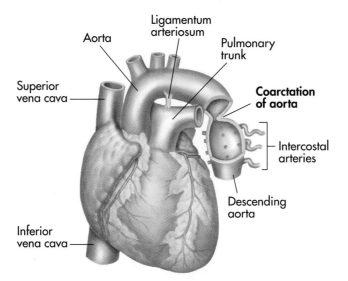

FIGURE 13-42
Coarctation of the aorta.
Modified from Canobbio, 1990.

PATENT DUCTUS ARTERIOSUS

Sometimes the ductus arteriosus, which is patent in the fetal circulation, fails to close after birth. Blood flows through the ductus during systole and diastole, increasing the pressure in the pulmonary circulation and consequently the workload of the right ventricle. A small shunt can be asymptomatic; a larger one causes dyspnea on exertion. The neck vessels are dilated and pulsate, and the pulse pressure is wide. A harsh, loud, continuous murmur is often heard at the first to third intercostal spaces and the lower sternal border. It has a machinelike quality (Figure 13-43). This murmur is usually, but not always, unaltered by postural change, quite unlike the murmur of a venous hum.

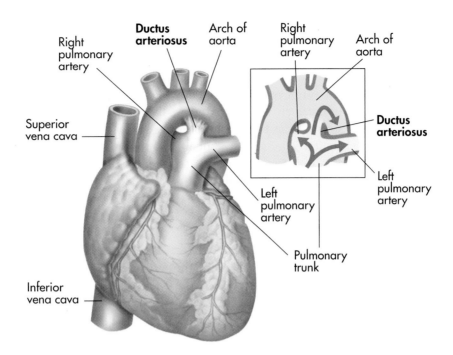

FIGURE 13-43

Patent ductus arteriosus.

Modified from Canobbio, 1990.

ATRIAL SEPTAL DEFECT

A congenital defect in the septum dividing the left and right atria causes a systolic ejection murmur that is diamond shaped, often loud, high in pitch, and harsh. It is heard best over the pulmonic area and not over the lesion, and may be accompanied by a brief, rumbling, early diastolic murmur. It does not usually radiate beyond the precordium. A systolic thrill may be felt over the area of the murmur, along with a palpable parasternal thrust. S_2 may be split fairly widely (Figure 13-44). Sometimes this murmur may not sound particularly impressive and, especially in an overweight child, may seem of little consequence. Still, if there is a palpable thrust and, on occasion, radiation through to the back, it is more apt to be significant.

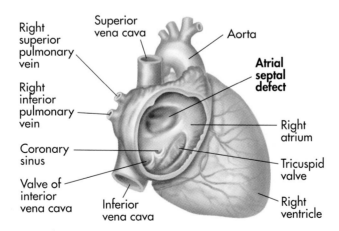

FIGURE 13-44

Atrial septal defect.

From Canobbio, 1990.

| DEXTROCARDIA AND SITUS INVERSUS | Congenital abnormality in the heart in the presence of situs inversus, a circumstance in which the heart and stomach are placed to the right and the liver to the left, is not very common; however, a right thoracic heart with normally placed stomach and liver should suggest congenital abnormality such as pulmonic stenosis, ventricular and atrial septal defects, and transposition of the great vessels. | As an affected infant matures, an unusually placed heart can change the clinical manifestations of disease by adulthood. For example, the substernal pressure of myocardial ischemia may be felt to the right of the precordium and may more often radiate into the right arm rather than to the left, the usual site when the heart is in its expected place. |

VESSEL DISORDERS

| CRANIAL ARTERITIS (GIANT CELL ARTERITIS) | Chronic generalized inflammatory disease of the branches of the aortic arch principally affects arteries of the carotid system and the temporal and occipital arteries. Temporal arteritis usually affects persons over the age of 50. Flulike symptoms (low-grade fever, malaise, anorexia) are accompanied by polymyalgia involving the trunk and proximal muscles. | Headache may be severe, there is throbbing in the temporal region on one or both sides, and the area over the temporal artery becomes red, swollen, tender, and nodulated. The temporal pulse may be variously strong, weak, or absent. Ocular symptoms, including loss of vision, are common. |

| ARTERIAL ANEURYSM | An aneurysm is a localized dilation of an artery caused by a weakness in the arterial wall (Figure 13-45). It is noticed as a pulsatile swelling along the course of an artery. Aneurysms occur most commonly in the aorta, although renal, femoral, and popliteal arteries are also common sites. A thrill or bruit may be evident over the aneurysm. | monly in the aorta, although renal, femoral, and popliteal arteries are also common sites. A thrill or bruit may be evident over the aneurysm. |

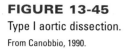
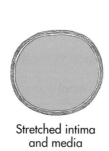
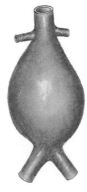

Stretched intima and media

FIGURE 13-45
Type I aortic dissection.
From Canobbio, 1990.

ARTERIOVENOUS FISTULA	An arteriovenous fistula is a pathologic communication between an artery and a vein. It may result in an aneurysmal dilation. A continuous bruit or thrill over the area of the fistula suggests its presence. Fistulas may be found in a variety of lo-	cations such as intracranially with a potential of intracranial hemorrhage (not uncommon), in the gastrointestinal tract (a not unusual source of gastrointestinal bleeding), and in the lungs (rare).
PERIPHERAL ATHEROSCLEROTIC DISEASE (ARTERIOSCLEROSIS OBLITERANS)	Occlusion of the blood supply to the extremities by atherosclerotic plaques causes symptoms that vary in severity. Intermittent claudication produces pain, ache, or cramp in the exercising muscle that receives a deficient blood supply. The amount of exercise necessary to cause the discomfort is predictable, occurring after the same distance walked each time. A brief rest relieves the pain.	The limb appears healthy, but pulses are weak or absent. Progressive occlusion results in severe ischemia, in which the foot or leg is painful at rest, cold, and numb, and skin changes occur (dry and scaling, with poor hair and nail growth). Edema seldom accompanies this disorder, but ulceration is common in severe disease, and the muscles may atrophy.
RAYNAUD PHENOMENON AND DISEASE	Idiopathic, intermittent spasm of the arterioles in the digits (occasionally in the nose and tongue) causes skin pallor. The vasospasm may last from minutes to hours. It can occur bilaterally, and the skin over the digits eventually appears smooth, shiny, and tight from loss of subcutaneous tissue. Ulcers may appear on tips of the digits. Raynaud disease occurs most frequently in young, otherwise healthy women in whom episodes recur	for at least 2 years with no evidence of underlying cause. Raynaud phenomenon is secondary to connective tissue diseases, neurogenic lesions, drug intoxication, primary pulmonary hypertension, and trauma. It is rare in childhood, and although it has been associated with immunologic abnormalities in this age-group, there is no evidence of serious prognostic significance.
ARTERIAL EMBOLIC DISEASE	Dilation of the left atrium because of mitral regurgitation can lead to atrial fibrillation and clot formation within the atrium. If the clot is unstable, emboli	may be disbursed throughout the arterial system, giving rise to occlusion of small arteries and necrosis of the tissue supplied by that vessel (Figure 13-46).

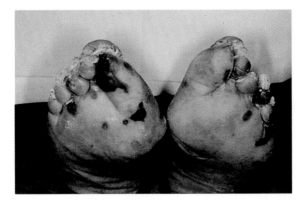

FIGURE 13-46

Embolic phenomenon.

Courtesy Charles W. Bradley, DPM, MPA, and Caroline Harvey, DPM, California College of Podiatric Medicine, San Bruno, California.

VENOUS THROMBOSIS

Thrombosis can occur suddenly or gradually with varying severity of symptoms. It can be the result of trauma or prolonged immobilization. Clinical findings of thrombosis in a superficial vein include redness, thickening, and tenderness along the involved segment. Deep vein thrombosis in the femoral and pelvic circulations may be asymptomatic; and pulmonary embolism, sometimes fatal, may occur without warning. Signs and symptoms suggestive of deep vein thrombosis include tenderness along the iliac vessels and the femoral canal, in the popliteal space, and over the deep calf veins; slight swelling that may be distinguished only by measuring and comparing the upper and lower legs bilaterally, minimal ankle edema, low-grade fever, and tachycardia. Homans sign can be helpful but is not absolutely reliable in suggesting deep vein thrombosis.

JUGULAR VENOUS PRESSURE DISORDERS

TRICUSPID REGURGITATION

With severe tricuspid regurgitation, the v wave is much more prominent and occurs earlier, often merging with the C wave (Figure 13-47). Concomitant physical findings might include a holosystolic murmur in the tricuspid region, a pulsatile liver, and peripheral edema (see Table 13-13).

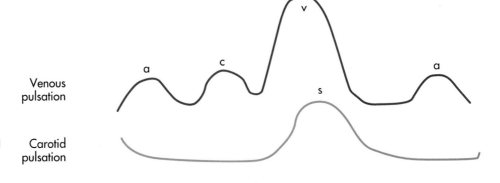

FIGURE 13-47
Diagram of pulsation in tricuspid regurgitation.

ATRIAL FIBRILLATION

With atrial fibrillation, the a wave is absent and the pulse is typically irregular. Therefore, there are only two venous pulsations for each arterial pulsation, and the time interval between v waves is variable.

CARDIAC TAMPONADE

The jugular venous pressure is particularly helpful for evaluating patients with pericardial disease. With cardiac tamponade, the Y-descent is abolished and the jugular venous pressure is markedly elevated (15 to 25 cm H_2O). Additionally, the JVP fails to fall with inspiration as it usually does and may actually increase (Kussmaul sign). Other physical findings may include tachycardia and pulsus paradoxus (decrease in systolic blood pressure greater than 15 mm Hg with inspiration) (see Box 13-9 and Figure 13-39.)

CONSTRICTIVE PERICARDITIS

In constrictive pericarditis, the jugular venous pressure is elevated, just as with cardiac tamponade, but there is a prominent Y-descent. Additional physical findings in constrictive pericarditis may include signs of severe right heart failure such as ascites and severe peripheral edema (Figure 13-48).

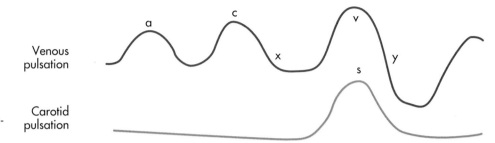

FIGURE 13-48
Diagram of pulsation in constrictive pericarditis.

CHILDREN

ACUTE RHEUMATIC FEVER

Acute rheumatic fever is a systemic connective tissue disease that occurs after a streptococcal pharyngitis or skin infection; it is characterized by a variety of major and minor manifestations (Box 13-14). It may result in serious cardiac valvular involvement of the mitral or aortic valve. Often the same valve is both stenotic and regurgitant. The tricuspid and pulmonic valves may be, but are not often, affected. The major physical findings may include the murmurs of mitral regurgitation and aortic insufficiency, cardiomegaly, the friction rub of pericarditis, congestive heart failure, a migratory polyarthritis (most frequently in the larger joints), chorea (at times without other manifestations), a transient erythema marginatum (pink margins with pale centers), and, rarely in recent years, firm, painless subcutaneous nodules, particularly on, but not limited to, the elbows, knees, and wrists. Although there has been a marked diminution in the incidence of rheumatic fever in the last 20 years, there is a recent worrisome resurgence. Children between the ages of 5 and 15 years are most commonly affected. Prevention—adequate treatment for streptococcal pharyngitis or skin infections—is the best therapy.

BOX 13-14 **Revised Jones Criteria for Guidance in the Diagnosis of Rheumatic Fever**

Major Manifestations	Minor Manifestations
Carditis	*Clinical*
Polyarthritis	Previous rheumatic fever or rheumatic heart disease
Chorea	Arthralgia
Erythema marginatum	Fever
Subcutaneous nodules	*Laboratory*
	Acute phase reactions: erythrocyte sedimentation rate, C-reactive protein, leukocytosis
	Prolonged P-R interval on ECG

Supporting Evidence of Streptococcal Infection

- Increased titer of antistreptolysin antibodies (antistreptolysin O in particular)
- Positive throat culture for group A streptococcus
- Recent scarlet fever

The presence of two major or one major and two minor manifestations suggests a high probability of acute rheumatic fever, if supported by evidence of a preceding group A streptococcal infection. You should never make the diagnosis on the basis of laboratory findings and two minor manifestations alone.

From the American Heart Association, 1984.

KAWASAKI DISEASE

Kawasaki disease is an acute illness of uncertain cause, affecting the young, and males more often than females. The manifestations are general and are typified by fever lasting a few days to 3 weeks and by the effects of a systemic vasculitis with conjunctival injection, strawberry tongue, edema of the hands and feet, some lymphadenopathy, and polymorphous nonvesicular rashes, among a wide variety of other findings. The critical concern, however, is cardiac involvement. As the disease progresses and as the vasculitis takes hold, aneurysms of the coronary artery may develop, sometimes very early, some times later. Other arteries may be involved, and early death may be the result of myocardial infarction, rupture of an aneurysm, or generalized vasculitis of the smaller vessels of the heart. An aneurysm may rupture even years later. Effective therapy requires early diagnosis and treatment in the first few days of the illness with high-dose intravenous gamma globulin. Corticosteroids are not given because they may exaggerate aneurysmal dilations.

OLDER ADULTS

ATHEROSCLEROTIC HEART DISEASE

Atherosclerotic heart disease may cause myocardial insufficiency, angina pectoris, dysrhythmias, and congestive heart failure.

MITRAL INSUFFICIENCY

Mitral insufficiency is usually silent and painless until it produces sudden heart failure, stroke, or dysrhythmias. It also occurs after infarction involving the mitral chordae, along with tachycardia, pallor, a variety of alterations in the heart sounds, occasional pericardial friction rub, various murmurs, and dysrhythmias.

ANGINA	The definition of angina is "pain." With reference to the heart, it indicates a substernal pain or intense pressure radiating at times to the neck, jaws, and the arms, particularly the left. It is often accompanied by shortness of breath, fatigue,	diaphoresis, faintness, and syncope. Although angina is listed as a common abnormality in the elderly, it can occur, of course, in much younger men and women.
SENILE CARDIAC AMYLOIDOSIS	Amyloid deposits in the heart cause heart failure. Electrocardiography or echocardiography shows a small, thickened left	ventricle, and the right ventricle may also be thickened. The contractility of the heart may at times be reduced.
AORTIC SCLEROSIS	The elderly, and even some persons of middle age, may develop thickening and calcification of the aortic valves. The result need not be a significant obstruction	to left ventricular outflow, but, regardless of severity, there may be a midsystolic (ejection) murmur.
ARTERIOSCLEROSIS OBLITERANS OF THE EXTREMITIES	This is an age-related progressive arterial disease paralleling the development of atherosclerosis elsewhere. The particular and sole specific symptom is intermittent claudication, pain, spasm, or weakness in a muscle at work, especially during walk-	ing, that is almost immediately relieved by rest. It is severe enough to force the patient to stop and to sit because it is too painful to continue or the muscle gives way and the patient falls.
VENOUS ULCERS	These ulcers are generally found on the medial or lateral aspects of the lower limbs, most often in the elderly. Induration, edema, and hyperpigmentation are common associated findings. Heart fail-	ure, hypoalbuminemia, and nutritional deficiency may be factors adding to the result of the aging of the veins. Peripheral neuropathy and diabetes mellitus, as well as arterial disease, may be causal.

More information at Mosby   *http://www1.mosby.com/physexam_seidel*

CHAPTER 14

BREASTS AND AXILLAE

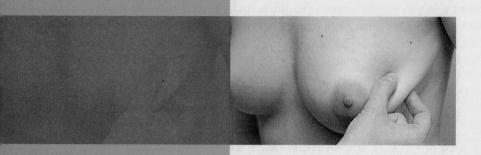

ANATOMY AND PHYSIOLOGY

The breasts are paired mammary glands located on the anterior chest wall, superficial to the pectoralis major and serratus anterior muscles (Figure 14-1). In women the breast extends from the second or third rib to the sixth or seventh rib, and from the sternal margin to the midaxillary line. The nipple is located centrally, surrounded by the areola. The male breast consists of a small nipple and areola overlying a thin layer of breast tissue that is indistinguishable by palpation from surrounding tissue.

The female breast is composed of glandular and fibrous tissue and subcutaneous and retromammary fat. The glandular tissue is arranged into 15 to 20 lobes per breast that radiate about the nipple. Each lobe is composed of 20 to 40 lobules, which consist of the milk-producing acini cells that empty into lactiferous ducts. These cells are small and inconspicuous in the nonpregnant, nonlactating woman. A lactiferous duct drains milk from each lobe onto the surface of the nipple.

The layer of subcutaneous fibrous tissue provides support for the breast. Suspensory ligaments (Cooper ligaments) extend from the connective tissue layer through the breast and attach to the underlying muscle fascia, providing further support for the breast. The muscles forming the floor of the breast are the pectoralis major, pectoralis minor, serratus anterior, latissimus dorsi, subscapularis, external oblique, and rectus abdominis.

Vascular supply to the breast is primarily through branches of the internal mammary artery and the lateral thoracic artery. This network provides most of the blood supply to the deeper tissues of the breast and to the nipple. The intercostal arteries assist in supplying the more superficial tissues.

The subcutaneous and retromammary fat that surrounds the glandular tissue composes most of the bulk of the breast. The proportions of each of the component tissues vary with age, nutritional status, pregnancy, lactation, and genetic predisposition.

For the purposes of examination the breast is divided into five segments: four quadrants and a tail (Figure 14-2). The greatest amount of glandular tissue lies in the upper outer quadrant. Breast tissue extends from this quadrant into the axilla, forming the tail of Spence. In the axillae the mammary tissue is in direct contact with the axillary lymph nodes.

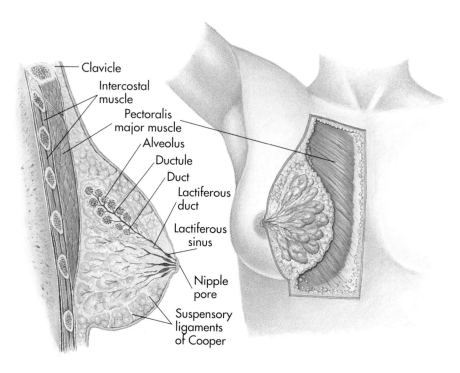

FIGURE 14-1
Anatomy of the breast, showing position and major structures.

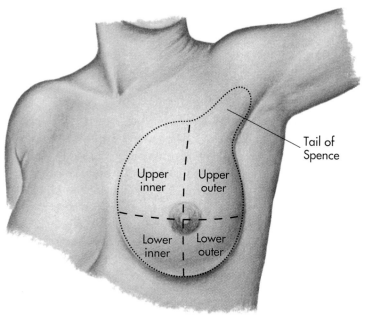

FIGURE 14-2
Quadrants of the left breast and axillary tail of Spence.

The nipple, onto which the lactiferous ducts empty, is located centrally on the breast and is surrounded by the pigmented areola. The nipple is composed of epithelium that is infiltrated with circular and longitudinal smooth muscle fibers. Contraction of the smooth muscle, induced by tactile, sensory, or autonomic stimuli, produces erection of the nipple and causes the lactiferous ducts to empty. The process of erection is supported by venous stasis in the erectile vascular tissue. Tiny sebaceous glands may be apparent on the areola surface (Montgomery tubercles or follicles). Some hair follicles may be found about the circumference of the areola. Supernumerary nipples or breast tissue is sometimes present along the mammary ridge that extends from the axilla during embryonic development (see Figure 14-10).

TABLE 14-1 Patterns of Lymph Drainage

Area of Breast	Drainage
Superficial	
Upper outer quadrant	Scapular, brachial, intermediate nodes toward axillary nodes
Medial portion	Internal mammary chain toward opposite breast and abdomen
Deep	
Posterior chest wall and portion of the arm	Posterior axillary nodes (subscapular)
Anterior chest wall	Anterior axillary nodes (pectoral)
Upper arm	Lateral axillary nodes (brachial)
Retroareolar area	Interpectoral (Rotter) nodes into the axillary chain
Areola and Nipple	Midaxillary, subclavicular, and supraclavicular nodes

Each breast contains a lymphatic network that drains the breast radially and deeply to underlying lymphatics. Superficial lymphatics drain the skin, and deep lymphatics drain the mammary lobules. Table 14-1 summarizes the patterns of lymph drainage.

The complex of lymph nodes, their locations, and direction of drainage are illustrated in Figure 14-3. The axillary nodes are more superficial and are therefore more accessible and relatively easy to palpate when enlarged. The anterior axillary (pectoral) nodes are located along the lower border of the pectoralis major inside the lateral axillary fold. The midaxillary (central) nodes are high in the axilla close to the ribs. The posterior axillary (subscapular) nodes lie along the lateral border of the scapula and deep in the posterior axillary fold, whereas the lateral axillary (brachial) nodes can be felt along the upper humerus.

CHILDREN AND ADOLESCENTS

The breast evolves in structure and function throughout life. Childhood and preadolescence represent a latent phase of breast development during which only minimal branching of primary ducts occurs. Thelarche (breast development) represents an early sign of puberty in adolescent girls. The developmental process has been classified and described in a number of ways. Tanner's five stages of developing sexual maturity, discussed in Chapter 5 (Growth and Measurement), is the classification most commonly used.

In using the Tanner charts to stage breast development, it is important to note certain temporal relationships. It is unusual for the onset of menses to occur before stage III. About 25% of females begin menstruation at stage III. Approximately 75% are menstruating at stage IV and are beginning a reasonably regular menstrual cycle. Some 10% of young women do not begin to menstruate until stage V. The average interval from the appearance of the breast bud (stage II) to menarche is 2 years. Stage IV may not occur in as many as 25% of all adolescents and may be only minimal in another 25%. It is also important to remember that breasts develop at different rates in the individual, which can result in asymmetry.

PHYSICAL VARIATIONS

As adolescents develop, they may wonder about their breast size. Asian women generally have smaller breasts than white women, but data are lacking regarding breast size in other groups.

Data from Algaratnam, Wong, 1985.

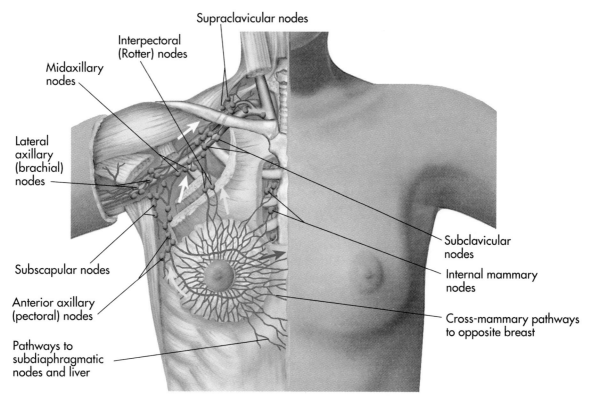

FIGURE 14-3
Lymphatic drainage of breast.

PREGNANT WOMEN

Striking changes occur in the breasts during pregnancy. In response to luteal and placental hormones, the lactiferous ducts proliferate and the alveoli increase extensively in size and number, which may cause the breasts to enlarge two to three times their prepregnancy size. The increase in glandular tissue displaces connective tissue and, as a result, the tissue becomes softer and looser. Toward the end of pregnancy as epithelial secretory activity increases, colostrum is produced and accumulates in the acini cells (alveoli).

The areolae become more deeply pigmented and their diameter increases. The nipples become more prominent, darker, and more erectile. Montgomery tubercles often develop as sebaceous glands hypertrophy.

Mammary vascularization increases, causing veins to engorge and become visible as a blue network beneath the surface of the skin.

LACTATING WOMEN

In the first few days after delivery, small amounts of colostrum are secreted from the breasts. Colostrum contains more protein and minerals than mature milk does. Colostrum also contains antibodies and other host resistance factors. Milk production to replace colostrum begins 2 to 4 days after delivery in response to surging prolactin levels, declining estrogen levels, and the stimulation of sucking. As the alveoli and lactiferous ducts fill, the breasts may become full and tense. This, combined with tissue edema and a delay in effective ejection reflexes, produces breast engorgement.

At the termination of lactation, involution occurs over a period of about 3 months. Breast size decreases without loss of lobular and alveolar components; the breasts rarely return to their prelactation size.

| OLDER ADULTS | Before menopause there is a moderate decrease in glandular tissue and some decomposition of alveolar and lobular tissue. After menopause, glandular tissue continues to atrophy gradually and is replaced by fat deposited in the breasts. The inframammary ridge at the lower edge of the breast thickens. The breasts tend to hang more loosely from the chest wall because of these tissue changes and the relaxation of the suspensory ligaments. The nipples become smaller, flatter, and lose some erectile ability. |

The skin may take on a relatively dry, thin texture. Loss of hair in the axillae may also occur.

REVIEW OF RELATED HISTORY

PRESENT PROBLEM

- Breast discomfort
  - Temporal sequence: onset gradual or sudden; length of time symptom has been present; does symptom come and go or is it always present
  - Relationship to menses: timing, severity
  - Character: stinging, pulling, burning, drawing, stabbing, aching, throbbing; unilateral or bilateral; localization; radiation
  - Associated symptoms: lump or mass, discharge from nipple
  - Contributory factors: skin irritation under breasts from tissue-to-tissue contact or from rubbing of brassiere; strenuous activity; recent injury to breast
  - Medications: nonprescription or prescription
- Breast mass or lump
  - Temporal sequence: length of time since lump first noted; does lump come and go or is it always present; relationship to menses
  - Symptoms: tenderness or pain (characterize as described previously), dimpling or change in contour
  - Changes in lump: size, character, relationship to menses (timing or severity)
  - Associated symptoms: nipple discharge or retraction, tender lymph nodes
  - Medications: nonprescription or prescription
- Nipple discharge
  - Character: onset gradual or sudden, duration, color, consistency, odor, amount
  - Associated symptoms: nipple retraction; breast lump or discomfort
  - Associated factors: relationship to menses or other activity; recent injury to breast
  - Medications: nonprescription or prescription; contraceptives; phenothiazines, digitalis, diuretics, steroids

PAST MEDICAL HISTORY

- Previous breast disease: cancer, fibroadenomas, fibrocystic disease
- Surgeries: breast biopsies, aspirations, implants, reductionplasties; oophorectomy
- Menstrual history: age at menarche or menopause; cycle length, duration and amount of flow, regularity; associated breast symptoms (nipple discharge; pain or discomfort)
- Pregnancy: age at each pregnancy, length of each pregnancy, date of delivery or termination
- Lactation: number of children breast-fed; duration of time for breast-feeding; date of termination of last breast-feeding; medications used to suppress lactation
- Past use of hormonal medications: name and dosage, reason for use (contraception, menstrual control, menopausal symptom relief), length of time on hormones, date of termination

FAMILY HISTORY

- Breast cancer: which relative (particularly mother or sister); type of cancer; age at time of occurrence; treatment and results

■ Other breast disease in female and male relatives: type of disease; age at time of occurrence; treatment and results

PERSONAL AND SOCIAL HISTORY

■ Age
■ Any changes in breast characteristics: pain, tenderness, lumps, discharge, skin changes, size or shape changes
■ Changes in the breast that occur with the menstrual cycle: tenderness, swelling, pain, enlarged nodes
■ Date of first day of last menstrual period
■ Menopause: onset, course, associated problems, residual problems
■ Breast support used with strenuous exercise or sports activities
■ Amount of caffeine intake
■ Breast self-examination: frequency; at what time in the menstrual cycle; have woman describe her procedure
■ Risk factors for breast cancer (see the Risk Factors box on breast cancer below)
■ Risk factors for benign breast disease (see the Risk Factors box on benign breast disease below)
■ Mammography history
■ Medications: Nonprescription or prescription, particularly oral contraceptives or other hormones: name, dosage, length of time taking
■ Use of alcohol

RISK FACTORS   **Breast Cancer**

- Age (80% of cases occur after age 50 years; no plateau effect with aging)
- Gender: Female
- Personal history of breast cancer
- Family history of breast cancer (mother, sister, daughter, or two or more close relatives such as cousins or aunts)
- Previous breast biopsies for benign breast disease (atypical hyperplasia)
- Laboratory evidence of specific genetic mutations that increase susceptibility to breast cancer (e.g., mutations in BRCA1 and BRCA2)
- Increased breast tissue density on mammogram (women age 45 or older with ≥75% dense tissue)
- Early menarche (before age 12)
- Late menopause (after age 50)
- Nulliparity
- Late age at birth of first child (after age 30)
- Estrogen replacement therapy after menopause (risk not yet known)

RISK FACTORS   **Benign Breast Disease**

- Early menarche (before age 12)
- Late menopause (after age 50)
- Nulliparity or low parity
- Late age at birth of first child (after age 30)
- High socioeconomic status
- Caffeine consumption (controversial)

PREGNANT WOMEN

■ Sensations: fullness, tingling, tenderness
■ Use of supportive brassiere
■ Knowledge and information about breast-feeding
■ Plans to breast-feed, experience, expectations (all women should be encouraged to consider breast-feeding because of the positive health benefits for the newborn)

LACTATING WOMEN

- Cleaning procedures for breasts: use of soap products that can remove natural lubricants, frequency of use; nipple preparations (not generally helpful)
- Use of nursing brassiere
- Nipples: tenderness, pain, cracking, bleeding; retracted; related problems with feeding; exposure to air
- Associated problems: engorgement, leaking breasts, plugged duct (localized tenderness and lump), fever, infection; treatment and results; infant with oral candidal infection
- Nursing routine: length of feeding, frequency, rotation of breasts, positions used
- Breast milk pumping device(s) used, frequency of use
- Cultural beliefs
- Food and environmental agents that can affect breast milk (e.g., chocolate, photography chemicals)
- Medications that can cross the milk-blood barrier (e.g., cimetidine, clemastine, thiouracil). All medications, prescription and nonprescription, should be evaluated for potential side effects in the newborn.

OLDER ADULTS

- Skin irritation under pendulous breasts from tissue-to-tissue contact or from rubbing of brassiere; treatment
- Hormone therapy during or since menopause: name and dosage of medication; duration of therapy

---

BOX 14-1   **Breast Self-Examination**

Breast self-examination (BSE) should be done once a month so that you become familiar with the usual appearance and feel of your breasts. Familiarity makes it easier to notice any changes in the breast from one month to another. Early discovery of a change from what is "normal" is the main idea behind BSE.

If you menstruate, the best time to do BSE is 2 or 3 days after your period ends, when your breasts are least likely to be tender or swollen. If you no longer menstruate, pick a day, such as the first day of the month, to remind yourself it is time to do BSE.

Here is how to do BSE:

1. Stand before a mirror. Inspect both breasts for anything unusual, such as any discharge from the nipples, puckering, dimpling, or scaling of the skin.

The next two steps are designed to emphasize any change in the shape or contour of your breasts. As you do them, you should be able to feel your chest muscles tighten.

2. Watching closely in the mirror, clasp hands behind your head and press hands forward.
3. Next, press hands firmly on hips and bow slightly toward your mirror as you pull your shoulders and elbows forward.

Some women do the next part of the examination in the shower. Fingers glide over soapy skin, making it easy to appreciate the texture underneath.

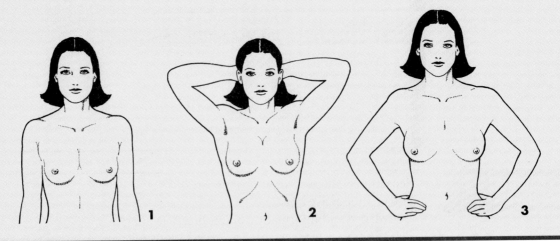

1   2   3

EXAMINATION AND FINDINGS

EQUIPMENT

- Flashlight with transilluminator
- Ruler
- Small pillow or folded towel
- Glass slide and cytologic fixative, if nipple discharge is present

Adequate lighting is essential for revealing shadows and subtle variations in skin color and texture. Adequate exposure is also essential, requiring that the patient be disrobed to the waist. Draping one breast while examining the other to protect the patient's modesty is more a disservice than a consideration, because simultaneous observation of both breasts is necessary to detect minor differences between them that may be significant. Modesty is a concern, however, and you or the patient may be uncomfortable at first. A matter-of-fact and composed approach with attention to the patient as a person will go a long way in reassuring the patient of your regard and sensitivity.

Breast Self-Examination

Take a few extra minutes during this examination to have the patient demonstrate how she does her breast self-examination. This gives you an opportunity to review the process and rationale for self-examination with her, and to instruct her in the correct techniques if necessary (Box 14-1). It would be appropriate at this time to review the accepted recommendations for early breast cancer detection (Box 14-2).

BOX 14-1 **Breast Self-Examination—cont'd**

4. Raise your left arm. Use three or four fingers of your right hand to explore your left breast firmly, carefully, and thoroughly. Beginning at the outer edge, press the flat part of your fingers in small circles, moving the circles slowly around the breast. Gradually work toward the nipple. Be sure to cover the entire breast. Pay special attention to the area between the breast and the armpit, including the armpit itself. Feel for any unusual lump or mass under the skin.

5. Gently squeeze the nipple and look for a discharge. Repeat the exam on your right breast.
6. Steps 4 and 5 should be repeated lying down. Lie flat on your back, left arm over your head and a pillow or folded towel under your left shoulder. This position flattens the breast and makes it easier to examine. Use the same circular motion described earlier.

   Repeat on your right breast.

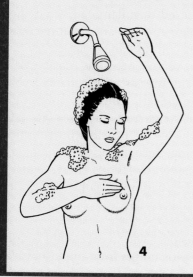

4

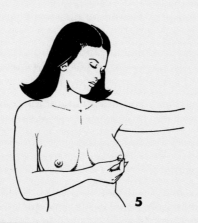

5

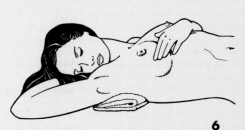

6

BOX 14-2   Screening for Breast Cancer

Breast cancer is the most common type of cancer among women in the United States and is the second leading cause of cancer death in women. Early detection through screening is important for timely treatment and prevention of death. Authorities do not completely agree on the frequency and timing of screening recommendations; all currently agree that breast self-examination (BSE), clinical breast examination (CBE), and mammography are the appropriate screening activities, used in conjunction.

The following is a summary of the various recommendations:

BSE: monthly

CBE: over age 40 years: annually
        under age 40 years: annually or 1-3 years

Mammogram:
   Women at average risk
      over age 50: annually or 1-2 years
      ages 40-49: every 1-2 years
   Women at high risk
      begin age 35 or before age 40 years

INSPECTION

Breast

With the patient in a sitting position with arms hanging loosely at the sides, inspect each breast and compare them for size, symmetry, contour, skin color and texture, venous patterns, and lesions. Perform this portion of the examination for both women and men. With female patients, lift the breasts with your fingertips, inspecting the lower and lateral aspects to determine whether there are any changes in the color or texture of the skin.

Women's breasts vary somewhat in shape, from convex to pendulous or conical, and frequently, one breast is somewhat smaller than the other (Figure 14-4). Men's breasts are generally even with the chest wall, although some men, particularly those who are overweight, have breasts with a convex shape.

The skin texture should appear smooth and the contour should be uninterrupted. Retractions and dimpling signify the contraction of fibrotic tissue that occurs with carcinoma. Alterations in contour are best seen on bilateral comparison of one breast with the other. A peau d'orange appearance of the skin indicates edema of the breast caused by blocked lymph drainage in advanced or inflammatory carcinoma (Figure 14-5). The skin appears thickened with enlarged pores and accentuated skin markings. Healthy skin may look similar if the pores of the skin are large.

Venous patterns should be bilaterally similar. Venous networks may be visible, although these are usually pronounced only in the breasts of pregnant or obese women. If these are bilateral, there is no cause for concern. However, unilateral venous patterns can be produced by dilated superficial veins from increased blood flow to a malignancy. This finding should alert you to the need for further investigation.

Other markings and nevi that are long-standing, unchanging, or nontender are of little concern. Changes or the recent appearance of any lesions always signal the need for closer investigation. A film mammogram, xerogram, or biopsy is indicated.

Nipple and Areola

Inspect the areolae and nipples in both men and women. The areola should be round or oval and bilaterally equal or nearly equal. The color ranges from pink to black. In light-skinned women the areola usually turns brown with the first pregnancy and remains dark. In women with dark skin, the areola is brown before pregnancy. A pep-

MNEMONICS

FIVE Ds RELATED TO NIPPLES

D *D*ischarge
D *D*epression or inversion
D *D*iscoloration: pregnancy
D *D*ermatologic changes: Paget disease
D *D*eviation: compare opposite side

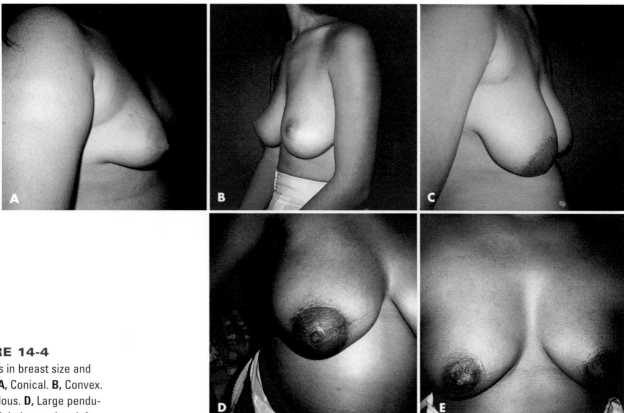

FIGURE 14-4

Variations in breast size and contour. **A,** Conical. **B,** Convex. **C,** Pendulous. **D,** Large pendulous. **E,** Right larger than left.

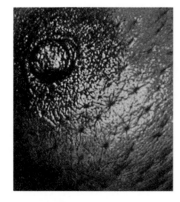

FIGURE 14-5

Peau d'orange appearance from edema.

From Gallager, 1978.

pering of nontender, nonsuppurative Montgomery tubercles is considered an expected finding (Figure 14-6). The surface should be otherwise smooth. The peau d'orange skin associated with carcinoma is often seen first in the areola.

The nipples should be bilaterally equal or nearly equal in size. Most nipples are everted, but one or both nipples may be inverted (Figure 14-7). In these instances, ask if there is a lifetime history of inversion. Recent unilateral inversion or retraction of a previously everted nipple suggests malignancy.

Simultaneous bilateral inspection is necessary to detect nipple retraction or deviation. Retraction is seen as a flattening, withdrawal, or inversion of the nipple and indicates inward pulling by inflammatory or malignant tissue (Figure 14-8). The fibrotic tissue of carcinoma can also change the axis of the nipple, causing it to point in a direction different from that of the other nipple.

The nipples should be a homogenous color and match that of the areolae. Their surface may be either smooth or wrinkled, but should be free of crusting, cracking, or discharge. Variations in areola color will be apparent (Figure 14-9).

Supernumerary nipples, which are more common in black women than in white women, appear as one or more extra nipples located along the embryonic mammary ridge (the "milk line") (Figure 14-10). These nipples and areolae may be pink or brown, are usually small, and are commonly mistaken for moles (Figure 14-11). Infrequently, some glandular tissue may accompany these nipples. In some cases, supernumerary nipples may be associated with congenital renal or cardiac anomalies, particularly in whites.

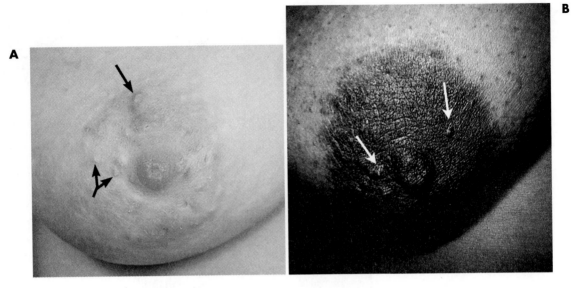

FIGURE 14-6
Montgomery tubercles. **A,** Light-skinned woman. **B,** Dark-skinned woman.

A from Mansel, Bundred, 1995.

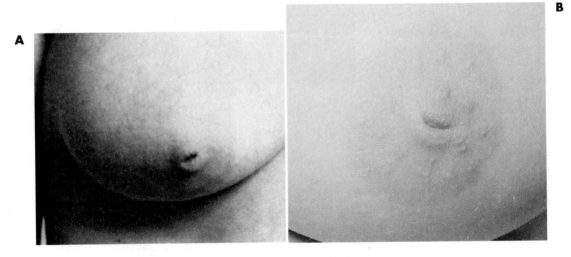

FIGURE 14-7
A, Simple nipple inversion with lifetime history. **B,** Acquired nipple inversion.

B from Mansel, Bundred, 1995.

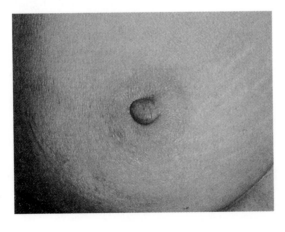

FIGURE 14-8
Nipple retraction laterally and swelling behind right nipple in Asian woman with breast cancer.

From Mansel, Bundred, 1995.

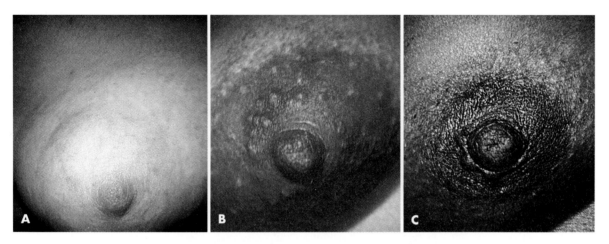

FIGURE 14-9
Variations in color of areola. **A**, Pink. **B**, Brown. **C**, Black.

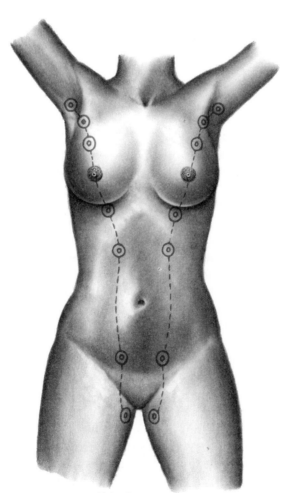

FIGURE 14-10
Supernumerary nipples and tissue may arise along the "milk line," an embryonic ridge.
From Thompson et al, 1997.

G.J.Wassilchenko

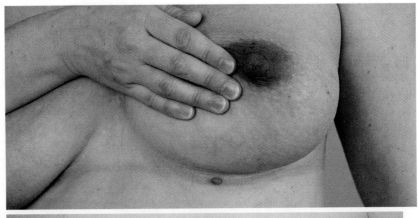

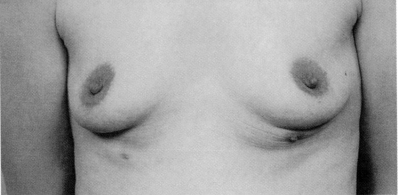

FIGURE 14-11
A, Supernumerary nipple without glandular tissue. **B,** Supernumerary breast and nipple on left side and supernumerary nipple alone on right side.
B from Mansel, Bundred, 1995.

REINSPECTION IN VARIED POSITIONS

Reinspect the woman's breasts with the patient in the following positions:
- Seated with arms over the head: this adds tension to the suspensory ligaments, accentuates dimpling, and may reveal variations in contour and symmetry (Figure 14-12, *A*).
- Seated with hands pressed against hips (or alternatively have the patient push her palms together): This contracts the pectoral muscles, which can reveal deviations in contour and symmetry (Figure 14-12, *B* and *C*).
- Seated and leaning forward from the waist: This also causes tension in the suspensory ligaments. The breasts should hang equally. This maneuver can be particularly helpful in assessing the contour and symmetry of large breasts, since the breasts fall away from the chest wall and hang freely. As the patient leans forward, support her by the hands (Figure 14-12, *D*).

For all patient positions, the breasts should appear bilaterally equal, with an even contour and absence of dimpling, retraction, or deviation.

PALPATION

Breast

After a thorough inspection, systematically palpate the breasts, axillae, and supraclavicular regions. Palpation of male breasts can be brief but should not be omitted.

Methods. Have the patient sit with arms hanging freely at the sides. Palpate all four quadrants of the breast, feeling for lumps or nodules (Box 14-3). Use your finger pads because they are more sensitive than your fingertips.

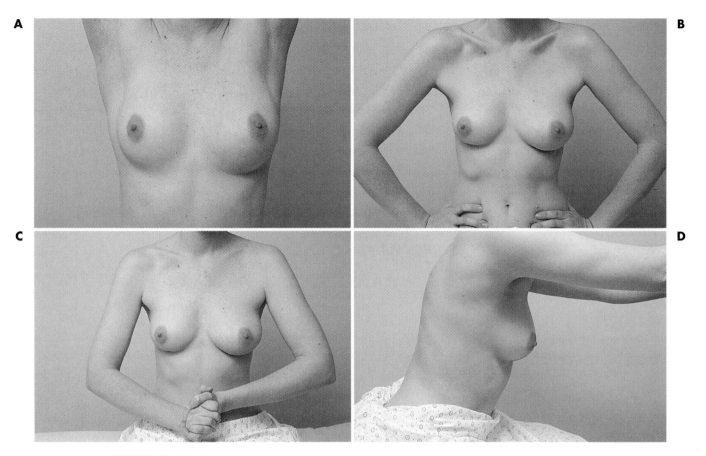

FIGURE 14-12

Inspect the breasts in the following positions. **A,** Arms extended overhead. **B,** Hands pressed against hips. **C,** Pressing hands together (an alternate way to flex the pectoral muscles). **D,** Leaning forward from the waist.

BOX 14-3 **Documenting Breast Masses**

If a breast mass is felt, characterize it by its location, size, shape, consistency, tenderness, mobility, delineation of borders, and retraction (see Figures 14-17 and 14-18, p. 503). Transillumination can be used to confirm the presence of fluid in certain masses. These characteristics are not diagnostic by themselves, but, in conjunction with a thorough history, they provide a great deal of clinical information for correlation with findings from diagnostic testing.

Any and all breast masses or lumps that you encounter should be described by the following characteristics:

Location:	Which quadrant; distance from nipple; depict in illustration
Size:	In centimeters: length, width, thickness
Shape:	Round, discoid, lobular, stellate; regular or irregular
Consistency:	Firm, soft, hard
Tenderness:	To what degree
Mobility:	Movable (in what directions) or fixed to overlying skin or subadjacent fascia
Borders:	Discrete or poorly defined
Retraction:	Presence or absence of dimpling; altered contour

All new solitary or dominant masses must be investigated with further diagnostic testing.

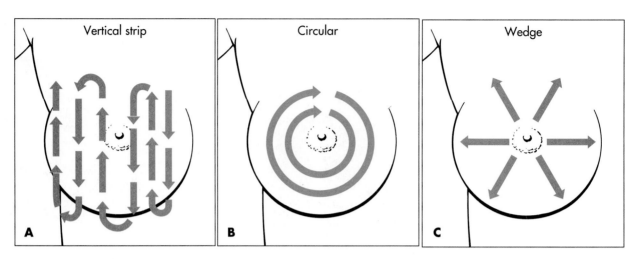

FIGURE 14-13
Various methods for palpation of the breast. **A,** Palpate from top to bottom in vertical strips. **B,** Palpate in concentric circles. **C,** Palpate out from the center in wedge sections.
From Belcher, 1993.

Palpate systematically, pushing gently but firmly, toward the chest with your fingers rotating in a clockwise or counterclockwise pattern. Figure 14-13 illustrates three methods that are commonly used for palpation. Many methods are used; any are acceptable, as long as every part of the breast is palpated. In the vertical strip technique, begin at the top of the breast and palpate, first downward, then upward, working your way down over the entire breast. In the concentric circle technique, begin at the outermost edge of the breast and spiral your way inward toward the nipple. To use the wedge method, palpate from the center of the breast in radial fashion, returning to the areola to begin each spoke. Regardless of the method used, be sure to also palpate the breast tissue that lies beneath the nipple.

It is essential to include the tail of Spence in palpation, because most malignancies occur in the upper outer quadrant of the breast. Early lesions can be very tiny and may be detected only through meticulous technique. The exact sequence you select for palpation is not critical, but it is essential to develop a systematic approach that always begins and ends at a fixed point. This will help ensure that all portions of the breast are examined. Do a complete light palpation and then repeat the examination with deeper, heavier palpation.

Press firmly enough to get a good sense of the underlying tissue, but not so firmly that the tissue is compressed against the rib cage, as this can give a false impression of a mass. In women, a firm transverse ridge of compressed tissue (the inframammary ridge) may be felt along the lower edge of the breast. It is easy to mistake this for a breast mass.

Try not to lift your fingers off the breast as you move from one point to another. For large breasts it may be helpful to immobilize the inferior surface of the breast with one hand while examining the superior surface with the other hand (Figure 14-14).

Males. In most men, expect to feel a thin layer of fatty tissue overlying muscle. Obese men may have a somewhat thicker fatty layer, giving the appearance of breast enlargement. A firm disk of glandular tissue can be felt in some men.

Females. The breast tissue of adult women will feel dense, firm, and elastic. Expected variations include the lobular feel of glandular tissue (this feels like tiny granular bumps widely dispersed throughout the breast tissue) and the fine, granular feel of breast tissue in older women. A cyclical pattern of breast enlargement, increased nodularity, and tenderness is a common response to hormonal changes

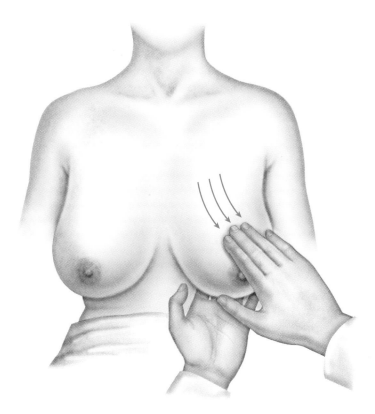

FIGURE 14-14
Palpating large breasts.

during the menstrual cycle. Be aware of where the woman is in her cycle, because these changes are most likely to occur premenstrually and during menses. They are least noticeable during the week after menstrual flow.

Tail of Spence

Palpate the tail of Spence in each breast (Figure 14-15). With the patient still in a seated position, have her raise her arms over her head, and palpate the tail as it enters the axilla, gently compressing the tissue between your thumb and fingers.

Additional Positions

Continue palpation (always gently) with the patient in the supine position. Have her raise one arm behind her head and place a small pillow or folded towel under that shoulder to spread the breast tissue more evenly over the chest wall (Figure 14-16). Palpate that breast, compressing the breast tissue between your fingers and the chest wall, using a rotary motion with your fingers. Repeat palpation with the woman's arm at her side. Breast tissue shifts with the change in arm position and allows palpation of a different portion of the breast overlying the ribs. Repeat these maneuvers for the other breast. If a breast mass is felt, note its characteristics and palpate its dimensions, consistency, and mobility (Figures 14-17 and 14-18; see also Box 14-3 on p. 499).

Nipple

The nipple should be palpated on both male and female patients. Compress the nipple between your thumb and index finger and inspect for discharge (Figure 14-19). Do this gently because pinching can cause tissue trauma. Palpation may cause erection of the nipple and puckering of the areola. If discharge appears, note its color and try to determine the origin by massaging radially around the areola while watching for the discharge through the ductal opening on the nipple surface (Figure 14-20). Prepare a smear of the discharge for cytologic examination. Spread a small amount on the glass slide and spray it with the cytologic fixative.

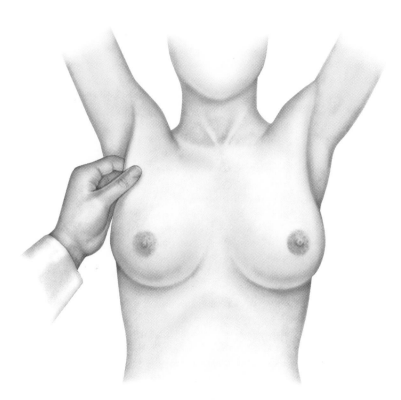

FIGURE 14-15
Palpating the tail of Spence.

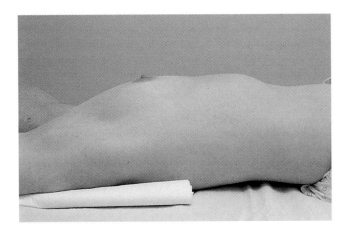

FIGURE 14-16
Supine position for palpation.

Lymph Nodes

Palpate for lymph nodes in both male and female patients. To palpate the axillae, have the patient seated with arms flexed at the elbow. If you begin on the right, support the right lower arm with your right hand while examining the right axilla with your left hand, as shown in Figure 14-21. With the palmar surface of your fingers, reach deeply into the axillary hollow, pushing firmly but not too aggressively upward. Then bring your fingers downward so that you gently roll the soft tissues against the chest wall and muscles of the axilla. Be sure to explore all sections of the axilla—the apex, the central or medial aspect along the rib cage, the lateral aspect along the upper surface of the arm, the anterior wall along the pectoral muscles, and the posterior wall along the border of the scapula. Then do a mirror image of this maneuver for the right axilla.

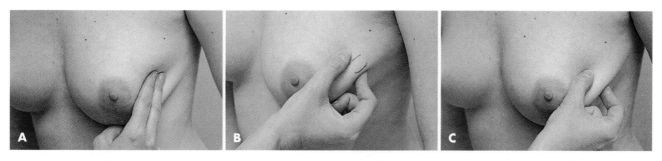

FIGURE 14-17
A, Palpating for consistency of a breast lesion. **B,** Palpating for delineation of borders of breast mass.
C, Palpating for mobility of breast mass.

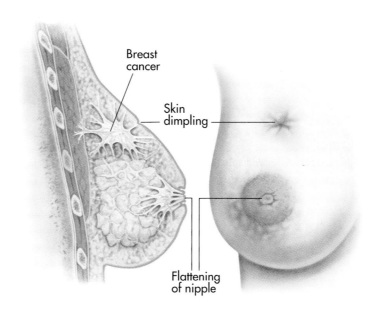

FIGURE 14-18
Clinical signs of cancer: nipple
retraction and dimpling of skin.

Breast
cancer

Skin
dimpling

Flattening
of nipple

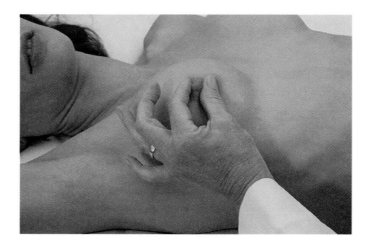

FIGURE 14-19
Palpation of the nipple.
From Thompson, Wilson, 1996.

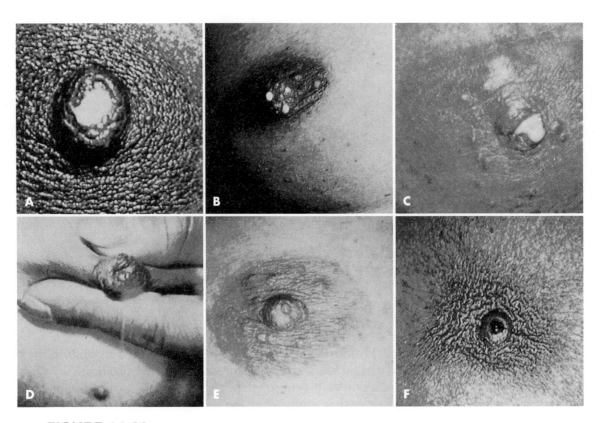

FIGURE 14-20
Types of nipple discharge. **A,** Milky discharge. **B,** Multicolored sticky discharge. **C,** Purulent discharge.
D, Watery discharge. **E,** Serous discharge. **F,** Serosanguinous discharge.
From Gallagher, 1978.

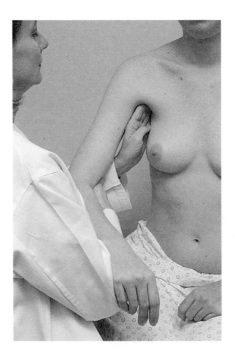

FIGURE 14-21
Palpation of the axilla for lymph
nodes.

| BOX 14-4 | Examining the Patient Who Has Had a Mastectomy |

The patient who has had a mastectomy has special examination needs. In addition to examining the unaffected breast in the usual manner, you must examine the mastectomy site, with particular attention to the scar. If malignancy recurs, it may be at the scar site. Be aware that a woman who has had a mastectomy may feel uncomfortable removing her brassiere and prosthesis if she wears one. (See "An Approach to Sensitive Issues," Chapter 1, pp. 18-21.)

Inspect the mastectomy site and axilla for any visible signs of swelling, lumps, thickening, redness, color change, rash, or irritation to the scar. Note muscle loss or lymphedema that may be present, depending on the type and extent of the surgical procedure.

Palpate the surgical scar with two fingers, using small, circular motions to assess for swelling, lumps, thickening, or tenderness. Then palpate the chest wall using three or four fingers in a sweeping motion across the area, being sure not to miss any spots. Remember to use your finger pads and not your fingertips.

If the patient has had breast reconstruction, augmentation, or a lumpectomy, perform breast examination in the usual manner, with particular attention to any scars and new tissue.

Finally, palpate for lymph nodes in the axillary and supraclavicular areas.

Remember to have this patient demonstrate her (or his) breast self-examination procedures. Regular monthly breast self-examination is an essential component of continuing health care for these individuals

Nodes are not usually palpable in the adult. Palpable nodes may be the result of an inflammatory or malignant process. Nodes that are detected should be described according to location, size, shape, consistency, tenderness, fixation, and delineation of borders. (See Chapter 8, Lymphatic System.)

The supraclavicular area also should be palpated for the presence of enlarged nodes. Hook your fingers over the clavicle and rotate them over the entire supraclavicular area. Have the patient turn his or her head toward the side being palpated and raise the same shoulder, allowing your fingers to reach more deeply into the fossa. You can also have the patient bend the head forward to relax the sternocleidomastoid muscle. These nodes are considered to be sentinel nodes (Virchow nodes), so any enlargement is highly significant. Virchow nodes are the first sign of invasion of the lymphatics by abdominal or thoracic carcinoma.

INFANTS

The breasts of many well infants, male and female, are enlarged for a relatively brief time during the newborn period. The enlargement may be noted at birth and is the result of passively transferred maternal estrogen. If you squeeze the breast bud gently, a small amount of clear or milky white fluid, commonly called "witch's milk," is sometimes expressed. The enlargement is rarely more than 1 to 1.5 cm in diameter and can be easily palpated behind the nipple. Usually disappearing within 2 weeks, it rarely lasts beyond 3 months of age.

ADOLESCENTS

The right and left breasts of the adolescent female may not develop at the same rate. Reassure the girl that this asymmetry is common and that her breasts are developing appropriately. Chapter 5, Growth and Measurement, describes the stages of breast development. Breast tissue of the adolescent female feels homogenous, dense, firm, and elastic. Although malignancy in this age-group is rare, routine examination provides an excellent opportunity for reassurance and education. Starting breast self-examination early can also help establish a healthful habit for life.

Many males at puberty have transient unilateral or bilateral subareolar masses. These are firm, sometimes tender, and are often a source of great concern to the patient and his parents. Reassure them that these breast buds will most likely disappear, usually within a year. They seldom enlarge to a point of cosmetic difficulty.

Occasionally, however, pubescent males experience gynecomastia, an unusual and unexpected enlargement that is readily noticeable. Fortunately, it is usually temporary and benign and resolves spontaneously. If the enlargement is extreme, it can be corrected surgically for psychologic or cosmetic reasons. In rare instances, biopsy is required to rule out the presence of cancer.

Adolescent breast symptoms ranging from galactorrhea to pain and cysts. Male gynecomastia can be associated with the use of either illicit or prescription drugs. Symptoms resolve after the drugs are discontinued.

PREGNANT WOMEN

Many changes in the breasts occur during pregnancy. Most become obvious during the first trimester. The woman may experience a sensation of fullness with tingling, tenderness, and a bilateral increase in size. It is important to ascertain that the woman is providing adequate support for her breasts with a properly fitting brassiere. As her breasts continue to enlarge, she may need to alter the size and style of the brassiere.

Generally, the nipples enlarge and are more erectile. As the pregnancy progresses, the nipples sometimes become flattened or inverted. A crust caused by dried colostrum can be evident on the nipple. The colostrum, a clear viscous discharge that begins as early as the sixth week of gestation, becomes yellow and more viscous in later pregnancy. The areola begins to broaden and darken, and Montgomery tubercles may appear (Figure 14-22).

Palpation reveals a generalized coarse nodularity, and the breasts feel lobular because of hypertrophy of the mammary alveoli. Dilated subcutaneous veins may create a network of blue tracing across the breasts.

During the second trimester, vascular spiders may develop on the upper chest, arms, neck, and face as a result of elevated levels of circulating estrogen. The spiders are bluish in color and do not blanch with pressure. Striae may be evident on the breasts as a result of stretching as they increase in size.

LACTATING WOMEN

During the period of lactation it is important to assess whether the breasts are adequately supported with a properly fitting brassiere. Palpate the breasts to determine the degree of softness. Full breasts, which are firm, dense, and slightly enlarged, may become engorged. Engorged breasts feel hard and warm and are enlarged, shiny, and painful. Engorgement is not an unusual condition in the first 24 to 48 hours after the breasts fill with milk. However, its development later may signal the onset of mastitis.

Clogged milk ducts are a relatively common occurrence in lactating women. A clogged duct may result from either inadequate emptying of the breast or a brassiere that is too tight. The clogged duct will create a tender spot on the breast that may feel lumpy and hot. Frequent nursing and/or expression of the milk, along with local application of heat, will help open the duct. A clogged duct left unattended will probably result in the development of mastitis.

Examine the nipples for signs of irritation (redness and tenderness) and for blisters or petechiae, which are precursors of overt cracking. If the nipples are already cracked, they will be sore and may be bleeding. There is no correlation between color of the nipple and nipple damage from breast-feeding, which has to do with placement of the nipple in the infant's mouth. Lighter-colored nipples are no more prone to damage than are darker nipples.

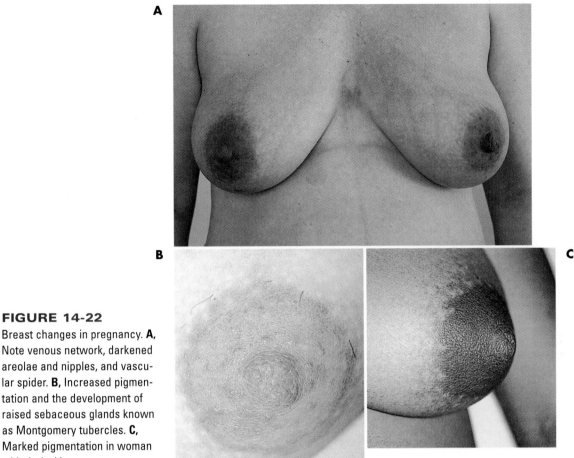

FIGURE 14-22
Breast changes in pregnancy. **A,** Note venous network, darkened areolae and nipples, and vascular spider. **B,** Increased pigmentation and the development of raised sebaceous glands known as Montgomery tubercles. **C,** Marked pigmentation in woman with dark skin.

B and **C** from Symonds, Macpherson, 1994.

After pregnancy and lactation, there is regression of most of these changes. The areolae and nipples tend to retain their darker color, and the breasts become less firm than in their prepregnant state.

OLDER ADULTS

The breasts in postmenopausal women may appear flattened, elongated, and suspended more loosely from the chest wall as the result of glandular tissue atrophy and relaxation of the suspensory ligaments. The lobular feel of glandular tissue is replaced by a finer, granular feel on palpation. The inframammary ridge thickens and can be felt more easily. The nipples become smaller and flatter.

Postmenopausal women should be encouraged to continue monthly breast self-examination. Because the breasts are no longer subject to hormonal changes of menstruation, these women should choose a convenient date and regularly examine their breasts on this date. Hormone replacement therapy can result in fluid-filled breast cysts, which can be painful.

FEMALES

Breasts: moderate size, conical shape, left slightly larger than right. No skin lesions; contour smooth without dimpling or retraction; venous patterns symmetric. Nipples symmetric without discharge; Montgomery tubercles bilaterally. Tissue dense, particularly in upper quadrants. No palpable masses. No supraclavicular, infraclavicular, or axillary lymphadenopathy.

MALES

Breasts: small, bilaterally symmetric with male contour. No skin or nipple lesions; no nipple discharge. Tissue smooth without palpable masses. No palpable supraclavicular, infraclavicular, or axillary lymph nodes.

For additional sample documentation, see Chapter 24, Recording Information.

SUMMARY OF EXAMINATION | Breasts and Axillae

Females

1. Inspect with patient seated and arms hanging loosely at the sides. Inspect both breasts and compare them for the following (p. 494).
   - Size
   - Symmetry
   - Contour
   - Retractions or dimpling
   - Skin color and texture
   - Venous patterns
   - Lesions
   - Supernumerary nipples
2. Inspect both areolae and nipples and compare them for the following (pp. 494-495):
   - Shape
   - Symmetry
   - Color
   - Smoothness
   - Size
   - Nipple inversion, eversion, or retraction
3. Reinspect breasts with the patient in the following positions (p. 498):
   - Arms extended over head
   - Hands pressed on hips or hands pushed together in front of chest
   - Seated and leaning over
   - In recumbent position
4. With patient seated, palpate breasts systematically in all four quadrants and the tail of Spence and over areolae for lumps or nodules (pp. 498-500); if breasts are large, perform bimanual palpation (p. 500).
5. Palpate nipples; compress gently to observe for discharge (p. 501).
6. Palpate for lymph nodes in the apex, medial and lateral aspects, anterior and posterior walls of the axilla, and the supraclavicular area (p. 502).
7. Continue palpation of breast tissue with patient supine, one arm behind head and towel under shoulder (p. 501).

Males

1. Inspect breasts for the following (p. 494):
   - Symmetry
   - Enlargement
   - Surface characteristics
2. Inspect both areolae and nipples and compare them for the following (pp. 494-500):
   - Shape
   - Symmetry
   - Color
   - Smoothness
   - Size
   - Nipple inversion, eversion, or retraction
3. Palpate breasts and over areolae for lumps or nodules (pp. 498-500).
4. Palpate nipple; compress to observe for discharge (p. 501).
5. Palpate for lymph nodes in the apex, medial and lateral aspects, anterior and posterior walls of the axilla, and the supraclavicular area (p. 502).

COMMON ABNORMALITIES

FIBROCYSTIC DISEASE	Benign cyst formation caused by ductal enlargement is associated with a long follicular or luteal phase of the menstrual cycle. The lesions are filled with fluid and are usually bilateral and multiple. Characteristically the cysts are tender and	painful with an increase in these symptoms premenstrually. Fibrocystic disease occurs most commonly in women between the ages of 30 and 55. Table 14-2 details the differences between fibrocystic disease, fibroadenoma, and breast cancer.
FIBROADENOMA	This benign neoplasm accounts for the majority of breast tumors in young women. Fibroadenomas are generally asymptomatic and do not change premenstrually. A sudden change in the size	of an existing fibroadenoma may signal a malignant change. Biopsy is often performed to rule out carcinoma (Table 14-2).

TABLE 14-2	Differentiating Signs and Symptoms of Breast Masses		
DIFFERENTIAL DIAGNOSIS	**Fibrocystic Disease**	**Fibroadenoma**	**Cancer**
Age range	20-49	15-55	30-80
Occurrence	Usually bilateral	Usually bilateral	Usually unilateral
Number	Multiple or single	Single; may be multiple	Single
Shape	Round	Round or discoid	Irregular or stellate
Consistency	Soft to firm; tense	Firm, rubbery	Hard, stonelike
Mobility	Mobile	Mobile	Fixed
Retraction signs	Absent	Absent	Often present
Tenderness	Usually tender	Usually nontender	Usually nontender
Borders	Well delineated	Well delineated	Poorly delineated; irregular
Variation with menses	Yes	No	No

MALIGNANT BREAST TUMORS

Peak incidence of malignancy is between ages 40 and 60, with two thirds of malignant breast tumors occurring in women under age 65. About 80% of patients with breast cancer have a painless lump in the breast as the initial symptom. Metastases occur through the lymph and vascular systems. The following findings are associated with breast cancer: mass or thickening in breast; marked asymmetry of breasts; prominent unilateral veins; discolorations (erythema or ecchymosis); peau d'orange; ulcerations; dimpling, puckering, or retraction of skin or areola; fixed inversion or deviation in position of the nipple; crusting or erosion of the nipple or areola; or change in surface characteristics (e.g., moles or scars) (Table 14-2 and Figure 14-23).

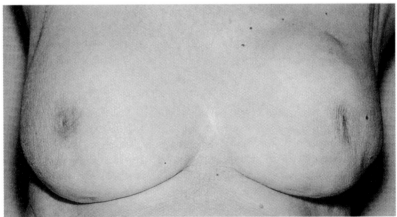

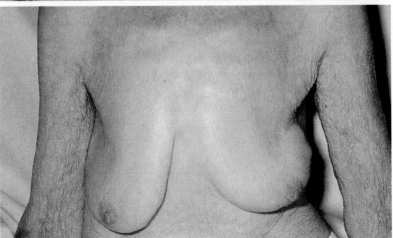

FIGURE 14-23
A, Patient with lump and nipple retraction in left breast. **B,** Patient with altered nipple height resulting from breast cancer in left breast.

From Mansel, Bundred, 1995.

FAT NECROSIS

Fat necrosis is a response to local injury. It is felt as a firm irregular mass, often appearing as an area of discoloration (Figure 14-24).

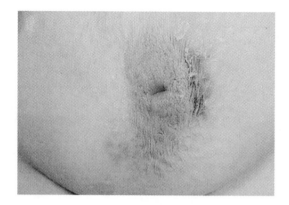

FIGURE 14-24

Fat necrosis presenting as a hard mass in the breast following an episode of trauma sufficient to cause bruising.

From Mansel, Bundred, 1995.

INTRADUCTAL PAPILLOMAS AND PAPILLOMATOSIS

These 2- to 3-cm tumors of the subareolar ducts may occur singly or in multiples. Papillomas are a common cause of serous or bloody nipple discharge. They need to be excised and examined to rule out malignancy.

PAGET DISEASE

Paget disease of the breast is a surface manifestation of underlying ductal carcinoma. A red, scaling, crusty patch forms on the nipple, areola, and surrounding skin. The lesion appears eczematous but, unlike eczema, occurs unilaterally (Figure 14-25).

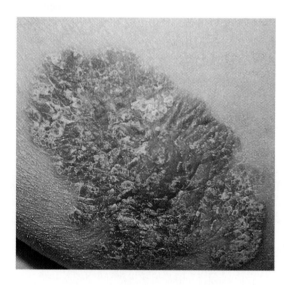

FIGURE 14-25

Paget disease.

From Habif, 1996.

ADULT GYNECOMASTIA

Gynecomastia is a smooth, firm, mobile, tender disk of breast tissue located behind the areola in males. It may be unilateral or bilateral. In adult men it can be caused by hormone imbalance; testicular, pituitary, or hormone-secreting tumors; liver failure; and antihypertensive medications or those containing estrogens or steroids (Figure 14-26).

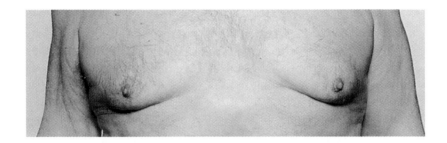

FIGURE 14-26
Adult gynecomastia.
From Mansel, Bundred, 1995.

RETENTION CYSTS

Inflammation of the sebaceous glands in the areola results in retention cysts. They may become tender and suppurative.

GALACTORRHEA

Lactation not associated with child-bearing is most commonly caused by drugs, especially phenothiazines, tricyclic antidepressants, some antihypertensive agents, and estrogens. Intrinsic causes of galactorrhea include prolactin-secreting tumors, pituitary tumors, hypothyroidism (Figure 14-27), Cushing syndrome, and hypoglycemia.

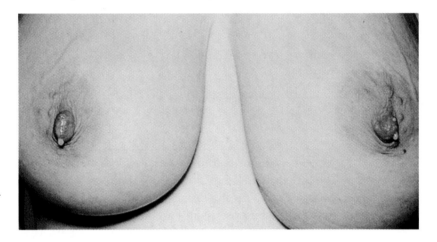

FIGURE 14-27
Galactorrhea produced by a prolactin-secreting pituitary tumor.
From Mansel, Bundred, 1995.

CHILDREN

GYNECOMASTIA

Enlargement of breast tissue in boys is caused by puberty, hormonal imbalance, testicular or pituitary tumors, and medications containing estrogens or steroids (Figure 14-28).

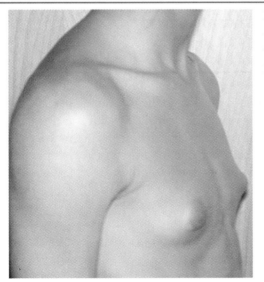

FIGURE 14-28
Prepubertal gynecomastia, small and subareolar.
Courtesy Wellington Hung, MD, Children's National Medical Center, Washington, DC.

PREMATURE
THELARCHE

Prepubertal breast enlargement of un-known cause in girls can occur in the ab-sence of other signs of sexual matura-tion. The degree of enlargement varies from very slight to fully developed breasts. It usually occurs bilaterally, with the breasts continuing to enlarge slowly throughout childhood until full develop-ment is reached during adolescence (Fig-ure 14-29).

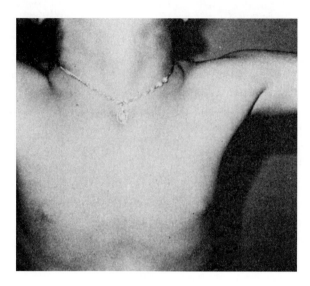

FIGURE 14-29
Premature thelarche.
Courtesy Wellington Hung, MD, Children's National Medical Center, Washington, DC.

LACTATING WOMEN

MASTITIS

Mastitis is inflammation and infection of the breast tissue characterized by sudden onset of swelling, tenderness, erythema, and heat, which is usually accompanied by chills, fever, and increased pulse rate. Most infections are staphylococcal, often *Staphylococcus aureus.* Mastitis is most common in lactating women after milk is established, usually the second to third week after delivery; however, it may occur at any time. Mastitis is not an indi-cation to discontinue breast-feeding. Abscess formation can result, which pre-sents as discharge of pus (suppuration) and a large hardened mass with an area of fluctuation, erythema, and heat. The underlying pus-filled abscess may impart a bluish tinge to the skin.

OLDER ADULTS

MAMMARY DUCT
ECTASIA

Mammary duct ectasia occurs most fre-quently in menopausal women. The sub-areolar ducts become blocked with desquamating secretory epithelium, ne-crotic debris, and chronic inflammatory cells. This condition is frequently bilat-eral and is characterized by pain, tender-ness, periods of inflammation, and a nip-ple discharge that is spontaneous, sticky, multicolored, and from multiple ducts. Nipple retraction may occur. There is no known association with malignancy.

Remember to check   Mosby   *http://www1.mosby.com/physexam_seidel*

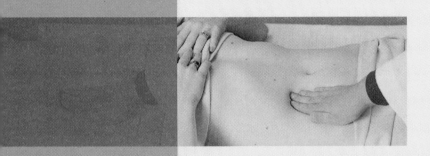

CHAPTER 15

ABDOMEN

ANATOMY AND PHYSIOLOGY

The abdominal cavity contains several of the body's vital organs (Figure 15-1). The peritoneum, a serous membrane, lines the cavity and forms a protective cover for many of the abdominal structures. Double folds of the peritoneum around the stomach constitute the greater and lesser omentum. The mesentery, a fan-shaped fold of the peritoneum, covers most of the small intestine and anchors it to the posterior abdominal wall.

ALIMENTARY TRACT   The alimentary tract is a tube approximately 27 ft long that runs from the mouth to the anus and includes the esophagus, stomach, small intestine, and large intestine. It functions to ingest and digest food; absorb nutrients, electrolytes, and water; and excrete waste products. Food and the products of digestion are moved along the length of the digestive tract by peristalsis, which is under autonomic nervous system control.

The esophagus is a collapsible tube about 10 in long, connecting the pharynx to the stomach. Passing just posterior to the trachea, the esophagus descends through the mediastinal cavity, travels through the diaphragm, and enters the stomach at the cardiac orifice.

The flask-shaped stomach lies transversely in the upper abdominal cavity, just below the diaphragm. It consists of three sections: the fundus, which lies above and to the left of the cardiac orifice; the middle two thirds, or body; and the pylorus, the most distal portion that narrows and terminates in the pyloric orifice. The stomach secretes hydrochloric acid and digestive enzymes that break down fats and proteins. Pepsin acts to digest proteins, whereas gastric lipase acts on emulsified fats. Very little absorption takes place in the stomach.

The small intestine, about 21 ft long, begins at the pyloric orifice. Coiled in the abdominal cavity, it joins the large intestine at the ileocecal valve. The first 12 in of the small intestine, the duodenum, forms a C-shaped curve around the head of the pancreas. The common bile duct and pancreatic duct open into the duodenum at the duodenal papilla, about 3 in below the pylorus of the stomach. The next 8 ft of intestine is the jejunum, which gradually becomes larger and thicker. The ileum makes up

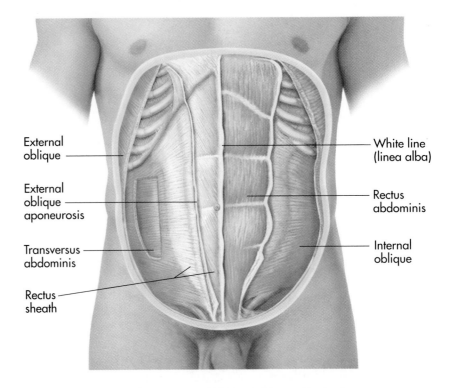

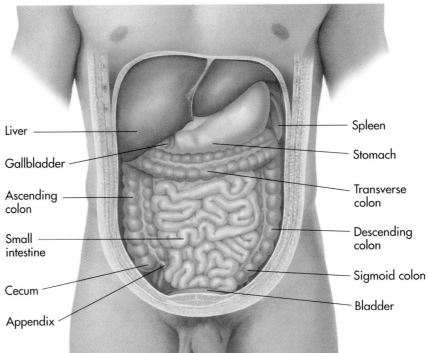

FIGURE 15-1
Anatomic structures of the abdominal cavity.

the remaining 12 ft of the small intestine. The ileocecal valve between the ileum and large intestine prevents backward flow of fecal material.

Digestion is completed in the small intestine through the action of pancreatic enzymes, bile, and several small intestine enzymes. Nutrients are absorbed through the walls of the small intestine, whose functional surface area is enormously increased by its circular folds and villi.

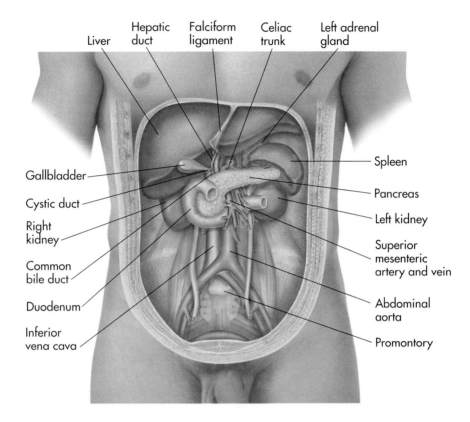

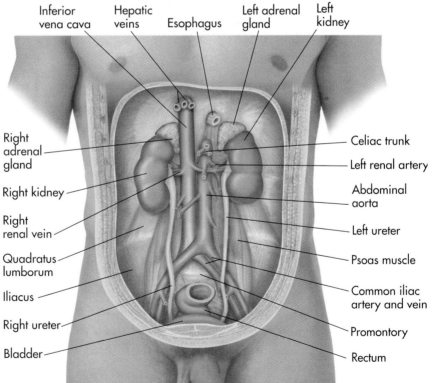

FIGURE 15-1—cont'd
Anatomic structures of the abdominal cavity.

The large intestine begins at the cecum, a blind pouch about 2 to 3 in long. The ileal contents empty into the cecum through the ileocecal valve, and the vermiform appendix extends from the base of the cecum. The ascending colon rises from the cecum along the right posterior abdominal wall to the undersurface of the liver, where it turns toward the midline (the hepatic flexure), becoming the transverse colon. The transverse colon crosses the abdominal cavity toward the spleen, turning downward at the splenic flexure. The descending colon continues along the left abdominal wall to the rim of the pelvis, where it turns medially and inferiorly to form the S-shaped sigmoid colon. The rectum extends from the sigmoid colon to the muscles of the pelvic floor, where it continues as the anal canal and terminates at the anus.

The large intestine is about $4\frac{1}{2}$ to 5 ft long, with a diameter of $2\frac{1}{2}$ in. Water absorption takes place here. Mucous glands secrete large quantities of alkaline mucus that lubricate the intestinal contents and neutralize acids formed by intestinal bacteria. Live bacteria decompose undigested food residue, unabsorbed amino acids, cell debris, and dead bacteria through a process of putrefaction.

LIVER

The liver lies in the right upper quadrant of the abdomen, just below the diaphragm. Its inferior surface almost embraces the gallbladder, stomach, duodenum, and hepatic flexure of the colon. The heaviest organ in the body, the liver weighs about 3 lb in the adult. It is composed of four lobes containing lobules, the functional units. Each lobule is made up of liver cells radiating around a central vein. Branches of the portal vein, hepatic artery, and bile duct embrace the periphery of the lobules. Bile secreted by the liver cells drains from the bile ducts into the hepatic duct, which joins the cystic duct from the gallbladder to form the common bile duct.

The hepatic artery transports blood to the liver directly from the aorta, and the portal vein carries blood from the digestive tract and spleen to the liver. Repeated branching of both vessels makes the liver a highly vascularized organ. Three hepatic veins carry blood from the liver and empty into the inferior vena cava.

The liver plays an important role in the metabolism of carbohydrates, fats, and proteins. Glucose is converted and stored as glycogen until, in response to varying levels of insulin and regulator hormones, it is reconverted and released again as glucose. The liver also has the capacity to convert amino acids to glucose (gluconeogenesis). Fats, arriving at the liver in the form of fatty acids, are oxidized to two carbon components in preparation for entry into the tricarboxylic acid cycle. Cholesterol is used by the liver to form bile salts. Synthesis of fats from carbohydrates and proteins also occurs in the liver. Proteins are broken down to amino acids through hydrolysis, and their waste products are converted to urea for excretion.

Other functions of the liver include storage of several vitamins and iron, detoxification of potentially harmful substances, production of antibodies, conjugation and excretion of steroid hormones, and the production of prothrombin, fibrinogen, and other substances for blood coagulation. The liver is responsible for the production of the majority of proteins circulating in the plasma. It serves a vital role as an excretory organ through the synthesis of bile, the secretion of organic wastes into bile, and the conversion of fat-soluble wastes to water-soluble material for renal excretion.

GALLBLADDER

The gallbladder is a saclike, pear-shaped organ about 4 in long, lying recessed in the inferior surface of the liver. Its function is to concentrate and store bile from the liver. In response to cholecystokinin, a hormone produced in the duodenum, the gallbladder releases bile into the cystic duct, which, with the hepatic duct, forms the common bile duct. Contraction of the gallbladder propels bile among the common duct and into the duodenum at the duodenal papilla. Composed of cholesterol, bile salts, and pigments, bile serves to maintain the alkaline pH of the small intestine to permit emulsification of fats so that absorption can be accomplished.

PANCREAS

The pancreas lies behind and beneath the stomach, with its head resting in the curve of the duodenum and its tip extending across the abdominal cavity to almost touch the spleen. As part of the pancreas' function as an exocrine gland, the acinar cells of the pancreas produce digestive juices containing inactive enzymes for the breakdown of proteins, fats, and carbohydrates. Collecting ducts empty the juice into the pancreatic duct (duct of Wirsung), which runs the length of the organ. The pancreatic duct empties into the duodenum at the duodenal papilla, alongside the common bile duct. Once introduced into the duodenum, the digestive enzymes are activated. As an endocrine gland, islet cells scattered throughout the pancreas produce the hormones insulin and glucagon. These are secreted directly into the blood to regulate the body's level of glucose. Insulin, the major anabolic hormone of the body, also serves several other vital functions.

SPLEEN

The spleen is in the left upper quadrant, lying above the left kidney and just below the diaphragm. White pulp (lymphoid tissue) constitutes most of the organ and functions as part of the reticuloendothelial system to filter blood and to manufacture lymphocytes and monocytes. The red pulp of the spleen contains a capillary network and venous sinus system that allow for the storage and release of blood, permitting the spleen to accommodate up to several hundred milliliters at once.

KIDNEYS, URETERS, AND BLADDER

The two kidneys, the excretory organs responsible for the removal of water-soluble waste, are located in the retroperitoneal space of the upper abdomen. Each extends from about the vertebral level of T12 to L3. The right kidney is usually slightly lower than the left, presumably because of the large, heavy liver just above it. Both kidneys are imbedded in fat and fascia, which anchor and protect these organs. Each contains more than 1 million nephrons, the structural and functional units of the kidneys. The nephrons are composed of a tuft of capillaries, the glomerulus, a proximal convoluted tubule, the loop of Henle, and a distal convoluted tubule. The distal tube empties into a collecting tubule.

Each kidney receives about one eighth of the cardiac output through its renal artery. The glomeruli filter blood at a rate of about 125 ml per minute in the adult male and about 110 ml per minute in the adult female. Most of the filtered material, including electrolytes, glucose, water, and small proteins, is actively resorbed in the proximal tubule. Some organic acids are also actively secreted in the distal tubule. Urinary volume is carefully controlled by antidiuretic hormone (ADH) to maintain a constant total body fluid volume. Urine passes into the renal pelvis via the collecting tubules and then into the ureter. Peristaltic waves move it on to a reservoir, the urinary bladder, which has a capacity of about 400 to 500 ml in the adult.

The kidney also serves as an endocrine gland responsible for the production of renin, which is important for the ultimate control of aldosterone secretion. It is the primary source of erythropoietin production in adults, thus influencing the body's red cell mass. In addition to synthesizing several prostaglandins, the kidney produces the biologically active form of vitamin D.

MUSCULATURE AND CONNECTIVE TISSUES

The muscles that form and protect the abdominal cavity are composed of the rectus abdominis muscles anteriorly and the internal and external oblique muscles laterally. The linea alba, a tendinous band, is located in the midline of the abdomen between the rectus abdominis muscles. It extends from the xiphoid process to the symphysis pubis and contains the umbilicus. The inguinal ligament (Poupart ligament) extends from the anterior superior spine of the ilium to the pubis on each side.

VASCULATURE

The abdominal portion of the descending aorta travels from the diaphragm through the abdominal cavity, just to the left of midline. At about the level of the umbilicus the aorta branches into the two common iliac arteries. The splenic and renal arteries, which supply their respective organs, also branch off within the abdomen.

INFANTS

The pancreatic buds, liver, and gallbladder all begin to form during week 4 of gestation, by which time the intestine already exists as a single tube. The motility of the gastrointestinal tract develops in a cephalocaudal direction, permitting amniotic fluid to be swallowed by 16 weeks of gestation. Production of meconium, an end product of fetal metabolism, begins shortly thereafter. By 36 to 38 weeks of gestation, the gastrointestinal tract is capable of adapting to extrauterine life. However, its elasticity, musculature, and control mechanisms continue to develop, reaching adult levels of function at 2 to 3 years of age.

During gestation, the liver begins to form blood cells at about week 6, synthesize glycogen by week 9, and produce bile by week 12. The liver's role as a metabolic and glycogen storage organ accounts for its large size at birth. Its growth during infancy is not as rapid as skeletal growth, but it remains the heaviest organ in the body.

Pancreatic islet cells are developed by 12 weeks of gestation and begin producing insulin. The spleen is active in blood formation during fetal development and the first year of life. After that time, the spleen aids in the destruction of blood cells and the formation of hemoglobin.

Nephrogenesis begins during the second embryologic month. By 12 weeks the kidney is able to produce urine, and the bladder expands as a sac. Development of new nephrons ceases by 36 weeks of gestation. After birth the kidney increases in size incrementally because of enlargement of the more than 1 million existing nephrons and adjoining tubules—a process that parallels body growth. The glomerular filtration rate is approximately 0.5 ml/min before 34 weeks of gestation and gradually increases in a linear fashion to 125 ml/min.

PREGNANT WOMEN

As the uterus enlarges, the muscles of the abdominal wall stretch and ultimately lose some tone (Figure 15-2). During the third trimester the rectus abdominis muscles may separate, allowing abdominal contents to protrude at the midline.

After pregnancy, the muscles gradually regain tone, although separation of the rectus abdominis muscles (diastasis recti) may persist. The umbilicus flattens or protrudes. The abdominal contour changes when lightening occurs (about 2 weeks before term in a nullipara), and the fetal presenting part descends into the true pelvis. Striae may form as the skin is stretched. A line of pigmentation at the midline (linea nigra) often develops (Figure 15-3). Abdominal muscles have less tone and are less active.

Upward displacement of the stomach occurs later in pregnancy. In about 15% to 20% of pregnant women, herniation through the diaphragm by the upper portion of the stomach can occur after the seventh or eighth month; this is more common in older, obese, and multiparous women. Increased progesterone production causes a decrease in tone and motility of the smooth muscles, which results in delayed emptying

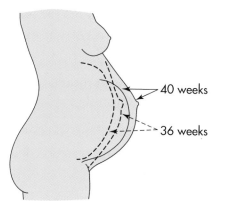

FIGURE 15-2
Contour changes in the abdomen
during pregnancy.
From Lowdermilk, Perry, Bobak, 1997.

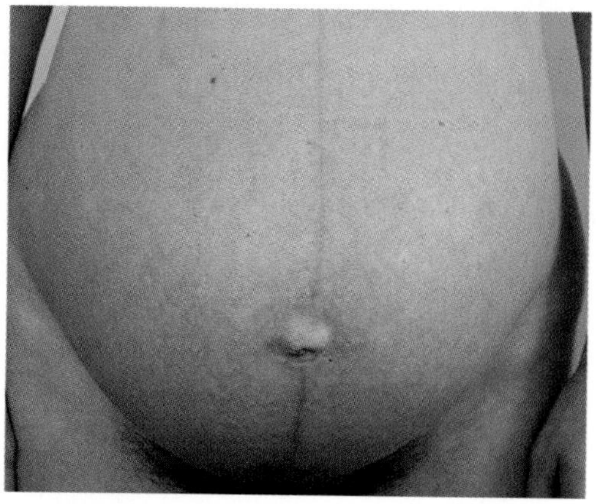

FIGURE 15-3
Linea nigra in the third trimester of pregnancy.

time of the stomach. Incompetence of the pyloric sphincter may result in alkaline reflux of duodenal contents into the stomach. Heartburn is a common complaint.

The gallbladder may become distended, accompanied by decreased emptying time and change in tone. The combination of gallbladder stasis and secretion of lithogenic bile increases formation of cholesterol crystals in the development of gallstones. Gallstones are more frequent in the second and third trimesters.

The kidneys enlarge slightly (by about 1 to 2 cm in length) during pregnancy. The renal pelvis and ureters dilate from the effects of estrogen and progesterone, pressure from the enlarging uterus, and an increase in blood volume. Dilation of the ureter is more common on the right side than on the left, because it is probably affected by displacement of the uterus to the right by an enlarged right ovarian vein. The ureters also elongate and form single and double curves of varying sizes and angulation. These changes lead to urinary stasis. Renal function is most efficient if the woman lies in the lateral recumbent position, which helps prevent compression of the vena cava and aorta. These changes can last up to 12 weeks after delivery.

The bladder has increased sensitivity and compression during pregnancy, which may lead to frequency and urgency of urination during the first and third trimesters. After the fourth month the increase in uterine size, hyperemia, and hyperplasia of muscle and connective tissue cause elevation of the bladder trigone and thickening of the posterior margin, which produce a marked deepening and widening of the trigone by the end of the pregnancy. During the third trimester, compression may also result from the descent of the fetus into the pelvis; this, in turn, causes a sense of urgency even if there is only a small amount of urine in the bladder.

The colon is displaced laterally upward and posteriorly, peristaltic activity may decrease, and water absorption is increased. As a result, bowel sounds are diminished, and constipation and flatus are more common. The appendix is displaced upward and laterally so that it is high and to the right, away from the McBurney point. Blood flow to the pelvis increases, as does venous pressure, contributing to hemorrhoid formation.

In the postpartum period the uterus involutes rapidly. Immediately after delivery the uterus is approximately the size of a 20-week pregnancy (at the level of the umbilicus). By the end of the first week, it is about the size of a 12-week pregnancy, palpable at the symphysis pubis. The muscles of the pelvic floor and the pelvic supports gradually regain their tone during the postpartum period and may require 6 to 7 weeks to recover. Stretching of the abdominal wall during pregnancy may result in persistent striae and diastasis of the rectus muscles.

OLDER ADULTS

The process of aging brings about changes in the functional abilities of the gastrointestinal tract. Motility of the intestine is the most severely affected; secretion and absorption are affected to a lesser degree. Altered motility may be caused in part by age-related changes in neurons of the central nervous system and by changes in collagen properties that increase the resistance of the intestinal wall to stretching. Reduced circulation to the intestine often follows other system changes associated with hypoxia and hypovolemia. Thus functional abilities of the intestine can decrease secondary to adverse changes occurring elsewhere in the older adult.

As a result of epithelial atrophy, the secretion of both digestive enzymes and protective mucus in the intestinal tract is decreased. Particular elements of the mucosal cells show a lesser degree of differentiation and are associated with reduction in secretory ability. These cells are also more susceptible to both physical and chemical agents, including ingested carcinogens. Bacterial flora of the intestine can undergo both qualitative and quantitative changes and become less biologically active. These changes may impair digestive ability and manifest food intolerances in the older adult.

Liver size decreases after age 50, which parallels the decrease in lean body mass. Hepatic blood flow decreases as a result of the decline in cardiac output associated with aging. The liver loses some ability to metabolize certain drugs.

The size of the pancreas is unaffected by aging, although the main pancreatic duct and its branches widen. With aging there is an increase in fibrous tissue and fatty deposition with acinar cell atrophy. However, the large reserve of the organ results in no significant physiologic changes. The functional reserve of the pancreas may be reduced, although this can occur as a result of delayed gastric emptying rather than pancreatic changes.

There may be an increase of biliary lipids, specifically the phospholipids and cholesterol. This can result in the formation of gallstones.

REVIEW OF RELATED HISTORY

PRESENT PROBLEM

- Abdominal pain
  - Onset and duration: when it began; sudden or gradual; persistent, recurrent, intermittent
  - Character: dull, sharp, burning, gnawing, stabbing, cramping, aching, colicky
  - Location: of onset, change in location over time, radiating to another area, superficial or deep
  - Associated symptoms: vomiting, diarrhea, constipation, passage of flatus, belching, jaundice, change in abdominal girth
  - Relationship to: menstrual cycle, abnormal menses, urination, defecation, inspiration, change in body position, food or alcohol intake, stress, time of day, trauma
  - Recent stool characteristics: color, consistency, odor, frequency
  - Urinary characteristics: frequency, color, volume congruent with fluid intake, force of stream, ease of starting stream, ability to empty bladder
  - Medications: prescription or nonprescription; high doses of aspirin, acetaminophen; steroids; nonsteroidal antiinflammatory drugs
- Indigestion
  - Character: feeling of fullness, heartburn, discomfort, excessive belching, flatulence, loss of appetite, severe pain
  - Location: localized or general, radiates to arms or shoulders

- Association with: food intake, timing of food intake, amount, type; date of last menstrual period
- Onset of symptoms: time of day or night, sudden or gradual
- Symptom relieved by antacids, rest, activity
- Medications: prescription or nonprescription; antacids
- Nausea: associated with vomiting; particular stimuli (odors, activities, time of day, food intake); date of last menstrual period
- Medications: prescription or nonprescription; antiemetics
- Vomiting
  - Character: nature (color, fresh blood or coffee grounds, undigested food particles), quantity, duration, frequency, ability to keep any liquids or food in stomach
  - Relationship to: previous meal, change in appetite, diarrhea or constipation, fever, weight loss, abdominal pain, medications, headache, nausea, date of last menstrual period
  - Medications: prescription or nonprescription; antiemetics
- Diarrhea
  - Character: watery, copious, explosive; color; presence of blood, mucus, undigested food, oil, or fat; odor; number of times per day, duration; change in pattern
  - Associated symptoms: chills, fever, thirst, weight loss, abdominal pain or cramping, fecal incontinence
  - Relationship to: timing and nature of food intake, stress
  - Travel history
  - Medications: prescription or nonprescription; laxatives or stool softeners; antidiarrheals
- Constipation
  - Character: presence of bright blood, black or tarry appearance of stool; diarrhea alternating with constipation; accompanied by abdominal pain or discomfort
  - Pattern: last bowel movement, pain with passage of stool, change in pattern or size of stool
  - Diet: recent change in diet, inclusion of high-fiber foods
  - Medications: prescription or nonprescription; laxatives, stool softeners, diuretics; iron
- Fecal incontinence
  - Character: stool characteristics, timing in relation to meals, number of episodes per day; occurring with or without warning sensation
  - Associated with: use of laxatives, presence of underlying disease (cancer, inflammatory bowel disease, diverticulitis, colitis, proctitis, diabetic neuropathy)
  - Relationship to: fluid and dietary intake, immobilization
  - Medications: prescription or nonprescription; laxatives, stool softeners, iron, diuretics
- Jaundice
  - Onset and duration
  - Color of stools or urine
  - Associated with abdominal pain, chills, fever
  - Exposure to hepatitis
  - Medications: prescription or nonprescription; high doses of acetaminophen
- Dysuria
  - Character: location (suprapubic, at end of urethra), pain or burning, frequency or volume changes

- Exposure to: tuberculosis, fungal or viral infection, parasitic infection, bacterial infection
    - Increased frequency of sexual intercourse
- Urinary frequency
    - Change in usual pattern and/or volume
    - Associated with dysuria or other urinary characteristics: urgency, hematuria, incontinence, nocturia
    - Change in urinary stream; dribbling
    - Medications: prescription or nonprescription; diuretics
- Urinary incontinence
    - Character: amount and frequency, constant or intermittent, dribbling versus frank incontinence
    - Associated with: urgency, previous surgery, coughing, sneezing, walking up stairs, nocturia, menopause
    - Medications: prescription or nonprescription; diuretics
- Hematuria
    - Character: color (bright red, rusty brown, cola-colored); present at beginning, end, or throughout voiding
    - Associated symptoms: flank or costovertebral pain, passage of wormlike clots, pain on voiding
    - Alternate possibilities: ingestion of foods containing red vegetable dyes (may cause red urinary pigment); ingestion of laxatives containing phenolphthalein
    - Medications: prescription or nonprescription; aspirin
- Chyluria (milky urine)
    - Exposure to parasitic infections through travel
    - Exposure to tuberculosis
    - Medications: prescription or nonprescription

PAST MEDICAL HISTORY

- Gastrointestinal disorder: peptic ulcer, polyps, inflammatory bowel disease, intestinal obstruction, pancreatitis
- Hepatitis or cirrhosis of the liver
- Abdominal or urinary tract surgery or injury
- Urinary tract infection: number, treatment

RISK FACTORS	Persons at Risk for Viral Hepatitis		
Hepatitis A	**Hepatitis B**	**Hepatitis C**
Household/sexual contacts of infected persons	Drug users who inject	Drug users who inject
International travelers	Sexually active heterosexuals	Health care workers
Person living in American Indian reservation, Alaska native villages and other regions with endemic hepatitis A	Homosexual men	Hemodialysis patients
	Infants/children of immigrants from disease-endemic areas	Low socioeconomic level
	Low socioeconomic level	Sexual/household contacts of infected persons
During outbreaks: day care center employees or attendees; homosexually active men; drug users who inject	Sexual/household contacts of infected persons	Sexually active heterosexuals
	Infant of infected mothers	Transfusion recipients
	Health care workers	
	Hemodialysis patients	

CDC, September 1997
www.cdc.gov/nciod/diseases/hepatitis

- Major illness: cancer, arthritis (steroids or aspirin use), kidney disease, cardiac disease
- Blood transfusions
- Hepatitis vaccine

FAMILY HISTORY

- Familial Mediterranean fever (periodic peritonitis)
- Gallbladder disease
- Kidney disease: renal stone, polycystic disease, renal tubular acidosis, renal or bladder carcinoma
- Malabsorption syndrome: cystic fibrosis, celiac disease
- Hirschsprung disease, aganglionic megacolon
- Polyposis: Peutz-Jeghers syndrome, familial multiple polyposis
- Colon cancer

PERSONAL AND SOCIAL HISTORY

- Nutrition: 24-hour recall intake, food preferences and dislikes, ethnic foods frequently eaten, religious food restrictions, food intolerances, life-style effects on food intake, weight gain or loss*
- First day of last menstrual period
- Alcohol intake: frequency and usual amounts
- Recent stressful life events: physical and psychologic changes
- Exposure to infectious diseases: hepatitis, flu; travel history
- Trauma: through type of work, physical activity, abuse
- Use of alcohol
- Use of street drugs

INFANTS

- Birth weight (less than 1500 g at higher risk for necrotizing enterocolitis)
- Passage of first meconium stool within 24 hours
- Jaundice: in newborn period, exchange transfusions, phototherapy, breast-fed infant, appearing later in first month of life
- Vomiting: increasing in amount or frequency, forceful or projectile, failure to gain weight, insatiable appetite, blood in emesis (pyloric stenosis or gastroesophageal reflux)
- Diarrhea, colic, failure to gain weight, weight loss, steatorrhea (malabsorption syndrome)
- Apparent enlargement of abdomen (with or without pain), constipation, or diarrhea

CHILDREN

- Constipation: toilet training methods; diet; soiling; diarrhea; abdominal distention; pica; size, shape, consistency, and time of last stool; rectal bleeding; painful passage of stool
- Abdominal pain: splinting of abdominal movement, resists movement, keeps knees flexed

PREGNANT WOMEN

- Urinary symptoms: frequency, urgency, nocturia (common in early and late pregnancy); burning, dysuria, odor (signs of infection)
- Abdominal pain: weeks of gestation (pregnancy can alter the usual location of pain)
- Fetal movement
- Contractions: onset, frequency, duration, intensity; accompanying symptoms; lower back pain; leakage of fluid, vaginal bleeding

*NOTE: For nutrition and eating disorders history, see Chapter 6, pp. 141-148.

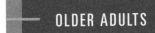

- Urinary symptoms: nocturia, change in stream, dribbling, frank incontinence
- Change in bowel patterns, constipation, diarrhea, incontinence
- Dietary habits: inclusion of fiber in diet, change in ability to tolerate certain foods, change in appetite

EXAMINATION AND FINDINGS

EQUIPMENT

- Stethoscope
- Centimeter ruler and nonstretchable measuring tape
- Marking pen

PREPARATION

To perform the abdominal examination satisfactorily, you will need a good source of light, full exposure of the abdomen, warm hands with short fingernails, and a comfortable, relaxed patient. Have the patient empty his or her bladder before the examination begins. A full bladder interferes with accurate examination of nearby organs and makes the examination uncomfortable for the patient. Place the patient in a supine position with arms at sides. The patient's abdominal musculature should be as relaxed as possible to allow access to the underlying structures. It may be helpful to place a small pillow under the patient's head and another small pillow under the slightly flexed knees. Drape a towel over the patient's chest for warmth and privacy. Ask the patient to breathe slowly through the mouth. Make your approach slow and gentle, avoiding sudden movements. Ask the patient to point to any tender areas, and examine those last.

Landmarks

For the purposes of examination, the abdomen can be divided into either four quadrants or nine regions. To divide the abdomen into quadrants, draw an imaginary line from the sternum to the pubis, through the umbilicus. Draw a second imaginary line perpendicular to the first, horizontally across the abdomen through the umbilicus (Figure 15-4). The nine regions are created by two imaginary horizontal lines, one across the lowest edge of the costal margin and the other across the edge of the iliac crest, and by two vertical lines bilaterally from the midclavicular line to the middle of the Poupart ligament, approximating the lateral borders of the rectus abdominis muscles (Figure 15-5). Choose one of these mapping methods and use it consistently. Quadrants are the more common of the two methods. Box 15-1 lists the contents of the abdomen in each of the quadrants and regions. Become accustomed to mentally visualizing the underlying organs and structures in each of the zones as you proceed with the examination.

Certain other anatomic landmarks are useful in describing the location of pain, tenderness, and other findings. These landmarks are illustrated in Figure 15-6.

INSPECTION

Surface Characteristics

Begin by inspecting the abdomen from a seated position at the right side of the patient. This position allows a tangential view that enhances shadows and contouring. Observe the skin color and surface characteristics. The skin of the abdomen is subject to the same expected variations in color and surface characteristics as the rest of the body. The skin may be somewhat paler if it has not been exposed to the sun. Tanning lines are often visible on light-colored skin. A fine venous network is often visible. Above the umbilicus, venous return should be toward the head; below the umbilicus

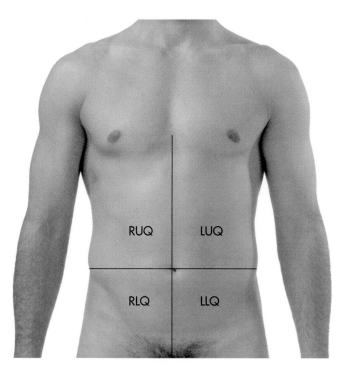

FIGURE 15-4

Four quadrants of the abdomen.

From Thompson, Wilson, 1996.

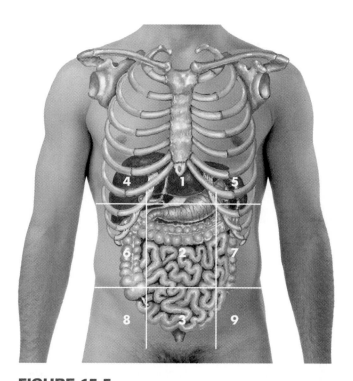

FIGURE 15-5

Nine regions of the abdomen. 1, Epigastric; 2, umbilical; 3, hypogastric (pubic); 4 and 5, right and left hypochondriac; 6 and 7, right and left lumbar; 8 and 9, right and left inguinal.

From Thompson, Wilson, 1996.

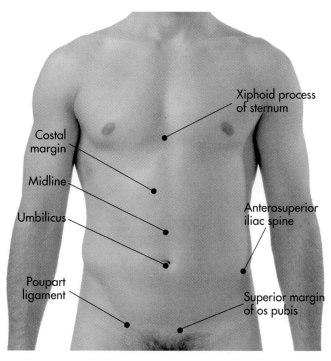

FIGURE 15-6

Landmarks of the abdomen.

From Thompson, Wilson, 1996.

BOX 15-1   **Landmarks for Abdominal Examination**

Anatomic Correlates of the Four Quadrants of the Abdomen

Right Upper Quadrant (RUQ)	**Left Upper Quadrant (LUQ)**
Liver and gallbladder	Left lobe of liver
Pylorus	Spleen
Duodenum	Stomach
Head of pancreas	Body of pancreas
Right adrenal gland	Left adrenal gland
Portion of right kidney	Portion of left kidney
Hepatic flexure of colon	Splenic flexure of colon
Portions of ascending and transverse colon	Portions of transverse and descending colon
Right Lower Quadrant (RLQ)	**Left Lower Quadrant (LLQ)**
Lower pole of right kidney	Lower pole of left kidney
Cecum and appendix	Sigmoid colon
Portion of ascending colon	Portion of descending colon
Bladder (if distended)	Bladder (if distended)
Ovary and salpinx	Ovary and salpinx
Uterus (if enlarged)	Uterus (if enlarged)
Rights spermatic cord	Left spermatic cord
Right ureter	Left ureter

Anatomic Correlates of the Nine Regions of the Abdomen

4 Right Hypochondriac	**1 Epigastric**	**5 Left Hypochondriac**
Right lobe of liver	Pyloric end of stomach	Stomach
Gallbladder	Duodenum	Spleen
Portion of duodenum	Pancreas	Tail of pancreas
Hepatic flexure of colon	Portion of liver	Splenic flexure of colon
Portion of right kidney		Upper pole of left kidney
Suprarenal gland		Suprarenal gland
6 Right Lumbar	**2 Umbilical**	**7 Left Lumbar**
Ascending colon	Omentum	Descending colon
Lower half of right kidney	Mesentery	Lower half of left kidney
Portion of duodenum and jejunum	Lower part of duodenum	Portions of jejunum and ileum
	Jejunum and ileum	
8 Right Inguinal	**3 Hypogastric (Pubic)**	**9 Left Inguinal**
Cecum	Ileum	Sigmoid colon
Appendix	Bladder	Left ureter
Lower end of ileum	Uterus (in pregnancy)	Left spermatic cord
Right ureter		Left ovary
Right spermatic cord		
Right ovary		

From Barkauskas et al, 1998.

it should be toward the feet (Figure 15-7, *A*). To determine the direction of venous return, use the following procedure. Place the index finger on each hand side by side over a vein. Press laterally, separating the fingers and milking empty a section of vein. Release one finger and time the refill. Release the other finger and time the refill. The flow of venous blood is in the direction of the faster filling. Flow patterns are altered in some disease states (Figure 15-7, *B* and *C*).

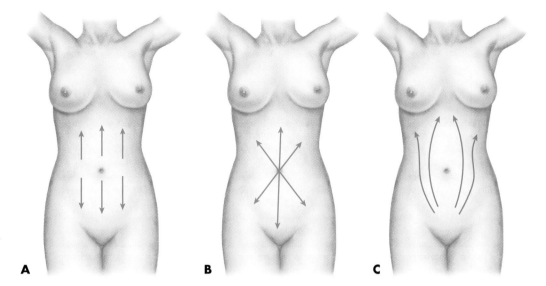

FIGURE 15-7
Abdominal venous patterns.
A, Expected. **B,** Portal hypertension. **C,** Inferior vena cava obstruction.

Unexpected findings include generalized color changes such as jaundice or cyanosis. A glistening taut appearance suggests ascites. Inspect for bruises and localized discoloration. Areas of redness may indicate inflammation. A bluish periumbilical discoloration (Cullen sign) suggests intraabdominal bleeding. Striae often result from pregnancy or weight gain. Striae of recent origin are pink or blue in color but turn silvery white over time. Abdominal tumor or ascites that stretches the skin also produces striae. The striae of Cushing disease remain purplish.

Inspect for any lesions, particularly nodules. Lesions are of particular importance since gastrointestinal diseases often produce secondary skin changes. A pearl-like enlarged umbilical node may signal intraabdominal lymphoma. Skin and gastrointestinal lesions may arise from the same cause or occur without relationship to one another.

Note any scars and draw their location, configuration, and relative size on an illustration of the abdomen. If the cause of a scar was not explained during the history, now is a good time to pursue that information. The presence of scarring should alert you to the possibility of internal adhesions.

Contour

Inspect the abdomen for contour, symmetry, and surface motion, using tangential lighting to illuminate contour and visible peristalsis. Contour is the abdominal profile from the rib margin to the pubis, viewed on the horizontal plane. The expected contours can be described as flat, rounded, or scaphoid (Figure 15-8). A flat contour is common in well-muscled, athletic adults. The rounded or convex contour is characteristic of young children, but in adults it is the result of subcutaneous fat or poor muscle tone from inadequate exercise. The abdomen should be evenly rounded with the maximum height of convexity at the umbilicus. The scaphoid or concave contour is seen in thin adults.

Note the location and contour of the umbilicus. It should be centrally located without displacement upward, downward, or laterally. The umbilicus may be inverted or protrude slightly, but it should be free of inflammation, swelling, or bulges that may indicate a hernia.

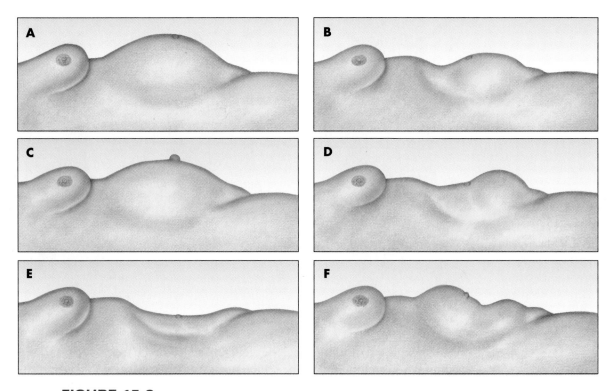

FIGURE 15-8
Abdominal profiles. **A,** Fully rounded or distended, umbilicus inverted. **B,** Distended lower half. **C,** Fully rounded or distended, umbilicus everted. **D,** Distended lower third. **E,** Scaphoid. **F,** Distended upper half.

Inspect for symmetry from a seated position at the patient's side, and then move to a standing position behind the patient's head. Contralateral areas of the abdomen should be symmetric in appearance and contour. Look for any distention or bulges.

Generalized symmetric distention may occur as a result of obesity, enlarged organs, and fluid or gas. Distention from the umbilicus to the symphysis can be caused by an ovarian tumor, pregnancy, uterine fibroids, or a distended bladder. Distention of the upper half, above the umbilicus, can mean carcinoma, pancreatic cyst, or gastric dilation. Asymmetric distention or protrusion may indicate hernia, tumor, cysts, bowel obstruction, or enlargement of abdominal organs.

Ask the patient to take a deep breath and hold it. The contour should remain smooth and symmetric. This maneuver lowers the diaphragm and compresses the organs of the abdominal cavity, which may cause previously unseen bulges or masses to appear. Next ask the patient to raise his or her head from the table. This contracts the rectus abdominis muscles, which produces muscle prominence in thin or athletic adults. Superficial abdominal wall masses may become visible. If a hernia is present, the increased abdominal pressure may cause it to protrude.

An incisional hernia is caused by a defect in the abdominal musculature that develops after a surgical incision. The hernia will protrude in the area of the surgical scar. Protrusion of the navel indicates an umbilical hernia. The adult type develops during pregnancy, in long-standing ascites, or when intrathoracic pressure is repeatedly increased, as occurs in chronic respiratory disease. Hernias may also occur in the midline of the epigastrium (hernia of the linea alba). This type of hernia contains a bit of fat and is felt as a small, tender nodule. Most hernias are reducible, meaning that the contents of the hernial sac are easily replaced. If not, the hernia is nonreducible or incarcerated. A nonreducible hernia in which the blood supply to the protruded contents is obstructed is *strangulated* and requires immediate surgical intervention.

In addition to hernias, separation of the rectus abdominis muscles (diastasis recti) may become apparent when the patient raises his or her head from the table. Diastasis recti is often caused by pregnancy or obesity. The condition is of little clinical significance.

Movement

With the patient's head again resting on the table, inspect the abdomen for movement. Smooth, even movement should occur with respiration. Males exhibit primarily abdominal movement with respiration, whereas females show mostly costal movement. Limited abdominal motion associated with respiration in adult males may indicate peritonitis or disease. Surface motion from peristalsis is seen as a rippling movement across a section of the abdomen. Usually not visible in either males or females, it indicates a definite abnormality, most often an intestinal obstruction. Pulsation in the upper midline is often visible in thin adults. Marked pulsation may occur as the result of increased pulse pressure or abdominal aortic aneurysm.

AUSCULTATION

Once inspection is completed, the next step is auscultation. This technique is used to assess bowel motility and to discover vascular sounds. Unlike the usual sequence, auscultation of the abdomen always precedes percussion and palpation, because these may alter the frequency and intensity of bowel sounds.

Bowel Sounds

Place the diaphragm of a warmed stethoscope on the abdomen and hold it in place with very light pressure. Some practitioners say they prefer to use the bell. In reality, they tend to pull the skin tight with the bell and, in effect, make a diaphragm. A cold stethoscope, like cold hands, may initiate contraction of the abdominal muscles. Listen for bowel sounds and note their frequency and character. They are usually heard as clicks and gurgles that occur irregularly and range from 5 to 35 per minute. Loud prolonged gurgles called borborygmi ("stomach growling") are sometimes heard. Increased bowel sounds may occur with gastroenteritis, early intestinal obstruction, or hunger. High-pitched tinkling sounds suggest intestinal fluid and air under pressure, as in early obstruction. Decreased bowel sounds occur with peritonitis and paralytic ileus. The absence of bowel sounds is established only after 5 minutes of continuous listening. Auscultate all four quadrants to make sure that no sounds are missed and to localize specific sounds.

Vascular Sounds

Listen with the bell of the stethoscope in the epigastric region and each of the four quadrants for bruits in the aortic, renal, iliac, and femoral arteries (Figure 15-9). Listen with the diaphragm for friction rubs over the liver and spleen. Friction rubs are high pitched and are heard in association with respiration. Although friction rubs in the abdomen are rare, they indicate inflammation of the peritoneal surface of the organ from tumor, infection, or infarct.

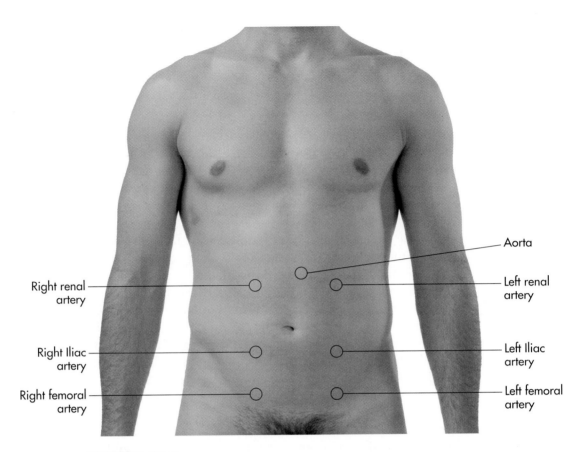

FIGURE 15-9
Sites to auscultate for bruits: renal arteries, iliac arteries, aorta, and femoral arteries.
From Thompson, Wilson, 1996.

Auscultate with the bell of the stethoscope in the epigastric region and around the umbilicus for a venous hum, which is soft, low pitched, and continuous. A venous hum occurs with increased collateral circulation between portal and systemic venous systems.

PERCUSSION

Percussion (generally indirect) is used to assess the size and density of the organs in the abdomen and to detect the presence of fluid (as with ascites), air (as with gastric distention), and fluid-filled or solid masses. Percussion is used either independently or concurrently with palpation while specific organs are evaluated, and it can validate palpatory findings. For simplicity, percussion and palpation are discussed separately; however, either approach is acceptable.

First percuss all quadrants or regions of the abdomen for a sense of overall tympany and dullness (Table 15-1). Tympany is the predominant sound because air is present in the stomach and intestines. Dullness is heard over organs and solid masses. A distended bladder produces dullness in the suprapubic area. Develop a systematic route for percussion, as shown in Figure 15-10.

Liver Span
Now go back and percuss individually the liver, spleen, and stomach. Begin liver percussion at the right midclavicular line over an area of tympany. (Always begin with an area of tympany and proceed to an area of dullness, because that sound change is easier to detect than the change from dullness to tympany.) Percuss upward along the

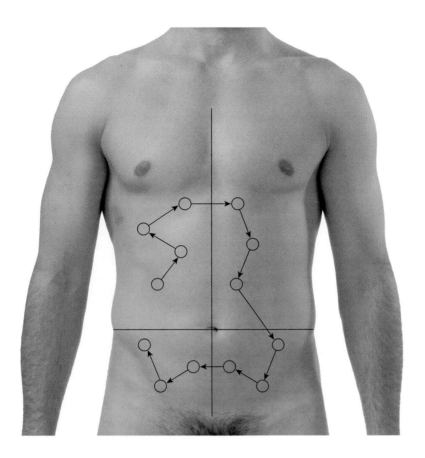

FIGURE 15-10

Systematic route for abdominal percussion.

From Thompson, Wilson, 1996.

TABLE 15-1	**Percussion Notes of the Abdomen**	
Note	**Description**	**Location**
Tympany	Musical note of higher pitch than resonance	Over air-filled viscera
Hyperresonance	Pitch lies between tympany and resonance	Base of left lung
Resonance	Sustained note of moderate pitch	Over lung tissue and sometimes over the abdomen
Dullness	Short, high-pitched note with little resonance	Over solid organs adjacent to air-filled structures

Adapted from AH Robins Co.

midclavicular line, as shown in Figure 15-11, to determine the lower border of the liver. The area of liver dullness is usually heard at the costal margin or slightly below it. Mark the border with a marking pen. A lower liver border that is more than 2 to 3 cm (¾ to 1 in) below the costal margin may indicate organ enlargement or downward displacement of the diaphragm because of emphysema or other pulmonary disease.

To determine the upper border of the liver, begin percussion on the right midclavicular line at an area of lung resonance. Continue downward until the percussion tone changes to one of dullness, which marks the upper border of the liver. Mark the location with the pen. The upper border usually begins at the fifth to seventh intercostal space. An upper border below this may indicate downward displacement or liver atrophy. Dullness extending above the fifth intercostal space suggests upward displacement from abdominal fluid or masses.

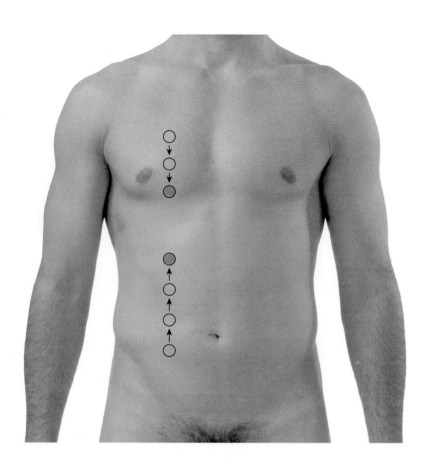

FIGURE 15-11
Liver percussion route.
From Thompson, Wilson, 1996.

Measure the distance between the marks to estimate the vertical span of the liver. The usual span is approximately 6 to 12 cm ($2\frac{1}{2}$ to $4\frac{1}{2}$ in). A span greater than this may indicate liver enlargement, whereas a lesser span suggests atrophy. Age and sex influence liver size. Obviously, the liver will be larger in adults than in children. Liver span is usually greater in males and tall individuals than in females and short people. Interestingly, in the early years of life, the liver tends to be somewhat larger in the female, but usually by about 2 years of age, the liver of the male will be larger. Of course, individuals at every age vary, and the generalization will not hold true in all cases.

Although percussion provides the most accurate clinical measure of liver size, the measure remains only a gross estimate. Errors in estimating liver span can occur when the dullness of pleural effusion or lung consolidation obscures the upper liver border, leading to overestimation of size. Similarly, gas in the colon may produce tympany in the right upper quadrant and obscure the dullness of the lower liver border, leading to underestimation of liver size.

Liver Descent

To assess the descent of the liver, ask the patient to take a deep breath and hold it while you percuss upward again from the abdomen at the right midclavicular line. The area of lower border dullness should move downward 2 to 3 cm. This maneuver will guide subsequent palpation of the organ.

Additional Liver Assessment

If liver enlargement is suspected, additional percussion maneuvers can provide further information. Percuss upward and then downward over the right midaxillary line. Liver dullness is usually detected in the fifth to seventh intercostal space. Dullness beyond those limits suggests a problem. You can also percuss along the midsternal line to estimate the midsternal liver span. Percuss upward from the abdomen and downward from the lungs, marking the upper and lower borders of dullness. The usual span at the midsternal line is 4 to 8 cm (1½ to 3 in). Spans exceeding 8 cm suggest liver enlargement.

It is best to report the size of the liver in two ways: by liver span as determined from percussing the upper and lower borders and by the extent of liver projection below the costal margin. When the size of a patient's liver is important in assessing the clinical condition, projection below the costal margin alone will not provide enough comparative information.

Spleen

The spleen is percussed just posterior to the midaxillary line on the left side. Percuss in several directions as shown in Figure 15-12, beginning at areas of lung resonance. A small area of splenic dullness may be heard from the sixth to the tenth rib. A large area of dullness suggests spleen enlargement; however, a full stomach or feces-filled intestine may mimic the dullness of splenic enlargement. Percuss the lowest intercostal space in the left anterior axillary line before and after the patient takes a deep breath. The area should remain tympanic. With splenic enlargement, tympany changes to dullness as the spleen is brought forward and downward with inspiration. Remember that it is not possible to distinguish between the dullness of the posterior flank and that of the spleen. In addition, the dullness of a healthy spleen is often obscured by the tympany of colonic air.

Gastric Bubble

Finally, percuss for the gastric air bubble in the area of the left lower anterior rib cage and left epigastric region. The tympany produced by the gastric bubble is lower in pitch than the tympany of the intestine.

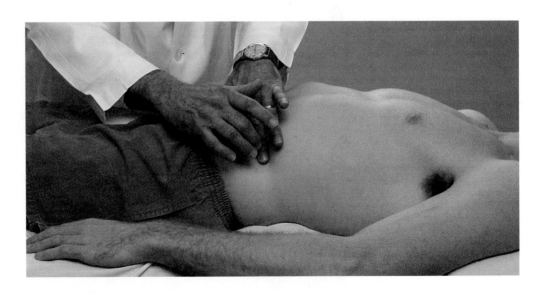

FIGURE 15-12
Percussion of the spleen.

PALPATION

Palpation is used to assess the organs of the abdominal cavity and to detect muscle spasm, masses, fluid, and areas of tenderness. The abdominal organs are evaluated for size, shape, mobility, consistency, and tension. Stand at the patient's side (usually the right) with the patient in the supine position. Make certain that the patient is comfortable and that the abdomen is as relaxed as possible; bending the patient's knees may help relax the muscles. Your hands should be warm to avoid producing muscle contraction, which will hinder further examination. Ticklishness may also create a problem (Box 15-2).

Light Palpation

Begin with a light, systematic palpation of all four quadrants, initially avoiding any areas that have already been identified as problem spots. Lay the palm of your hand lightly on the abdomen, with the fingers extended and approximated (Figure 15-13). With the palmar surface of your fingers, depress the abdominal wall no more than 1 cm, using a light and even pressing motion. Avoid short, quick jabs. The abdomen should feel smooth, with a consistent softness. The patient's abdomen may tense if you press too deeply, if your hands are cold, if the patient is ticklish, or if inflammation is present. Guarding should alert you to move cautiously through the remainder of the examination.

Light palpation is particularly useful in identifying muscular resistance and areas of tenderness. A large mass or distended structure may be appreciated on light palpation as a sense of resistance. If resistance is present, try to determine whether it is voluntary or involuntary in the following way: Place a pillow under the patient's

---

BOX 15-2	**Examining the Abdomen in a Ticklish Patient**

The ticklishness of a patient can sometimes make it difficult for you to palpate the abdomen satisfactorily. However, there are ways to overcome this problem. Ask the patient to perform self-palpation, and place your hands over the patient's fingers, not quite touching the abdomen itself. After a time, let your fingers drift slowly onto the abdomen while still resting primarily on the patient's fingers. You can still learn a good deal, and ticklishness might not be so much of a problem. You might also use the diaphragm of the stethoscope (making sure it is warm enough) as a palpating instrument. This serves as a starting point, and again your fingers can drift over the edge of the diaphragm and palpate without eliciting an excessively ticklish response. Applying a stimulus to another, less sensitive part of the body with your nonpalpating hand can also decrease a ticklish response. In some instances a patient's ticklishness cannot be overcome, and you just have to palpate as best you can.

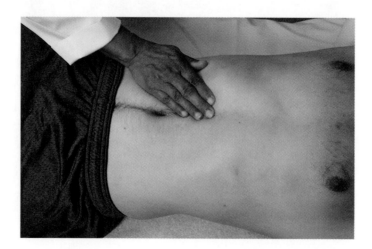

FIGURE 15-13

Light palpation of the abdomen. With fingers extended and approximated, press in no more than 1 cm.

From Thompson, Wilson, 1996.

knees and ask the patient to breathe slowly through the mouth as you feel for relaxation of the rectus abdominis muscles on expiration. If the tenseness remains, it is probably an involuntary response to localized or generalized rigidity. Rigidity is a boardlike hardness of the abdominal wall overlying areas of peritoneal irritation.

Specific zones of peritoneal irritation may be identified through cutaneous hypersensitivity (Figure 15-14). To evaluate hypersensitivity, gently lift a fold of skin away from the underlying muscle or stimulate the skin with a pin or other object and have the patient describe the local sensation (Figure 15-15). In the event of hypersensitivity, the patient will perceive pain or an exaggerated sensation in response to this maneuver.

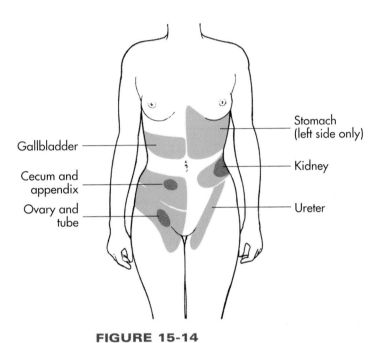

FIGURE 15-14
Areas of cutaneous hypersensitivity.

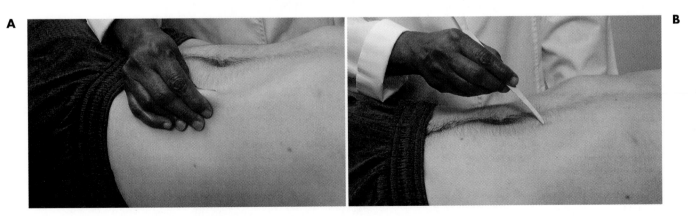

FIGURE 15-15
Testing for cutaneous hypersensitivity. **A,** Lift a fold of skin away from underlying muscle or,
B, stimulate the skin with a sharp point or a broken tongue blade.
From Thompson, Wilson, 1996.

Moderate Palpation

Continue palpation of all four quadrants with the same hand position as for light palpation, exerting moderate pressure as an intermediate step to gradually approach deep palpation. Tenderness not elicited on gentle palpation may become evident with deeper pressure. An additional maneuver of moderate palpation is performed with the side of your hand (Figure 15-16). This maneuver is useful in assessing organs that move with respiration, specifically the liver and spleen. Palpate during the entire respiratory cycle; as the patient inspires, the organ is displaced downward, and you may be able to feel it as it bumps gently against your hand.

Deep Palpation

Deep palpation is necessary to thoroughly delineate abdominal organs and to detect less obvious masses. Use the palmar surface of your extended fingers, pressing deeply and evenly into the abdominal wall (Figure 15-17). Palpate all four quadrants, moving the fingers back and forth over the abdominal contents. (The abdominal wall may also slide back and forth as you do this.) Often you are able to feel the borders of the rectus abdominis muscles, the aorta, and portions of the colon. Tenderness not elicited with light or moderate palpation may become evident. Deep pressure may also evoke tenderness in the healthy person over the cecum, sigmoid colon, aorta, and in the midline near the xiphoid process.

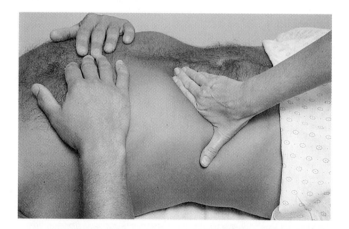

FIGURE 15-16
Moderate palpation using the side of the hand.

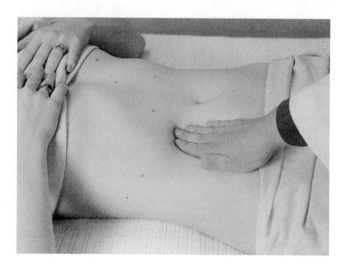

FIGURE 15-17
Deep palpation of the abdomen. Press deeply and evenly with the palmar surface of extended fingers.
From Thompson, Wilson, 1996.

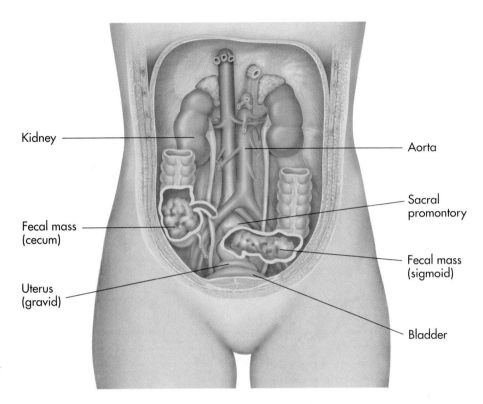

FIGURE 15-18
Abdominal structures frequently felt as "masses."

Kidney

Fecal mass (cecum)

Uterus (gravid)

Aorta

Sacral promontory

Fecal mass (sigmoid)

Bladder

Masses

Identify any masses and note the characteristics: location, size, shape, consistency, tenderness, pulsation, mobility, and movement with respiration. To determine if a mass is superficial (located in the abdominal wall) or intraabdominal, have the patient lift his or her head from the examining table, thus contracting the abdominal muscles. Masses in the abdominal wall will continue to be palpable, whereas those located in the abdominal cavity will be more difficult to feel, since they are obscured by abdominal musculature. The presence of feces in the colon, often mistaken for an abdominal mass, can be felt as a soft, rounded, boggy mass in the cecum and in the ascending, descending, or sigmoid colons. Other structures that are sometimes mistaken for masses are the lateral borders of the rectus abdominis muscles, the uterus, aorta, sacral promontory, and common iliac artery (Figure 15-18). If you can mentally visualize the placement of the abdominal structures, it will be easier to distinguish between what you know ought to be there and an unexpected finding.

Umbilical Ring

Palpate the umbilical ring and around the umbilicus. The area should be free of bulges, nodules, and granulation. The umbilical ring should be round and free of irregularities. Note whether it is incomplete or soft in the center, which suggests the potential for herniation. The umbilicus may be either slightly inverted or everted, but it should not protrude.

Bimanual Technique

If deep palpation is difficult because of obesity or muscular resistance, you can use a bimanual technique with one hand atop the other as shown in Figure 15-19. Exert pressure with the top hand while concentrating on sensation with the other hand. Some examiners prefer to use the bimanual technique for all patients.

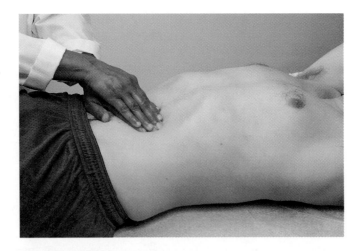

FIGURE 15-19
Deep bimanual palpation.
From Thompson, Wilson, 1996.

A

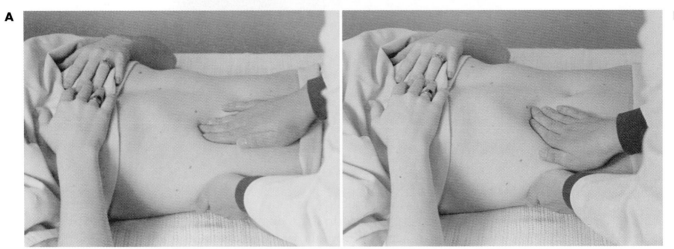

B

FIGURE 15-20
A, Palpating the liver. Fingers are extended, with tips on right midclavicular line below the level of liver tenderness and pointing toward the head. **B,** Alternate method for liver palpation with fingers parallel to the costal margin.
From Thompson, Wilson, 1996.

Palpation of Specific Structures

Liver. Place your left hand under the patient at the eleventh and twelfth ribs, pressing upward to elevate the liver toward the abdominal wall. Place your right hand on the abdomen, fingers pointing toward the head and extended so the tips rest on the right midclavicular line below the level of liver dullness, as shown in Figure 15-20, *A*. As an alternative, you can place your right hand parallel to the right costal margin, as shown in Figure 15-20, *B*. In either case, press your right hand gently but deeply in and up. Have the patient breathe regularly a few times and then take a deep breath. Try to feel the liver edge as the diaphragm pushes it down to meet your fingertips. Ordinarily, the liver is not palpable, although it may be felt in some thin persons even when no pathologic condition exists. If the liver edge is felt, it should be firm, smooth, even, and nontender. Feel for nodules, tenderness, and irregularity. If the liver is palpable, repeat the maneuver medially and laterally to the costal margin to assess the contour and surface of the liver.

Alternate techniques. An alternate technique is to hook your fingers over the right costal margin below the border of liver dullness, as shown in Figure 15-21. Stand on

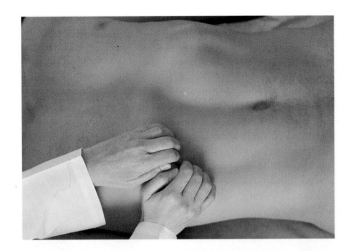

FIGURE 15-21
Palpating the liver with fingers hooked over the costal margin.

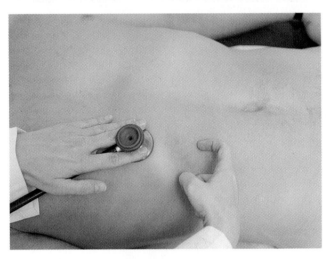

FIGURE 15-22
Scratch technique for auscultating the liver. With stethoscope over the liver, lightly scratch the abdominal surface, moving toward the liver. The sound will be intensified over the liver.

the patient's right side facing his or her feet. Press in and up toward the costal margin with your fingers and ask the patient to take a deep breath. Try to feel the liver edge as it descends to meet your fingers.

If the abdomen is distended or the abdominal muscles tense, the usual techniques for determining the lower liver border may be unproductive. At such a point, the scratch test may be useful (Figure 15-22). This technique uses auscultation to detect the differences in sound transmission over solid and hollow organs. Place the stethoscope over the liver and with the finger of your other hand scratch the abdominal surface lightly, moving toward the liver border. When you encounter the liver, the sound you hear in the stethoscope will be intensified.

To check for liver tenderness when the liver is not palpable, use indirect fist percussion. Place the palmar surface of one hand over the lower right rib cage, and then strike your hand with the ulnar surface of the fist of your other hand as shown in Figure 15-23. The healthy liver is not tender to percussion.

Gallbladder. Palpate below the liver margin at the lateral border of the rectus abdominis muscle for the gallbladder. A healthy gallbladder will not be palpable. A palpable, tender gallbladder indicates cholecystitis, whereas nontender enlargement suggests common bile duct obstruction. If you suspect cholecystitis, have the patient take a deep breath during deep palpation. As the inflamed gallbladder comes in contact with the examining fingers, the patient will experience pain and abruptly halt inspiration (Murphy sign).

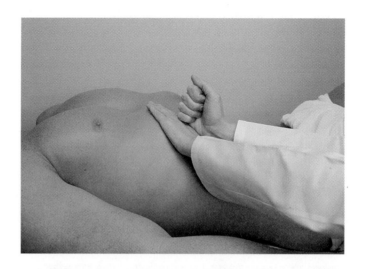

FIGURE 15-23
Fist percussion of the liver.

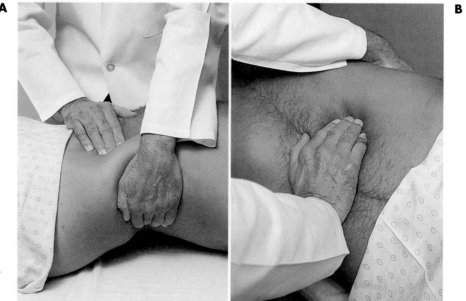

FIGURE 15-24
A, Palpating the spleen. Press upward with the left hand at the patient's left costovertebral angle. Feel for the spleen with the right hand below the left costal margin. **B,** Palpating the spleen with the patient lying on the side. Press inward with left hand and tips of the right fingers.

Spleen. While still standing on the patient's right side, reach across with your left hand and place it beneath the patient over the left costovertebral angle. Press upward with that hand to lift the spleen anteriorly toward the abdominal wall. Place the palmar surface of your right hand with fingers extended on the patient's abdomen below the left costal margin (Figure 15-24, *A*). Use findings from percussion as a guide. Press your fingertips inward toward the spleen as you ask the patient to take a deep breath. Try to feel the edge of the spleen as it moves downward toward your fingers. The spleen is not usually palpable in an adult; if you can feel it, it is probably enlarged (Box 15-3). Be sure to palpate with your fingers below the costal margin so that you will not miss the lower edge of an enlarged spleen. Be gentle in palpation to avoid rupturing an enlarged spleen.

Repeat the palpation while the patient is lying on the right side with hips and knees flexed (Figure 15-24, *B*). Still standing on the right side, press inward with your left hand to assist gravity in bringing the spleen forward and to the right. Press inward with the fingertips of your right hand and feel for the edge of the spleen. Again, you will not usually feel it; if you can, it is probably enlarged.

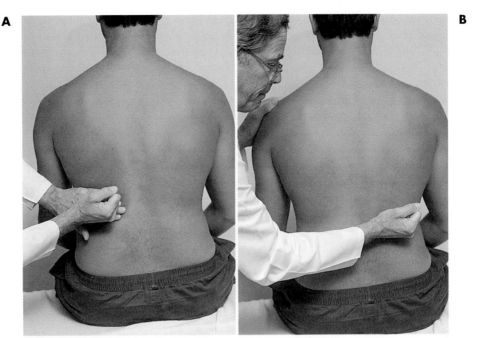

FIGURE 15-25
Fist percussion of the costovertebral angle for kidney tenderness. **A,** Indirect percussion. **B,** Direct percussion.

BOX 15-3 | **An Enlarged Spleen or an Enlarged Left Kidney?**

When an organ is palpable below the left costal margin, it may be difficult to differentiate an enlarged spleen from an enlarged left kidney. Percussion should help distinguish between the organs. The percussion note over an enlarged spleen is dull since the spleen displaces bowel. The usual area of splenic dullness will be increased downward and toward the midline. The percussion note over an enlarged kidney is resonant because the kidney is deeply situated behind the bowel. In addition, the edge of the spleen is sharper than that of the kidney. A palpable notch along the medial border suggests an enlarged spleen rather than an enlarged kidney.

Kidneys. To assess each kidney for tenderness, ask the patient to assume a sitting position. Place the palm of your hand over the right costovertebral angle and strike your hand with the ulnar surface of the fist of your other hand. Repeat the maneuver over the left costovertebral angle (Figure 15-25, *A*). Direct percussion with the fist over each costovertebral angle may also be used (Figure 15-25, *B*). The patient should perceive the blow as a thud, but it should not cause tenderness or pain. For efficiency of time and motion, assessment for kidney tenderness is usually performed while examining the back rather than the abdomen.

Left kidney. Ask the patient to lie supine. Standing on the patient's right side, reach across with your left hand as you did in spleen palpation and place it over the left flank. Place your right hand at the patient's left costal margin. Have the patient take a deep breath and then elevate the left flank with your left hand and palpate deeply (because of the retroperitoneal position of the kidney) with your right hand (Figure 15-26). Try to feel the lower pole of the kidney with your fingertips as the patient inhales. The left kidney is ordinarily not palpable.

Another approach is to "capture" the kidney. Move to the patient's left side and position your hands as before, with the left hand over the patient's left flank and the right hand at the left costal margin. Ask the patient to take a deep breath. At the height of inspiration, press the fingers of your two hands together to capture the kidney between the fingers. Ask the patient to breathe out and hold the exhalation while you

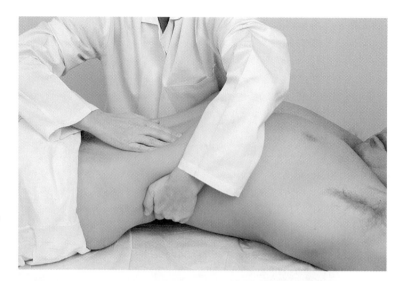

FIGURE 15-26
Palpating the left kidney. Elevate the left flank with the left hand. Palpate deeply with the right hand.

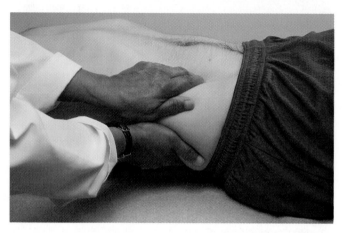

FIGURE 15-27
Capture technique for palpating the kidney (right kidney). As the patient takes a deep breath, press the fingers of both hands together. As the patient exhales, slowly release the pressure and feel for the kidney to slip between the fingers.

From Thompson, Wilson, 1996.

slowly release your fingers. If you have captured the kidney you may feel it slip beneath your fingers as it moves back into place. Although the patient may feel the capture and release, the maneuver should not be painful. Again, a left kidney is seldom palpable.

Right kidney. Stand on the patient's right side, placing one hand under the patient's right flank and the other hand at the right costal margin. Perform the same maneuvers as you did for the left kidney (Figure 15-27). Because of the anatomic position of the right kidney, it is more frequently palpable than the left kidney. If it is palpable, it should be smooth, firm, and nontender. It may be difficult to distinguish the kidney from the liver edge. The liver edge tends to be sharp, whereas the kidney is more rounded. The liver also extends more medially and laterally and cannot be captured.

Aorta. With the patient in the supine position, palpate deeply slightly to the left of the midline and feel for the aortic pulsation. If the pulsation is prominent, try to determine the direction of pulsation. A prominent lateral pulsation suggests an aortic aneurysm. Although the aortic pulse may be felt, particularly in thin adults, the pulse should be in an anterior direction.

If you are unable to feel the pulse on deep palpation, an alternate technique may help. Place the palmar surface of your hands with fingers extended on the midline. Press the fingers deeply inward on each side of the aorta and feel for the pulsation. In thin individuals, you can use one hand, placing the thumb on one side of the aorta and the fingers on the other side (Figure 15-28).

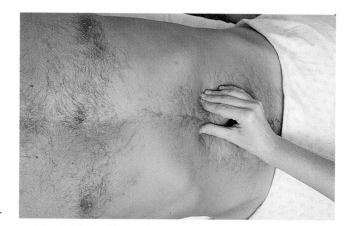

FIGURE 15-28
Palpating the aorta. Place the thumb on one side of the aorta and the fingers on the other side.

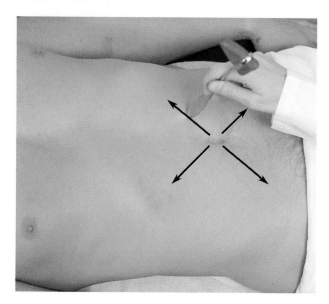

FIGURE 15-29
Examination of the superficial abdominal reflexes. One of several approaches is illustrated. Stroke the upper abdominal area upward, away from the umbilicus, and the lower abdominal area downward, away from the umbilicus.

Urinary bladder. The urinary bladder is not palpable in a healthy patient unless the bladder is distended with urine. When the bladder is distended, you can feel it as a smooth, round, tense mass. You can determine the distended bladder outline with percussion; a distended bladder will elicit a lower percussion note than the surrounding air-filled intestines.

Abdominal reflexes. With the patient supine, stroke each quadrant of the abdomen with the end of a reflex hammer or tongue blade edge. The upper abdominal reflexes are elicited by stroking upward and away from the umbilicus, and lower abdominal reflexes are elicited by stroking downward and away from the umbilicus (Figure 15-29). With each stroke, expect to see contraction of the rectus abdominis muscles and pulling of the umbilicus toward the stroked side. A diminished reflex may be present in patients who are obese or whose abdominal muscles have been stretched during pregnancy. Absence of the reflex may indicate a pyramidal tract lesion.

ADDITIONAL PROCEDURES

Ascites Assessment

Ascites may be suspected in patients who have protuberant abdomens or who have flanks that bulge in the supine position. Percuss for areas of dullness and resonance with the patient supine. Since ascites fluid settles with gravity, expect to hear dullness in the dependent parts of the abdomen and tympany in the upper parts where the relatively lighter bowel has risen. Mark the borders between tympany and dullness.

Shifting dullness. Test for shifting dullness to help ascertain the presence of fluid. Have the patient lie on one side and again percuss for tympany and dullness and mark the borders. In the patient without ascites, the borders will remain relatively constant. In ascites, the border of dullness shifts to the dependent side (approaches the midline) as the fluid resettles with gravity (Figure 15-30).

Fluid wave. Another maneuver is to test for a fluid wave. This procedure requires three hands, so you will need assistance from the patient or another examiner (Figure 15-31). With the patient supine, ask him or her or another person to press the edge of the hand and forearm firmly along the vertical midline of the abdomen. This positioning helps stop the transmission of a wave through adipose tissue. Place your hands on each side of the abdomen and strike one side sharply with your fingertips. Feel for the impulse of a fluid wave with the fingertips of your other hand. An easily detected fluid wave suggests ascites, but be cautioned that the findings of this maneuver are not conclusive. A fluid wave can sometimes be felt in people without ascites and, conversely, may not occur in people with early ascites.

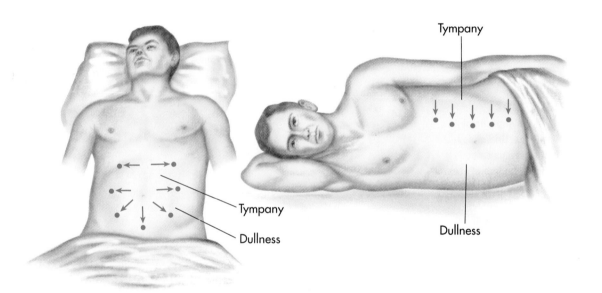

FIGURE 15-30
Testing for shifting dullness. Dullness shifts to the dependent side.

FIGURE 15-31
Testing for fluid wave. Strike one side of the abdomen sharply with the fingertips. Feel for the impulse of a fluid wave with the other hand.

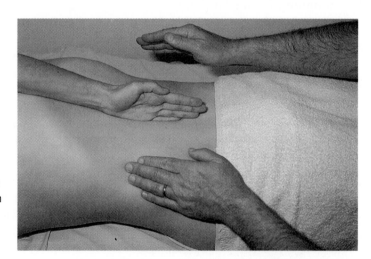

Auscultatory percussion. Auscultatory percussion has been suggested as an additional maneuver for detecting ascites. Have the patient void and then stand for 3 minutes to allow fluid to gravitate to the pelvis. Hold the diaphragm of the stethoscope immediately above the symphysis pubis in the midline with one hand. With the other hand, apply finger-flicking percussion to three or more sites from the costal margin perpendicularly downward toward the pelvis. In the healthy person the percussion note is first dull and then changes sharply to a loud note at the pelvic border. In patients with ascites the percussion note changes above the pelvic border at the fluid level.

Puddle sign. Another maneuver allows you to test for fluid pooling (puddle sign). Ask the patient to assume the knee-chest position and maintain that position for several minutes to allow any fluid to pool by gravity. Percuss the umbilical area for dullness to determine the presence of fluid (Figure 15-32). The area will remain tympanic if no fluid is present.

None of these maneuvers is specific or reliable, and generally all have been replaced by sonographic examination of the abdomen. Their importance is now largely historical.

Pain Assessment

Abdominal pain is a common complaint, but one that is frequently difficult to evaluate. How bad is the pain? Is there an underlying physical cause? Has there been recent trauma? Pain that is severe enough to make the patient unwilling to move, accompanied by nausea and vomiting, and marked by areas of localized tenderness generally has an underlying physical cause. While examining the abdomen, keep your eyes on the patient's face. The facial response is as important in your evaluation as the patient's verbal response to questions about the quality and degree of pain. Ask the patient to cough or take a deep breath. Assess the patient's willingness to jump or to walk. Is the pain exacerbated? A time-honored test is to ask the patient, "Do you want something to eat?" It is unlikely that hunger will persist in the face of acute intraabdominal infection (Box 15-4).

Common causes of abdominal pain are described in Table 15-2. Careful assessment of the quality (Table 15-3) and location of pain (Box 15-5) can usually narrow the possible causes, allowing you to select additional diagnostic studies with greater efficiency. Findings associated with peritoneal irritation are summarized in Box 15-6. Table 15-4 delineates symptoms found in other body systems that help direct the abdominal examination.

SMELL THE VOMITUS

A variety of odors from vomitus are possible:
- fetid (gastrointestinal obstruction)
- kerosene (hydrocarbon ingestion)
- violets (sometimes from turpentine)
- garlic (arsenic)

MNEMONICS

FEATURES OF PERITONITIS:
"PERITONITIS"

P *Pain: front, back, sides, shoulders*

E *Electrolytes fall, shock ensues*

R *Rigidity or rebound of anterior abdominal wall*

I *Immobile abdomen and patient*

T *Tenderness (rebound)*

O *Obstruction*

N *Nausea and vomiting*

I *Increasing pulse, decreasing blood pressure*

T *Temperature falls then rises*

I *Increasing girth of abdomen*

S *Silent abdomen (no bowel sounds)*

From Shipman, 1984.

FIGURE 15-32

Testing for pooling abdominal fluid. Percuss the umbilical area for dullness.

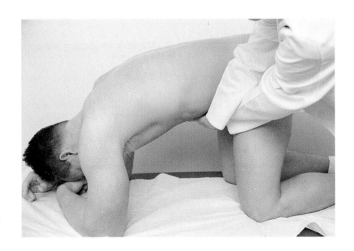

TABLE 15-2	Common Conditions Producing Abdominal Pain*	
Condition	**Usual Pain Characteristics**	**Possible Associated Findings**
Appendicitis	Initially periumbilical or epigastric; colicky; later becomes localized to RLQ, often at McBurney point	Guarding, tenderness; + iliopsoas and + obturator signs, RLQ skin hyperesthesia; anorexia, nausea, or vomiting after onset of pain; low-grade fever; + Aaron, Rovsing, Markle, and McBurney signs†
Cholecystitis	Severe, unrelenting RUQ or epigastric pain; may be referred to right subscapular area	RUQ tenderness and rigidity, + Murphy sign, palpable gallbladder, anorexia, vomiting, fever, possible jaundice
Pancreatitis	Dramatic, sudden, excruciating LUQ, epigastric, or umbilical pain; may be present in one or both flanks; may be referred to left shoulder	Epigastric tenderness, vomiting, fever, shock; + Grey Turner sign; + Cullen sign: both signs occur 2-3 days after onset
Perforated gastric or duodenal ulcer	Abrupt RUQ; may be referred to shoulders	Abdominal free air and distention with increased resonance over liver; tenderness in epigastrium or RUQ; rigid abdominal wall, rebound tenderness
Diverticulitis	Epigastric, radiating down left side of abdomen especially after eating; may be referred to back	Flatulence, borborygmi, diarrhea, dysuria, tenderness on palpation
Intestinal obstruction	Abrupt, severe, spasmodic; referred to epigastrium, umbilicus	Distention, minimal rebound tenderness, vomiting, localized tenderness, visible peristalsis; bowel sounds absent (with paralytic obstruction) or hyperactive high pitched (with mechanical obstruction)
Volvulus	Referred to hypogastrium and umbilicus	Distention, nausea, vomiting, guarding; sigmoid loop volvulus may be palpable
Leaking abdominal aneurysm	Steady throbbing midline over aneurysm; may radiate to back, flank	Nausea, vomiting, abdominal mass, bruit
Biliary stones, colic	Episodic, severe, RUQ, or epigastrium lasting 15 min to several hours; may be referred to subscapular area, especially right	RUQ tenderness, soft abdominal wall, anorexia, vomiting, jaundice, subnormal temperature
Salpingitis	Lower quadrant, worse on left	Nausea, vomiting, fever, suprapubic tenderness, rigid abdomen, pain on pelvic examination
Ectopic pregnancy	Lower quadrant; referred to shoulder; with rupture is agonizing	Hypogastric tenderness, symptoms of pregnancy, spotting, irregular menses, soft abdominal wall, mass on bimanual pelvic exam. Ruptured: shock, rigid abdominal wall, distention; + Kehr, Cullen signs
Pelvic inflammatory disease	Lower quadrant, increases with activity	Tender adnexa and cervix, cervical discharge, dyspareunia
Ruptured ovarian cyst	Lower quadrant, steady, increases with cough or motion	Vomiting, low-grade fever, anorexia, tenderness on pelvic examination
Renal calculi	Intense; flank, extending to groin and genitals; may be episodic	Fever, hematuria; + Kehr sign
Splenic rupture	Intense; LUQ, radiating to left shoulder; may worsen with foot of bed elevated	Shock, pallor, lowered temperature
Peritonitis	Onset sudden or gradual; pain generalized or localized, dull or severe and unrelenting; guarding; pain on deep inspiration	Shallow respiration; + Blumberg, Markle, and Ballance signs; reduced bowel sounds, nausea and vomiting; + obturator and illiopsoas tests

*+, Positive; *RLQ,* right lower quadrant; *RUQ,* right upper quadrant; *LUQ,* left upper quadrant.
†See Table 15-5 for explanation of signs.

BOX 15-4 Clues in Diagnosing Abdominal Pain

There are all types of rules for telling whether pain in the abdomen has significance. A few of them follow:

- Patients may give a "touch-me-not" warning—that is, to not touch in a particular area; however, these patients may not actually have pain if their faces seem relaxed and unconcerned, even smiling. When you touch they might recoil, but the unconcerned face persists. (Actually, this sign is helpful in other areas of the body, as well as the abdomen.)
- Patients with an organic cause for abdominal pain are generally not hungry. A negative response to the "Do you want something to eat?" question is probable, particularly with appendicitis or intraabdominal infection.
- Ask the patient to point a finger to the location of the pain. If it is not directed to the navel but goes immediately to a fixed point, there is a great likelihood that this has significant physical importance. The farther from the navel the pain, the more likely it will be organic in origin (Apley rule). If the finger goes to the navel and the patient seems otherwise well to you, you should include psychogenic causes in the list of differential diagnoses.
- Patients with nonspecific abdominal pain may keep their eyes closed during abdominal palpation, whereas patients with organic disease usually keep their eyes open.

TABLE 15-3 Quality and Onset of Abdominal Pain

Characteristic	Possible Related Condition
Burning	Peptic ulcer
Cramping	Biliary colic, gastroenteritis
Colic	Appendicitis with impacted feces; renal stone
Aching	Appendiceal irritation
Knifelike	Pancreatitis
Gradual onset	Infection
Sudden onset	Duodenal ulcer, acute pancreatitis, obstruction, perforation

BOX 15-5 Some Causes of Pain Perceived in Anatomic Regions

Right Upper Quadrant

Duodenal ulcer
Hepatitis
Hepatomegaly
Pneumonia
Cholecystitis

Right Lower Quadrant

Appendicitis
Salpingitis
Ovarian cyst
Ruptured ectopic pregnancy
Renal/ureteral stone
Strangulated hernia
Meckel diverticulitis
Regional ileitis
Perforated cecum

Periumbilical

Intestinal obstruction
Acute pancreatitis
Early appendicitis
Mesenteric thrombosis
Aortic aneurysm
Diverticulitis

Left Upper Quadrant

Ruptured spleen
Gastric ulcer
Aortic aneurysm
Perforated colon
Pneumonia

Left Lower Quadrant

Sigmoid diverticulitis
Salpingitis
Ovarian cyst
Ruptured ectopic pregnancy
Renal/ureteral stone
Strangulated hernia
Perforated colon
Regional ileitis
Ulcerative colitis

Modified from Judge et al, 1988.

BOX 15-6 **Findings in Peritoneal Irritation**

Involuntary rigidity of abdominal muscles
- Tenderness and guarding
- Absent bowel sounds
- Positive obturator test (p. 550)
- Positive iliopsoas test (p. 549)
- Rebound tenderness (Blumberg sign and McBurney sign, p. 549)
- Abdominal pain on walking
- Positive heel jar test (Markle sign, Table 15-5)
- Positive Rovsing sign (Table 15-5)

TABLE 15-4 **Symptoms or Signs Elicited in Other Systems That May Relate to the Abdominal Examination**

Symptom or Sign	Possible Pathologic Condition	Symptom or Sign	Possible Pathologic Condition
Shock	Acute pancreatitis, ruptured tubal pregnancy	Flank tenderness	Renal inflammation, pyelonephritis
Mental status deficit	Hemorrhage—duodenal ulcer		Renal stone
	Abdominal epilepsy		Renal infarct
Hypertension	Aortic dissection		Renal vein thrombosis
	Abdominal aortic aneurysm	Leg edema	Iliac obstruction, pelvic mass
	Renal infarction		
	Glomerulonephritis		Renal disease
	Vasculitis	Lymphadenopathy	Renal vein thrombosis
Orthostatic hypotension	Hypovolemia—blood loss, fluid loss		Hepatitis
			Lymphoma
Pulse deficit	Aortic dissection	Jaundice	Mononucleosis
	Aortic aneurysm or thrombosis		Liver-biliary disease
Bruits	Aortic dissection	Dark yellow to brown urine	Excessive hemolysis
	Aortic aneurysm		Liver-biliary disease
	Dissection or aneurysm of arteries—splenic, renal, or iliac		Blood resulting from kidney stone, infarct, glomerulonephritis, or pyelonephritis
Low-output cardiac symptoms—atrial fibrillation	Ischemia of mesentery		
Valvular disease, congestive heart failure	Embolus	Fever (39.4° C [103° F]) and chills	Peritonitis
			Pelvic infection
Pleural effusion	Esophageal rupture		Cholangitis
	Pancreatitis	White blood cell count >10,000 mm^3 or shift to left (more than 80% polymorphonuclear cells) >20,000 mm^3	Pyelonephritis
	Ovarian tumor		Appendicitis (95%)
			Acute cholecystitis (90%)
			Localized peritonitis
			Bowel strangulation
			Bowel infarction

From Barkauskas et al, 1998.

Rebound Tenderness

The following maneuver is considered crude and unnecessary by many examiners, since light percussion produces a mild localized response in the presence of peritoneal inflammation. If the patient is experiencing abdominal pain, this maneuver can be used to determine peritoneal irritation (Box 15-6). Place the patient in the supine position. Hold your hand at a 90-degree angle to the abdomen with the fingers extended, then press gently and deeply into a region remote from the area of dis-

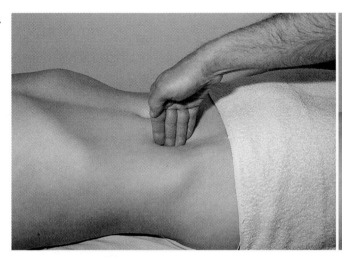
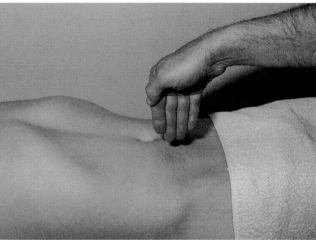

FIGURE 15-33
Testing for rebound tenderness. **A,** Press deeply and gently into the abdomen; then, **B,** rapidly withdraw the hands and fingers.

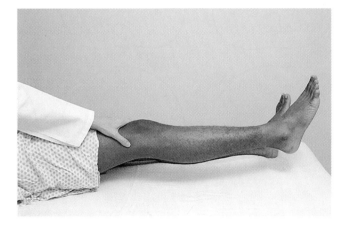

FIGURE 15-34
Iliopsoas muscle test. The patient raises the leg from the hip while the examiner pushes downward against it.

comfort. Rapidly withdraw your hand and fingers (Figure 15-33). The return to position (rebound) of the structures that were compressed by your fingers causes a sharp stabbing pain at the site of peritoneal inflammation (positive Blumberg sign). Rebound tenderness over the McBurney point in the lower right quadrant suggests appendicitis (positive McBurney sign). The maneuver for rebound tenderness should be performed at the end of the examination, because a positive response produces pain and muscle spasm that can interfere with any subsequent examination.

Iliopsoas Muscle Test

A patient with a positive iliopsoas sign will experience lower quadrant pain. Perform this test when you suspect appendicitis, since an inflamed appendix may cause irritation of the lateral iliopsoas muscle. Ask the patient to lie supine and then place your hand over the lower thigh. Ask the patient to raise the leg, flexing at the hip, while you push downward against the leg (Figure 15-34). An alternate technique is to position the patient on the left side and ask that the right leg be raised from the hip while you press downward against it. A third technique is to hyperextend the leg by drawing it backward while the patient is lying on the right side.

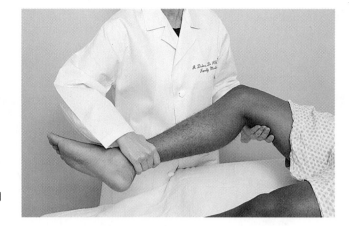

FIGURE 15-35
Obturator muscle test. With the right leg flexed at the hip and knee, rotate the leg laterally and medially.

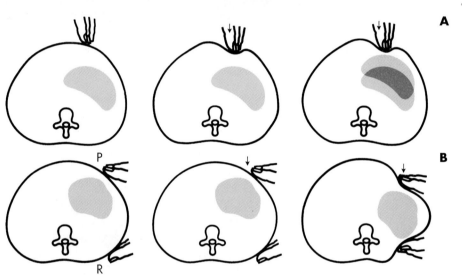

FIGURE 15-36
Ballottement technique.
A, Single-handed ballottement. Push inward at a 90-degree angle. If the object is freely movable, it will float upward to touch the fingertips. **B,** Bimanual ballottement; P, pushing; R, receiving hand.
From GI series, 1981, AH Robbins Co.

Obturator Muscle Test

Perform this test when you suspect a ruptured appendix or a pelvic abscess, since these conditions can cause irritation of the obturator muscle. Pain in the hypogastric region is a positive sign, indicating irritation of the obturator muscle. The patient should be supine for this test. Ask the patient to flex the right leg at the hip and knee to 90 degrees. Hold the leg just above the knee, grasp the ankle, and rotate the leg laterally and medially (Figure 15-35).

Ballottement

Ballottement is a palpation technique used to assess a floating mass, such as the head of a fetus. To perform abdominal ballottement with one hand, place your extended fingers, hand, and forearm at a 90-degree angle to the abdomen. Push in toward the mass with the fingertips (Figure 15-36, *A*). If the mass is freely movable, it will float upward and touch the fingertips as fluid and other structures are displaced by the maneuver.

To perform bimanual ballottement, place one hand on the anterior abdominal wall and one hand against the flank. Push inward on the abdominal wall while palpating with the flank hand to determine the presence and size of the mass (Figure 15-36, *B*).

TABLE 15-5	Abdominal Signs Associated with Common Abnormalities	
Sign	**Description**	**Associated Conditions**
Aaron	Pain or distress occurs in the area of the patient's heart or stomach on palpation of McBurney point	Appendicitis
Ballance	Fixed dullness to percussion in left flank, and dullness in right flank that disappears on change of position	Peritoneal irritation
Blumberg	Rebound tenderness	Peritoneal irritation; appendicitis
Cullen	Ecchymosis around umbilicus	Hemoperitoneum; pancreatitis; ectopic pregnancy
Dance	Absence of bowel sounds in right lower quadrant	Intussusception
Grey Turner	Ecchymosis of flanks	Hemoperitoneum; pancreatitis
Kehr	Abdominal pain radiating to left shoulder	Spleen rupture; renal calculi; ectopic pregnancy
Markle (heel jar)	Patient stands with straightened knees, then raises up on toes, relaxes, and allows heels to hit floor, thus jarring body. Action will cause abdominal pain if positive	Peritoneal irritation; appendicitis
McBurney	Rebound tenderness and sharp pain when McBurney point is palpated	Appendicitis
Murphy	Abrupt cessation of inspiration on palpation of gallbladder	Cholecystitis
Romberg-Howship	Pain down the medial aspect of the thigh to the knees	Strangulated obturator hernia
Rovsing	Right lower quadrant pain intensified by left lower quadrant abdominal palpation	Peritoneal irritation; appendicitis

Abdominal Signs

"Classic" abdominal pain signs have often been given the name of the person who first described them. Some of the most common are included in Table 15-5.

INFANTS AND CHILDREN

The infant's abdomen should be examined if possible during a time of relaxation and quiet. It is often best to do this at the start of the overall examination, especially before initiating any procedure that might cause distress (Figure 15-37). Sucking a bottle or pacifier may help relax the infant. The parent's lap makes the best examining surface, much better than having the child lie fixed and supine on a table. Sit facing the parent, knees touching, and conduct the abdominal examination entirely on the parent's lap. This works well during the first several months, and often the first 2 to 3 years, of life. The infant will be most secure.

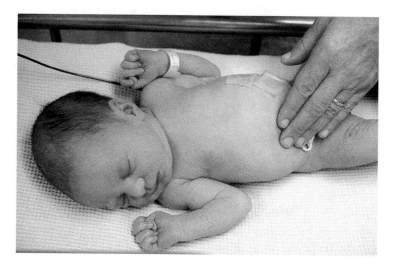

FIGURE 15-37
Positioning to examine the infant's abdomen.

INSPECTION

Inspect the abdomen, noting its shape, contour, and movement with respiration. It should be rounded and dome-shaped, because the abdominal musculature has not fully developed. Note any localized fullness. Abdominal and chest movements should be synchronous, with a slight bulge of the abdomen at the beginning of respiration. Note whether the abdomen protrudes above the level of the chest or is scaphoid. A distended or protruding abdomen can result from feces, a mass, or organ enlargement. A scaphoid abdomen suggests that the abdominal contents are displaced into the thorax.

Note any pulsations over the abdomen. Pulsations in the epigastric area are common in newborns and infants. Superficial veins are usually visible in the thin infant. However, distended veins across the abdomen are an unexpected finding suggestive of vascular obstruction or abdominal distention or obstruction. If any distended veins are present, identify the direction of blood flow. Spider nevi may indicate liver disease.

Inspect the umbilical cord of the newborn, counting the number of vessels. Two arteries and one vein should be present. A single umbilical artery should alert you to the possibility of congenital anomalies. Any intestinal structure present in the umbilical cord or protruding into the umbilical area and visible through a thick transparent membrane suggests an omphalocele.

The umbilical stump area should be dry and odorless. Inspect it for discharge, redness, induration, and skin warmth. Once the stump has separated, serous or serosanguinous discharge may indicate a granuloma when no other signs of infection are present. Inspect all folds of skin in the umbilicus for a nodule of granulomatous tissue.

Note any protrusion through the umbilicus or rectus abdominis muscles when the infant strains. The umbilicus is usually inverted. An umbilical hernia, the protrusion of omentum and intestine through the umbilical opening, forming a visible and palpable bulge, is a common finding in infants (Figure 15-38).

The umbilicus often everts with increased abdominal pressure, for example, with coughing or sneezing. Umbilical hernias can be very large and impressive. It is ordinarily easy to reduce them temporarily by pushing the contents back into a more appropriate intraabdominal position. Usually, however, they pop right out again. The

> ### UMBILICAL CORD
> A thick umbilical cord suggests a well-nourished fetus; a thin cord suggests otherwise.

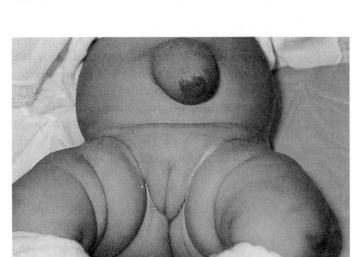

FIGURE 15-38
Umbilical hernia in an infant.

apparent size is not cause for alarm, and generally it pays to temporize. Measure the diameter of the umbilical opening rather than the protruding contents to determine the size. The maximum size is generally reached by 1 month of age, and the hernia will generally close spontaneously by 1 to 2 years of age. Diastasis rectus abdominis, a separation 1 to 4 cm wide in the midline usually between the xiphoid and the umbilicus, is a common finding when the rectus abdominis muscles do not approximate each other. Ordinarily, there is no need to repair this. Herniation through the rectus abdominis muscles, however, is a problem.

If the infant is vomiting frequently, use tangential lighting and observe the abdomen at eye level for peristaltic waves. Peristalsis is not usually visible. Peristaltic waves may sometimes be seen in thin, malnourished infants, but their presence usually suggests an intestinal obstruction, such as pyloric stenosis.

AUSCULTATION AND PERCUSSION

The procedures of auscultation and percussion of the abdomen do not differ from those used for adults. Peristalsis is detected when metallic tinkling is heard every 10 to 30 seconds, and bowel sounds should be present within 1 to 2 hours after birth. Since a scaphoid abdomen suggests a diaphragmatic hernia in the newborn, auscultate the chest for bowel sounds. No bruits or venous hums should be detected on abdominal auscultation.

Renal bruits are associated with renal artery stenosis and rarely with renal arteriovenous fistula. The bruit of stenosis has a high frequency and is soft; the bruit of arteriovenous fistula is continuous. Both are hard to hear. Try first with the patient held upright or sitting, listening at the posterior flank; and then try with the patient supine, listening over the abdomen.

The abdomen may produce more tympany on percussion than is found in adults, because infants swallow air when feeding or crying. As with adults, tympany in a distended abdomen is usually the result of gas, whereas dullness may indicate fluid or a solid mass. The upper edge of the liver should be detected within 1 cm of the fifth intercostal space at the right midclavicular line. Until 2 years of age females have a slightly larger liver span than males. The mean range of liver spans in infants and children is as follows:

AGE	LIVER SPAN (CM)
6 months	2.4-2.8
12 months	2.8-3.1
24 months	3.5-3.6
3 years	4.0
4 years	4.3-4.4
5 years	4.5-4.8
6 years	4.8-5.1
8 years	5.1-5.6
10 years	5.5-6.1

PALPATION

Palpate the abdomen with the infant's feet slightly elevated and knees flexed to promote relaxation of the abdominal musculature (Box 15-7). Begin with superficial palpation to detect the spleen, liver, and masses close to the surface. The spleen is usually palpable 1 to 2 cm below the left costal margin during the first few weeks after birth. A detectable spleen tip at the left costal margin is a common finding in well infants and young children. Any increase in spleen size may indicate blood dyscrasias or septicemia.

BOX 15-7 **Palpating an Infant's Abdomen**

The abdomen of an infant can seem very tiny in relation to the size of your hand. One technique for palpating a very small abdomen is as follows: Place your right hand gently on the abdomen with the thumb at the right upper quadrant and the index finger at the left upper quadrant. Press very gently at first, only gradually increasing pressure (never too vigorously) as you palpate over the entire abdomen.

ENLARGED LIVER

An infant of a mother with poorly controlled diabetes may more often than not have an "enlarged" liver, a finding that, by itself, presents no problem.

PALPATE WITH CAUTION!

Once a mass is felt near the kidney, do not repeatedly or aggressively palpate the mass. Such palpation could cause the release of cells that have metastatic potential.

MNEMONICS

INTUSSUSCEPTION IN INFANTS: "A B C D E F"

A Abdominal or anal "sausage"

B Blood from the rectum (red currant jelly)

C Colic: babies draw up their legs

D Distention, dehydration, and shock

E Emesis

F Face pale

From Shipman, 1984.

Liver Palpation

To assess the liver, superficially palpate at the right midclavicular line 3 to 4 cm below the costal margin. As the infant inspires, wait to feel a narrow mass tap your finger. Gradually move your fingers up the midclavicular line until the sensation is felt. The liver edge is usually palpable just below the right costal margin in the newborn. The liver edge may be palpable at 1 to 3 cm below the right costal margin in infants and toddlers. Estimation of true liver size can be accomplished only by percussing the upper border, as well as palpating the lower edge. Together the techniques provide an estimate of liver span, rather than just a projection of size below the costal margin. Hepatomegaly is present when the liver is more than 3 cm below the right costal margin, suggesting infection, cardiac failure, or liver disease.

Deep Palpation

Deep palpation is then performed in all quadrants. The location, size, shape, tenderness, and consistency of any masses should be noted. Transillumination should be used to distinguish cystic masses from solid masses. Fluid-filled masses will transilluminate, whereas solid masses will not. When pulsations are seen, palpate the aorta for any sign of enlargement. Fixed masses that are laterally mobile, pulsatile, or located along the vertebral column should be investigated further with special studies. If any suspicion of a neoplasm exists, limit palpation of the mass, because manipulation may cause injury or spread of malignancy.

A sausage-shaped mass in the left lower quadrant may indicate feces in the sigmoid colon associated with constipation. A midline suprapubic mass suggests Hirschsprung disease, in which feces fill the rectosigmoid colon. A sausage-shaped mass in the left or right upper quadrant may indicate intussusception. The olive-shaped mass of pyloric stenosis can often be detected with deep palpation in the right upper quadrant immediately after the infant vomits. It may be helpful to sit the infant in your lap, folding the upper body gently against your palpating hand, bringing the pyloric mass into opposition with your hand. Almost all other palpable masses in the abdomen of the newborn are renal in origin.

In the infant and toddler the bladder can usually be palpated and percussed in the suprapubic area. Determine the size of the bladder to detect any sign of distention. A distended bladder, felt as a firm, central dome-shaped structure in the lower abdomen, may indicate urethral obstruction or central nervous system defects.

Palpate the femoral arteries as described in Chapter 13 (Heart and Blood Vessels).

Tenderness or pain on palpation may be difficult to detect in the infant. However, pain and tenderness are assessed by such behaviors as change in the pitch of crying, facial grimacing, rejection of the opportunity to suck, and drawing the knees to the abdomen with palpation. When an infant will not stop crying, seize the quiet mo-

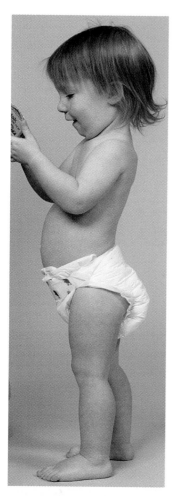

FIGURE 15-39
Potbellied stance of a toddler.

ment in the respiratory cycle to palpate in order to distinguish between a hard and soft abdomen. The abdomen should be soft during inspiration. If the abdomen remains hard with a noticeable rigidity or resistance to pressure during both respiratory phases, peritoneal irritation may be present. It is often necessary to delay examination of a distressed infant for a little while, waiting for a quieter moment, unless there is reason for urgency.

The abdomen of the young child protrudes slightly, giving a potbellied appearance when the child is standing, sitting, and supine (Figure 15-39). After age 5, the contour of the child's abdomen, when supine, may become convex and will not extend above an imaginary line drawn from the xiphoid process to the symphysis pubis. Respirations will continue to be abdominal until the child is 6 to 7 years old. Abdominal respiration beyond this age suggests thoracic problems. Restricted abdominal respiration in young children can be caused by peritoneal irritation or an acute abdomen. Diastasis rectus abdominis ordinarily resolves by 6 years of age.

The upper edge of the liver should be detected by percussion at the sixth intercostal space. The lower edge of the liver may be palpated either at, or 1 to 2 cm below, the right costal margin.

Palpate the abdomen of a child who is ticklish with a firm rather than feathery touch. If that is unsuccessful, place the child's hand under the palm of your examining hand, leaving your fingers free to palpate. Localization of abdominal tenderness or pain may be difficult in the young child who cannot verbalize about the site or character of pain. Distract the child with a toy, or question the child about a favorite activity as you begin palpating in the abdominal region believed most distant from the area of pain. Observe for changes in facial expression and for constriction of the pupils during palpation to identify the location of greatest pain. Check for rebound tenderness and make the same observations of the child's facial expression and pupils. As with adults, check rebound tenderness cautiously. Too vigorous an approach may be cruel and inhumane. Once a child has experienced palpation that is too intense, a subsequent examiner has little chance for easy access to the abdomen.

ADOLESCENTS

The techniques of abdominal examination of the adolescent are the same as those used for adults. Do not overlook the possibility of pregnancy as a cause of a mass in the lower abdomen, even in young adolescent females.

PREGNANT WOMEN

Uterine changes that can be detected on pelvic examination are discussed in Chapter 16 (Female Genitalia). Bowel sounds will be diminished as a result of decreased peristaltic activity. Striae and a midline band of pigmentation (linea nigra) may be present. Gastrointestinal complaints of nausea and vomiting are common in the first trimester. Constipation is a common occurrence, and hemorrhoids often develop later in pregnancy.

Assessment of the abdomen of pregnant women includes uterine size estimation for gestational age, fetal growth, position of the fetus, monitoring of fetal well-being, and the presence of uterine contractions. Evaluation techniques for fetal well-being, such as ultrasound examination and electronic fetal monitoring, are not reviewed in this text.

GESTATIONAL AGE

Before assessment of the abdomen, calculation is performed to determine the estimated date of delivery or confinement (EDC). One of the most common methods is to use the Naegele rule: add 7 days to the first day of the last normal menstrual period and count back 3 months.

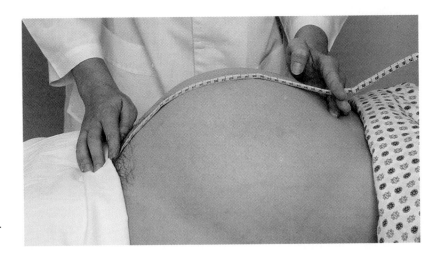

FIGURE 15-40
Measurement of fundal height from the symphysis to the superior fundus uterus.

The average duration of pregnancy is considered to be 280 days, or 40 weeks. The pregnancy is then divided into trimesters, each of which is slightly more than 13 weeks, or 3 calendar months. However, the clinically appropriate unit of measure is weeks of gestation completed. Weeks of gestation completed can be easily calculated by using an obstetric wheel that provides information (depending on its design) such as time of ovulation, implantation, EDC, and weeks and days of gestation.

Assessment of the abdomen of pregnant women includes measurement of fundal height. This technique provides an estimate for the length of the pregnancy and growth of the fetus. To measure fundal height, perform the following steps:

- Have the patient empty her bladder before the procedure.
- Ask the patient to lie supine.
- With a nonstretchable tape measure, measure from the upper part of the pubis symphysis to the superior fundus uterus over the middle portion of the fundus (Figure 15-40). The measurement is recorded in centimeters.
- The same person should perform the measurement each time to decrease chances of individual variations.

This measurement is most accurate between 20 and 30 weeks of gestation when the fundal height in centimeters may be equal to the gestational age in weeks. When the two do not vary more than 3 cm between 20 and 30 weeks, the assessment of dating the pregnancy will be accurate. A 1 cm increase per week in fundal height is an expected pattern. Twin pregnancy or other conditions that enlarge the uterus should be suspected if during the second trimester the uterine size is larger than usually occurs during the expected week of gestation. If the uterine size is smaller than is expected, the possibility of intrauterine growth retardation should be considered.

During the second and third trimesters, the McDonald rule can also been used to estimate the duration of the pregnancy from fundal height measurement. Using the McDonald rule, divide the height of the fundus (in centimeters) by 3.5; the resultant figure is said to equal the duration of pregnancy in lunar months.

Factors that can affect the accuracy of the fundal height measurement are obesity, amount of amniotic fluid, myomata, multiple gestation, fetal size and attitude, and position of the uterus.

FETAL WELL-BEING

Assessment of fetal well-being includes, but is not limited to, measurement of fetal heart rate (FHR) and fetal movements. To determine the fetal heart rate, count the FHR or impulse for 1 minute (using a Doppler or fetoscope), and compare it with the mother's pulse during that time. Also note the quality and rhythm of the fetal heart rate. Charting of the results is usually done using a two-line figure in which the point of intersection is the umbilicus and the four quadrants are the maternal abdomen. Use an "X" or the FHR obtained to identify the point on the maternal abdomen in which the maximal impulse was heard (see example below):

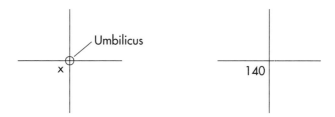

Kick counts can be used as an indicator of fetal well-being. Instruct the woman to note the pattern of movement over a given time. If the pattern shows a decrease or if movement ceases, the woman should notify her health care professional. Different techniques for monitoring fetal movements exist. One way is the Cardiff fetal movement (FM) count in which the pregnant woman notes FM beginning at 9 AM until the tenth movement is felt. The time interval is recorded on a graph. A change in the usual pattern may indicate fetal distress. It may be necessary to modify this system based on the woman's schedule. Begin FM recording based on the woman's situation. If there are no identifiable risks of uteroplacental insufficiency, start recording between 34 and 36 weeks' gestation. If there are risk factors, monitoring should start as early as 28 weeks. Remember that there are no universally accepted FM counting criteria. Individual assessment of circumstances is necessary. Another method includes maternal perception of one to two clusters of fetal movements in a 30 to 60 minute period (Fai et al, 1996). If no monitoring technique is used, the occurrence of three or fewer FMs in 1 hour while the woman is in left lateral position, at rest, or after ingestion of fluids signals the need for further evaluation of fetal well-being.

FETAL POSITION

Assessment of fetal position can be performed using the four steps of the Leopold maneuvers (Figure 15-41). After positioning the woman supine with her head slightly elevated and knees slightly flexed, place a small towel under her right hip. If you are right-handed, stand at the woman's right side facing her and perform the first three steps, then turn and face her feet for the last step; if you are left-handed, stand on the woman's left for the first three steps, then turn and face her feet for the last step. The maneuvers are performed as follows:

1. Place hands over the fundus and identify the fetal part (Figure 15-41, *A*). The head feels round, firm, and freely movable, and is detectable by ballottement. The buttocks feel softer and less mobile and regular.
2. With the palmar surface of your hand, locate the back of the fetus by applying gentle but deep pressure (Figure 15-41, *B*). The back feels smooth and convex, whereas the small parts (the feet, hands, knees, and elbows) will feel more irregular.
3. With the right hand if you are right-handed or with the left if you are left-handed, using the thumb and third finger, gently grasp the presenting part over the symphysis pubis (Figure 15-41, *C*). The head will feel firm and, if not engaged, will be movable from side to side and easily displaced upward. If the buttocks are presenting, they will feel softer and irregular. If the presenting part is not engaged, the fourth step is used.

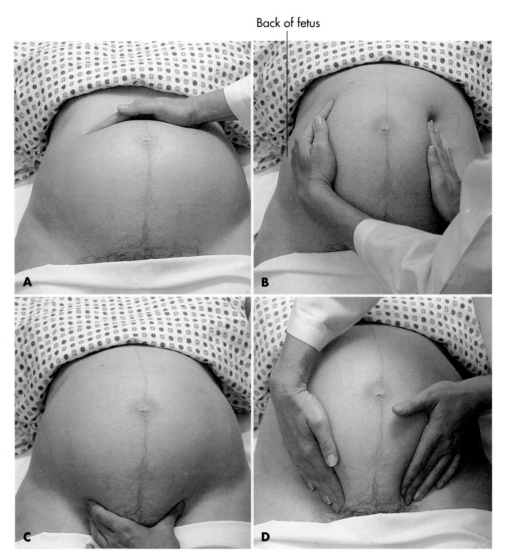

Back of fetus

FIGURE 15-41

Leopold maneuvers. **A,** First maneuver. Place hand(s) over fundus and identify the fetal part. **B,** Second maneuver. Use the palmar surface of one hand to locate the back of the fetus. Use the other hand to feel the irregularities, such as hands and feet. **C,** Third maneuver. Use thumb and third finger to grasp presenting part over the symphysis pubis. **D,** Fourth maneuver. Use both hands to outline the fetal head. With a head presenting deep in the pelvis, only a small portion may be felt.

4. Turn and face the woman's feet and use two hands to outline the fetal head (Figure 15-41, *D*). If the head is presenting and is deep into the pelvis, only a small portion may be felt. Palpation of the cephalic prominence (the part of the fetus that prevents descent of the examiner's hand) on the same side as the small parts suggests that the head is flexed and the vertex presenting. This is the optimal position. Palpation of the cephalic prominence on the same side as the back suggests that the presenting part is extended.

When recording the information obtained from the abdominal palpation, include the presenting part (that is, vertex if the head, or breech if the buttocks), the lie (the relationship of the long axis of the fetus to the long axis of the mother) as either longitudinal or vertical, and the attitude of the fetal head if it is the presenting part (flexed or extended). With experience, you will also be able to estimate the weight of the fetus.

Twins are a variation, often suspected when there is the presence of two fetal heart tones or on abdominal palpation when a second set of fetal parts is detected. Diagnosis is made by ultrasound examination. The technique for abdominal palpation in twin pregnancy is depicted in Figure 15-42.

The FHR can also be used to estimate position of the fetus. The areas of maximal intensity of the FHR and the position of the fetus are depicted in Figure 15-43.

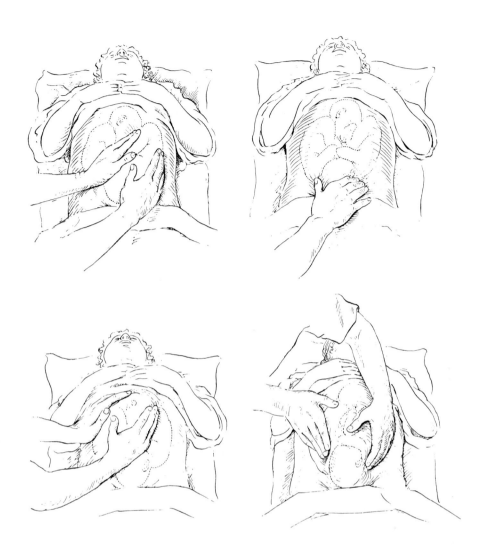

FIGURE 15-42
Abdominal palpation of twin
pregnancy.
From Wilson, Carrington, 1987.

FIGURE 15-43
Areas of maximal intensity of
FHR for differing positions: RSA,
right sacrum anterior; ROP, right
occipitoposterior; RMA, right
mentum anterior; ROA, right occipitoanterior; LSA, left sacrum
anterior; LOP, left occipitoposterior; LMA, left mentum anterior;
and LOA, left occipitoanterior.
A, Presentation is breech if FHR
is heard above umbilicus. **B,** Presentation is vertex if FHR is
heard below umbilicus.
From Lowdermilk, Perry, Bobak, 1997.

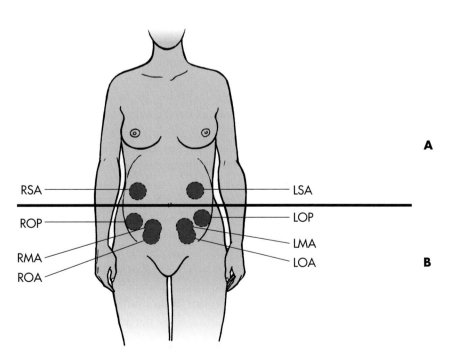

CONTRACTIONS

Uterine contractions begin as early as the third month of gestation. These contractions are a natural condition of pregnancy and are called Braxton Hicks contractions. They may go unnoticed by the woman but may become painful at times, especially as the pregnancy progresses and with increased gravidity.

Uterine contractions can be assessed with abdominal palpation, but more accuracy is obtained through use of electronic monitoring equipment, either indirectly through the abdominal wall or directly with the placement of an intrauterine pressure catheter. Assessment through abdominal palpation is helpful when equipment is not available to determine the onset or course of labor, either preterm or term. Practice is needed to determine the difference between mild, moderate, and strong contractions. Place the fingertips on the abdomen so that you are able to detect the contraction and relaxation of the uterus, and keep them there throughout the entire contraction, including the period of relaxation.

The strength of the contraction is classified as follows:
- Mild: slightly tense fundus that is easy to indent with the fingertips
- Moderate: firm fundus that is difficult to indent with the fingertips
- Strong: rigid or hard, boardlike fundus or one that does not indent with fingertips

The duration of the contraction is measured in seconds from the beginning until relaxation occurs. The frequency of contractions is measured from the beginning of one contraction to the beginning of the next. The frequency of contractions is assessed for regularity (at regular intervals, such as every 5 minutes, or at irregular or sporadic intervals). Each woman's experience of the discomfort created by the contracting uterus varies because of physiologic makeup, past experiences, cultural influences, expectations, prenatal education, support, and other factors. Her sense of the event should not be discounted based on physiologic and subjective measures.

OLDER ADULTS

The techniques of examination are the same as those used for younger adults. The abdominal wall of the older adult becomes thinner and less firm as a result of the loss of connective tissue and muscle mass that accompanies aging. Palpation therefore may be relatively easier and yield more accurate findings. A pulsating abdominal aortic aneurysm may be more readily palpable than it is in younger patients. Deposition of fat over the abdominal area is common, despite concurrent loss of fatty tissue over the extremities. The abdominal contour is often rounded as a result of loss of muscle tone.

The only modifications in examination techniques require some common sense. Use judgment in determining whether a patient is able to assume a particular position, such as the kneeling position, to test for fluid pooling in assessing ascites. Similarly, remember that rotation of joints, such as with the obturator muscle test, may cause discomfort in patients who have decreased muscle flexibility or joint tenderness.

Be aware that respiratory changes can produce corresponding findings in the abdominal examination. The liver of patients with hyperexpanded lungs may be displaced downward. In this case, both the upper and lower borders of the liver may be detected 1 to 2 cm below the usual markers, but the liver span should still be between 6 and 12 cm. On the other hand, with the decrease in liver size after age 50, you may find that the midclavicular liver span is somewhat less.

With decreased intestinal motility associated with aging, intestinal disorders are common in older adults, so be particularly sensitive to patient complaints and related findings in this regard. Constipation is a frequent complaint, and you are more likely

MNEMONICS

*CAUSES OF CONSTIPATION:
"CONSTIPATED"*

C *C*ongenital: Hirschsprung disease

O *O*bstruction

N *N*eoplasms

S *S*tricture of colon

T *T*opical: painful hemorrhoids or fissure

I *I*mpacted feces

P *P*rolapse of the rectum

A *A*norexia and depression

T *T*emperature high, dehydration results

E *E*ndocrine: hypothyroidism

D *D*iet, diverticulitis, and drugs

From Shipman, 1984.

to feel stool in the sigmoid colon. Accompanying complaints of gas and a sensation of bloatedness may be reflected in increased tympany on percussion. Fecal impaction is a common finding in older adults with severe or chronic constipation.

Obstruction may be a problem with older adults, occurring as a result of hypokalemia, myocardial infarction, and infections such as pneumonia, septicemia, peritonitis, and pancreatitis. Vomiting, distention, diarrhea, and constipation can signal obstruction.

The incidence of gastrointestinal cancer increases with age, with various symptoms that depend on the site of the tumor. Symptoms vary from dysphagia to nausea, vomiting, anorexia, and hematemesis to changes in stool frequency, size, consistency, or color. See Chapter 18 (Anus, Rectum, and Prostate) for a discussion of rectal digital examination, an important step in the detection of colon cancer.

Pain perception may be altered as part of the aging process, and older patients may exhibit atypical pain symptoms, including less severe or totally absent pain with disease states that characteristically produce pain in younger adults. Therefore evaluation of pain in the older adult must take into account concurrent symptoms and accompanying findings.

SAMPLE DOCUMENTATION

Abdomen: rounded and symmetrical with white striae adjacent to umbilicus in all quadrants. A well healed 5-cm white surgical scar evident in right lower quadrant. No areas of visible pulsations or peristalsis. Active bowels sounds audible in all four quadrants. Percussion tones tympanic over epigastrium and resonant over remainder of abdomen. Liver span 8 cm at right midclavicular line. On inspiration, liver edge firm, smooth and nontender. No splenomegaly. Musculature soft and relaxed to light palpation. No masses or areas of tenderness to deep palpation. Superficial reflexes intact. No costovertebral angle tenderness.

For additional sample documentation see Chapter 24, Recording Information.

SUMMARY OF EXAMINATION   **Abdomen (Patient Supine)**

1. Inspect the abdomen for the following (pp. 524-529):
   - Skin characteristics
   - Venous return patterns
   - Contour
   - Symmetry
   - Surface motion
2. Inspect abdominal muscles as patient raises head to detect presence of the following (pp. 528-529):
   - Masses
   - Hernia
   - Separation of muscles
3. Auscultate with stethoscope diaphragm for the following (p. 529):
   - Bowel sounds in all four quadrants
   - Friction rubs over liver and spleen
4. Auscultate with bell of stethoscope for the following (p. 530):
   - Venous hums in epigastric area and around umbilicus
   - Bruits over aorta and renal and femoral arteries
5. Percuss the abdomen for the following (pp. 530-534):
   - Tone in all four quadrants
   - Liver borders to estimate span
   - Splenic dullness in left midaxillary line
   - Gastric air bubble
6. Lightly palpate in all quadrants for the following (pp. 534-536):
   - Muscular resistance
   - Tenderness
   - Masses
7. Deeply palpate all quadrants for the following (pp. 536-543):
   - Bulges and masses around the umbilicus and umbilical ring
   - Liver border in right costal margin
   - Gallbladder below liver margin at lateral border of the rectus muscle
   - Spleen in left costal margin
   - Right and left kidneys
   - Aortic pulsation in midline
   - Other masses
8. Elicit the abdominal reflexes (p. 543).
9. With patient sitting, percuss the left and right costovertebral angles for kidney tenderness (p. 541).

COMMON ABNORMALITIES

ALIMENTARY TRACT

HIATAL HERNIA WITH ESOPHAGITIS

A hiatal hernia occurs when a part of the stomach has passed through the esophageal hiatus in the diaphragm into the chest cavity. The condition is very common and occurs most often in women and older adults. It is associated with obesity, pregnancy, ascites, and the use of tight-fitting belts and clothes; muscle weakness is a primary factor in developing this condition. A hiatal hernia is clinically significant when accompanied by acid reflux, producing esophagitis. Patients complain of epigastric pain and/or heartburn that worsens with lying down and is relieved by sitting up or with antacids, of water brash (the mouth fills with fluid from the esophagus), and of dysphagia. Incarceration of the hernia can occur, requiring surgical intervention. Symptoms of incarceration include sudden onset of vomiting, pain, and complete dysphagia.

DUODENAL ULCER

The most common form of peptic ulcer disease, duodenal ulcer, is a chronic circumscribed break in the duodenal mucosa that scars with healing (Figure 15-44). The ulcers may occur as a result of infection with *Helicobacter pylori* and cause increased gastric acid secretion. The condition occurs approximately twice as often in men as in women. Duodenal ulcers occur on both the anterior and posterior walls; anterior wall ulcers may produce tenderness on palpation of the abdomen. Patients generally complain of localized epigastric pain that occurs when the stomach is empty and that is relieved by food or antacids. Upper gastrointestinal bleeding can occur as a result of ulceration, producing symptoms that include hematemesis, melena, dizziness or syncope, decreased blood pressure, increased pulse rate, and decreased hematocrit level. Perforation of the duodenum is a life-threatening event that requires immediate surgical intervention. The patient exhibits signs of an acute abdomen. Anterior ulcers are more likely to perforate, whereas posterior ulcers are more likely to bleed.

A   **B**

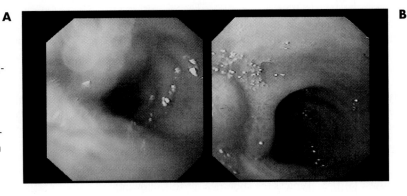

FIGURE 15-44

Peptic ulcer. **A** and **B**, Two endoscopic views of the duodenum demonstrate the grayish-white base of an ulcer crater. **B** also demonstrates slightly erythematous, boggy tissue at the margin of the ulcer.

From Zitelli, Davis, 1997.

CROHN DISEASE

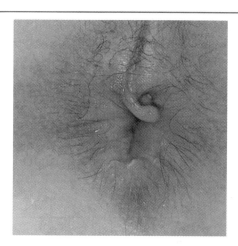

FIGURE 15-45

Crohn disease. Note a scar from previous incision and drainage. Perianal skin tags are common in Crohn disease and a good clue to diagnosis.

From Zitelli, Davis, 1997.

Crohn disease is a chronic inflammatory disorder of the gastrointestinal tract that produces ulceration, fibrosis, and malabsorption. Inflammation may occur anywhere along the gastrointestinal tract; the terminal ileum and colon are the most common sites. There is no clear evidence that dietary, psychologic, or environmental factors cause the disease. On colonoscopy the mucosa has a characteristic cobblestone appearance. Fissure and fistula formation, sometimes extending to the skin, is common (Figure 15-45). Patients exhibit chronic diarrhea, compromised nutritional status, and often other systemic manifestations such as arthritis, iritis, and erythema nodosum (Table 15-6).

TABLE 15-6	Comparison of Crohn Disease and Ulcerative Colitis		
Disease	**Pathologic Conditions**		**Characteristics**
Crohn disease	Inflammation, transmural bowel wall thickens, lumen narrows; mucosa ulcerated, cobblestone appearance (Figure 15-46); mesenteric fibrosis		Cramping diarrhea, mild bleeding, occurs anywhere in GI tract; fissure, fistula, abscess formation; periumbilical colic; malabsorption; folate deficiency
Ulcerative colitis	Inflammation confined to mucosa; starts in rectum, progresses through colon; vascular engorgement of submucosa; mucosa ulcerated and denuded with granulation tissue (Figure 15-47); minimal fibrosis		Mild to severe symptoms; bloody, watery diarrhea; no localized peritoneal signs; weight loss, fatigue, general debility; may progress to carcinoma of colon

DIFFERENTIAL DIAGNOSIS

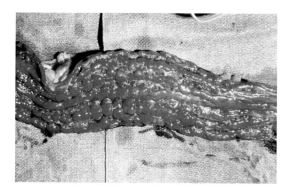

FIGURE 15-46

Crohn disease showing deep ulcers and fissures, creating "cobblestone" effect.

From Doughty, Jackson, 1993.

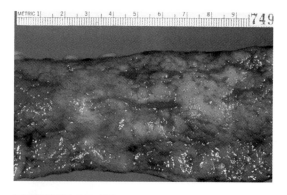

FIGURE 15-47

Ulcerative colitis showing severe mucosal edema and inflammation with ulcerations and bleeding.

From Doughty, Jackson, 1993.

ULCERATIVE COLITIS	Ulcerative colitis is a chronic inflammatory disorder of the colon and rectum that produces mucosal friability and areas of ulceration; fibrosis is minimal. The etiologic factor is unknown, but immunologic and genetic factors have been implicated. The condition is not caused by psychosomatic mechanisms. Ulcerative colitis is characterized by bloody, frequent, watery diarrhea, with patients reporting as many as 20 to 30 diarrheal	stools per day. Patients may also exhibit weight loss, fatigue, and general debilitation. Ulcerative colitis may range from mild to severe, depending on the degree of involvement of the colon. The condition may remain in remission for years after an acute phase of the illness. Active chronic ulcerative colitis predisposes an individual to carcinoma of the colon (Table 15-6).
STOMACH CANCER	Gastric carcinomas are most commonly found in the lower half of the stomach. These neoplasms arise from epithelial cells of the mucous membrane. In early stages, the growth is confined to the mucosa and submucosa, but as the disease progresses, the muscular layer of the stomach will also be involved. Metastases, local and distant, are common.	Symptoms may be vague and nonspecific, and include loss of appetite, feeling of fullness, weight loss, dysphagia, and persistent epigastric pain. Physical examination may reveal tenderness in the midepigastrium, an enlarged liver, positive supraclavicular nodes, and ascites. An epigastric mass is not palpable until late stages of the disease.
DIVERTICULOSIS	Inflammation of existing diverticula produces left lower quadrant pain, anorexia, nausea, vomiting, and altered bowel habits, usually constipation. The pain usually becomes localized at the site of	the inflammatory process (Figure 15-48). The abdomen may be distended and tympanic with decreased bowel sounds and localized tenderness.

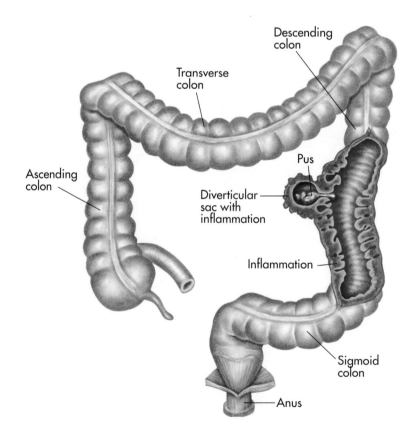

FIGURE 15-48

Diverticulosis (diverticulitis).

From Doughty, Jackson, 1993.

COLON CANCER	Carcinoma of the colon usually occurs in the rectum, sigmoid, and lower descending colon; but it may also appear in the proximal colon. The earliest sign is usually occult blood in the stool detectable by guaiac testing. The patient often gives	a history of changes in the frequency or character of stool. There are few early physical findings unless a lesion is felt on rectal examination (see Chapter 18, Anus, Rectum, and Prostate). A tumor may be palpable in the right or left lower quadrant.

HEPATOBILIARY SYSTEM

HEPATITIS	Hepatitis is an inflammatory process of the liver characterized by diffuse or patchy hepatocellular necrosis. The condition is most commonly caused by viral infection, alcohol, drugs, or toxins. Symptoms include jaundice, hepatomegaly, anorexia, abdominal and gastric discomfort, clay-colored stools, and tea-colored urine. Liver function tests are abnormal. Systemic infection may produce small focal areas of hepatic necrosis and inflammation, termed reactive hepatitis.	Reactive hepatitis causes minor liver function abnormalities and is usually asymptomatic. Acute viral hepatitis is caused by at least five distinct agents (Table 15-7). Hepatitis D occurs only in persons infected with hepatitis B, either as a co-infection in acute hepatitis B, or as a superinfection in chronic hepatitis B. Hepatitis E (epidemic) is a self-limited type of hepatitis that may occur after natural disasters because of fecal-contaminated water or food.
CIRRHOSIS	Cirrhosis is characterized by destruction of the liver parenchyma. The liver is initially often enlarged with a firm nontender border on palpation, but as scarring progresses, the liver mass is reduced, and it generally cannot be palpated. Associated symptoms include ascites, jaun-	dice, prominent abdominal vasculature, cutaneous spider angiomas, dark urine, light-colored stools, and spleen enlargement. The patient often complains of fatigue, and in late stages muscle wasting may be evident.
LIVER CARCINOMA	Invasion of the liver by malignant cells produces liver enlargement and a hard, irregular border on palpation. Nodules may be present and palpable, and the	liver may be either tender or nontender. Associated symptoms can include ascites, jaundice, anorexia, fatigue, dark urine, and light-colored stools.
CHOLELITHIASIS	Stone formation in the gallbladder is responsible for most gallbladder diseases. Many patients are asymptomatic; however, symptoms of indigestion, colic, and mild	transient jaundice are not unusual. The condition commonly produces episodes of acute cholecystitis and pancreatitis.
GALLBLADDER CANCER	Invasion of the gallbladder by malignant cells results in abdominal pain, jaundice,	and weight loss. A mass may be palpable in the upper abdomen.

TABLE 15-7 | **Comparison Viral Hepatitis Infections***

Type	Mode of Transmission	Prevalence	Clinical Sequelae	Prevention
Hepatitis A virus (HAV)	Fecal-oral; food/water-borne outbreaks; blood-borne (rare)	125,000-200,000 acute infections/year; 33% of Americans have evidence of past infection (immunity)	Prolonged or relapsing hepatitis (15%); no chronic infection; 100 deaths/year	Vaccine; immune globulin before and after exposure; good hygiene and sanitation
Hepatitis B virus (HBV)	Bloodborne; sexual; perinatal	140,000-320,000 acute infection/year; 1-1.25 million Americans chronically infected	Chronic infection (6%-10%); 150 death/year from acute infection; 5,000-6,000 deaths/year from chronic liver disease including primary liver cancer	Vaccine; screen pregnant women and treat infected infants; screen blood/organ/tissue donors
Hepatitis C virus (HCV)	Bloodborne, sexual, perinatal	28,000-180,000 acute infection/year; 3.5 million Americans chronically infected	Chronic infection (85%); chronic liver disease (70%); 8,000-10,000 deaths/year from chronic liver disease	No vaccine; screen blood/organ/tissue donors
Hepatitis D virus (HDV, delta agent)	Bloodborne, sexual; perinatal (rare) HDV infection can be acquired either as a co-infection with HBV or as a superinfection of persons with chronic HBV infection	6,000-13,000 acute infections/year; 70,000 Americans chronically infected. In U.S. and countries with a low prevalence of chronic HBV infection, HDV prevalence is generally low. In countries with moderate and high levels of chronic HBV prevalence, the prevalence of HDV infection is highly variable	Chronic HBV carriers who acquire HDV superinfection usually develop chronic HDV infection, with evidence of chronic liver diseases with cirrhosis (70%-80%); 1,000 deaths/year from chronic liver disease	No vaccine; co-infection can be prevented with either preexposure or postexposure prophylaxis for HBV. However, no products exist to prevent HDV superinfection of persons with chronic HBV infection. Prevention of HDV superinfection depends primarily on education to reduce risk behaviors
Hepatitis E virus (HEV, epidemic)	Fecal-oral route and fecally contaminated drinking water; nosocomial transmission, presumably by person-to-person contact, has been reported	Accounts for >50% of acute sporadic hepatitis in both children and adults in some high endemic areas. Low prevalence in U.S. and other nonendemic areas (<2%). U.S. cases are in travelers returning from high HEV-endemic areas	May account for some cases of unclassified chronic hepatitis	No vaccine; clean water supply; hygienic practices for travelers to endemic countries: avoiding drinking water (and beverages with ice) of unknown purity, uncooked shellfish, and uncooked fruits or vegetables that are not peeled or prepared by the traveler

*Source CDC, 1997; figures cited are for the United States unless otherwise indicated
www.cdc.gov/ncidod/diseases/hepatitis/index.htm. September, 1997.

| CHOLECYSTITIS | Cholecystitis is an inflammatory process of the gallbladder that may be either acute or chronic. Acute cholecystitis has associated stone formation (cholelithiasis) in 90% of all cases, causing obstruction and inflammation. Acute cholecystitis without stones results from any condition that affects the regular emptying and filling of the gallbladder, such as immobilization or sudden starvation. The primary symptom of acute cholecystitis is | pain in the right upper quadrant with radiation around the midtorso to the right scapular region. The pain is abrupt and severe, and lasts for 2 to 4 hours. Chronic cholecystitis refers to repeated attacks of acute cholecystitis in a gallbladder that is scarred and contracted. These patients will exhibit fat intolerance, flatulence, nausea, anorexia, and nonspecific abdominal pain and tenderness of the right hypochondriac region. |

PANCREAS

CHRONIC PANCREATITIS	Chronic inflammation of the pancreas produces constant unremitting abdomi-	nal pain, epigastric tenderness, weight loss, steatorrhea, and glucose intolerance.
PANCREAS CANCER	Invasion of the pancreas by malignant cells results in abdominal pain that radiates from the epigastrium to the upper	quadrants or back, weight loss, anorexia, and jaundice.

SPLEEN

| SPLEEN RUPTURE | The spleen is the most commonly injured organ in abdominal trauma because of its anatomic location. The mechanism of injury can be either blunt or penetrating but is more often blunt, for example, from motor vehicle accidents. The symptoms of splenic rupture | are pain in the left upper quadrant with radiation to the left shoulder (positive Kehr sign), hypovolemia, and peritoneal irritation. Diagnosis is made by positive paracentesis or splenic scan. Surgical intervention may be required. |

KIDNEYS

GLOMERULO-NEPHRITIS	Inflammation of the capillary loops of the renal glomeruli usually produces nonspecific symptoms. The patient com-	plains of nausea, malaise, and arthralgias. Hematuria may occur. Pulmonary infiltrates may be present.
HYDRONEPHROSIS	Hydronephrosis is the dilation of the renal pelvis from back pressure of urine that cannot flow past an obstruction in	the ureter. The patient experiences hematuria, pyuria, and fever, if secondary infection is present.
PYELONEPHRITIS	Infection of the kidney and renal pelvis is characterized by flank pain, bacteriuria, pyuria, dysuria, nocturia, and frequency.	Costovertebral angle tenderness may be evident.
RENAL ABSCESS	Renal abscess is a localized infection within the cortex of the kidney. The patient may complain of chills, fever, and	aching flanks. Fist percussion produces costovertebral angle tenderness.

RENAL CALCULI	Renal calculi are stones formed in the pelvis of the kidney from a physiochemical process; calculus formation is associated with obstruction and infections in the urinary tract. Renal calculi are composed of calcium salts, uric acid, cystine, and struvite. Any situation leading to an alkaline urine is conducive to stone formation, because uric acid, calcium, and	phosphate are all more soluble in a low pH. Urine temperature, ionic strength, and concentration also affect stone formation. The condition is much more prevalent in men than in women. Symptoms include fever, hematuria, and flank pain that may extend to the groin and genitals.
ACUTE RENAL FAILURE	This is the sudden, severe impairment of renal function causing an acute uremic episode. The impairment may be prerenal, renal, or postrenal. Urine output	may be normal, decreased, or absent. The patient may show signs of either fluid overload or deficit.
CHRONIC RENAL FAILURE	Chronic renal failure is a slow, insidious, and irreversible impairment of renal function. Uremia usually develops gradually.	The patient may experience oliguria or anuria and have signs of fluid overload.
RENAL ARTERY EMBOLI	Numerous small or a few major emboli can occlude the renal artery, causing either acute or chronic renal failure. The condition may be a silent event or a full-	blown syndrome of flank pain and tenderness, hematuria, hypertension, fever, and decreased renal function.
MALODOROUS URINE	Many (but not all) diseases or disorders signaled by malodorous urine are inborn	errors of metabolism (Box 15-8).

BOX 15-8   Diseases and Conditions Signaled by Malodorous Urine

- Maple syrup — Maple syrup urine disease
- Mousy, musty — Phenylketonuria
- Dead fish — Fish odor syndrome (Trimethylaminuria)
- Cat's urine — Cat syndrome (similar to Werdnig-Hoffman disease)
- Yeastlike, celery — Oasthouse urine disease (methionine)
- Fishy, musty — Tyrosinemia/tyrosinosis
- Rancid butter — Rancid butter syndrome (hypermethioninemia)
- Ammonia — Urea-splitting bacteria (especially *Proteus*)
- Rotting fish — Uremia (di-, tri-methylamines)
- Stale water — Acute tubular necrosis
- Violets — Turpentine ingestion
- Medicinal — Antibiotics: penicillin, cephalosporins

Adapted from Wilson MEH, 1997; and Mace et al., 1976.

INFANTS

INTUSSUSCEPTION	The prolapse of one segment of the intestine into another causes intestinal obstruction. Intussusception commonly occurs in infants between 3 and 12 months old. The cause is unknown. Symptoms include acute intermittent abdominal pain, abdominal distention, vomiting, and passage at first of normal brown stool. Subsequent stools are mixed with blood and mucus with a red currant jelly appearance. A sausage-shaped mass	may be palpated in the right or left upper quadrant, whereas the lower quadrant feels empty (positive Dance sign). Intussusception in an infant can be dramatic in onset. The apparently well child starts crying suddenly and excruciatingly, sometimes awakening from sleep. The child is inconsolable, sometimes doubling up with pain. The episode can cease abruptly, but the symptoms will most likely recur.
PYLORIC STENOSIS	Hypertrophy of the circular muscle of the pylorus leads to obstruction of the pyloric sphincter during the first month after birth. Symptoms include regurgitation progressing to projectile vomiting (vigorous, shoots out of the mouth, and	carries a short distance), feeding eagerly (even after a vomiting episode), failure to gain weight, and signs of dehydration. A small rounded tumor is often palpable in the right upper quadrant, particularly after the infant vomits.
MECONIUM ILEUS	Meconium ileus is a lower intestinal obstruction, caused by thickening and hardening of meconium in the lower intestine. Identified by the failure to pass	meconium in the first 24 hours after birth and by abdominal distention, it is often the first manifestation of cystic fibrosis.
BILIARY ATRESIA	Biliary atresia is a congenital obstruction or absence of some or all of the bile duct system. Symptoms include jaundice that usually becomes apparent at 2 to 3 weeks	of age, hepatomegaly, abdominal distention, poor weight gain, and pruritus. Stools become lighter in color and urine darkens.
MECKEL DIVERTICULUM	An outpouching of the ileum varies in size from a small appendiceal process to a segment of bowel several inches long, often in the proximity of the ileocecal valve. It is the most common congenital anomaly of the gastrointestinal tract. The	symptoms, if any, are those of intestinal obstruction or diverticulitis. In many cases, there is bright or dark red rectal bleeding with little abdominal pain, although symptoms like those of acute appendicitis are not uncommon.
GASTROESOPHAGEAL REFLUX	Relaxation or incompetence of the lower esophagus persisting beyond the newborn period produces gastroesophageal reflux. Symptoms include regurgitation	and vomiting, which can be severe enough to cause weight loss and failure to thrive, respiratory problems from aspiration, and bleeding from esophagitis.
NECROTIZING ENTEROCOLITIS	An inflammatory disease of the gastrointestinal mucosa, necrotizing enterocolitis is associated with prematurity and immaturity of the gastrointestinal tract.	Signs include abdominal distention, occult blood in stool, and respiratory distress. The condition is often fatal, complicated by perforation and septicemia.

CHILDREN

NEUROBLASTOMA

A common solid malignancy in early childhood, neuroblastoma frequently appears as a mass in the adrenal medulla of the young child, but a mass may occur anywhere along the craniospinal axis. A firm, fixed, nontender, irregular and nodular abdominal mass that crosses the midline is often found. Symptoms include malaise, loss of appetite, weight loss, and protrusion of one or both eyes. Other symptoms arise from compression of the mass or metastasis to adjacent organs.

WILMS TUMOR (NEPHROBLASTOMA)

Nephroblastoma, the most common intraabdominal tumor of childhood, usually appears at 2 to 3 years of age. It is a firm, nontender mass deep within the flank, only slightly movable and not usually crossing the midline. It is sometimes bilateral. Painless enlargement of the abdomen is the usual sign; however, a low-grade fever and hypertension may be present.

HIRSCHSPRUNG DISEASE (CONGENITAL AGANGLIONIC MEGACOLON)

The primary absence of parasympathetic ganglion cells in a segment of the colon interrupts the motility of the intestine. The absence of peristalsis causes feces to accumulate proximal to the defect, leading to an intestinal obstruction. Symptoms include failure to thrive, constipation, abdominal distention, and episodes of vomiting and diarrhea. The newborn may fail to pass meconium in the first 24 to 48 hours after birth. Symptoms in older infants and young children are generally intestinal obstruction or severe constipation.

PREGNANT WOMEN

HYDRAMNIOS (POLYHYDRAMNIOS)

Hydramnios is an excessive quantity of amniotic fluid, which can range from 2000 ml of fluid to as much as 15 L. Chronic hydramnios is a gradual accumulation of excess amniotic fluid, whereas acute hydramnios is a very sudden increase over a few days. Hydramnios is common in twin pregnancies; however, in other pregnancies it is associated with an increased incidence of fetal malformations, especially of the central nervous system and gastrointestinal tract. There is usually difficulty in palpating fetal small parts and in hearing fetal heart tones. A large uterus and tense uterine wall may also be present. Symptoms are primarily due to pressure on the surrounding organs from the distended uterus and include dyspnea, edema, and pain. Hydramnios may lead to perinatal mortality from premature labor and fetal abnormalities.

OLDER ADULTS

FECAL INCONTINENCE

Fecal incontinence in the elderly is associated with three major causes: fecal impaction, underlying disease, and neurogenic disorders. The most common cause, *fecal impaction,* is associated with immobilization and poor fluid and dietary intake. Typically these patients will have an "overflow incontinence" or a soft stool that oozes around the impaction. *Underlying diseases* such as cancer, inflammatory bowel disease, diverticulitis, colitis, proctitis, or diabetic neuropathy may all have fecal incontinence as a presenting symptom. Overuse of laxatives may also be a cause of incontinence. *Neurogenic disorders* take two forms: local or cognitive. Local refers to any process that causes the degeneration of the mesenteric plexus and lower bowel, resulting in a lax sphincter muscle, diminished sacral reflex, and decreased puborectal muscle tone. Cognitive neurogenic disorders usually result from stroke or dementia. These patients are unable to recognize rectal fullness and have an inability to inhibit intrinsic rectal contraction. Their stools are normally formed and occur in a set pattern, usually after a meal. Incontinence in the elderly patient is diagnosed through digital rectal examination, abdominal films, history, and assessment of cognitive abilities.

URINARY INCONTINENCE

MNEMONICS

REVERSIBLE CAUSES OF URINARY INCONTINENCE: "DRIP"

D *Delirium*

  Dehydration

R *Retention*

  Restricted mobility

I *Impaction*

  Infection

P *Polyuria*

  Pharmaceuticals

  Psychologic

From Penninger, 1993.

The most common types of urinary incontinence in the elderly are stress, urge, overflow, and functional. *Stress incontinence* is a leakage of urine due to increased intraabdominal pressure that can occur from coughing, laughing, exercise, or lifting heavy things. Causes of stress incontinence include weakness of bladder neck supports and anatomic damage to the urethral sphincter, both often associated with childbirth. *Urge incontinence* is the inability to hold urine once the urge to void occurs. Causes of this abnormality can be local genitourinary conditions such as infection or tumor or central nervous system disorders such as stroke. Reflex incontinence, a type of urge incontinence, is caused by uninhibited bladder contractions and no urge to void. *Overflow incontinence* is a mechanical dysfunction resulting from an overdistended bladder. This type of incontinence has many causes: anatomic obstruction by prostatic hypertrophy and strictures; neurologic abnormalities that impair detrusor contractility, such as multiple sclerosis; or spinal lesions. With *functional incontinence* there is an intact urinary tract, but other factors such as cognitive abilities, immobility, or musculoskeletal impairments lead to incontinence. Assessment of the incontinent patient can often be accomplished through a thorough history, physical examination, and urinary analysis. Note that many elderly patients will have more than one type of incontinence at any given time (Table 15-8).

TABLE 15-8	**Urinary Incontinence**	
Condition	**History**	**Physical Findings**
Stress incontinence	Small volume incontinence with cough, sneezing, laughing, running; history of prior pelvic surgery	Pelvic floor relaxation; cystocele, rectocele; lax urethral sphincter; loss of urine with provocative testing; atrophic vaginitis; postvoid residual <100 ml
Urge incontinence	Uncontrolled urge to void; large volume incontinence; history of central nervous system disorders such as stroke, multiple sclerosis, parkinsonism	Unexpected findings only as related to CNS disorder; postvoid residual <100 ml
Overflow incontinence	Small volume incontinence, dribbling, hesitancy. In men symptoms of enlarged prostate; nocturia, dribbling, hesitance, deceased force and caliber of stream	Distended bladder; prostate hypertrophy; stool in rectum, fecal impaction; postvoid residual >100 ml
	In neurogenic bladder: history of bowel problems, spinal cord injury, or multiple sclerosis	Evidence of spinal cord disease or diabetic neuropathy; lax sphincter; gait disturbance
Functional incontinence	Change in mental status; impaired mobility; new environment. Medications: hypnotics, diuretics, anticholinergic agents, alpha-adrenergic agents, calcium-channel blockers	Impaired mental status; impaired mobility. Impaired mental status or unexpected findings only as related to other physical conditions

Check it out— *http://www1.mosby.com/physexam_seidel*

CHAPTER 16

FEMALE GENITALIA

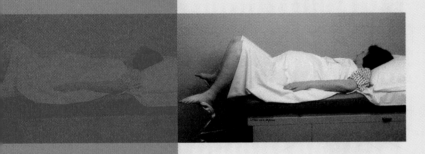

ANATOMY AND PHYSIOLOGY

The vulva, or external genital organs, includes the mons pubis, labia majora, labia minora, clitoris, vestibular glands, vaginal vestibule, vaginal orifice, and urethral opening (Figure 16-1). The symphysis pubis is covered by a pad of adipose tissue called the mons pubis or mons veneris, which in the postpubertal female is covered with coarse terminal hair. Extending downward and backward from the mons pubis are the labia majora, two folds of adipose tissue covered by skin. The labia majora vary in appearance, depending on the amount of adipose tissue present. The outer surfaces of the labia majora are also covered with hair in the postpubertal female.

Lying inside and usually hidden by the labia majora are the labia minora, two hairless, flat, reddish folds. The labia minora meet at the anterior of the vulva, where each labium divides into two lamellae, the lower pair fusing to form the frenulum of the clitoris and the upper pair forming the prepuce. Tucked in between the frenulum and the prepuce is the clitoris, a small bud of erectile tissue, the homologue of the penis and a primary center of sexual excitement. Posteriorly, the labia minora meet as two ridges that fuse to form the fourchette.

The labia minora enclose the area designated as the vestibule, which contains six openings: the urethra, the vagina, two ducts of Bartholin glands, and two ducts of Skene glands. The lower two thirds of the urethra lies immediately above the anterior vaginal wall and terminates in the urethral meatus at the midline of the vestibule just above the vaginal opening and below the clitoris. Skene ducts drain a group of urethral glands and open onto the vestibule on each side of the urethra. The ductal openings may be visible.

The vaginal opening occupies the posterior portion of the vestibule and varies in size and shape. Surrounding the vaginal opening is the hymen, a connective tissue membrane that may be circular, crescentic, or fimbriated. After the hymen tears and becomes permanently divided, the edges either disappear or cicatrize, leaving hymenal tags. Bartholin glands, located posteriorly on each side of the vaginal orifice, open onto the sides of the vestibule in the groove between the labia minora and the

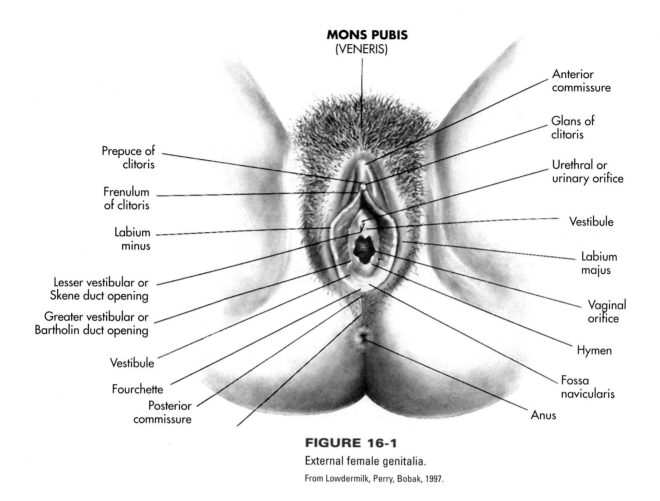

FIGURE 16-1

External female genitalia.

From Lowdermilk, Perry, Bobak, 1997.

hymen. The ductal openings are not usually visible. During sexual excitement, Bartholin glands secrete mucus into the introitus for lubrication.

The pelvic floor consists of a group of muscles that form a supportive sling for the pelvic contents. The muscle fibers insert at various points on the bony pelvis and form functional sphincters for the vagina, rectum, and urethra (Figure 16-2).

INTERNAL GENITALIA

The vagina is a musculomembranous tube that is transversely rugated during the reproductive phase of life. It inclines posteriorly at an angle of approximately 45 degrees with the vertical plane of the body (Figure 16-3). The anterior wall of the vagina is separated from the bladder and urethra by connective tissue called the vesicovaginal septum. The posterior vaginal wall is separated from the rectum by the rectovaginal septum. Usually the anterior and posterior walls of the vagina lie in close proximity, with only a small space between them. The upper end of the vagina is a blind vault into which the uterine cervix projects. The pocket formed around the cervix is divided into the anterior, posterior, and lateral fornices. These are of clinical importance since the internal pelvic organs can be palpated through their thin walls. The vagina carries menstrual flow from the uterus, serves as the terminal portion of the birth canal, and is the receptive organ for the penis during sexual intercourse.

The uterus sits in the pelvic cavity between the bladder and the rectum. It is an inverted, pear-shaped, muscular organ that is relatively mobile (Figure 16-4). The uterus is covered by the peritoneum and lined by the endometrium, which is shed

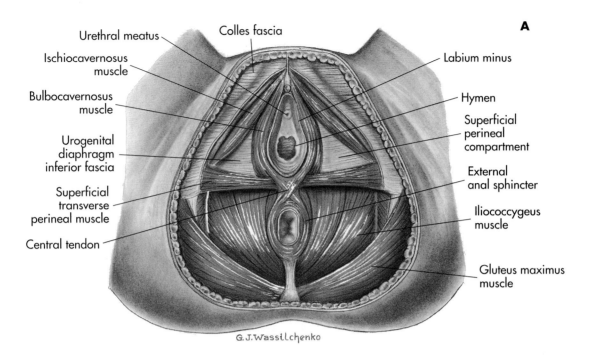

A, Urethral meatus, Colles fascia, Ischiocavernosus muscle, Bulbocavernosus muscle, Urogenital diaphragm inferior fascia, Superficial transverse perineal muscle, Central tendon, Labium minus, Hymen, Superficial perineal compartment, External anal sphincter, Iliococcygeus muscle, Gluteus maximus muscle

G.J.Wassilchenko

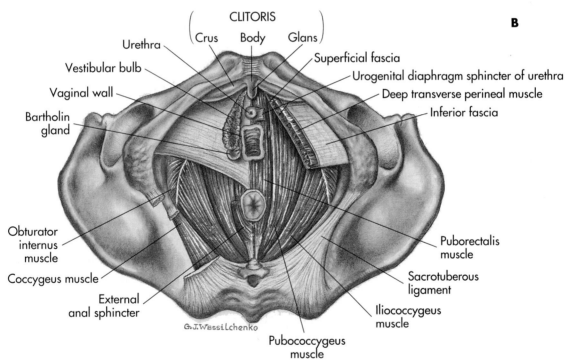

B, CLITORIS (Crus, Body, Glans), Urethra, Vestibular bulb, Vaginal wall, Bartholin gland, Superficial fascia, Urogenital diaphragm sphincter of urethra, Deep transverse perineal muscle, Inferior fascia, Obturator internus muscle, Coccygeus muscle, External anal sphincter, Puborectalis muscle, Sacrotuberous ligament, Iliococcygeus muscle, Pubococcygeus muscle

G.J.Wassilchenko

FIGURE 16-2

A, Superficial musculature of the perineum. **B,** Deep musculature of the perineum.

From Thompson et al, 1997.

during menstruation. The rectouterine cul-de-sac (pouch of Douglas) is a deep recess formed by the peritoneum as it covers the lower posterior wall of the uterus and upper portion of the vagina, separating it from the rectum. The uterus is flattened anteroposteriorly and usually inclines forward at a 45-degree angle, although it may be anteverted, anteflexed, retroverted, or retroflexed. In nulliparous women the size is

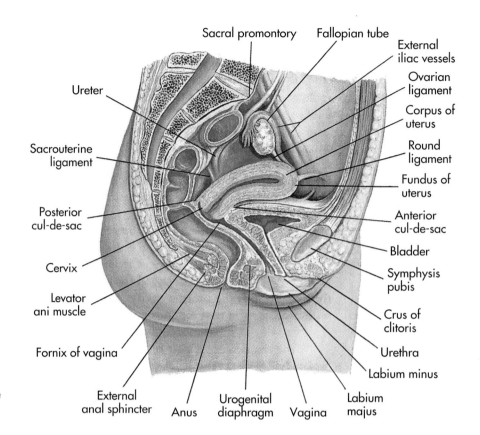

FIGURE 16-3
Midsagittal view of the female pelvic organs.

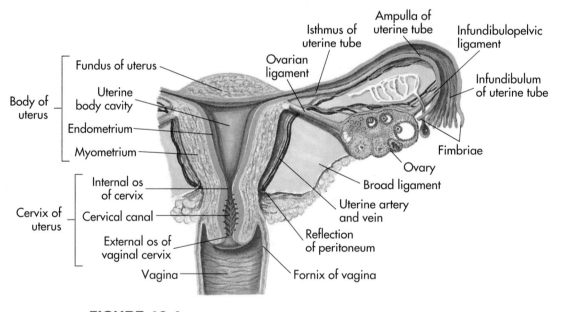

FIGURE 16-4
Cross-sectional view of internal female genitalia and pelvic contents.

approximately 5.5 to 8 cm long, 3.5 to 4 cm wide, and 2 to 2.5 cm thick. The uterus of a parous woman may be larger by 2 to 3 cm in any of the dimensions. The non-pregnant uterus weighs approximately 60 to 90 g (Figure 16-5).

The uterus is divided anatomically into the corpus and cervix. The corpus consists of the fundus, which is the convex upper portion between the points of insertion

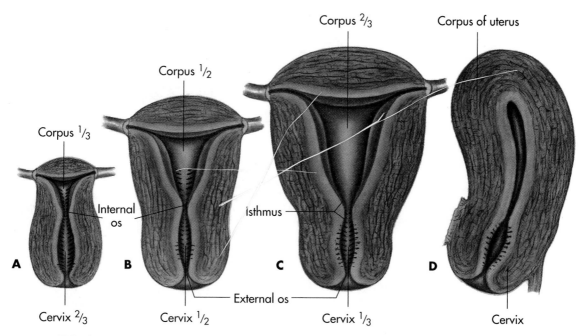

FIGURE 16-5
Comparative sizes of uteri at various stages of development. **A**, Prepubertal. **B**, Adult nulliparous. **C**, Adult multiparous. **D**, Lateral view, adult multiparous. The fractions give the relative proportion of the size of the corpus and the cervix.

of the fallopian tubes; the main portion or body; and the isthmus, which is the constricted lower portion adjacent to the cervix. The cervix extends from the isthmus into the vagina. The uterus opens into the vagina via the external cervical os.

The adnexae of the uterus are composed of the fallopian tubes and ovaries. The fallopian tubes insert into the upper portion of the uterus and extend laterally to the ovaries. Each tube ranges from 8 to 14 cm long and is supported by a fold of the broad ligament called the mesosalpinx. The isthmus end of the fallopian tube opens into the uterine cavity. The fimbriated end opens into the pelvic cavity, with a projection that extends to the ovary and captures the ovum. Rhythmic contractions of the tubal musculature transport the ovum to the uterus.

The ovaries are a pair of oval organs resting in a slight depression on the lateral pelvic wall at the level of the anterosuperior iliac spine. The ovaries are approximately 3 cm long, 2 cm wide, and 1 cm thick in the adult woman during the reproductive years. Ovaries secrete estrogen and progesterone, which have several functions, including controlling the menstrual cycle (Figure 16-6 and Table 16-1) and supporting pregnancy.

The internal genitalia are supported by four pairs of ligaments: the cardinal, uterosacral, round, and broad ligaments.

THE BONY PELVIS

The pelvis is formed from four bones—two innominate (each consisting of ilium, ischium, and pubis), the sacrum, and the coccyx (Figure 16-7). The bony pelvis is important in accommodating a growing fetus during pregnancy and the birth process. The four pelvic joints—the symphysis pubis, the sacrococcygeal, and the two sacroiliac joints—usually have little movement. During pregnancy, increased levels of the circulating hormones estrogen and relaxin contribute to the strengthening and elasticity

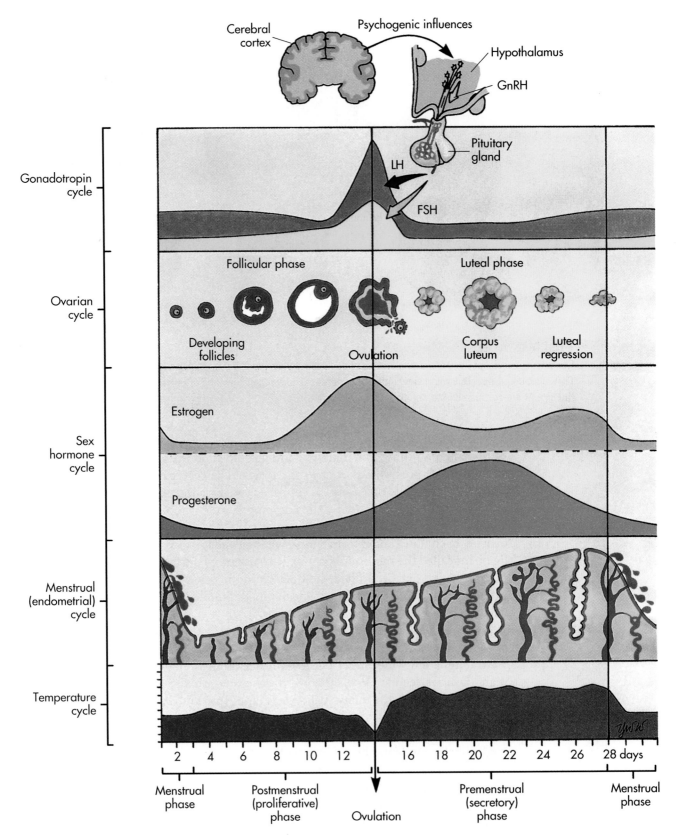

FIGURE 16-6

Female menstrual cycle. Diagram shows the interrelationship of the cerebral, hypothalmic, pituitary, and uterine functions throughout a standard 28-day menstrual cycle. The variations in basal body temperature are also shown.

From Thibodeau and Patton, 1996.

TABLE 16-1	The Menstrual Cycle

Phase		Process Description
Menstrual Phase: Days 1 to 4		
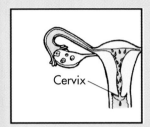	Ovary	Estrogen levels begin to rise, preparing follicle and egg for next cycle.
	Uterus	Progesterone stimulates endometrial prostaglandins that cause vasoconstriction; upper layers of endometrium shed.
	Breast	Cellular activity in the alveoli decreases; breast ducts shrink.
	Central nervous system (CNS) hormones	FSH and LH levels decrease.
	Symptom	Menstrual bleeding may vary, depending on hormones and prostaglandins.
Postmenstrual, preovulatory phase: Days 5 to 12		
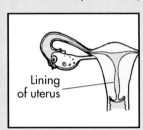	Ovary	Ovary and maturing follicle produce estrogen. *Follicular phase*—egg develops within follicle.
	Uterus	*Proliferative phase*—uterine lining thickens.
	Breast	Parenchymal and proliferation (increased cellular activity) of breast ducts occurs.
	CNS hormone	FSH stimulates ovarian follicular growth.
Ovulation: Day 13 or 14		
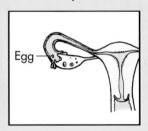	Ovary	Egg is expelled from follicle into abdominal cavity and drawn into the uterine (fallopian) tube by fimbriae and cilia; follicle closes and begins to form corpus luteum. Fertilization of egg may occur in outer one third of tube if sperm are unimpeded.
	Uterus	End of proliferative phase; progesterone causes further thickening of the uterine wall.
	CNS hormones	LH and estrogen levels increase rapidly; LH surge stimulates release of egg.
	Symptom	Mittelschmerz may occur with ovulation; cervical mucus is increased and is stringy and elastic (spinnbarkeit).
Secretory phase: Days 15 to 20		
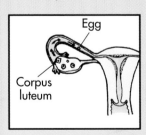	Ovary	Egg (ovum) is moved by cilia into the uterus.
	Uterus	After the egg is released, the follicle becomes a corpus luteum; secretion of progesterone increases and predominates.
	CNS hormones	LH and FSH decrease.
Premenstrual, luteal phase: Days 21 to 28		
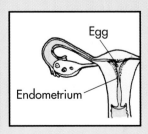	Ovary	If implantation does not occur, the corpus luteum degenerates. Progesterone production decreases, and estrogen production drops and then begins to rise as a new follicle develops.
	Uterus	Menstruation starts around day 28, which begins day 1 of the menstrual cycle.
	Breast	Alveolar breast cells differentiate into secretory cells
	CNS hormones	Increased levels of GnRH cause increased secretion of FSH.
	Symptoms	Vascular engorgement and water retention may occur.

From Edge and Miller, 1994.

of pelvic ligaments and softening of the cartilage. As a result, the pelvic joints separate slightly, allowing some mobility. Later in pregnancy, the symphysis pubis separates appreciably, which may cause discomfort when walking. Protrusion of the abdomen as the uterus grows causes the pelvis to tilt forward, placing additional strain on the back and sacroiliac joints.

The pelvis is divided into two parts. The shallow upper section is considered the false pelvis, which consists mainly of the flared-out iliac bones. The true pelvis is the lower curved bony canal, including the inlet, cavity, and outlet, through which the fetus must pass during birth. The upper border of the outlet is at the level of the ischial spines, which project into the pelvic cavity and serve as important landmarks during labor. The lower border of the outlet is bounded by the pubic arch and the ischial tuberosities (Figure 16-8).

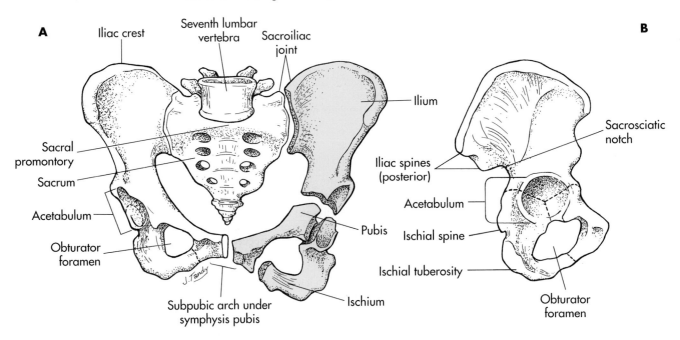

FIGURE 16-7

Adult female pelvis. **A,** Anterior view. The three embryonic parts of the left innominate bone are lightly shaded. **B,** External view of right innominate bone (fused).

From Lowdermilk, Perry, Bobak, 1997.

FIGURE 16-8

Female pelvis. **A,** Cavity of the false pelvis is a shallow basin above the inlet; the true pelvis is a deeper cavity below the inlet. **B,** Cavity of the true pelvis is an irregularly curved canal (*arrows*).

From Lowdermilk, Perry, Bobak, 1997.

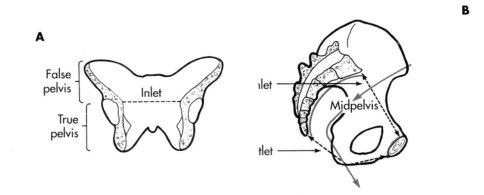

<table>
<tr><td>

INFANTS AND CHILDREN

</td><td>

The vagina of the female infant is a small narrow tube with fewer epithelial layers than that of the adult. The uterus is approximately 35 mm long, with the cervix constituting about two thirds of the entire length of the organ. The ovaries are tiny and functionally immature. The labia minora are relatively avascular, thin, and pale. The labia majora are hairless and nonprominent. The hymen is a thin diaphragm just inside the introitus, usually with a crescent-shaped opening in the midline. The clitoris is small.

During childhood the genitalia, except for the clitoris, grow incrementally at varying rates. Anatomic and functional development accelerates with the onset of puberty and the accompanying hormonal changes.

</td></tr>
</table>

ADOLESCENTS

During puberty the external genitalia increase in size and begin to assume adult proportions. The clitoris becomes more erectile and the labia minora more vascular. The labia majora and mons pubis become more prominent and begin to develop hair, often occurring simultaneously with breast development. Growth changes and secondary sex characteristic developments that occur during puberty are discussed in Chapter 5, Growth and Measurement.

If the hymen is intact, the vaginal opening is about 1 cm. The vagina lengthens, and the epithelial layers thicken. The vaginal secretions become acidic.

The uterus, ovaries, and fallopian tubes increase in size and weight. The uterine musculature and vascular supply increase. The endometrial lining thickens in preparation for the onset of menstruation (menarche), which usually occurs between the ages of 8 and 16 years. Just before menarche, vaginal secretions increase. Functional maturation of the reproductive organs is reached during puberty.

PREGNANT WOMEN

The high levels of estrogen and progesterone that are necessary to support pregnancy are responsible for uterine enlargement during the first trimester. After the third month, uterine enlargement is primarily the result of mechanical pressure of the growing fetus. As the uterus enlarges, the muscular walls strengthen and become more elastic. As the uterus becomes larger and more ovoid, it rises out of the pelvis into the abdominal cavity. Uterine weight at term, excluding the fetus and placenta, will usually have increased more than tenfold, to a weight of about 1000 g.

Hormonal activity (relaxin and progesterone) is responsible for the softening of the pelvic cartilage and strengthening of the pelvic ligaments. As a consequence, the pelvic joints separate slightly, allowing some mobility, which results in the characteristic "waddle" gait. There is also an increase in back pain.

During pregnancy an increase in uterine blood flow and lymph causes pelvic congestion and edema. As a result, the uterus, cervix, and isthmus soften, and the cervix takes on a bluish color. The softness and compressibility of the isthmus result in exaggerated uterine anteflexion during the first 3 months of pregnancy, causing the fundus to press on the urinary bladder.

The vaginal changes are similar to the cervical changes and result in the characteristic violet color. Both the mucosa of the vaginal walls and the connective tissue thicken, and smooth muscle cells hypertrophy. These changes result in an increased length of the vaginal walls, so that at times they can be seen protruding from the vulvar opening. The papillae of the mucosa have a hobnailed appearance. The vaginal secretions increase and have an acidic pH due to an increase in lactic acid production by the vaginal epithelium. Figure 16-9 compares the changes that occur in a woman experiencing her first pregnancy with a woman who has experienced more than one.

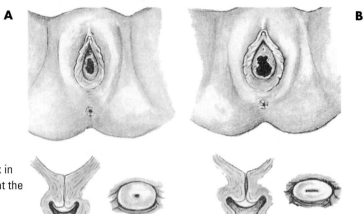

FIGURE 16-9

Comparison of vulva and cervix in **A**, nullipara, and **B**, multipara at the same stage of pregnancy.

From Lowdermilk, Perry, Bobak, 1997.

OLDER ADULTS

Concurrent with endocrine changes, ovarian function diminishes during a woman's 40s, and menstrual periods begin to cease between 40 and 55 years of age, although fertility may continue. Menopause is conventionally defined as 1 year with no menses. Just as menarche in the adolescent is one aspect of puberty, so menopause is only one aspect of this transitional phase of the life cycle. During this time, estrogen levels decrease, causing the labia and clitoris to become smaller. The labia majora also become flatter as body fat is lost. Pubic hair turns gray and is usually more sparse. Other hormone levels change as well. Both adrenal androgens and ovarian testosterone levels markedly decrease after menopause, which may account in part for decreases in libido and muscle mass and strength.

The vaginal introitus gradually constricts. The vagina narrows, shortens, and loses its rugation; and the mucosa becomes thin, pale, and dry, which may result in dyspareunia. The cervix becomes smaller and paler. The uterus decreases in size, and the endometrium thins.

The ovaries also decrease to approximately 1 to 2 cm. Follicles gradually disappear, and the surface of the ovary convolutes. Ovulation usually ceases about 1 to 2 years before menopause.

The ligaments and connective tissue of the pelvis sometimes lose their elasticity and tone, thus weakening the supportive sling for the pelvic contents. The vaginal walls may lose some of their structural integrity.

Menopause has systemic effects, which include an increase in body fat and intraabdominal deposition of body fat (tendency toward male pattern of body fat distribution). Levels of total and low-density lipoprotein cholesterol increase. Thermoregulation is altered, which produces the hot flushes associated with menopause. After menopause, women experience an increased risk of cardiovascular disease. Postmenopausal hormone replacement (estrogen with or without progestin) is prescribed to reduce the impact of menopausal symptoms and sequelae.

REVIEW OF RELATED HISTORY

PRESENT PROBLEM

- Abnormal bleeding
  - Character: shortened interval between periods (less than 19-21 days), lengthened interval between periods (more than 37 days), amenorrhea, prolonged menses (more than 7 days), bleeding between periods
  - Change in flow: nature of change, number of pads or tampons used in 24 hours (tampons/pads soaked?), presence of clots
  - Temporal sequence: onset, duration, precipitating factors, course since onset
  - Associated symptoms: pain, cramping, abdominal distention, pelvic fullness, change in bowel habits, weight loss or gain
  - Medications: prescription or nonprescription; oral contraceptives
- Pain
  - Temporal sequence: date and time of onset, sudden versus gradual onset, course since onset, duration, recurrence
  - Character: specific location, type, and intensity of pain
  - Associated symptoms: vaginal discharge or bleeding, gastrointestinal symptoms, abdominal distention or tenderness, pelvic fullness
  - Association with menstrual cycle: timing, location, duration, changes
  - Relationship to body functions and activities: voiding, eating, defecation, flatus, exercise, walking up stairs, bending, stretching, sexual activity
  - Aggravating or relieving factors
  - Previous medical care for this problem
  - Efforts to treat
  - Medications: prescription or nonprescription
- Vaginal discharge
  - Character: amount, color, odor, consistency, changes in characteristics
  - Occurrence: acute or chronic
  - Douching habits
  - Clothing habits: use of cotton or ventilated underwear and pantyhose, tight pants or jeans
  - Presence of discharge or symptoms in sexual partner
  - Use of condoms
  - Associated symptoms: itching; tender, inflamed, or bleeding external tissues; dyspareunia; dysuria or burning on urination; abdominal pain or cramping; pelvic fullness
  - Efforts to treat: antifungal vaginal cream
  - Medications: prescription or nonprescription; oral contraceptives, antibiotics
- Premenstrual symptoms complaint
  - Symptoms: headaches, weight gain, edema, breast tenderness, irritability or mood changes
  - Frequency: every period?
  - Interference with activities of daily living
  - Relief measures
  - Aggravating factors
  - Medications: prescription or nonprescription
- Menopausal symptoms complaint
  - Age at menopause or currently experiencing
  - Symptoms: menstrual changes, mood changes, tension, hot flashes
  - Postmenopausal bleeding

- General feelings about menopause: self-image, effect on intimate relationships
- Mother's experience with menopause
- Medications: hormone replacement therapy; related side effects: breast tenderness, bloating, vaginal bleeding; other medications prescription or nonprescription
- Infertility
  - Length of time attempting pregnancy, sexual activity pattern, knowledge of fertile period in menstrual cycle
  - Abnormalities of vagina, cervix, uterus, fallopian tubes, ovaries
  - Contributing factors: stress, nutrition, chemical substances
  - Partner factors: see Chapter 17, Male Genitalia
  - Diagnostic evaluation to date
- Urinary symptoms: dysuria, burning on urination, frequency, urgency
  - Character: acute or chronic; frequency of occurrence; last episode; onset; course since onset; feel like bladder is empty or not after voiding; pain at start, throughout, or at cessation of urination
  - Description of urine: color, presence of blood or particles, clear or cloudy
  - Associated symptoms: vaginal discharge or bleeding, abdominal pain or cramping, abdominal distention, pelvic fullness, flank pain
  - Medications: prescription or nonprescription

RISK FACTORS   Cervical Cancer

- Age between 40 and 50 years
- Personal history of cervical dysplasia
- Personal history of infection with human papilloma virus (HPV 16, 18, 33, 35, 45) or herpes simplex virus (HSV-2),
- Early age at first sexual intercourse
- Multiple lifetime sexual partners or partner(s) with multiple partners
- HIV +
- Smoking
- Multiple pregnancies

Data from American Cancer Society, 1997

RISK FACTORS   Ovarian Cancer

- Age between 40 and 60 years
- Taking fertility drugs
- Early menarche (before age 12)
- Late menopause (after age 50)
- Personal history of the following:
  - Ovarian dysfunction, anovulation, or spontaneous abortions
  - Cancer of the breast or endometrium or inherited gene mutations (BRCA1, BRCA2)
  - Irradiation of pelvic organs
- Family history of ovarian or breast cancer
- Infertility or nulliparity
- Exposure to talc or asbestos

Data from American Cancer Society, 1997.

RISK FACTORS **Endometrial Cancer**

- Postmenopause
- Early menarche (before age 12)
- Late menopause (after age 50)
- Unopposed estrogen replacement therapy
- Infertility or nulliparity
- Obesity (+30 lb = 3× risk; +50 lb = 10× risk)
- Taking tamoxifen
- Prior pelvic irradiation
- Personal history of breast or ovarian cancer or inherited gene mutations (BRCA1, BRCA2)
- Personal history of endometrial hyperplasia, diabetes, hypertension, liver disease
- Family history of endometrial breast of colon cancer
- High socioeconomic status

Data from American Cancer Society, 1997

PAST MEDICAL HISTORY

- Menstrual history
  - Age of menarche
  - Date of last normal menstrual period: first day of last cycle
  - Number of days in cycle and regularity of cycle
  - Character of flow: amount (number of pads or tampons used in 24 hours), duration, presence and size of clots
  - Dysmenorrhea: characteristics, duration, frequency (occurs with each cycle?), relief measures
  - Intermenstrual bleeding or spotting: amount, duration, frequency, timing in relation to phase of cycle
  - Intermenstrual pain: severity, duration, timing; association with ovulation
  - Premenstrual symptoms: headaches, weight gain, edema, breast tenderness, irritability or mood changes, frequency (occur with every period?), interference with activities of daily living, relief measures
- Sexual history
  - Current sexual activity: number of current and previous partners; number of their partners; gender of partner(s)
  - Method(s) of contraception: current and past; satisfaction with
  - Use of barrier protection for sexually transmitted diseases (STDs)
  - Prior STDs
  - Satisfaction with relationship(s)
- Obstetric history
  - G: Gravity: total number of pregnancies
  - T: number of term pregnancies
  - P: number of preterm pregnancies
  - A: number of abortions, spontaneous or induced
  - L: number of living children
  - Complications of pregnancy, delivery, abortion, or with fetus or neonate
- Menopausal history
  - Age of menopause or currently experiencing
  - Associated symptoms: menstrual changes, mood changes, tension, hot flashes
  - Postmenopausal bleeding

- Birth control measures during menopause
- General feelings about menopause: self-image, effect on intimate relationships
- Mother's experience with menopause
- Medications: hormone replacement therapy; related side effects: breast tenderness, bloating, vaginal bleeding; other medications prescription or nonprescription
- Gynecologic history
  - Prior Papanicolaou (Pap) smears and results
  - Prior abnormal Pap smears, when, how treated, follow-up
  - Recent gynecologic procedures
  - Past gynecologic procedures or surgery (tubal ligation, hysterectomy, oophorectomy, laparoscopy, cryosurgery, conization)
  - Sexually transmitted diseases
  - Pelvic inflammatory disease
  - Vaginal infections
  - Diabetes
  - Cancer of reproductive organs

FAMILY HISTORY

- Diabetes
- Cancer of reproductive organs
- Mother received diethylstilbestrol (DES) while pregnant with patient
- Multiple pregnancies
- Congenital anomalies

PERSONAL AND SOCIAL HISTORY

- Cleansing routines: use of sprays, powders, perfume, antiseptic soap, deodorants, or ointments
- Contraceptive history
  - Current method: length of time used, effectiveness, consistency of use, side effects, satisfaction with method
  - Previous methods: duration of use for each, side effects, and reasons for discontinuing each
- Douching history
  - Frequency: length of time since last douche; number of years douching
  - Method
  - Solution used
  - Reason for douching
- Sexual history
  - Difficulties, concerns, problems
  - Satisfaction with current practices, habits, and sexual relationship(s)
  - Number of partners
  - Sexual preference
- Date of last pelvic examination
- Date of last Pap smear and results
- Use of street drugs

INFANTS AND CHILDREN

Usually no special questions are required unless there is a specific complaint from the parent or child.
- Bleeding
  - Character: onset, duration, precipitating factor if known, course since onset

- Age of mother at menarche
- Associated symptoms: pain, change in crying of infant, child fearful of parent or other adults
- Parental suspicion about insertion of foreign objects by child
- Parental suspicion about possible sexual abuse
- Pain
  - Character: type of pain, onset, course since onset, duration
  - Specific location
  - Associated symptoms: vaginal discharge or bleeding, urinary symptoms, gastrointestinal symptoms, child fearful of parent or other adults
  - Contributory problems: use of bubble bath, irritating soaps, or detergents; parental suspicion about insertion of foreign objects by child or about possible sexual abuse
- Vaginal discharge
  - Relationship to diapers: use of powder or lotions, how frequently diapers are changed
  - Associated symptoms: pain, bleeding
  - Contributory problems: parental suspicion about insertion of foreign objects by child or about possible sexual abuse

ADOLESCENTS

As the older child matures, you should ask her the same questions that you ask any adult woman. You should not assume that youthful age precludes sexual activity or any of the related concerns. While taking the history, it is necessary at some point to talk with the child alone while the parent is out of the room. Your questions should be posed in a gentle, matter-of-fact, and nonjudgmental manner.

PREGNANT WOMEN

- Expected date of delivery (EDC) or weeks of gestation
- Previous obstetric history: GPTAL, prenatal complications
- Previous birth history: length of gestation at birth, birth weight, fetal outcome, length of labor, fetal presentation, type of delivery, complications (natal and postnatal)
- Previous menstrual history: see menstrual history in past medical history
- Surgical history: prior uterine surgery
- Family history: diabetes mellitus, twins
- Involuntary passage of fluid, which may result from rupture of membranes (ROM); determine onset, duration, color, odor, amount, and if still leaking
- Bleeding
  - Character: onset, duration, precipitating factor if known (e.g., intercourse, trauma), course since onset, amount
  - Associated symptoms
  - Pain: type (e.g., sharp or dull, intermittent or continuous), onset, location, duration
- Gastrointestinal symptoms: nausea, vomiting, heartburn

OLDER ADULTS

- See past medical history: menopausal history
- Symptoms associated with age-related physiologic changes: itching, urinary symptoms, dyspareunia
- Changes in sexual desire or behavior: in self or partner(s)

EXAMINATION AND FINDINGS

EQUIPMENT

- Drapes
- Speculum
- Gloves
- Water-soluble lubricant
- Lamp
- Sterile cotton swabs
- Glass slides
- Wooden or plastic spatula
- Cervical brush devices
- Cytologic fixative
- Culture plates or media
- DNA probe kits for chlamydia and gonorrhea, if needed

PREPARATION

The pelvic examination may be accompanied by some anxiety on the part of both the patient and a novice examiner. Although most women express lack of enthusiasm in anticipation of a pelvic examination, most do not experience anxiety. Marked anxiety before an examination may be a sign that something is not quite right. Before beginning you should find out the source of the anxiety. It could be a bad experience either in a patient's personal life (child abuse, sexual assault) or during a previous pelvic examination; it could be the lack of familiarly with what she can expect during the examination; it could be worry about possible findings or their meaning. Don't assume you know—use your skills and ask. It is your job to minimize the patient's apprehension and discomfort. Explain in general terms what you are going to do. Maintain eye contact with the patient, both before and, as much as possible, during the examination. Some women from various cultural or ethnic groups may not return eye contact as a show of respect. Be sensitive to cultural variations in behavior. If the patient has not seen the equipment before, show it to her, and explain its use.

Assure the patient that you will explain to her what you are doing as the examination proceeds. Let her know that you will be as gentle as possible, and to let you know if she feels any discomfort.

Make sure that the room is a comfortable temperature and that privacy is ensured. The door should be securely closed and should be opened only with permission of both the patient and examiner. The examination table should be positioned so that the patient faces away from it during the examination. A drawn curtain can ensure that any door opening will not expose the patient. Ideally, examiners of either sex will be accompanied by a female assistant. A female assistant, particularly for male examiners, is often required by policy and protects both the examiner and patient. Some patients may be reluctant to reveal confidential and sensitive material in the presence of an observer.

Have the patient empty her bladder before the examination. Bimanual examination is extremely uncomfortable for the woman if her bladder is full. A full bladder also makes it difficult to palpate the pelvic organs.

POSITIONING

Assist the patient into the lithotomy position on the examining table. (If a table with stirrups is not available or if the woman is unable to assume the lithotomy position, the examination can be performed in other positions (see pp. 612-620). Help the woman stabilize her feet in the stirrups and slide her buttocks down to the edge of the examining table. Place your hand at the edge of the table and instruct her to move

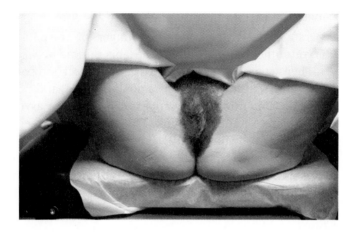

FIGURE 16-10
Draped patient in dorsal lithotomy position.

down until she touches your hand. If the patient is not positioned correctly, you will have difficulty with the speculum examination.

DRAPING AND GLOVING

The patient can be draped in such a way that allows minimal exposure. A good method is to cover her knees and symphysis, depressing the drape between her knees. This allows you to see the woman's face (and she, yours) throughout the examination (Figure 16-10).

Once the patient is positioned and draped, make sure that any equipment is nearby and in easy reach. Arrange the examining lamp so that the external genitalia are clearly visible. Wash your hands and put gloves on both hands. Remember that once you have touched any of the patient's genital skin, your glove is potentially "contaminated." Do not touch any surfaces or instruments that will not be discarded or immediately disinfected until you remove or change your gloves. This includes lights, drawers, door handles, counter surfaces, examining table surfaces, fixative and specimen bottles and jars, and patient records. Change gloves as often as you need to. Some clinicians prefer to double or triple glove at the beginning of an examination and then remove a glove when a clean hand is needed.

Ask the woman to separate or drop open her knees. Never try to spread her legs forcibly or even gently. The pelvic examination is an intrusive procedure, and you may need to wait a moment until the woman is ready. Tell her that you are going to begin, then start with a neutral touch on her lower thigh, moving your examining hand along the thigh without breaking contact, to the external genitalia.

EXTERNAL EXAMINATION

Inspection and Palpation

Sit at the end of the examining table and inspect and palpate the external genitalia. Look at the hair distribution and notice the surface characteristics of the mons pubis and labia majora. The skin should be smooth and clean, the hair free of nits or lice.

Labia Majora

The labia majora may be gaping or closed and may appear dry or moist. They are usually symmetric and may be either shriveled or full. The tissue should feel soft and homogeneous. Labial swelling, redness, or tenderness, particularly if unilateral, may be indicative of a Bartholin gland abscess. Look for excoriation, rashes, or lesions, which suggest an infectious or inflammatory process. If any of these signs are present, ask the woman if she has been scratching. Observe for discoloration, varicosities, obvious stretching, or signs of trauma or scarring.

Labia Minora

Separate the labia majora with the fingers of one hand and inspect the labia minora. Use your other hand to palpate the labia minora between your thumb and second finger. Then separate the labia minora and inspect and palpate the inside of the labia minora, clitoris, urethral orifice, vaginal introitus, and perineum (Figure 16-11).

The labia minora may appear symmetric or asymmetric, and the inner surface should be moist and dark pink. The tissue should feel soft, homogeneous, and without tenderness (Figure 16-12). Look for inflammation, irritation, excoriation, or caking of discharge in the tissue folds, which suggests vaginal infection or poor hygiene. Discoloration or tenderness may be the result of traumatic bruising. Ulcers or vesicles may be signs of a sexually transmitted disease. Feel for irregularities or nodules.

Clitoris

Inspect the clitoris for size. Generally the clitoris is about 2 cm or less in length and 0.5 cm in diameter. Enlargement may be a sign of a masculinizing condition. Observe also for atrophy, inflammation, or adhesions.

Urethral Orifice

The urethral orifice appears as an irregular opening or slit. It may be close to or slightly within the vaginal introitus and is usually in the midline. Inspect for dis-

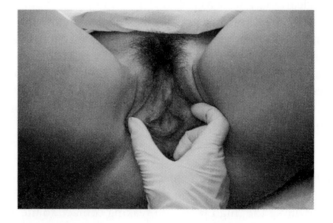

FIGURE 16-11
Separation of the labia.
From Edge, Miller, 1994.

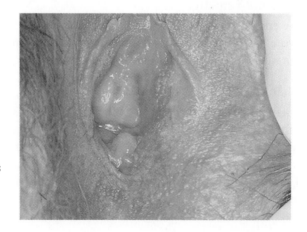

FIGURE 16-12
Normal vulva with finely textured papular sebaceous glands on the inner labia majora and labia minora.
From Morse, Moreland, Holmes, 1996.

charge, polyps, caruncles, and fistulas. Signs of irritation, inflammation, or dilation suggest repeated urinary tract infections or insertion of foreign objects. Ask questions about any findings at a later time—not during the pelvic examination when the woman feels most vulnerable.

Vaginal Introitus

The vaginal introitus can be a thin vertical slit or a large orifice with irregular edges from hymenal remnants (myrtiform caruncles). The tissue should be moist. Look for swelling, discoloration, discharge, lesions, fistulas, or fissures.

Skene and Bartholin Glands

With the labia still separated, examine the Skene and Bartholin glands. Tell the woman you are going to insert one finger in her vagina and that she will feel you pressing forward with it. With your palm facing upward, insert the index finger of the examining hand into the vagina as far as the second joint of the finger. Exerting upward pressure, milk the Skene glands by moving the finger outward. Do this on both sides of the urethra, and then directly on the urethra (Figure 16-13). Look for dis-

---

BOX 16-1   **Genital Self-Examination for Women**

Genital self-examination (GSE) is now recommended for anyone who is at risk for contracting a sexually transmitted disease (STD). This includes sexually active persons who have had more than one sexual partner or whose partner has had other partners. The purpose of GSE is to detect any signs or symptoms that might indicate the presence of a sexually transmitted disease. Many people who have an STD do not know that they have one, and some STDs can remain undetected for years. GSE should become a regular part of routine self-health care practices.

You should explain and demonstrate the following procedure to your patients and give them the opportunity to perform a GSE under your guidance.

Instruct the patient to start by examining the area that the public hair covers. Patients may want to use a mirror and position it so that they can see their entire genital area. The pubic hair should then be spread apart with the fingers, and the woman should carefully look for any bumps, sores, or blisters on the skin. Bumps and blisters may be red or light colored or resemble pimples. Also instruct the patient to look for warts, which may look similar to warts on other parts of the body. At first they may be small, bumpy spots. Left untreated, however, they could develop a fleshy, cauliflower-like appearance (see Figure 16-43).

Next, instruct the patient to spread the outer vaginal lips apart and look closely at the hood of the clitoris. She should gently pull the hood up to see the clitoris and again look for any bumps, blisters, sores, or warts. Then both sides of the inner vaginal lips should be examined for the same signs.

Have the patient move on to examine the area around the urinary and vaginal openings, looking for any bumps, blisters, sores, or warts (see Figure 16-47). Some signs of STDs may be out of view—in the vagina or near the cervix. Therefore if patients believe that they have come in contact with an STD, they should see their health care provider even if no signs or symptoms are discovered during self-examination.

Also educate patients about other symptoms associated with STDs, specifically, pain or burning on urination, pain in the pelvic area, bleeding between menstrual periods, or an itchy rash around the vagina. Some STDs may cause a vaginal discharge. Because most women have a vaginal discharge from time to time, they should try to be aware of what their "normal" discharge looks like. Discharge caused by an STD will be different from the usual. It may be yellow and thicker and have an odor.

Instruct patients that if they have any of the above signs or symptoms, they should see a health care provider.

Modified from Genital Self-Examination: GSE guide, Research Triangle Park, NC, 1989, Burroughs Wellcome Co. (Instructional pamphlets available.)

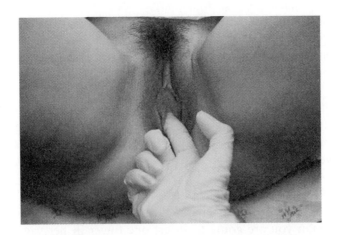

FIGURE 16-13
Palpation of Skene glands.
From Edge, Miller, 1994.

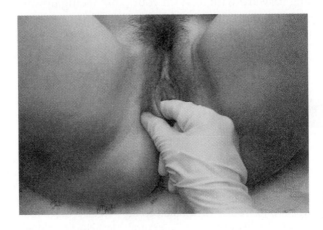

FIGURE 16-14
Palpation of Bartholin glands.
From Edge, Miller, 1994.

charge and note any tenderness. If a discharge occurs, note its color, consistency, and odor, and obtain a culture. Discharge from the Skene glands or urethra usually indicates an infection, most frequently but not necessarily gonococcal.

Maintaining labial separation and with your finger still in the vaginal opening, tell the patient that she will feel you pressing around the entrance to the vagina. Palpate the lateral tissue between your index finger and thumb. Palpate the entire area, paying particular attention to the posterolateral portion of the labia majora where the Bartholin glands are located. Note any swelling, tenderness, masses, heat, or fluctuation. Observe for discharge from the opening of the Bartholin gland duct. Palpate and observe bilaterally, since each gland is separate (Figure 16-14). Note the color, consistency, and odor of any discharge, and obtain a specimen for culture. Swelling that is painful, hot to the touch, and fluctuant is indicative of an abscess of the Bartholin gland. The abscess is usually gonococcal or staphylococcal in origin and is pus filled. A nontender mass is indicative of a Bartholin cyst, which is the result of chronic inflammation of the gland.

Muscle Tone

It usually is not necessary to test muscle tone unless the woman has told you about signs of weak muscle tone (e.g., urinary incontinence or the sensation of something "falling out"). To test, ask the patient to squeeze the vaginal opening around your finger, explaining that you are testing muscle tone. Some nulliparous women can squeeze fairly tightly, some multiparous women less so. Then ask the patient to bear

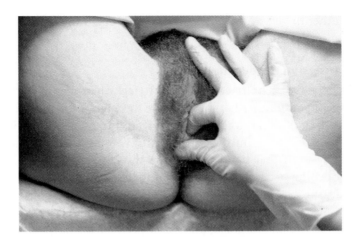

FIGURE 16-15
Palpating the perineum

down as you watch for bulging and urinary incontinence. Bulging of the anterior wall and urinary incontinence indicate the presence of a cystocele. Bulging of the posterior wall indicates a rectocele. Uterine prolapse is marked by protrusion of the cervix or uterus on straining.

Perineum

Inspect and palpate the perineum. The perineal surface should be smooth; episiotomy scarring may be evident in women who have borne children. The tissue will feel thick and smooth in the nulliparous woman. It will be thinner and rigid in multiparous women. In either case, it should not be tender. Look for inflammation, fistulas, lesions, or growths (Figure 16-15).

Anus

The anal surface is more darkly pigmented, and the skin may appear coarse. It should be free of scarring, lesions, inflammation, fissures, lumps, skin tags, or excoriation. If you touch the anus or perianal skin, be sure to change your gloves so that you do not introduce bacteria into the vagina during the internal examination.

INTERNAL EXAMINATION

Preparation

It is essential that you become familiar with how the speculum operates *before* you begin the examination, so that you do not inadvertently hurt the woman through mishandling of the instrument. Chapter 3, Examination Techniques and Equipment, details the proper use of the speculum. Become familiar with both the reusable stainless steel and the disposable plastic specula, because the mechanism of action is somewhat different.

Lubricate the speculum (and the gloved fingers) with water only if you plan to obtain cytologic or any other studies, since gel lubricant interferes with specimen analysis. Otherwise, water-soluble lubricant may be used. Since studies may be indicated only after visualization of the vaginal walls and cervix, most clinicians routinely lubricate only with water. An added advantage of using water as a lubricant is that a cold speculum can be warmed by rinsing in warm (but not hot) water. A speculum can also be warmed by holding it in your hand (if it is warm) or under the lamp for a few minutes.

Select the appropriate size speculum (see Chapter 3), and hold it in your hand with the index finger over the top of the proximal end of the anterior blade and the other fingers around the handle. This position controls the blades as the speculum is inserted into the vagina.

Insertion of Speculum

Tell the patient that she is going to feel you touching her again, and gently insert a finger of your other hand just inside the vaginal introitus and apply pressure downward. Ask the woman to breathe slowly and to try to consciously relax her muscles or the muscles of her buttocks. Wait until you feel the relaxation (Figure 16-16, *A*). Use the fingers of that hand to separate the labia minora very widely so that the hymenal opening becomes clearly visible. Then slowly insert the speculum along the path of least resistance, often slightly downward, avoiding trauma to the urethra and vaginal walls. Some clinicians insert the speculum blades at an oblique angle; others prefer to keep the blades horizontal. In either case avoid touching the clitoris, catching pubic hair, or pinching labial skin (Figure 16-16, *B* and *C*).

Insert the speculum the length of the vaginal canal. While maintaining gentle downward pressure with the speculum, open it by pressing on the thumb piece. Sweep the speculum slowly upward until the cervix comes in to view. Gently reposition the speculum, if necessary, to locate the cervix. Adjust the light source.

Once the cervix is visualized, manipulate the speculum so that the cervix is well exposed between the anterior and posterior blades. Lock the speculum blades into place to stabilize the distal spread of the blades, and adjust the proximal spread as needed (Figure 16-16, *D*).

Cervix

Color. Inspect the cervix for color, position, size, surface characteristics, discharge, and size and shape of the os. The cervix should be pink, with the color evenly distributed. A bluish color indicates increased vascularity, which may be a sign of pregnancy. Symmetric, circumscribed erythema around the os is an expected finding that indicates exposed columnar epithelium from the cervical canal. However, beginning practitioners should consider any reddened areas as an unexpected finding, especially if patchy or if the borders are irregular. A pale cervix is associated with anemia.

Position. The position of the cervix correlates with the position of the uterus. A cervix that is pointing anteriorly indicates a retroverted uterus; one pointing posteriorly indicates an anteverted uterus. A cervix in the horizontal position indicates a uterus in midposition. The cervix should be located in the midline. Deviation to the right or left may indicate a pelvic mass, uterine adhesions, or pregnancy. The cervix may protrude 1 to 3 cm into the vagina. Projection greater than 3 cm may indicate a pelvic or uterine mass. The cervix of a woman of childbearing age is usually 2 to 3 cm in diameter. An enlarged cervix is generally indicative of a cervical infection.

Surface characteristics. The surface of the cervix should be smooth. Some squamocolumnar epithelium of the cervical canal may be visible as a symmetric reddened circle around the os (Figure 16-17). Nabothian cysts may be observed as small, white or yellow, raised, round areas on the cervix. These are retention cysts of the endocervical glands and are considered to be an expected finding. An infected nabothian cyst becomes swollen with fluid and distorts the shape of the cervix, giving it an irregular appearance. Look for friable tissue, red patchy areas, granular areas, and white patches that could indicate cervicitis, infection, or carcinoma.

Discharge. Note any discharge. Determine whether the discharge comes from the cervix itself, or whether it is vaginal in origin and has only been deposited on the cervix. Usual discharge is odorless; may be creamy or clear; may be thick, thin, or

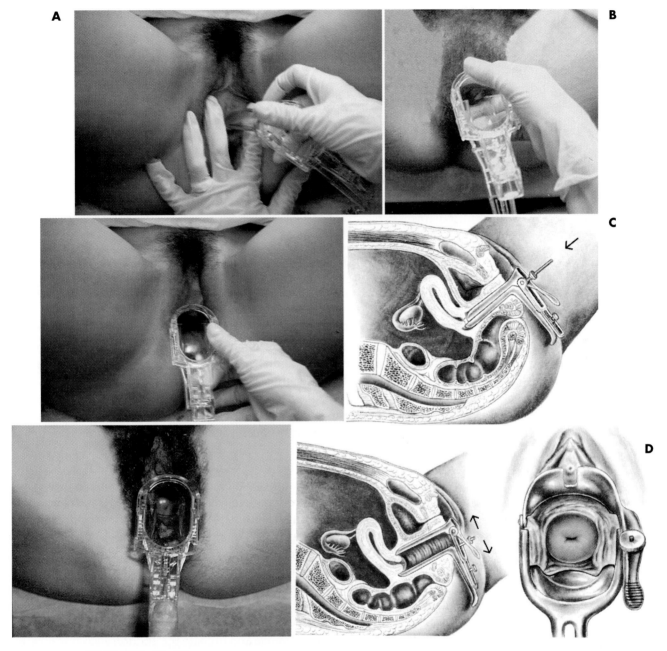

FIGURE 16-16

Examination of the internal genitalia with a speculum. Begin by inserting a finger and applying downward pressure to relax the vaginal muscles. **A,** Gently insert the closed speculum blades into the vagina. **B,** Direct the speculum along the path of least resistance. **C,** Insert the speculum the length of the vaginal canal. **D,** Speculum is in place, locked, and stabilized. Note cervix in full view.

Photos for **A** and **C** from Edge, Miller, 1994.

stringy; and is often heavier at midcycle or immediately before menstruation. The discharge of a bacterial or fungal infection will more likely have an odor and will vary in color from white to yellow, green, or gray.

Size and shape. The os of the nulliparous woman is small, round, or oval. The os of a multiparous woman is usually a horizontal slit or may be irregular and stellate.

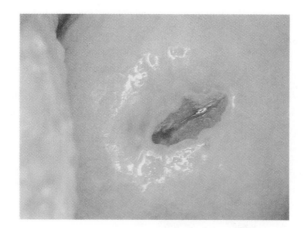

FIGURE 16-17
Normal cervix. The squamo-columnar junction and lower part of the endocervical canal are seen.
From Morse, Moreland, Holmes, 1996.

Trauma from induced abortion or difficult removal of an intrauterine device may change the shape of the os to a slit (Figure 16-18). Obtain specimens for Pap smear, culture, or other laboratory analysis.

Obtaining Vaginal Smears and Cultures

Very often during the speculum examination, you will be obtaining vaginal specimens for smears and cultures. Vaginal specimens are obtained while the speculum is in place in the vagina, but after the cervix and its surrounding tissue have been inspected. Collect specimens as indicated for Pap smear, sexually transmitted disease screening, and wet mount. Label the specimen with the patient's name and a description of the specimen (e.g., cervical smear, vaginal smear, and culture). Be sure to follow Standard Precautions for the safe collection of human secretions.

Papanicolaou smear. Brushes are now being used in conjunction with, or instead of, the conventional spatula to improve the quality of cells obtained. The cylindric-type brush (e.g., a Cytobrush) collects endocervical cells only. First, collect a sample from the ectocervix with a spatula (Figure 16-19). Insert the longer projection of the spatula into the cervical os. Rotate it 360 degrees, keeping it flush against the cervical tissue. Withdraw the spatula, and spread the specimen on a glass slide. A single light stroke with each side of the spatula is sufficient to thin the specimen out over the slide. Immediately spray with cytologic fixative and label the slide as the ectocervical specimen. Then introduce the brush device into the vagina and insert it into the cervical os until only the bristles closest to the handle are exposed (Figure 16-20). Slowly rotate one half to one full turn. Remove and prepare the endocervical smear by rolling and twisting the brush with moderate pressure across a glass slide. Fix the specimen with spray and label as the endocervical specimen. Warn the patient that she may have blood spotting after this procedure.

The paintbrush-type brush (e.g., Cervex-brush) is used for collecting both ectocervical and endocervical cells at the same time (Figure 16-20). This brush utilizes flexible plastic bristles, which are reported to cause less blood spotting after the examination. Introduce the brush into the vagina and insert the central long bristles into the cervical os until the lateral bristles bend fully against the ectocervix. Maintain gentle pressure and rotate the brush by rolling the handle between the thumb and forefinger three to five times to the left and right. Withdraw the brush, and transfer the sample to a glass slide with two single paint strokes: Apply first one side of the bristle, turn the brush over, and paint the slide again in exactly the same area. Apply fixative and label as the ectocervical and endocervical specimen.

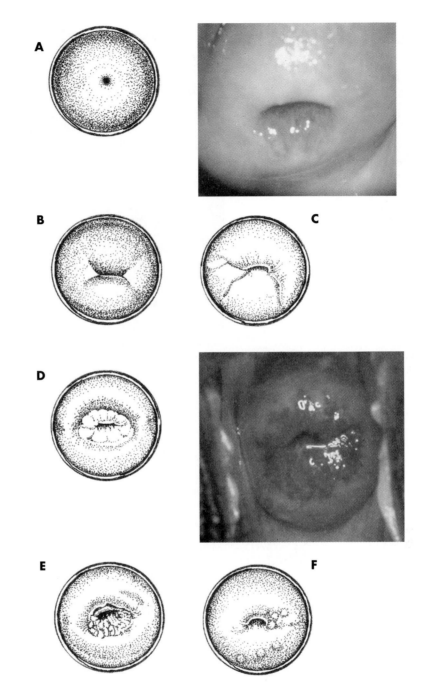

FIGURE 16-18

Common appearances of the cervix. **A,** Normal nulliparous cervix. The surface is covered with pink squamous epithelium that is uniform in consistency. The os is small and round. A small area of ectropion is visible inferior to the os. **B,** Parous cervix. Note slit appearance of os. **C,** Multigravidous, lacerated. **D,** Everted. Columnar mucosal cells usually found in the endocervical canal have extended out into the surface of the cervix, creating a circular raised erythematous appearance. Note the normal nonpurulent cervical mucus. This normal variant is not to be confused with cervicitis. **E,** Eroded. **F,** Nabothian cysts.

Photos from Zitelli, Davis, 1996; **A** courtesy C. Stevens, and **D** courtesy E. Jerome, MD.

Gonococcal culture specimen. Immediately after the Pap smear is obtained, introduce a sterile cotton swab into the vagina and insert it into the cervical os (Figure 16-21). Hold it in place for 10 to 30 seconds. Withdraw the swab and spread the specimen in a large Z pattern over the culture medium, rotating the swab at the same time. Label the tube or plate, and follow agency routine for transporting and warming the specimen. If indicated, an anal culture can be obtained after the vaginal speculum has been removed. Insert a fresh, sterile cotton swab about 2.5 cm into the rectum and rotate it full circle. Hold it in place for 10 to 30 seconds. Withdraw the swab and prepare the specimen as described for the vaginal culture.

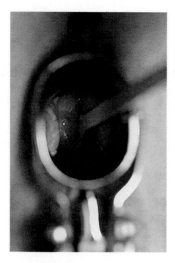

FIGURE 16-19

Scrape the cervix with the bifid end of the spatula for obtaining Pap smear.

From Symonds, Macpherson, 1994.

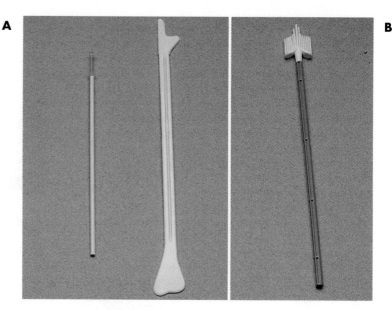

FIGURE 16-20

Implements used to obtain a Pap smear. **A,** Cytobrush and spatula. **B,** Cervex-brush.

A courtesy International Cytobrush, Inc., Florida. **B** courtesy Unimar, Connecticut.

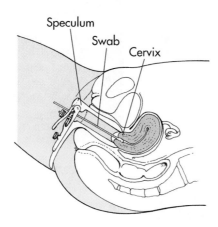

FIGURE 16-21

Obtaining a cervical specimen by inserting a swab into the cervical os.

From Grimes, 1991.

DNA probe for chlamydia and gonorrhea. This test involves the construction of nucleic acid sequence (called a probe) that will match to a sequence in the DNA or RNA of the target tissue. The results are rapid and sensitive. Use a Dacron swab (with plastic or wire shaft) when collecting your specimen, as wooden cotton-tipped applicators may interfere with the test results. Also be sure to check the expiration date so as not to use out of date materials. Insert the swab into the cervical os and rotate the swab in the endocervical canal for 30 seconds to ensure adequate sampling and absorption by the swab. Avoid contact with the vaginal mucous membranes, which would contaminate the specimen. Remove the swab and place it the tube containing the specimen reagent.

Wet mount and potassium hydroxide (KOH) procedures. In a woman with vaginal discharge, these microscope examinations can demonstrate the presence of *Trichomonas vaginalis,* bacterial vaginosis, or candidiasis. For the wet mount obtain a specimen of vaginal discharge using a swab. Smear the sample on a glass slide and add a drop of normal saline. Place a coverslip on the slide, and view under the microscope. The presence of trichomonads indicates *T. vaginalis.* The presence of bacteria-filled epithelial cells (clue cells) indicates bacterial vaginosis. On a separate glass slide place a specimen of vaginal discharge, apply a drop of aqueous 10% KOH, and put a coverslip in place. The presence of fishy odor (the "whiff test") suggests bacterial vaginosis. The KOH dissolves epithelial cells and debris and facilitates visualization of the mycelia of a fungus. View under the microscope for the presence of mycelial fragments, hyphae, and budding yeast cells, which indicates candidiasis.

Withdrawal of Speculum

Unlock the speculum and remove it slowly and carefully, so that you can inspect the vaginal walls. Note color, surface characteristics, and secretions. The color should be about the same pink as the cervix, or a little lighter. Reddened patches, lesions, or pallor indicates a local or systemic pathologic condition. The surface should be moist, smooth or rugated, and homogeneous. Look for cracks, lesions, bleeding, nodules, and swelling. Secretions that may be expected are usually thin, clear or cloudy, and odorless. Secretions indicative of infection are often profuse; may be thick, curdy, or frothy; appear gray, green, or yellow; and may have a foul odor.

As the speculum is withdrawn, the blades will tend to close themselves. Avoid pinching the cervix and vaginal walls. Maintain downward pressure of the speculum to avoid trauma to the urethra. Hook your index finger over the anterior blade as it is removed. Keep one thumb on the handle lever and control closing of the speculum. Make sure that the speculum is fully closed when the blades pass through the hymenal ring. Note the odor of any vaginal discharge that has pooled in the posterior blade and obtain a specimen, if you have not already done so. Deposit the speculum in the proper container.

BIMANUAL EXAMINATION

Inform the woman that you are now going to examine her internally with your fingers. Change your gloves or remove the outer glove and lubricate the index and middle fingers of your examining hand. Insert the tips of the gloved index and middle fingers into the vaginal opening and press downward, again waiting for the muscles to relax. Gradually and gently insert your fingers their full length into the vagina. Palpate the vaginal wall as you insert your fingers. It should be smooth, homogeneous, and nontender. Feel for cysts, nodules, masses, or growths.

Be careful where you place your thumb during the bimanual examination. You can tuck it into the palm of your hand, but that will cut down on the distance you can insert your fingers. Be aware of where the thumb is and keep it from touching the clitoris, which can produce discomfort (Figure 16-22).

Cervix

Locate the cervix with the palmar surface of your fingers, feel its end, and run your fingers around its circumference to feel the fornices. Feel the size, length, and shape, which should correspond with your observations from the speculum examination. The consistency of the cervix in a nonpregnant woman will be firm, like the tip of the nose; during pregnancy the cervix is softer. Feel for nodules, hardness, and roughness. Note the position of the cervix as discussed in the speculum examination. The cervix should be in the midline and may be pointing anteriorly or posteriorly.

Grasp the cervix gently between your fingers and move it from side to side. Observe the patient for any expression of pain or discomfort with movement. The cervix should move 1 to 2 cm in each direction without more than minimal discomfort.

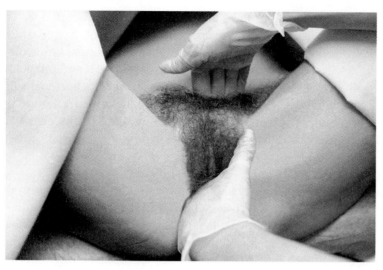
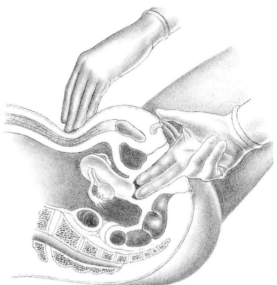

FIGURE 16-22
Bimanual palpation of the uterus.

Painful cervical movement suggests a pelvic inflammatory process such as acute pelvic inflammatory disease or a ruptured tubal pregnancy.

Uterus

Position. Palpate the uterus. Place the palmar surface of your other hand on the abdominal midline, midway between the umbilicus and the symphysis pubis. Place the intravaginal fingers in the anterior fornix. Slowly slide the abdominal hand toward the pubis, pressing downward and forward with the flat surface of your fingers. At the same time, push inward and upward with the fingertips of the intravaginal hand while you push downward on the cervix with the backs of your fingers. Think of it as trying to bring your two hands together as you press down on the cervix. If the uterus is anteverted or anteflexed (the position of most uteri), you will feel the fundus between the fingers of your two hands at the level of the pubis (Figure 16-23, *A* and *B*).

If you do not feel the uterus with the previous maneuver, place the intravaginal fingers together in the posterior fornix, with the abdominal hand immediately above the symphysis pubis. Press firmly downward with the abdominal hand while you press against the cervix inward with the other hand. A retroverted or retroflexed uterus should be felt with this maneuver (Figure 16-23, *C* and *D*).

If you still cannot feel the uterus, move the intravaginal fingers to each side of the cervix. Keeping contact with the cervix, press inward and feel as far as you can. Then slide your fingers so that one is on top of the cervix and one is underneath. Continue pressing inward while moving your fingers to feel as much of the uterus as you can. When the uterus is in the midposition, you will not be able to feel the fundus with the abdominal hand (Figure 16-23, *E*).

Confirm the location and position of the uterus by comparing your inspection findings with your palpation findings. The uterus should be located in the midline regardless of its position. Deviation to the right or left is indicative of possible adhesions, pelvic masses, or pregnancy. Knowing the position of the uterus is essential

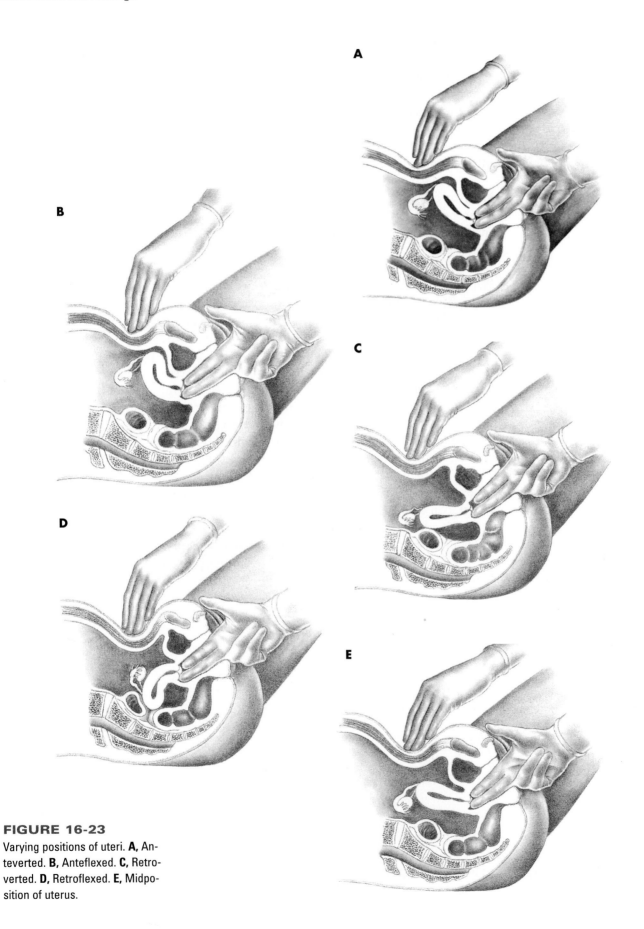

FIGURE 16-23
Varying positions of uteri. **A,** Anteverted. **B,** Anteflexed. **C,** Retroverted. **D,** Retroflexed. **E,** Midposition of uterus.

before performing any intrauterine procedure, including insertion of an intrauterine contraceptive device.

Size, shape, and contour. Palpate the uterus for size, shape, and contour. It should be pear shaped and 5.5 to 8 cm long, although it is larger in all dimensions in multiparous women. A uterus larger than expected in a woman of childbearing age is indicative of pregnancy or tumor. The contour should be rounded, and walls should feel firm and smooth in the nonpregnant woman. The contour smoothness will be interrupted by pregnancy or tumor.

Mobility. Gently move the uterus between the intravaginal hand and abdominal hand to assess for mobility and tenderness. The uterus should be mobile in the anteroposterior plane. A fixed uterus indicates adhesions. Tenderness on movement suggests a pelvic inflammatory process or ruptured tubal pregnancy.

Adnexa and Ovaries

Palpate the adnexal areas and ovaries. Place the fingers of your abdominal hand on the right lower quadrant. With the intravaginal hand facing upward, place both fingers in the right lateral fornix. Press the intravaginal fingers deeply inward and upward toward the abdominal hand, while at the same time sweeping the flat surface of the fingers of the abdominal hand deeply inward and obliquely downward toward the symphysis pubis. Palpate the entire area by firmly pressing the abdominal hand and intravaginal fingers together. Repeat the maneuver on the left side (Figure 16-24).

The ovaries, if palpable, should feel firm, smooth, ovoid, and approximately $3 \times 2 \times 1$ cm in size. The healthy ovary is slightly to moderately tender on palpation. Marked tenderness, enlargement, and nodularity are unexpected. Usually no other structures are palpable except for round ligaments. Fallopian tubes are usually not palpable, so a problem may exist if they are felt. You are also palpating for adnexal masses, and if any are found they should be characterized by size, shape, location, consistency, and tenderness.

The adnexa are frequently difficult to palpate because of their location and position and the presence of excess adipose tissue in some women. If you are unable to feel anything in the adnexal areas with thorough palpation, you can assume that no abnormality is present, provided no clinical symptoms exist.

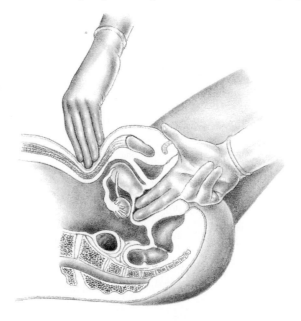

FIGURE 16-24

Bimanual palpation of adnexa. Sweep abdominal fingers downward to capture ovary.

| BOX 16-2 | Examining the Woman Who Has Had a Hysterectomy |

Examination of a woman who has had a hysterectomy is essentially no different from the usual procedure. The same examination steps and sequence are followed, with minor variation in what you are assessing. Getting an accurate history before the examination will assist you in knowing what to look for. Determine whether the surgical approach was vaginal or abdominal, whether the woman had a total or partial hysterectomy (i.e., whether she still has fallopian tubes and ovaries), the reason for the hysterectomy, bladder or bowel changes since the surgery, and the presence of menopausal symptoms.

Examine the external genitalia for atrophy, skin changes, decreased resilience, and discharge. In these patients, specimens for gonococci or chlamydia are often taken at the vestibule rather than internally. On speculum examination, the cervix will be absent. In the woman who had a vaginal hysterectomy, the surgical scar (vaginal cuff) will be visible at the end of the vaginal canal and will be an identifiable white or pink suture line in the posterior fornix. A Pap smear should be taken from this suture line with the blunt end of the spatula. Be sure to label the specimen as vaginal cells; otherwise the report may be sent back as incomplete or unsatisfactory because of a lack of endocervical cell sample. Assess the walls, mucosa, and secretions as you ordinarily would. The vaginal canal of a woman who has had a total hysterectomy might show the same changes as those that occur with menopause (such as a decrease in rugae and secretions), especially if the woman is not receiving hormone replacement therapy. Examine for a cystocele or rectocele. Stress incontinence may be a problem, so observe for this when having the patient bear down.

On bimanual examination the uterus will obviously not be present; further findings will depend on whether the hysterectomy was total or partial. If partial, proceed with the examination as usual, assessing the ovaries and surrounding area. If the hysterectomy was total, assess the adnexal area for masses, adhesions, or tenderness. The bladder and bowel may feel more prominent than usual.

RECTOVAGINAL EXAMINATION

Preparation

The rectovaginal exploration is an important part of the total pelvic examination. It allows you to reach almost 2.5 cm (1 in) higher into the pelvis, which enables you to better evaluate the pelvic organs and structures. It is an uncomfortable examination for the patient, however, and she may ask you to omit it. Nevertheless, it is important to perform, and you should explain to the woman why it is necessary.

As you complete the bimanual examination, withdraw your examining fingers, change gloves, and lubricate fingers. Tell the patient that she may feel the urgency of a bowel movement. Assure her that she will not have one, and ask her to breathe slowly and consciously try to relax her sphincter, rectum, and buttocks, since tightening the muscles makes the examination more uncomfortable for her.

Anal Sphincter

Place your index finger in the vagina, then press your middle finger against the anus and ask the patient to bear down. As she does, slip the tip of the finger into the rectum just past the sphincter. Palpate the area of the anorectal junction and just above it. Ask the woman to tighten and relax her anal sphincter. Observe sphincter tone. An extremely tight sphincter may be the result of anxiety about the examination, may be caused by scarring, or may indicate spasticity caused by fissures, lesions, or inflammation. A lax sphincter suggests neurologic deficit, whereas an absent sphincter may result from improper repair of third-degree perineal laceration after childbirth or trauma.

Rectal Walls and Rectovaginal Septum

Slide both your vaginal and rectal fingers in as far as they will go, then ask the woman to bear down. This will bring an additional centimeter within reach of your fingers. Rotate the rectal finger to explore the anterior rectal wall for masses, polyps, nodules, strictures, irregularities, and tenderness. The wall should feel smooth and uninterrupted. Palpate the rectovaginal septum along the anterior wall for thickness, tone, and nodules. You may feel the uterine body and occasionally the uterine fundus in a retroflexed uterus.

Uterus

Press firmly and deeply downward with the abdominal hand just above the symphysis pubis while you position the vaginal finger in the posterior vaginal fornix, and press strongly upward against the posterior side of the cervix. Palpate as much of the posterior side of the uterus as possible, confirming your findings from the vaginal examination regarding location, position, size, shape, contour, consistency, and tenderness of the uterus. This maneuver is particularly useful in evaluating a retroverted uterus (Figure 16-25).

Adnexa

If you were unable to palpate the adnexal areas on bimanual examination or if the findings were questionable, repeat the adnexal examination using the same maneuvers described in the bimanual examination.

Stool

As you withdraw your fingers, rotate the rectal finger to evaluate the posterior rectal wall just as you did earlier for the anterior wall. Gently remove your examining fingers and observe for secretions and stool. Note the color and presence of any blood. Prepare a specimen for occult blood testing. Unless the woman is unable to, let her wipe off the lubricating gel herself. She can do a more thorough and comfortable job. Be sure to provide tissues and an appropriate disposal receptacle.

Completion

Assist the woman into a sitting position and give her the opportunity to regain her equilibrium and composure. Provide a sanitary pad if she is menstruating. Share with her the findings and ask her to voice her feelings about the examination. This conversation may be brief, but it should never be avoided. Some clinicians prefer to leave the room and give the woman the opportunity to dress before discussing findings.

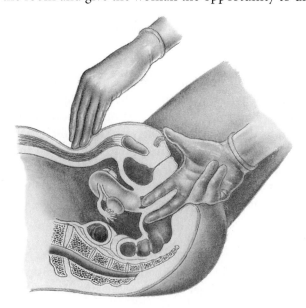

FIGURE 16-25
Rectovaginal palpation.

INFANTS

The appearance of the external genitalia can help in the assessment of gestational age in the newborn. Examination is conducted with the infant's legs held in a frog position. The labia majora appear widely separated, and the clitoris is prominent up to 36 weeks of gestation, but by full term the labia majora completely cover the labia minora and clitoris.

The newborn's genitalia reflect the influence of maternal hormones. The labia majora and minora may be swollen, with the labia minora often more prominent. The hymen is often protruding, thick, and vascular, and it may simulate an extruding mass. These are all transient phenomena and will disappear in a few weeks (Figure 16-26).

The clitoris may appear relatively large; this usually has no significance. True hypertrophy is not common; however, an enlarged clitoris must always suggest adrenal hyperplasia when seen in the newborn.

The central opening of the hymen is usually about 0.5 cm in diameter. It is important to determine the presence of an opening. However, make no effort to stretch the hymen. An imperforate hymen is rare but can cause difficulty later on, including hydrocolpos in the child and hematocolpos in the adolescent.

Malformations in the external genitalia are often difficult to define. If the baby was a breech delivery, her genitalia may be swollen and bruised for many days after delivery. Any ambiguous appearance or unusual orifice in the vulvar vault or perineum must be expeditiously explored before the infant is inappropriately assigned a gender.

A mucoid whitish vaginal discharge is frequently seen during the newborn period and sometimes as late as 4 weeks after birth. The discharge is occasionally mixed with blood. This is the result of passive hormonal transfer from the mother and is an expected finding.

Thin but difficult-to-separate adhesions between the labia minora are often seen during the first few months or even years of life. Sometimes they completely

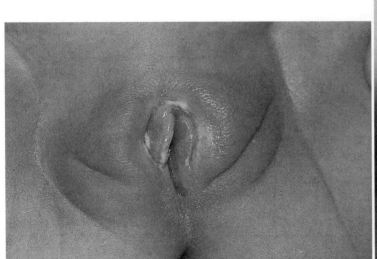
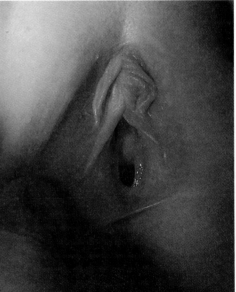

FIGURE 16-26

Normal appearance of the female genitalia. **A,** Genitalia of a newborn girl. The labia majora are full, and the thickened labia minora protrude between them. **B,** Genitalia of a 2-year-old girl. The labia majora are flattened, and the labia minora and hymen are thin and flat.

From Zitelli, Davis, 1996; **A** courtesy Ian Holzman, M.D., New York.

cover the vulvar vestibule. There may be just the smallest of openings through which urine can escape. These may require separation, perhaps by the gentlest of teasing or the application of estrogen creams.

Vaginal discharges in infants and young children may occur as the result of irritation from the diaper or powder. These discharges are usually mucoid.

CHILDREN

Indications for Examination

The extent of the gynecologic examination depends on the child's age and complaints. For the well child the examination includes only inspection and palpation of the external genitalia. The internal vaginal examination is performed on a young child only when there is a specific problem such as bleeding, discharge, trauma, or suspected sexual abuse. Bubble bath vaginitis is common in young girls and does not require an internal examination. Speculum examination on a young child requires special equipment and an experienced and knowledgeable gynecologist or pediatrician.

The young child usually cooperates with examination of the external genitalia if your approach is very matter of fact. The very young child can lie in the parent's lap, with the parent holding her legs in a frog position. The preschool child can be placed on the examining table, lying back against the head of the table, which should be raised about 30 degrees. The parent can help the child hold her legs up in a frog position.

A school-age child will not like the examination but is likely to cooperate if you take the time to reassure her that you will only look at and touch the outside. You might have the child help by taking her hand and first having her touch herself. She should be positioned on the table on her back with her knees flexed and drawn up. The examination should be approached with the same degree of respect, explanation, and caution as with the adult woman.

It is appropriate to have another person chaperone during examination of the genitalia. However, the older child should be consulted about this arrangement.

Inspection and Palpation

Inspect the perineum, all the structures of the vulvar vestibule, and the urethral and vaginal orifices by separating the labia with the thumb and forefinger of one hand.

Adequate visualization of the interior of the vagina and the hymenal opening can be difficult in prepubertal girls. A technique that can be helpful is that of anterior labial traction. Firmly grasp both labia majora (not the minora) with the thumb and index finger of each hand, then gently but firmly pull the labia forward and slightly to the side. Gentle but firm traction will not cause discomfort. A previously obscured hymenal opening almost always becomes visible with this technique, as does the interior of the vagina, nearly to the cervix. Most foreign bodies are visible with this method. With the help of an assistant, a swab is easily inserted through the hymenal opening to obtain cultures if needed.

Bartholin and Skene glands are usually not palpable; if they are, enlargement exists. This indicates infection, which is most often (but not always) gonococcal. Ask the girl to cough and observe the hymen. An imperforate hymen will bulge, whereas one with an opening will not.

Discharge

A vaginal discharge often irritates the perineal tissues, causing redness and perhaps excoriation. Other sources of perineal irritation are bubble baths, soaps, detergents, and urinary tract infections. Carefully question the parent for a history of hematuria,

---

BOX 16-3 **Evaluation of Masturbation in Children**

Masturbation is a common, healthy, self-discovery activity in children. Parents sometimes express concern about their child's masturbation activity. The following guidelines can help you determine when such activity might be a cause for concern.

Healthy Activity	**Needs Further Assessment**
Occasional	Frequent, compulsive
Discreet, private	No regard for privacy
Not preferred over other activity or play	Often preferred over other activity or play
No physical signs or symptoms	Produces genital discomfort, irritation, or physical signs
External stimulation of genitalia only	Involves penetration of the genital orifices; includes bizarre practices or rituals

From Haka-Ikse, Mian, 1993.

BOX 16-4 **"Red Flags" for Sexual Abuse**

The following signs and symptoms in children or adolescents should raise your suspicion for sexual abuse. Remember, however, that any sign or symptom by itself is of limited significance; it may be related to sexual abuse, or it may be from another cause altogether. This is an area in which good clinical judgment is imperative. Each sign or symptom must be considered in context with the particular child's health status, stage of growth and development, and entire history:

- Evidence of general physical abuse or neglect
- Evidence of trauma and/or scarring in genital, anal, and perianal areas
- Unusual changes in skin color or pigmentation in genital or anal area
- Presence of sexually transmitted disease (oral, anal, genital)
- Anorectal problems such as itching, bleeding, pain, fecal incontinence, poor anal sphincter tone, bowel habit dysfunction
- Genitourinary problems such as rash or sores in genital area, vaginal odor, pain (including abdominal pain), itching, bleeding, discharge, dysuria, hematuria, urinary tract infections, enuresis
- Behavioral manifestations such as use of sexually provocative mannerisms, excessive masturbation, unusual or inappropriate sexual knowledge or experience
- Significant behavioral changes such as problems with school, dramatic weight changes, depression

Modified from Koop, 1988.

---

dysuria, or other symptoms that would indicate urinary tract infection. A foul odor is more likely indicative of a foreign body (particularly in preschool children), especially if a secondary infection is present. Vaginal discharge may also result from trichomonal, gonococcal, or monilial infection.

Injuries

Swelling of vulvar tissues, particularly if accompanied by bruising or foul-smelling discharge, should alert you to the possibility of sexual abuse, which unfortunately is common in our society (Box 16-4). It must always be suspected if a young child has a sexually transmitted disease or if there is injury to the external genitalia. Injuries to the softer structure of the external genitalia are *not* caused by bicycle seats. A straddle injury from a bicycle seat is generally evident over the symphysis pubis where the structures are more fixed. The injuries resulting from sexual molestation are generally more posterior and may involve the perineum grossly.

Such findings cannot be ignored, and careful questioning of the parent or custodian is mandatory.

SMELL THE VAGINAL DISCHARGE

If sexual abuse is suspected, it is helpful to be aware of the characteristic odor of semen.

> **BOX 16-5** **Causes of Genital Bleeding in Children**
>
> Vaginal bleeding during childhood is *always* clinically important, and requires further evaluation. Common causes in children include the following:
> - Genital lesions
>   - Vaginitis
>   - Foreign body
>   - Trauma
>   - Tumors
> - Endocrine changes
>   - Estrogen ingestion
>   - Precocious puberty
>   - Hormone-producing ovarian tumor

Bleeding

Vaginal bleeding in children is often the result of injury, manipulation with foreign bodies, or sexual abuse. Occasionally there may be an ovarian tumor or carcinoma of the cervix. Remember, too, that some girls begin menstruation well before the expected time (Box 16-5).

RECTAL EXAMINATION

On occasion a rectal examination may be indicated to determine the presence or absence of the uterus or the presence of foreign bodies in the vagina. The rectal examination is performed with the patient lying on her back, feet held together, knees bent up on the abdomen. Place one hand on the child's knees to steady her, slipping the gloved examining finger into the rectum. Most examiners prefer the index finger, but this is not mandatory. Once your finger is introduced, you may release the legs and use your free hand to simultaneously palpate the abdomen. If the child is old enough to cooperate, have her pant like a puppy to relax the muscles. Foreign bodies will be palpable, as will the cervix. The ovaries are not usually felt. There may be bleeding and even a transient mild rectal prolapse after the examination, so be sure to warn the parent of this.

ADOLESCENTS

The adolescent requires the same examination and positioning as the adult. Ask whether this is the young woman's first gynecologic examination. The first examination is perhaps the most important, because it will set the stage for how she views future examinations. Take all the time necessary to explain to her what you will be doing. Use models or illustrations to show her what will happen and what you will look for. An adolescent should be allowed the privacy, if she desires, of having the examination without her parent present. This can also provide an opportunity to talk with her in private. An interview without the parent may be necessary to obtain an accurate sexual history, including sexual abuse, and to discuss sexual play (Box 16-6).

Choose the appropriate size speculum. A pediatric speculum with blades that are 1 to 1.5 cm wide can be used and should cause minimal discomfort. If the adolescent is sexually active, a small adult speculum may be used.

As the girl goes through puberty, you will see the maturational changes of sexual development (see Chapter 5, Growth and Measurement, Figure 5-21). Just before menarche there is a physiologic increase in vaginal secretions. The hymen may or may not be stretched across the vaginal opening. By menarche the opening should be at least 1 cm wide. As the adolescent matures, the findings are the same as those for the adult.

BOX 16-6	**Evaluation of Sexual Play in Adolescents**

Adolescents need strong support and guidance as they experiment with independence, the search for identity, and a healthy gender role. In adolescence, sexual play and exploration may encompass the full range of sexual behavior. The critical factors in determining the significance of any sexual activity to the healthy development of sexuality are whether it fits the religious and moral codes of the youth and family and whether there is a power imbalance in the relationship. The following guidelines can help you determine whether activity is part of healthy development or requires further assessment.

Healthy Activity	Needs Further Assessment
Discreet, private	No regard for privacy
Mutual consent	One adolescent does not freely consent
No power imbalance	Power imbalance
No threats or violence	Actual or implied threats of violence
Infrequent	Frequent, compulsive
Age-appropriate language and sexual knowledge	Language beyond age-appropriate level of sexual knowledge
Does not result in injury	Causes injury
Basic, rudimentary sexual activity	Explicit, graphic, and detailed sexual activity
	Attempted or actual penetration of genital orifices

From Haka-Ikse, Mian, 1993.

PREGNANT WOMEN

The gynecologic examination for the pregnant woman follows the same procedure as that for the nonpregnant adult woman. In early pregnancy you can feel a softening of the isthmus, while the cervix is still firm. In the second month of pregnancy the cervix, vagina, and vulva acquire their bluish color from increased vascularity. The cervix itself softens and will feel more like lips rather than like the firmness of the nose tip. The fundus flexes easily on the cervix. There is slight fullness and softening of the fundus near the site of implantation or a lateral bulge or soft prominence with cornual implantation. These findings are summarized in Box 16-7. You will notice increased vaginal secretions as a result of increased vascularity. None of these findings is perfectly sensitive or specific for detecting pregnancy, and they should not replace human chorionic gonadotropin testing.

Pelvic Size

The size of the bony pelvis is estimated during one of the prenatal visits, in addition to the routine vaginal, bimanual, and rectovaginal examinations. It is usually performed during the third trimester to increase the accuracy of measurement and the comfort of the woman.

Since the bones are covered with varying amounts of soft tissue and are not directly accessible, the measurements are only approximations. Firm pressure is needed to obtain the most accurate measurements. More direct ways to measure the pelvis are through computed tomography, ultrasound, or x-ray examination. However, the last is rarely used in pregnancy.

Four pelvic types are found in women—gynecoid, android, anthropoid, and platypelloid (Table 16-2). Pelvic measurements vary depending on the type of pelvis the woman has and, to some degree, on muscle and tissue strength. The select clinical measurements that are described in Table 16-3 may help guide the practitioner in safe labor management but should not be used to predict labor outcome.

PHYSICAL VARIATIONS

Black and white women differ in their percentage of pelvic types. Both have a similar percentage of the gynecoid type, but white women more often have the android type, and black women more often have the anthropoid type.

> **BOX 16-7** **Early Signs of Pregnancy**
>
> The following are physical signs that occur early in pregnancy. These signs, along with internal ballottement, palpation of fetal parts, and positive test results for urine or serum HCG, are probable indicators of pregnancy. They are considered "probable" because clinical conditions other than pregnancy can cause any one of them. Their occurrence together, however, creates a strong case for the presence of a pregnancy.
>
> | Sign | Finding | Approximate Weeks of Gestation |
> |------|---------|-------------------------------|
> | Goodell | Softening of the cervix | 4-6 |
> | Hegar | Softening of the uterine isthmus | 6-8 |
> | McDonald | Fundus flexes easily on the cervix | 7-8 |
> | Braun von Fernwald | Fullness and softening of the fundus near the site of implantation | 7-8 |
> | Piskacek | Palpable lateral bulge or soft prominence of one uterine cornu | 7-8 |
> | Chadwick | Bluish color of the cervix, vagina, and vulva | 8-12 |

TABLE 16-2   **Comparison of Pelvic Types**

	Gynecoid (50% of Women)	Android (23% of Women)	Anthropoid (24% of Women)	Platypelloid (3% of Women)
Brim	Slightly ovoid or transversely rounded	Heart shaped, angulated	Oval, wider anteroposteriorly	Flattened anteroposteriorly, wide transversely
	○ Round	♥ Heart	○ Oval	○ Flat
Depth	Moderate	Deep	Deep	Shallow
Side walls	Straight	Convergent	Straight	Straight
Ischial spines	Blunt, somewhat widely separated	Prominent, narrow interspinous diameter	Prominent, often with narrow interspinous diameter	Blunted, widely separated
Sacrum	Deep, curved	Slightly curved, terminal portion often beaked	Slightly curved	Slightly curved
Subpubic arch	Wide	Narrow	Narrow	Wide
Usual mode of delivery	Vaginal Spontaneous Occiput anterior position	Caesarian Vaginal Difficult with forceps	Vaginal Forceps/spontaneous occiput posterior or occiput anterior position	Vaginal Spontaneous

From Lowdermilk, Perry, Bobak, 1997.

Uterus Size

Early uterine enlargement may not be symmetric. Determination of the size of the uterus can be used to estimate gestational age. There is a lack of consensus about the accuracy of estimates of the size of the uterus at the various weeks; however, some estimate should be made. The size of various fruits is a common, though not reliable, means for describing the size of the uterus in early pregnancy. Centimeters are more accurate units of measurement and should be used for as soon as possible. Table 16-4 provides estimates of uterine size.

TABLE 16-3   Obstetric Measurements for Estimating Pelvic Size

Name of Measurement	Expected Measurement	Distance Measured
Pelvic Inlet		
If the pelvis is abnormal, the AP (anteroposterior) diameter is often shortened.		
Diagonal conjugate: the most important clinical measurement for estimating the AP diameter of the pelvic inlet (Figure 16-27)	12.5-13 cm	From the symphysis pubis (inferior border) to the sacral promontory
Obstetric conjugate: the AP diameter of the pelvic inlet obtained only by x-ray techniques or estimated from the diagonal conjugate (there may be a discrepancy) (Figure 16-28)	Diagonal conjugate minus 1.5 to 2 cm, depending on the pubic arch; about 11 cm or >11 cm radiographically	From the symphysis pubis (posterior border) to the sacral promontory
Midplane		
Direct measurement is not possible; if the ischial spines are prominent, the side walls converge, or the concavity of the sacrum is shallow, contraction is suspected.		
Transverse diameter or interspinous diameter: can only be estimated (Figure 16-29)	10.5 cm	The narrowest transverse diameter in the midplane between the interspinous processes
Outlet		
Accessible for measurement		
Biischial diameter, intertuberous diameter, or transverse diameter of the outlet: provides information on the adequacy of the pelvic outlet; two techniques can be used (Figures 16-30 and 16-31)	>8 cm	From the interior border of one ischial tuberosity to the other

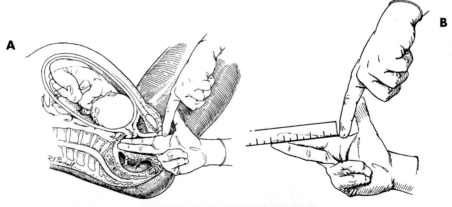

FIGURE 16-27

Measuring the diagonal conjugate. **A,** Insert the fingers until the tips reach the sacral promontory. With a finger of the other hand against the inferior border of the symphysis, mark where the symphysis pubis meets the hand. **B,** Compare the hand distance with a ruler to determine the diameter of the diagonal conjugate. **C,** Correct hand position shown with an anatomic model.

Photo from Symonds, Macpherson, 1994.

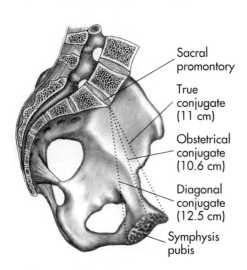

Sacral promontory

True conjugate (11 cm)

Obstetrical conjugate (10.6 cm)

Diagonal conjugate (12.5 cm)

Symphysis pubis

FIGURE 16-28
Estimate the obstetric conjugate using the diagonal conjugate. The diagonal conjugate varies in length depending on the height and inclination of the symphysis pubis.

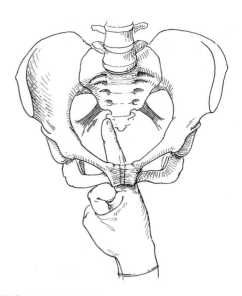

FIGURE 16-29
Estimating the transverse (interspinous) diameter. Insert the two examining fingers into the vagina and locate the ischial spines. If the spines are prominent, they may project into the pelvis similar to spikes. If they are flush with the pelvic walls, you might locate them by identifying the sacrospinous ligament and following it anteriorly to the spines. Estimate the distance between the ischial spines by moving your fingers from side to side.

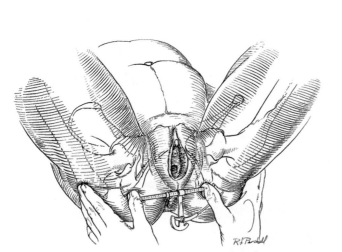

FIGURE 16-30
Determining the biischial diameter. Measure the distance between the tuberosities using the Thom pelvimeter; position it centrally and extend the tips of the crossbar until they touch the ischial tuberosities.

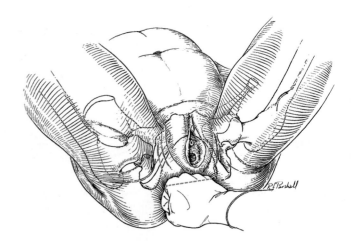

FIGURE 16-31
Alternate technique for determining the biischial diameter. First, measure your closed fist to determine its width; then place your fist against the perineum between the ischial tuberosities. Determine the distance between the tuberosities compared with your fist.

TABLE 16-4	Estimates of Uterine Size in Early Pregnancy		
Weeks of Gestation	Uterine Length (cm)	Uterine Width (cm)	
6	7.3-9.1	3.9	
8	8.8-10.8	5.0	
10	10.2-12.5	6.1	
12	11.7-14.2	7.1	
14	13.2-15.9	8.2	

From Fox, 1985.

Changes in fundal height at the various weeks of gestation are shown in Figure 16-32, along with some changes that are detectable on examination. Abdominal measurements are discussed in Chapter 15 (Abdomen), and breast and skin changes in pregnancy are discussed in Chapter 14 (Breasts and Axillae).

Cervical Dilation and Length

Other pregnancy conditions that are assessed during the pelvic examination include cervical dilation and effacement. Information about the fetus includes the position and station of the presenting part. Dilation involves the opening of the cervical canal to allow for the passage of the fetus. The process is measured in centimeters and progresses from a closed os (internal) to 10 cm, which is full or complete dilation. The time may vary among women between centimeters of dilation, depending on the parity of the woman, weeks of gestation (some dilation may be present late in pregnancy), and progress of labor.

Effacement refers to the thinning of the cervix that results when myometrial activity pulls the cervix upward, allowing the cervix to become part of the lower uterine segment during prelabor or early labor. The cervix is reduced in length. Ultrasonographic methods estimate its length at 3 to 4 cm at the end of the third trimester. It gradually thins to only a few millimeters (paper thin). Effacement should be recorded in centimeters. Effacement usually precedes cervical dilation in the primipara and often occurs with dilation in the multipara.

Station

Station is the relationship of the presenting part to the ischial spines of the mother's pelvis. Vaginal examination and palpation are performed during labor to estimate the descent of the presenting part. The measurement is determined by centimeters above and below the ischial spines and is recorded by plus signs and minus signs (Figure 16-33). For example, the station at 1 cm below the spines is recorded as a +1, at the spines as a 0, and at 1 cm above the spines as a −1. Record (in centimeters) the routine cervical examination findings for dilation, cervical length, and station, in that order.

Fetal Head Position

The position of the fetal head can be determined by vaginal examination once dilation has begun. Insert your fingers anteriorly into the posterior aspect of the vagina and then move your fingers upward over the fetal head as you turn them, locating the sagit-

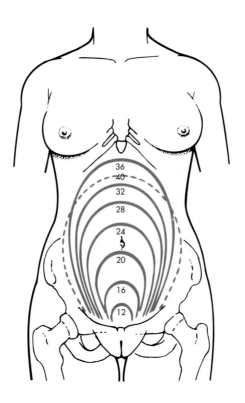

FIGURE 16-32

Changes in fundal height with pregnancy. *Weeks 10-12,* Uterus within pelvis; fetal heartbeat can be detected with Doppler. *Week 12,* Uterus palpable just above symphysis pubis. *Week 16,* Uterus palpable halfway between symphysis and umbilicus; ballottement of fetus is possible by abdominal and vaginal examination. *Week 20,* Uterine fundus at lower border of umbilicus; fetal heartbeat can be auscultated with fetoscope. *Weeks 24-26,* Uterus changes from globular to avoid shape; fetus palpable. *Week 28,* Uterus approximately halfway between umbilicus and xiphoid; fetus easily palpable. *Week 34,* Uterine fundus just below xiphoid. *Week 40,* Fundal height drops as fetus begins to engage in pelvis.

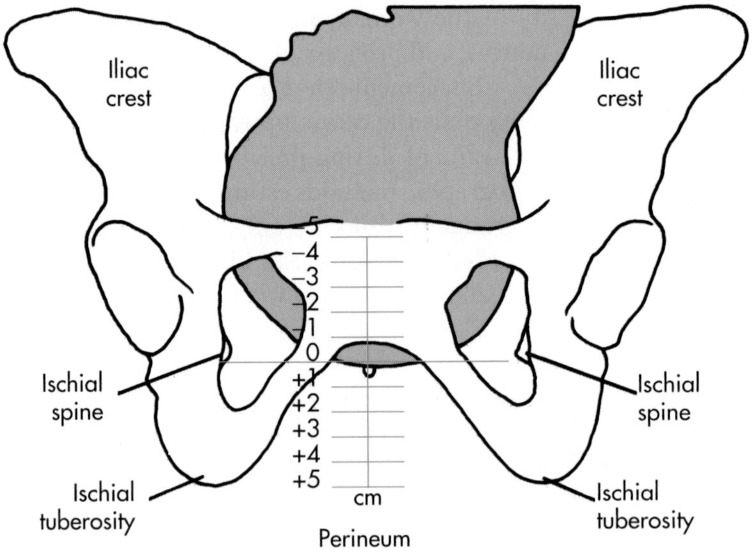

FIGURE 16-33

Stations of presenting part (degree of descent). Silhouette shows head of infant approaching station +1.

Courtesy Ross Products Division, Abbott Laboratories Inc., Columbus, Ohio. From Lowdermilk, Perry, Bobak, 1997.

tal suture with the posterior and anterior fontanels at either end (Figure 16-34, *A*). The position of the fontanels is determined by examining the anterior aspect of the sagittal suture and then using a circular motion to pass alongside the head until the other fontanel is felt and differentiated (Figure 16-34, *B*). The position of the face and breech are easier to determine, because the various parts are more distinguishable.

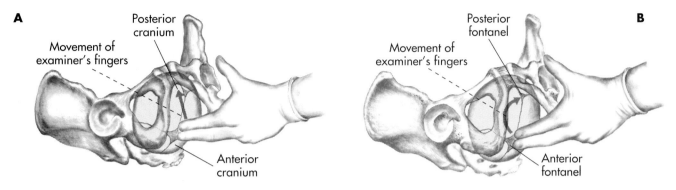

FIGURE 16-34
A, Locating the sagittal suture on vaginal examination. **B**, Differentiating the fontanels on vaginal examination.

Other Pregnancy-Associated Changes

The uterus may become more anteflexed during the first 3 months from softening of the isthmus. As a result, the fundus may press on the urinary bladder, causing the woman to experience urinary frequency.

Early uterine enlargement may not be symmetric, and you may feel deviation of the uterus to one side and an irregularity in its contour at the site of implantation. This uterine irregularity occurs around week 8 to 10 (Piskacek sign).

Changes in fundal height at the various weeks of gestation are shown in Figure 16-32, along with some changes that are detectable on examination. Breast and skin changes that occur with pregnancy are discussed in Chapter 14 (Breasts and Axillae).

OLDER ADULTS

The temptation with older women is to defer the examination *because* of their age. This is not appropriate. The examination procedure for the older adult is the same as that for the adult of childbearing age, with a few modifications for comfort. The older woman may require more time and assistance to assume the lithotomy position. She may need assistance from another individual to help hold her legs, since they may tire easily when the hip joints remain in abduction for an extended period. Patients with orthopnea will need to have their head and chest elevated during examination. You may need to use a smaller speculum, depending on the degree of introital constriction that occurs with aging.

Note that the labia appear flatter and smaller, corresponding with the degree of loss of subcutaneous fat elsewhere on the body. The skin is drier and shinier than that of a younger adult, and the pubic hair is gray and may be sparse. The clitoris is smaller than that of a younger adult.

The urinary meatus may appear as an irregular opening or slit. It may be located more posteriorly, very near or within the vaginal introitus, as a result of relaxed perineal musculature.

The vaginal introitus may be constricted and may admit only one finger. In some multiparous older women, the introitus may gape, with the vaginal walls rolling toward the opening.

The vagina is narrower and shorter, and you will see and feel the absence of rugation. The cervix is smaller and paler than in younger women, and the surrounding fornices may be smaller or absent. The cervix may seem less mobile if it protrudes less far into the vaginal canal. The os may be smaller but should still be palpable.

The uterus diminishes in size and may not be palpable, and the ovaries are rarely palpable because of atrophy. Ovaries that are palpable should be considered suspicious for tumor, and additional workup, such as ultrasonography, to exclude cancer is required.

The rectovaginal septum will feel thin, smooth, and pliable. Anal sphincter tone may be somewhat diminished. Since the pelvic musculature relaxes, look particularly for stress incontinence and prolapse of the vaginal walls or uterus.

As with younger women, as you inspect and palpate you are evaluating for signs of inflammation (older women are particularly susceptible to atrophic vaginitis), infection, trauma, tenderness, growths, masses, nodules, enlargement, irregularity, and changes in consistency.

WOMEN WITH DISABILITIES*

Preparing for the Examination

The disabled woman or clinician can do a number of things to promote a comfortable pelvic examination experience:

- Each disability affects each person differently. Therefore it is important for clinicians to educate themselves about relevant aspects of a woman's disability. A clinician's sensitivity in asking only pertinent questions about the disability will increase the woman's comfort and cooperation.
- When speaking with a disabled patient, clinicians should remember to speak directly to the patient. Often people will address a disabled person's friend, an attendant, or an interpreter instead of speaking directly to the person.
- The communication system used by a hearing-impaired or speech-impaired woman (e.g., a sign language interpreter, word board, or talk box) should be discussed at the onset of the visit.
- Since it is not necessary for a woman to remove all her clothes for the pelvic examination, she can wear an easily removable skirt or pair of pants. A button-up or zipper shirt will facilitate the breast examination. By only partially undressing, a woman can conserve time and energy.
- Removing or rearranging the furnishings in the examination room will provide the space needed for a woman to negotiate her wheelchair or for an interpreter to be seen.
- The paper covering can be taken off the examination table if it is a bother during transfers and positioning.
- Obstetric or foot stirrups can be padded or equipped with a strap to increase the patient's comfort and safety.
- If a urine sample is required, a disabled woman with a mobility impairment (e.g., spinal cord injury, polio, or cerebral palsy) should be given the option of bringing a urine sample with her.
- Equipment such as obstetric stirrups, a high-low examination table, or a particularly wide examination table can be obtained to facilitate safer, easier transfers and positioning.
- Specialized educational materials (e.g., braille or taped information or three-dimensional anatomic models) can be acquired to make information accessible to sensory-impaired patients.

Alternative Positions for the Pelvic Examination

A number of alternatives in positioning for the pelvic examination are possible. A disabled woman is the best judge of which position will work for her and how to use as-

*Modified from Ferreyra, Hughes, 1982.

sistants most effectively. These decisions should be made by the patient and the clinician together.

An assistant will help the disabled woman and the clinician facilitate a comfortable, thorough pelvic examination. For example, the assistant may help the woman position herself on the examination table. At least one assistant should be available throughout the examination in addition to the clinician. The assistant might be a staff member or an attendant or friend of the disabled patient.

The positions described in the following pages do not represent an all-inclusive list. They are meant to be used flexibly, depending on each woman's specific needs. This information will be useful to women (and men) with a wide variety of disabilities. The disabilities may include the following:

Amputation	Muscular diseases
Arthritis	Multiple sclerosis
Blindness or visual impairment	Poliomyelitis
Cerebral palsy	Scoliosis
Deafness or hearing impairment	Short stature
Spina bifida	Stroke
Spinal cord injury	

Many disabled women cannot comfortably assume the traditional (lithotomy) pelvic examination position, which requires a woman to be on her back, knees bent, legs spread apart, with her feet placed in metal stirrups at the foot of the examination table. As a result of a disability, a woman may experience one or more conditions that will require the use of an alternative position. The conditions may include the following:

Joint stiffness and inflammation	Muscle weakness
Paralysis	Spasticity
Lack of muscle control	Lack of balance
Pain (hip, back, etc.)	Muscular contractions

Some nondisabled women may experience one or more of these conditions, resulting in a need for an alternative position, just as some disabled women may wish to use the traditional pelvic examination position.

Knee-chest position. In the knee-chest position, the woman lies on her side with both knees bent, with her top leg brought closer to her chest (Figure 16-35). A variation of this position would allow the woman to lie with her bottom leg straightened while the top leg is still bent close to her chest. The speculum can be inserted with the handle pointed in the direction of the woman's abdomen or back. Because the woman is lying on her side, the clinician should be sure to angle the speculum toward the small of the patient's back and not straight up toward her head. Once the speculum has been removed, the woman will need to roll onto her back.

The assistant may provide support for the patient while she is on the examination table, help the woman straighten her bottom leg if she prefers the variation of this position, or support the patient in rolling onto her back for the bimanual examination. If the patient cannot spread her legs, the assistant may help her elevate one leg.

The knee-chest position does not require the use of stirrups. It is particularly good for a woman who feels most comfortable and balanced lying on her side.

Diamond-shaped position. In the diamond-shaped position the woman lies on her back with her knees bent so that both legs are spread flat and her heels meet at the foot of the table (Figure 16-36). The speculum must be inserted with the handle up. The bimanual examination can be easily performed from the side or foot of the table.

POSITIONING
The diamond-shaped position can also be used with children.

The assistant may help the patient support herself on the table and hold her feet together in alignment with her spine to maintain this position. A woman may be more comfortable using pillows or an assistant to elevate her thighs and/or use a pillow under the small of the back.

The diamond-shaped position does not require the use of stirrups. A woman must be able to lie flat on her back to use this position.

Obstetric stirrups position. In the obstetric stirrups position the woman lies on her back near the foot of the table with her legs supported under the knee by obstetric stirrups (Figure 16-37). The speculum can be inserted with the handle down. The bimanual examination can be performed from the foot of the table.

The patient may want assistance in putting her legs into the stirrups. The stirrups can be padded to increase comfort and reduce irritation. A strap can be attached

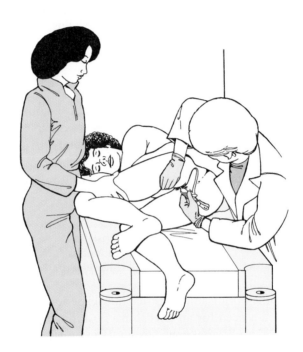

FIGURE 16-35
The knee-chest position.

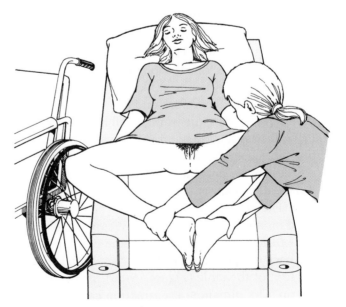

FIGURE 16-36
The diamond-shaped position.

to each stirrup to hold a woman's legs securely in place if the woman prefers this increased support.

Obstetric stirrups provide much more support than the traditionally used foot stirrups. This position allows a woman who has difficulty using the foot stirrups to assume the traditional pelvic examination position.

M-shaped position. In the M-shaped position the woman lies on her back, knees bent and apart, feet resting on the examination table close to her buttocks (Figure 16-38). The speculum must be inserted with the handle up. The bimanual examination can be performed from the foot of the table.

If the woman feels her legs are not completely stable on the examination table, an assistant may support her feet or knees. If a woman has bilateral leg amputations, assistants may elevate her legs to simulate this position.

The M-shaped position does not require the use of stirrups. This position allows the patient to lie with her entire body supported by the table.

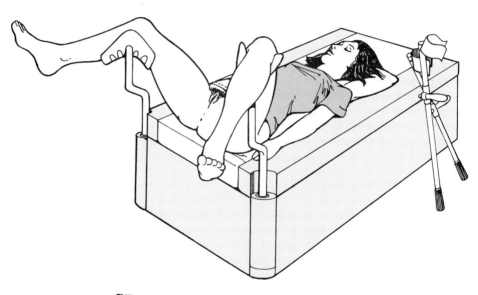

FIGURE 16-37
The obstetric stirrups position.

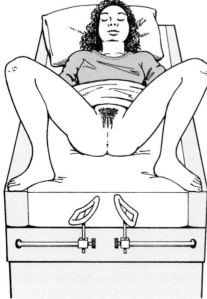

FIGURE 16-38
The M-shaped position.

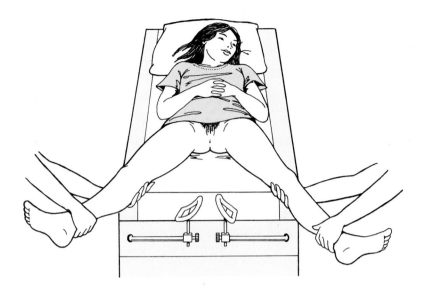

FIGURE 16-39
The V-shaped position.

V-shaped position. In the V-shaped position the woman lies on her back with her straightened legs spread out wide to either side of the table (Figure 16-39). If a woman is able to put one foot in the stirrup, a variation of this position would allow the woman to hold one leg out straight and keep one foot in a stirrup. The speculum must be inserted with the handle up, and the bimanual examination can be performed from the side or foot of the table.

At least one and possibly two assistants are needed to enable the woman to maintain this position. The assistants should support each straightened leg at the knee and ankle. The patient may be more comfortable if her legs are slightly elevated or if a pillow is used under the small of her back or tailbone.

The V-shaped position may or may not require stirrups. The patient must be able to lie comfortably on her back to use this position.

The Visually Impaired Woman

A woman with a visual impairment will probably want to assume a foot-stirrup position for the pelvic examination (Figure 16-40). Before the examination, the clinician can ask the patient if she would like to examine the speculum, swab, or other instruments that will be used during the examination. If three-dimensional genital models are available, they can be used to acquaint the woman with her anatomy as well as the examination process. During the examination, a woman may feel more at ease if continuous tactile or verbal contact is maintained, for example, a hand on her leg or a clinician narrating what is taking place during the examination. Clinicians or assistants should remember to identify themselves on entering the examination room and inform the woman if it is necessary for them to leave.

Some visually impaired women will want to be oriented to their surroundings, whereas others may not. Each woman should be encouraged to specify the kind of orientation and mobility assistance she needs. Staff members should verbally describe and assist the woman in locating where she should put her clothes, where the various furnishings are positioned, where and how to take a urine sample if one is needed, how she can approach the examination table, and how to position herself on the table and put her feet in the stirrups.

A red-tipped white cane and guide dog are mobility aids used by many visually impaired people. If a woman is accompanied by a guide dog, do not pet or distract

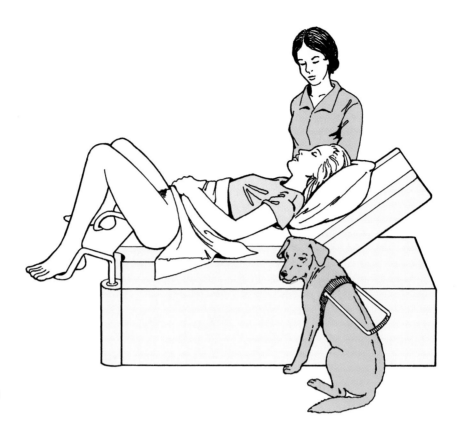

FIGURE 16-40
Positioning the visually impaired woman.

the dog. The dog is trained to respond only to its mistress. A woman may prefer to keep her guide dog or white cane nearby in the examination room. Do not move either of these items without the patient's permission.

The Hearing-Impaired Woman

A woman with a hearing impairment will most likely want to assume the foot-stirrup position (Figure 16-41). Her head may be elevated so that she can see the clinician and/or interpreter. The drape that is used to cover the woman's body below her waist should be eliminated or kept low between her legs. Before the examination, a patient may wish to examine the instruments that will be used during the examination. If three-dimensional genital models are available, they can be used to acquaint the client with her anatomy, as well as review the examination process. Some patients may wish to view the examination with a mirror while it is happening.

The patient should choose which form of communication she wishes to use during her examination: a sign language interpreter, lip reading, or writing. Although a patient may use an interpreter throughout most of the visit, she may decide not to use the interpreter during the actual examination. Many patients will feel more comfortable with a female interpreter. If an interpreter is used, the woman and the clinician should decide where the interpreter should stand. The interpreter may stand by the clinician at the foot of the table or, for more privacy, she may stand nearer the patient at the head of the table. When working with an interpreter, the clinician should speak directly to the patient at a regular speed instead of to the interpreter. If a woman wishes to lip read, the clinician should be careful not to move her face out of sight of the patient without first explaining what she is doing. The clinician should always look directly at the patient and enunciate her words clearly when the woman prefers lip reading.

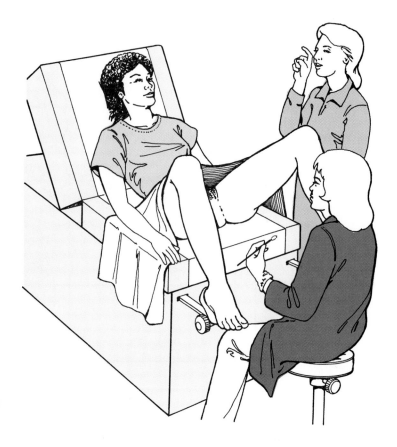

FIGURE 16-41
Positioning the hearing-impaired woman.

Getting on the Examination Table

The patient is the expert in transferring from the wheelchair or in using assistants to climb onto the examination table. Transfers are relatively simple if the woman, assistants, and clinician all understand the method that will best suit the woman's disability, the room space, and the examination table (Box 16-8).

Transfer Methods

Pivot transfer. Standing in front of the woman, the assistant takes the woman's knees between her knees, grasps the woman around the back and under the arms, raises her to a vertical position, and then pivots the patient from her wheelchair to the table. The examination table must be low enough for the patient to sit on; therefore, a hydraulic high-low table may be needed when using this transfer method.

Cradle transfer. While bending or squatting beside the woman, the assistant puts one arm under both of the woman's knees and the other arm around her back and under her armpits. The assistant stands and carries the woman to the table. Two assistants can be used if they grasp each other's arms behind the patient's back and under her knees, if one assistant cannot do it alone. It is important that both assistants work together.

Two-person transfer. In all two-person transfers, the assistants must be careful to work together to lift the woman over the arms of her wheelchair from a sitting position onto the examination table. A stronger, taller person should always lift the upper half of the patient's body. There are two ways to perform a two-person transfer.

BOX 16-8 | **Transfer Guidelines**

Guidelines for the Lifter

- The patient should direct the transfer and positioning process.
- Assistants should not overestimate their ability to lift.
- Keep in mind that not all nonambulatory women need assistance.
- Assistants should keep their backs straight, remember to bend their knees, and lift with their legs.
- It may be helpful to perform a test lift or practice the transfer by lifting the woman just over her wheelchair before attempting a complete transfer.
- Assistants who feel that they may drop a patient during a transfer should not panic. It is important, whenever possible, to explain to the woman what is happening to reassure her throughout the situation. Assistants will usually have time to lower the patient safely to the floor until they can get additional help.

Guidelines for the Disabled Patient

- The patient should explain clearly which transfer method she prefers and direct the clinician and assistants during the process.
- Assistants can help by preparing equipment. Since many people are not familiar with wheelchairs or supportive devices, the patient may need to explain to the clinicians and assistants how they can handle belongings. Women who use wheelchairs should explain how to apply the brakes, detach the footrests and armrests, or turn off the motor of an electric wheelchair. If the woman wears adaptive devices such as leg braces or supportive undergarments, she should explain how to remove them if necessary and where to put them.
- Women who use urinary equipment should direct assistants in the moving or straightening of catheter tubing. The patient may wish to unstrap her leg bag and place it on the table beside her or across her abdomen for proper drainage. Assistants should be reminded not to pull on the tubing or allow kinks to develop.
- The patient should inform the clinician and assistants when she is comfortable and balanced, after the transfer is completed.
- All parties should be aware of jewelry, clothing, tubing, or equipment, which might catch or otherwise interfere with the transfer.

Method 1 requires the patient to fold her arms across her chest. The assistant standing behind her kneels down, putting her elbows under the patient's armpits, and grasps the patient's opposite wrists. The second assistant lifts and supports the woman under her knees.

Method 2 can be used if the patient cannot fold her arms. The assistant standing behind the patient puts her hands together if possible so there is less likelihood of losing hold of the patient. The second assistant lifts and supports the woman under her knees.

Equipment. Some disabled women use a slide board, which forms a bridge from the wheelchair to the examination table for the client to slide across. For this method to work, the table and chair must be approximately the same height. Most examination tables, however, are quite a bit higher than most wheelchairs. Some examining rooms have high-low examination tables. These tables can be adjusted to the height that will facilitate the safest and easiest transfer. A wider table can also make transfers and positioning easier, even if it is not adjustable in height.

Special Concerns for Physical Examination of the Disabled Patient

Bowel and bladder concerns, specifically spasticity, hypersensitivity, and hyperreflexia, are conditions common to many disabled persons and should be given special attention during the examination process.

Bowel and bladder concerns. Some disabled women do not have voluntary bladder or bowel movements (e.g., women with spinal cord injuries or spina bifida). A woman's bladder or bowel routine could affect the pelvic examination.

A woman's bowel movement routine may require the same type of physical stimulation that she will experience during the speculum, bimanual, or rectal examination. A bowel movement can occur during the pelvic examination.

If a woman is catheterized, it is not necessary to remove the catheter, as it will not interfere with the pelvic examination in any way. An indwelling catheter need not be removed during the examination unless it is not working and another catheter is available for insertion.

The two types of indwelling catheters are the urethral, which is inserted directly into the woman's urethra, and the suprapubic, which is inserted directly into the bladder through a surgically made opening below her navel. Both allow urine drainage through tubing into a leg bag. The leg bag, usually attached to a woman's leg by a strap, should be empty at the start of the examination so it need not be drained later.

If a woman uses an intermittent catheterization system, she urinates by manually opening her bladder sphincter at regular intervals during the day. Tactile stimulation in her pelvic area during the examination could cause her bladder sphincter to open and she will become incontinent. The patient may consider scheduling her pelvic examination appointment around her urinary schedule.

Autonomic hyperreflexia. Autonomic hyperreflexia, also called hyperflexia or dysreflexia, describes a set of symptoms common to people with a spinal cord injury. It is often due to stimulation of the bowel, bladder, or skin below the spinal lesion. Common symptoms may include high blood pressure, sweating, blotchy skin, nausea, or goosebumps. A spinal cord-injured person may experience one or more of these symptoms to some degree during a bowel movement, for example.

Some causes of hyperreflexia that may occur during the pelvic examination include reactions to a cold hard examination table or cold stirrups, insertion and manipulation of the speculum, pressure during the bimanual or rectal examination, or tactile contact with hypersensitive areas (e.g., swabbing the cervix). Causes of hyperreflexia that may but are not necessarily related to the pelvic examination include urinary blockage due to a malfunctioning catheter, bowel blockage, skin irritation, or extreme temperature change.

Before starting the examination, the disabled woman and the clinician should discuss the patient's hyperreflexic symptoms. If the woman has experienced a pelvic examination since her injury, she will be able to identify which symptoms are common and which are uncommon. If a woman experiences uncommon hyperreflexic symptoms during the examination, her blood pressure must be reduced while the source of the stimulation is found and removed (e.g., removal of the speculum). Most

Although our discussion focuses on measures to assist in the pelvic examination of a woman with a disability, remember that much of this information is applicable to, and many of these measures can be adapted for, examination of any patient with a disability. Furthermore, the transfer techniques can be used in any situation in which a patient has a limitation of mobility.

people with a spinal cord injury will experience a drop in blood pressure if brought from supine to a sitting position. If the blood pressure does not decrease and the stimulus has been removed, or the hyperreflexic symptoms persist, leading to a throbbing headache or nasal obstruction, this should be considered an emergency and an experienced clinician should be called. A patient experiencing any degree of hyperreflexia should not be left alone.

Once the hyperreflexia ceases, the woman and the clinician should decide whether to continue the examination. If the examination is continued and hyperreflexia recurs, another examination should be scheduled. As always, the disabled woman is the expert on her own symptoms and reactions.

Hypersensitivity. Before the examination, the patient may want to inform the clinician of any hypersensitive areas of her body to help prevent possible discomfort or spasms during the examination. Some women may experience variable responses to ordinary tactile stimulation, such as spasms or pain. Often, sensitive areas can be avoided or an extra amount of lubricative jelly can be used to decrease friction or pressure.

Spasticity. Spasms may be a common aspect of a woman's disability. Ranging from slight tremors to quick, violent contractions, spasms may occur during a transfer, while assuming an awkward or uncomfortable position, or from stimulation of the skin with the speculum. If spasm occurs during the pelvic examination, the assistant should gently support the area (usually leg, arm, or abdominal region) to avoid any injury to the patient. Spasms should be allowed to resolve before the examination is continued.

A feeling of physical security can decrease spasm intensity and/or frequency. A disabled woman who experiences spasms should never be left alone on the examination table. A spasm could pose a serious danger to her. An assistant should stand near the examination table and maintain physical contact with the patient to provide a feeling of safety.

GENITALIA

External: Female hair distribution; no masses, lesions, or swelling. Urethral meatus intact without erythema or discharge. Perineum intact with a healed episiotomy scar present. No lesions.

Internal: Vaginal mucosa pink and moist with rugae present. No unusual odors. Discharge scant and white. Cervix pink with horizontal slit, midline; no lesions or discharge.

Bimanual: Cervix smooth, firm, mobile, without motion tenderness. Uterus midline, anteverted, firm smooth and nontender; not enlarged. Ovaries not palpable. No adnexal tenderness.

Rectovaginal: Sphincter tone, intact; anal ring smooth and intact. No masses or tenderness. Rectovaginal septum intact. Stool brown, occult blood tested negative.

For additional sample documentation see Chapter 24, Recording Information.

SUMMARY OF EXAMINATION Female Genitalia

The patient is in the lithotomy position for the following:

External Genitalia

1. Inspect the pubic hair characteristics and distribution (p. 589).
2. Inspect and palpate the labia for the following (p. 589-590):
   - Symmetry color
   - Caking of discharge
   - Inflammation
   - Irritation or excoriation
   - Swelling
3. Inspect the urethral meatus and vaginal opening for the following (pp. 590-591):
   - Discharge
   - Lesions or caruncles
   - Polyps
   - Fistulas
5. Milk the Skene glands (p. 591).
6. Palpate the Bartholin glands (p. 592).
7. Inspect and palpate the perineum for the following (p. 593):
   - Smoothness
   - Tenderness inflammation
   - Fistulas
   - Lesions or growths
8. Inspect for bulging and urinary incontinence as the patient bears down (p. 593).
9. Inspect the perineal area and anus for the following (p. 593):
   - Skin characteristics
   - Lesions
   - Fissures or excoriation
   - Inflammation

Internal Genitalia
Speculum Examination

1. Insert the speculum along the path of least resistance (p. 594).
2. Inspect the cervix for the following (pp. 594-595):
   - Color
   - Position
   - Size
   - Surface characteristics
   - Discharge
   - Size and shape of os
3. Collect necessary specimens for culture and Pap smears (pp. 596-599).

4. Inspect vaginal walls for the following (p. 599):
   - Color
   - Surface characteristics
   - Secretions

Bimanual Examination

1. Insert the index and middle fingers of one hand into the vagina and place the other hand on the abdominal midline (p. 599)
2. Palpate the vaginal walls for the following (p. 599):
   - Smoothness
   - Tenderness
   - Lesions (cysts, nodules, or masses)
3. Palpate the cervix for the following (pp. 599-600):
   - Size shape and length
   - Position
   - Mobility
4. Palpate the uterus for the following (pp. 600-602):
   - Location
   - Position
   - Size shape and contour
   - Mobility
   - Tenderness
5. Palpate the ovaries for the following (p. 602):
   - Size
   - Shape
   - Consistency
   - Tenderness
6. Palpate adnexal areas for masses and tenderness (p. 602).

Rectovaginal Examination

1. Insert the index finger into the vagina and the middle finger into the anus (p. 603).
2. Assess sphincter tone (p. 603).
3. Palpate the rectovaginal septum for the following (p. 603-604):
   - Thickness
   - Tone
   - Nodules
4. Palpate the posterior aspect of the uterus (p. 604).
5. Palpate the anterior and posterior rectal wall for the following (p. 604):
   - Masses, polyps, or nodules
   - Strictures, other irregularities, tenderness
6. Note characteristics of feces when the gloved finger is removed (p. 604).

COMMON ABNORMALITIES

PREMENSTRUAL SYNDROME (PMS)	Premenstrual syndrome usually begins in a woman's late 20s and increases in incidence and severity as menopause approaches. It is characterized by edema, headache, weight gain, and behavioral	disturbances such as irritability, nervousness, dysphoria, and lack of coordination. Symptoms occur 5 to 7 days before menses and subside with onset of menses.
INFERTILITY	The inability to conceive over a period of 1 year of unprotected regular intercourse has many causes, including both male and female conditions. Contributing factors in the woman include abnormalities of the vagina, cervix, uterus, fallopian tubes, and ovaries. Male infertility can be caused by insufficient, nonmotile, or im-	mature sperm; ductal obstruction of sperm; and transport-related factors. Factors influencing both women and men include stress, nutrition, chemical substances, chromosomal abnormalities, certain disease processes, sexual and relationship problems, and immunologic response.

ENDOMETRIOSIS

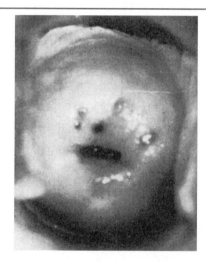

The presence and growth of endometrial tissue outside the uterus cause pelvic pain, dysmenorrhea, and heavy or prolonged menstrual flow. On bimanual examination tender nodules may be palpable along the uterosacral ligaments. Diagnosis is confirmed by laparoscopy (Figure 16-42).

FIGURE 16-42

Superficial endometriosis of the ectocervix, resembling hemorrhagic Nabothian cysts.

From Gardner, 1962.

LESIONS FROM SEXUALLY TRANSMITTED DISEASES

CONDYLOMA
ACUMINATUM
(GENITAL WARTS)

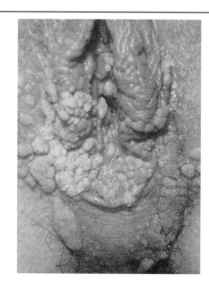

Warty lesions on the labia, within the vestibule, or in the perianal region are the result of human papillomavirus (HPV) infection. Venereal warts are sexually transmitted (Figure 16-43). They are generally flesh-colored, whitish pink to reddish brown, discrete, soft growths. They may occur singly or in clusters and may enlarge to form cauliflower-like masses.

FIGURE 16-43

Condyloma acuminatum.

From Morse, Moreland, Holmes, 1996.

MOLLUSCUM CONTAGIOSUM

Caused by a poxvirus, this usually benign skin infection may be transmitted by sexual contact. The incubation period is from 2 to 7 weeks. The lesions are white or flesh-colored, dome-shaped papules that are round or oval (Figure 16-44). The surface has a characteristic central umbilication from which a thick creamy core can be expressed. The lesions may last from several months to several years. Diagnosis is usually based on the clinical appearance of the lesions. Direct microscopic examination of stained material from the core will reveal typical "molluscum bodies" within the epithelial cell.

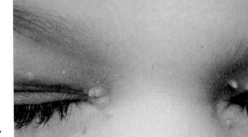

FIGURE 16-44
Molluscum contagiosum. Note that these have occurred around the eyes.

Courtesy Walter Tunnesen, MD, Chapel Hill, NC.

CONDYLOMA LATUM

Lesions of secondary syphilis appear about 6 to 12 weeks after infection. They are flat, round, or oval papules covered by a gray exudate (Figure 16-45).

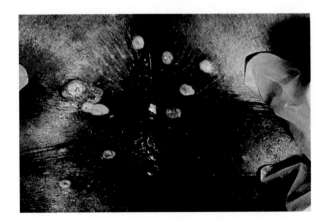

FIGURE 16-45
Condyloma latum.

Courtesy Antoinette Hood, MD, University of Indiana School of Medicine, Indianapolis.

SYPHILITIC CHANCRE (PRIMARY SYPHILIS)

A syphilitic chancre is a firm, painless ulcer. Most chancres in women develop internally and often go undetected (Figure 16-46).

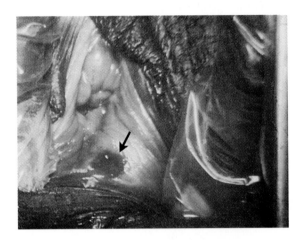

FIGURE 16-46
Primary syphilitic chancre in vagina.
From Habif, 1996.

HERPES LESIONS

Genital herpes is a sexually transmitted disease that produces small red vesicles. The lesions may itch and are usually painful. Initial infection is often extensive, whereas recurrent infection is usually confined to a small localized patch on the vulva, perineum, vagina, or cervix (Figures 16-47 and 16-48).

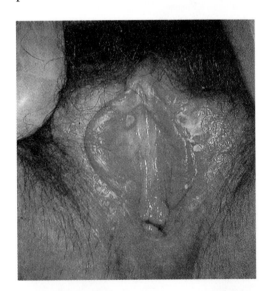

FIGURE 16-47
Herpes lesions. Scattered erosions covered with exudate.
From Habif, 1996.

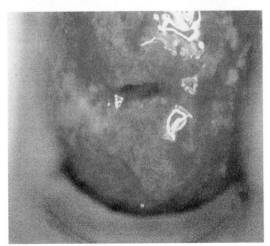

FIGURE 16-48
Herpetic cervicitis. Erythema, purulent exudate, and erosions are present on the cervix.
From Morse, Moreland, Holmes, 1996.

VULVA AND VAGINA

INFLAMMATION OF BARTHOLIN GLAND

Inflamed Bartholin glands are commonly, but not always, caused by gonococcal infection. It may be acute or chronic. Acute inflammation produces a hot, red, tender, fluctuant swelling that may drain pus. Chronic inflammation results in a nontender cyst on the labium (Figure 16-49).

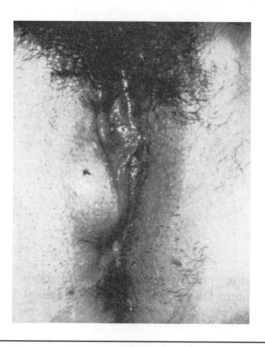

FIGURE 16-49
Inflammation of Bartholin glands.
From Kaufman, Faro, 1994.

CYSTOCELE

A cystocele is a hernial protrusion of the urinary bladder through the anterior wall of the vagina, sometimes even exiting the introitus. The bulging can be seen and felt as the woman bears down. More severe degrees of cystocele are accompanied by urinary stress incontinence (Figure 16-50).

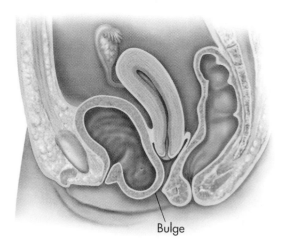

Bulge

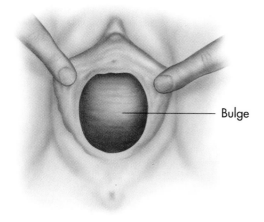

Bulge

FIGURE 16-50
Cystocele.

RECTOCELE

Hernial protrusion of part of the rectum through the posterior wall of the vagina is called rectocele or proctocele. Bulging can be observed and felt as the woman bears down (Figure 16-51).

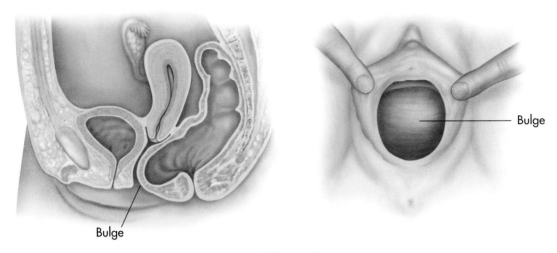

FIGURE 16-51
Rectocele.

CARCINOMA

Vaginal cancer in young women may be related to in utero DES exposure. Findings include vaginal discharge, lesions, and masses; and there may be a history of spotting, pain, and change in urinary habits. Cancer of the vulva appears as an ulcerated or raised red lesion on the vulva (Figure 16-52).

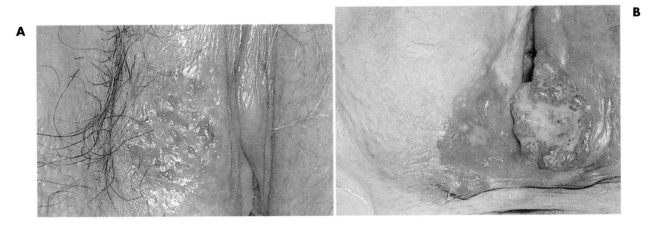

FIGURE 16-52
A, Basal cell carcinoma of the vulva. **B,** Ulcerative squamous cell carcinoma of the vulva.
From Symonds, Macpherson, 1994.

URETHRAL CARUNCLE   A bright red polypoid growth that protrudes from the urethral meatus, most urethral caruncles cause no symptoms (Figure 16-53).

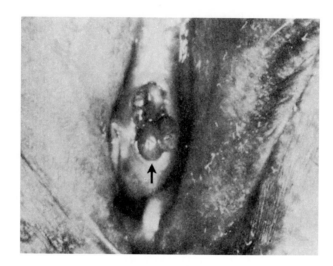

FIGURE 16-53
Urethral caruncle, a red fleshy lesion at the urethral meatus.
From Kaufman, Faro, 1994.

VAGINAL INFECTIONS   Vaginal infections often produce a vaginal discharge and may be accompanied by urinary and other symptoms. However, symptoms may be entirely absent. Vaginal infections can be sexually transmitted, although candidal infections can result from antibiotics, oral contraceptives, and systemic disease (Table 16-5).

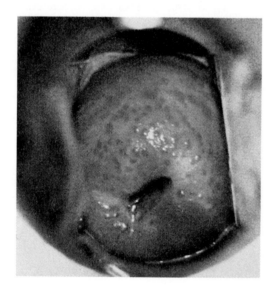

FIGURE 16-54
Trichomonas. The vaginal mucosa is inflamed and often speckled with petechial lesions. In adolescents, petechial hemorrhages may also be found on the cervix, resulting in the so-called strawberry cervix.
From Zitelli, Davis, 1996.

TABLE 16-5	Vaginal Discharges and Infections		
Condition	**History**	**Physical Findings**	**Diagnostic Tests**
Physiologic vaginitis	Increase in discharge No foul odor, itching or edema	Clear or mucoid discharge; pH < 4.5	Wet mount: up to 3-5 WBCs; epithelial cells
Bacterial vaginosis (*Gardnerella vaginalis*)	Foul-smelling discharge; complains of "fishy odor"	Homogenous thin, white or gray discharge; pH > 4.5	+KOH "whiff" test; wet mount: + Clue cells (Figure 16-55, *A*)
Candida vulvovaginitis (*Candida albicans*)	Pruritic discharge; itching of labia; itching may extend to thighs	White, curdy discharge; pH 4.0-5.0; cervix may be red; may have erythema of perineum and thighs	KOH prep: mycelia, budding, branching yeast, pseudohypha (Figure 16-55, *B*)
Trichomoniasis (*Trichomonas vaginalis*)	Watery discharge foul odor; dysuria and dyspareunia with severe infection	Profuse, frothy, greenish discharge; pH 5.0-6.6; red friable cervix with petechiae ("strawberry" cervix) (Figure 16-54)	Wet mount: Round or pear-shaped protozoa; motile "gyrating" flagella (Figure 16-55, *C*)
Gonorrhea (*Neisseria gonorrhoeae*)	Partner with sexually transmitted disease (STD); often asymptomatic or may have symptoms of pelvic inflammatory disease (PID)	Purulent discharge from cervix; Skene/Bartholin inflammation; cervix and vulva may be inflamed	Gram stain Culture DNA probe
Chlamydia (*Chlamydia trachomatis*)	Partner with nongonococcal urethritis; often asymptomatic; may complain of spotting after intercourse or urethritis	+/− purulent discharge; cervix may or may not be red or friable	DNA probe
Atrophic vaginitis	Dyspareunia; vaginal dryness; perimenopausal or postmenopausal	Pale thin vaginal mucosa; pH > 4.5	Wet mount: folded clumped epithelial cells
Allergic vaginitis	New bubble bath, soap, douche, or other hygiene products	Foul smell, erythema, pH < 4.5	Wet mount: WBCs
Foreign body	Red and swollen vulva; vaginal discharge; history of use of tampon, condom, or diaphragm	Bloody or foul-smelling discharge	Wet mount: WBCs

WBC, white blood cell; *KOH*, potassium hydroxide

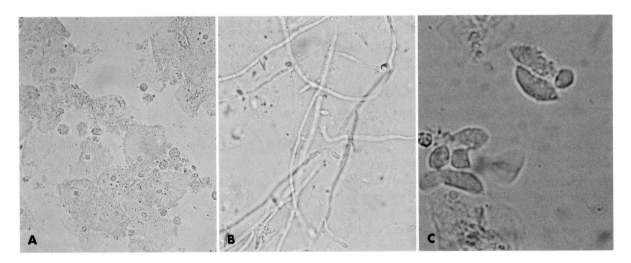

FIGURE 16-55
Microscopic differentiation of vaginal infections. **A,** Bacterial vaginosis: "clue cells." **B,** Candida vulvovaginitis: "budding, branching hyphae." **C,** Trichomoniasis: "motile trichomonads."
From Zitelli, Davis, 1996.

DIFFERENTIAL DIAGNOSIS

CERVIX

LACERATIONS

Cervical lacerations are caused by trauma, most often childbirth. Lacerations can produce lateral transverse, bilateral transverse, or stellate scarring (Figure 16-56).

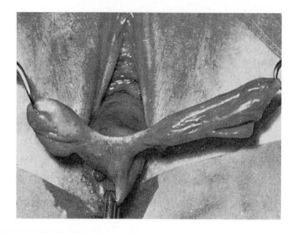

FIGURE 16-56
Severely lacerated cervix with hypertrophy and prolapse.
From Willson et al, 1987.

INFECTED NABOTHIAN CYSTS

Enlarged fluid-filled retention cysts often distort the shape of the cervix. Infected nabothian cysts vary in size and may occur singly or in multiples.

CERVICAL POLYP

Cervical polyps are bright red, soft, and fragile. They usually arise from the endocervical canal (Figure 16-57).

A

B

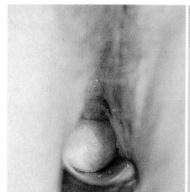
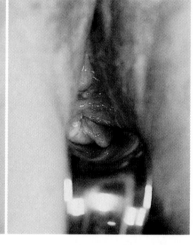
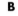

FIGURE 16-57
A, Fibroid polyp protruding through the external cervical os. **B,** Small endocervical polyp.
From Symonds, Macpherson, 1994.

CERVICAL CARCINOMA

Cervical cancer produces a hard granular surface at or near the cervical os. The lesion can evolve to form an extensive irregular cauliflower growth that bleeds easily. Early lesions are indistinguishable from ectropion (Figure 16-58).

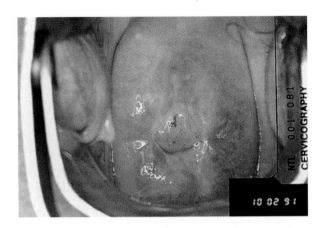

FIGURE 16-58
The lesion is predominantly around the external os.
From Symonds, Macpherson, 1994.

ECTROPION

Columnar epithelium from the cervical canal appears as shiny red tissue around the os that may bleed easily. Ectropion is not an abnormality, but because it is indistinguishable from early cervical carcinoma, further diagnostic studies (Pap smear, biopsy) must be performed for differential diagnosis.

UTERUS

UTERINE PROLAPSE

The uterus prolapses as the result of weakening of the supporting structures of the pelvic floor, often occurring concurrently with a cystocele and rectocele. The uterus becomes progressively retroverted and descends into the vaginal canal (Figure 16-59). In first-degree prolapse the cervix remains within the vagina; in second-degree prolapse the cervix is at the introitus; in third-degree prolapse the cervix and vagina drop outside the introitus (Figure 16-60).

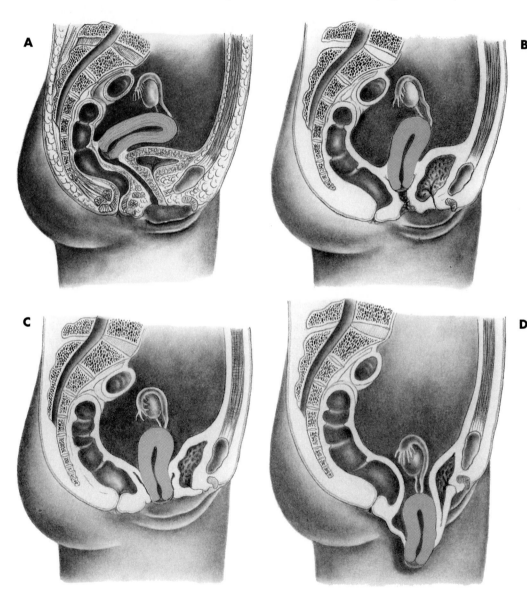

FIGURE 16-59
Uterine prolapse. **A,** Expected uterine position. **B,** First-degree prolapse of the uterus. **C,** Second-degree prolapse of the uterus. **D,** Complete prolapse of the uterus.

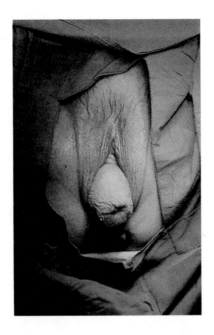

FIGURE 16-60

A third-degree prolapse of the uterus and vaginal walls.

From Symonds, Macpherson, 1994.

UTERINE BLEEDING

Abnormality in menstrual bleeding and inappropriate uterine bleeding are common gynecologic problems (Table 16-6). The following terms associated with menstrual bleeding can be found in the Glossary: *amenorrhea, dysfunctional uterine bleeding, hypermenorrhea, hypomenorrhea, menorrhagia, metrorrhagia, oligomenorrhea, postmenopausal bleeding, polymenorrhea,* and *spotting.*

TABLE 16-6	Types of Uterine Bleeding and Associated Causes
Type	**Common Causes**
Midcycle spotting	Midcycle estradiol fluctuation associated with ovulation
Delayed menstruation with excessive bleeding	Anovulation or threatened abortion
Frequent bleeding	Chronic PID, endometriosis, DUB, anovulation
Profuse menstrual bleeding	Endometrial polyps, DUB, adenomyosis, submucous leiomyomas, IUD
Intermenstrual or irregular bleeding	Endometrial polyps, DUB, uterine or cervical cancer, oral contraceptives
Postmenopausal bleeding	Endometrial hyperplasia, estrogen therapy, endometrial cancer

Modified from Thompson et al, 1997.
DUB, Dysfunctional uterine bleeding; *IUD,* intrauterine device; *PID,* pelvic inflammatory disease.

MYOMAS
(LEIOMYOMAS,
FIBROIDS)

Myomas are common, benign, uterine tumors that appear as firm, irregular nodules in the contour of the uterus. They may occur singly or in multiples and vary greatly in size. The uterus may become enlarged (Figure 16-61).

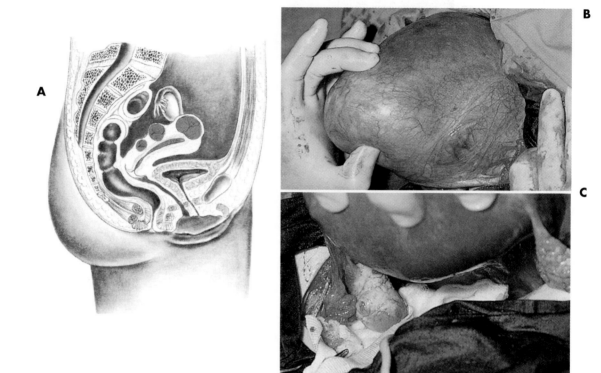

FIGURE 16-61
Myomas of the uterus (fibroids). **A,** Common location of myomas. **B,** Multiple uterine fibroids. **C,** Multiple uterine fibroids with enlarged ovaries resulting from multiple small cysts.
B and **C** from Symonds, Macpherson, 1994.

ENDOMETRIAL
CARCINOMA

Endometrial cancer occurs most often in postmenopausal women, particularly those receiving estrogen therapy. The symptom is postmenopausal bleeding.

ADNEXA

OVARIAN CYSTS AND TUMORS

Ovarian growths can occur unilaterally or bilaterally. Cysts tend to be smooth and sometimes compressible, whereas tumors feel more solid and nodular; nei-ther is usually tender. A ruptured ovarian cyst will produce symptoms similar to those of ruptured tubal pregnancy (Figure 16-62).

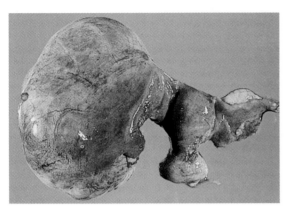

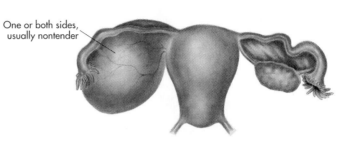

One or both sides, usually nontender

FIGURE 16-62
Ovarian cyst.
Photo from Symonds, Macpherson, 1994.

OVARIAN CARCINOMA

Ovarian cancer is difficult to detect and often asymptomatic at first. An ovary that is enlarged should be considered suspicious for cancer, and further diagnostic tests are required.

RUPTURED TUBAL PREGNANCY

A ruptured tubal pregnancy causes marked pelvic tenderness, with tenderness and rigidity of the lower abdomen. Motion of the cervix produces pain. A tender, unilateral adnexal mass may indicate the site of the pregnancy. Tachycardia and shock reflect the hemorrhage into the peritoneal cavity and cardiovascular collapse. This is a surgical emergency (Figure 16-63).

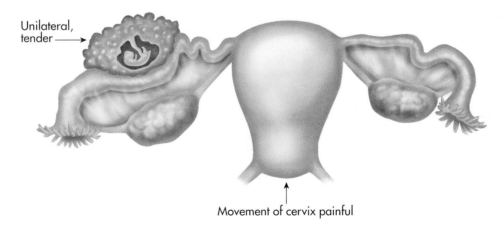

Unilateral, tender

Movement of cervix painful

FIGURE 16-63
Ruptured tubal pregnancy.

PELVIC
INFLAMMATORY
DISEASE (PID)

Often caused by gonococcal and chlamydial infection, PID may be acute or chronic. Acute PID produces very tender, bilateral adnexal areas; the patient guards and usually cannot tolerate bimanual examination. The symptoms of chronic PID are bilateral, tender, irregular, and fairly fixed adnexal areas (Figure 16-64).

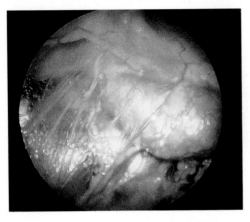 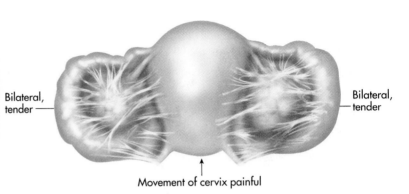

Bilateral, tender

Bilateral, tender

Movement of cervix painful

FIGURE 16-64
Pelvic inflammatory disease. Photo shows sheet of fine adhesions covering tubes and ovary, which is buried beneath the tubes.
Photo from Symonds, Macpherson, 1994.

SALPINGITIS

Inflammation or infection of the fallopian tube is often associated with PID. Salpingitis causes lower quadrant pain with tenderness on bimanual examination (Figure 16-65).

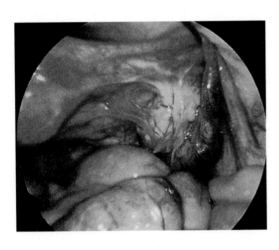 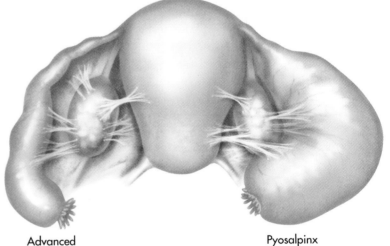

Advanced

Pyosalpinx

FIGURE 16-65
Salpingitis. Photo shows acute salpingitis with adhesions. Dye has been instilled into the grossly swollen fallopian tube on the right. Dense adhesions obscure the ovary.
Photo from Morse, Moreland, Holmes, 1996.

INFANTS AND CHILDREN

AMBIGUOUS GENITALIA

Certain conditions of the labia and clitoris may indicate ambiguous genitalia. For example, partially fused labia suggest the presence of a scrotum; a urinary meatus that is not located behind the clitoris may indicate the presence of a penis (Figure 16-66).

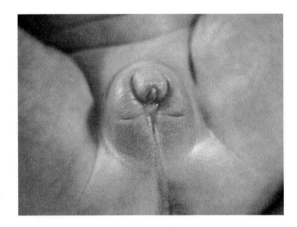

FIGURE 16-66
Ambiguous genitalia.
Courtesy Patrick C. Walsh, MD, The Johns Hopkins School of Medicine, Baltimore.

HYDROCOLPOS

Vaginal secretions can collect behind an imperforate hymen. Hydrocolpos may be manifested by a small midline lower abdominal mass or a small cystic mass between the labia. The condition may resolve spontaneously or may require surgical intervention.

VULVOVAGINITIS

Vaginal discharge that is accompanied by warm, erythematous, and swollen vulvar tissues is termed vulvovaginitis. Possible causes include sexual abuse; trichomonal, monilial, or gonococcal infection; secondary infection from a foreign body; and nonspecific infection from bubble baths, diaper irritation, urethritis, and injury (Figure 16-67).

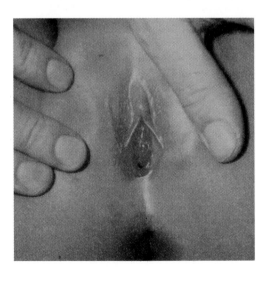

FIGURE 16-67
Nonspecific inflammation characteristic of chemical irritant vulvovaginitis.
From Zitelli, Davis, 1996.

PREGNANT WOMEN

PREMATURE RUPTURE OF MEMBRANES

The spontaneous premature rupture of the membranes (PROM) in a preterm pregnancy carries a high risk of perinatal morbidity and mortality, as well as maternal morbidity and mortality. The cause of PROM is not known; however, certain conditions such as infection and hydramnios have been implicated. Some health care professionals also consider the rupture of membranes before the onset of labor in a term pregnancy to be premature rupture if labor does not begin in 12 hours. Symptoms include the passage of fluid from the vagina. Management depends on the weeks of gestation and the condition of the mother and fetus.

PROLAPSE OF THE UMBILICAL CORD

When the presenting part of the fetus does not fill the pelvic inlet, a loop of cord may advance with the presenting part. Prolapse of the cord usually occurs with rupture of the membranes. Predisposing factors are premature labor, a fetus in breech presentation or transverse position, hydramnios, a high or floating presenting part (not engaged), and multiple pregnancy. The symptoms may be obvious, such as a loop of cord protruding from the vagina or the palpation of the pulsating cord on vaginal examination. The presence of variable decelerations in fetal heart rate is also associated with cord compression. Unless immediate measures are taken to relieve compression of the cord and deliver the fetus, death of the fetus can result.

BLEEDING

There are many causes for bleeding during pregnancy. In early pregnancy, bleeding may be due to "unknown" causes of little consequence or to a potentially life-threatening condition such as an ectopic pregnancy. Late in pregnancy, causes of bleeding may range from benign conditions such as cervical changes to a potentially life-threatening abruptio placentae. Whatever the cause, bleeding in pregnancy should be investigated thoroughly with a careful history and physical assessment. However, women who are bleeding in labor or have a suspected placenta previa should not be examined without preparation for emergency cesarean section.

VULVAR VARICOSITIES

Vulvar varicosities occur frequently during pregnancy. The varicosities may involve both the vulva and the rectal area. Pressure from the pregnant uterus and possibly hereditary factors contribute to the formation of the varicosities.

ATROPHIC VAGINITIS

Atrophy of the vagina is caused by lack of estrogen. The vaginal mucosa is dry and pale, although it may become reddened and develop petechiae and superficial erosions. The accompanying vaginal discharge may be white, gray, yellow, green, or blood-tinged. It can be thick or watery, and although it varies in amount, the discharge is rarely profuse (Figure 16-68).

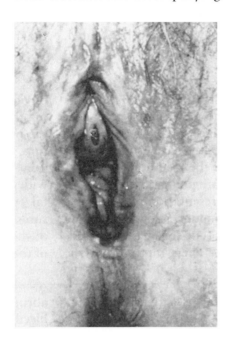

FIGURE 16-68
Advanced postmenopausal atrophy of the vulva in a 72-year-old woman.
From Kaufman, Faro, 1994.

URINARY
INCONTINENCE

See the discussion in Chapter 15, Abdomen, pp. 571-572.

CHAPTER 17

MALE GENITALIA

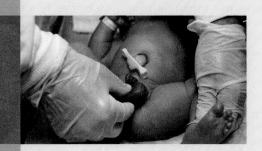

ANATOMY AND PHYSIOLOGY

The penis, testicles, epididymides, scrotum, prostate gland, and seminal vesicles constitute the male genitalia (Figure 17-1).

The physiologic function of the penis is to serve as the final excretory organ for urine and, when erect, as the means of introducing sperm into the vagina. The penis consists of the two corpora cavernosa, which form the dorsum and sides, and the corpus spongiosum, which contains the urethra. The corpus spongiosum expands at its distal end to form the glans penis. The urethral orifice is a slitlike opening located approximately 2 mm ventral to the tip of the glans (Figures 17-2 and 17-3). The skin of the penis is thin, redundant to permit erection, and free of subcutaneous fat. It is generally more darkly pigmented than body skin. Unless the patient has been circumcised, the prepuce (foreskin) covers the glans. In the uncircumcised male, smegma is formed by the secretion of sebaceous material by the glans and the desquamation of epithelial cells from the prepuce. It appears as a cheesy white material on the glans and in the fornix of the foreskin.

The scrotum, like the penis, is generally more darkly pigmented than body skin. A septum divides the scrotum into two pendulous sacs, each containing a testis, epididymis, spermatic cord, and a muscle layer that allows the scrotum to relax or contract (Figure 17-4). Testicular temperature is controlled by altering the distance of the testes from the body through muscular action. Spermatogenesis requires maintenance of temperatures lower than 37° C.

The testicles are responsible for the production of both spermatozoa and testosterone. The adult testis is ovoid and measures approximately 4 × 3 × 2 cm. The epididymis is a soft, comma-shaped structure located on the posterolateral and upper aspect of the testis in 90% of males. It provides for storage, maturation, and transit of sperm. The vas deferens begins at the tail of the epididymis, ascends the spermatic cord, travels through the inguinal canal, and unites with the seminal vesicle to form the ejaculatory duct.

The prostate gland, which resembles a large chestnut and is approximately the size of a testis, surrounds the urethra at the bladder neck. The physiologic function of

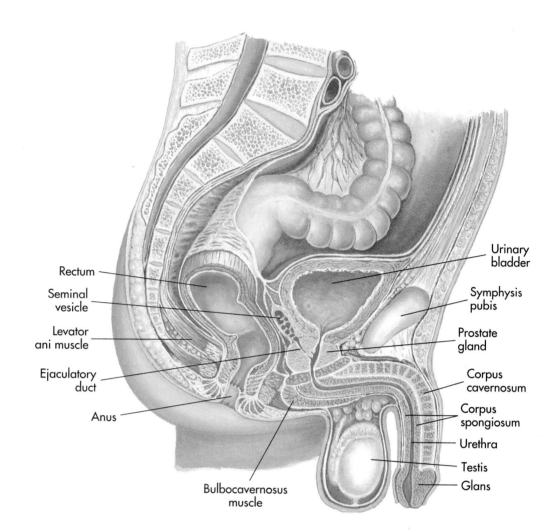

Rectum

Seminal
vesicle

Levator
ani muscle

Ejaculatory
duct

Anus

Bulbocavernosus
muscle

Urinary
bladder

Symphysis
pubis

Prostate
gland

Corpus
cavernosum

Corpus
spongiosum

Urethra

Testis

Glans

FIGURE 17-1
Male pelvic organs.

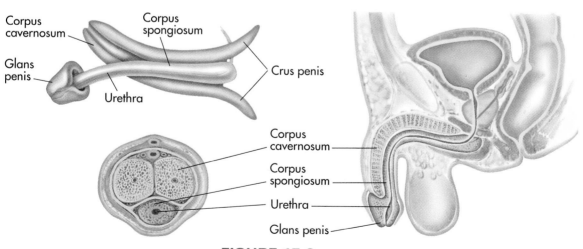

Corpus
cavernosum

Corpus
spongiosum

Glans
penis

Urethra

Crus penis

Corpus
cavernosum

Corpus
spongiosum

Urethra

Glans penis

FIGURE 17-2
Anatomy of the penis.

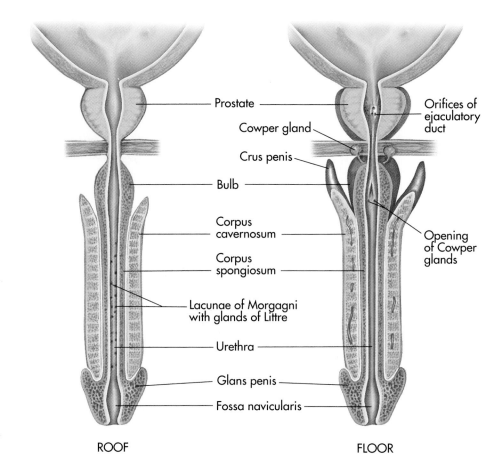

FIGURE 17-3
Anatomy of urethra and penis.
From Lowdermilk, Perry, Bobak, 1997.

ROOF   FLOOR

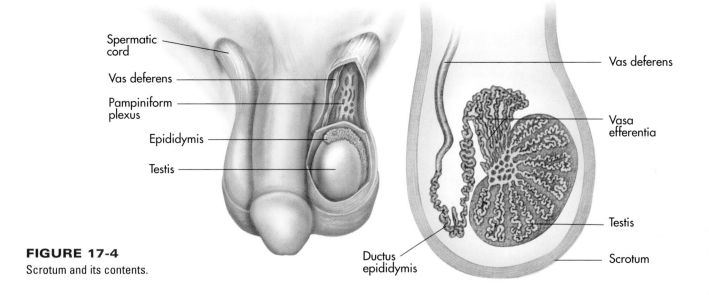

FIGURE 17-4
Scrotum and its contents.

the prostate and its secretions is not completely understood. It produces the major volume of ejaculatory fluid, which contains fibrinolysin. This enzyme liquifies the coagulated semen, a process that may be important for satisfactory sperm motility. The seminal vesicles extend from the prostate onto the posterior surface of the bladder.

SEXUAL PHYSIOLOGY

Erection

Erection of the penis occurs when the two corpora cavernosa become engorged with blood, generally 20 to 50 ml. Increased blood supply is produced by increased arterial dilation and decreased venous outflow; both processes are under the control of the autonomic nervous system.

Erection is a neurovascular reflex that can be induced by psychogenic and local reflex mechanisms. Local reflex mechanisms involve spinal reflex arcs that are initiated by tactile stimuli. Psychogenic erection can be initiated by any type of sensory input—auditory, visual, tactile, or imaginative stimuli. Cortical input can also serve to suppress sexual arousal.

Orgasm

Orgasm is a complex, pleasurable sensation accompanying ejaculation, which is the emission of secretions from the vas deferens, epididymides, prostate, and seminal vesicles. Orgasm is followed by constriction of the vessels supplying blood to the corpora cavernosa and gradual detumescence.

INFANTS AND CHILDREN

The external genitalia are identical for male and female at 8 weeks' gestational age, but by 12 weeks of gestation sexual differentiation has occurred. Any fetal insult during 8 or 9 weeks of gestation may lead to major anomalies of the external genitalia. Minor morphologic abnormalities arise from injury after that period of development.

During the third trimester, the testes descend from the retroperitoneal space through the inguinal canal to the scrotum. At full term, one or both testes may still lie within the inguinal canal, with the final descent into the scrotum occurring in the early postnatal period. Descent of the testicles may be arrested at any point, however, or may follow an abnormal path.

Small separations between the glans and the inner preputial epithelium begin during the third trimester. Separation of the prepuce from the glans is usually incomplete at birth, however, and often remains so until the age of 3 to 4 years.

ADOLESCENTS

With the onset of puberty, sparse, downy, straight hair appears at the base of the penis; the scrotal skin reddens, thins, and becomes increasingly pendulous. The testes and penis begin enlarging. As maturation continues, the pubic hair darkens and extends over the entire pubic area, and the prostate gland enlarges. By the completion of puberty the pubic hair is curly, dense, and coarse and forms a diamond-shaped pattern from the umbilicus to the anus. The growth and development of the testes and scrotum are complete. The penis is enlarged in length and breadth. See Chapter 5, Growth and Measurement, for details of pubertal development.

OLDER ADULTS

Pubic hair becomes finer and less abundant with aging, and pubic alopecia may occur.

No change in the length of time necessary for the production of a mature spermatozoa occurs with aging. The viability of the sperm, however, probably decreases since the rate of conception declines with age. The ejaculatory volume may actually increase with age, perhaps because of decreased frequency of intercourse. The scrotum becomes more pendulous with aging, and the patient may complain about it.

Frequency of sexual activity usually declines with aging, although the rate of decline correlates most strongly with the frequency of sexual activity in youth—that is, the man who was highly active in youth is more likely to maintain a higher level of sexual activity during later years. Erection may develop more slowly, and orgasm may be less intense.

REVIEW OF RELATED HISTORY

PRESENT PROBLEM

- Difficulty achieving or maintaining erection
  - Pain with erection, prolonged painful erection
  - Constant or intermittent, with one or more sexual partners
  - Associated with alcohol ingestion or medication
  - Persistent erections unrelated to sexual stimulation
  - Curvature of penis in any direction with erection
  - Medications: prescription or nonprescription drugs that might interfere with sexual performance (diuretics, sedatives, antihypertensive agents, tranquilizers, estrogens, inhibitors of androgen synthesis)
- Difficulty with ejaculation
  - Painful or premature, efforts to treat the problem
  - Ejaculate color, consistency, odor, and amount
  - Medications: prescription or nonprescription
- Discharge or lesion on the penis
  - Character: lumps, sores, rash
  - Discharge: color, consistency, odor, tendency to stain underwear
  - Symptoms: itching, burning, stinging
  - Exposure to sexually transmitted disease: multiple partners, infection in partners, failure to use condom, history of prior sexually transmitted disease
  - Medications: prescription or nonprescription
- Infertility
  - Life-style factors that may increase temperature of scrotum: tight clothing, briefs, hot baths, employment in high-temperature environment (steel mill) or requiring prolonged sitting (truck driver)
  - Length of time attempting pregnancy, sexual activity pattern, knowledge of fertile period of woman's reproductive cycle
  - History of undescended testes
  - Diagnostic evaluation to date: semen analysis, physical examination, sperm antibody titers
  - Medications: nonprescription or prescription (testosterone, glucocorticoids, hypothalamic releasing hormone)
- Enlargement in inguinal area
  - Intermittent or constant, association with straining or lifting, duration, presence of pain
  - Change in size or character of mass; ability to reduce the mass; if unable to reduce it, how long since it could be reduced
  - Pain in the groin: character (tearing, sudden searing, or cutting pain), associated activity (lifting heavy object, coughing, or straining at stool)
  - Use of truss or other treatment
  - Medications: for pain; prescription or nonprescription
- Testicular pain or mass
  - Change in testicular size

RISK FACTORS **Carcinoma of the Male Genitalia**

Penile

- Lack of circumcision with failure to maintain good hygiene
- Condyloma acuminatum infection

Testicular

- Cryptorchidism with elevated testicular temperature

- Events surrounding onset: noted casually while bathing, after trauma, during a sporting event
- Irregular lumps, soreness, or heaviness of testes
- Medications: for pain; antibiotics; prescription or nonprescription

PAST MEDICAL HISTORY

- Surgery of genitourinary tract: undescended testes, hypospadias, epispadias, hydrocele, varicocele, hernia, prostate, sterilization
- Sexually transmitted diseases: single or multiple infections, specific organism (gonorrhea, syphilis, herpes, warts, chlamydia), treatment, effectiveness, residual problems
- Chronic illness: testicular or prostatic cancer, neurologic or vascular impairment, diabetes mellitus, arthritis, cardiac or respiratory disease

FAMILY HISTORY

- Infertility in siblings
- Hernias

PERSONAL AND SOCIAL HISTORY

- Employment risk of trauma to suprapubic region or genitalia, exposure to radiation or toxins
- Exercise: use of a protective device with contact sports
- Concerns about genitalia: size, shape, surface characteristics, texture
- Testicular self-examination practices
- Concerns about sexual practices: sexual partners (single or multiple), sexual lifestyle (heterosexual, homosexual, bisexual)
- Reproductive function: number of children, form of contraception used
- Use of alcohol
- Use of street drugs

INFANTS AND CHILDREN

- Maternal use of sex hormones or birth control pills during pregnancy
- Circumcised boy: complications from procedure
- Uncircumcised boy: hygiene measures, retractability of foreskin, interference with urinary stream
- Scrotal swelling with crying or bowel movement
- Congenital anomalies: hypospadias, epispadias, undescended testes, ambiguous genitalia
- Concerns with masturbation, sexual exploration
- Swelling, discoloration, or sores on the penis or scrotum, pain in the genitalia

ADOLESCENTS

- Knowledge of reproductive function, source of information about sexual activity and function
- Presence of nocturnal emissions, pubic hair, enlargement of genitalia, age at time of each occurrence
- Sexual activity, contraception used

OLDER ADULTS

- Change in frequency of sexual activity or desire: related to loss of spouse or other sexual partner; no sexual partner; sexually restrictive environment; depression; physical illness resulting in fatigue, weakness, or pain
- Change in sexual response: longer time required to achieve full erection, less forceful ejaculation, more rapid detumescence, longer interval between erections, prostatic surgery

EXAMINATION AND FINDINGS

EQUIPMENT

- Gloves
- Penlight for transillumination of any mass
- Drapes

Examination of the genitalia involves inspection, palpation, and transillumination of any mass found. The patient may be anxious about examination of his genitalia, so it is important to examine the genitalia carefully and completely but also expeditiously (Box 17-1). The patient may be lying or standing for this part of the examination (Figure 17-5).

INSPECTION AND PALPATION

Genital Hair Distribution

First inspect the genital hair distribution. Genital hair is more coarse than scalp hair. It should be abundant in the pubic region and may continue in a narrowing midline pattern to the umbilicus (the male escutcheon pattern). Depending on how the patient is positioned, it may be possible to note that the distribution continues around the scrotum to the anal orifice. The penis itself is not covered with hair, and the scrotum generally has scant amounts.

BOX 17-1 **Minimizing the Patient's Anxiety**

The physical examination is laden with anxiety-provoking elements for most people, but no part of the body is likely to arouse as much psychic discomfort for the male patient as examination of his genitals. Adolescents and men are often fearful of having an erection during the examination. Boys and adolescents may worry about whether their genitals are "normal," and misinformation on sexual matters (such as "the evils of masturbation") can add to their concerns. Your attitude and ability to communicate can reassure the apprehensive patient. Some important elements to remember:

- Know the language. It is inappropriate to talk down to anyone, but you and the patient must understand each other. You may not be entirely comfortable with some of the common words and phrases you may hear from the patients, but the common language may be appropriate in certain circumstances. You will not lose your dignity if you maintain your composure and you succeed in communicating effectively. Know the language and use it effectively, without apology, and in an undemeaning fashion.
- Never make jokes. Light, casual talk or jokes about the genitalia or sexual function are always inappropriate, no matter how well you know the patient. Feelings about one's own sexuality run deep and are frequently well masked. Do not pull at the edges of a mask you may not suspect is there.
- Remember that your face is easily seen by the patient when you are examining the genitalia. An unexpected finding may cause a sudden change in your expression. You must guard against what you communicate by the unspoken.
- You need not be defensive if you are a woman examining a man, any more than if you are a man examining a woman—an ordinary event historically. Here again, you communicate much by demeanor and hesitancy in speech. Do not be apologetic in any obvious or subtle way. Remember that you are a professional, fulfilling the responsibility of a professional.

Penis

Examine the penis. The dorsal vein should be apparent on inspection. If the patient is uncircumcised, retract the foreskin. It should retract easily, and a bit of white cheesy smegma may be seen over the glans. Occasionally the foreskin is tight and cannot be retracted. This condition is called phimosis (Figure 17-6) and may occur during the first 6 years of life. It is usually congenital but may result from recurrent infections or balanoposthitis (inflammation of the glans penis and prepuce). It may also be caused by previous unsuccessful efforts to retract the foreskin that have caused radial tearing of the preputial ring, resulting in adhesions of the foreskin to the glans. Balanitis, inflammation of the glans (Figure 17-7), occurs only in uncircumcised individuals and is often associated with phimosis. It may be caused by either bacterial or fungal infections and is most commonly seen in men with poorly controlled diabetes mellitus and a candidal infection.

If the patient is circumcised, the glans is exposed and appears erythematous and dry. No smegma will be present.

Urethral Meatus

Examine the external meatus of the urethra. The orifice should appear slitlike and be located on the ventral surface just millimeters from the tip of the glans. Press the glans

A **B**

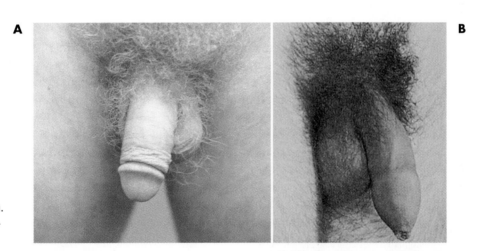

FIGURE 17-5
Appearance of male genitalia. **A,** Circumcised. **B,** Uncircumcised.

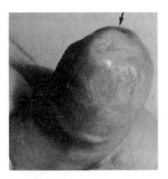

FIGURE 17-6
Phimosis.
From *400 Self-assessment picture tests in clinical medicine,* 1984. By permission of Mosby International.

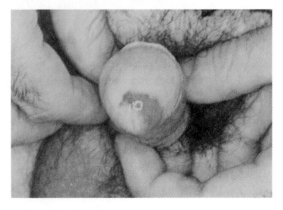

FIGURE 17-7
Balanitis.
From Lloyd-Davies et al, 1994.

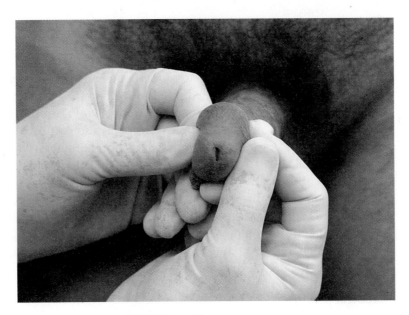

FIGURE 17-8
Examination of urethral orifice.

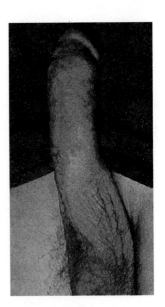

FIGURE 17-9
Priapism.
From Lloyd-Davies et al, 1994.

between thumb and forefinger to open the urethral orifice (Figure 17-8). You can certainly ask the patient to perform this procedure for you. The opening should be glistening and pink. Bright erythema or a discharge indicates inflammatory disease, whereas a pinpoint or round opening may result from meatal stenosis.

Penile Shaft

Palpate the shaft of the penis for tenderness and induration. Strip the urethra for any discharge by firmly compressing the base of the penis with your thumb and forefinger and moving them toward the glans. The presence of a discharge may well indicate a venereal infection. The texture of the flaccid penis should be soft and free of nodularity. Replace the foreskin after performing these maneuvers.

Rarely you may see a patient with a prolonged penile erection, called priapism (Figure 17-9). It is often painful. Although in the majority of cases the condition is idiopathic, it can occur in patients with leukemia or hemoglobinopathies such as sickle cell disease.

Scrotum

Inspect the scrotum (Figure 17-10). It should appear more deeply pigmented than the body skin, and the surface may be coarse. The scrotal skin is often reddened in red-haired individuals; however, reddened skin in other individuals may indicate an infectious process. The scrotum usually appears asymmetric, because the left testicle has a longer spermatic cord and therefore is often lower. The thickness of the scrotum definitely varies with temperature and age, and perhaps emotional state. Lumps in the scrotal skin are commonly caused by sebaceous cysts, also called epidermoid cysts. They appear as small lumps on the scrotum, but they may enlarge and discharge oily material (Figure 17-11).

Occasionally you may observe unusual thickening of the scrotum caused by edema, often with pitting. This does not generally imply disease related to the geni-

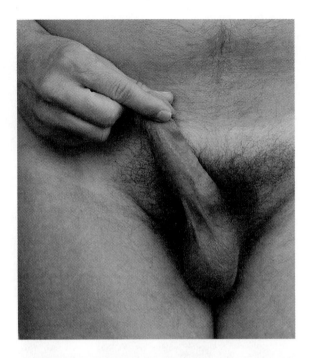

FIGURE 17-10
Inspection of scrotum and ventral surface of penis as the patient positions his penis.

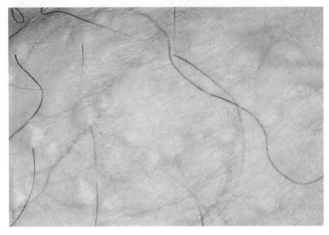

FIGURE 17-11
Sebaceous glands on the scrotum.
From Morse, Moreland, and Holmes, 1996.

talia but is more likely a consequence of general fluid retention associated with cardiac, renal, or hepatic disease.

Hernia

Examine for evidence of a hernia. Figure 17-16 (p. 660) shows the anatomy of the region and the three common types of hernias. With the patient standing, ask him to bear down as if having a bowel movement. While he is straining, inspect the area of the inguinal canal and the region of the fossa ovalis. After asking the patient to relax again, insert your examining finger into the lower part of the scrotum and carry it upward along the vas deferens into the inguinal canal (Figure 17-12). Which finger you use depends on the size of the patient. In the young child the little finger is appropriate; in the adult the index or middle finger is generally used. You should be able to feel the oval external ring. Ask the patient to cough. If a hernia is present, you should feel the sudden presence of a viscus against your finger. The hernia is described as indirect if it lies within the inguinal canal. It may also come through the external canal and even pass into the scrotum. This type of hernia occurs more frequently in young

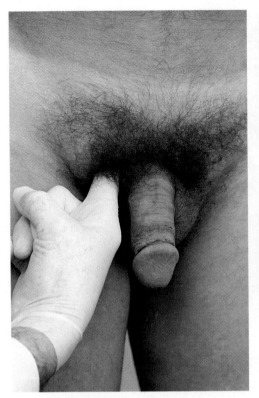

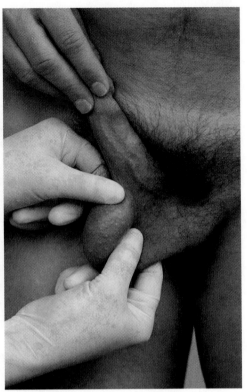

FIGURE 17-12
Checking for inguinal hernia; gloved finger inserted through inguinal canal.

FIGURE 17-13
Palpating contents of the scrotal sac.

men and is the most common of the abdominal hernias. Since an indirect hernia on one side strongly suggests the possibility of bilateral herniation, be sure to examine both sides thoroughly. If the viscus is felt medial to the external canal, it probably represents a direct inguinal hernia.

Testes

The testes should be palpated using the thumb and first two fingers. They should be sensitive to gentle compression but not tender, and they should feel smooth and rubbery and be free of nodules (Figure 17-13). In some diseases such as syphilis and diabetic neuropathy, a testis may be totally insensitive to painful stimuli. Irregularities in texture or size may indicate an infection, cyst, or tumor.

The epididymis, located on the posterolateral surface of the testis, should be smooth, discrete, larger cephalad, and nontender. You may be able to feel the appendix epididymidis as an irregularity on the cephalad surface.

Next palpate the vas deferens. It has accompanying arteries and veins, but they cannot be precisely identified by palpation. The vas deferens itself feels smooth and discrete; it should not be beaded or lumpy in its course as you palpate from the testicle to the inguinal ring. The presence of such unexpected findings might indicate diabetes or old inflammatory changes, especially tuberculosis.

All patients, but especially boys and young men, should be taught the techniques of self-examination of the genitalia (Box 17-2).

BOX 17-2 Genital Self-Examination for Men

Since testicular tumors are the most common cancer occurring in young men, all male patients should be instructed in the technique of genital self-examination (GSE). The patient should obviously be made aware of the rationale. GSE is also recommended for anyone who is at risk for contracting a sexually transmitted disease. This includes sexually active persons who have had more than one sexual partner or whose partner has had other partners. In these cases the purpose of GSE is to detect any signs or symptoms that might indicate the presence of a sexually transmitted disease (STD). Many people who have an STD do not know they have one, and some STDs can remain undetected for years. GSE should become a regular part of routine self-health care practices.

You should explain and demonstrate the following procedure to your patients and give them the opportunity to perform a GSE with your guidance.

Instruct the patient to hold the penis in his hand and examine the head. If not circumcised, he should pull back the foreskin to expose the head. Inspection and palpation of the entire head of the penis should be performed in a clockwise motion, while the patient carefully looks for any bumps, sores, or blisters on the skin. Bumps and blisters may be red or light colored, or may resemble pimples. Have the patient also look for genital warts, which may look similar to warts on other parts of the body. At first they may be small bumpy spots. Left untreated, they could develop a fleshy cauliflower-like appearance. The urethral meatus should also be examined for any discharge.

Next the patient will examine the entire shaft and look for the same signs and symptoms. Instruct him to separate the pubic hair at the base of the penis and carefully examine the skin underneath. Make sure he includes the underside of the shaft in the examination; a mirror may be helpful.

Instruct the patient to move on to the scrotum and examine it. He should hold each testicle gently and inspect and palpate the skin for the same signs, including the underneath of the scrotum. The patient should also be alert to any lump, swelling, soreness, or irregularities in the testicle. (Suggest to the patient that self-examination of the scrotum at home be performed while bathing, since the warmth is likely to make the scrotal skin less thick.)

Educate the patient about other symptoms associated with STDs, specifically, pain or burning on urination or discharge from the penis. The discharge may vary in color, consistency, and amount.

If the patient has any of the above signs or symptoms, he should see a health care provider.

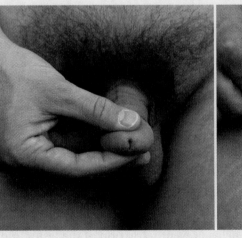
Self-examination of penis.

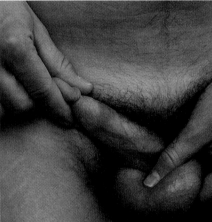
Self-examination of scrotum.

Modified from Burroughs Wellcome Co, 1989. (Instructional pamphlets available.)

Cremasteric Reflex

Finally, evaluate the cremasteric reflex. Stroke the inner thigh with a blunt instrument such as the handle of the reflex hammer, or for a child, with your finger. The testicle and scrotum should rise on the stroked side (see Chapter 20, Neurologic System).

Examination of the prostate is detailed in Chapter 18, Anus, Rectum, and Prostate.

INFANTS

Examine the genitalia of the newborn for congenital anomalies, incomplete development, and sexual ambiguity. Inspect the penis for size, placement of the urethral opening, and any anomalies. The nonerect length of the penis at birth is 2 to 3 cm. Transitory erection of the penis during infancy is common, and the penis should have a straight projection. A small penis (microphallus) may indicate other organ anomalies. The small penis must also be differentiated from the unusually large clitoris found in pseudohermaphroditism. A hooked, downward bowing of the penis suggests a chordee.

INSPECTION AND PALPATION

Inspect the glans penis of the neonate. The foreskin in the uncircumcised infant is commonly tight, but it should retract enough to permit a good urinary stream. Do not retract the foreskin more than necessary to see the urethra, especially if the neonate will not be circumcised. Do not force, because this can tear the prepuce from the glans, causing binding adhesions to form between the prepuce and the glans. Mobility of the foreskin increases with time, and it should be fully retractable by 3 or 4 years of age. The slitlike urethral meatus should be located near the tip. Inspect the glans of the circumcised infant for ulcerations, bleeding, and inflammation (Box 17-3). The urinary stream should be strong with good caliber. Dribbling or a reduced force or caliber of the urinary stream may indicate stenosis of the urethral meatus. On occasion, hypospadias may be associated with a sex chromosomal abnormality 47XXY or 47XYY.

Inspect the scrotum for size, shape, rugae, the presence of testicles, and any anomalies (Figure 17-14). The scrotum of the premature infant may appear underdeveloped, without rugae, and without testes, whereas the full-term neonate should have a loose, pendulous scrotum with rugae and a midline raphe. The proximal end of the scrotum should be the widest area. The scrotum in infants usually appears large compared with the rest of the genitalia. Edema of the external genitalia is common, especially after a breech delivery. A deep cleft in the scrotum (bifid scrotum) is usually associated with other genitourinary anomalies or ambiguous genitalia.

When examining the scrotum, particularly in the young, make certain that your hands are warm and your touch is gentle. The cremasteric reflex—known as the yo-yo reflex—in which the scrotal contents retract, is a response to cold hands and abrupt handling. Before you palpate the scrotum, place the thumb and index finger of one hand over the inguinal canals at the upper part of the scrotal sac. This maneuver helps prevent retraction of the testes into the inguinal canal or abdomen. Palpate each side of the scrotum to detect the presence of the testes or other masses. The testicle of the newborn is approximately 1 cm in diameter.

If either of the testicles is not palpable, place a finger over the upper inguinal ring and gently push toward the scrotum. You may feel a soft mass in the inguinal canal. Try to push it toward the scrotum and palpate it with your thumb and index finger. If the testicle can be pushed into the scrotum, it is considered a descended testicle, even though it retracts to the inguinal canal. A testicle that is either palpable in

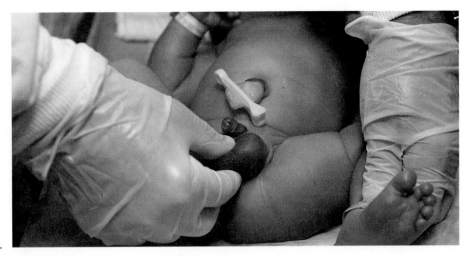

FIGURE 17-14
Palpating the scrotum of an infant.

BOX 17-3 | **Circumcision**

There has been much discussion recently about the appropriateness of routine circumcision; some persons believe it is not medically indicated. However, attitudes vary and are highly personal. Recent evidence suggesting that circumcision prevents urinary tract infections in infants has received much attention. Nonetheless, this potential advantage must be weighed against the risks inherent in any operative procedure. Although a definitive answer may not yet be available, circumcision will continue to be performed on many children, frequently on the basis of religious prescription.

---

the inguinal canal but cannot be pushed into the scrotum or not palpable at all is considered an undescended testicle.

Palpate over the internal inguinal canal with the flat part of your fingers. Roll the spermatic cord beneath the fingers to feel the solid structure going through the ring. If the feeling of smoothness disappears as you palpate, the peritoneum is passing through the ring, indicating an invisible hernia. An apparent bulge in the inguinal area suggests a visible hernia. Palpation may elicit a sensation of crepitus.

Transillumination

When any mass other than the testicle or spermatic cord is palpated in the scrotum, determine if it is filled with fluid, gas, or solid material. It will most likely be a hernia or hydrocele. Attempt to reduce the size of the mass by pushing it back through the external inguinal canal. If a bright penlight transilluminates the mass and there is no change in size when reduction is attempted, it most likely contains fluid (hydrocele with a closed tunica vaginalis). A mass that does not transilluminate but does change in size when reduction is attempted is probably a hernia. A mass that neither changes in size nor transilluminates may represent an incarcerated hernia, which is a surgical emergency.

CHILDREN

The external genitalia of the toddler and preschooler are examined as described for infants. Preschoolers may have developed a sense of modesty, so you should explain what you are doing and quickly complete the examination. Reassure the child that he is developing appropriately whenever such reassurance is possible.

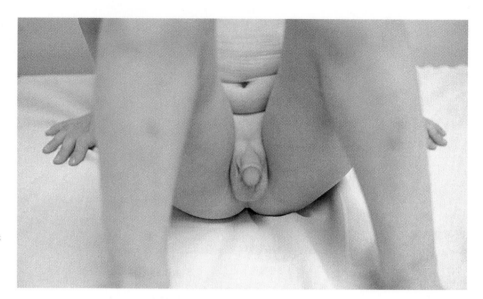

FIGURE 17-15
Position of child to push testicles into the scrotum. An alternative maneuver is to seat the child in tailor position.

INSPECTION AND PALPATION

Inspect the penis for size, lesions, swelling, inflammation, and malformation. Retract the foreskin in the uncircumcised boy without forcing it, and inspect the glans for lesions, discharge, and the location and appearance of the urethral meatus. It is important not to force the retraction of the foreskin, because forced retraction may contribute to the formation of binding adhesions. Some adherence of the prepuce to the glans may continue even until 6 years of age. The penis may appear relatively small if obscured by fat in obese boys.

The scrotum is inspected for size, shape, color, and the presence of testicles or other masses. Well-formed rugae indicate that the testes have descended during infancy, even if the testes are not apparent in the scrotum. Palpate the scrotum to identify the testes and epididymides. The testes should be about 1 cm in size.

Some testes are very retractile and therefore hard to find. Warm hands, a warm room, and a gentle approach will help. If the patient is old enough to cooperate, ask him to sit in tailor position with legs crossed, or have the child sit on a chair with the heels of his feet on the chair seat and his hands on his knees. Either position places pressure on the abdominal wall that will help push the testicles into the scrotum. If an inguinal hernia exists, this maneuver is also useful in eliciting that finding (Figure 17-15). A scrotum that remains small, flat, and undeveloped is a good indication of cryptorchidism (undescended testes).

A hard, enlarged, painless testicle may indicate a tumor. Acute swelling in the scrotum with discoloration can result from torsion of the spermatic cord or orchitis. Acute painful swelling without discoloration and a thickened or nodular epididymis suggests epididymitis. An enlarged penis without enlargement of the testes occurs with precocious puberty, adrenal hyperplasia, and some central nervous system lesions.

ADOLESCENTS

The examination of older children and adolescents is the same as for adults. Because of their modesty and great sensitivity to development, this portion of the physical examination is usually performed last. The degree of maturation should be classified for the pubic hair, penile size, and the development of testes and scrotum according to the stages described by Tanner (Chapter 5, Growth and Measurement). The adolescent male may need to be reassured that his genital development is proceeding as expected. If he has an erection during the examination, explain that this is a common response to touch and that it is not a problem.

SUMMARY OF EXAMINATION   Male Genitalia

The following steps are performed with the patient lying or standing.

1. Inspect the pubic hair characteristics and distribution (p. 650).
2. Retract the foreskin if the patient is uncircumcised (p. 651).
3. Inspect the glans of the penis with foreskin retracted, noting the following (p. 651):
   - Color
   - Smegma
   - External meatus of urethra
   - Urethral discharge
4. Palpate the penis, noting the following (p. 652):
   - Tenderness
   - Induration
5. Strip the urethra for discharge (p. 652).
6. Inspect the scrotum and ventral surface of the penis for the following (p. 652):
   - Color
   - Texture
   - Asymmetry
   - Unusual thickening
   - Presence of hernia
7. Transilluminate any masses in the scrotum (p. 657)
8. Palpate the inguinal canal for a direct or indirect hernia (p. 653).
9. Palpate the testes, epididymides, and vasa deferentia for the following (p. 654):
   - Consistency
   - Size
   - Tenderness
   - Bleeding, lumpiness, or nodules
10. Palpate for inguinal lymph nodes (pp. 221, 231, 236).
11. Elicit the cremasteric reflex bilaterally (p. 656).

COMMON ABNORMALITIES

HERNIA

An abdominal hernia is the protrusion of a peritoneal-lined sac through some defect in the abdominal wall. Figure 17-16 shows the anatomy of the region and the three common types of pelvic hernias. Table 17-1 explains the distinguishing characteristics. Hernias occur because there is a potential space for protrusion of some abdominal organ, commonly the bowel but occasionally the omentum. These hernias arise along the course that the testicle traveled as it exited the abdomen and entered the scrotum during intrauterine life. Femoral hernias occur at the fossa ovalis, where the femoral artery exits the abdomen, and are more common in females than males. A strangulated hernia is a nonreducible hernia in which the blood supply to the protruded tissue is compromised; this condition requires prompt surgical intervention.

TABLE 17-1 Distinguishing Characteristics of Hernias

	Indirect Inguinal	Direct Inguinal	Femoral
Incidence	Most common type of hernia; both sexes are affected; often patients are children and young males	Less common than indirect inguinal; occurs more often in males than females; more common in those over age 40	Least common type of hernia; occurs more often in females than males; rare in children
Occurrence	Through internal inguinal ring; can remain in canal, exit the external ring, or pass into scrotum; may be bilateral	Through external inguinal ring; located in region of Hesselbach triangle; rarely enters scrotum	Through femoral ring, femoral canal, and fossa ovalis
Presentation	Soft swelling in area of internal ring; pain on straining; hernia comes down canal and touches fingertip on examination	Bulge in area of Hesselbach triangle; usually painless; easily reduced; hernia bulges anteriorly, pushes against side of finger on examination	Right side presentation more common than left; pain may be severe; inguinal canal empty on examination

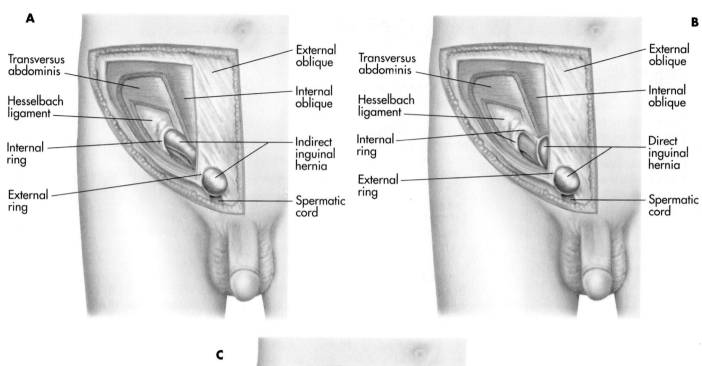

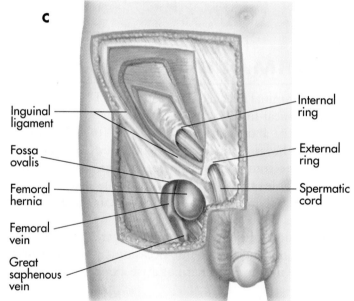

FIGURE 17-16

Anatomy of region of common pelvic hernias. **A,** Indirect inguinal hernia. **B,** Direct inguinal hernia. **C,** Femoral hernia.

PENIS

PARAPHIMOSIS

Paraphimosis is the inability to replace the foreskin to its usual position after it has been retracted behind the glans. Impairment of local circulation can lead to edema or gangrene of the glans (Figure 17-17).

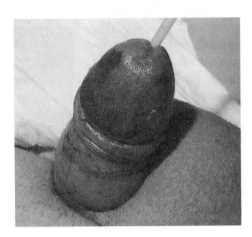

FIGURE 17-17

Paraphimosis.

Courtesy Patrick C. Walsh, MD, The Johns Hopkins University School of Medicine, Baltimore.

HYPOSPADIAS

Hypospadias is a congenital defect in which the urethral meatus is located on the ventral surface of the glans, penile shaft, or the perineal area. If the orifice is ventral but within the substance of the glans, it is termed primary hypospadias. An orifice along the ventral shaft of the penis is termed secondary hypospadias, and one located at the base of the penis is termed tertiary hypospadias (Figure 17-18). Rarely, the orifice may appear on the dorsal surface, a condition called epispadias.

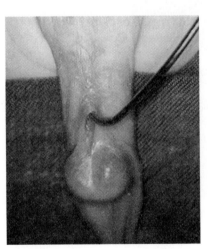

FIGURE 17-18

Hypospadias.

From *400 Self-assessment picture tests in clinical medicine*, 1984. By permission of Mosby International.

SYPHILITIC CHANCRE

The lesion of primary syphilis generally occurs 2 weeks after exposure. It is most commonly located on the glans, is painless, and has indurated borders with a clear base. Scrapings from the ulcer show spirochetes when examined microscopically (Figure 17-19).

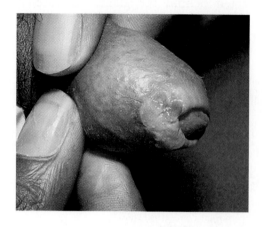

FIGURE 17-19
Syphilitic chancre.
Courtesy Antoinette Hood, MD, Indiana University School of Medicine, Indianapolis.

HERPES

Venereal herpes is a viral infection that appears as superficial vesicles. The lesions may be located on the glans, on the penile shaft, or at the base of the penis. They are frequently quite painful, and at the time of primary infection are often associated with inguinal lymphadenopathy and systemic symptoms including fever (Figure 17-20).

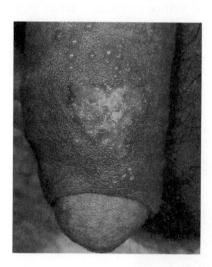

FIGURE 17-20
Genital herpes.
From Habif, 1996.

CONDYLOMA ACUMINATUM (GENITAL WARTS)

A soft, reddish lesion that arises because of infection with a papovavirus is called condyloma acuminatum. The lesions are commonly present on the prepuce, glans penis, and penile shaft; but they may be present within the urethra as well. The lesions may undergo malignant degeneration to squamous cell carcinoma (Figure 17-21).

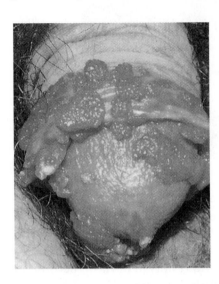

FIGURE 17-21
Condyloma acuminatum (genital warts).

From *Diagnostic picture tests in clinical medicine,* 1984. By permission of Mosby International.

LYMPHOGRANULOMA VENEREUM

Lymphogranuloma venereum is a sexually transmitted disease caused by a chlamydial organism. Although the lesions appear on the genitalia, symptoms may be systemic. The initial lesion is a painless erosion at or near the coronal sulcus (Figure 17-22). Subsequently local lymph nodes become involved; unless the infection is treated, draining sinus tracts may form. If lymphatic drainage is blocked, penile and scrotal lymphedema may ensue.

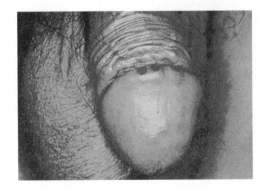

FIGURE 17-22
Lymphogranuloma venereum.

Reprinted from Meheus, Ursi, *Sexually transmitted diseases,* Kalamazoo, Michigan, The Upjohn Company, 1982, with permission.

MOLLUSCUM CONTAGIOSUM

Molluscum contagiosum is a sexually transmitted disease caused by a poxvirus. The lesions are pearly gray, often umbilicated, smooth, and dome shaped, with discrete margins. They occur most commonly on the glans penis (Figure 17-23).

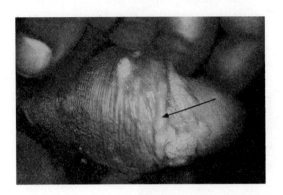

FIGURE 17-23

Molluscum contagiosum *(arrow)*, with condyloma acuminatum (genital warts).

Reprinted from Meheus , Ursi, *Sexually transmitted diseases*, Kalamazoo, Michigan, The Upjohn Company, 1982, with permission.

PEYRONIE DISEASE

A disorder of unknown cause, Peyronie disease is characterized by a fibrous band in the corpus cavernosum. It is generally unilateral and results in deviation of the penis during erection. Depending on the extent of the fibrous band, the condition may make erection painful and intromission impossible. No treatment has been altogether successful. Vitamin E therapy has recently become popular, and corticosteroid injection has also been used. Occasionally surgery is required to remove the fibrous band (Figure 17-24).

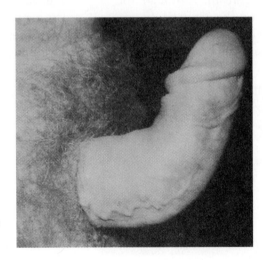

FIGURE 17-24

Peyronie disease.

Courtesy Patrick C. Walsh, MD, The Johns Hopkins University School of Medicine, Baltimore.

PENILE CARCINOMA

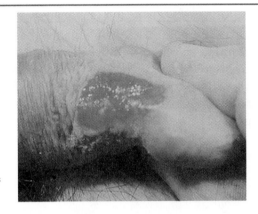

FIGURE 17-25
Carcinoma of the penis.
Courtesy Patrick C. Walsh, MD, The Johns Hopkins University School of Medicine, Baltimore.

Cancer of the penis is generally squamous and tends to occur in uncircumcised men who practice poor hygiene. It often appears as a painless ulceration that, unlike a syphilitic chancre, fails to heal. The lesions are often extensive by the time help is sought, either because of fear or because the lesion is unnoticed under the foreskin (Figure 17-25).

SCROTUM

HYDROCELE

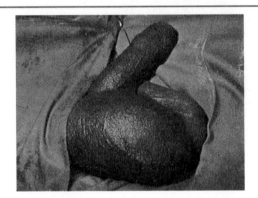

FIGURE 17-26
Hydrocele.
From Lloyd-Davies et al, 1994.

The nontender, smooth, firm mass of the hydrocele results from fluid accumulation in the tunica vaginalis. Unless it has been present for a long time and is very large and taut, palpation of a hydrocele should reveal that it is confined to the scrotum and does not enter the inguinal canal. The mass will transilluminate. This condition is common in infancy. If the tunica vaginalis is not patent, the hydrocele will generally disappear spontaneously in the first 6 months of life (Figure 17-26).

SPERMATOCELE

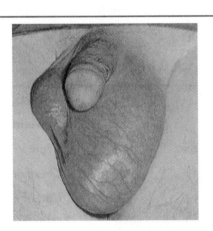

FIGURE 17-27
Spermatocele.
From Lloyd-Davies, et al, 1994.

A spermatocele is a cystic swelling occurring on the epididymis. It is not as large as a hydrocele, but it does transilluminate (Figure 17-27).

VARICOCELE

An abnormal tortuosity and dilation of veins of the pampiniform plexus within the spermatic cord is termed a varicocele. It is most common on the left side and may be associated with pain. It occurs in boys and young men and may be associated with reduced fertility, probably from increased venous pressure and elevated testicular temperature. The condition, often visible only when the patient is standing, is classically described as "bag of worms" (Figure 17-28).

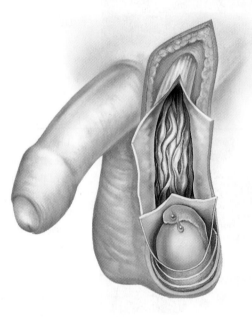

FIGURE 17-28
Varicocele.

ORCHITIS

An acute inflammation of the testis, orchitis is uncommon except as a complication of mumps in the adolescent or adult. It is generally unilateral and results in testicular atrophy in 50% of the cases (Figure 17-29).

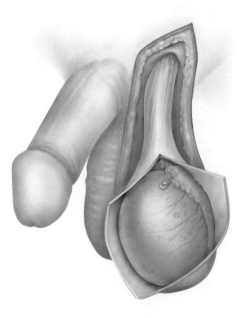

FIGURE 17-29
Orchitis.

EPIDIDYMITIS

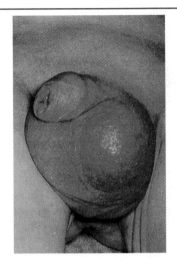

FIGURE 17-30
Epididymitis.
From Lloyd-Davies, et al, 1994.

Inflammation of the epididymis is often seen in association with a urinary tract infection. The epididymis is exquisitely tender, and the overlying scrotum may be markedly erythematous. Scrotal elevation may relieve the pain. A major consideration in the differential diagnosis is testicular torsion, a surgical emergency (Table 17-2). Systemic symptoms such as fever and examination of the urine for white blood cells and bacteria may help to distinguish between these two conditions. Occasionally chronic epididymitis may occur as a consequence of tuberculosis. In the chronic form, the epididymis feels firm and lumpy, and may be slightly tender, and the vasa deferentia may be beaded (Figure 17-30).

TABLE 17-2	**Acute Testicular Swelling**	
	Torsion	**Epididymitis**
Cause	Twisting of testis on spermatic cord	Bacterial infection (STD or UTI)
Age	Newborn to adolescence	Adolescence to adulthood
Onset of pain	Acute	More gradual
Vomiting	Common	Uncommon
Anorexia	Common	Uncommon
Fever	Uncommon	Possible
Dysuria	Uncommon	Possible
Supporting findings	Absence of cremasteric reflex on side of acute swelling Scrotal discoloration	Urethral discharge History of recent sexual activity Fever Pyuria Thickened or nodular epididymis

TESTICULAR TORSION   Testicular torsion is a surgical emergency occurring most commonly in adolescents. It has an acute onset and is often accompanied by nausea and vomiting. On examination, the testicle is exquisitely tender, and scrotal discoloration is often present (Table 17-2).

TESTICULAR TUMOR

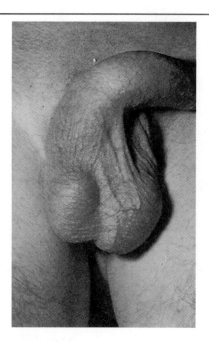

FIGURE 17-31
Testicular tumor.
From *400 Self-assessment pictures tests in clinical medicine*, 1984.

A neoplasm arising from the testicle appears as an irregular, nontender mass fixed on the testis. It does not transilluminate. It may be associated with inguinal lymphadenopathy. Testicular tumor tends to occur in young men and is the most common tumor in males ages 15 to 30. Most testicular tumors are malignant (Figure 17-31).

KLINEFELTER SYNDROME

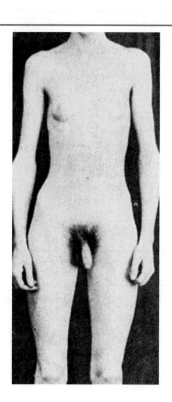

FIGURE 17-32
Klinefelter syndrome.
From Wilson, Walsh, 1979.

Klinefelter syndrome is a congenital anomaly associated with XXY chromosomal inheritance. It is associated with hypogonadism, including a small scrotum, female distribution of pubic hair, and, in some cases, gynecomastia (Figure 17-32).

INFANTS

AMBIGUOUS GENITALIA

This is a condition in which the examiner is uncertain whether the newborn has a very small penis with hypospadias or an enlarged clitoris. There may be partial fusion of the labioscrotal fold or a bifid scrotum. Testes cannot be palpated. The infant should have prompt chromosomal studies performed (Figure 17-33).

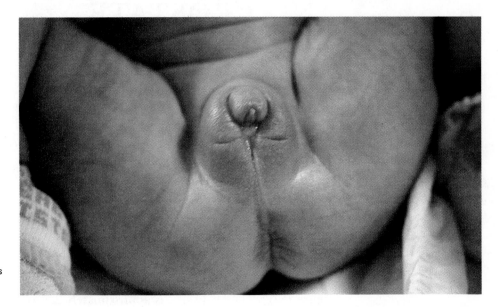

FIGURE 17-33
Ambiguous genitalia in infant.
Courtesy Patrick C. Walsh, MD, The Johns Hopkins University School of Medicine, Baltimore.

CHAPTER 18

ANUS, RECTUM, AND PROSTATE

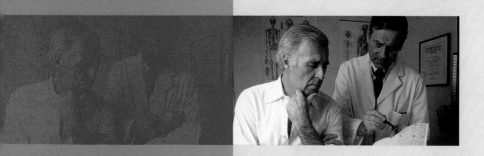

ANATOMY AND PHYSIOLOGY

The rectum and anus form the terminal portions of the gastrointestinal (GI) tract (Figure 18-1). The anal canal is approximately 2.5 to 4 cm long and opens onto the perineum. The tissue visible at the external margin of the anus is moist, hairless mucosa. Juncture with the perianal skin is characterized by increased pigmentation and, in the adult, the presence of hair.

The anal canal is normally kept securely closed by concentric rings of muscle, the internal and external sphincters. The internal ring of smooth muscle is under involuntary autonomic control. The urge to defecate occurs when the rectum fills with feces, which causes reflexive stimulation that relaxes the internal sphincter. Defecation is controlled by the striated external sphincter, which is under voluntary control. The lower half of the canal is supplied with somatic sensory nerves, making it sensitive to painful stimuli, whereas the upper half is under autonomic control and is relatively insensitive. Therefore conditions of the lower anus cause pain, whereas those of the upper anus may not.

Internally the anal canal is lined by columns of mucosal tissue (columns of Morgagni) that fuse to form the anorectal junction. The spaces between the columns are called crypts, into which anal glands empty. Inflammation of the crypts can result in fistula or fissure formation. Anastomosing veins cross the columns, forming a ring called the zona hemorrhoidalis. Internal hemorrhoids result from dilation of these veins. The lower segment of the anal canal contains a venous plexus that drains into the inferior rectal veins. Dilation of this plexus results in external hemorrhoids.

The rectum lies superior to the anus and is approximately 12 cm long. Its proximal end is continuous with the sigmoid colon. The distal end, the anorectal junction, is visible on proctoscopic examination as a sawtooth-like edge, but it is not palpable. Above the anorectal junction, the rectum dilates and turns posteriorly into the hollow of the coccyx and sacrum, forming the rectal ampulla, which stores flatus and feces. The rectal wall contains three semilunar transverse folds (Houston valves), with as yet poorly defined function. The lowest of these folds can be palpated by the examiner.

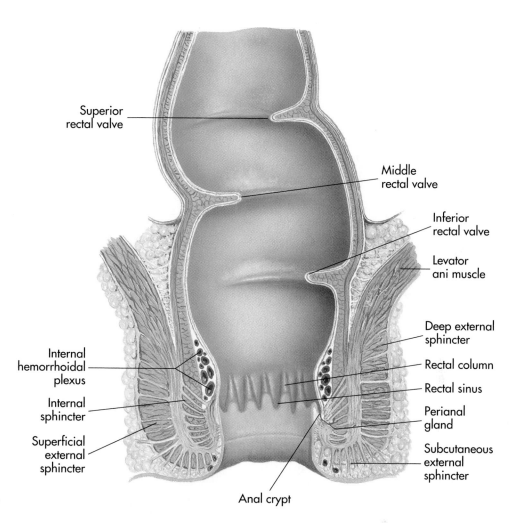

FIGURE 18-1

Anatomy of the anus and rectum.

In males the prostate gland is located at the base of the bladder and surrounds the urethra. It is composed of muscular and glandular tissue and is approximately $4 \times 3 \times 2$ cm. The posterior surface of the prostate gland is in close contact with the anterior rectal wall and is accessible by digital examination. It is convex and is divided by a shallow median sulcus into right and left lateral lobes. A third or median lobe, not palpable on examination, is composed of glandular tissue and lies between the ejaculatory duct and the urethra. It contains active secretory alveoli, which contribute to ejaculatory fluid. The seminal vesicles extend outward from the prostate (Figure 18-2).

In females the anterior rectal wall lies in contact with the vagina and is separated from it by the rectovaginal septum. See Chapter 16 (Female Genitalia) for a more detailed discussion.

INFANTS AND CHILDREN

At 7 weeks' gestation a portion of the caudal hindgut is divided by an anorectal septum into a urogenital sinus and a rectum. The urogenital sinus is covered by a membrane that develops into the anal opening by 8 weeks' gestation. Most anorectal malformations result from abnormalities in this partitioning process.

The first meconium stool is ordinarily passed within the first 24 to 48 hours after birth and indicates anal patency. Thereafter, it is common for newborns to have a stool after each feeding (the gastrocolic reflex). Both the internal and external sphincters are under involuntary reflexive control, because myelination of the spinal cord is incomplete.

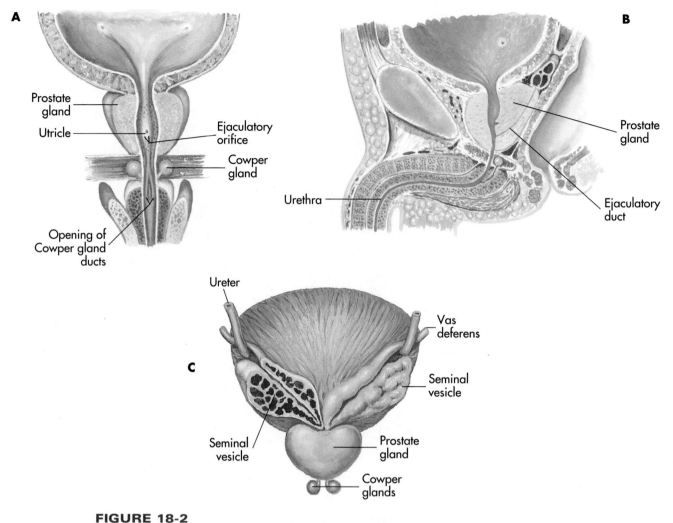

FIGURE 18-2
Anatomy of the prostate gland and seminal vesicles. **A,** Cross section. **B,** Lateral view. **C,** Posterior view.

By the end of the first year the infant may have one or two bowel movements daily. Control of the external anal sphincter is gradually achieved between the ages of 18 and 24 months.

In males the prostate is undeveloped, small, inactive, and not palpable on rectal examination. The prostate remains undeveloped until puberty, at which time androgenic influences prompt its growth and maturation. The initially minimal glandular component develops active secretory alveoli, and the prostate becomes functional.

PREGNANT WOMEN

In pregnancy, both pressure in the veins below the enlarged uterus and blood flow increase. Dietary habits and hormonal changes that decrease GI tract tone and motility produce constipation. These factors predispose pregnant women to the development of hemorrhoids. Labor, which results in pressure on the pelvic floor by the presenting part of the fetus and expulsive efforts of the woman, may also aggravate the condition, causing protrusion and inflammation of hemorrhoids during the puerperium.

OLDER ADULTS

Degeneration of afferent neurons in the rectal wall interferes with the process of relaxation of the internal sphincter in response to distention of the rectum. This can result in an elevated pressure threshold for the sensation of rectal distention in the older adult, with consequent retention of stool. Conversely, as the autonomically controlled internal sphincter loses tone, the external sphincter cannot by itself control the bowels, and the older adult may experience fecal incontinence.

In men the fibromuscular structures of the prostate gland atrophy, with loss of function of the secretory alveoli. However, the atrophy of aging is often obscured by benign hyperplasia of the glandular tissue. The muscular component of the prostate is progressively replaced by collagen.

REVIEW OF RELATED HISTORY

PRESENT PROBLEM

- Changes in bowel function
  - Character: number, frequency, consistency of stools; presence of mucus or blood; color (dark, bright red, black, light, or clay-colored); odor
  - Onset and duration: sudden or gradual, relation to dietary change, relation to stressful events
  - Accompanying symptoms: incontinence, flatus, pain, fever, nausea, vomiting, cramping, abdominal distention
  - Medications: iron, laxatives, stool softeners; prescription or nonprescription
- Anal discomfort: itching, pain, stinging, burning
  - Relation to body position and defecation
  - Straining at stool
  - Presence of mucus or blood
  - Interference with activities of daily living or sleep
  - Medications: hemorrhoid preparations; prescription or nonprescription
- Rectal bleeding
  - Color: bright or dark red, black
  - Relation to defecation
  - Amount: Spotting on toilet paper versus active bleeding
  - Accompanying changes in stool: color, frequency, consistency, shape, odor, presence of mucus
  - Associated symptoms: incontinence, flatus, rectal pain, abdominal pain or cramping, abdominal distention, weight loss
  - Medications: iron; prescription or nonprescription
- Males: changes in urinary function
  - History of enlarged prostate or prostatitis
  - Symptoms: hesitancy, urgency, nocturia, dysuria, change in force or caliber of stream, dribbling, urethral discharge

PAST MEDICAL HISTORY

- Hemorrhoids
- Spinal cord injury
- Males: prostatic hypertrophy or carcinoma
- Females: episiotomy or fourth-degree laceration during delivery

FAMILY HISTORY

- Rectal polyps
- Colon cancer (See the related Risk Factors box on p. 674).
- Prostatic cancer (See the related Risk Factors box, on p. 674).

> **RISK FACTORS   Colorectal Cancer**
>
> - Age over 40 (incidence peaks in ages 65 to 74)
> - Family history of colon cancer, familial polyposis, Gardner syndrome, Peutz-Jeghers syndrome
> - Personal history of colon polyps; Crohn disease; Gardner syndrome; ovarian, breast, or endometrial cancer; ulcerative colitis of more than 10 years' duration
> - Diet high in beef and animal fats, low in fiber
> - Exposure to asbestos, acrylics, and other carcinogens

> **RISK FACTORS   Prostate Cancer**
>
> - Age over 50 years
> - Race: black/African-American descent
> - Family history of prostate cancer
> - Diet high in animal fat

PERSONAL AND SOCIAL HISTORY

- Bowel habits and characteristics: timing, frequency, number, consistency, shape, color, odor
- Travel history: areas with high incidence of parasitic infestation, including zones in the United States
- Diet: inclusion of fiber foods (cereals, breads, nuts, fruits, vegetables) and concentrated high-fiber foods
- Risk factors for colorectal or prostatic cancer
- Use of alcohol

INFANTS AND CHILDREN

- Newborns: characteristics of stool
- Bowel movements accompanied by crying, straining, bleeding
- Feeding habits: types of foods, milk (bottle or breast for infants), appetite
- Age at which bowel control and toilet training were achieved
- Associated symptoms: episodes of diarrhea or constipation; tenderness when cleaning after a stool; perianal irritations; weight loss; nausea, vomiting; incontinence in toilet-trained child (association with convulsions)
- Congenital anomaly: imperforate anus, myelomeningocele, aganglionic megacolon

PREGNANT WOMEN

- Weeks' gestation and estimated date of delivery
- Exercise
- Fluid intake and dietary habits
- Medications: prenatal vitamins, iron

OLDER ADULTS

- Changes in bowel habits or character: frequency, number, color, consistency, shape, odor
- Associated symptoms: weight loss, rectal or abdominal pain, incontinence, flatus, episodes of constipation or diarrhea, abdominal distention, rectal bleeding
- Dietary changes: intolerance for certain foods, inclusion of fiber foods, regularity of eating habits, appetite
- Males: history of enlarged prostate, urinary symptoms (hesitancy, urgency, nocturia, dysuria, force and caliber of urinary stream, dribbling)

EXAMINATION AND FINDINGS

EQUIPMENT

- Gloves
- Water-soluble lubricant
- Penlight
- Drapes
- Fecal occult blood testing materials

PREPARATION

Although the rectal examination is generally uncomfortable and often embarrassing for the patient, it provides such important information that it is a mandatory part of every thorough examination. Be calm, slowly paced, and gentle in your touch. Explain what will happen step by step and let the patient know what to expect. A hurried or rough examination can cause unnecessary pain and sphincter spasm, and you can easily lose the trust and cooperation of the patient.

POSITIONING

EXAMINING PERSONS WITH DISABILITIES

The measures discussed in Chapter 16, Female Genitalia, would be applicable to both men and women for this examination.

The rectal examination can be performed with the patient in any of these positions: knee-chest, left lateral with hips and knees flexed, or standing with the hips flexed and the upper body supported by the examining table. In adult males, the latter two positions are satisfactory for most purposes and allow adequate visualization of the perianal and sacrococcygeal areas. In women the rectal examination is most often performed as part of the rectovaginal examination while the woman is in the lithotomy position (see Chapter 16, Female Genitalia).

Ask the patient to assume one of the examining positions, guiding gently with your hands when necessary. Use drapes but retain good visualization of the area. Glove one or both hands.

SACROCOCCYGEAL AND PERIANAL AREAS

Inspect the sacrococcygeal (pilonidal) and perianal areas. The skin should be smooth and uninterrupted. Inspect for lumps, rashes, inflammation, excoriation, scars, pilonidal dimpling, and tufts of hair at the pilonidal area. Fungal infection and pinworm infestation can cause perianal irritation. Fungal infection is more common in adults with diabetes, and pinworms are more common in children. Palpate the area. The discovery of tenderness and inflammation should alert you to the possibility of a perianal abscess, anorectal fistula or fissure, pilonidal cyst, or pruritus ani.

ANUS

Spread the patient's buttocks apart and inspect the anus. The use of a penlight or gooseneck lamp can assist in visualization. The skin around the anus will appear coarser and more darkly pigmented. Look for skin lesions, skin tags or warts, external hemorrhoids, fissures, and fistulas. Ask the patient to bear down. This will make fistulas, fissures, rectal prolapse, polyps, and internal hemorrhoids more readily apparent. Clock referents are used to describe the location of anal and rectal findings: 12:00 is in the ventral midline and 6:00 is in the dorsal midline.

SPHINCTER

IN PAIN?

The patient with a really acute problem will often shift uncomfortably from side to side when sitting.

Lubricate your index finger and press the pad of it against the anal opening (Figure 18-3, A). Ask the patient to bear down to relax the external sphincter. As relaxation occurs, slip the tip of the finger into the anal canal (Figure 18-3, B). Warn the patient that there may be a feeling of urgency for a bowel movement, assuring him or her that it will not happen. Ask the patient to tighten the external sphincter around your finger (Figure 18-4, A), noting its tone; it should tighten evenly with no discomfort to the patient. A lax sphincter may indicate neurologic deficit. An extremely tight sphincter can result from scarring, spasticity caused by a fissure or other lesion, inflammation, or anxiety about the examination.

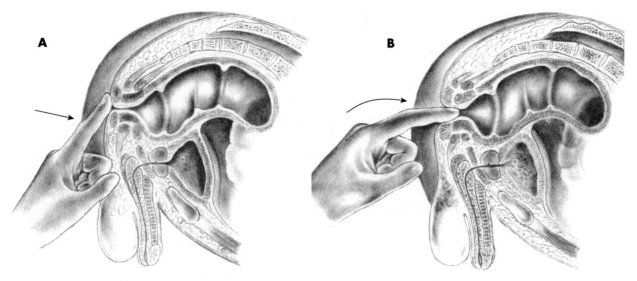

FIGURE 18-3
A, Correct procedure for introducing finger into rectum. Press pad of finger against the anal opening. **B,** As external sphincter relaxes, slip the fingertip into the anal canal. Note that patient is in the hips-flexed position.

An anal fistula or fissure may produce such extreme tenderness that you are not able to complete the examination without local anesthesia. Rectal pain is almost always indicative of a local disease. Look for irritation, rock hard constipation, rectal fissures, or thrombosed hemorrhoids. Always inquire about previous episodes of pain.

ANAL RING

Rotate your finger to examine the muscular anal ring (Figure 18-4, *B*). It should feel smooth and exert even pressure on the finger. Note any nodules or irregularities.

LATERAL AND POSTERIOR RECTAL WALLS

Insert your finger farther and palpate in sequence the lateral and posterior rectal walls, noting any nodules, masses, irregularities, polyps, or tenderness (Figure 18-4, *C*). The walls should feel smooth, even, and uninterrupted. Internal hemorrhoids are not ordinarily felt unless they are thrombosed. The examining finger can palpate a distance of about 6 to 10 cm into the rectum.

BIDIGITAL PALPATION

Bidigital palpation with the thumb and index finger can sometimes reveal more information than palpating with the index finger alone. To perform bidigital palpation, lightly press your thumb against the perianal tissue and bring your index finger toward the thumb. This technique is particularly useful for detecting a perianal abscess.

ANTERIOR RECTAL WALL AND PROSTATE

Rotate the index finger to palpate the anterior rectal wall as above. In males, you can palpate the posterior surface of the prostate gland (Figure 18-5). Tell the patient that he may feel the urge to urinate but that he will not. Note the size, contour, consistency, and mobility of the prostate. The gland should feel like a pencil eraser—firm, smooth, and slightly movable—and it should be nontender. A healthy prostate has a diameter of about 4 cm, with less than 1 cm protrusion into the rectum. Greater protrusion denotes prostatic enlargement, which should be noted and the amount of protrusion recorded. Prostate enlargement is classified by the amount of projection into the rectum: grade I is 1 to 2 cm of protrusion; grade II, 2 to 3 cm; grade III, 3 to 4 cm; and grade IV, more than 4 cm. The sulcus may be obliterated when the lobes are hypertrophied or neoplastic. A rubbery or boggy consistency is indicative of benign hyper-

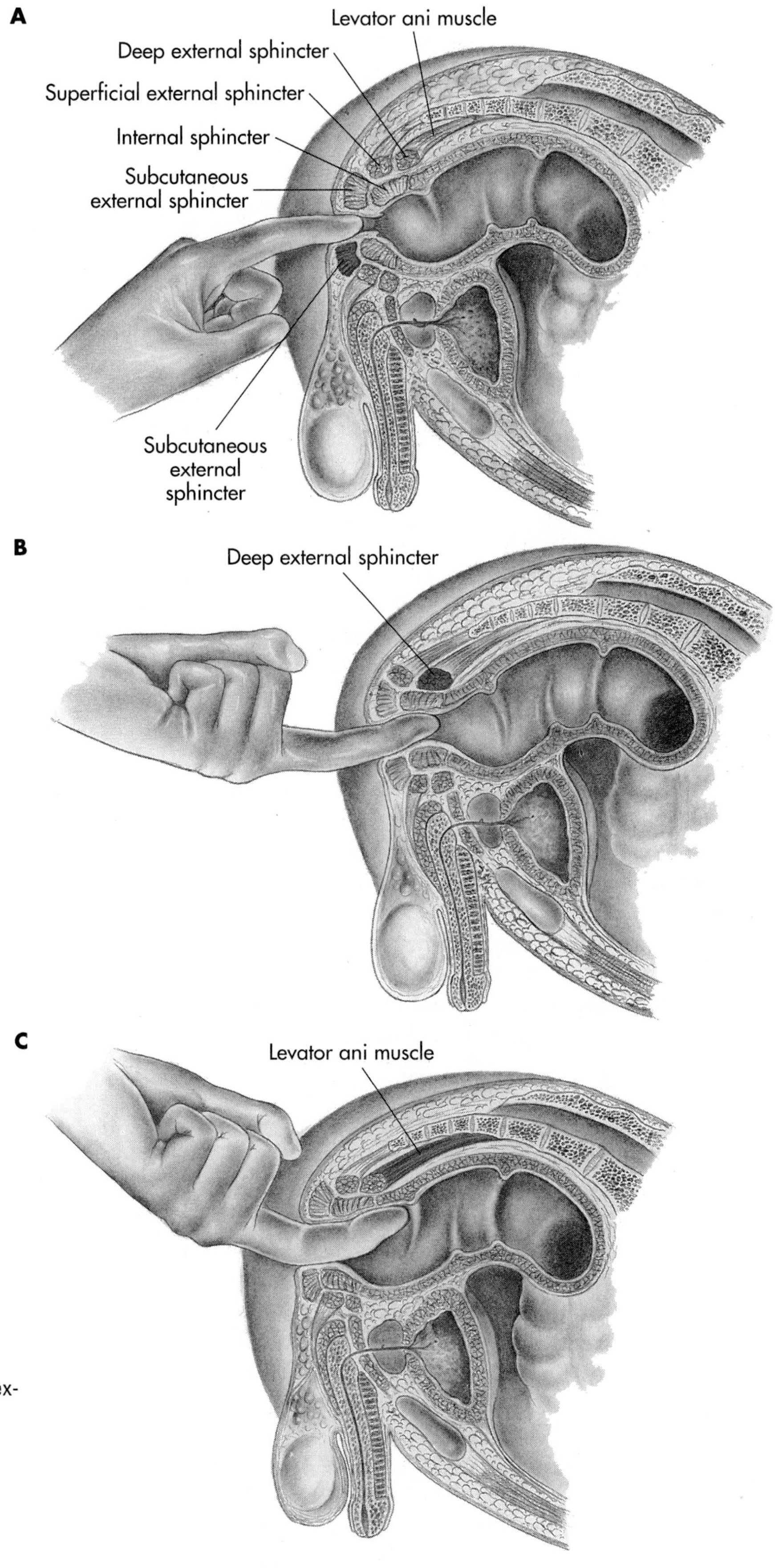
A
Levator ani muscle
Deep external sphincter
Superficial external sphincter
Internal sphincter
Subcutaneous external sphincter
Subcutaneous external sphincter
B
Deep external sphincter
C
Levator ani muscle

FIGURE 18-4
A, Palpation of subcutaneous external sphincter. Feel it tighten around the examining finger. **B,** Palpation of deep external sphincter. **C,** Palpation of the posterior rectal wall.

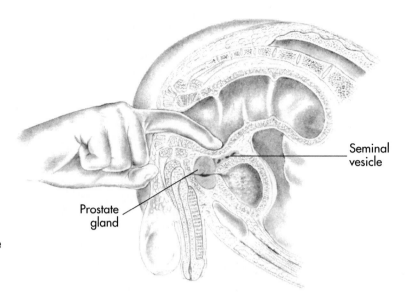

Seminal
vesicle

Prostate
gland

FIGURE 18-5
Palpation of the posterior surface
of the prostate gland. Feel for the
lateral lobes and median sulcus.

trophy, whereas stony hard nodularity may indicate carcinoma, prostatic calculi, or chronic fibrosis. Fluctuant softness suggests prostatic abscess. Identify the lateral lobes and the median sulcus. The prostatic lobes should feel symmetric. The seminal vesicles are not palpable unless they are inflamed.

Palpation of the prostate can force secretions through the urethral orifice. Any secretions that appear on the meatus should be cultured and examined microscopically. Specimen preparation techniques are described in Chapter 16 (Female Genitalia).

UTERUS AND CERVIX

In females a retroflexed or retroverted uterus is usually palpable through rectal examination. The cervix may be palpable through the anterior rectal wall (see Chapter 16, Female Genitalia). Do not mistake these structures or a tampon for a tumor.

After palpating the anterior wall in females and the prostate in males, ask the patient to bear down. This allows you to reach a few centimeters farther into the rectum. Because the anterior rectal wall is in contact with the peritoneum, you may be able to detect the tenderness of peritoneal inflammation and the nodularity of peritoneal metastases. The nodules, called shelf lesions, are palpable just above the prostate in males and in the cul-de-sac of females.

STOOL

Slowly withdraw your finger and examine it for any fecal material, which should be soft and brown (Box 18-2). Note any blood or pus. Very light tan or gray stool could indicate obstructive jaundice, whereas tarry black stool should make you suspect upper intestinal tract bleeding. A more subtle blood loss can result in a virtually unchanged color of the stool, but even a small amount will yield a positive test for occult blood (Box 18-3). Test any fecal material for blood using a chemical guaiac procedure.

Proctoscopy is indicated if there is persistent anal or rectal bleeding, any interruption in the smooth contour of the rectal wall on palpation, persistent pain with negative findings on rectal examination, or unexplained persistent stool changes.

INFANTS AND CHILDREN

Rectal examination is not automatically performed on infants and children unless there is a particular problem. An examination is required whenever there is any symptom that suggests an intraabdominal or pelvic problem, a mass or tenderness, bladder distention, bleeding, or rectal or bowel abnormalities. Deviation from the expected stool pattern in infants demands investigation (Table 18-1).

BOX 18-1 Screening for Prostate Cancer

Screening for prostate cancer is controversial, with recommendations varying among the major authorities. The following summarizes some of the various recommendations

Digital Rectal Examination (DRE)

Although most authorities agree on using DRE as part of periodic health screening for men over age 50, its role in screening for prostate cancer is not clear. Those authorities that do advocate DRE recommend it (in conjunction with PSA testing) as part of the periodic health examination in men over age 50 who are at average risk and in men over age 40 who are at higher risk (black; family history of prostate cancer).

Prostate-Specific Antigen (PSA)

PSA is a glycoprotein that is specific to the prostate but not to prostate cancer. It is produced by all types of prostate tissue whether healthy, hyperplastic, or malignant; therefore whether to screen asymptomatic men for prostate cancer with PSA testing is controversial. Screening can detect tumors at a more favorable stage, but there are no data indicating that PSA screening decreases mortality from prostate cancer.

Some authorities do not recommend use of PSA for routine screening. Those that do recommend it in conjunction with DRE as described previously (over age 50 for average-risk men; over age 40 for high-risk men)

PSA results under 4 ng/ml are usually considered normal. Results over 10 ng/ml are considered high; results between 4 and 10 ng/ml are considered borderline. The higher the PSA level the more likely the presence of prostatic cancer. However, men with prostate cancer can have a negative or borderline PSA level. A negative PSA and a negative DRE make the presence of cancer unlikely.

New types of PSA tests have been developed that may be useful when the usual PSA result is borderline:

PSA density (PSAD) is calculated by dividing the PSA number by the prostate volume (measured by TRUS, see below).

Age-specific ranges maybe useful as older men have higher PSA levels than younger men, even in the absence of cancer.

PSA velocity measures how quickly the PSA level rises over time. Serial testing may be appropriate for managing borderline results.

Free PSA ratio indicates how much PSA circulates unbound and how much is bound. For PSA results in the borderline range, a low free PSA ratio increases the chance that prostate cancer is present and suggests the need for biopsy.

Biopsy

Biopsy of the prostate tissue is recommended when the PSA level is high. Results in the borderline range may be an indication for biopsy if the DRE is abnormal. Biopsy also may be used when the Free PSA ratio is low, in the presence of borderline PSA results.

Transurethral Ultrasonography (TRUS)

TRUS is used when the PSA is borderline and the DRE is normal. TRUS may be able to indicate areas of the prostate that require biopsy. It can also be used to determine prostate volume, which can be used in the calculation of PSA density.

BOX 18-2 Stool Characteristics in Disease

Changes in the shape, content, or consistency of the stool suggest that some disease process is present. Stool characteristics can sometimes point to the type of disorder present; therefore you should be familiar with the following characteristics and associated disorders:

- Intermittent, pencil-like stools suggest a spasmodic contraction in the rectal area.
- Persistent, pencil-like stools indicate permanent stenosis from scarring or from pressure of a malignancy.
- Pipestem stools and ribbon stools indicate lower rectal stricture.
- A large amount of mucus in the fecal matter is characteristic of intestinal inflammation and mucous colitis.
- Small flecks of blood-stained mucus in liquid feces are indicative of amebiasis.
- Fatty stools are seen in patients with pancreatic disorders and malabsorption syndromes.
- Stools the color of aluminum (caused by a mixture of melena and fat) occur in tropical sprue, carcinoma of the hepatopancreatic ampulla, and children treated with sulfonamides for diarrhea.

It is imperative that you respect the child's modesty and apprehension. Careful explanation of each step in the process is necessary for the child who is old enough to understand.

Routinely inspect the anal region and perineum, examining the surrounding buttocks for redness, masses, and evidence of change in firmness. Inspect for swollen, tender perirectal protrusion, abscesses, and possibly rectal fistulae. A variety of problems can be discovered by this inspection. Shrunken buttocks suggests a chronic debilitating disease. Asymmetric creases occur with congenital dislocation of the hips.

BOX 18-3 **Common Causes of Rectal Bleeding**

There are numerous reasons that blood can appear in the feces, ranging from benign, self-limiting events to serious, life-threatening disease. Following are some common causes:

- Anal fissures
- Anaphylactoid purpura
- Aspirin-containing medications
- Bleeding disorders
- Coagulation disorders
- Colitis
- Dysentery, acute and amebic
- Esophageal varices
- Familial telangiectasia
- Foreign body trauma
- Hemorrhoids
- Hiatal hernia
- Hookworm
- Intussusception
- Iron poisoning
- Meckel diverticulum
- Neoplasms of any kind
- Oral steroids
- Peptic ulcers, acute and chronic
- Polyps, single or multiple
- Regional enteritis
- Strangulated hernia
- Swallowed blood
- Thrombocytopenia
- Volvulus

TABLE 18-1 **Sequence and Description of Stools in Infants**

Infants	Type of Stool
Newborn	Meconium: greenish-black, viscous, contains occult blood; first stool is sterile; passed within 24 hours by 94% of newborns
3-6 days old	Transitional: thin, slimy, brown to green
Breast-fed	Mushy, loose, golden yellow; frequency varies from after each feeding to every few days; nonirritating to skin
Formula-fed	Light yellow, characteristic foul odor, irritating to skin

Data from Lowdermilk, Perry, Bobak, 1997.

Perirectal redness and irritation are suggestive of pinworms, *Candida,* or other irritants of the diaper area. Rectal prolapse results from constipation, diarrhea, or sometimes severe coughing or straining. Hemorrhoids are rare in children, and their presence suggests a serious underlying problem such as portal hypertension. Small flat flaps of skin around the rectum (condylomas) may be syphilitic in origin. Sinuses, tufts of hair, and dimpling in the pilonidal area may indicate lower spinal deformities.

Lightly touch the anal opening, which should produce anal contraction (described by practitioners as an "anal wink"). Lack of contraction may indicate a lower spinal cord lesion.

Examine the patency of the anus and its position in all newborn infants. To determine patency, insert a lubricated catheter no more than 1 cm into the rectum. Patency is usually confirmed by passage of meconium. Occasionally a perianal fistula may be confused with an anal orifice. Be careful in making this judgment. Sometimes the anal orifice can seem appropriate, yet there may be atresia just inside or a few centimeters within the rectum. Rectal examination or insertion of a catheter does not always provide definitive assessment, and radiologic studies may be necessary. If there is no evidence of stool in the newborn, suspect rectal atresia, Hirschsprung disease (congenital megacolon), or cystic fibrosis.

Perform the rectal examination in infants and young children with the child lying on his or her back. You may hold the child's feet together and flex the knees and hips on the abdomen with one hand, using the gloved index finger of your other hand for the examination (Figure 18-6). Some examiners are reluctant to use the index fin-

NEWBORN RECTAL EXAMINATION

When attempting to perform a digital rectal examination on a newborn, use your pinky finger and don't force.

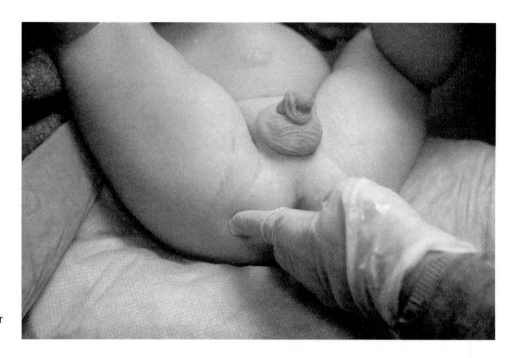

FIGURE 18-6
Positioning the infant or child for rectal examination.

ger because of its size, choosing instead the fifth finger. However, even with the smallest of adult fingers, some bleeding and transient prolapse of the rectum often occur right after examination. Always warn the parents of this possibility.

Assess the tone of the rectal sphincter. It should feel snug but neither too tight nor too loose. A very tight sphincter can cause enough tension to produce a stenosis, which leads to stool retention and pain during a bowel movement. A lax sphincter is associated with lesions of the peripheral spinal nerves or spinal cord, *Shigella* infection, and previous fecal impactions.

Feel for feces in the rectum. Chronic constipation in children with mental deficiency or emotional problems is often associated with a rectum distended with feces. A consistently empty rectum in the presence of constipation is a clue to the diagnosis of Hirschsprung disease. A fecal mass in the rectum accompanying diarrhea suggests overflow diarrhea. Stool recovered on the examining finger should be tested for occult blood.

A rectal examination in the young female gives good access to information about the cervix and uterus (see Chapter 16, Female Genitalia). The ovaries are not usually palpable on rectal examination.

In boys the prostate is usually not felt. A palpable prostate in preadolescent boys suggests precocious puberty or some virilizing disease.

The rectum can be further evaluated for suspected fissures, fistulae, or polyps by using a small proctoscope or even a wide-mouth speculum on the otoscope.

Rectal examination should be a usual part of the physical examination for adolescents. The same procedures and guidelines that are used for adults apply to adolescents. Be especially sensitive to a first examination, and spend additional time explaining what to expect. Illustrations and models can be very helpful.

PREGNANT WOMEN

The examination of the rectum provides information about rectovaginal musculature and more specific information about the cervix and uterus (see Chapter 16, Female Genitalia). During pregnancy the stool color may be dark green or black due to the consumption of iron preparations. Iron may also cause diarrhea or constipation. Assessment for hemorrhoids should include both external and internal evaluation. Hemorrhoids are usually not found early in pregnancy. However, late in pregnancy they may be an expected variation. Evaluate hemorrhoids for their size, extent, location (internal or external), discomfort to the patient, and for signs of infection or bleeding.

OLDER ADULTS

The examination procedure and findings for the older adult are much the same as those for the younger adult. The older patient may be more limited in ability to assume a position other than the left lateral. Sphincter tone may be somewhat decreased. Older adults commonly experience fecal impaction resulting from constipation. Older males are far more likely to have an enlarged prostate, which will be felt as smooth, rubbery, and symmetric. The median sulcus may or may not be obliterated. Older adults are more likely to have polyps and are at higher risk for carcinoma, making the rectal examination particularly important in this age group.

SAMPLE DOCUMENTATION

Anus, rectum, prostate: Perianal area intact without lesions. An external skin tag is visible at 6 o'clock. No fissures or fistulas. Sphincter tightens evenly. Prostate is symmetric, smooth, firm, nontender, without enlargement of nodules. Rectal walls free of masses. Moderate amount of soft stool present; occult blood test negative.

For additional sample documentation see Chapter 24, Recording Information.

SUMMARY OF EXAMINATION — Anus, Rectum, and Prostate

1. Inspect the sacrococcygeal and perianal area for the following (p. 675):
   - Skin characteristics
   - Lesions
   - Pilonidal dimpling and/or tufts of hair
   - Inflammation
   - Excoriation
2. Inspect the anus for the following (p. 675):
   - Skin characteristics and tags
   - Lesions, fissures, hemorrhoids, or polyps
   - Fistulas
   - Prolapse
3. Insert finger and assess sphincter tone (p. 675).
4. Palpate the muscular ring for the following (p. 676):
   - Smoothness
   - Evenness
5. Palpate the lateral, posterior, and anterior rectal walls for the following (p. 676):
   - Nodules, masses, or polyps
   - Tenderness
   - Irregularities
6. In males, palpate the posterior surface of the prostate gland through the anterior rectal wall for the following (pp. 676-678):
   - Size
   - Contour
   - Consistency
   - Mobility
7. In females, palpate the cervix and uterus through the anterior rectal wall for the following (p. 678):
   - Size
   - Shape
   - Position
   - Smoothness
   - Mobility
8. Have the patient bear down and palpate deeper for the following (p. 678):
   - Tenderness
   - Nodules
9. Withdraw the finger and examine fecal material for the following (p. 678):
   - Color
   - Consistency
   - Blood or pus
   - Occult blood by chemical test

COMMON ABNORMALITIES

ANUS, RECTUM, AND SURROUNDING SKIN

PILONIDAL CYST OR SINUS

Most pilonidal cysts and sinuses are first diagnosed in young adults, although they are usually a congenital anomaly. Located in the midline, superficial to the coccyx and lower sacrum, the cyst or sinus is seen as a dimple with a sinus tract opening. The opening may contain a tuft of hair and be surrounded by erythema. A cyst may be palpable. The condition is usually asymptomatic, but it is sometimes complicated by an abscess, secondary infection, or fistula.

PERIANAL AND PERIRECTAL ABSCESSES

These abscesses appear as an area of swelling with variable degrees of erythema of the anus, both internally and externally. The abscess is painful and tender, and usually the patient has a fever (Figure 18-7).

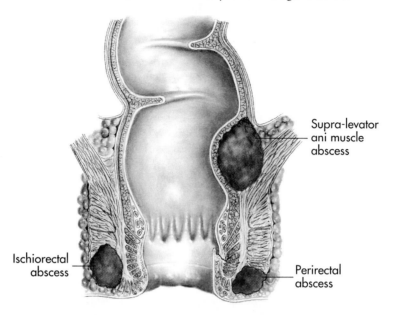

FIGURE 18-7
Perianal and perirectal abscesses. Common sites of abscess formation.

ANORECTAL FISSURE AND FISTULA

A tear in the anal mucosa (*fissure*) appears most often in the posterior midline, although it can also occur in the anterior midline. The fissure is usually caused by traumatic passage of large, hard stools. A sentinel skin tag may be seen at the lower edge of the fissure. There may be ulceration through which muscles of the internal sphincter are seen. The patient may have symptoms of pain, itching, or bleeding. The internal sphincter is spastic. Examination is painful and may require local anesthesia (Figure 18-8).

An *anorectal fistula* is an inflammatory tract that runs from the anus or rectum and opens onto the surface of the perianal skin or other tissue. It is caused by drainage of a perianal or perirectal abscess. Serosanguinous or purulent drainage may appear with compression of the area. The external opening is usually seen as elevated red granular tissue.

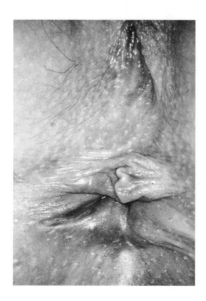

FIGURE 18-8
Lateral and fissure in adult.
Courtesy Gershon Efron, MD, Sinai Hospital of Baltimore.

PRURITUS ANI

Chronic inflammation of perianal skin results in excoriation, thickening, and pigmentation. The patient complains of burning or itching that may interfere with sleep. It is commonly caused by fungal infection in adults and by parasites in children.

HEMORRHOIDS

External hemorrhoids are varicose veins that originate below the anorectal line and are covered by anal skin. They may cause itching and bleeding with defecation. Usually not visible at rest, they can protrude on standing and straining at stool. If not reduced, they can become edematous and thrombosed and may require surgical removal. Thrombosed hemorrhoids appear as blue, shiny masses at the anus. Hemorrhoidal skin tags, which can appear at the site of resolved hemorrhoids, are fibrotic or flaccid and painless (Figure 18-9, *A*).

Internal hemorrhoids are varicose veins that originate above the anorectal junction and are covered by rectal mucosa. They produce soft swellings that are not palpable on rectal examination and are not visible unless they prolapse through the anus. They do not cause discomfort unless they are thrombosed, prolapsed, or infected. Bleeding may occur with or without defecation. Daily bleeding may be sufficient to cause anemia. Proctoscopy is usually required for diagnosis (Figure 18-9, *B*).

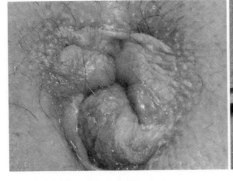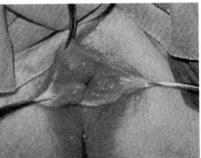

FIGURE 18-9
A, Prolapsed hemorrhoids.
B, Primary internal hemorrhoids.
Courtesy Gershon Efron, MD, Sinai Hospital of Baltimore.

POLYPS

Occurring anywhere in the intestinal tract, polyps are a relatively common finding. They may be adenomas or inflammatory in origin and can occur singly or in profusion. Polyps are usually evidenced by rectal bleeding, and it is not uncommon to find a polyp protruding through the rectum. They are sometimes palpable on rectal examination as soft nodules and can be either pedunculated (on a stalk) or sessile (closely adhering to the mucosal wall). However, because of their soft consistency, polyps may be difficult to feel on palpation. Proctoscopy is usually required for diagnosis, and biopsy may be performed to distinguish them from carcinoma (Figure 18-10).

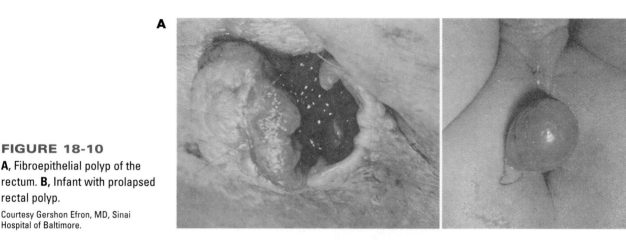

FIGURE 18-10
A, Fibroepithelial polyp of the rectum. **B,** Infant with prolapsed rectal polyp.
Courtesy Gershon Efron, MD, Sinai Hospital of Baltimore.

RECTAL CARCINOMA	Cancer of the rectum is usually felt as a sessile polypoid mass with nodular raised edges and areas of ulceration. The consistency is often stony, and the contour is irregular. Rectal carcinoma is often asymptomatic, so routine rectal examination is essential for adults.
INTRAPERITONEAL METASTASES	Malignant metastases may develop in the pelvis anterior to the rectum. These can be felt as a hard, nodular shelf at the tip of the examining finger.
RECTAL PROLAPSE	The rectal mucosa, with or without the muscular wall, prolapses through the anal ring as the patient strains at stool. A prolapse of the mucosa is pink and looks like a doughnut or rosette. Complete prolapse involving the muscular wall is larger, red, and has circular folds. Rectal prolapse in children is associated with cystic fibrosis (Figure 18-11).

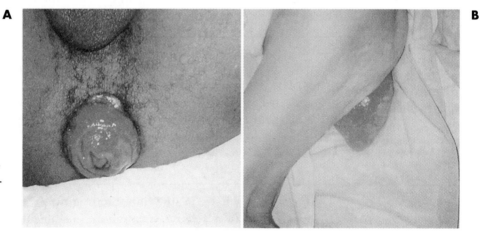

FIGURE 18-11
Prolapse of the rectum. **A,** Complete prolapse. **B,** Complete prolapse in an elderly patient.
Courtesy Gershon Efron, MD, Sinai Hospital of Baltimore.

PROSTATE

PROSTATITIS

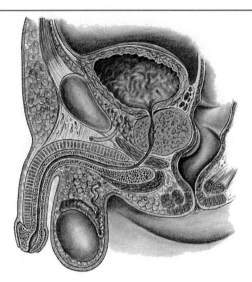

FIGURE 18-12
Prostatitis.

In *acute prostatitis* the prostate is enlarged, acutely tender, and often asymmetric. The patient may also have urethral discharge and fever. An abscess may develop, which is felt as a fluctuant mass in the prostate. The seminal vesicles are often involved and may be dilated and tender on palpation (Figure 18-12).

Chronic prostatitis is usually asymptomatic. However, the prostate may feel boggy, enlarged, and tender or have palpable areas of fibrosis that simulate neoplasm.

CHILDREN

ENTEROBIASIS (ROUNDWORM, PINWORM)	The adult nematode (parasite) lives in the rectum or colon and emerges onto perianal skin to lay eggs while the child sleeps. The patient experiences intense itching of the perianal area, and perianal irritation often results from scratching. The parents often describe unexplained	irritability in the infant or child, especially at night. The nematodes can be seen on microscopic examination. To obtain a specimen, press the sticky side of cellulose tape against the perianal folds and then press the tape on a glass slide.
IMPERFORATE ANUS	A variety of anorectal malformations can occur during fetal development (Figure 18-13). The rectum may end blindly, be stenosed, or have a fistulous connection to the perineum, urinary tract, or, in females, the vagina. The condition is usu-	ally diagnosed by rectal examination and confirmed by lack of passage of stool within the first 48 hours of life (Figures 18-14 and 18-15). Radiographic confirmation may be necessary.

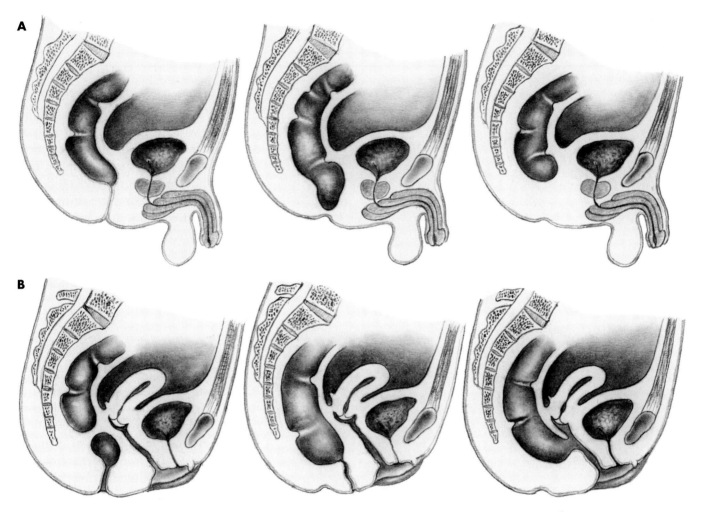

FIGURE 18-13

Imperforate anus: various anorectal malformation. **A,** *Left to right,* Congenital anal stenosis, anal membrane atresia, anal agenesis. **B,** *Left to right,* Rectal atresia, retroperineal fistula, rectovaginal fistula.

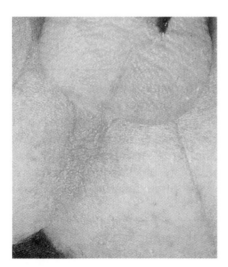

FIGURE 18-14

Imperforate anus.

From *Diagnostic picture tests in clinical medicine,*
1984. By permission of Mosby International.

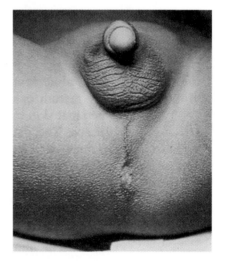

FIGURE 18-15

Rectal atresia.

Courtesy Gershon Efron, MD, Sinai Hospital of
Baltimore.

BENIGN PROSTATIC HYPERTROPHY

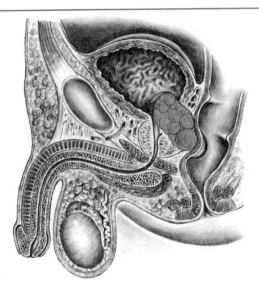

FIGURE 18-16
Benign prostatic hypertrophy.

Benign prostatic hypertrophy (BPH) is common in men over age 50. The gland begins to grow at adolescence, continuing to enlarge with advancing age. Growth of the prostate parallels the increased incidence of BPH. Urinary symptoms include hesitancy, decreased force and caliber of stream, dribbling, incomplete emptying of the bladder, frequency, urgency, nocturia, and dysuria. On rectal examination the prostate feels smooth, rubbery, symmetric, and enlarged. The median sulcus may or may not be obliterated (Figure 18-16).

PROSTATIC CARCINOMA

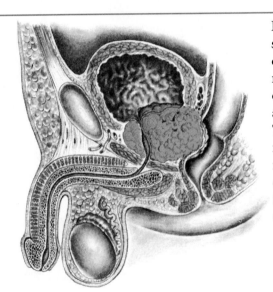

FIGURE 18-17
Carcinoma of prostate.

Rare before age 50, the incidence of prostatic cancer increases with age. Early carcinoma is asymptomatic. As the malignancy advances, symptoms of urinary obstruction occur. On rectal examination a hard, irregular nodule may be palpable. The prostate feels asymmetric, and the median sulcus is obliterated as the carcinoma enlarges. Prostatic calculi and chronic inflammation produce similar findings, and biopsy is required for differential diagnosis (Figure 18-17).

Remember to check *http://www1.mosby.com/physexam_seidel*

CHAPTER 19

MUSCULOSKELETAL SYSTEM

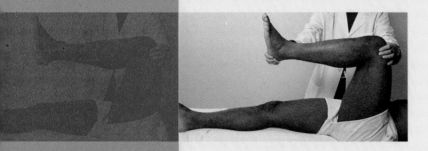

The musculoskeletal system provides the stability and mobility necessary for physical activity. Physical performance requires bones, muscles, and joints that function smoothly and effortlessly. Because the musculoskeletal system serves as the body's main line of defense against external forces, injuries are common, and all have the potential for producing permanent disability. Numerous disease processes, including metabolic disorders, affect the musculoskeletal system and can ultimately cause disability.

Disorders that affect the musculoskeletal system may also arise from the neurologic system. For example, delay in an expected muscle response can be caused by pain from a bone or muscle injury, or it may be the result of a cerebellar defect. A careful neurologic examination will help differentiate the cause.

ANATOMY AND PHYSIOLOGY

The musculoskeletal system is a bony structure with its joints held together by ligaments, attached to muscles by tendons, and cushioned by cartilage (Figures 19-1 and 19-2). In addition to giving structure to the soft tissues of the body and allowing movement, the functions of the musculoskeletal system include protecting vital organs, providing storage space for minerals, producing blood cells (hematopoiesis), and resorbing and reforming itself.

Most joints are diarthrodial—freely moving articulations that are enclosed by a capsule of fibrous articular cartilage, ligaments, and cartilage covering the ends of the opposing bones. A synovial membrane lines the articular cavity and secretes the serous lubricating synovial fluid. Bursae develop in the spaces of connective tissue between tendons, ligaments, and bones to promote ease of motion at points where friction would otherwise occur. Table 19-1, p. 695, describes the classification of joints.

The variability in size and strength of muscles among individuals is influenced by genetic constitution, nutrition, and exercise. At all ages, muscles increase in size with use and shrink with inactivity. Individual muscles must have intact neurologic innervation to function and to move joints through their full range of motion.

Text continued on p. 695.

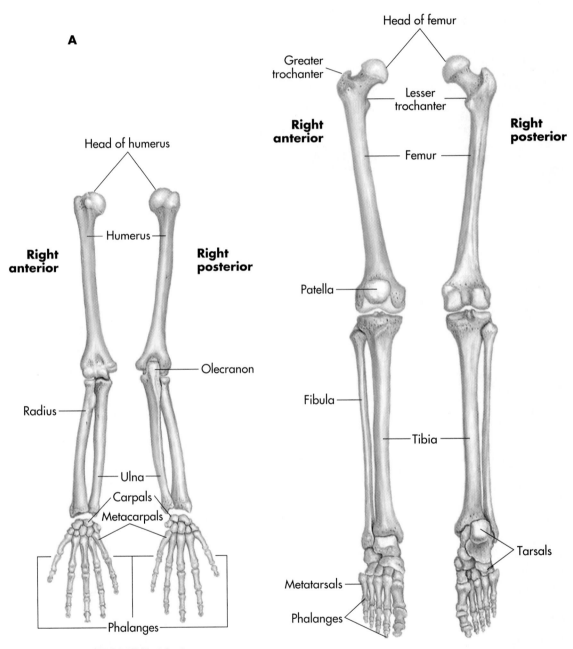

FIGURE 19-1

A, Bones of the upper and lower extremities.

B   **Anterior**   **Posterior**

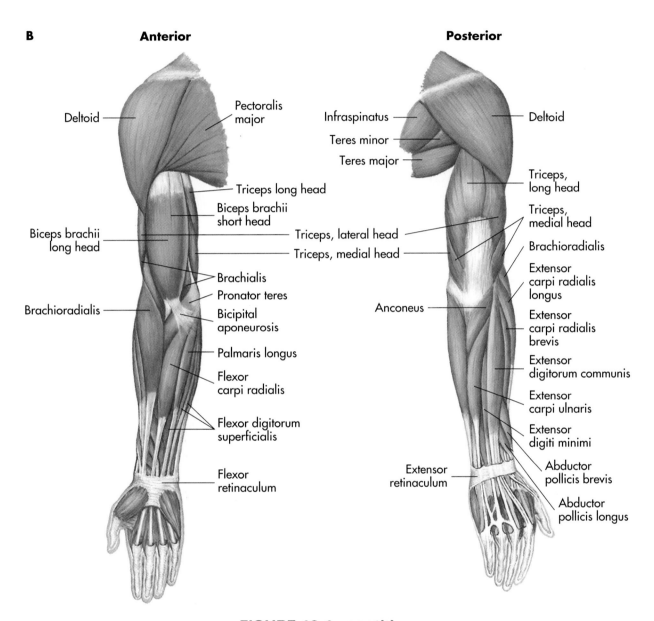

Deltoid

Pectoralis
major

Infraspinatus

Deltoid

Teres minor

Teres major

Triceps,
long head

Triceps long head

Biceps brachii
short head

Biceps brachii
long head

Triceps, lateral head

Triceps,
medial head

Triceps, medial head

Brachioradialis

Brachialis

Extensor
carpi radialis
longus

Pronator teres

Brachioradialis

Bicipital
aponeurosis

Anconeus

Extensor
carpi radialis
brevis

Palmaris longus

Extensor
digitorum communis

Flexor
carpi radialis

Extensor
carpi ulnaris

Flexor digitorum
superficialis

Extensor
digiti minimi

Extensor
retinaculum

Abductor
pollicis brevis

Flexor
retinaculum

Abductor
pollicis longus

FIGURE 19-1—cont'd
B, Muscles of the upper extremities.

C

Anterior

Posterior

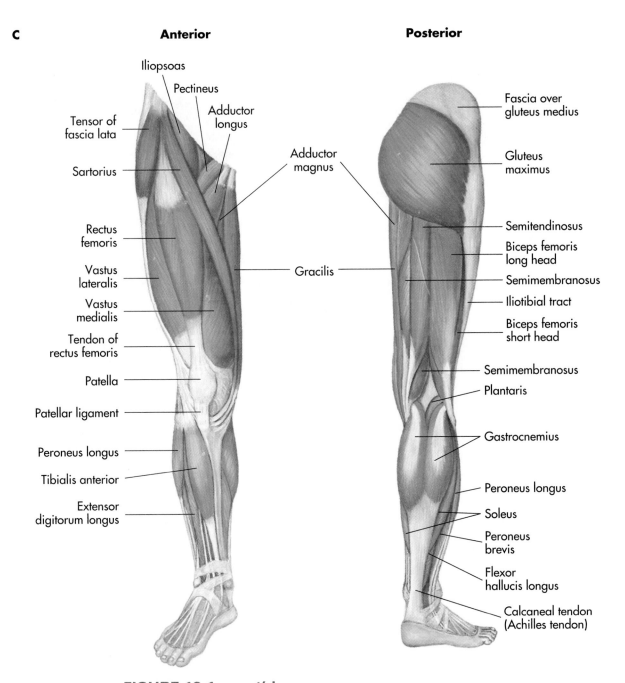

Iliopsoas

Pectineus

Adductor longus

Tensor of fascia lata

Sartorius

Adductor magnus

Rectus femoris

Vastus lateralis

Gracilis

Vastus medialis

Tendon of rectus femoris

Patella

Patellar ligament

Peroneus longus

Tibialis anterior

Extensor digitorum longus

Fascia over gluteus medius

Gluteus maximus

Semitendinosus

Biceps femoris long head

Semimembranosus

Iliotibial tract

Biceps femoris short head

Semimembranosus

Plantaris

Gastrocnemius

Peroneus longus

Soleus

Peroneus brevis

Flexor hallucis longus

Calcaneal tendon (Achilles tendon)

FIGURE 19-1—cont'd

C, Muscles of the lower extremities.

A   **Anterior**   **Posterior**   **B**

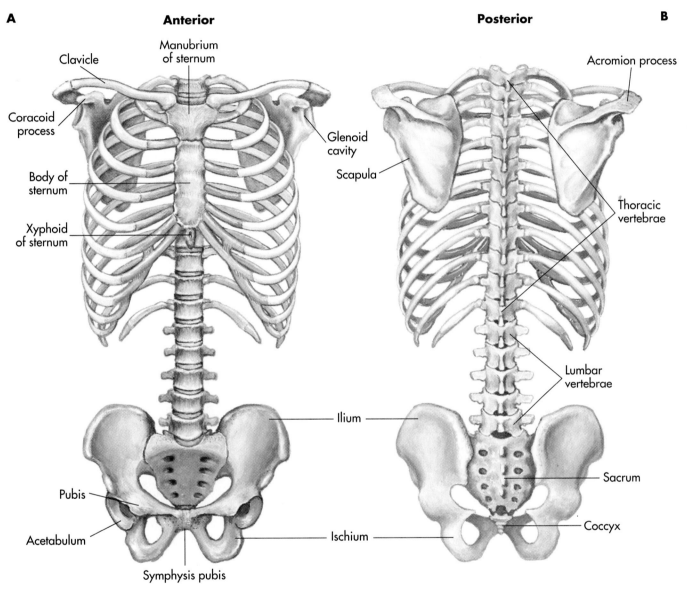

FIGURE 19-2
A, Bones of the trunk, anterior view. **B,** Bones of the trunk, posterior view.

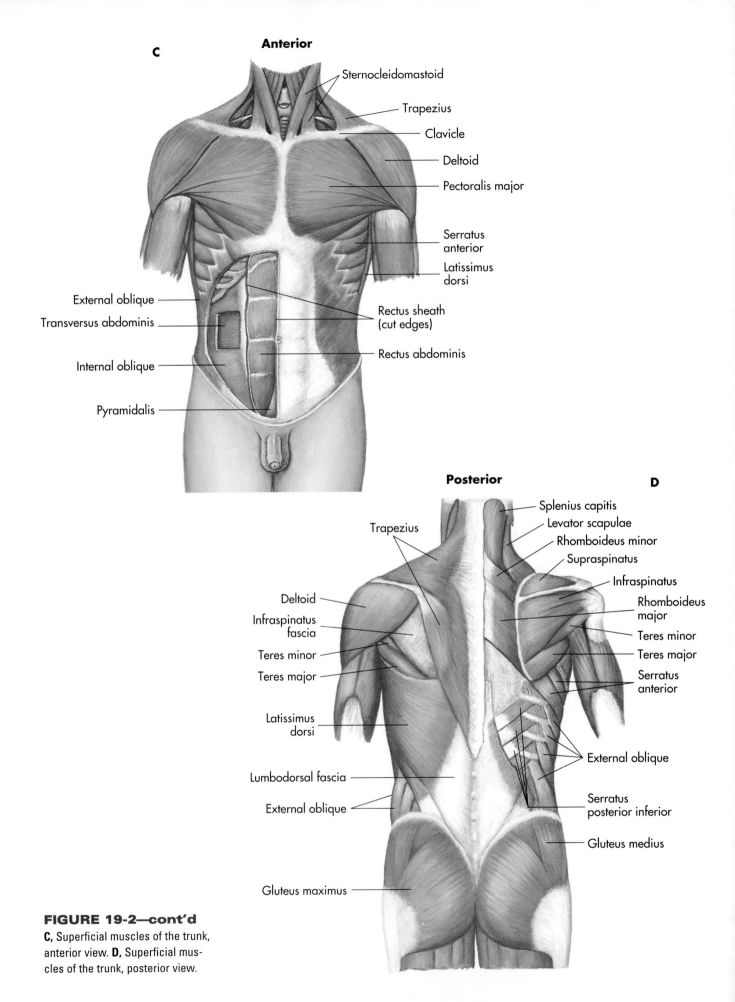

Anterior

C

Sternocleidomastoid

Trapezius

Clavicle

Deltoid

Pectoralis major

Serratus anterior

Latissimus dorsi

External oblique

Transversus abdominis

Internal oblique

Pyramidalis

Rectus sheath (cut edges)

Rectus abdominis

Posterior

D

Splenius capitis

Levator scapulae

Rhomboideus minor

Supraspinatus

Infraspinatus

Rhomboideus major

Teres minor

Teres major

Serratus anterior

External oblique

Serratus posterior inferior

Gluteus medius

Trapezius

Deltoid

Infraspinatus fascia

Teres minor

Teres major

Latissimus dorsi

Lumbodorsal fascia

External oblique

Gluteus maximus

FIGURE 19-2—cont'd
C, Superficial muscles of the trunk, anterior view. **D,** Superficial muscles of the trunk, posterior view.

TABLE 19-1	Classification of Joints	
Type of Joint	**Example**	**Description**
Synarthrosis		No movement is permitted
Suture	Cranial sutures	United by thin layer of fibrous tissue
Synchondrosis	Joint between the epiphysis and diaphysis of long bones	A temporary joint in which the cartilage is replaced by bone later in life
Amphiarthrosis		Slightly movable joint
Symphysis	Symphysis pubis	Bones are connected by a fibrocartilage disk
Syndesmosis	Radius-ulna articulation	Bones are connected by ligaments
Diarthrosis (synovial)		Freely movable; enclosed by joint capsule, lined with synovial membrane
Ball and socket	Hip	Widest range of motion, movement in all planes
Hinge	Elbow	Motion limited to flexion and extension in a single plane
Pivot	Atlantoaxis	Motion limited to rotation
Condyloid	Wrist between radius and carpals	Motion in two planes at right angles to each other, but no radial rotation
Saddle	Thumb at carpal-metacarpal joint	Motion in two planes at right angles to each other, but no axial rotation
Gliding	Intervertebral	Motion limited to gliding

HEAD AND SPINE

The temporomandibular joint consists of the articulation between the mandible and the temporal bone in the cranium. Each is located in the depression just anterior to the tragus of the ear. The hinge action of the joint opens and closes the mouth, whereas the gliding action permits lateral movement, protrusion, and retraction of the mandible (Figures 19-3 and 19-4). See Chapter 9, Head and Neck, for a description of the fused bones of the cranium.

The spine is composed of cervical, thoracic, lumbar, and sacral vertebrae. Except for the sacral vertebrae, they are separated from each other by fibrocartilaginous disks. Each disk has a nucleus of fibrogelatinous material that cushions the vertebral bodies (Figure 19-5). The vertebrae form a series of joints that glide slightly over each others' surfaces, permitting movement on several axes. The cervical vertebrae are the most mobile. Flexion and extension occur between the skull and C1, whereas rotation occurs between C1 and C2. The sacral vertebrae are fused and, with the coccyx, form the posterior portion of the pelvis.

UPPER EXTREMITIES

The glenohumoral joint (shoulder) consists of the articulation between the humerus and the glenoid fossa of the scapula. The acromion and coracoid processes and the ligament between them form the arch surrounding and protecting the joint. The shoulder is a ball and socket joint that permits movement of the humerus on many axes (Figure 19-6).

Two additional joints adjacent to the glenohumeral joint complete the articulation of the shoulder girdle. The acromioclavicular joint consists of the articulation between the acromion process and the clavicle, and the sternoclavicular joint consists of the articulation between the manubrium of the sternum and the clavicle.

The elbow consists of the articulation of the humerus, radius, and ulna. Its three contiguous surfaces are enclosed in a single synovial cavity, with the ligaments of the radius and ulna protecting the joint. A bursa lies between the olecranon and the skin (Figure 19-7). The elbow is a hinge joint, permitting movement of the humerus and ulna on one plane (flexion and extension).

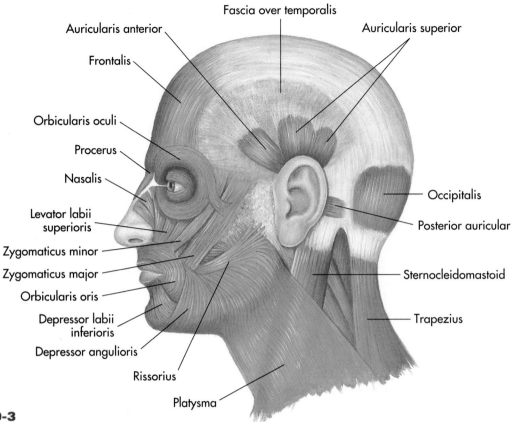

FIGURE 19-3
Muscles of the face and head, left lateral view.

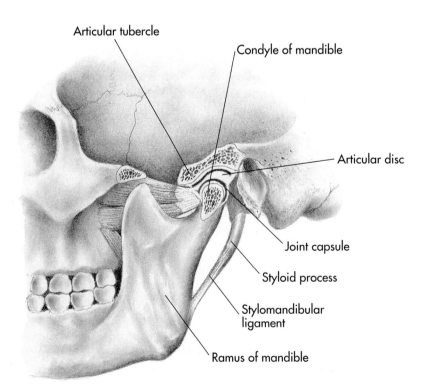

FIGURE 19-4
Structures of the temporomandibular joint.

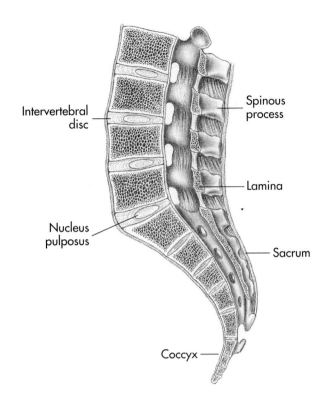

FIGURE 19-5

Structures of vertebral joints.

From Thompson et al, 1997.

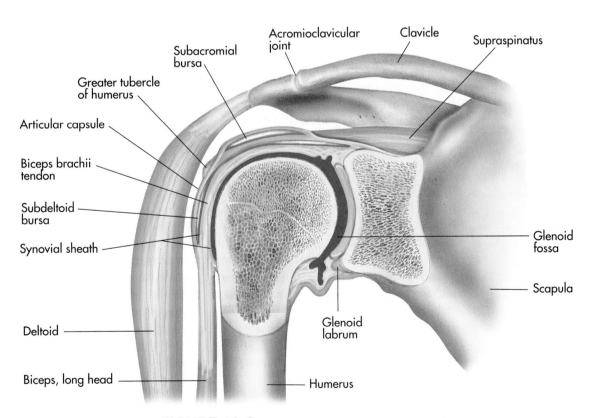

FIGURE 19-6

Structures of glenohumeral and acromioclavicular joints.

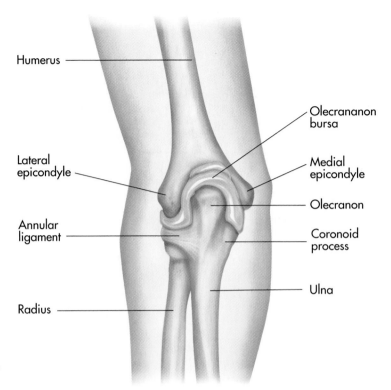

Humerus

Olecrananon bursa

Lateral epicondyle

Medial epicondyle

Olecranon

Annular ligament

Coronoid process

Ulna

Radius

FIGURE 19-7
Structures of the left elbow joint, posterior view.

The forearm joints consist of the articulations between the radius and ulna at both the proximal and distal locations. They are important for pronation and supination.

The radiocarpal joint (wrist) consists of the articulation of the radius and the carpal bones. Additional articulations occur between the proximal and distal row of carpal bones. An articular disk separates the ulna and carpal bones, and the joint is protected by ligaments and a fibrous capsule. The wrist is a condyloid joint, permitting movement in two planes (flexion, extension, radial, and ulnar movement). The hand has articulations between the carpals and metacarpals, metacarpals and proximal phalanges, and middle and distal phalanges. The metacarpophalangeal joints are condyloid (Figure 19-8).

LOWER EXTREMITIES The joint of the hip consists of the articulation between the acetabulum and the femur. The depth of the acetabulum in the pelvic bone and the joint, which is supported by three strong ligaments, helps stabilize and protect the head of the femur in the joint capsule. Three bursae reduce friction in the hip. The hip is a ball and socket joint, permitting movement of the femur on many axes (Figure 19-9).

The knee consists of the articulation of the femur, tibia, and patella. Fibrocartilaginous disks (medial and lateral menisci), which cushion the tibia and femur, are attached to the tibia and the joint capsule. Collateral ligaments give medial and lateral stability to the knee. Two cruciate ligaments cross obliquely within the knee, adding anterior and posterior stability. Several bursae reduce friction. The suprapatellar bursa separates the patella, quadriceps tendon, and muscle from the femur. The knee is a hinge joint permitting movement (flexion and extension) between the femur and tibia on one plane (Figure 19-10).

The tibiotalar joint (ankle) consists of the articulation of the tibia, fibula, and talus. It is protected by ligaments on the medial and lateral surfaces. The tibiotalar joint is a hinge joint that permits flexion and extension (dorsiflexion and plantar flexion) in one plane. Additional joints in the ankle, the talocalcaneal joint (subtalar) and

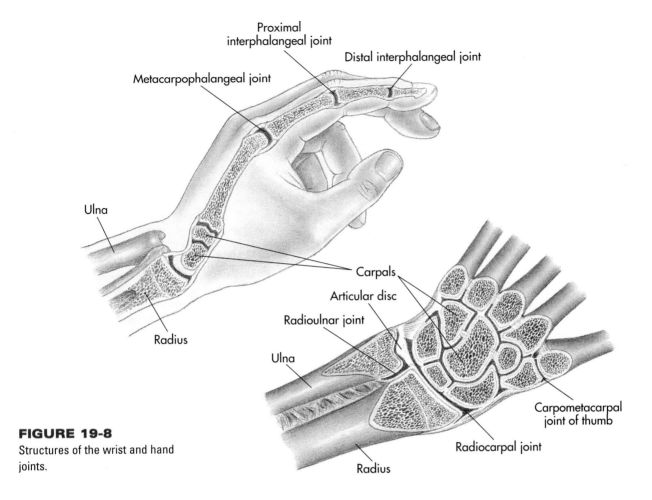

FIGURE 19-8
Structures of the wrist and hand joints.

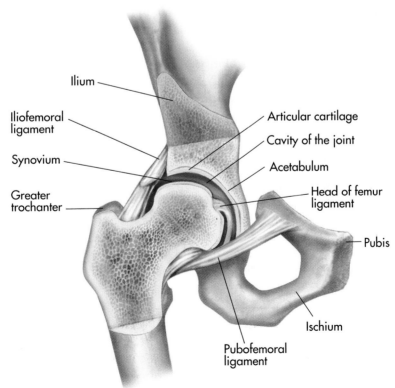

FIGURE 19-9
Structures of the hip.

From Thompson et al, 1997.

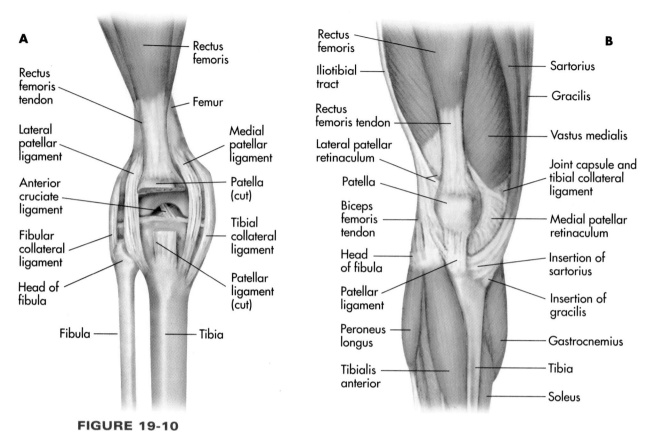

FIGURE 19-10
Structures of the knee, anterior view. **A**, Bones and ligaments of the joint. **B**, Muscles attaching at the knee.

transverse tarsal joint, permit a pivot or rotation movement (pronation and supination) of the joint. Articulations of the foot between the tarsals and metatarsals, the metatarsal and proximal phalanges, and the middle and distal phalanges are condyloid (Figure 19-11).

INFANTS AND CHILDREN

During fetal development the skeletal system emerges from embryologic connective tissues to form cartilage that calcifies and eventually becomes true bone. Throughout infancy and childhood, long bones increase in diameter by the apposition of new bone tissue around the bone shaft. Increased length of long bones results from the proliferation of cartilage at the growth plates (epiphyses). In the smaller bones, such as the carpals, ossification centers form in calcified cartilage. There is a specific sequence and timing of bone growth and ossification during childhood. Ligaments are stronger than bone until adolescence; therefore injuries to long bones and joints are more likely to result in fractures than in sprains.

The number of muscle fibers an individual ultimately develops is established during fetal life. Muscle fibers lengthen during childhood as the skeletal system grows.

ADOLESCENTS

Rapid growth during Tanner Stage III (p. 119) results in decreased strength in the epiphyses, as well as general decreased strength and flexibility, leading to greater potential for injury. Bone growth is completed at about age 20, when the last epiphysis closes and becomes firmly fused to the shaft. However, peak bone mass is not achieved until about age 35 in both genders.

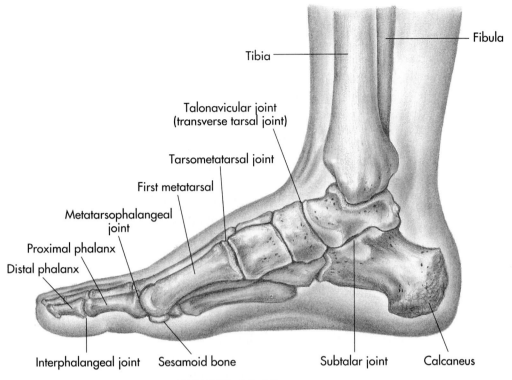

FIGURE 19-11
Bones and joints of the ankle and foot.

PREGNANT WOMEN

Increased levels of circulating hormones contribute to the elasticity of ligaments and softening of the cartilage in the pelvis at about 12 to 20 weeks. This results in increased mobility of the sacroiliac, sacrococcygeal, and symphysis pubis joints.

To compensate for the enlargement of the uterus during later pregnancy, progressive lordosis occurs in an effort to shift the center of gravity back over the lower extremities. The ligaments and muscles of the lower spine may become stressed, leading to lower back pain.

Painful muscle cramps, usually in the gastrocnemius, thigh, or gluteal muscles, occur during the second half of pregnancy in more than 25% of pregnant women. They are more likely to occur at night or after awakening and initiating muscle activity. The cause is unknown.

OLDER ADULTS

PHYSICAL VARIATIONS

Women's bones are less dense than those of men, and black women have denser bones than white, Asian, and Native American women; consequently you will rarely see serious osteoporosis in black women. Black women's bone density is similar to that of white males.

With aging, the skeletal system undergoes an alteration in the equilibrium between bone deposition and bone resorption, and resorption dominates. The loss of bone density affects the entire skeleton, but the long bones and the vertebrae are particularly vulnerable. Weight-bearing bones may become predisposed to fractures. Bony prominences become more apparent with the loss of subcutaneous fat. Cartilage around joints deteriorates.

The muscle mass also undergoes alteration, as increased amounts of collagen collect in the tissues initially, followed by fibrosis of connective tissue. Tendons become less elastic. This results in a reduction of total muscle mass, tone, and strength. A progressive decrease in reaction time, speed of movements, agility, and endurance also occurs.

A sedentary lifestyle and any health problem that contributes to reduced physical activity promote and hasten the musculoskeletal changes associated with aging. Routine exercise and a well-balanced diet help slow the progression of these changes.

REVIEW OF RELATED HISTORY

PRESENT PROBLEM

- Joint complaints
  - Character: stiffness or limitation of movement, change in size or contour, swelling or redness, constant pain or pain with particular motion, unilateral or bilateral involvement, interference with daily activities, joint locking or giving way
  - Associated events: time of day, activity, specific movements, injury, strenuous activity, weather
  - Temporal factors: change in frequency or character of episodes, better or worse as day progresses, nature of onset (slow versus rapid)
  - Efforts to treat: exercise, rest, weight reduction, physical therapy, heat, ice, splints
  - Medications: salicylates, nonsteroidal antiinflammatory drugs, antirheumatics, corticosteroids; prescription or nonprescription
- Muscular complaints
  - Character: limitation of movement, weakness or fatigue, paralysis, tremor, tic, spasms, clumsiness, wasting, aching or pain
  - Precipitating factors: injury, strenuous activity, sudden movement, stress
  - Efforts to treat: heat, ice, splints, rest
  - Medications: muscle relaxants, salicylates, nonsteroidal antiinflammatory drugs; prescription or nonprescription
- Skeletal complaints
  - Character: difficulty with gait or limping; numbness, tingling, or pressure sensation; pain with movement, crepitus; deformity or change in skeletal contour
  - Associated event: injury, recent fractures, strenuous activity, sudden movement, stress; postmenopause
  - Efforts to treat: rest, splints
  - Medications: hormone replacement therapy, calcium; prescription or nonprescription
- Injury
  - Sensation at time of injury: click, tearing, numbness, tingling, catching, locking, grating, snapping, warmth or coldness
  - Mechanism of injury: direct trauma, overuse, sudden change of direction, forceful contraction, overstretch
  - Pain: location, type, onset (sudden or gradual), aggravating or alleviating factors, position of comfort
  - Swelling: location, timing (with activity or injury)
- Back pain
  - Abrupt or gradual onset
  - Character: tearing, burning, or steady ache; tingling or numbness; location and distribution (unilateral or bilateral), radiation to buttocks, groin or legs; triggered by coughing or sneezing and sudden movements
  - Associated event: trauma, occupational and nonoccupational lifting heavy weights, long distance driving, sports activities
  - Efforts to treat: rest, avoid standing or sudden movements
  - Medications: muscle relaxants, analgesics

PAST MEDICAL HISTORY

- Trauma: nerves, soft tissue, bones, joints; residual problems; bone infection
- Surgery on joint or bone
- Chronic illness: cancer, arthritis, osteoporosis, renal or neurologic disorder
- Skeletal deformities or congenital anomalies

FAMILY HISTORY
- Congenital abnormalities of hip or foot
- Scoliosis or back problems
- Arthritis: rheumatoid, osteoarthritis, ankylosing spondylitis, gout
- Genetic disorders: osteogenesis imperfecta, dwarfing syndrome, rickets, hypophosphatemia, hypercalciuria

PERSONAL AND SOCIAL HISTORY
- Employment: past and current, lifting and potential for unintentional injury, safety precautions, use of spinal support, chronic stress on joints
- Exercise: extent, type, and frequency; stress on specific joints; overall conditioning; sport (level of competition, type of shoes and athletic gear)
- Functional abilities: personal care (eating, bathing, dressing, grooming, elimination); other activities (housework, walking, climbing stairs, caring for pet)
- Weight: recent gain, overweight or underweight for body frame
- Height: maximum height achieved, any changes
- Nutrition: amount of calcium, vitamin D, calories, and protein
- Tobacco use
- Alcohol use

RISK FACTORS **Sports Injury**

- Poor physical conditioning
- Failure to warm up muscles adequately
- Intensity of competition
- Collision and contact sports participation
- Rapid growth
- Overuse of joints

RISK FACTORS **Osteoporosis**

- Race (white, Asian, Native American)
- Northwestern European descent
- Blonde or red hair, freckles
- Light body frame, thin
- Family history of osteoporosis
- Nulliparous
- Menopause before age 45
- Postmenopause
- Constant dieting
- Calcium intake <500 mg/day
- Scoliosis, rheumatoid arthritis
- Metabolic disorders (diabetes, hypercortisolism, hyperthyroidism)
- Drugs that decrease bone density (thyroxine, steroids, heparin)
- Poor teeth
- Previous fractures
- Cigarette smoking
- Heavy alcohol use

RISK FACTORS **Osteoarthritis**

- Obesity
- Family history of osteoarthritis
- Lax ligaments with postural joint abnormality
- Age over 40 years

INFANTS AND CHILDREN

- Birth history
  - Presentation, large for gestational age, birth injuries (may result in fractures or nerve damage)
  - Low birth weight, premature, resuscitated, required special ventilator support (may result in anoxia leading to muscle tone disorders)
- Fine and gross motor developmental milestones, appropriate for chronologic age
- Quality of movement: spasticity, flaccidity, cog wheel rigidity
- Leg pain
  - Character: localized or generalized; in muscle or joint; limitation of movement; associated with movement, trauma, or growth spurt
  - Onset: age, sudden or gradual, at night with rest, after activity
  - Participation in organized sports

PREGNANT WOMEN

- Muscle cramps: nature of onset, frequency and time of occurrence, muscle(s) involved, efforts to treat
- Back pain
  - Weeks of gestation, associated with multiple pregnancy, efforts to treat
  - Associated symptoms: uterine tightening, nausea, vomiting, fever, malaise (could signify musculoskeletal discomfort if not from another condition)
  - Type of shoes (heels may increase lordosis)

OLDER ADULTS

- Weakness
  - Onset: sudden or gradual, localized or generalized, occurred with activity or after sustained activity
  - Associated symptoms: stiffness of joints, muscle spasms or tension, any particular activity, dyspnea
- Increases in minor injuries: stumbling, falls, limited agility; association with poor vision
- Change in ease of movement: loss of ability to perform sudden movements, change in exercise endurance, pain, stiffness, localized to particular joints or generalized
- Nocturnal muscle spasm: frequency, associated back pain, numbness or coldness of extremities
- History of injuries or excessive use of a joint or group of joints, claudication, known joint abnormalities
- Previous fractures

EXAMINATION AND FINDINGS

EQUIPMENT

PHYSICAL VARIATIONS

What appears to be lumbar lordosis in black women is usually due to a larger gluteal prominence. X-ray evidence indicates that the incidence of actual lordosis does not differ between black and white women.

- Skin-marking pencil
- Goniometer
- Tape measure
- Reflex hammer

Begin your examination of the musculoskeletal system by observing the gait and posture when the patient enters the examining room. Note how the patient walks, sits, rises from sitting position, takes off a coat, and responds to other directions given during the examination.

As you give specific attention to bones, joints, and muscles, the body surface must be exposed and viewed with good lighting. Position the patient to provide the greatest stability to the joints. Examine each region of the body for limb and trunk

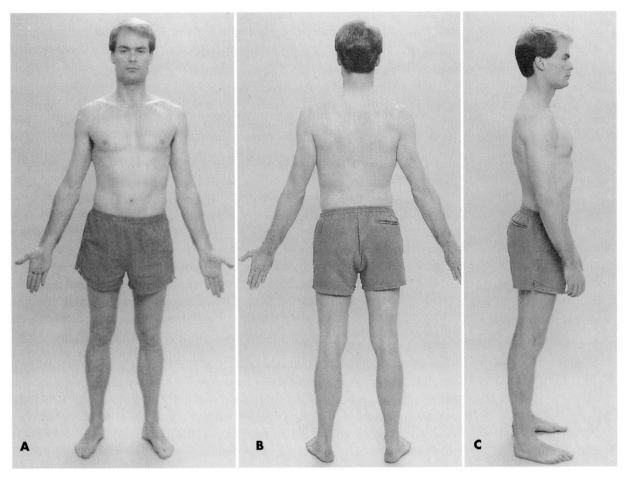

FIGURE 19-12
Inspection of overall body posture. Note the even contour of the shoulders, level scapulae and iliac crests, alignment of the head over the gluteal folds, and symmetry and alignment of extremities.
A, Anterior view. **B,** Posterior view. **C,** Lateral view: The occiput, shoulders, buttocks, and heels should be able to touch the wall the patient stands against.

stability, muscular strength and function, and joint function. Position the extremities uniformly as you examine and look for asymmetry.

INSPECTION

Inspect the anterior, posterior, and lateral aspects of the patient's posture (Figure 19-12). Observe the patient's ability to stand erect, the symmetry of the body parts, and the alignment of extremities. Note any lordosis, kyphosis, or scoliosis.

Inspect the skin and subcutaneous tissues overlying the muscles, cartilage, bones, and joints for discoloration, swelling, and masses.

Observe the extremities for overall size, gross deformity, bony enlargement, alignment, contour, and symmetry of length and position. Expect to find bilateral symmetry in length, circumference, alignment, and the position and number of skin folds.

Inspect the muscles for gross hypertrophy or atrophy, fasciculations, and spasms. Muscle size should approximate symmetry bilaterally, without atrophy or hypertrophy. Bilateral symmetry should not be defined as absolute, since there is no perfect symmetry. For example, the dominant forearm is expected to be larger in athletes who play racquet sports and in manual laborers. Fasciculation occurs after injury to a muscle's motor neuron. Muscle wasting occurs after injury as a result of pain, disease of the muscle, or damage to the motor neuron.

PALPATION

Palpate all bones, joints, and surrounding muscles. Note any heat, tenderness, swelling, fluctuation of a joint (associated with effusion), crepitus, and resistance to pressure. No discomfort should occur when you apply pressure to bones or joints. Muscle tone should be firm, not hard or doughy. Spasticity is an increase in muscle tone. Palpate inflamed joints last. Synovial thickening can sometimes be felt in joints that are close to the skin surface when the synovium is edematous or hypertrophied because of inflammation. Crepitus can be felt when two irregular bony surfaces rub together as a joint moves, when two rough edges of a broken bone rub together, or with the movement of a tendon inside the tendon sheath when tenosynovitis is present.

RANGE OF MOTION

Examine both the active and passive range of motion for each major joint and its related muscle groups. Adequate space for the patient to move each muscle group and joint through its full range is necessary and may be provided by pulling the examining table away from the wall if appropriate. Instruct the patient in moving each joint through its range of motion as detailed under examination of specific joints and muscles. Pain, limitation of motion, spastic movement, joint instability, deformity, and contracture suggest a problem with the joint, related muscle group, or nerve supply.

Ask the patient to relax and allow you to passively move the same joints until the end of the range is felt. Do not force the joint if there is pain or muscle spasm. Passive range of motion often exceeds active range of motion by 5 degrees. Range of motion with active and passive maneuvers should be equal between contralateral joints. Discrepancies between active and passive range of motion may indicate true muscle weakness or a joint disorder. No crepitation or tenderness with movement should be apparent. Spastic muscles are harder to put through the range of motion. Measurements may vary if the muscle tested relaxes with gentle persistence.

When a joint appears to have an increase or limitation in its range of motion, a goniometer is used to precisely measure the angle. Begin with the joint in the fully extended or neutral position, and then flex the joint as far as possible. Measure the angles of greatest flexion and extension, comparing these with the expected flexion and extension values (Figure 19-13).

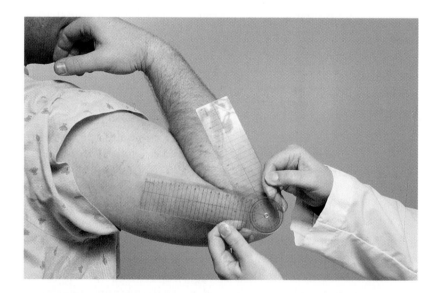

FIGURE 19-13
Use of goniometer to measure joint range of motion.

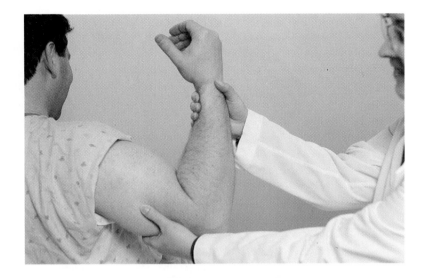

FIGURE 19-14
Evaluation of muscle strength: flexion of the elbow against opposing force.

TABLE 19-2	Assessing Muscle Strength			
		Scales		
Muscle Function Level		**Grade**	**% Normal**	**Lovett Scale**
No evidence of contractility		0	0	0 (zero)
Slight contractility, no movement		1	10	T (trace)
Full range of motion, gravity eliminated*		2	25	P (poor)
Full range of motion against gravity		3	50	F (fair)
Full range of motion against gravity, some resistance		4	75	G (good)
Full range of motion against gravity, full resistance		5	100	N (normal)

From Barkauskas et al, 1998.
*Passive movement.

MUSCLE STRENGTH

Evaluating the strength of each muscle group, which is also considered part of the neurologic examination, is usually integrated with examination of the associated joint for range of motion. Ask the patient to first contract the muscle you indicate by extending or flexing the joint and then to resist when you apply opposing force against that muscle contraction (Figure 19-14). Do not allow the patient to move the joint. Compare the muscle strength bilaterally. Expect muscle strength to be bilaterally symmetric with full resistance to opposition. Full muscle strength requires complete active range of motion.

Variations in muscle strength are graded from no voluntary contraction to full muscle strength, using one of the scales in Table 19-2. When muscle strength is grade 3 or less, disability is present; activity cannot be accomplished in a gravity field, and external support is necessary to perform movements. Weakness may result from disuse atrophy, pain, fatigue, or overstretching.

SPECIFIC JOINTS AND MUSCLES

Temporomandibular Joint

Locate the temporomandibular joints with your fingertips placed just anterior to the tragus of each ear. Allow your fingertips to slip into the joint space as the patient's mouth opens, and gently palpate the joint space (Figure 19-15). An audible or palpable snapping or clicking in the temporomandibular joints is not unusual, but pain, crepitus, locking, or popping may indicate temporomandibular joint dysfunction.

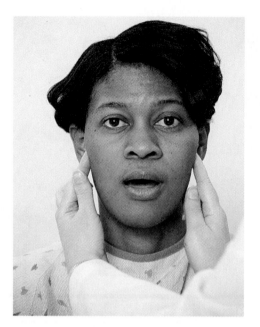

FIGURE 19-15
Palpation of the temporomandibular joint.

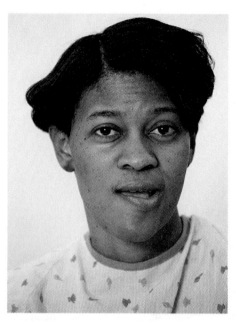

FIGURE 19-16
Lateral range of motion in the temporo-mandibular joint.

Range of motion is examined by asking the patient to perform the following movements:

- Open and close the mouth. Expect a space of 3 to 6 cm between the upper and lower teeth when the jaw is open.
- Laterally move the lower jaw to each side. The mandible should move 1 to 2 cm in each direction (Figure 19-16).
- Protrude and retract the chin. Both movements should be possible.

Strength of the temporalis and masseter muscles is evaluated by asking the patient to clench the teeth while you palpate the contracted muscles and apply opposing force. Cranial nerve V is simultaneously tested with this maneuver.

Cervical Spine

Inspect the patient's neck, from both an anterior and a posterior position, observing for alignment of the head with the shoulders and symmetry of the skin folds and muscles. Expect the cervical spine to be straight with the head erect and in appropriate alignment. No asymmetric skin folds should be apparent.

Palpate the posterior neck, cervical spine, and paravertebral, trapezius, and sternocleidomastoid muscles. The muscles should have good tone and be symmetric in size, with no palpable tenderness or muscle spasm.

Evaluate range of motion in the cervical spine by asking the patient to perform the following movements (Figure 19-17):

- Bend the head forward, chin to the chest. Expect flexion of 45 degrees.
- Bend the head backward, chin toward the ceiling. Expect hyperextension of 45 degrees.
- Bend the head to each side, ear to each shoulder. Expect lateral bending of 40 degrees.
- Turn the head to each side, chin to shoulder. Expect rotation of 70 degrees.

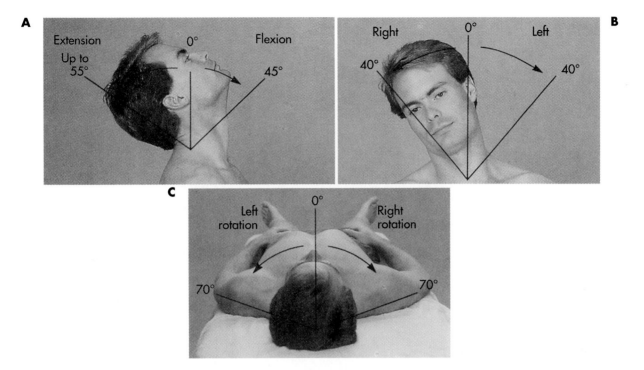

FIGURE 19-17
Range of motion of the cervical spine. **A,** Flexion and hyperextension. **B,** Lateral bending. **C,** Rotation.

FIGURE 19-18
Examining the strength of the sternocleidomastoid and trapezius muscles. **A,** Flexion with palpation of the sternocleidomastoid muscle. **B,** Extension against resistance. **C,** Rotation against resistance.

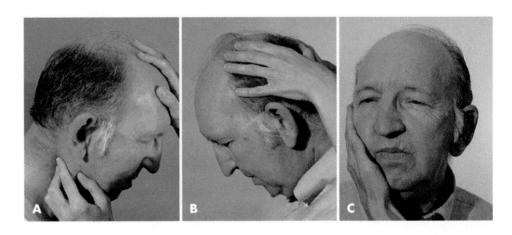

The strength of the sternocleidomastoid and trapezius muscles is evaluated with the patient maintaining each of the above positions while you apply opposing force. With rotation, cranial nerve XI is simultaneously tested (Figure 19-18).

Thoracic and Lumbar Spine

Major landmarks of the back include each spinal process of the vertebrae (C7 and T1 are usually most prominent), the scapulae, iliac crests, and paravertebral muscles (Figure 19-19). Expect the head to be positioned directly over the gluteal cleft and the vertebrae to be straight as indicated by symmetric shoulder, scapular, and iliac crest heights. The curves of the cervical and lumbar spines should be convex. The knees and feet should be in alignment with the trunk, pointing directly forward.

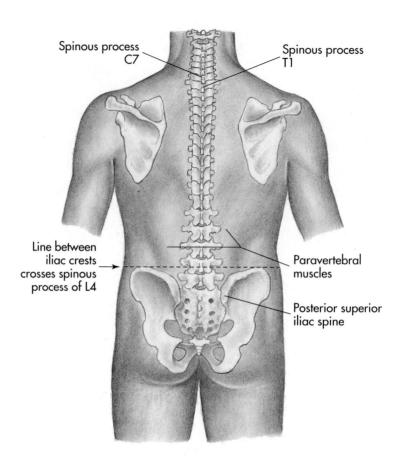

FIGURE 19-19
Landmarks of the back.

Lordosis is common in patients who are markedly obese or pregnant. The appearance of lordosis in black women may result from their more prominent gluteal muscle. Kyphosis may be observed in aging adults. A sharp angular deformity, a gibbus, is associated with a collapsed vertebra from osteoporosis (Figure 19-20).

With the patient standing erect, palpate along the spinal processes and paravertebral muscles (Figure 19-21). Percuss for spinal tenderness, first by tapping each spinal process with one finger, and then by rapping each side of the spine along the paravertebral muscles with the ulnar aspect of your fist. No muscle spasm or spinal tenderness with palpation or percussion should be elicted.

Ask the patient to slowly bend forward and touch the toes while you observe from behind. Inspect the spine for unexpected curvature. (A mark with the skin pencil on each spinal process will enhance the inspection, especially if a curvature is suspected.) The patient's back should remain symmetrically flat as the concave curve of the lumbar spine becomes convex with forward flexion. A lateral curvature or rib hump should make you suspect scoliosis (Figure 19-22). Then have the patient rise but remain bent at the waist to fully extend the back. Reversal of the lumbar curve should be apparent.

Range of motion is evaluated by asking the patient to perform the following movements:

- Bend forward at the waist and try to touch the toes. Expect flexion of 75 to 90 degrees (Figure 19-23, *A*).
- Bend back at the waist as far as possible. Expect hyperextension of 30 degrees (Figure 19-23, *B*).

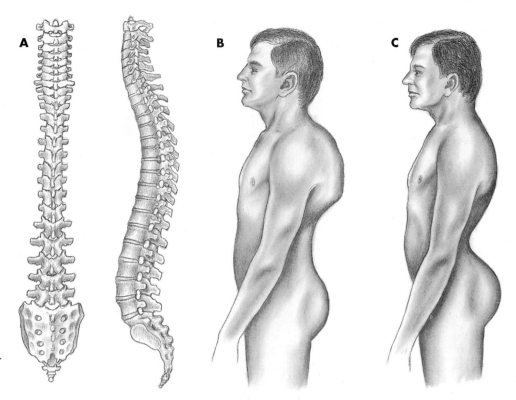

FIGURE 19-20
Deviations in spinal column curvatures. **A,** Expected spine curvatures. **B,** Kyphosis. **C,** Lordosis.
From Thompson et al, 1997.

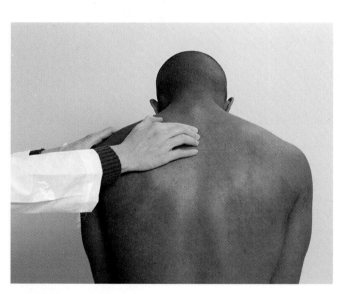

FIGURE 19-21
Palpation of the spinal processes of the vertebrae.

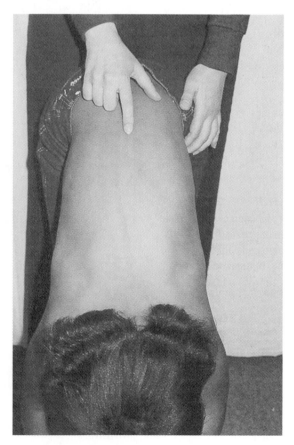

FIGURE 19-22
Inspection of the spine for lateral curvature and lumbar convexity.

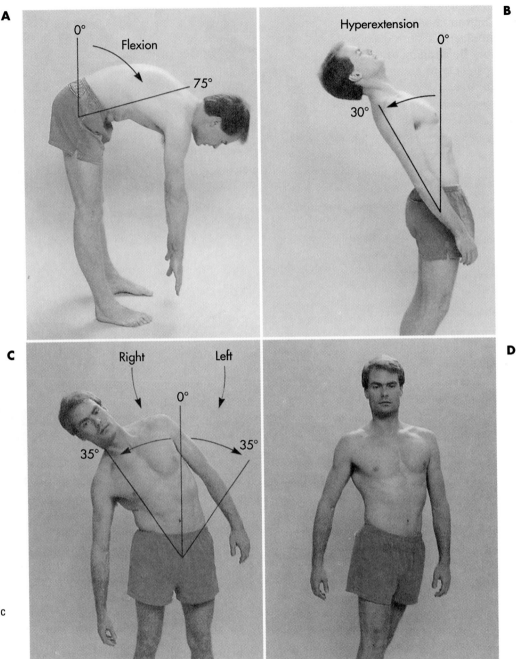

FIGURE 19-23
Range of motion of the thoracic and lumbar spine. **A,** Flexion. **B,** Hyperextension. **C,** Lateral bending. **D,** Rotation of the upper trunk.

- Bend to each side as far as possible. Expect lateral bending of 35 degrees bilaterally (Figure 19-23, *C*).
- Swing the upper trunk from the waist in a circular motion front to side to back to side, while you stabilize the pelvis. Expect rotation of the upper trunk 30 degrees forward and backward (Figure 19-23, *D*).

Shoulders

Inspect the contour of the shoulders, the shoulder girdle, the clavicles and scapulae, and the area muscles. There should be symmetry of size and contour of all shoulder

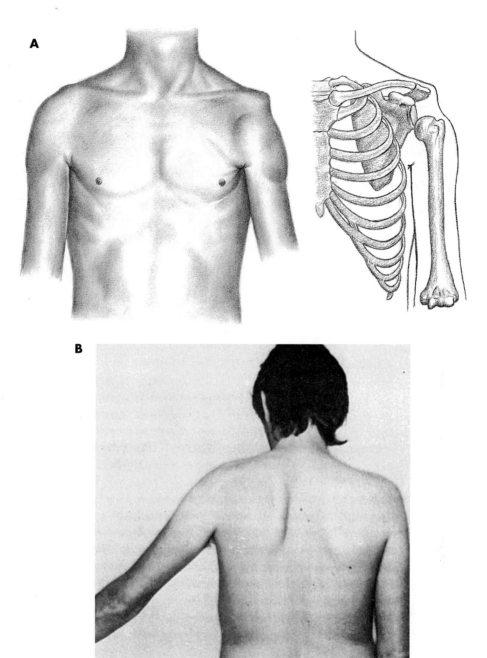

FIGURE 19-24
Contour changes of the shoulder.
A, With dislocation. **B,** Winging
of the scapula with abduction of
the arm.

B, from DePalma, 1983.

structures. When the shoulder contour is asymmetric and one shoulder has hollows in the rounding contour, suspect a shoulder dislocation. Ask the patient to stand close to a wall and push against it with both hands. Observe for a winged scapula, an outward prominence of the scapula, indicating injury to the nerve of the anterior serratus muscle (Figure 19-24).

Palpate the sternoclavicular joint, acromioclavicular joint, clavicle, scapulae, coracoid process, greater tubercle of the humerus, biceps groove, and area muscles.

Examine the range of motion by asking the patient to perform the following movements:

- Shrug the shoulders. Expect the shoulders to rise symmetrically.
- Raise both arms forward and straight up over the head. Expect forward flexion of 180 degrees (Figure 19-25, *A*).

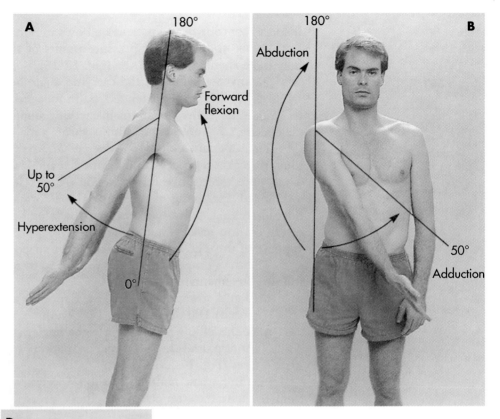

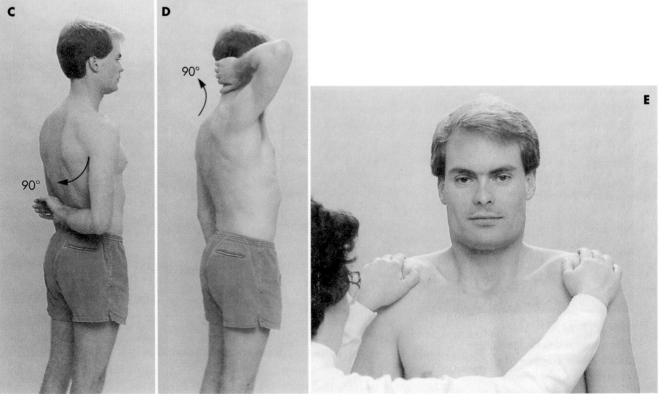

FIGURE 19-25

Range of motion of the shoulder. **A,** Forward flexion and hyperextension. **B,** Abduction and adduction.
C, Internal rotation. **D,** External rotation. **E,** Shrugged shoulders.

- Extend and stretch both arms behind the back. Expect hyperextension of 50 degrees (Figure 19-25, A).
- Lift both arms laterally and straight up over the head. Expect shoulder abduction of 180 degrees.
- Swing each arm across the front of the body. Expect adduction of 50 degrees (Figure 19-25, B).
- Place both arms behind the hips, elbows out. Expect internal rotation of 90 degrees (Figure 19-25, C).
- Place both arms behind the head, elbows out. Expect external rotation of 90 degrees (Figure 19-25, D).

Have the patient maintain shrugged shoulders, forward flexion, and abduction while you apply opposing force to evaluate the strength of the shoulder girdle muscles. Cranial nerve XI is simultaneously evaluated with the shrugged shoulders maneuver (Figure 19-25, E).

Elbows

Inspect the contour of the patient's elbows in both flexed and extended positions. Subcutaneous nodules along pressure points of the extensor surface of the ulna may indicate rheumatoid arthritis (Figure 19-26).

Note any deviations in the carrying angle between the humerus and radius while the arm is passively extended, palm forward. The carrying angle is usually 5 to 15 degrees laterally. Variations in carrying angle are cubitus valgus, a lateral angle exceeding 15 degrees, and cubitus varus, a medial carrying angle (Figure 19-27).

Flex the patient's elbow 70 degrees and palpate the extensor surface of the ulna, the olecranon process, and the medial and lateral epicondyles of the humerus. Then palpate the groove on each side of the olecranon process for tenderness, swelling, and thickening of the synovial membrane (Figure 19-28). A boggy, soft, or fluctuant swelling, point tenderness at the lateral epicondyle or along the grooves of the olecranon process and epicondyles, and increased pain with pronation and supination of the elbow should cause you to suspect epicondylitis or tendinitis.

The elbow's range of motion is examined by asking the patient to perform the following movements:

- Bend and straighten the elbow with the elbow fully extended at 0 degrees. Expect flexion of 160 degrees and full extension of 180 degrees (Figure 19-29, A).
- With the elbow flexed at a right angle, rotate the hand from palm side down to palm side up. Expect pronation of 90 degrees and supination of 90 degrees (Figure 19-29, B).

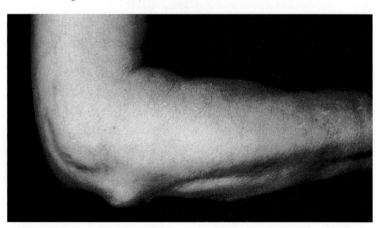

FIGURE 19-26

Subcutaneous nodules on the extensor surface of the forearm near the elbow.

Reprinted from the Clinical Slide Collection of the Rheumatic Diseases, copyright 1991. Used by permission of the American College of Rheumatology.

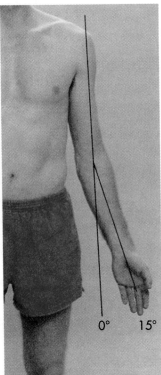

FIGURE 19-27
Expected carrying angle of the arm, at 5 to 15 degrees.

FIGURE 19-29
Range of motion of the elbow.
A, Flexion and extension.
B, Pronation and supination.

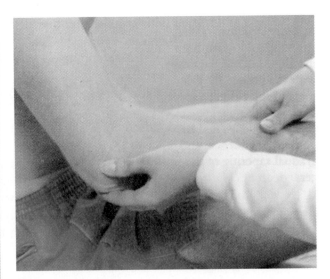

FIGURE 19-28
Palpation of the olecranon process grooves.

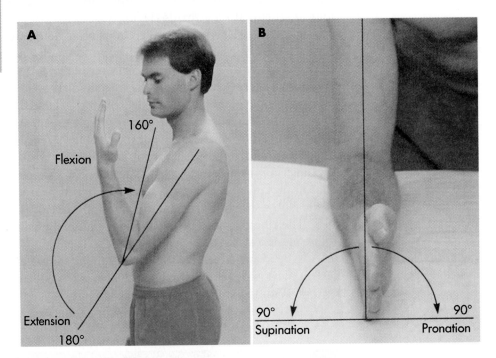

Have the patient maintain flexion and extension while you apply opposing force to evaluate the strength of the elbow muscles.

Hands and Wrists

Inspect the dorsal and palmar aspects of the hands, noting the contour, position, shape, number, and completeness of digits. Note the presence of palmar and phalangeal creases. The palmar surface of each hand should have a central depression with a prominent, rounded mound (thenar eminence) on the thumb side of the hand and a less prominent hypothenar eminence on the little finger side of the hand. Expect the fingers to fully extend when in close approximation to each other and to be aligned with the forearm. The lateral finger surfaces should gradually taper from the proximal to the distal aspects (Figure 19-30).

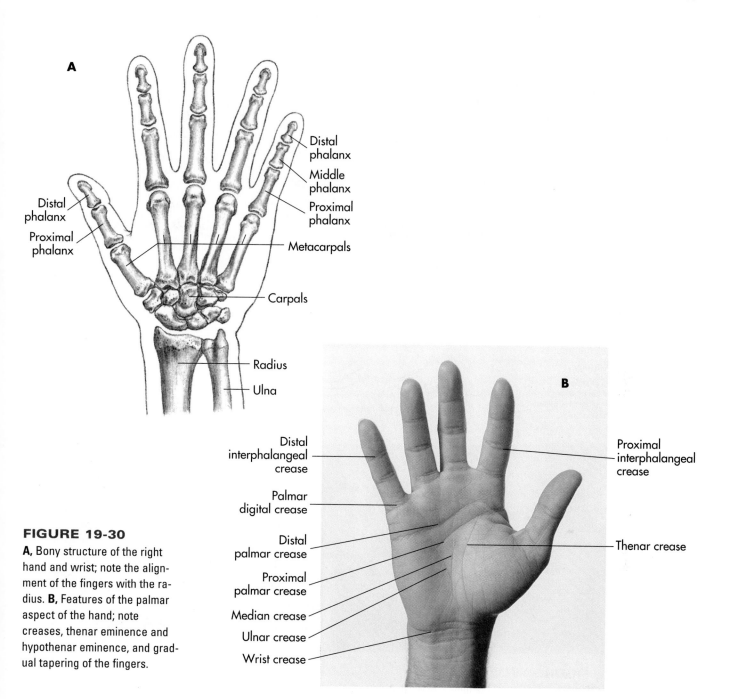

FIGURE 19-30

A, Bony structure of the right hand and wrist; note the alignment of the fingers with the radius. **B,** Features of the palmar aspect of the hand; note creases, thenar eminence and hypothenar eminence, and gradual tapering of the fingers.

Deviation of the fingers to the ulnar side and swan neck or boutonniere deformities of the fingers usually indicate rheumatoid arthritis (Figure 19-31).

Palpate each joint in the hand and wrist. Palpate the interphalangeal joints with your thumb and index finger. The metacarpophalangeal joints are palpated with both thumbs. Palpate the wrist and radiocarpal groove with your thumbs on the dorsal surface and your fingers on the palmar aspect of the wrist (Figure 19-32). Joint surfaces should be smooth, without nodules, swelling, bogginess, or tenderness. A firm mass over the dorsum of the wrist may be a ganglion.

Bony overgrowths in the distal interphalangeal joints, which are felt as hard, nontender nodules usually 2 to 3 mm in diameter but sometimes encompassing the entire joint, are associated with osteoarthritis. When located along the distal inter-

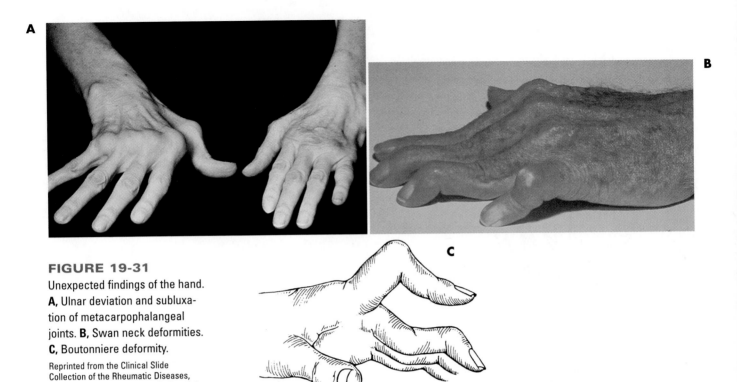

FIGURE 19-31

Unexpected findings of the hand.
A, Ulnar deviation and subluxation of metacarpophalangeal
joints. **B,** Swan neck deformities.
C, Boutonniere deformity.

Reprinted from the Clinical Slide
Collection of the Rheumatic Diseases,
copyright 1991. Used by permission of the
American College of Rheumatology.

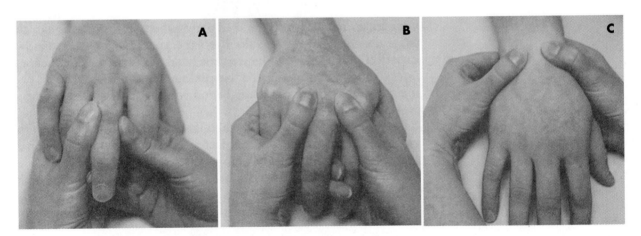

FIGURE 19-32

Palpation of joints of the hand and wrist. **A,** Interphalangeal joints. **B,** Metacarpophalangeal joints.
C, Radiocarpal groove and wrist.

phalangeal joints, they are called Heberden nodes; those along the proximal interphalangeal joints are called Bouchard nodes. Painful, fusiform swelling of the proximal interphalangeal joints causes spindle-shaped fingers, which are associated with
the acute stage of rheumatoid arthritis (Figure 19-33). Cystic, round, nontender
swellings along tendon sheaths or joint capsules that are more prominent with flexion may indicate ganglia.

With your index or middle finger, strike the median nerve where it passes
through the carpal tunnel, under the flexor retinaculum and volar carpal ligament
(Figure 19-34). A tingling sensation radiating from the wrist to the hand along the median nerve is a positive *Tinel* sign, which is associated with carpal tunnel syndrome.

A
B
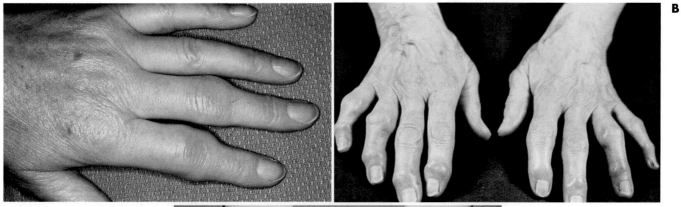

C
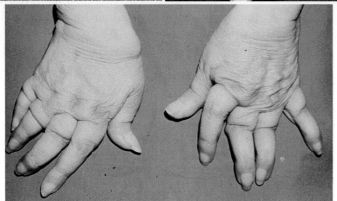

FIGURE 19-33

Unexpected findings of the fingers. **A,** Fusiform swelling or spindle-shaped enlargement of the proximal interphalangeal joints. **B,** Degenerative joint disease; Heberden nodes at the distal interphalangeal joints and Bouchard nodes at the proximal interphalangeal joints. **C,** Telescoping digits with hypermobile joints.

Reprinted from the Clinical Slide Collection of the Rheumatic Diseases, copyright 1991. Used by permission of the American College of Rheumatology.

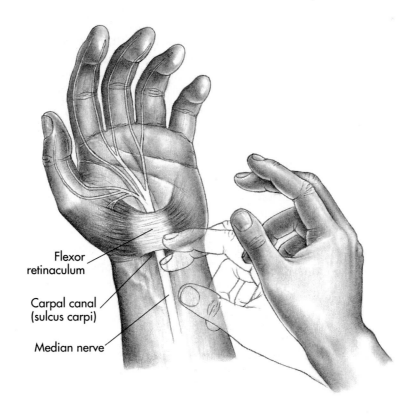

Flexor retinaculum

Carpal canal (sulcus carpi)

Median nerve

FIGURE 19-34

Elicitation of the Tinel sign.

Examine the range of motion of the hand and wrist by asking the patient to perform these movements:

- Bend the fingers forward at the metacarpophalangeal joint; then stretch the fingers up and back at the knuckle. Expect metacarpophalangeal flexion of 90 degrees and hyperextension as much as 20 degrees (Figure 19-35, *A*).
- Touch the thumb to each fingertip and to the base of the little finger; make a fist. All movements should be possible (Figure 19-35, *B* and *C*).
- Spread the fingers apart and then touch them together. Both movements should be possible (Figure 19-35, *D*).
- Bend the hand at the wrist up and down. Expect flexion of 90 degrees and hyperextension of 70 degrees (Figure 19-35, *E*).
- With the palm side down, turn each hand to the right and left. Expect radial motion of 20 degrees and ulnar motion of 55 degrees (Figure 19-35, *F*).

Have the patient maintain wrist flexion and hyperextension while you apply opposing force to evaluate strength of the wrist muscles. To evaluate hand strength, have the patient grip two of your fingers tightly. To avoid painful compression from an overzealous squeeze, offer your two fingers of one hand side by side in the handshake position. Finger extension, abduction, and adduction positions may also be used to evaluate hand strength.

Hips

Inspect the hips anteriorly and posteriorly while the patient stands. Using the major landmarks of the iliac crest and the greater trochanter of the femur, note any asymmetry in the iliac crest height, the size of the buttocks, or the number and level of gluteal folds.

Palpate the hips and pelvis with the patient supine (Figure 19-36). No instability, tenderness, or crepitus is expected.

Examine the hips' range of motion by asking the patient to perform the following movements:

- While supine, raise the leg with the knee extended above the body. Expect up to 90 degrees of hip flexion (Figure 19-37, *A*).
- While either standing or prone, swing the straightened leg behind the body without arching the back. Expect hip hyperextension of 30 degrees or less (Figure 19-37, *B*).
- While supine, raise one knee to the chest while keeping the other leg straight. Expect hip flexion of 120 degrees (Figure 19-37, *C*).
- While supine, swing the leg laterally and medially with knee straight. With the adduction movement, passively lift the opposite leg to permit the examined leg full movement. Expect some degree of both abduction and adduction (Figure 19-37, *D*).
- While supine, flex the knee and rotate the leg inward toward the other leg. Expect internal rotation of 40 degrees (Figure 19-37, *E*).
- While supine, place the lateral aspect of the foot on the knee of the other leg; move the flexed knee toward the table. Expect 45 degrees of external rotation (Patrick test) (Figure 19-37, *F*).

Have the patient maintain flexion of the hip with the knee in flexion and extension while you apply opposing force to evaluate strength of hip muscles. Muscle strength can also be evaluated during abduction and adduction, as well as by resistance to uncrossing the legs while seated.

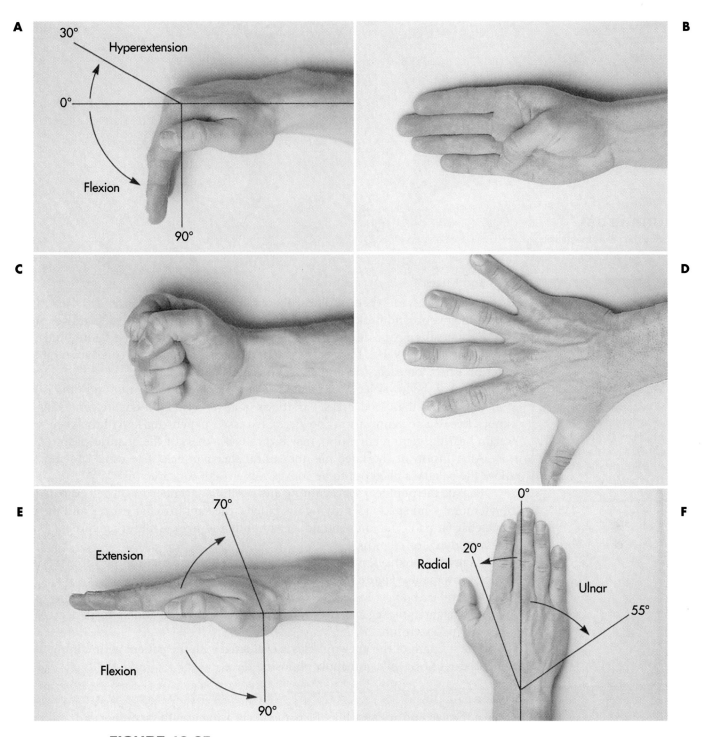

FIGURE 19-35
Range of motion of the hand and wrist. **A,** Metacarpophalangeal flexion and hyperextension. **B,** Finger flexion: thumb to each fingertip and to the base of the little finger. **C,** Finger flexion: fist formation. **D,** Finger abduction. **E,** Wrist flexion and hyperextension. **F,** Wrist radial and ulnar movement.

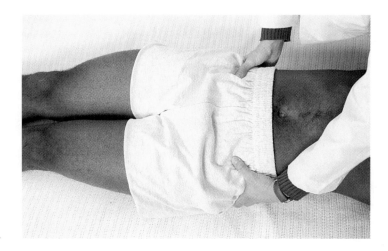

FIGURE 19-36
Palpating the pelvis for stability.

Legs and Knees

Inspect the knees and their popliteal spaces in both flexed and extended positions, noting the major landmarks: tibial tuberosity, medial and lateral tibial condyles, medial and lateral epicondyles of the femur, adductor tubercle of the femur, and the patella (see Figure 19-10). Inspect the extended knee for its natural concavities on the anterior aspect, on each side, and above the patella.

Observe the lower leg alignment. The angle between the femur and tibia is expected to be less than 15 degrees. Variations in lower leg alignment are genu valgum (knock knees) and genu varum (bowlegs). Excessive hyperextension of the knee with weight bearing, genu recurvatum, may indicate weakness of the quadriceps muscles.

An effusion of the knee fills the suprapatellar pouch. The usual indentation above the patella is filled out to be convex rather than concave.

Palpate the popliteal space, noting any swelling or tenderness. Then palpate the tibiofemoral joint space, identifying the patella, the suprapatellar pouch, and the infrapatellar fat pad. The joint should feel smooth and firm, without tenderness, bogginess, nodules, or crepitus.

Examine the knees' range of motion by asking the patient to perform the following movements (Figure 19-38):

- Bend each knee. Expect 130 degrees of flexion.
- Straighten the leg and stretch it. Expect full extension and up to 15 degrees of hyperextension.

The strength of the knee muscles is evaluated with the patient maintaining flexion and extension while you apply opposing force.

Feet and Ankles

Inspect the feet and ankles while the patient is bearing weight (standing and walking) and sitting. Landmarks of the ankle include the medial malleolus, the lateral malleolus, and the Achilles tendon. Expect smooth and rounded malleolar prominences, prominent heels, and prominent metatarsophalangeal joints. Calluses and corns indicate chronic pressure or irritation.

Observe the contour of the feet and the position, size, and number of toes. The feet should be in alignment with the tibias. Pes varus (in-toeing) and pes valgus (out-toeing) are common alignment variations. Weight bearing should be on the midline of the foot, on an imaginary line from the heel midline to between the second and third toes. Deviations in forefoot alignment (metatarsus varus or metatarsus valgus), heel pronation, and pain or injury often cause a shift in weight-bearing position (Figure 19-39).

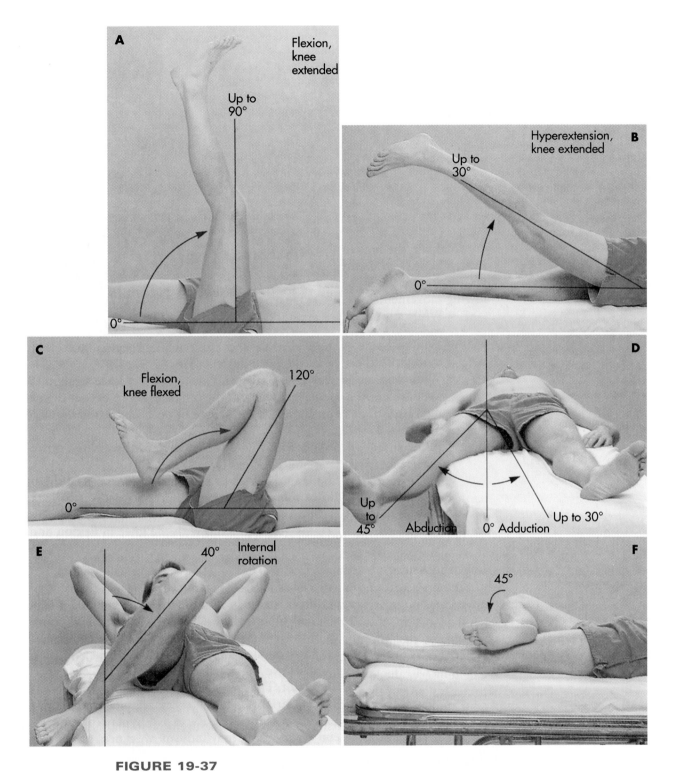

FIGURE 19-37
Range of motion of the hip. **A,** Hip flexion, leg extended. **B,** Hip hyperextension, knee extended.
C, Hip flexion, knee flexed. **D,** Abduction. **E,** Internal rotation. **F,** External rotation.

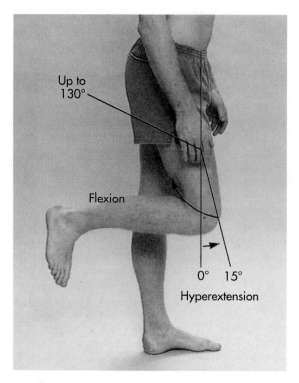

FIGURE 19-38
Range of motion of the knee: flexion and extension.

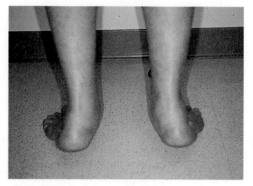

FIGURE 19-39
Pronation of heel. Notice that weight bearing is not through the midline of the foot.
Courtesy Charles W. Bradley, DPM, MPA, and Caroline Harvey, DPM, California College of Podiatric Medicine.

Expect the foot to have a longitudinal arch, although the foot may flatten with weight-bearing. Common variations include pes planus, a foot that remains flat even when not bearing weight, and pes cavus, a high instep (Figure 19-40). Pes cavus may be associated with claw toes.

The toes should be straight forward, flat, and in alignment with each other. Several common deviations of the toes can occur (Figure 19-41). Hyperextension of the metatarsophalangeal joint with flexion of the toe's proximal joint is called *hammer toe*. A flexion deformity at the distal interphalangeal joint is called a *mallet toe*. *Claw toe* is hyperextension of the metatarsophalangeal joint with flexion of the toe's proximal and distal joints. *Hallux valgus* is lateral deviation of the great toe that may cause overlapping with the second toe. A bursa often forms at the pressure point and, if it becomes inflamed, forms a painful bunion.

Heat, redness, swelling, and tenderness are signs of an inflamed joint, possibly caused by rheumatoid arthritis, septic joint, fracture, or tendonitis. An inflamed metatarsophalangeal joint of the great toe should make you suspect gouty arthritis. A draining tophus may occasionally be present.

Palpate the Achilles tendon and the anterior surface of the ankle. A thickened Achilles tendon may indicate hyperlipidemia. Using the thumb and fingers of both hands, compress the forefoot, palpating each matatarsophalangeal joint.

The range of motion of the foot and ankle is assessed by asking the patient to perform the following movements while sitting:

- Point the foot toward the ceiling. Expect dorsiflexion of 20 degrees (Figure 19-42, *A*).

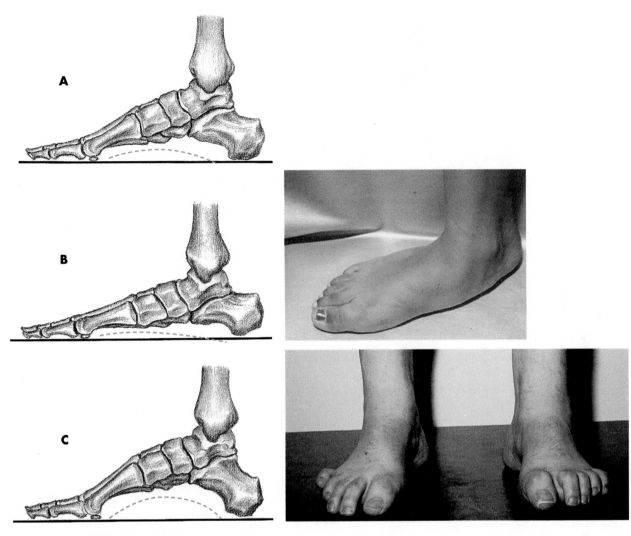

FIGURE 19-40
Variations in the longitudinal arch of the foot. **A,** Expected arch. **B,** Pes planus (flatfoot). **C,** Pes cavus (high instep).

Photos for **B** and **C** courtesy Charles W. Bradley, DPM, MPA, and Caroline Harvey, DPM, California College of Podiatric Medicine.

- Point the foot toward the floor. Expect plantar flexion of 45 degrees.
- Bending the foot at the ankle, turn the sole of the foot toward and then away from the other foot. Expect inversion of 30 degrees and eversion of 20 degrees (Figure 19-42, *B*).
- Rotating the ankle, turn the foot away from and then toward the other foot while the examiner stabilizes the leg. Expect abduction of 10 degrees and adduction of 20 degrees (Figure 19-42, *C*).
- Bend and straighten the toes. Expect flexion and extension, especially of the great toes.

Have the patient maintain dorsiflexion and plantar flexion while you apply opposing force to evaluate strength of the ankle muscles. Abduction and adduction of the ankle and flexion and extension of the great toe may also be used to evaluate muscle strength.

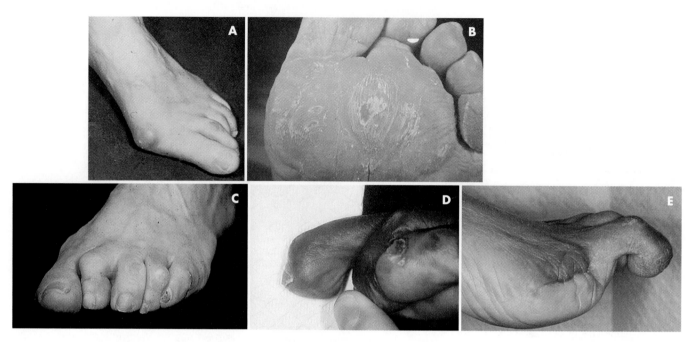

FIGURE 19-41

Unexpected findings of the feet. **A,** Hallux valgus with bunion. **B,** Protruding metatarsal heads with callosities. **C,** Hammer toes. **D,** Mallet toe. **E,** Claw toes.

Courtesy Charles W. Bradley, DPM, MPA, and Caroline Harvey, DPM, California College of Podiatric Medicine.

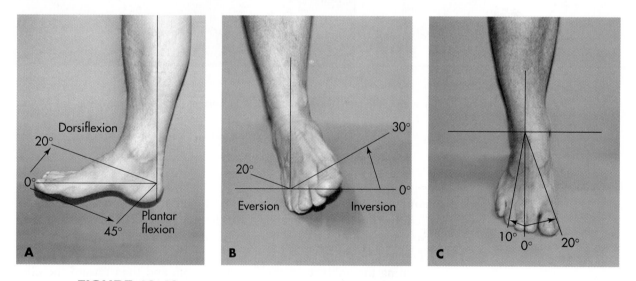

FIGURE 19-42

Range of motion of the foot and ankle. **A,** Dorsiflexion and plantar flexion. **B,** Inversion and eversion. **C,** Abduction and adduction.

ADDITIONAL PROCEDURES

Various other procedures for further evaluation of specific joints of the musculoskeletal system are performed when problems are detected with routine procedures (Box 19-1).

Limb Measurement

When a difference in length or circumference of matching extremities is suspected, measure and compare the size of both extremities. Leg length is measured from the anterior superior iliac spine to the medial malleolus of the ankle, crossing the knee on the medial side (Figure 19-43, *A*). Arm length is measured from the acromion process through the olecranon process to the distal ulnar prominence. The circumference of the extremities is measured in centimeters at the same distance on each limb from a major landmark (Figure 19-43, *B*). Serious athletes who use the dominant arm almost exclusively in their activities (pitchers and tennis players) may have some discrepancy in circumference. For most people, no more than a 1 cm discrepancy in length and circumference between matching extremities should be found.

BOX 19-1	Special Procedures for Assessment of the Musculoskeletal System

Procedure	Condition Detected
Limb measurement	Asymmetry in limb size
Straight leg raising	L4, L5, S1 nerve root irritation
Bragard stretch test	L4, L5, S1 nerve root irritation
Femoral stretch test	L1, L2, L3 and L4 nerve root irritation
Ballottement	Effusion or excess fluid in knee
Bulge sign	Excess fluid in knee
McMurray test	Torn meniscus in knee
Drawer test	Anteroposterior instability in knee
Varus/valgus stress test	Mediolateral instability in knee
Lachman test	Anterior cruciate ligament integrity
Apley test	Torn meniscus in knee
Thomas test	Flexion contracture of hip
Trendelenburg sign	Weak hip abductor muscles

A 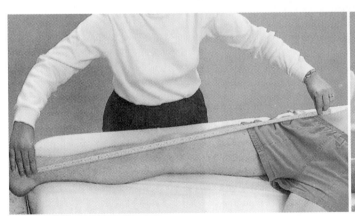   B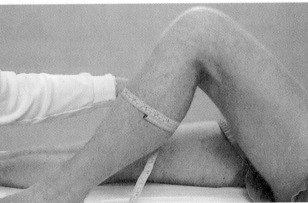

FIGURE 19-43
Measuring **A,** limb length, and **B,** leg circumference.

Lower Spine Assessment

The *straight leg raising test* is used to test for nerve root irritation or lumbar disk herniation at the L4, L5, and S1 levels. Have the patient lie supine with the neck slightly flexed. Ask the patient to raise the leg, keeping the knee extended (see Figure 19-37, *A*). No pain should be felt below the knee with leg raising. *Lasegue* sign is positive when the patient is unable to raise the leg more than 30 degrees without pain. Flexion of the knee often eliminates the pain with leg raising. Repeat the procedure on the unaffected leg. Crossover pain in the affected leg with this maneuver is more supportive of the finding of tension on the nerve roots.

The *Bragard stretch test* also tests for lumbar disk herniation at the L4, L5, and S1 levels. Have the patient lie supine with the neck slightly flexed. Hold the patient's lower leg and raise it slowly with the knee extended until the patient feels pain. Lower the leg slightly and briskly dorsiflex the foot. Pain will be produced if the nerve is inflamed (Figure 19-44).

The *sitting knee extension test* is used to evaluate sciatic nerve tenderness. While the patient is sitting, ask the patient to extend the leg at the knee. Pain with extension or attempts to lean backward to reduce tension on the nerve is a positive sign of sciatic nerve tenderness.

The *Femoral stretch test* or hip extension test is used to detect inflammation of the nerve root at the L1, L2, L3, and sometimes L4 level. Have the patient lie prone and extend the hip. No pain is expected. The presence of pain on extension is a positive sign of nerve root irritation (Figure 19-45).

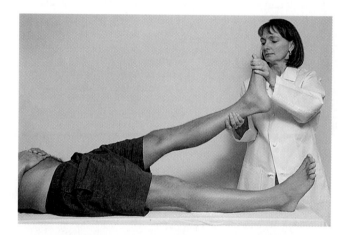

FIGURE 19-44
Bragard stretch test for lumbar nerve root irritation.

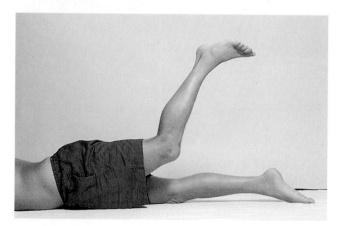

FIGURE 19-45
Femoral stretch test for high lumbar nerve root irritation.

Knee Assessment

Ballotement is used to determine the presence of excess fluid or an effusion in the knee. With the knee extended, apply downward pressure on the suprapatellar pouch with the web or the thumb and forefinger of one hand, and then push the patella sharply downward against the femur with a finger of your other hand. If an effusion is present, a tapping or clicking will be sensed when the patella is pushed against the femur. Release the pressure against the patella, but keep your finger lightly touching it. If an effusion is present, the patella will float out as if a fluid wave were pushing it (Figure 19-46).

Examination for the *bulge sign* is also used to determine the presence of excess fluid in the knee. With the patient's knee extended, milk the medial aspect of the knee upward two or three times, and then tap the lateral side of the patella. Observe for a bulge of returning fluid to the hollow area medial to the patella (Figure 19-47).

The *McMurray test* is used to detect a torn meniscus. Have the patient lie supine and flex one knee completely with the foot flat on the table near the buttocks. Maintain that flexion with your thumb and index finger, stabilizing the knee on either side of the joint space. Hold the heel with your other hand, and rotate the foot and lower

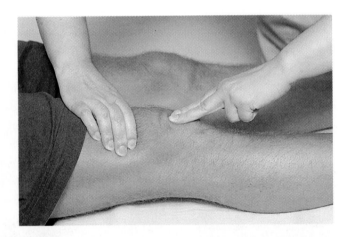

FIGURE 19-46
Procedure for ballottement examination of the knee.

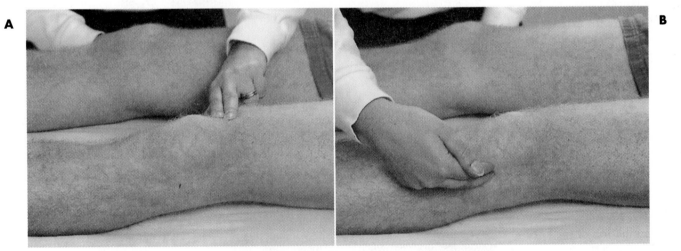

FIGURE 19-47
Testing for the bulge sign in examination of the knee. **A,** Milk the medial aspect of the knee two or three times. **B,** Then tap the lateral side of the patella.

leg to a lateral position. Extend the patient's knee to a 90-degree angle, noting any palpable or audible click or limited extension of the knee. Return the knee to full flexion, and repeat the procedure, rotating the foot and lower leg to a medial position (Figure 19-48). A palpable or audible click in the knee or lack of extension is a positive sign.

The *drawer test* is used to identify instability of the knee on the anteroposterior plane. Have the patient lie supine and flex the knee 45 to 90 degrees, placing the foot flat on the table. Place both hands on the lower leg and try to push the lower leg forward and backward (Figure 19-49). Excessive anterior or posterior movement of the knee is an unexpected finding, indicating injury to the anterior cruciate ligament or posterior cruciate ligament.

The *Lachman test* is used to evaluate anterior cruciate ligament integrity. With the patient supine, flex the knee 20 to 30 degrees. Place one hand above the knee to stabilize the femur, and place the other hand around the proximal tibia. While stabilizing the femur, pull the tibia anteriorly. Attempt to have the patient relax the hamstring muscles for an optimal test. Increased laxity compared to the uninjured side indicates injury to the ligament.

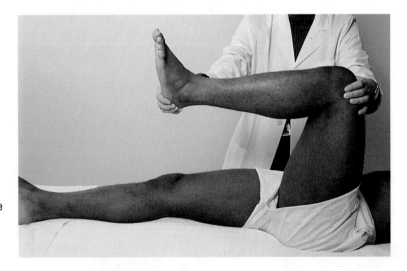

FIGURE 19-48
Procedure for examination of the knee with the McMurray test. Knee is flexed after lower leg was rotated to medial position.

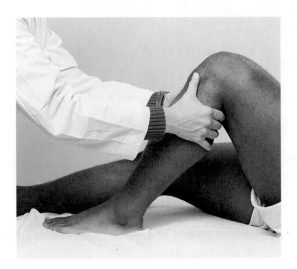

FIGURE 19-49
Examination of the knee with the drawer test for anterior and posterior stability.

The *varus and valgus stress test* is used to identify knee instability in the mediolateral plane. Have the patient lie supine and extend the knee. Stabilize the femur with one hand and hold the ankle with your other hand. Try to abduct the knee. Excessive laxity is felt as joint opening. Laxity in this position indicates injury to both the cruciate and collateral ligaments. Then repeat the abduction and adduction movements with the patient's knee flexed to 30 degrees. No excessive medial or lateral movement of the knee is expected (Figure 19-50).

When the patient complains of a knee locking, use the *Apley test* to detect a meniscal tear. Have the patient lie prone and flex the knee to 90 degrees. Place your hand on the heel of the foot and press firmly, opposing the tibia to the femur. Then rotate the lower leg externally and internally (Figure 19-51). Be cautious and do not cause the patient excess pain. Any clicks, locking, or pain in the knee is a positive Apley sign.

Hip Assessment

The *Thomas test* is used to detect flexion contractures of the hip that may be masked by excessive lumbar lordosis. Have the patient lie supine and fully extend one leg flat on the examining table and flex the other leg with the knee to the chest. Observe the patient's ability to keep the extended leg flat on the examining table (Figure 19-52). Lifting the extended leg off the examining table indicates a hip flexion contracture in the extended leg.

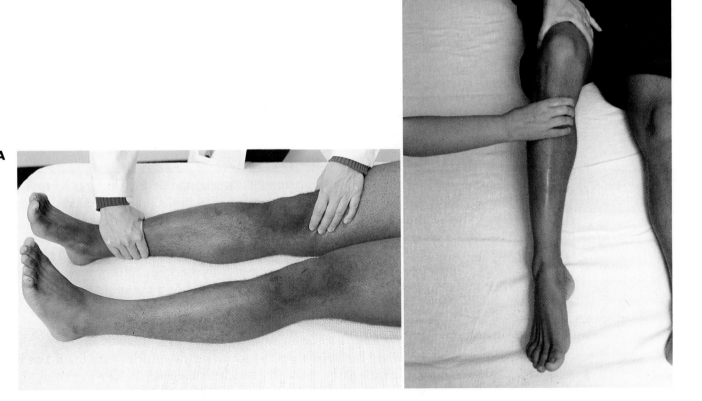

FIGURE 19-50
Varus and valgus stress test of the knee. **A,** With knee extended. **B,** With knee flexed.

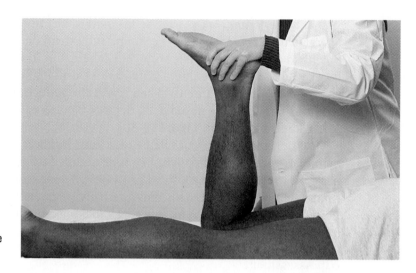

FIGURE 19-51
Examination of the knee with the Apley test.

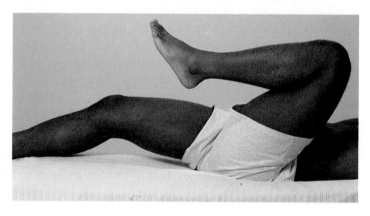

FIGURE 19-52
Procedures for examination of the hip with the Thomas test. Note the elevation of the extended leg off the examining table.

The *Trendelenburg test* is a maneuver to detect weak hip abductor muscles. Ask the patient to stand and balance first on one foot and then the other. Observing from behind, note any asymmetry or change in the level of the iliac crests. When the iliac crest drops on the side of the lifted leg, the hip abductor muscles on the weight-bearing side are weak (Figure 19-53).

INFANTS

Genetic and fetal insults can produce musculoskeletal anomalies. The fetus is exposed to various postural pressures that can be manifested in the infant as reduced extension of extremities and torsions of various bones.

Fully undress the infant and observe the posture and spontaneous generalized movements. (Use a warming table when examining newborns.) No localized or generalized muscular twitching is expected. Inspect the back for tufts of hair, dimples, discolorations, cysts, or masses near the spine. A mass near the spine that transilluminates should cause you to suspect a meningocele or myelomeningocele.

From about age 2 months, the infant should be able to lift the head and trunk from the prone position, giving you an indication of forearm strength. Assess the curvature of the spine and the strength of the paravertebral muscles with the infant in sitting position. Kyphosis of the thoracic and lumbar spine will be apparent in sitting position until the infant can sit without support (Figure 19-54).

Inspect the extremities, noting symmetric flexion of arms and legs. The axillary, gluteal, femoral, and popliteal creases should be symmetric, and the limbs should be freely movable. No unusual proportions of asymmetry of limb length or circumfer-

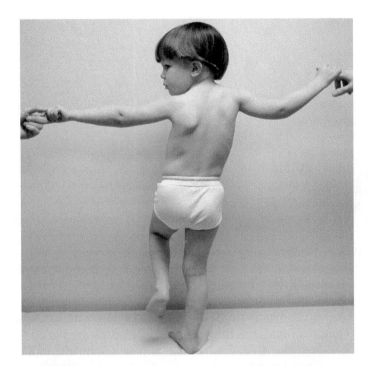

FIGURE 19-53
Test for the Trendelenburg sign. Note any asymmetry in the level of the iliac crests with weight bearing.

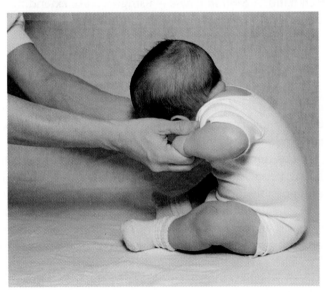

FIGURE 19-54
Kyphosis, expected convex curvature of the newborn spine.

ence, constricted annular bands, or other deformities should be noted. Unequal limb length and circumference have been associated with intraabdominal neoplasms.

Place the newborn in a fetal position to observe how that may have contributed to any asymmetry of flexion, position, or shape of the extremities. Newborns have some resistance to full extension of the elbows, hips, and knees. Movements should be symmetric.

All babies are flat-footed, and many newborns have a slight varus curvature of the tibias (tibial torsion) or forefoot adduction (metatarsus adductus) from fetal positioning. The midline of the foot may bisect the third and fourth toes, rather than the second and third toes. The forefoot should be flexible, straightening with abduction. It is necessary to follow apparent problems carefully, but it is seldom necessary to intervene. As growth and development take place, the expected body habitus is usually achieved.

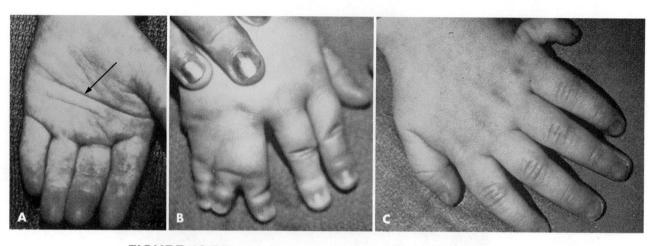

FIGURE 19-55
Anomalies of the newborn's hand. **A,** Simian crease. **B,** Syndactyly. **C,** Polydactyly.
Courtesy Mead Johnson, Evansville, Illinois.

The hands should open periodically with the fingers fully extended. When the hand is fisted, the thumb should be positioned inside the fingers. Open the fist and observe the dermatoglyphic features, noting the palmar and phalangeal creases on each hand. A *Simian crease*—a single crease extending across the entire palm—is associated with Down syndrome. Count the fingers and toes, noting polydactyly or syndactyly (Figure 19-55).

Palpate the clavicles and long bones for fractures, dislocations, crepitus, masses, and tenderness. One of the most easily missed findings in the newborn is a fractured clavicle. It is embarrassing to have a parent ask what that lump is on the baby's collar bone. It is the callus that forms as the healing clavicle shapes and remolds itself. The tell-tale bony irregularity and crepitus may well have been detected during the neonatal examination.

Position the baby with the trunk flexed, and palpate each spinal process. Feel the shape of each, noting whether it is thin and well formed, as expected, or whether it is split, possibly indicating a bifid defect (Figure 19-56).

Palpate the muscles to evaluate muscle tone, grasping the muscle to estimate its firmness. Observe for spasticity or flaccidity, and when detected, determine if it is localized or generalized. Use passive range of motion to examine joint mobility.

The *Barlow-Ortolani maneuver* to detect hip dislocation or subluxation should be performed each time you examine the infant during the first year of life. Position yourself at the supine infant's feet, and flex the hips and knees to 90 degrees. Grasp a leg in each of your hands with your thumb on the inside of each thigh, the base of the thumb on each knee, and your fingers gripping the outer thigh with fingertips resting on the greater trochanter (Figure 19-57). First, adduct the thighs to the maximum so that your thumbs touch. Apply downward pressure on the femur, not too vigorously, in an attempt to disengage the femoral head from the acetabulum. Next, slowly abduct the thighs while maintaining axial pressure. With the fingertips on the greater trochanter, exert a lever movement in the opposite direction so that your fingertips press the head of the femur back toward the acetabulum center. If the head of the femur slips back into the acetabulum with a palpable clunk when pressure is exerted, suspect hip subluxation or dislocation. Asymmetric gluteal folds and abduction of the hips limited to less than 160 degrees may also indicate developmental dysplasia of the hip with hip dislocation (Figure 19-58).

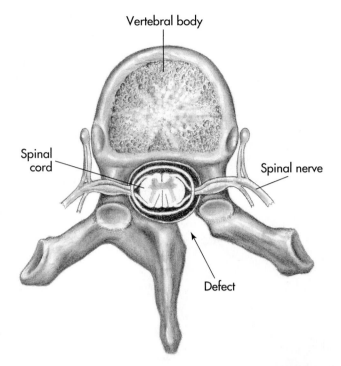

FIGURE 19-56
Bifid defect of the vertebra identified by palpation.

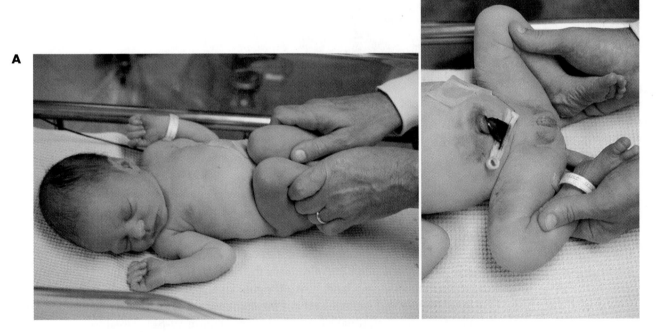

FIGURE 19-57
Barlow-Ortolani maneuver to detect hip dislocation. **A,** Phase I, adduction. **B,** Phase II, abduction.

The test for the *Allis sign* is also used to detect hip dislocation or a shortened femur. With the infant supine on the examining table, flex both knees, keeping the feet flat on the table and the femurs aligned with each other. Position yourself at the child's feet, and observe the height of the knees (Figure 19-59). When one knee appears lower than the other, the Allis sign is positive.

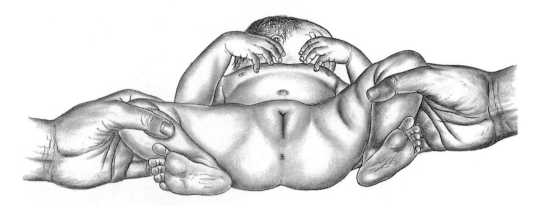

FIGURE 19-58
Signs of hip dislocation: limitation of abduction and asymmetric gluteal folds.

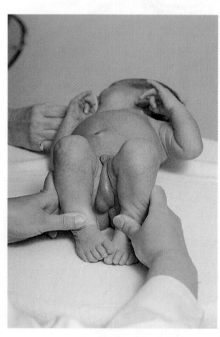

FIGURE 19-59
Examination for the Allis sign: unequal upper leg length would indicate a positive sign.

Muscle strength is evaluated by holding the infant upright with your hands under the axillae (Figure 19-60). Adequate shoulder muscle strength is present if the infant maintains the upright position. If the infant begins to slip through your fingers, muscle weakness is present.

Tibial torsion is evaluated with the child prone on the examining table. Flex one knee 90 degrees and align the midline of the foot parallel to the femur. Using the thumb and index finger of one hand, grasp the medial and lateral malleoli of the ankle, placing your thumb and index finger on the same side of the leg. If your thumbs are not parallel to each other, tibial torsion is present (Figure 19-61). Tibial torsion, a residual effect of fetal positioning, is expected to resolve after 6 months of weight bearing.

CHILDREN

Watching young children during play or while they are with the parent as the history is taken can provide a great deal of information about the child's musculoskeletal system. If the child has been able to pick up and play with toys, moving in unconstrained fashion without evidence of limitation, the laying on of hands is still necessary but may not reveal any additional information. Suggest activities that will enhance your observations. The function of joints, range of motion, bone stability, and muscle strength can be adequately evaluated by observing the child climb, jump, hop, rise from a sitting position, and manipulate toys or other objects.

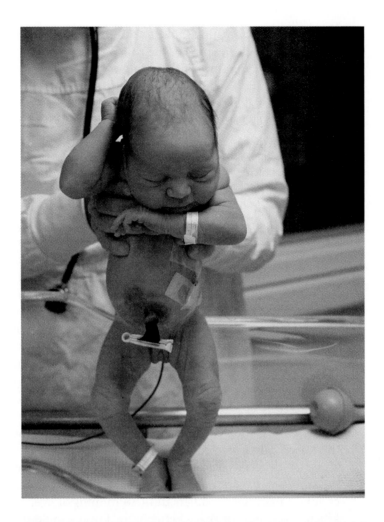

FIGURE 19-60
Evaluation of shoulder muscle
strength in the newborn.

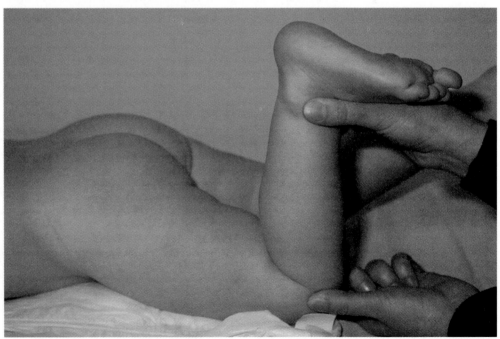

FIGURE 19-61
Examination for tibial torsion.

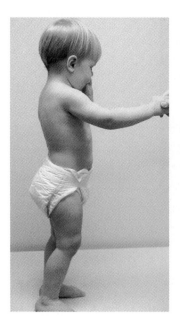

FIGURE 19-62
Lumbar curvature of the toddler's spine.

Position the young child to observe motor development and musculoskeletal function. Inspect the spine of the child while he or she is standing. Young children will have a lumbar curvature of the spine and a protuberant abdomen (Figure 19-62). Observe the toddler's ability to sit, creep, and grasp and release objects during play. Knowledge of the expected sequence of motor development will facilitate your examination (Table 19-3).

The motor development of black infants is often advanced over that of white infants; thus black children under 3 years of age may reach the milestones outlined in Table 19-3 before white children. White children start to catch up with black children around 3 years of age. As you inspect the bones, joints, and muscles, pay particular attention to the alignment of the legs and feet, because developmental stresses are placed on the musculoskeletal system. Remember to observe the wear of the child's shoes and ask about his or her favorite sitting posture. The reverse tailor position places stress on the joints of the hips, knees, and ankles. This could lead to future problems in lower limb alignment, such as femoral anteversion (Figure 19-63).

Inspect the longitudinal arch of the foot and the position of the feet with weight bearing. The longitudinal arch of the foot is obscured by a fat pad until about 3 years of age, and after that time, it should be apparent when it is not bearing weight. Metatarsus adductus should be resolved. The feet of the toddler will often pronate slightly inward until about 30 months of age. After that time, weight bearing should shift to the midline of the feet.

Bowleg (genu varum) is evaluated with the child standing, facing you, knees at your eye level. Measure the distance between the knees when the medial malleoli of the ankles are together. Genu varum is present if a space of 2.5 cm (1 in) exists between the knees. The expected 10- to 15-degree angle at the tibiofemoral articulation increases with genu varum but remains bilaterally symmetric. On future examinations, note any increase in the angle or increased space between the knees. Genu varum is a common finding of toddlers until 18 months of age. Asymmetry of the tibiofemoral articulation angle or space between the knees should not exceed 4 cm (1½ in).

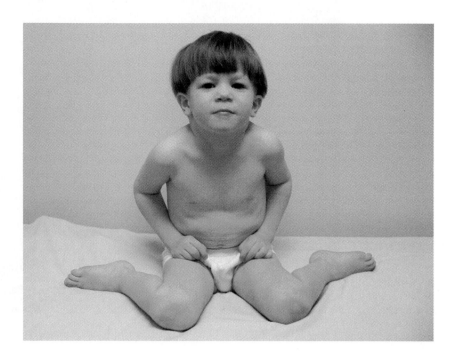

FIGURE 19-63
Reverse tailor sitting position.

TABLE 19-3	Expected Motor Development Sequence in Children, Birth to 9 Years of Age	
Age	**Fine Motor Development**	**Gross Motor Development**
1 month		Turns head to side; keeps knees tucked under abdomen; gross head lag and rounded back when pulled to sitting position
2 months		Holds head in same plane as rest of body; can raise head and hold position
3 months	When supine, puts hands together; holds hands in front of face	Raises head to 45 degrees; may turn from prone to side position; slight head lag when pulled to sitting position
4 months	Grasps rattle; hands held together	Actively lifts head, looks around; rolls from prone to supine position; no head lag when pulled to sitting position; attempts to bear weight when held standing up
5 months	Can reach and pick up object; plays with toes	Able to push up from prone position with forearms and maintain position; rolls over prone to supine to prone; back straight when sitting
6 months	Drops object to reach for another offered; holds rattle or spoon	Sits, posture shaky, uses tripod position; raises abdomen off table when prone; when standing, supports almost full weight
7 months	Transfers object between hands; holds object in each hand	Sits alone, uses hands for support; bounces in standing position; pulls feet to mouth
8 months	Begins thumb-finger grasping	Sits without support
9 months	Bangs objects together	Begins creeping, abdomen off floor; stands holding on when placed in position
10 month	Points with one finger; picks up small objects	Pulls self to standing position, unable to let self down; walks holding on to stable objects
11 months		Walks around room holding on to objects; stands securely, holding on with one hand
12 months	Feeds self with cup and spoon fairly well; offers toy and releases it	Sits from standing posture; twists and turns, maintaining posture; stands without support momentarily
15 months	Puts raisin into bottle; takes off shoes; pulls toys	Walks alone well; seats self in chair
18 months	Holds crayon, scribbles spontaneously	Walks up and down steps holding one hand, some running ability
2 years	Turns doorknob; takes off shoes and socks; builds 2-block tower	Walks up stairs alone, two feet on each step; walks backward; kicks ball
30 months	Builds 4-block tower; feeds self more neatly; dumps raisin from bottle	Jumps from object; throws ball overhand; walking more stable
3 years	Unbuttons front buttons; copies vertical line within 30 degrees; copies circle; builds 8-block tower	Walks up stairs alternating feet; walks down steps two feet on each step; pedals tricycle; jumps in one place; performs broad jump
4 years	Copies cross; buttons large buttons	Walks down stairs alternating feet; balances on one foot for 5 seconds
5 years	Dresses self with minimal assistance; colors within lines; draws 3-part human	Hops on one foot; catches bounced ball 2 of 3 times; heel-toe walking
6 years	Copies square; draws 6-part human	Jumps, tumbles, skips, hops; walks straight line; skips rope with practice; rides bicycle; heel-toe walking backward
7 years	Prints well, begins to write script	Skips and plays hopscotch; running and climbing more coordinated
8 years	Mature handwriting skill	Movements more graceful
9 years		Eye-hand coordination developed

Modified from Bowers, Thompson, 1992.

BOX 19-2 | **Screening Musculoskeletal Examination for Child and Adolescent Sports Participation***

- Observe posture and general muscle contour bilaterally
- Observe gait
- Ask patient to walk on tiptoes and heels
- Observe patient hop on each foot
- Ask patient to duck walk four steps with knees completely bent
- Inspect spine for curvature and lumbar extension, fingers touching toes with knees straight
- Palpate shoulder and clavicle for dislocation
- Check the following joints for range of motion: neck, shoulder, elbow, forearm, hands, fingers, and hips
- Test knee ligaments for drawer sign

*See Appendix B for detailed guidelines.

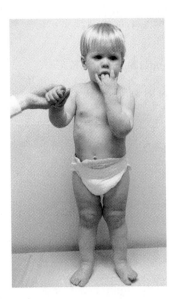

FIGURE 19-64
Genu valgum (knock knee) in the young child.

Knock knee (genu valgum) is also evaluated with the child standing, facing you, knees at your eye level. Measure the distance between the medial malleoli of the ankles with the knees together. Genu valgum is present if a space of 2.5 cm (1 in) exists between the medial malleoli. As with genu varum, the tibiofemoral articulation angle will increase with genu valgum. On future examinations, note any increase in the angle or increased space between the ankles. Genu valgum is a common finding of children between 2 and 4 years of age (Figure 19-64). Asymmetry of the tibiofemoral articulation angle or a space between the medial malleoli should not exceed 5 cm (2 in).

Subluxation of the head of the radius is often called nursemaid's elbow. Tugging on a child's arm while removing clothing or lifting a child by grabbing the hand can lead to this dislocation. The injury is relatively easy to cause and fortunately easy to reduce, but it is better to prevent it. A toddler should not dangle in the air suspended by an adult's grasp on the hand.

Palpate the bones, muscles, and joints, paying particular attention to asymmetric body parts. Use passive range of motion to examine a joint and muscle group if some limitation of movement is noted while the child is playing.

Ask the child to stand, rising from a supine position. The child with good muscle strength will rise to a standing position without using the arms for leverage. Generalized muscle weakness is indicated by the *Gower sign* in which the child rises from a sitting position by placing hands on the legs and pushing the trunk up (Figure 19-65).

ADOLESCENTS

Examine older children and adolescents with the same procedures used for adults. Remember to use caution when examining sports-related injuries.

The spine should be smooth with balanced concave and convex curves. No lateral curvature or rib hump with forward flexion should be apparent. The shoulders and scapulae should be level with each other within ½ in, and a distance between the scapulae of 3 to 5 in is usual. Adolescents may have slight kyphosis and rounded shoulders with an interscapular space of 5 or 6 in.

PREGNANT WOMEN

Postural changes with pregnancy are common. The growing fetus shifts the woman's center of gravity forward, leading to increased lordosis and a compensatory forward cervical flexion (Figure 19-66). Stooped shoulders and large breasts exaggerate the spinal curvature. Increased mobility and instability of the sacroiliac joints and symphisis pubis as the ligaments become less tense contribute to the "waddling" gait of late pregnancy.

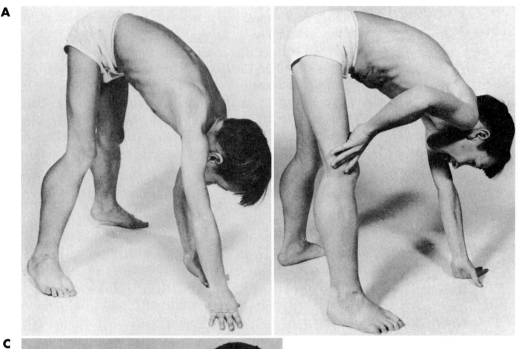

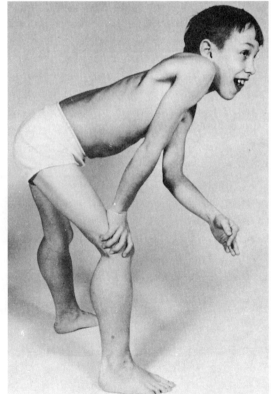

FIGURE 19-65

Gower sign of generalized muscle weakness. **A,** Maneuvers to position supported by both arms and legs. **B,** Pushes off floor to rest hand on knee. **C,** Then pushes self upright.

From Swaiman, Wright, 1982.

During pregnancy, expected increases in the lumbosacral curve and anterior flexion of the head in the cervicodorsal region become apparent. To assess for lumbosacral hyperextension, ask the woman to bend forward at the waist toward her toes. Palpate the distance between the L4 and S1 spinal processes. As the woman rises to standing, from full flexion to full extension, note when the distance between L4 and S1 becomes fixed. If it becomes fixed before the spine is fully extended, the woman will be hyperextended when walking, possibly resulting in lower back pain.

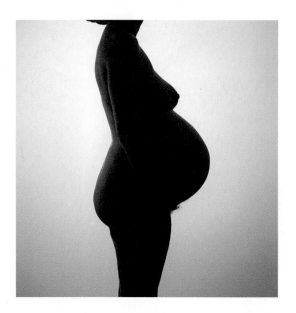

FIGURE 19-66
Postural changes with pregnancy.

Carpal tunnel syndrome is experienced by some women during the last trimester because of the associated fluid retention during pregnancy. The symptoms abate after delivery.

OLDER ADULTS

The older adults should be able to participate in the physical examination as described for the adult, but the response to your requests may be more slow and deliberate. Fine and gross motor skills required to perform activities of daily living such as dressing, grooming, climbing steps, and writing will provide an evaluation of the patient's joint muscle agility (see the Functional Assessment box). Joint and muscle agility have tremendous extremes among older adults (Figure 19-67).

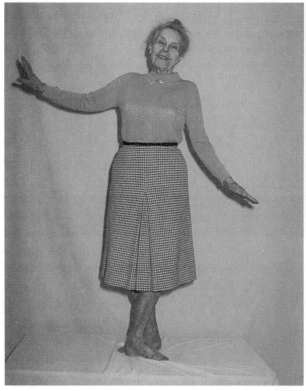

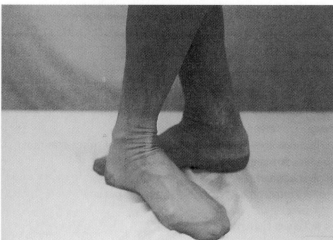

FIGURE 19-67
Agility in the older adult. Note the flexibility and ability to balance of this 83-year-old woman.

The patient's posture may display increased dorsal kyphosis, accompanied by flexion of the hips and knees. The head may tilt backward to compensate for the increased thoracic curvature (see Figure 19-20, *B*). The extremities may appear to be relatively long if the trunk has diminished in length. The base of support may be broader with the feet more widely spaced, and the patient may hold the arms away from the body to aid balancing.

The reduction in total muscle mass is often related to atrophy, either from disuse, as in patients with arthritis, or from loss of nervous innervation, as in patients with diabetic neuropathy.

FUNCTIONAL ASSESSMENT

Musculoskeletal Assessment

Activity to Observe	Indicators of Weakened Muscle Groups
Rising from lying to sitting position	Rolling to one side and pushing with arms to raise to elbows; grabbing a siderail or table to pull to sitting
Rising from chair to standing	Pushing with arms to supplement weak leg muscles; upper torso thrusts forward before body rises
Walking	Lifting leg farther off floor with each step; shortened swing phase; foot may fall or slide forward; arms held out for balance or move in rowing motion
Climbing steps	Holding handrail for balance; pulling body up and forward with arms; uses stronger leg
Descending steps	Lowering weakened leg first; often descends sideways holding rail with both hands; may watch feet
Picking up item from floor	Leaning on furniture for support; bending over at waist to avoid bending knees; uses one hand on thigh to assist with lowering and raising torso
Tying shoes	Using footstool to decrease spinal flexion
Putting on and pulling up trousers or stockings	Difficulty may indicate decreased shoulder and upper arm strength; these activities often performed in sitting position until clothing is pulled up
Putting on sweater	Putting sleeve on weaker arm or shoulder first; uses internal or external shoulder rotation to get remaining arm in sleeve
Zipping dress in back	Difficulty with this indicates weakened shoulder rotation
Combing hair	Difficulty indicates problems with grasp, wrist flexion, pronation and supination of forearm, and elbow rotation
Pushing chair away from table while seated	Standing and easing chair back with torso; difficulty indicates problems with upper arm, shoulder, lower arm strength, and wrist motion
Buttoning button or writing name	Difficulty indicates problem with manual dexterity and finger-thumb opposition

Modified from Bowers, Thompson, 1992.

SUMMARY OF EXAMINATION   Musculoskeletal System

The following steps are performed with the patient standing, sitting, and walking.

1. Inspect the skeleton and extremities and compare sides for the following (p. 705):
   - Alignment
   - Contour and symmetry of body parts
   - Size
   - Gross deformity
2. Inspect the skin and subcutaneous tissues over muscles and joints for the following (p. 705):
   - Color
   - Number of skin folds
   - Swelling
   - Masses
3. Inspect muscles and compare contralateral sides for the following (p. 705):
   - Size
   - Symmetry
   - Fasciculations or spasms
4. Palpate all bones, joints, and surrounding muscles for the following (p. 706):
   - Muscle tone
   - Heat
   - Tenderness
   - Swelling
   - Crepitus
5. Test each major joint for active and passive range of motion and compare contralateral sides (p. 706).
6. Test major muscle groups for strength and compare contralateral sides (p. 707).

Joints That Deserve Particular Attention
Temporomandibular Joint
1. Test range of motion by having the patient perform the following (pp. 707-708):
   - Opening and closing mouth
   - Moving jaw laterally to each side
   - Protruding and retracting jaw
2. Palpate the joint space for clicking, popping, and pain (p. 707).
3. Test strength of temporalis muscles with the patient's teeth clenched (p. 708).

Cervical Spine
1. Inspect the neck for the following (p. 708):
   - Alignment
   - Symmetry of skin folds and muscles
2. Test range of motion by the following maneuvers (pp. 708-709):
   - Forward flexion (45°)
   - Hyperextension (55°)
   - Lateral bending (40°)
   - Rotation (70°)

3. Test strength of sternocleidomastoid and trapezius muscles (cranial nerve XI, spinal accessory) (p. 709).

Thoracic and Lumbar Spine
1. Inspect the spine for alignment (pp. 709-710).
2. Palpate the spinal processes and paravertebral muscles (p. 710).
3. Percuss for spinal tenderness (p. 710).
4. Test range of motion by the following maneuvers (pp. 710-712):
   - Forward flexion (75°)
   - Hyperextension (30°)
   - Lateral bending (35°)
   - Rotation

Shoulders
1. Inspect shoulders and shoulder girdle for contour (p. 712-713).
2. Palpate the joint spaces and bones of the shoulders (p. 713).
3. Test range of motion by the following maneuvers (pp. 713-715):
   - Shrugging the shoulders
   - Forward flexion (180°) and hyperextension (up to 50°)
   - Abduction (180°) and adduction (50°)
   - Internal and external rotation (90°)
4. Test muscle strength by the following maneuvers (p. 715):
   - Shrugged shoulders
   - Forward flexion
   - Abduction
   - Medial and lateral rotation

Elbows
1. Inspect the elbows in flexed and extended position for the following (p. 715):
   - Contour
   - Carrying angle (5-15°)
2. Palpate the extensor surface of the ulna, olecranon process, and the medial and lateral epicondyles of the humerus (p. 715).
3. Test range of motion by the following maneuvers (pp. 715-716):
   - Flexion (160°)
   - Extension (180°)
   - Pronation and supination (90°)

Hands and Wrists
1. Inspect the dorsum and palm of hands for the following (pp. 716-717):
   - Contour
   - Position
   - Shape
   - Number and completeness of digits

SUMMARY OF EXAMINATION   Musculoskeletal System—cont'd

2. Palpate each joint in the hand and wrist (pp. 717-718).
3. Strike the median nerve to test for the Tinel sign (p. 718):
4. Test range of motion by the following maneuvers (p. 720):
   - Metacarpophalangeal flexion (90°) and hyperextension (30°)
   - Thumb opposition
   - Forming a fist
   - Finger adduction and abduction
   - Wrist extension, hyperextension (70°), and flexion (90°)
   - Radial (20°) and ulnar motion (55°)
5. Test muscle strength by the following maneuvers (p. 720):
   - Wrist extension and hyperextension
   - Hand grip

Hips

1. Inspect the hips for symmetry and level of gluteal folds (p. 720).
2. Palpate hips and pelvis for the following (p. 720):
   - Instability
   - Tenderness
   - Crepitus
3. Test range of motion by the following maneuvers (p. 720):
   - Flexion (120°), extension (90°) and hyperextension (30°)
   - Adduction (30°) and abduction (45°)
   - Internal rotation (40°)
   - External rotation (45°)

4. Test muscle strength of hips with the following maneuvers (p. 720):
   - Knee in flexion and extension
   - Abduction and adduction
5. Inspect for flexion contractures with the Thomas test (p. 731).
6. Inspect for weak hip abductor muscles with the Trendelenburg test (p. 732).

Legs and Knees

1. Inspect the knees for natural concavities (p. 722).
2. Palpate the popliteal space and joint space (p. 722).
3. Test range of motion by flexion (130°) and extension (0-15°) (p. 722).
4. Test the strength of muscles in flexion and extension (p. 722).

Feet and Ankles

1. Inspect the feet and ankles during weight bearing and non-weight bearing for the following (pp. 722, 724):
   - Contour
   - Alignment with tibias
   - Size
   - Number of toes
2. Palpate the Achilles tendon and each metatarsal joint (p. 724).
3. Test range of motion by the following maneuvers (pp. 724-725):
   - Dorsiflexion (20°) and plantar flexion (45°)
   - Inversion (30°) and eversion (20°)
   - Flexion and extension of the toes
4. Test strength of muscles in plantar flexion and dorsiflexion (p. 725).

COMMON ABNORMALITIES

ANKYLOSING
SPONDYLITIS

A hereditary, chronic inflammatory disease, ankylosing spondylitis initially affects the lumbar spine and sacroiliac joints. Larger joints of the shoulders, hips, and knees may be affected later. The inflamed intervertebral disks become infiltrated with vascular connective tissue that ossifies. The disease progresses to eventual fusion and deformity of the entire spine. The disease develops predominantly in males during early adulthood (Figure 19-68).

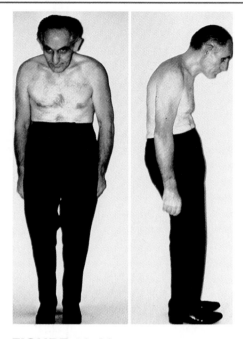

FIGURE 19-68

Gross postural changes in man affected by ankylosing spondylitis.

Reprinted from the Clinical Slide Collection of the Rheumatic Diseases, copyright 1991. Used by permission of the American College of Rheumatology

LUMBOSACRAL
RADICULOPATHY

Lumbosacral radiculopathy is herniation of a lumbar disk that irritates the corresponding nerve root and results in muscle weakness, paresthesia, and pain in the distribution of the nerve root dermatome. Disk herniation is generally caused by degenerative changes of the disk, most commonly occurring at the L4 and L5 nerve roots. The greatest incidence occurs between 31 and 50 years of age. The condition is commonly associated with lifting heavy objects while the arms are extended and the spine is flexed, such as occurs when bending to lift a child weighing more than 25 pounds. Common symptoms include low back pain with radiation to the buttocks and posterior thigh or down the leg in the distribution of the dermatome of the nerve root. Tenderness over the paraspinal musculature may also be present. Pain may be unilateral, bilateral, or alternating sides. Sneezing and coughing often induce or aggravate the pain. Pain relief is often achieved by lying down.

CARPAL TUNNEL
SYNDROME

Compression on the median nerve caused by thickening of its flexor tendon sheath often results from microtrauma, repetitive motion of the arms and hands, or vibration. It is also associated with rheumatoid arthritis, gout, hypothyroidism, and the hormonal changes of pregnancy and menopause. The symptoms of numbess, burning, and tingling in the hands often occur at night, but they can also be elicited by rotational movements of the wrist. Pain may also occur in the arms. Weakness of the hand and flattening of the thenar eminence of the palm may result. The disorder is three times more common in women. For a discussion of the Tinel sign, see p. 718 (Figure 19-69).

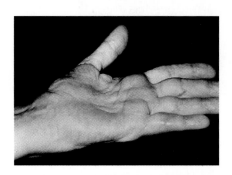

FIGURE 19-69

Carpal tunnel syndrome with thenar atrophy.

Reprinted from the Clinical Slide Collection of the Rheumatic Diseases, copyright 1991. Used by permission of the American College of Rheumatology.

GOUT

Gout is a hereditary overproduction or decreased excretion of uric acid and urate salts. Urate salts are deposited in the joints, ear cartilage, and kidneys to lower the uric acid blood serum level. The joint classically affected is the proximal phalanx of the great toe, although other joints of the wrists, hands, ankles, and knees are sometimes affected. Symptoms include a red, hot, swollen joint; exquisite pain; limited range of motion; tophi; and mild fever. The disease primarily affects men over age 40 (Figure 19-70).

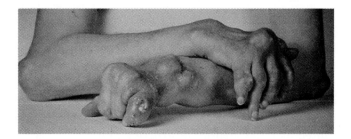

FIGURE 19-70

Gout with many tophi present on the hands, wrists, and in both olecranon bursae.

Reprinted from the Clinical Slide Collection of the Rheumatoid Diseases, copyright 1991. Used by permission of the American College of Rheumatology.

TEMPOROMANDIBU-
LAR JOINT SYNDROME

Temporomandibular joint (TMJ) syndrome is painful jaw movement caused by congenital anomalies, malocclusion, trauma, arthritis, and other joint diseases. There is unilateral facial pain that usually worsens with joint movement and may be referred to any point on the face or neck. Most patients have a muscle spasm, and many have clicking, popping, or crepitus in the affected joint.

OSTEOMYELITIS

Osteomyelitis, an infection in the bone, usually results from an open wound or systemic infection. Purulent matter spreads through the cortex of the bone and into the soft tissues. Signs of infection include edema, erythema, warmth at the site, tenderness, pain with movement, and generalized signs such as spiking fevers, headache, and nausea.

BURSITIS

Bursitis is an inflammation of a bursa resulting from constant friction between the skin and tissues around the joint. Common sites include the shoulder, elbow, hip, and knee. Signs include limitation of motion caused by swelling, pain on movement, point tenderness, and an erythematous, warm site (Figure 19-71).

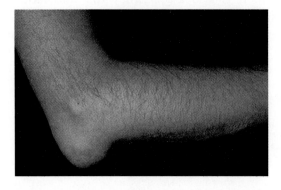

FIGURE 19-71

Olecranon bursitis.

Reprinted from the Clinical Slide Collection of the Rheumatic Diseases, copyright 1991. Used by permission of the American College of Rheumatology.

PAGET DISEASE (OSTEITIS DEFORMANS)

An inflammatory focal disorder of the bone, Paget disease appears in persons over 45 years of age. Excessive bone resorption and excessive bone formation produce a mosaic pattern of lamellar bone. Bowed tibias, misshapen pelvis or skull, shortened thorax, and frequent fractures occur. The bones of the skull are often affected, which can produce symptoms of vertigo, headache, and progressive deafness from involvement of the ossicles or neural elements. The cause in unknown, although a slow-acting virus is suspected.

OSTEOARTHRITIS

A noninflammatory disorder of movable joints, osteoarthritis results in deterioration and abrasion of cartilage and the formation of new bone at joint surfaces (Table 19-4). The incidence increases as people age, with 90% of people over age 60 years affected.

RHEUMATOID ARTHRITIS

Rheumatoid arthritis is a chronic, systemic, inflammatory disorder of joints that can occur at any age. The cause is unknown but may be associated with infection, autoimmunity, trauma, stress, or familial predisposition. Deformities are caused by inflammatory destruction and the remodeling of articular surfaces by muscle mechanical forces. The sexual predilection is 3:1, females to males (Table 19-4). The disease has a lower incidence in Asian and Hispanic groups than in white and black groups.

TABLE 19-4	Comparison of Osteoarthritis and Rheumatoid Arthritis	
Signs and Symptoms	**Osteoarthritis**	**Rheumatoid Arthritis**
Onset	Insidious	Gradual or sudden (24-48 hr)
Duration of stiffness	Few minutes, localized, but short "gelling" after prolonged rest	Often hours, most pronounced after rest
Pain	On motion, with prolonged activity, relieved by rest	Even at rest, may disturb sleep
Weakness	Usually localized and not severe	Often pronounced, out of proportion with muscle atrophy
Fatigue	Unusual	Often severe, with onset 4-5 hr after rising
Emotional depression and lability	Unusual	Common, coincides with fatigue and disease activity, often relieved if in remission
Tenderness localized over afflicted joint	Common	Almost always, most sensitive indicator of inflammation
Swelling	Effusion common, little synovial reaction	Fusiform soft tissue enlargement, effusion common, synovial proliferation and thickening
Heat, erythema	Unusual	Sometimes present
Crepitus, crackling	Coarse to medium on motion	Medium to fine
Joint enlargement	Mild with firm consistency	Moderate to severe

DIFFERENTIAL DIAGNOSIS

Modified from McCarty, 1993.

SPORTS INJURIES

Trauma to the musculoskeletal system results in a variety of injuries to muscles, bones, and supportive joint structures. The injury may be the result of an acute incident or overuse and repetitive trauma.

MUSCLE STRAIN

A muscle can become strained from stretching, tearing, or forceful contraction beyond its functional capacity. Severity ranges from a mild intrafibrinous tear to a total rupture of a single muscle. Signs include temporary weakness, numbness, and contusion.

SPRAIN

Stretching or tearing a supporting ligament of a joint by forced movement beyond its normal range can cause a sprain. Severe sprains may result in total rupture of ligaments and permanent joint instability if not treated. Signs include pain, marked swelling, hemorrhage, and loss of function.

DISLOCATION

Dislocation is the complete separation of the contact between two bones in a joint, often caused by pressure or force pushing the bone out of the joint. Signs include deformity and inability to use the extremity or joint as usual.

FRACTURE

A fracture is a partial or complete break in the continuity of a bone resulting from trauma (direct, indirect, twisting, or crushing). Muscle contractions and spasms lead to shortening of tissues around the bone, thus causing deformity. Other signs include edema, pain, loss of function, color changes, and paresthesia.

TENOSYNOVITIS

An inflammation of the synovium-lined sheath around a tendon, tenosynovitis results from repetitive actions associated with occupational or sports activities.

Common sites include the shoulder, knee, heel, and wrist. Signs include point tenderness, edema, pain with movement, and a weak grasp.

INFANTS AND CHILDREN

MYELOMENINGOCELE, SPINA BIFIDA

Congenital neural tube defects, with incomplete closure of the vertebral column, permit the meninges and some-

times the spinal cord to protrude into a saclike structure (Figure 19-72).

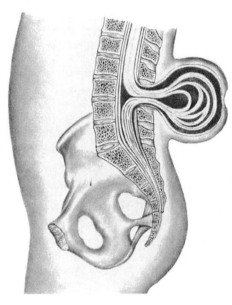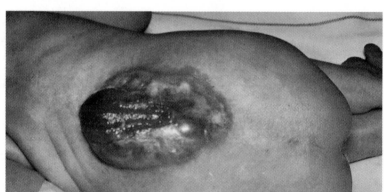

FIGURE 19-72
Myelomeningocele.
Drawing from Wong, 1995. Photo from Zitelli, Davis, 1996; courtesy Christine L. Williams, New York Medical College.

CLUBFOOT (TALIPES EQUINOVARUS)

Clubfoot is a fixed congenital defect of the ankle and foot. The most common combination of position deformities in-

cludes inversion of the foot at the ankle and plantar flexion, with the toes lower than the heel (Figure 19-73).

FIGURE 19-73
Clubfoot deformity, talipes equinovarus (bilateral deviation).
From Zitelli, Davis, 1996.

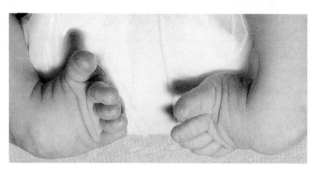

METATARSUS ADDUCTUS (METATARSUS VARUS)

The most common congenital foot deformity, metatarsus adductus can be either fixed or flexible. This defect is caused by intrauterine positioning. Medial adduction of the toes and forefoot results from angulation at the tarsometatarsal joint. The lateral border of the foot is convex, and a crease is sometimes apparent on the medial border of the foot. The heel and ankle are uninvolved (Figure 19-74).

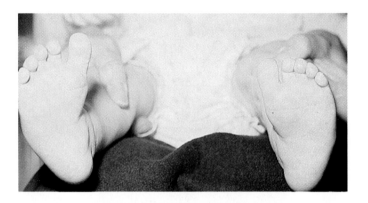

FIGURE 19-74
Bilateral metatarsus adductus. Viewed from plantar aspect showing rounding of the lateral border of the feet.
From Zitelli, Davis, 1996.

DEVELOPMENTAL DYSPLASIA OF THE HIP

Developmental dysplasia of the hip is a common congenital defect with varying degrees of involvement. Females are affected more than males by a 6:1 ratio. Acetabular dysplasia arises from delay in ossification of the acetabulum, which is oblique and shallow, but the femoral head remains in the acetabulum. Subluxation is an incomplete dislocation in which the femoral head remains in contact with the acetabulum, but the joint ligaments and capsule are stretched, which allows displacement of the femoral head. Dislocation indicates that the femoral head loses contact completely with the acetabular capsule and is displaced over the fibrocartilaginous rim.

HYPOPHOSPHATEMIC RICKETS

An X-linked dominant genetic disorder, hypophosphatemic rickets results in impaired bone mineralization. The kidneys inadequately reabsorb phosphorus in the proximal tubules, leading to an excess urinary excretion of phosphorus. No signs of the disorder are apparent at birth or for the first few months of life. Children develop linear growth retardation, genu varum, and spontaneous tooth abscesses because of faulty dentin formation. The lower limb deformity is accompanied by muscle weakness and a decreased energy level.

CLEIDOCRANIAL
DYSPLASIA

Cleidocranial dysplasia is an autosomal dominant disorder with deficient ossification of the bones of the cranium, clavicles, and pelvis. Complete or partial absence of the clavicles results in excessive forward movement of the shoulders. It is accompanied by defective ossification of the cranium, with large fontanels and delayed closing of the sutures (Figure 19-75.) The defective symphysis pubis results in a waddling gait.

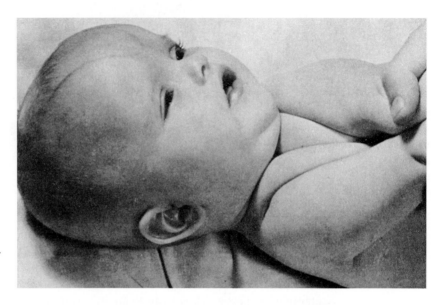

FIGURE 19-75
Cleidocranial dysplasia: congenital absence of the clavicles.
From Swaiman, Wright, 1982.

EPIPHYSEAL
OSTEOCHONDRITIS

A disorder of repetitive trauma to the epiphysis, epiphyseal osteochondritis results in compression microfractures and vascular insufficiency. Necrosis of the entire epiphysis may occur. *Legg-Calvé-Perthes disease* is one form affecting the hip, most commonly occurring in children ages 2 to 10 years; a limp is the presenting symptom. Another form of the disorder, *Osgood-Schlatter disease,* affects the knee. It most commonly occurs in children ages 9 to 15 years. Symptoms include pain and swelling of the tibial tuberosity.

MUSCULAR
DYSTROPHY

Muscular dystrophy is a group of genetic disorders involving gradual degeneration of the muscle fibers. The disorders are characterized by progressive weakness and muscle atrophy or pseudohypertrophy from fatty infiltrates. Some forms cause mild disability, and these patients can expect a normal life span. Other types produce severe disability, deformity, and death.

SCOLIOSIS

Scoliosis is a physical deformity with a concave curvature of the anterior vertebral bodies, convex posterior curves, and lateral rotation of the thoracic spine. In severe deformities the patient has uneven shoulder and hip levels, and the rotational deformity causes a rib hump and flank asymmetry on forward flexion. Physiologic alterations in the spine, chest, and pelvis result (Figure 19-76). Structural scoliosis most commonly affects girls and progresses during early adolescence and has no known cause. Functional scoliosis may also occur because of a leg length discrepancy.

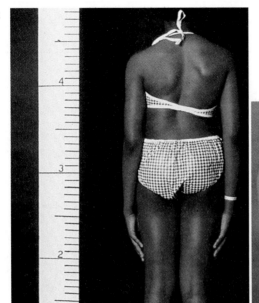
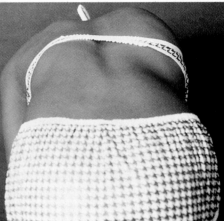

FIGURE 19-76
Scoliosis, lateral curvature of the spine, with increased convexity to the right. **A,** Scapular asymmetry is easily discernible in the upright position. **B,** Forward flexion reveals a mild rib hump deformity.

From Zitelli, Davis, 1996.

RADIAL HEAD SUBLUXATION	Radial head subluxation, also known as nursemaid's elbow, is a dislocation injury caused by jerking the arm upward while the elbow is flexed. This injury is common in children 1 to 4 years of age. The	child complains of pain in the elbow and wrist, refuses to move the arm, and holds it slightly flexed and pronated. Supination motion is resisted.
FEMORAL ANTEVERSION	With femoral anteversion the femurs twist medially with the patella facing inward. Increased internal rotation of the hip of more than 70 degrees and decreased external hip rotation contribute to or result from the condition. In-toeing of the feet increases up to 5 to 6 years of	age and gradually decreases, and to compensate, the tibias may twist laterally to permit correct positioning of the feet (Figure 19-77). Femoral anteversion is often associated with reverse tailor sitting. It is more common in females.

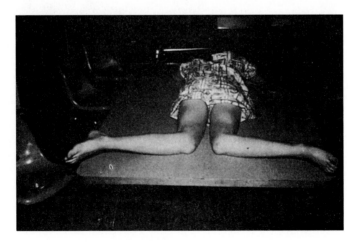

FIGURE 19-77
Femoral anteversion.
From Mann, Coughlin, 1993.

OLDER ADULTS

OSTEOPOROSIS

Osteoporosis is a silent progressive disease in which a decrease in bone mass occurs because bone resorption is more rapid than bone deposition. The bones become fragile and susceptible to spontaneous fractures; the presenting symptom is usually an acute, painful fracture. The most common fracture sites are hip, vertebrae, and wrist. In the spine wedge compression fractures lead to kyphotic bowing of the spine. Affected persons lose height, have a bent spine, and appear to sink into their hips. Women are more commonly affected, with a 4:1 ratio to men. It is most common in postmenopausal women (Figure 17-78).

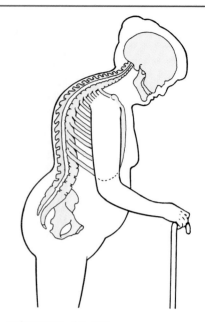

FIGURE 19-78
Hallmark of osteoporosis: dowager hump.

DUPUYTREN CONTRACTURE

Dupuytren contracture affects the palmar fascia of one or more fingers and tends to be bilateral. Although the cause is unknown, there appears to be a hereditary component. A gradual increase in incidence occurs with age. It is also seen with increased frequency in patients with diabetes, alcoholic liver disease, and epilepsy (Figure 19-79).

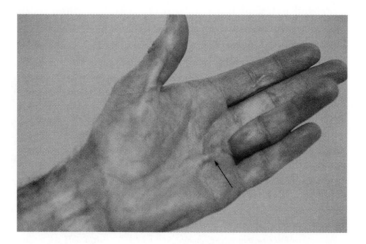

FIGURE 19-79
Dupuytren contracture.

Check it out— *http://www1.mosby.com/physexam_seidel*

CHAPTER 20

NEUROLOGIC SYSTEM

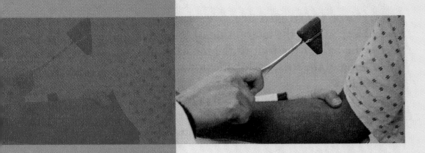

The nervous system, with its central and peripheral divisions, maintains and controls all body functions by its voluntary and autonomic responses. Evaluation of motor, sensory, autonomic, cognitive, and behavioral elements makes neurologic assessment one of the most complex portions of the physical examination.

ANATOMY AND PHYSIOLOGY

The central nervous system (brain and spinal cord) is the main network of coordination and control for the body (Figure 20-1). The peripheral nervous system, composed of motor and sensory nerves and ganglia outside the central nervous system, carries information to and from the central nervous system. The autonomic nervous system regulates the internal environment of the body, over which a person has no voluntary control. It has two divisions, each tending to balance the impulses of the other. The sympathetic division prods the body into action during times of physiologic and psychologic stress. The parasympathetic division functions in a complementary and a counterbalancing manner to conserve body resources and maintain day-to-day body functions such as digestion and elimination.

The intricate interrelationship of the nervous system permits the body to perform the following:

- Receive sensory stimuli from the environment
- Identify and integrate the adaptive processes needed to maintain current body functions
- Orchestrate body function changes required for adaptation and survival
- Integrate the rapid responsiveness of the central nervous system with the more gradual responsiveness of the endocrine system
- Control cognitive and voluntary behavioral processes
- Control subconscious and involuntary body functions

The brain and spinal cord are protected by the skull and vertebrae, the meninges, and cerebrospinal fluid. Three layers of meninges surround the brain and spinal cord, assisting in the production and drainage of cerebrospinal fluid (Figure 20-2). Cerebrospinal fluid circulates between an interconnecting system of ventricles in the brain and around the brain and spinal cord, serving as a shock absorber.

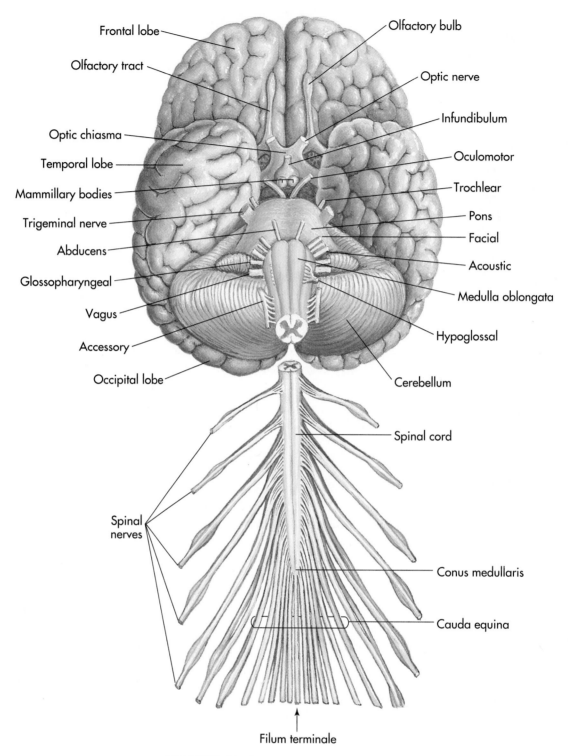

FIGURE 20-1

Base view of brain and cross-section of spinal cord.

A

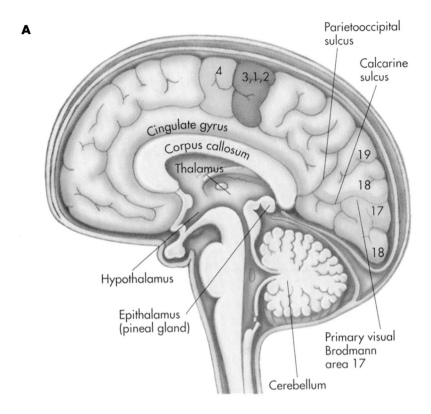

Parietooccipital sulcus

Calcarine sulcus

4

3,1,2

Cingulate gyrus

Corpus callosum

Thalamus

19

18

17

18

Hypothalamus

Epithalamus (pineal gland)

Primary visual Brodmann area 17

Cerebellum

B

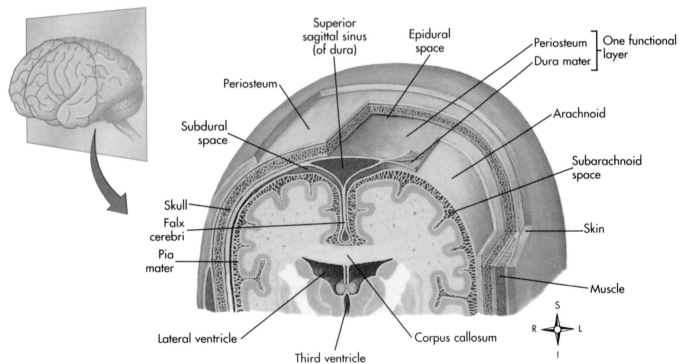

Superior sagittal sinus (of dura)

Epidural space

Periosteum
Dura mater
} One functional layer

Periosteum

Arachnoid

Subdural space

Subarachnoid space

Skull

Falx cerebri

Skin

Pia mater

Muscle

Lateral ventricle

Third ventricle

Corpus callosum

S
R L
I

FIGURE 20-2

Cross-sectional view of brain and meningeal layers. **A,** Functional areas of the cerebral cortex, midsagittal view. **B,** Frontal section of the superior portion of the head, as viewed from the front. Both bony and membranous coverings of the brain can be seen.

A, From McCance, Huether, 1998. **B,** From Thibodeau, Patton, 1996.

BRAIN

The brain receives its blood supply from the two internal carotid arteries, two vertebral arteries, and the basilar artery (Figure 20-3). Blood drains from the brain through venous sinuses that empty into the internal jugular veins. The three major units of the brain are the cerebrum, the cerebellum, and the brainstem.

Cerebrum

Two cerebral hemispheres, each divided into lobes, form the cerebrum. The gray outer layer, the cerebral cortex, houses the higher mental functions and is responsible

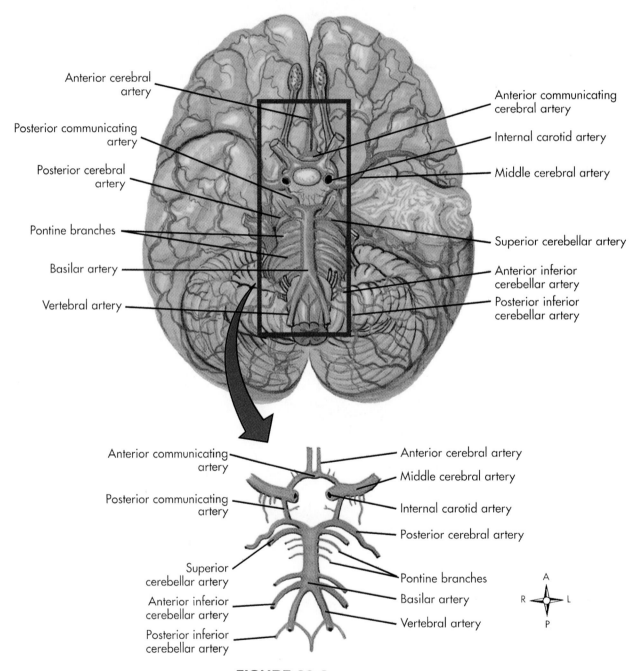

FIGURE 20-3

Arterial blood supply to the brain.

From Thibodeau, Patton, 1996.

for general movement, visceral functions, perception, behavior, and the integration of these functions. Commissural fibers interconnect the counterpart areas in each hemisphere, unifying the cerebrum's higher sensory and motor function (Figure 20-4 and Figure 4-1).

The *frontal lobe* contains the motor cortex associated with voluntary skeletal movement and fine repetitive motor movements.

The *parietal lobe* is primarily responsible for processing sensory data as it is received. It assists with the interpretation of tactile sensations (temperature, pressure, pain, size, shape, texture, and two-point discrimination), as well as visual, gustatory, olfactory, and auditory sensations. Recognition of body parts and awareness of body position (proprioception) are dependent on the parietal lobe.

The *occipital lobe* contains the primary vision center and provides interpretation of visual data.

The *temporal lobe* is responsible for the perception and interpretation of sounds and determination of their source. It is also involved in the integration of taste, smell, and balance.

The *limbic system* mediates certain patterns of behavior (primitive behaviors, visceral response to emotional and biologic rhythms) that determine survival, such as mating, aggression, fear, and affection. Interference with the physiology of the limbic system results in distorted perception and inappropriate behavior.

Cerebellum

The cerebellum aids the motor cortex of the cerebrum in the integration of voluntary movement. It processes sensory information from the eyes, ears, touch receptors, and musculoskeleton. Integrated with the vestibular system, the cerebellum utilizes the sensory data for reflexive control of muscle tone, equilibrium, and posture.

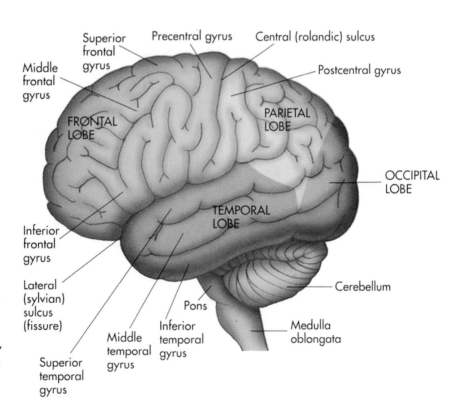

FIGURE 20-4

Lobes and principle fissures of the cerebral cortex, cerebellum, and brainstem (left hemisphere, lateral view).

From McCance, Huether, 1998.

Brainstem

The brainstem is the pathway between the cerebral cortex and the spinal cord, and it controls many involuntary functions. Its structures include the medulla oblongata, pons, midbrain, and diencephalon. The nuclei of the 12 cranial nerves arise from these structures (Figure 20-5 and Table 20-1). The thalamus is the major integrating center for perception of various sensations (along with the cortical processing for interpretation), serving as the relay center between the basal ganglia and cerebellum.

Cranial Nerves

Cranial nerves are peripheral nerves that arise from the brain rather than the spinal cord. Each nerve has motor or sensory functions, and four cranial nerves have parasympathetic functions (Table 20-2).

Basal Ganglia

The basal ganglia or cerebral nuclei function as the extrapyramidal system pathway and processing station between the cerebral motor cortex and the upper brainstem. They contribute input from visual, labyrinthine, and proprioceptive sources that allow gross intentional movement without conscious thought, by exerting a fine tuning effect on motor movements.

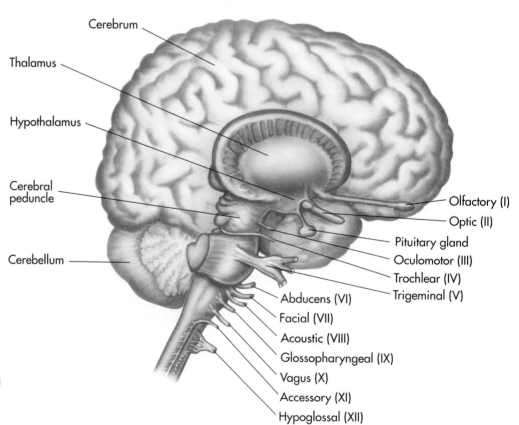

FIGURE 20-5

Structures of the diencephalon and location of the cranial nerve roots.

From Rudy, 1984.

TABLE 20-1   Structures of the Brainstem and Their Function

Structure	Function
Medulla oblongata CN IX-XII	Respiratory, circulatory, and vasomotor activities; houses respiratory center Reflexes of swallowing, coughing, vomiting, sneezing, and hiccupping Relay center for major ascending and descending spinal tracts that decussate at the pyramid
Pons CN V-VIII	Reflexes of pupillary action and eye movement Regulates respiration; houses a portion of the respiratory center Controls voluntary muscle action with corticospinal tract pathway
Midbrain CN III-IV	Reflex center for eye and head movement Auditory relay pathway Corticospinal tract pathway
Diencephalon CN I-II	Relays impulses between cerebrum, cerebellum, pons, and medulla (Figure 20-5)
Thalamus	Conveys all sensory impulses (except olfaction) to and from cerebrum before their distribution to appropriate associative sensory areas Integrates impulses between motor cortex and cerebrum, influencing voluntary movements and motor response Controls state of consciousness, conscious perceptions of sensations, and abstract feelings
Epithalamus	Houses the pineal body Sexual development and behavior
Hypothalamus	Major processing center of internal stimuli for autonomic nervous system Maintains temperature control, water metabolism, body fluid osmolarity, feeding behavior, and neuroendocrine activity
Pituitary gland	Hormonal control of growth, lactation, vasoconstriction, and metabolism

TABLE 20-2   The Cranial Nerves and Their Function

Cranial Nerves	Function
Olfactory (I)	Sensory: smell reception and interpretation
Optic (II)	Sensory: visual acuity and visual fields
Oculomotor (III)	Motor: raise eyelids, most extraocular movements Parasympathetic: pupillary constriction, change lens shape
Trochlear (IV)	Motor: downward, inward eye movement
Trigeminal (V)	Motor: jaw opening and clenching, chewing and mastication Sensory: sensation to cornea, iris, lacrimal glands, conjunctiva, eyelids, forehead, nose, nasal and mouth mucosa, teeth, tongue, ear, facial skin
Abducens (VI)	Motor: lateral eye movement
Facial (VII)	Motor: movement of facial expression muscles except jaw, close eyes, labial speech sounds (b, m, w, and rounded vowels) Sensory: taste—anterior two thirds of tongue, sensation to pharynx Parasympathetic: secretion of saliva and tears
Acoustic (VIII)	Sensory: hearing and equilibrium
Glossopharyngeal (IX)	Motor: voluntary muscles for swallowing and phonation Sensory: sensation of nasopharynx, gag reflex, taste—posterior one third of tongue Parasympathetic: secretion of salivary glands, carotid reflex
Vagus (X)	Motor: voluntary muscles of phonation (guttural speech sounds) and swallowing Sensory: sensation behind ear and part of external ear canal Parasympathetic: secretion of digestive enzymes; peristalsis; carotid reflex; involuntary action of heart, lungs, and digestive tract
Spinal accessory (XI)	Motor: turn head, shrug shoulders, some actions for phonation
Hypoglossal (XII)	Motor: tongue movement for speech sound articulation (l, t, n) and swallowing

Modified from Rudy, 1984.

SPINAL CORD AND SPINAL TRACTS

The *spinal cord* begins at the foramen magnum and is a continuation of the medulla oblongata, terminating at L1 or L2 of the vertebral column. Fibers, grouped into tracts, run through the spinal cord carrying sensory, motor, and autonomic impulses between higher centers in the brain and the body. The myelin-coated white matter of the spinal cord contains the ascending and descending tracts (Figure 20-6). The gray matter, which contains the nerve cell bodies, is arranged in a butterfly shape with anterior and posterior horns.

The *descending spinal tracts* originate in the brain and convey impulses to various muscle groups with inhibitory or facilitatory actions. They also have a role in the control of muscle tone and posture. The pyramidal tract is the great motor pathway that carries impulses for voluntary movement, especially those requiring skill.

The *ascending spinal tracts* mediate various sensations. They facilitate the sensory signals necessary for complex discrimination tasks and are capable of transmitting precise information about the type of stimulus and its location. The posterior (dorsal) column spinal tract carries the fibers for the discriminatory sensations of touch, deep pressure, vibration, position of the joints, stereognosis, and two-point discrimination. The spinothalamic tracts carry the fibers for the sensations of light and crude touch, pressure, temperature, and pain.

Upper motor neurons, all originating and terminating within the central nervous system, make up the descending pathways from the brain to the spinal cord. Their primary role is influencing and modifying spinal reflex arcs and circuits. The lower motor neurons originate in the anterior horn of the spinal cord and terminate in the muscle fibers. Cranial nerves are also lower motor neurons and have a direct influence on muscles they innervate.

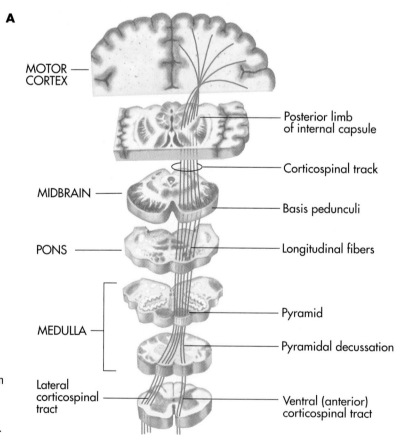

A

MOTOR CORTEX

Posterior limb of internal capsule

Corticospinal track

MIDBRAIN

Basis pedunculi

PONS

Longitudinal fibers

Pyramid

MEDULLA

Pyramidal decussation

Lateral corticospinal tract

Ventral (anterior) corticospinal tract

FIGURE 20-6

Tracts of the spinal cord.
A, Pathway of spinal tracts from spinal cord to motor cortex. Note decussation of the pyramids at the level of the medulla.

Spinal Nerves

Thirty-one pairs of spinal nerves arise from the spinal cord and exit at each intervertebral foramen (Figure 20-7). The sensory and motor fibers of each spinal nerve supply and receive information in a specific body distribution called a dermatome (Figure 20-8). The anterior branches of several spinal nerves combine to form nerve plexi, so that a spinal nerve may lose its individuality to some extent. The spinal nerve may also complement the effort of an anatomically related nerve or even help compensate for some loss of function. A multitude of peripheral nerves originate from these nerve plexi (Figure 20-9).

Within the spinal cord, each spinal nerve separates into ventral and dorsal roots. The motor fibers of the ventral root carry impulses from the spinal cord to the muscles and glands of the body. The sensory fibers of the dorsal root carry impulses from sensory receptors of the body to the spinal cord. From here the impulses travel to the brain for interpretation by the cerebral sensory cortex. The impulse may alternatively initiate a reflex action when it synapses immediately with the motor fiber after a stimulus such as a tap on a stretched muscle tendon. In this case, the impulse is transmitted outward by the motor neuron in the anterior horn of the spinal cord via the spinal nerve and peripheral nerve of the skeletal muscle, stimulating a brisk contraction (Figure 20-10, p. 768). Such a reflex is dependent on intact afferent nerve fibers, functional synapses in the spinal cord, intact motor nerve fibers, functional neuromuscular junctions, and competent muscle fibers.

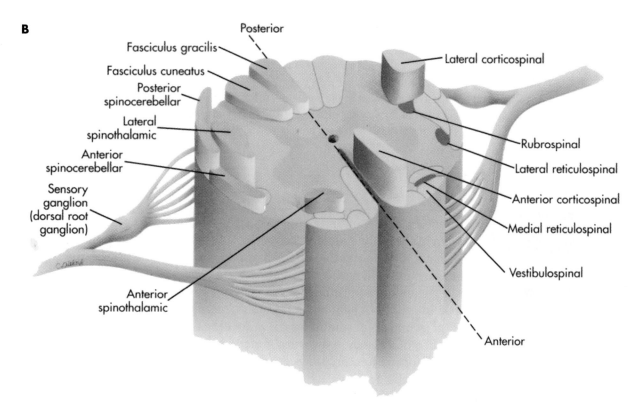

FIGURE 20-6—cont'd
B, Major ascending (sensory) tracts, shown here only on the left, are highlighted in blue. Major descending (motor) tracts, shown here only on the right, are highlighted in red.
A, Modified from Rudy, 1984. **B,** From Thibodeau, Patton, 1996.

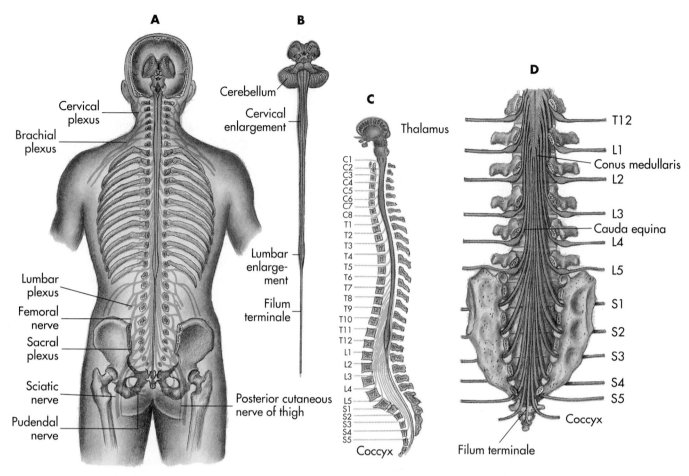

FIGURE 20-7

Location of exiting spinal nerves in relation to the vertebrae. **A**, Posterior view. **B**, Anterior view of brainstem and spinal cord. **C**, Lateral view showing relationship of spinal cord to vertebrae. **D**, Enlargement of caudal area with group of nerve fibers composing the cauda equina.

From Rudy, 1984.

INFANTS AND CHILDREN

The major portion of brain growth occurs in the first year of life, along with myelinization of the brain and nervous system. Any intruding event (infection, biochemical imbalance, or trauma) that upsets brain development and growth during this period can have profound effects on eventual brain function.

The following primitive reflexes are present in the newborn: yawn, sneeze, hiccup, blink at bright light and loud sound, pupillary constriction with light, and withdrawal from painful stimuli. As the brain develops, some primitive reflexes are inhibited when more advanced cortical functions and voluntary control take over.

Motor maturation proceeds in a cephalocaudal direction. Motor control of the head and neck develops first, followed by the trunk and extremities. Motor development is a succession of integrated milestones, each leading to more complex and independent function (see Table 19-3). There is an orderly sequence to development, but considerable variation in timing exists in children. Many capabilities may be developing simultaneously in any one child.

Brain growth continues until 12 to 15 years of age.

PHYSICAL VARIATIONS

The timing of motor development varies considerably in children. Black children are more advanced than white children, at least until the age of 3 years.

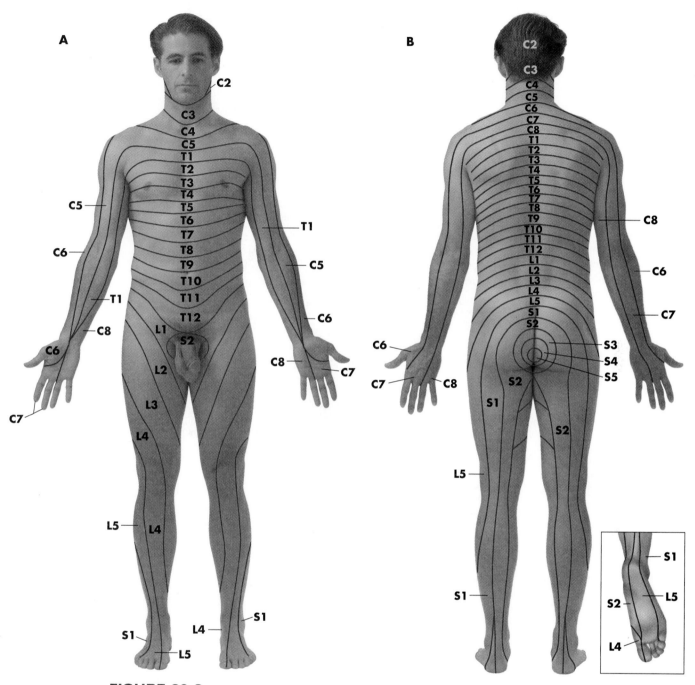

FIGURE 20-8

Dermatomes of the body, the area of body surface innervated by particular spinal nerves; C1 usually has no cutaneous distribution. **A,** Anterior view. **B,** Posterior view. It appears that there is a distinct separation of surface area controlled by each dermatome, but there is almost always overlap between spinal nerves.

A

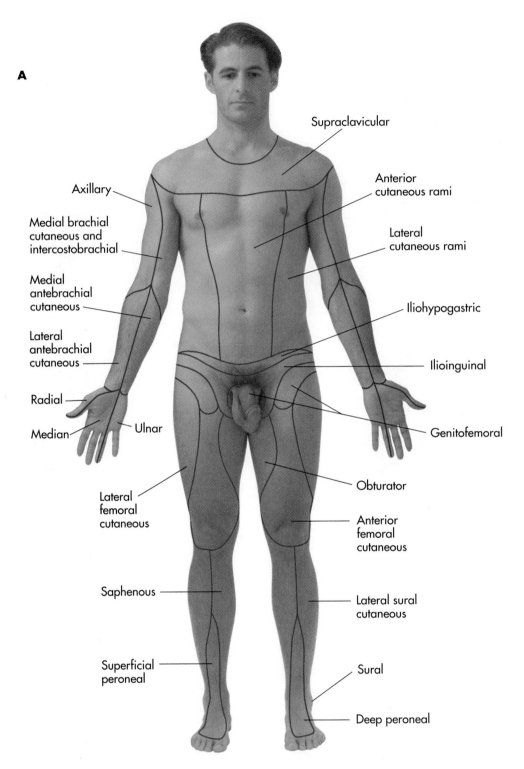

FIGURE 20-9

Area of sensory innervation by certain peripheral nerves. **A,** Anterior view.

B

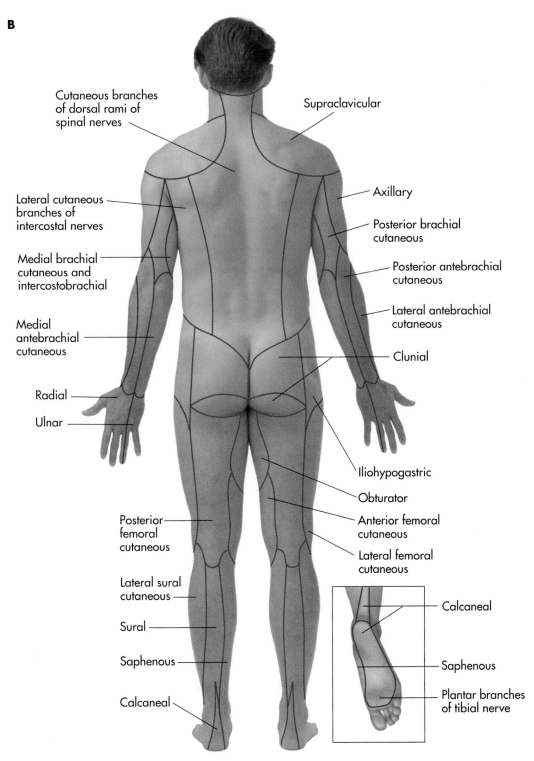

Cutaneous branches
of dorsal rami of
spinal nerves

Supraclavicular

Axillary

Posterior brachial
cutaneous

Lateral cutaneous
branches of
intercostal nerves

Posterior antebrachial
cutaneous

Medial brachial
cutaneous and
intercostobrachial

Lateral antebrachial
cutaneous

Medial
antebrachial
cutaneous

Clunial

Radial

Ulnar

Iliohypogastric

Obturator

Anterior femoral
cutaneous

Posterior
femoral
cutaneous

Lateral femoral
cutaneous

Lateral sural
cutaneous

Calcaneal

Sural

Saphenous

Saphenous

Plantar branches
of tibial nerve

Calcaneal

FIGURE 20-9—cont'd
B, Posterior view.

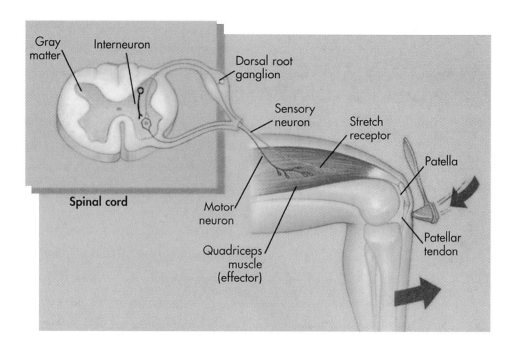

FIGURE 20-10
Cross section of spinal cord showing simple reflex arc.
From Thibodeau, Patton, 1996.

PREGNANT WOMEN	Hypothalamic-pituitary neurohormonal changes occur with pregnancy; however, specific alterations in the neurologic system are not well identified. More common physiologic alterations that may occur during pregnancy are contraction or tension headaches (worsened by postural changes and new situational problems) and acroparaesthesia (numbness and tingling of the hands) due to postural kinking of blood vessels at the thoracic outlet. This may be confused with carpal tunnel syndrome. During the first trimester, women increase their naptime and sleeptime, but they may not feel rested even with increased sleep. Late in pregnancy women have more frequent night awakening and less sleep time.
OLDER ADULTS	The changes that occur with aging are more physiologic than anatomic. The number of cerebral neurons is thought to decrease by 1% a year beginning at 50 years of age. However, the vast number of reserve cells inhibits the appearance of clinical signs. The velocity of nerve impulse conduction declines 10% between 30 and 90 years of age, so responses to various stimuli take longer. Sensory perceptions of touch and pain stimuli may also be diminished.

REVIEW OF RELATED HISTORY

PRESENT PROBLEM

- Seizures or convulsions
  - Sequence of events (independent observer's report): aura, fall to ground, shrill cry, motor activity, transition phase, change in color of face or lips, pupil changes or eye deviations, loss of consciousness, postictal phase, total length of seizure activity
    - Character of symptoms
    - Aura: irritability, tension, confusion, blurred vision, mood changes, focal motor seizure activity, gastrointestinal distress
    - Level of consciousness: loss, impairment, duration
    - Automatism: eyelid fluttering, chewing, lip smacking, swallowing

- Muscle tone: flaccid, stiff, tense, twitching; where spasm began and moved through the body; change in character of motor activity during seizure
  - Postictal behavior: weakness, paralysis, confusion, drowsiness, headaches, muscle aching, time sleeping after seizure; any lateralization of signs
- Relationship of seizure to time of day, meals, fatigue, emotional stress, excitement, menses, and discontinuing medications or poor compliance with medications; activity before attack
- Frequency of seizures; age at first seizure
- Medications: anticonvulsant; prescription and nonprescription; initiation of medication that hastens catabolism of anticonvulsant

- Pain
  - Onset: sudden or progressive, associated with injury
  - Quality and intensity: deep or superficial; aching, boring, throbbing, sharp or stabbing, burning, pressing, stinging, cramping, gnawing, prickling, shooting; duration and constancy
  - Location or path: along distribution of one or more peripheral nerves or a more general distribution; radiating from one part to another
  - Associated manifestations: crying, decreased activities, sweating, muscle rigidity, tremor, impaired mental processes or concentration, weakness
  - Efforts to treat
  - Medications: opioids and nonsteroidal antiinflammatories; prescription or nonprescription

- Gait coordination
  - Balance: sensation of listing when walking to doorway
  - Falling: fall one way, backward, forward, consistent direction; associated with looking up
  - Legs simply give way
  - Associated problems: rheumatoid arthritis of cervical spine, ataxia, stroke, seizure, arthritis in knees, arrhythmias, sensory changes
  - Medications: phenytoin, pyrimethamine, etoposide, vinblastine; prescription or nonprescription

- Weakness or paresthesia
  - Onset: with initiation of or following sustained activity, time before symptoms begin, rapid or slow
  - Character: generalized or specific body area affected; progressively ascending or transient; proximal or distal extremities, unilateral or bilateral; hypersensitivity to touch or burning sensation
  - Associated symptoms: tingling, limb feels encased in tight bandage, pain, shortness of breath, stiffness of joints, spasms, muscle tension, sensory deficits; loss of urinary or anal control
  - Concurrent chronic illness such as HIV infection, nutritional or vitamin deficiency
  - Medications: zidovudine, diaminodiphenylsulfone, dideoxyinosine, amphotericin B; prescription or nonprescription

PAST MEDICAL HISTORY

- Trauma: head, spinal cord, or localized injury; central nervous system insult; birth trauma; cerebrovascular accident
- Meningitis, encephalitis, plumbism
- Deformities, congenital anomalies
- Cardiovascular, circulatory problem: hypertension, aneurysm, stroke
- Neurologic disorder, brain surgery, residual effects

FAMILY HISTORY

- Hereditary disorders: neurofibromatosis, Huntington chorea, muscular dystrophy, Tay-Sachs disease
- Alcoholism
- Mental retardation
- Epilepsy or seizure disorder, headaches
- Alzheimer disease
- Learning disorders
- Weakness or gait disorders
- Medical or metabolic disorder: thyroid disease, hypertension, diabetes mellitus

PERSONAL AND SOCIAL HISTORY

- Environmental or occupational hazards: exposure to lead, arsenic, insecticides, organic solvents, other chemicals; operate farm or other dangerous equipment; work at heights or in water
- Hand, eye, and foot dominance; family patterns of dexterity and dominance
- Ability to care for self: hygiene, activities of daily living, finances, communication, shopping; ability to fulfill work expectations
- Sleeping or eating patterns; weight loss or gain; anxiety
- Use of alcohol
- Use of street drugs, especially mood-altering drugs

INFANTS

- Prenatal history: mother's health, medications taken, infections, exposure to TORCH (toxoplasmosis, other [syphilis, tuberculosis], rubella, cytomegalovirus, herpes) infections, feelings of well-being, toxemia, bleeding, history of trauma or stress, persistent vomiting, hypertension, drug or alcohol use
- Birth history: Apgar score, gestational age, birth weight, presentation, use of instruments, prolonged or precipitate labor, fetal distress
- Respiratory status at birth: breathed immediately, need for oxygen, continuous apnea, cyanosis, resuscitative efforts, need for ventilator
- Neonatal health: jaundice (from blood type incompatibility or breast feeding), infections, seizures, irritability, sucking and swallowing poorly coordinated
- Congenital anomalies, multiple handicapping conditions

CHILDREN

- Developmental milestones
  - Age attained: smiling, head control in prone position, grasping, transferring objects between hands, rolling over, sitting, crawling, independent walking, toilet trained, similar pattern in siblings
  - Loss of previously achieved function: change in the child's rate of development; progress occurred as expected until a certain age with slow progress after that; or has always been slow to do things
- Performance of self-care activities: dressing, toileting, feeding
- Health problems
  - Headaches, unexplained vomiting, lethargy, personality changes
  - Seizure activity: association with fever, frequency, duration, character of movement
  - Any clumsiness, unsteady gait, progressive muscular weakness, unexplained falling, problems going up and down stairs, problems getting up after lying down on floor

PREGNANT WOMEN

- Weeks of gestation or EDC
- Convulsions/headache
  - Seizure activity: past history of seizures or pregnancy-induced hypertension; frequency, duration, character of movement

• Headache: onset, character, frequency, association with hypertension
• Nutritional status: dietary supplements such as prenatal vitamins, calcium; salt depletion

■ Pattern of increased stumbling, falls, or decreased agility; safety modifications in home
■ Interference with performance of daily living tasks, social withdrawal, feelings about symptoms
■ Hearing loss, vision deficit, or anosmia
■ Development of tremor: exacerbated by anxiety, relieved by alcohol
■ Fecal or urinary incontinence
■ Transient neurologic deficits (may indicate transient ischemic attacks)

RISK FACTORS   Cerebrovascular Accidents (Stroke)

■ Hypertension
■ Obesity
■ Sedentary life-style
■ Smoking tobacco products
■ Stress
■ Increased levels of serum cholesterol, lipoproteins, and triglycerides
■ Use of oral contraceptives in high-risk women
■ Family history of diabetes mellitus, cardiovascular disease, hypertension, and increased serum cholesterol levels.
■ Congenital cerebrovascular anomalies

EXAMINATION AND FINDINGS

EQUIPMENT

■ Penlight
■ Tongue blade
■ Sterile needles
■ Tuning forks, 200 to 400 Hz and 500 to 1000 Hz
■ Familiar objects—coins, keys, paper clip
■ Cotton wisp
■ 5.07 Monofilament
■ Reflex hammer
■ Vials of aromatic substances—coffee, orange, peppermint extract, oil of cloves
■ Vials of solutions—glucose, salt, lemon or vinegar, and quinine—with applicators
■ Test tubes of hot and cold water for temperature sensation testing
■ Denver Developmental Screening Test (for infants and children)

Because the neurologic examination is complex, the discussion is divided into four sections to give you an organized approach. These sections include cranial nerves, proprioception and cerebellar function, sensory function, and reflex function. Assessment of mental status is detailed in Chapter 4, Mental Status. Evaluation of muscle tone and strength, an integral part of the neurologic examination, is detailed in Chapter 19, Musculoskeletal System.

The neurologic system can be examined almost constantly while the rest of the body is explored. In fact, when the patient enters the room and you offer some suggestion as to where he or she might sit, the patient's response tells you a good deal about the functioning of the neurologic system. Your observation throughout the history and physical examination completes many aspects of the neurologic examina-

BOX 20-1 **Procedures of the Neurologic Screening Examination**

The shorter screening examination is commonly used for health visits when no known neurologic problem is apparent.

Cranial Nerves

Cranial nerves II through XII are routinely tested; however, taste and smell are not tested unless some aberration is found (pp. 772-777).

Proprioception and Cerebellar Function

One test is administered for each of the following: rapid rhythmic alternating movements, accuracy of movements, balance (Romberg test is given), and gait and heel-toe walking (pp. 778-782).

Sensory Function

Superficial pain and touch at a distal point in each extremity are tested; vibration and position senses are assessed by testing the great toe (pp. 783-786).

Deep Tendon Reflexes

All deep tendon reflexes are tested, excluding the plantar reflex and the test for clonus (pp. 788-789).

tion. By the time you begin to examine the neurologic status specifically, you should already be armed with clues to the system's state of health. When the history and examination findings have not yet revealed a potential neurologic problem, a neurologic screening examination may be performed, as shown in Box 20-1.

CRANIAL NERVES

An evaluation of the cranial nerves is an integral part of the neurologic examination. Ordinarily, taste and smell are not evaluated unless a problem is suspected. Quite often patients will not recognize that they have lost hearing in some ranges, certain taste sensations, or some visual aspects. Thus when a sensory loss is suspected, it is necessary to be compulsive about determining the extent of loss when testing the relevant cranial nerve.

Examination of some cranial nerves is described in detail in other chapters. The optic (II), oculomotor (III), trochlear (IV), and abducens (VI) nerves are tested in Chapter 10 (Eyes); the acoustic nerve (VIII) in Chapter 11 (Ears, Nose, and Throat); and the spinal accessory nerve (XI) in Chapter 19 (Musculoskeletal System). See Table 20-3 for a review of all cranial nerve examination procedures.

Cranial nerve function is expected to be intact, as described in Table 20-2 for each individual nerve. Unexpected findings indicate trauma or a lesion in the cerebral hemisphere or local injury to the nerve.

Olfactory (I)

Have available two or three vials of familiar aromatic odors. Use the least irritating aromatic substance (orange or peppermint extract) first so that the patient's perception of weaker odors is not impaired. To make sure the patient's nasal passages are patent, you should alternately occlude each naris as the patient inspires and expires.

The patient's eyes should be closed and one naris occluded. As you hold an opened vial under the nose, the patient should take a deep inspiration for the odor to reach the upper nose and swirl around the olfactory mucosa (Figure 20-11). Ask the patient to identify the odor. Repeat the process with the other naris occluded, using a different odor. Continue the process, comparing the patient's sensitivity and discriminatory ability from side to side, alternating the two or three odors. It is important to allow periods of rest between the offerings of different odors. Offering one odor after the other too quickly can confuse the olfactory sense.

MNEMONICS

CRANIAL NERVES: "ON OLD OLYMPUS' TOWERING TOPS A FINN AND GERMAN VIEWED SOME HOPS"

O *Olfactory*
O *Optic*
O *Oculomotor*
T *Trochlear*
T *Trigeminal*
A *Abducens*
F *Facial*
A *Acoustic*
G *Glossopharyngeal*
V *Vagal*
S *Spinal accessory*
H *Hypoglossal*

TABLE 20-3   Procedures for Cranial Nerve Examination

Cranial Nerve (CN)	Procedure
CN I (olfactory)	Test ability to identify familiar aromatic odors, one naris at a time with eyes closed.
CN II (optic)	Test vision with Snellen chart and Rosenbaum near vision chart. Perform ophthalmoscopic examination of fundi. Test visual fields by confrontation and extinction of vision.
CN III, IV, and VI (oculomotor, trochlear, and abducens)	Inspect eyelids for drooping. Inspect pupils' size for equality and their direct and consensual response to light and accommodation. Test extraocular eye movements.
CN V (trigeminal)	Inspect face for muscle atrophy and tremors. Palpate jaw muscles for tone and strength when patient clenches teeth. Test superficial pain and touch sensation in each branch. (Test temperature sensation if there are unexpected findings to pain or touch.) Test corneal reflex.
CN VII (facial)	Inspect symmetry of facial features with various expressions (smile, frown, puffed cheeks, wrinkled forehead, etc.) Test ability to identify sweet and salty tastes on each side of tongue.
CN VIII (acoustic)	Test sense of hearing with whisper screening tests or by audiometry. Compare bone and air conduction of sound. Test for lateralization of sound.
CN IX (glossopharyngeal)	Test ability to identify sour and bitter tastes. Test gag reflex and ability to swallow.
CN X (vagus)	Inspect palate and uvula for symmetry with speech sounds and gag reflex. Observe for swallowing difficulty. Evaluate quality of guttural speech sounds (presence of nasal or hoarse quality to voice).
CN XI (spinal accessory)	Test trapezius muscle strength (shrug shoulders against resistance). Test sternocleidomastoid muscle strength (turn head to each side against resistance).
CN XII (hypoglossal)	Inspect tongue in mouth and while protruded for symmetry, tremors, and atrophy. Inspect tongue movement toward nose and chin. Test tongue strength with index finger when tongue is pressed against cheek. Evaluate quality of lingual speech sounds (l, t, d, n).

Modified from Rudy, 1984.

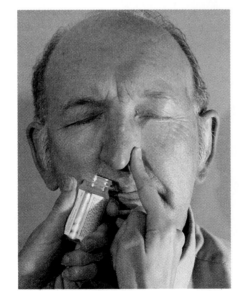

FIGURE 20-11

Examination of the olfactory cranial nerve. Occlude one naris, hold the vial with aromatic substance under the nose, and ask the patient to deeply inspire. The patient should discriminate between odors.

The patient should be able to perceive an odor on each side, usually identifying it. Inflammation of the mucous membranes, allergic rhinitis, and excessive tobacco smoking may all interfere with the ability to distinguish odors. The sense of smell may diminish with age. Anosmia, loss of sense of smell or inability to discriminate odors, can be caused by trauma to the cribriform plate or by an olfactory tract lesion.

Optic (II)

Visual acuity and visual fields are evaluated in Chapter 10, Eyes.

Oculomotor, Trochlear, and Abducens (III, IV, and VI)

Movement of the eyes through the six cardinal points of gaze, pupil size, shape, response to light and accommodation, and opening of the upper eyelids are all described in Chapter 10, Eyes.

When assessing patients with severe, unremitting headaches, the experienced examiner evaluates movement of the eyes for the presence or absence of lateral (temporal) gaze. The sixth cranial nerve is frequently one of the first functions to be lost in the presence of increased intracranial pressure.

Trigeminal (V)

Motor function is evaluated by observing the face for muscle atrophy, deviation of the jaw to one side, and fasciculations. Have the patient tightly clench the teeth as you palpate the muscles over the jaw, evaluating tone (Figure 20-12). Muscle tone over the face should be symmetric without fasciculations.

Three divisions of the nerve are evaluated for sharp, dull, and light touch sensation (Figure 20-13). While the patient's eyes are closed, touch each side of the face at the scalp, cheek, and chin areas, alternately using the sharp and smooth edge of a broken tongue blade, or a paper clip, making sure you do not use a predictable pattern. Ask the patient to report whether the sensation is sharp or dull. Then stroke the face in the same six areas with a cotton wisp or brush, asking the patient to tell when the stimulus is felt. A wooden applicator is used to test sensation over the buccal mucosa. There should be symmetric sensory discrimination over the face to all stimuli.

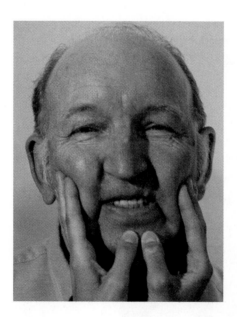

FIGURE 20-12

Examination of the trigeminal cranial nerve for motor function. Have the patient tightly clench the teeth, and then palpate the muscles over the jaw for tone.

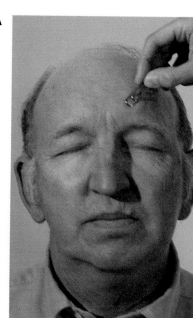

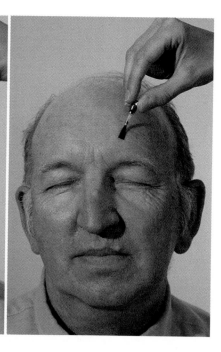

FIGURE 20-13

Examination of the trigeminal cranial nerve for sensory function. Touch each side of the face at the scalp, cheek, and chin areas alternately using no predictable pattern with, **A,** the point and rounded edge of a paper clip and, **B,** a brush. Ask the patient to discriminate between sensations.

If sensation is impaired, use test tubes filled with hot and cold water to evaluate temperature sensation. Ask the patient to tell you if hot or cold is felt as you touch the same six areas of the face. Contrast the sensory discrimination with temperature to the other primary sensations.

To test the corneal reflex, have the patient look up and away from you, as you approach from the side. (Contact lenses, if used, should be removed.) Avoiding the eyelashes and the conjunctiva, lightly touch the cornea of one eye with a cotton wisp. Repeat the procedure on the other cornea. A symmetric blink reflex to corneal stimulation should occur. Patients who wear contact lenses may have diminished or absent reflex.

Facial (VII)

Motor function is evaluated by observing a series of expressions you ask the patient to make: raise the eyebrows, squeeze the eyes shut, wrinkle the forehead, frown, smile, show the teeth, purse the lips to whistle, and puff out the cheeks (Figure 20-14). Observe for tics, unusual facial movements, and asymmetry of expression. Listen to the patient's speech and note any difficulties with enunciating labial sounds (*b, m,* and *p*). Muscle weakness is evidenced by one side of the mouth drooping, a flattened nasolabial fold, and lower eyelid sagging.

When evaluating taste, a sensory function of cranial nerves VII and IX, have available the four solutions, applicators, and a card listing the tastes. Make sure the patient cannot see the labels on the vials. Ask the patient to keep the tongue protruded and to point out the taste perceived on the card. Apply one solution at a time to the lateral side of the tongue in the appropriate taste bud region (Figure 20-15). Alternate the solutions, using a different applicator for each. Offer a sip of water after each stimulus. Each solution is used on both sides of the tongue to identify taste discrimination. The patient should identify each taste bilaterally when placed correctly on the tongue surface.

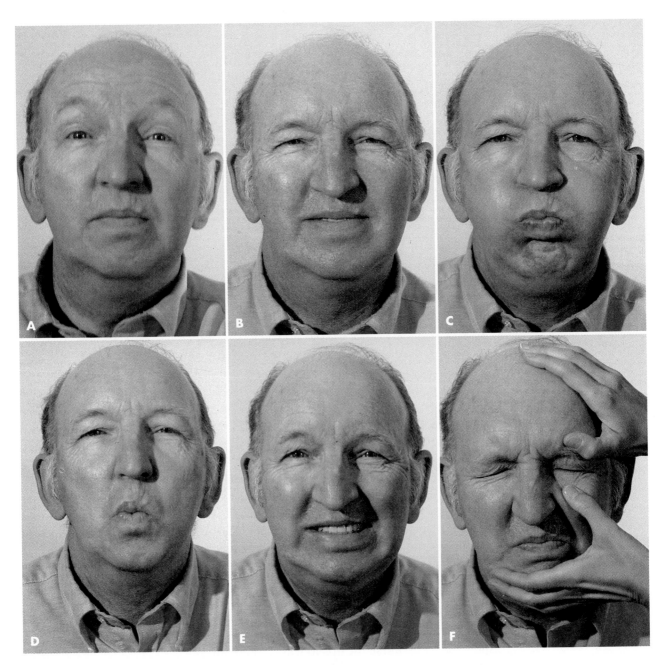

FIGURE 20-14

Examination of the facial cranial nerve for motor function. Ask the patient to, **A,** wrinkle the forehead by raising the eyebrows; **B,** smile; **C,** puff out the cheeks; **D,** purse the lips and blow out; **E,** show the teeth; and **F,** squeeze the eyes shut.

Acoustic (VIII)

Hearing is evaluated with an audiometer or the simple screening tests described in Chapter 11 (Ears, Nose, and Throat). Vestibular function is tested by the Romberg test (see p. 780). Other vestibular function tests are not routinely performed.

Glossopharyngeal (IX)

The sensory function of taste over the posterior third of the tongue is tested during cranial nerve VII evaluation. The glossopharyngeal nerve is simultaneously tested during evaluation of the vagus nerve for nasopharyngeal sensation (gag reflex) and the motor function of swallowing.

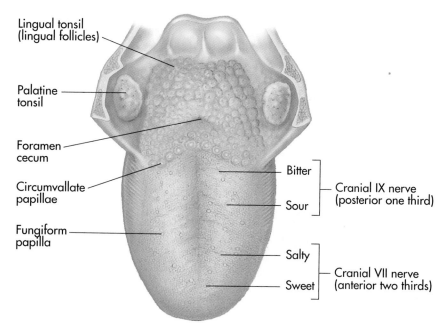

Lingual tonsil
(lingual follicles)

Palatine
tonsil

Foramen
cecum

Circumvallate
papillae

Fungiform
papilla

Bitter

Sour

Cranial IX nerve
(posterior one third)

Salty

Sweet

Cranial VII nerve
(anterior two thirds)

FIGURE 20-15

Location of the taste bud regions tested for the sensory function of the facial and glossopharyngeal cranial nerves.

Vagus (X)

To evaluate nasopharyngeal sensation, tell the patient you will be testing the gag reflex. Touch the posterior wall of the patient's pharynx with an applicator as you observe for upward movement of the palate and contraction of the pharyngeal muscles. The uvula should remain in the midline, and no drooping or absence of an arch on either side of the soft palate should be noted.

Motor function is evaluated by inspection of the soft palate for symmetry. Have the patient say "Ah," and observe the movement of the soft palate and uvula for asymmetry. If the vagus or glossopharyngeal nerve is damaged and the palate fails to rise, the uvula will deviate from the midline.

Have the patient sip and swallow water. This observation can be made while examining the thyroid gland. The patient should swallow easily, having no retrograde passage of water through the nose after the nasopharynx has closed off. Listen to the patient's speech, noting any hoarseness, nasal quality, or difficulty with guttural sounds.

Spinal Accessory (XI)

The size, shape, and strength of the trapezius and sternocleidomastoid muscles are evaluated in Chapters 9 (Head and Neck) and 19 (Musculoskeletal System).

Hypoglossal (XII)

Inspect the patient's tongue while at rest on the floor of the mouth and while protruded from the mouth (Figure 20-16). Note any fasciculations, asymmetry, atrophy, or deviation from the midline. Ask the patient to move the tongue in and out of the mouth, from side to side, curled upward as if to touch the nose, and curled downward as if to lick the chin. Test the tongue's muscle strength by asking the patient to push the tongue against the cheek as you apply resistance with an index finger. When listening to the patient's speech, no problems with lingual speech sounds (*l, t, d, n*) should be apparent.

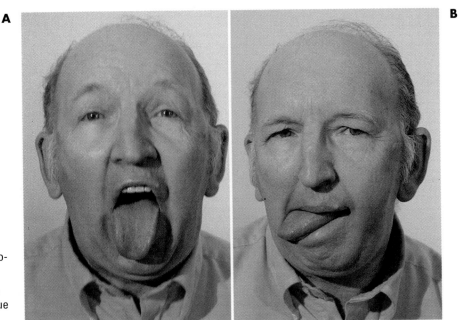

FIGURE 20-16

Examination of the hypoglossal cranial nerve. **A,** Inspect the protruded tongue for size, shape, symmetry, and fasciculation. **B,** Observe movement of the tongue from side to side.

PROPRIOCEPTION AND CEREBELLAR FUNCTION

Coordination and Fine Motor Skills

Rapid rhythmic alternating movements. Ask the seated patient to pat his or her knees with both hands, alternately turning up the palm and back of the hands, and increase the rate gradually (Figure 20-17, *A* and *B*). As an alternate procedure, have the patient touch the thumb to each finger on the same hand, sequentially from the index finger to the little finger and back. Test one hand at a time, increasing speed gradually (Figure 20-17, *C*).

Observe for stiff, slowed, nonrhythmic, or jerky clonic movements. The patient should smoothly execute these movements, maintaining rhythm with increasing speed.

Accuracy of movements. The finger-to-finger test is performed with the patient's eyes open. Ask the patient to use the index finger and alternately touch his or her nose and your index finger (Figure 20-18, *A* and *B*). Position your index finger about 18 inches from the patient and change the location of your finger several times during the test. Repeat the procedure with the other hand. The movements should be rapid, smooth, and accurate. Consistent past pointing (missing the examiner's index finger) may indicate cerebellar disease.

To perform the finger-to-nose test, ask the patient to close both eyes and touch his or her nose with the index finger of each hand. Alternate the hands used and increase speed gradually (Figure 20-18, *C*). Movement should be smooth, rapid, and accurate, even with increasing speed.

The heel-to-shin test is performed with the patient standing, sitting, or supine. Ask the patient to run the heel of one foot up and down the shin (from knee to ankle) of the opposite leg (Figure 20-18, *D*). Repeat the procedure with the other heel. The patient should move the heel up and down the shin in a straight line, without irregular deviations to the side.

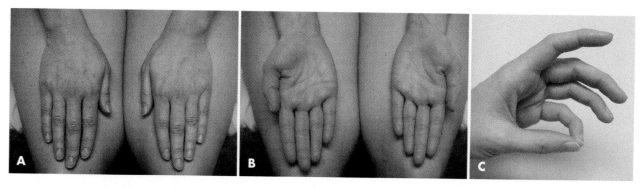

FIGURE 20-17

Examination of coordination with rapid alternating movements. **A** and **B,** Pat the knees with both hands, alternately using the palm and back of the hand. **C,** Touch the thumb to each finger of the hand in sequence from index finger to small finger and back.

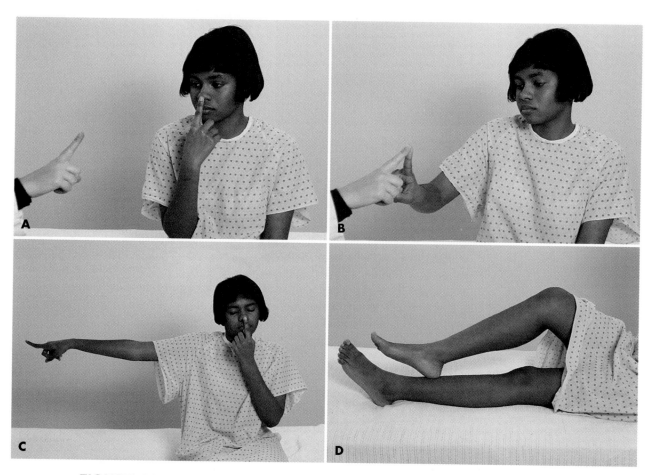

FIGURE 20-18

Examination of fine motor function. The patient, **A** and **B,** alternately touches own nose and the examiner's index finger with the index finger of one hand; **C,** alternately touches own nose with the index finger of each hand; and **D,** runs the heel of one foot down the shin or tibia of the other leg.

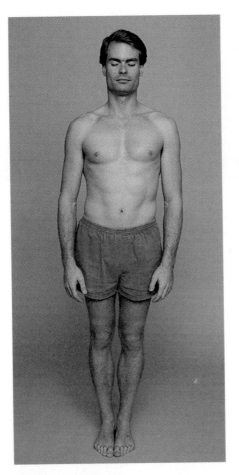

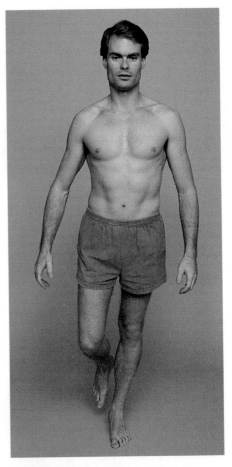

FIGURE 20-19
Evaluation of balance with the Romberg test.

FIGURE 20-20
Evaluation of balance with the patient hopping in place on one foot.

Balance

Equilibrium. Balance is initially evaluated with the Romberg test. Ask the patient (eyes open and then closed) to stand, feet together and arms at the sides (Figure 20-19). Stand close, prepared to catch the patient if he or she starts to fall. Slight swaying movement of the body is expected, but not to the extent that there is danger of falling. Loss of balance, a positive Romberg sign, indicates cerebellar ataxia, vestibular dysfunction, or sensory loss. If the patient staggers or loses balance with the Romberg test, postpone other tests of cerebellar function requiring balance.

To further evaluate balance, have the patient stand with feet slightly apart. Push the shoulders with enough effort to throw him or her off balance. Be ready to catch the patient if necessary. Recovery of balance should occur quickly.

Balance may also be tested with the patient standing on one foot. The patient's eyes should be closed, with arms held straight at the sides. Repeat the test on the opposite foot. Balance on each foot should be maintained for 5 seconds, but slight swaying is expected.

Have the patient (eyes open) hop in place first on one foot and then on the other (Figure 20-20). Note any instability, a need to continually touch the floor with the opposite foot, or a tendency to fall. The patient should hop on each foot for 5 seconds without loss of balance.

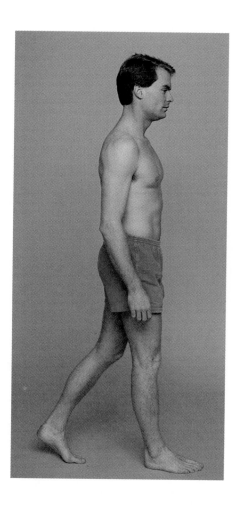

FIGURE 20-21

Evaluation of gait. Note the expected gait sequence and arm movements.

Gait. Observe the patient walk without shoes around the examining room or down a hallway, first with the eyes open and then closed. Observe the expected gait sequence, noting simultaneous arm movements and upright posture (Figure 20-21):

1. The first heel strikes the floor and then moves to full contact with the floor.
2. The second heel pushes off, leaving the ground.
3. Body weight is transferred from the first heel to the ball of its foot.
4. The leg swing is accelerated as weight is removed from the second foot.
5. The second foot is lifted and travels ahead of the weight-bearing first foot, swinging through.
6. The second foot slows in preparation for heel strike.

Note any shuffling, widely placed feet, toe walking, foot flop, leg lag, scissoring, loss of arm swing, staggering, or reeling. The patient should continuously sequence both stance and swing, step after step. The gait should have a smooth, regular rhythm and symmetric stride length. The trunk posture should sway with the gait phase, and arm swing should be smooth and symmetric. Figure 20-22 and Table 20-4 describe unexpected gait patterns.

Heel-toe walking will exaggerate any unexpected finding in gait evaluation. Have the patient walk a straight line, first forward and then backward, with eyes open and arms at the sides. Direct the patient to touch the toe of one foot with the heel of the other foot (Figure 20-23). Note any extension of the arms for balance, instability, a tendency to fall, or lateral staggering and reeling. Consistent contact between the heel and toe should occur, although slight swaying is expected.

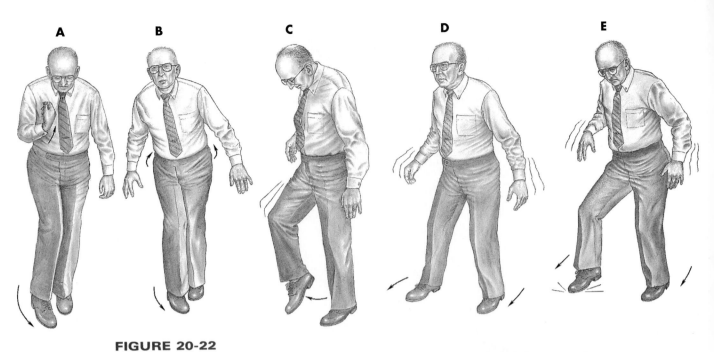

FIGURE 20-22

Unexpected gait patterns. **A**, Spastic hemiparesis. **B**, Spastic diplegia (scissoring). **C**, Steppage gait.
D, Cerebellar ataxia. **E**, Sensory ataxia.

TABLE 20-4	Characteristics of Unexpected Gait Patterns
Gait Pattern	**Characteristics**
Spastic hemiparesis	The affected leg is stiff and extended with plantar flexion of the foot. Movement of the foot results from pelvic tilting upward on the involved side. The foot is dragged, often scraping the toe, or it is circled stiffly outward and forward (circumduction). The affected arm remains flexed and adducted and does not swing (see Figure 20-22, *A*).
Spastic diplegia (scissoring)	The patient uses short steps, dragging the ball of the foot across the floor. The legs are extended, and the thighs tend to cross forward on each other at each step, due to injury to the pyramidal system (see Figure 20-22, *B*).
Steppage	The hip and knee are elevated excessively high to lift the plantar flexed foot off the ground. The foot is brought down to the floor with a slap. The patient is unable to walk on the heels (see Figure 20-22, *C*).
Dystrophic (waddling)	The legs are kept apart, and weight is shifted from side to side in a waddling motion due to weak hip abductor muscles. The abdomen often protrudes, and lordosis is common.
Tabetic	The legs are positioned far apart, lifted high and forcibly brought down with each step. The heel stamps on the ground.
Cerebellar gait (cerebellar ataxia)	The patient's feet are wide-based. Staggering and lurching from side to side are often accompanied by swaying of the trunk (see Figure 20-22, *D*).
Sensory ataxia	The patient's gait is wide-based. The feet are thrown forward and outward, bringing them down first on heels, then on toes. The patient watches the ground to guide his or her steps. A positive Romberg sign is present (see Figure 20-22, *E*).
Parkinsonian gait	The patient's posture is stooped and the body is held rigid. Steps are short and shuffling, with hesitation on starting and difficulty stopping (see Figure 20-34, *C*).
Dystonia	Jerky dancing movements appear nondirectional.
Ataxia	Uncontrolled falling occurs.
Antalgic limp	The patient limits the time of weight bearing on the affected leg to limit pain.

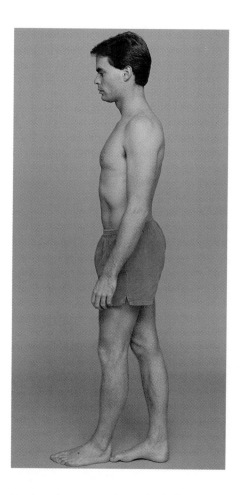

FIGURE 20-23
Evaluation of balance with heel-toe walking on a straight line.

SENSORY FUNCTION

Both primary and cortical discriminatory sensation are evaluated by having the patient identify various sensory stimuli. For the complete neurologic examination, each sense is tested in each major peripheral nerve. These sites should be routinely evaluated during the physical examination: hands, lower arms, abdomen, feet, and lower legs. Sensory discrimination of the face is determined with cranial nerve evaluation.

Each sensory discrimination procedure is tested with the patient's eyes closed. Use minimal stimulation initially, increasing it gradually until the patient becomes aware of it. A stronger stimulus is needed over the back, buttocks, and heavily cornified areas, where there are lower levels of sensitivity. Test contralateral areas of the body, and ask the patient to compare perceived sensations, side to side. With each type of sensory stimulus, there should be:

- Minimal differences side to side
- Correct interpretation of sensations (hot/cold, sharp/dull)
- Discrimination of the side of the body tested
- Location of sensation and whether proximal or distal to the previous stimuli

If evidence of sensory impairment is found, map the boundaries of the impairment by the distribution of major peripheral nerves or dermatomes. Loss of sensation can indicate spinal tract, brainstem, or cerebral lesions.

Primary Sensory Functions

Superficial touch. Touch the skin with a cotton wisp or with your fingertip, using light strokes. Do not depress the skin, and avoid stroking areas with hair (Figure 20-24, *A*). Have the patient point to the area touched or tell you when the sensation is felt.

Superficial pain. Alternating the sharp and smooth edge of a broken tongue blade or the point and hub of a sterile needle, touch the patient's skin in an unpredictable pattern. Allow 2 seconds between each stimulus to avoid a summative effect (Figure 20-24, *B*). Ask the patient to identify the sensation as sharp or dull and where it is felt. It is possible to combine evaluation of superficial pain and touch. Alternate use of the tongue blade or sterile needle and stroking with your fingertip to determine whether the patient can identify the change in sensation.

Temperature and deep pressure. Only when superficial pain sensation is not intact are temperature and deep pressure sensation tests performed. Roll test tubes of hot and cold water alternately against the skin, again in an unpredictable pattern, to evaluate temperature sensation. Ask the patient to indicate which temperature is perceived and where it is felt. Deep pressure sensation is tested by squeezing the trapezius, calf, or biceps muscle. The patient should experience discomfort.

Vibration. Place the stem of a vibrating tuning fork (the tuning fork with lower Hz has slower reduction of vibration) against several bony prominences, beginning at the most distal joints. The sternum, shoulder, elbow, wrist, finger joints, shin, ankle,

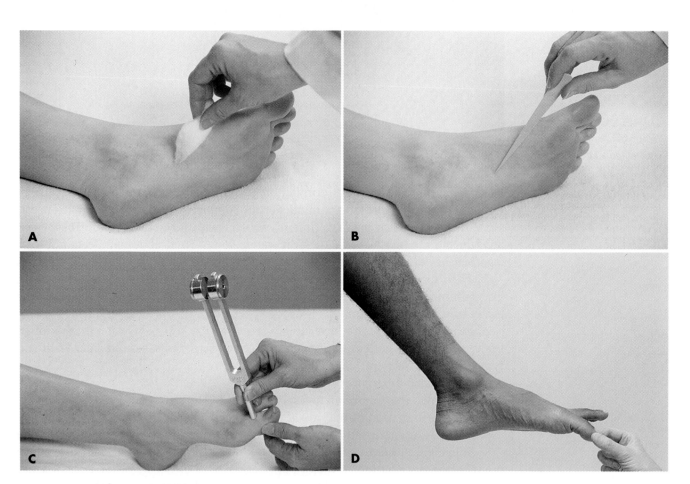

FIGURE 20-24
Evaluation of primary sensory function. **A,** Superficial tactile sensation; use a light stroke to touch the skin with a cotton wisp or brush. **B,** Superficial pain sensation; use the sharp and rounded edge of a broken tongue blade in a nonpredictable alternate pattern. **C,** Vibratory sensation; place the stem of a vibrating tuning fork against several bony prominences. **D,** Position sense of joints; hold the toe or finger by the lateral aspects in a raised or lowered position.

and toes may all be tested (Figure 20-24, *C*). A buzzing or tingling sensation should be felt. Ask the patient to tell you when and where the vibration is felt. Occasionally dampen the tines before application to see if the patient distinguishes a difference.

Position of joints. Hold the joint to be tested (great toe or finger) by the lateral aspects to avoid giving a clue about the direction moved. Beginning with the joint in neutral position, raise or lower the digit, and ask the patient to tell you which way it was moved. Return the digit to the neutral position before moving it in another direction (Figure 20-24, *D*). Repeat the procedure so that the great toe of each foot and a finger on each hand are tested.

Loss of sensory modalities may indicate peripheral neuropathy. Symmetric sensory loss indicates a polyneuropathy.

Cortical Sensory Functions

Cortical or discriminatory sensory functions test cognitive ability to interpret sensations associated with coordination abilities. Inability to perform these tests should make you suspect a lesion in the sensory cortex or the posterior columns of the spinal cord. The patient's eyes should be closed for these procedures.

Stereognosis. Hand the patient a familiar object (key, coin) to identify by touch and manipulation (Figure 20-25, *A*). Tactile agnosia, an inability to recognize objects by touch, suggests a parietal lobe lesion.

Two-point discrimination. Use two sterile needles and alternate touching the patient's skin with one point or both points simultaneously at various locations over the body (Figure 20-25, *B*). Find the distance at which the patient can no longer distinguish two points. Table 20-5 lists the minimal distances at which adults can discriminate two points on various parts of the body.

Extinction phenomenon. Simultaneously touch the cheek, hand, or other area on each side of the body with a sterile needle. Ask the patient to tell you how many stimuli there are and where they are. Both sensations should be felt.

Graphesthesia. With a blunt pen or an applicator stick, draw a letter or number on the palm of the patient's hand (Figure 20-25, *C*). Other body locations may also be used. Ask the patient to identify the figure. Repeat the procedure with a different figure on the other hand. The letter or number should be readily recognized.

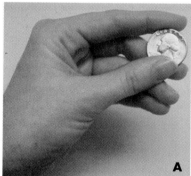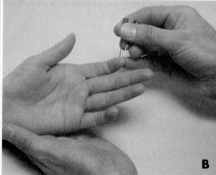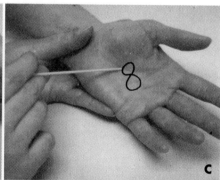

FIGURE 20-25

Evaluation of cortical sensory function. **A,** Stereognosis; patient identifies a familiar object by touch. **B,** Two-point discrimination; using two sterile needles, alternately place one or two points simultaneously on the skin, and ask the patient to determine if one or two sensations are felt. **C,** Graphesthesia; draw a letter or number on the body and ask the patient to identify it.

TABLE 20-5	Minimal Distances of Discriminating Two Points
Body Part	**Minimal Distance (mm)**
Tongue	1
Fingertips	2-8
Toes	3-8
Palms of hands	8-12
Chest and forearms	40
Back	40-70
Upper arms and thighs	75

From Barkauskas et al, 1998.

TABLE 20-6	Procedures for Testing the Integrity of Individual Spinal Tracts
Spinal Tracts	**Neurologic Tests**
Ascending Tracts	
Lateral spinothalamic	Superficial pain
	Temperature
Anterior spinothalamic	Superficial touch
	Deep pressure
Posterior column	Vibration
	Deep pressure
	Position sense
	Stereognosis
	Point location
	Two-point discrimination
Anterior and dorsal spinocerebellar	Proprioception
Descending Tracts	
Lateral and anterior corticospinal	Rapid rhythmic alternating movements
	Voluntary movement
	Deep tendon reflexes
	Plantar reflex
Medial and lateral reticulospinal	Posture and Romberg
	Gait
	Instinctual reactions

Point location. Touch an area on the patient's skin and withdraw the stimulus. Ask the patient to point to the area touched. No difficulty localizing the stimulus should be noted. This procedure is often performed simultaneously with superficial tactile sensation.

Table 20-6 provides a summary of procedures used to test the integrity of spinal tracts. Patterns of sensory loss are described in Box 20-2.

REFLEXES

Both superficial and deep tendon reflexes are used to evaluate the function of specific spine segmental levels (Table 20-7).

Superficial Reflexes

With the patient supine, stroke each quadrant of the abdomen with the end of a reflex hammer or tongue blade edge (see Chapter 15, Abdomen). A slight movement of the umbilicus toward each area of stimulation should be bilaterally equal. When abdominal reflexes are absent, either an upper or lower motor neuron disorder should be suspected.

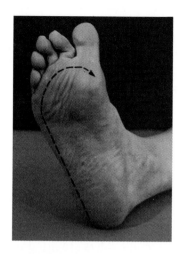

FIGURE 20-26

Plantar reflex indicating the direction of the stroke and the Babinski sign—dorsiflexion of the great toe with or without fanning of the toes.

Stroke the inner thigh of the male patient (proximal to distal) to elicit the cremasteric reflex. The testicle and scrotum should rise on the stroked side.

To elicit the plantar reflex, use a pointed object, stroke the lateral side of the foot from the heel to the ball, then curve across the ball of the foot to the medial side (Figure 20-26). Observe for plantar flexion, fanning of the toes, or dorsiflexion of the great toe with or without fanning of the other toes.

The patient should have plantar flexion of all toes. The Babinski sign is present when there is dorsiflexion of the great toe with or without fanning of the other toes. This is an expected response in children under 2 years of age, but it indicates pyramidal tract disease in other individuals. The ticklish patient may respond with some degree of Babinski sign, but this can be avoided with a firm touch.

BOX 20-2   **Patterns of Sensory Loss**

Injury or Defect and Description of Findings

Single peripheral nerve
- Sensory loss generally less than anatomic distribution of nerve; lost sensation in central portion with a zone of partial loss due to overlap with adjacent nerves. May lose all or selected modalities of sensation.

Multiple peripheral nerves (polyneuropathy)
- Sensory loss most severe over legs and feet or over hands (glove and stocking anesthesia). Change from expected to impaired sensation is gradual. Usually involves all modalities of sensation.

Multiple spinal nerve roots
- Usually incomplete loss of sensation in any area of the skin when one nerve root affected. When two or more nerve roots are completely divided, there is a zone of sensory loss surrounded by partial loss. Tendon reflexes may also be lost.

Complete transverse lesion of the spinal cord
- All forms of sensation are lost below the level of the lesion. Loss of pain, temperature, and touch sensation occurs one to two dermatomes below the lesion.

Partial spinal sensory syndrome (Brown-Sequard syndrome)
- Pain and temperature sensation occur one to two dermatomes below the lesion on the opposite side of the body from the lesion. Proprioceptive loss and motor paralysis occur on the lesion side of the body.

TABLE 20-7   **Superficial and Deep Tendon Reflexes**

Reflex	Spinal Level
Superficial	
Upper abdominal	T7, T8, and T9
Lower abdominal	T10 and T11
Cremasteric	T12, L1, and L2
Plantar	L4, L5, S1, and S2
Deep	
Biceps	C5 and C6
Brachioradial	C5 and C6
Triceps	C6, C7, and C8
Patellar	L2, L3, and L4
Achilles	S1 and S2

Modified from Rudy, 1984.

Deep Tendon Reflexes

Evaluation of deep tendon reflexes is performed with the patient relaxed, either sitting or lying down. Focus the patient's attention on an alternate muscle contraction, such as pulling clenched hands apart. Position the limb with slight tension on the tendon to be tapped. Palpate the tendon to locate the correct point for stimulation, rather than randomly tapping in the area. Hold the reflex hammer loosely between your thumb and index finger, and briskly tap the tendon with a flick of the wrist. At first you may strike too forcefully, but with practice you will learn to be more gentle.

Test each reflex, comparing responses on corresponding sides. Symmetric visible or palpable responses should be noted. Scoring of deep tendon reflex responses is shown in Table 20-8. Documentation of findings on a stick figure is illustrated in Chapter 24, Recording Information. Absent reflexes may indicate neuropathy or lower motor neuron disorder, whereas hyperactive reflexes suggest an upper motor neuron disorder. The characteristics of upper and lower motor neuron disorders are listed in Box 20-3.

Biceps reflex. Flex the patient's arm up to 45 degrees at the elbow. Palpate the biceps tendon in the antecubital fossa (Figure 20-27, *A*). Place your thumb over the tendon and your fingers under the elbow. Strike your thumb, rather than the tendon directly, with the reflex hammer. Contraction of the biceps muscle causes visible or palpable flexion of the elbow.

Brachioradial reflex. Flex the patient's arm up to 45 degrees and rest his or her forearm on your arm with the hand slightly pronated (Figure 20-27, *B*). Strike the brachioradial tendon (about 1 to 2 inches above the wrist) directly with the reflex hammer. Pronation of the forearm and flexion of the elbow should occur.

TABLE 20-8 | **Scoring Deep Tendon Reflexes**

Grade	Deep Tendon Reflex Response
0	No response
1+	Sluggish or diminished
2+	Active or expected response
3+	More brisk than expected, slightly hyperactive
4+	Brisk, hyperactive, with intermittent or transient clonus

BOX 20-3 | **Clinical Signs of Motor Neuron Lesions**

Upper Motor Neuron	Lower Motor Neuron
Muscle spasticity, possible contractures	Muscle flaccidity
Little or no muscle atrophy, but decreased strength	Loss of muscle tone and strength; muscle atrophy
Hyperactive deep tendon and abdominal reflexes; absent plantar reflex	Weak or absent deep tendon, plantar, and abdominal reflexes
No fasciculations	Fasciculations
Damage above level of brainstem will affect opposite side of body	Changes in muscles supplied by that nerve, usually a muscle on same side as the lesion
Paralysis of lower part of face, if involved	Bell palsy, if face involved; coordination unimpaired

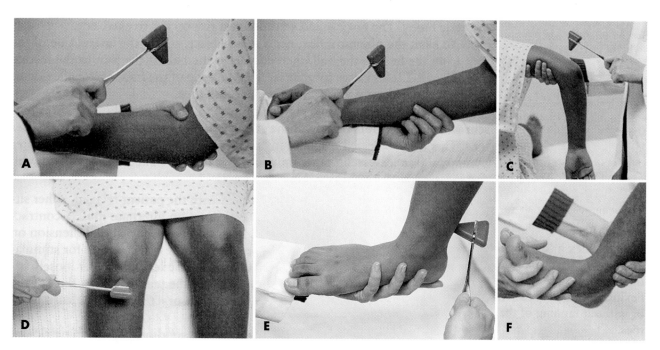

FIGURE 20-27
Location of tendons for evaluation of deep tendon reflexes. **A,** Biceps. **B,** Brachioradial. **C,** Triceps.
D, Patellar. **E,** Achilles. **F,** Evaluation of ankle clonus.

Triceps reflex. Flex the patient's arm at the elbow up to 90 degrees and rest the patient's hand against the side of the body. Palpate the triceps tendon and strike it directly with the reflex hammer, just above the elbow (Figure 20-27, *C*). Contraction of the triceps muscle causes visible or palpable extension of the elbow.

Patellar reflex. Flex the patient's knee up to 90 degrees, allowing the lower leg to hang loosely. Support the upper leg with your hand, not allowing it to rest against the edge of the examining table. Strike the patellar tendon just below the patella (Figure 20-27, *D*). Contraction of the quadriceps muscle causes extension of the lower leg.

Achilles reflex. With the patient sitting, flex the knee to 90 degrees and keep the ankle in neutral position, holding the heel of the foot in your hand. Alternatively, the patient may kneel on a chair with the toes pointing toward the floor. Strike the Achilles tendon at the level of the ankle malleoli (Figure 20-27, *E*). Contraction of the gastrocnemius muscle causes plantar flexion of the foot.

Clonus. Test for ankle clonus, especially if the reflexes are hyperactive. Support the patient's knee in partially flexed position and briskly dorsiflex the foot with your other hand, maintaining the foot in flexion (Figure 20-27, *F*). No rhythmic oscillating movements between dorsiflexion and plantar flexion should be palpated. Sustained clonus is associated with upper motor neuron disease.

ADDITIONAL PROCEDURES

Various other procedures for further evaluation of the neurologic system are performed when problems are detected with routine examination.

5.07 Monofilament

Use the 5.07 Monofilament to test for protective sensation on several sites of the foot in all patients with diabetes mellitus and peripheral neuropathy (Figure 20-28). While

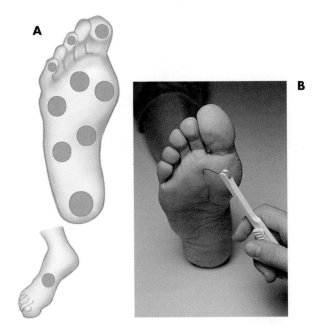

FIGURE 20-28
A, Sites for application of the 5.07 Monofilament to test for sensation. Indicate presence (+) or absence (−) of sensory perception. **B,** Application of the monofilament to the patient's foot with just enough pressure to bend the monofilament.

the patient's eyes are closed, apply the monofilament in a random pattern in several sites on the plantar surface of the foot and on one site of the dorsal surface. Do not test over calluses or broken skin. Do not repeat a test site. The monofilament should be applied to each site for 1.5 seconds. When the filament bends, adequate pressure is applied. Patients should feel the sensation in all sites. Loss of sensation to the touch of the monofilament is an indication of peripheral neuropathy, and the loss of protective pain sensation that alerts patients to skin breakdown and injury.

Meningeal Signs

A stiff neck or *nuchal rigidity* is a sign associated with meningitis and intracranial hemorrhage. With the patient supine, slip your hand under the head and raise it, flexing the neck. Try to make the patient's chin touch the sternum, but do not force it. Placing your hand under the shoulders and raising them slightly will help relax the neck, making the determination of true stiffness more accurate. Patients will generally not resist or complain of pain. Pain and a resistance to neck motion are associated with nuchal rigidity. Occasionally, painful swollen lymph nodes in the neck and superficial trauma may also cause pain and resistance to neck motion.

The *Brudzinski* sign may also be present when neck stiffness is assessed. Involuntary flexion of the hips and knees when flexing the neck is a positive Brudzinski sign for meningeal irritation.

The *Kernig* sign is evaluated by flexing the leg at the knee and hip when the patient is supine. Then attempt to straighten the leg. Pain in the lower back and resistance to straightening the leg at the knee constitute a positive Kernig sign, indicating meningeal irritation.

INFANTS

We ordinarily begin to suspect neurologic problems in the young because they are *not* doing something we expect them to do, rather than because we find a problem on physical examination. As in so much else, the major clues are discovered with an accurate and painstaking history.

The cranial nerves are not directly tested, but several observations made during the physical examination provide indirect evaluation (Table 20-9).

NEW AGE RANGE FOR ROLLING OVER

Change in sleep position from prone to the side or back as currently advised to reduce the risk of sudden infant death syndrome has an effect on the age at which infants roll over. Infants roll over at a later age than those that sleep in a prone position.

Data fromJantz, Blosser, Freuchting, 1997

Observe the infant's spontaneous activity for symmetry and smoothness of movement (Fig 20-29). Coordinated sucking and swallowing is also a function of the cerebellum. Hands are usually held in fists for the first 3 months of life, but not constantly; after 3 months they begin to open for longer periods. Purposeful movement (reaching and grasping for objects) begins at about 2 months of age. This progresses to taking objects with one hand at 6 months, transferring objects hand to hand at 7 months, and purposefully releasing objects by 10 months of age. There should be no tremors or constant overshooting of movements.

TABLE 20-9	**Indirect Cranial Nerve Evaluation in Newborns and Infants**
Cranial Nerves	**Procedures and Observations**
CN II, III, IV, and VI	Optical blink reflex: shine a light at the infant's open eyes. Observe the quick closure of the eyes and dorsal flexion of the infant's head. No response may indicate poor light perception.
	Gazes intensely at close object or face.
	Focuses on and tracks an object with both eyes.
	Doll's eye maneuver: see CN VIII.
CN V	Rooting reflex: touch one corner of the infant's mouth. The infant should open its mouth and turn its head in the direction of stimulation. If the infant has been recently fed, minimal or no response is expected (Figure 20-30).
	Sucking reflex: place your finger in the infant's mouth, feeling the sucking action. The tongue should push up against your finger with good strength. Note the pressure, strength, and pattern of sucking.
CN VII	Observe the infant's facial expression when crying. Note the infant's ability to wrinkle the forehead and the symmetry of the smile.
CN VIII	Acoustic blink reflex: loudly clap your hands about 30 cm from the infant's head; avoid producing an air current. Note the blink in response to the sound. No response after 2-3 days of age may indicate hearing problems. Infant will habituate to repeated testing.
	Moves eyes in direction of sound. Freezes position with high-pitched sound.
	Doll's eye maneuver: hold the infant under the axilla in an upright position, head held steady, facing you. Rotate the infant first in one direction and then in the other. The infant's eyes should turn in the direction of rotation and then the opposite direction when rotation stops. If the eyes do not move in the expected direction, suspect a vestibular problem or eye muscle paralysis.
CN IX and X	Swallowing and gag reflex.
CN XII	Coordinated sucking and swallowing ability.
	Pinch infant's nose; mouth will open and tip of tongue will rise in a midline position.

Modified from Thompson et al, 1997.

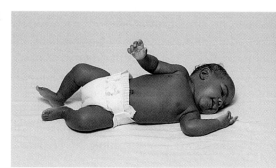
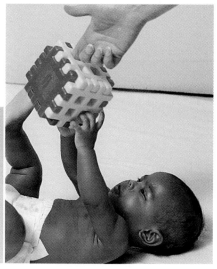

FIGURE 20-29
A, Note this infant's beginning effort to roll over. The asymmetric tonic neck reflex has disappeared (p.793). **B,** Observe purposeful movement such as reaching for the block.

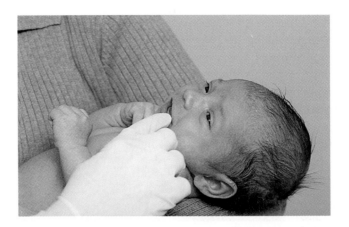

FIGURE 20-30

Demonstration of technique to elicit rooting reflex. Touch the corner of the infant's mouth and observe for movement of the head and opening of the mouth on the side of the stimulation.

TABLE 20-10	Primitive Reflexes Routinely Evaluated in Infants
Reflex (Appearance)	**Procedure and Findings**
Palmar grasp (birth)	Making sure the infant's head is in midline, touch the palm of the infant's hand from the ulnar side (opposite the thumb). Note the strong grasp of your finger. Sucking facilitates the grasp. It should be strongest between 1 and 2 months of age and disappear by 3 months (Figure 20-31, *A*).
Plantar grasp (birth)	Touch the plantar surface of the infant's feet at the base of the toes. The toes should curl downward. The reflex should be strong up to 8 months of age (Figure 20-31, *B*).
Moro (birth)	With the infant supported in semi-sitting position, allow the head and trunk to drop back to a 30-degree angle. Observe symmetric abduction and extension of the arms. Fingers fan out and thumb and index finger form a C. The arms then adduct in an embracing motion followed by relaxed flexion. The legs may follow a similar pattern of response. The reflex diminishes in strength by 3 to 4 months and disappears by 6 months (Figure 20-31, *C*).
Placing (4 days of age)	Hold the infant upright under the arms next to a table or chair. Touch the dorsal side of the foot to the table or chair edge. Observe flexion of the hips and knees and lifting of the foot as if stepping up on the table. Age of disappearance varies (Figure 20-31, *D*).
Stepping (between birth and 8 weeks)	Hold the infant upright under the arms and allow the soles of the feet to touch the surface of the table. Observe for alternate flexion and extension of the legs, simulating walking. It disappears before voluntary walking (Figure 20-31, *E*).
Asymmetric tonic neck or "fencing" (by 2 to 3 months)	With the infant lying supine and relaxed or sleeping, turn its head to one side so the jaw is over the shoulder. Observe for extension of the arm and leg on the side to which the head is turned and for flexion of the opposite arm and leg. Turn the infant's head to the other side, observing the reversal of the extremities' posture. This reflex diminishes at 3 to 4 months of age and disappears by 6 months. Be concerned if the infant never exhibits the reflex or seems locked in the fencing position. This reflex must disappear before the infant can roll over or bring its hands to its face (Figure 20-31, *F*).

A withdrawal of all limbs from a painful stimulus provides a measure of sensory integrity. Other sensory function is not routinely tested.

The patellar tendon reflexes are present at birth, and the Achilles and brachioradial tendon reflexes appear at 6 months of age. When deep tendon reflexes are tested, the examiner should use a finger to tap the tendon, rather than the reflex hammer. In each case, the muscle attached to the tendon struck should contract. Interpret findings as for adults; however, one to two beats of ankle clonus are common.

The plantar reflex is routinely performed as described in the adult examination. A positive Babinski sign, fanning of the toes and dorsiflexion of the great toe, is found until the infant is 16 to 24 months of age.

The posture and movement of the developing infant are routinely evaluated by primitive reflexes (Table 20-10) and are shown in Figure 20-31. Less commonly evaluated primitive reflexes are listed in Table 20-11. These reflexes appear and disappear

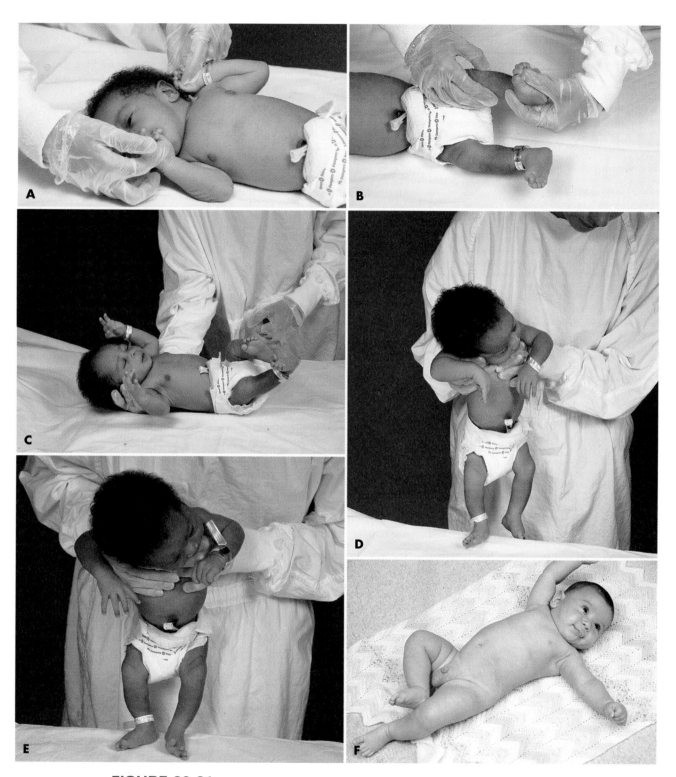

FIGURE 20-31
The preferred state of the infant for testing primitive reflexes is "quiet alert," neither hungry nor drowsy. Elicitation of the primitive reflexes. **A,** Palmar grasp. **B,** Plantar grasp. **C,** Moro reflex. **D,** Placing reflex. **E,** Stepping reflex. **F,** Asymmetric tonic neck reflex.

TABLE 20-11	Less Commonly Evaluated Primitive Reflexes in Infants
Reflex (Appearance)	**Procedure and Findings**
Glabella (birth)	With your index finger, briskly tap the bridge of the infant's nose between the eyes (glabella) when its eyes are open. Observe the sudden symmetric blinking of the eyes. The infant will blink for the first 4 to 5 taps.
Galant (trunk incurvature) (birth to 4 weeks)	Suspend the infant in prone position on one of your hands or on a flat surface. Stroke one side of the infant's back between the shoulders to the buttocks, about 4 to 5 cm from the spinal cord. Observe for the curvature of the trunk toward the side stroked. Repeat on the other side.
Landau (birth to 6 months)	Suspend the infant in prone position on both of your hands so that the infant's legs and arms are extending over both sides of your hand. Observe the infant's ability to lift its head and extend its spine on a horizontal plane. The reflex diminishes by 18 months of age and disappears by 3 years.
Parachute (4 to 6 months)	Hold the infant suspended in prone position and slowly lower it head first toward a surface. Observe the infant extend its arms and legs as if to protect itself. This reflex should not disappear.
Neck righting (3 months, after tonic neck disappears)	With the infant supine, turn its head to the side. Observe the infant turning its whole body in the direction the head is turned.

in a sequence corresponding with central nervous system development. Symmetry and smoothness of response are important observations. Posture and movement should also be inspected for any rhythmic twitching of the facial, extremity, and trunk musculature, as well as for any sustained asymmetric posturing. These signs, especially in paroxysmal episodes, are associated with seizure activity.

Muscle strength and tone are especially important to evaluate in the newborn and infant. Chapter 19, Musculoskeletal System, provides details related to this portion of the examination. Remember that the infant's neuromuscular development at the time of birth should be evaluated with the Dubowitz Clinical Assessment for gestational age (see Chapter 5, Growth and Measurement).

CHILDREN

The neurologic examination of the young child is done by observing the neuromuscular developmental progress and skills displayed during the examination. The Denver II is a useful tool to determine whether the child is developing as expected with fine and gross motor skills, language, and personal-social skills (see Appendix F).

Direct examination of cranial nerves requires some modifications in procedure according to the age of the child. Often a game is played to elicit the response. Table 20-12 describes the procedures.

Observe the young child at play, noting gait and fine motor coordination. The beginning walker exhibits a wide-based gait, whereas the older child walks with feet closer together, has better balance, and recovers more easily when unbalanced. Observe the child's skill in reaching for, grasping, and releasing toys. No tremors or constant overshooting movements should be apparent.

Heel-to-toe walking, hopping, and jumping are all coordination skills that develop in the young child. They can be evaluated by modifying the skill tested into a game for the child. Three pennies can be used to evaluate several aspects of the neurologic system, including vision, extraocular movements, and hearing (coin dropped on floor). Ask the child who is standing to pick a penny up off of the floor (tests vision and balance). Stick a moistened coin to the child's nose and ask the child to walk across the room (allows you to observe gait and any posturing). Have the child bal-

TABLE 20-12	Cranial Nerve Examination Procedures For Young Children	

Cranial Nerves	Procedures and Observations
CN II	If the child cooperates, the Snellen E or Picture Chart may be used to test vision.
	Visual fields may be tested, but the child may need the head immobilized.
CN III, IV, and VI	Have the child follow an object with the eyes, immobilizing the head if necessary. Attempt to move the object through the cardinal points of gaze.
CN V	Observe the child chewing a cookie or cracker, noting bilateral jaw strength.
	Touch the child's forehead and cheeks with cotton or string and watch the child bat it away.
CN VII	Observe the child's face when smiling, frowning, and crying.
	Ask the child to show his or her teeth.
	Demonstrate puffed cheeks and ask the child to imitate.
CN VIII	Observe the child turn to sounds such as a bell or whisper.
	Whisper a commonly used word behind the child's back and have him or her repeat the word.
	Perform audiometric testing.
CN IX and X	Elicit gag reflex
CN XI and XII	Instruct older child to stick out the tongue and shrug the shoulders or raise the arms.

Modified from Bowers, Thompson, 1992.

ance a penny on the nose and dorsum of each extended hand (tests the Romberg). (Freeman, 1997). The Denver II provides guidance for the ages at which you can expect these maneuvers to be accomplished and is standardized for most cultural groups.

Deep tendon reflexes are not routinely tested in a child who demonstrates appropriate development, because poor cooperation is often a problem. When reflexes are tested, use the same techniques described for adults; responses should be the same. Your index finger may also take the place of a reflex hammer, and may be less threatening to a child.

Evaluate light touch sensation by asking the child to close his or her eyes and point to where you touch or tickle. Have the child discriminate between rough and soft textures as an alternate procedure. Use the tuning fork to evaluate vibration sensation, asking the child to point to the area where the buzzing sensation is felt. Superficial pain sensation is not routinely tested in young children because of their fear of needles and sharp objects.

When checking cortical sensory integration, use geometric figures rather than numbers to evaluate graphesthesia. Draw each figure twice and ask the child if the figures are the same or different. (Make sure the child understands the terms *same* and *different*.) Some children will need a practice session with their eyes open to get good compliance with the examination.

Many of the techniques used in the adult neurologic examination are utilized for children, with some modifications for the child's level of understanding.

Because the child is still developing, there may be some unexpected findings in the school-age child that would be normal in younger children. These neurologic soft signs are nonfocal, functional neurologic findings that often provide subtle clues to an underlying central nervous system deficit or a neurologic maturation delay. Soft signs can be found in gross motor, fine motor, sensory, and reflex functional areas. Table 20-13 describes neurologic soft sign findings and the age at which you should become concerned if still present. Children with multiple soft signs are often found to have learning problems.

TABLE 20-13	Activities for Evaluating Neurologic Soft Signs in Children	
Activity	Soft Sign Findings	Latest Expected Age of Disappearance (Years)
Walking, running gait	Stiff-legged with a foot slapping quality, unusual posturing of the arms	3
Heel walking	Difficulty remaining on heels for a distance of 10 ft	7
Tip-toe walking	Difficulty remaining on toes for a distance of 10 ft	7
Tandem gait	Difficulty walking heel-to-toe, unusual posturing of arms	7
One-foot standing	Unable to remain standing on one foot longer than 5-10 sec	5
Hopping in place	Unable to rhythmically hop on each foot	6
Motor-stance	Difficulty maintaining stance (arms extended in front, feet together, and eyes closed), drifting of arms, mild writhing movements of hands or fingers	3
Visual tracking	Difficulty following object with eyes when keeping the head still; nystagmus	5
Rapid thumb-to-finger test	Rapid touching thumb to fingers in sequence is uncoordinated; unable to suppress mirror movements in contralateral hand	8
Rapid alternating movements of hands	Irregular speed and rhythm with pronation and supination of hands patting the knees	10
Finger-nose test	Unable to alternately touch examiner's finger and own nose consecutively	7
Right-left discrimination	Unable to identify right and left sides of own body	5
Two-point discrimination	Difficulty in localizing and discriminating when touched in one or two places	6
Graphesthesia	Unable to identify geometric shapes you draw in child's open hand	8
Stereognosis	Unable to identify common objects placed in own hand	5

PREGNANT WOMEN

Examination of pregnant women is the same as for the adult. Assessment of deep tendon reflexes during the initial examination can serve as a baseline evaluation.

OLDER ADULTS

Examination of the neurologic system of the older adult is identical to that of the adult. You may need to allow more time for performing maneuvers that require coordination and movement.

Medications can impair central nervous system function, causing slowed reaction time, tremors, and anxiety. Problems may develop because of the dosage, number, or interaction of medications prescribed or purchased over the counter.

The older adult may have markedly diminished senses of smell and taste. Sweet and salty tastes are usually impaired first. Other common cranial nerve changes include a reduced ability to differentiate colors, reduced upward gaze, slower adjustment to lighting changes, decreased corneal reflex, middle to high frequency hearing loss, and a reduced gag reflex (Crigger, Forbes, 1997).

Gait with advancing age is characterized by short, uncertain steps as proprioception declines. Shuffling may occur as speed, balance, and grace decrease with age. Legs may be flexed at the hips and knees (Figure 20-32).

Tactile and vibratory sensation, as well as position sense, are often impaired in the older adult. This patient may need stronger stimuli to detect sensation.

Changes in deep tendon reflexes occur with aging. The older adult usually has less brisk or even absent reflexes, with response diminishing in the lower extremities before the upper extremities are affected. The Achilles and plantar reflexes may be absent or difficult to elicit in some older adults. The superficial reflexes may also disappear. There is typically an increase in benign essential tremor with aging. Fine motor coordination and agility may be impaired.

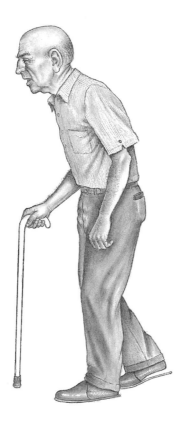

FIGURE 20-32
Short, uncertain steps are characteristic of gait with advancing age.

SUMMARY OF EXAMINATION   **Neurologic System**

Test Cranial Nerves I through XII
(pp. 772-778).

Cerebellar Function and Proprioception
1. Evaluate coordination and fine motor skills by the following (pp. 778-779):
   - Rapid rhythmic alternating movements
   - Accuracy of upper and lower extremity movements
2. Evaluate balance using the Romberg test (p. 780).
3. Observe the patient's gait (pp. 781-782).
   - Posture
   - Rhythm and sequence of stride and arm movements

Sensory Function
1. Test primary sensory responses to the following (pp. 783-784):
   - Superficial touch
   - Superficial pain
2. Test vibratory response to tuning fork over joints or bony prominences on upper and lower extremities (p. 784-785).
3. Evaluate perception of position sense with movement of the great toe or a finger (p. 785).
4. Assess ability to identify familiar object by touch and manipulation (p. 785).
5. Assess two-point discrimination (p. 785-786).
6. Assess ability to identify letter or number "drawn" on palm of hand (p. 785).
7. Assess ability to identify body area when touched (p. 786).

Superficial and Deep Tendon Reflexes
1. Test abdominal reflexes (pp. 543, 786).
2. Test the cremasteric reflex in male patients (p. 787).
3. Test the following deep tendon reflexes (pp. 788-789):
   - Biceps
   - Brachioradial
   - Triceps
   - Patellar
   - Achilles
4. Test for ankle clonus (p. 789).
5. Test the plantar reflex (p. 787).

COMMON ABNORMALITIES

DISORDERS OF THE CENTRAL NERVOUS SYSTEM

AIDS DEMENTIA COMPLEX (HIV ENCEPHALOPATHY)	A progressive dementia that is likely related to direct HIV infection of the brain, AIDS dementia complex may be difficult to distinguish from clinical depression in early stages. Insidious onset occurs, with headaches, loss of memory and concentration, and inability to follow complex instructions. Eventually global cognitive impairment occurs. Behavior changes in-	clude apathy related to work, recreation, and social activities. Motor findings include hyperreflexia; increased tone; slowed, rapid rhythmic movements; clumsiness and weakness in the arms and legs; and gait ataxia that mimics Huntington chorea and Parkinson disease. Fecal and urinary incontinence may also occur.
HUNTINGTON CHOREA	An autosomal hereditary, progressive degenerative disease, Huntington chorea is characterized by choreiform movements and mental deterioration progressing to	dementia. Symptoms usually appear between 30 and 40 years of age, and death occurs about 15 years later.
MULTIPLE SCLEROSIS	A debilitating, degenerative disorder of unknown cause, multiple sclerosis is characterized by multifocal demyelinated plaques throughout the white matter of the central nervous system. The onset of symptoms occurs between 20 and 40 years of age. Between remissions, acute episodes occur with varying types and	severity of symptoms. Symptoms include ocular disturbances such as diplopia, blurred vision, eye pain, and loss of visual acuity; muscle fatigue; facial palsy; numbness and tingling of the extremities; spastic weakness of the lower extremities; cerebellar ataxia; urinary incontinence; and depression or euphoric affect.
GENERALIZED SEIZURE DISORDER	A generalized seizure disorder is characterized by episodic, sudden, involuntary contractions of a group of muscles, resulting from excessive discharge of cerebral neurons. The disorder may be caused by systemic disease, head trauma, toxins, stroke, or hypoxic syndromes.	Disturbances in consciousness, behavior, sensation, and autonomic functioning often occur. Urinary and fecal incontinence may also accompany seizures. As many as 1% of the population have seizures, and 75% of new cases develop during childhood and adolescence.

MENINGITIS

> **SMELL THE CEREBROSPINAL FLUID**
>
> When a lumbar puncture is done in the event of a suspected meningitis, the odor of alcohol can indicate a cryptococcal infection.

An inflammatory process in the meninges, meningitis is caused by bacteria and viruses. Signs and symptoms include fever, chills, nuchal rigidity, headache, seizures, and vomiting, followed by alterations in level of consciousness. Young infants do not demonstrate nuchal rigidity until about 6 to 9 months of age, so this sign will not be present. Those infants affected will generally be very irritable and inconsolable and have fever, diarrhea, poor appetite, and toxic appearance. Bacterial meningitis is a life-threatening illness if not rapidly treated with appropriate antibiotics.

ENCEPHALITIS

Encephalitis is inflammation of the brain and spinal cord that also involves the meninges. The onset is often a mild, febrile viral illness. A quiescent stage often precedes the disturbance in central nervous system function and is characterized by headache, drowsiness, and confusion, eventually progressing to stupor and coma. Motor functions may also be impaired with severe paralysis or ataxia.

LYME DISEASE

Lyme disease is a multisystem infection caused by the *Borrelia burgdorferi* spirochete, which is carried by ticks. The disease has three stages of progression, with varying signs and symptoms in each patient. Neurologic signs may include headache, meningitis, encephalitis, polyneuritis, unilateral or bilateral facial paralysis, choreic movements, spastic paralysis, and ataxia. These signs may occur during early and/or late stages of the disease. Arthritis and acrodermatitis are signs associated with the third stage of the infection. Treatment with appropriate antibiotics will generally cure the infection, but some neurologic signs may be unresolved.

SPACE-OCCUPYING LESIONS (INTRACRANIAL TUMORS)

A space-occupying lesion is an abnormal growth of neural or nonneural tissue within the cranial cavity that may be primary or metastatic cancer. The lesion causes displacement of tissue and pressure on the cerebrospinal fluid circulation and may threaten function through the compression and destruction of tissues. Early signs and symptoms vary by the location of the tumor but often include headaches, vomiting, change in cognition, motor dysfunction, seizures, and personality changes. Peak ages of incidence are 3 to 12 years and 50 to 70 years.

CEREBROVASCULAR ACCIDENT (STROKE)

A sudden, focal neurologic deficit resulting from impaired circulation of the brain, cerebrovascular accident (CVA) is associated with cardiovascular disease. A thrombosis, embolism, or hemorrhage causes the circulation impairment. The most common site of lesions is within the distribution of the anterior circulation of the brain. General signs and symptoms include restlessness, lethargy, changes in level of consciousness, vital sign and pupil changes, nausea and vomiting, and impaired communication. Disability severity varies in survivors. See Table 20-14 for neurologic signs associated with CVA by location of lesion (Figure 20-33).

TABLE 20-14   Neurologic Signs Associated with CVA by Location

Artery Affected	Neurologic Signs
Internal Carotid Artery (Supplies the cerebral hemispheres and diencephalon by the ophthalmic and ipsilateral hemisphere arteries)	Unilateral blindness Severe contralateral hemiplegia and hemianesthesia Profound aphasia
Middle Cerebral Artery (Supplies structures of higher cerebral processes of communication; language interpretation; perception and interpretation of space, sensation, form, and voluntary movement)	Alterations in communication, cognition, mobility, and sensation Homonymous hemianopia Contralateral hemiplegia or hemiparesis
Anterior Cerebral Artery (Supplies medial surfaces and upper convexities of frontal and parietal lobes and medial surface of hemisphere, which includes motor and somesthetic cortex serving the legs)	Emotional lability Confusion, amnesia, personality changes Urinary incontinence Impaired mobility, with sensation greater in lower extremities than in upper Contralateral hemiplegia or hemiparesis
Posterior Cerebral Artery (Supplies medial and inferior temporal lobes, medial occipital lobe, thalamus, posterior hypothalamus, and visual receptive area)	Hemianesthesia Contralateral hemiplegia, greater in face and upper extremities than lower extremities Homonymous hemianopia Receptive aphasia Cortical blindness Memory deficits
Vertebral or Basilar Arteries (Supply the brainstem and cerebellum) Incomplete occlusion	Transient ischemic attacks Unilateral and bilateral weakness of extremities Diplopia, homonymous hemianopia Nausea, vertigo, tinnitus, and syncope Dysphagia Dysarthria Sometimes confusion and drowsiness
Anterior portion of pons	"Locked-in" syndrome—no movement except eyelids; sensation and consciousness preserved
Complete occlusion or hemorrhage	Coma Miotic pupils Decerebrate rigidity Respiratory and circulatory abnormalities Death
Posterior Inferior Cerebellar Artery (Supplies the lateral and posterior portion of the medulla)	Wallenberg syndrome Dysphagia, dysphonia Ipsilateral anesthesia of face and cornea for pain and temperature (touch preserved) Ipsilateral Horner syndrome Contralateral loss of pain and temperature sensation in trunk and extremities Ipsilateral decompensation of movement
Anterior Inferior and Superior Cerebellar Arteries (Supply the cerebellum)	Difficulty in articulation, swallowing, gross movements of limbs; nystagmus
Anterior Spinal Artery (Supplies the anterior spinal cord)	Flaccid paralysis, below level of lesion Loss of pain, touch, temperature sensation (proprioception preserved)
Posterior Spinal Artery (Supplies the posterior spinal cord)	Sensory loss, particularly proprioception, vibration, touch, and pressure (movement preserved)

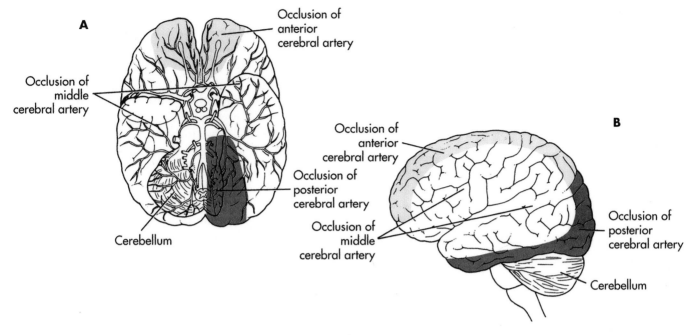

FIGURE 20-33
Areas of the brain affected by occlusion of the anterior, middle, and posterior cerebral artery branches. **A,** Inferior view. **B,** Lateral view.
From Rudy, 1984.

DISORDERS OF THE PERIPHERAL NERVOUS SYSTEM

MYASTHENIA GRAVIS

A neuromuscular disease involving the lower motor neurons and muscle fibers, myasthenia gravis is believed to be autoimmune in origin. It causes a defect in transmission at the neuromuscular junction. Nerve impulses do not pass on to the skeletal muscle at the myoneural junction. Symptoms begin either between 20 and 30 years of age or in late middle age. It is characterized by lower extremity weakness and abnormal fatigue in the muscles involved in ocular movement, facial expression, respiration, chewing, and swallowing. Patients may have a rapid decline in respiratory muscle function resulting in a life-threatening crisis.

GUILLAIN-BARRÉ SYNDROME

Guillain-Barré syndrome (acute idiopathic polyneuritis) is an acute polyneuropathy that commonly follows a nonspecific infection that occurred 10 to 14 days earlier and primarily affects the motor and autonomic peripheral nerves. Widespread inflammation or demyelination of the ascending or descending nerves leads to impaired conduction of nerve impulses between the nodes of Ranvier. It is characterized by ascending symmetric weakness (with sensation preserved) that increases in severity over days or weeks. Motor paralysis and respiratory muscle failure may result, requiring life support; however, 85% of patients eventually have full functional recovery after a recovery period lasting several weeks to months.

PERIPHERAL NEUROPATHY

MNEMONICS

CAUSES OF PERIPHERAL NEUROPATHY: "I'M DISTAL"

I   *Idiopathic, Inherited*
M   *Metabolic, Mechanical*
D   *Drugs*
I   *Infections*
S   *Sarcoidosis*
T   *Tumors*
A   *Autoimmune, Allergy*
L   *Lack of vitamins*
From Shipman, 1984.

Peripheral neuropathy is a disorder of the peripheral nervous system that results in motor and sensory loss in the distribution of one or more nerves. The most common cause is diabetes mellitus, but it may also be caused by toxins, such as kerosene, or vitamin B_{12} deficiency. In moderate to severe diabetic neuropathy, there is wasting of the foot muscles, absent ankle and knee reflexes, decreased or no vibratory sensation below the knees, and loss of pain or sharp touch sensation to the mid-calf level. Temperature sensation may be less impaired. The loss of pain sensation leads to the loss of a protective reflex or awareness of an injury. Loss of skin integrity can lead to ulceration and infection. In diabetes mellitus, this condition is compounded by impaired circulation that results in poor healing of skin ulcers and may result in amputation.

CHILDREN

CEREBRAL PALSY

A group of nonprogressive neuromuscular disorders of abnormal muscle tone and coordination, cerebral palsy results from insult to the cerebellum, basal ganglia, or motor cortex. Signs include delayed gross motor development, alterations in muscle tone, and abnormalities of posture, motor performance, and reflexes. The degree of disability produced depends on the extent of neurologic damage. Some patients can expect near-normal levels of functioning.

HIV ENCEPHALOPATHY

Progressive encephalopathy associated with AIDS in children is generally an advanced feature of the disease. It is associated with impaired brain growth due to cerebral atrophy, progressive motor dysfunction, regression or a plateau in developmental milestones, and generalized weakness with upper motor neuron signs. Less common findings include dysphagia, gait ataxia, and seizures.

RETT SYNDROME

Rett syndrome is a progressive encephalopathy of unknown cause that develops in girls after normal neurologic and mental development between 6 and 18 months of age. Characteristic signs include loss of voluntary hand movement, loss of previously acquired hand skills, hand wringing movements, gradual development of ataxia and rigidity of the legs, growth retardation, seizures, and loss of facial expression. There is deceleration of head growth between 5 and 48 months of age. The disorder is believed to account for substantial numbers of children with mental retardation. Children can survive several years in a helpless state.

PREGNANT WOMEN

MATERNAL OBSTETRIC PALSY

A number of different neuropathies result in weakness in the lower extremities because of mechanical compression of nerves during delivery. Femoral neuropathy results from compression of the lumbosacral plexus and peripheral nerves in the pelvic wall by the fetal head or forceps. Footdrop may result from compression of nerves in the lumbosacral trunk when the fetal brow presses against the mother's sacral ala. Compression of the common peroneal nerve between the leg holders and the fibula during delivery can also cause unilateral footdrop. If the axons are not crushed and degeneration of the nerves does not occur, these disorders are reversible.

OLDER ADULTS

PARKINSON DISEASE

Parkinson disease is a slowly progressive, degenerative neurologic disorder of the brain's dopamine neuronal systems. Patients may have as history of encephalitis, drug use, or cerebrovascular disease. There may be genetic, viral, vascular, toxic, and other unknown causes. The mean age at onset is 60 years; however, it sometimes occurs in young adults. Symptoms (often unilateral initially) begin with tremors at rest and with fatigue, disappearing with intended movement and sleep, respectively. The disorder progresses with tremor of the head, slowing of voluntary movements, and bilateral pillrolling of the fingers. Motor impairment causes delays in execution of movement, masked facial expression, and poor blink reflex. Muscular rigidity interferes with walking, leading to a gait of short, shuffling steps with the trunk in a forward flexion posture. Speech becomes slowed, slurred, and monotonous. Behavioral change and dementia occur in about 10% to 15% of patients (Figure 20-34).

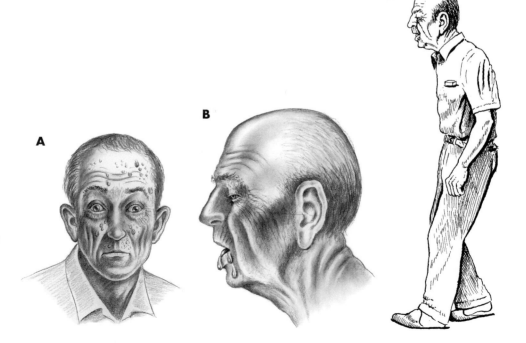

FIGURE 20-34
Characteristic features of Parkinson disease. **A,** Excessive sweating. **B,** Drooling with excess saliva. **C,** Gait with rapid, short, shuffling steps and reduced arm swinging.
From Rudy, 1984.

NORMAL PRESSURE HYDROCEPHALUS

Normal pressure hydrocephalus is a syndrome caused by noncommunicating hydrocephalus (dilated ventricles, but intracranial pressure is within expected ranges) that simulates degenerative diseases. Patients have a triad of signs including a gait disorder, psychomotor slowing, and incontinence. Patients may have progressive dementia with memory loss, mild bilateral upper motor neuron signs, and fecal and urinary incontinence. Some patients have a history of subarachnoid hemorrhage, traumatic brain injury, or meningitis. The condition is often correctable by a ventriculoperitoneal shunt.

CHAPTER 21

PUTTING IT ALL TOGETHER

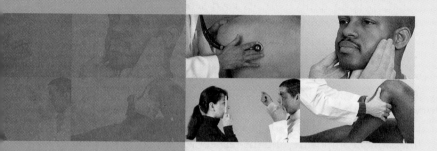

The relationship with the patient *mandates* the exercise of an art that, well done, leads to marvelous benefit. There is a powerful *therapeutic* effect in respectful attention to what the patient is saying (that is, using a true "listening ear"), careful exploration for hidden concerns, and explanation in unpatronizing, understandable terms. The enduring message is that you care, and that the patient is a full partner with you in the effort. This of itself helps in the relief of suffering. If you communicate well and if you and the patient can achieve a genuine alliance, you will find that you are of service and, happily, will feel much rewarded.

We have indicated "routines" for the taking of a history and the performance of a physical examination, and we have stressed your need to adopt a disciplined approach particular to your comfort. Discipline, however, does not suggest rigidity. Too great an adherence to routine may prevent the true story from emerging. That is why open-ended encouragement of the patient to speak of himself or herself, to tell the real story, can be so rewarding (Coles, 1989). It is helpful at a first meeting, if the situation allows, to sit back comfortably and to say, "Tell me about yourself", and to listen and to hear.

As a skillfully evoked story—the history—evolves, the absolute unity of mind and body and the power of an effective alliance with the patient become manifest. The physical examination, the "laying on of hands," complements the story and is essential to the confirmation of the alliance. Words and physical acts are all invested with pragmatic need *and* symbolic meaning and are all contributors to the conscious and subconscious requirements of an effective relationship. They ultimately make it possible to understand not only the objective biologic findings, the *disease*, but also the great variety of subjective findings that modify the experience of the disease and result in an *illness* being understood in human, *not scientific,* terms. Obviously, art and science are inextricable, and technologic expertise is a complement to, never a substitute for, skillful art. The computer cannot replace a good history and a competent physical examination.

GENERAL GUIDELINES

When you begin learning about a patient, you should not expect to proceed from A to Z on a rigid pathway. The information in this book is arranged by body systems, but the actual examination should be both flexible and disciplined. The history and physical examination are so interrelated that they need not be done in a particular sequence. The artistry of your effort arises from your ability to integrate the two procedures, according to the demand of the situation. Each of the steps in history taking and physical examination is an entity with its own sensitivity and specificity. You must understand the limits of each of those steps and how much information can be gained from them. Although you need to be always alert to deviations from the usual and the expected, you will learn when to omit steps that will yield information of little value. This is not being sloppy; it is using clinical judgment in adapting to circumstance. The steps blend into a fluid and comprehensible whole. The process of taking the history and performing the physical examination not only teaches you much about the patient, but also teaches the patient much about you—your personal discipline, your professional composure, and the respect you accord others (Box 21-1). You must not forget that the patient, who usually seeks your help because of a problem, may feel dependent and may be having some unease, anxiety, or even fear (Box 21-2). You can help allay these feelings simply by respecting them and not demeaning or ignoring them. Your explanations of what you will do next will help reassure the patient and alleviate anxiety. Always be honest about the possibility that a part of the examination may cause discomfort or pain; otherwise, you risk losing trust. If either you or the patient feels the need to have a third person in the room, you must certainly arrange it.

Always respect the patient's modesty. This does not mean that you do not ask the patient to undress, but rather that comfortable gowns and covers are available that can be shifted or removed from the area under examination while providing cover for other parts of the body. Doors and curtains should be closed, and it is best to leave the room when the patient undresses and prepares for the examination.

Early encounters with the human body generally result in some discomfort, sometimes revulsion, and often embarrassment. At times, sexual connotations cannot be ignored. There is also the thrilling privilege in taking on, at last, the responsibility for serving patients. Your comfort with the situation should never become so great that you forget that the experience may be much newer for the patient. Your own early reactions can provide insight into the patient's experience.

BOX 21-1	How to Ensure "Difficulty" with Patients

- Make them wait a long time, without explanation, particularly alone in the examining room
- Act busy and rushed
- Talk "medicalese"
- Be casual and superficial in offering reassurance, deflecting real concerns
- Skip the extra question that might reveal an underlying problem
- Ignore emotional responses to illness, such as anger, fear, uncertainty, guilt, and self-blame
- Ignore the stresses in a patient's life (and yours), the day-to-day pressures and needs that can overwhelm
- Convey your negative feelings or discomfort about a particular illness

Modified from Jellinek et al, 1991.

BOX 21-2	The Patient We Define as Difficult

We always want to do our best, and we always want our relationship with the patient to be positive. Sometimes, however, we find ourselves reacting negatively when patients are:

- Dependent, apparently needing insatiable, never-ending contact
- Denying, using denial to cope, being inattentive to instructions, not following through on treatment regimens
- Demanding, wanting preferential treatment, seeming always on the edge of a lawsuit, really often quite dependent, and often impressed with their self-determined status in society (the VIP)
- Rejecting, distrusting, always testing your competency and reliability

In all of these circumstances, it pays to learn what the patient's needs really are, to understand their insecurities, learn the available family and other social resources, and never put them down. Certainly, it is necessary to be as precise as possible, to keep all promises, to set firm limits on what you can do, and to try to retain an empathetic approach. The alliance with these patients can grow and mature, albeit sometimes painfully. It won't happen instantly. The advantage we have is that patients are more often than not, particularly when they are vulnerable, inclined to give us the chance to gain their trust and respect.

Suggested by Jellinek et al, 1990.

The invasion of a stranger's sensibilities can be most distracting to the student. You will learn a gentle, calm, and balanced demeanor. Your professional concern can be reassuring to the patient, but you must avoid inappropriate reassurance and premature expressions of concern over unexpected findings. Remember that while you examine the patient, he or she is also examining you, titrating his or her anxiety by your manner, your hesitations in speech, your changes in facial expression, your lingering over a part of the examination. In fact, many patients equate the gravity of the situation with the length of time you spend on part of the examination, whereas others equate length of time with thoroughness.

The patient should be told that you are a student and that you are apt to be a bit slower than the more experienced practitioner. You will naturally feel some pressure and uncertainty about your level of ability, but there is a half-life to this period of anxiety. Time, experience, and the appropriate observation of and supervision by preceptors will help build the foundation for your self-confidence.

At the beginning, when you are unaccustomed to the sequence of an examination, rely on guides such as those in this book. But do not hesitate to develop your own sequence of observations. There is no such thing as a "complete" examination. The goal is to perform an examination in which your observations are appropriate to the circumstance. This varies with the nature of the complaint and the age and gender of the patient.

The examination of a patient of any age is subject to variation. Because there is no "best way," you should develop your own approach, one that feels comfortable for you and ensures comfort for your patient. You need not take the history or perform the physical examination in the same sequence in which you will record them. Part of the history can be obtained while you are doing the physical examination, because as you discover certain findings, you will require more details than the earlier history may have elicited. Regardless of sequence, there are certain guidelines that should never be ignored (Box 21-3).

Once you have obtained basic information on the patient, you need to make an assessment about the urgency of the situation, determine whether the principal problems are new or long standing, decide which clues are most important, determine the extent of the problems and the number of body systems involved, and decide which of the possible clinical areas concerned are dominant.

BOX 21-3   Some Guidelines to an Appropriate Relationship with the Patient

- Dress neatly; always be well groomed.
- Address the patient respectfully and with the patient's name. Although a child's mother is a mother, she should not be addressed as such; she has a name.
- Patients are culturally diverse. Use the patient's language if at all possible; it is important that the patient understand you; if you must use colloquialisms to accomplish this, do so. DO NOT use complex medical terminology.
- Ensure comfort for the patient and, to the extent possible, for yourself.
- Be gentle.
- The setting should be quiet (radios and televisions should be turned off), comfortable, and well lighted (without glare).
- Avoid distraction and interruption (the telephone should not be allowed into the history and examining room unless there is an emergency).
- Adapt to the patient's circumstance; a person in traction will offer a different challenge from the 7-month-old baby on the parent's lap.
- Be flexible and avoid rigid adherence to a particular sequence. However, be certain that by the end of the examination you have made all the necessary observations.
- An examining table should allow you access to the patient from every side and be at a height that is convenient for both you and the patient. Because a table against the wall is an obstacle to examining the patient from every perspective, it is preferable to have the table away from the wall.
- Have the patient free of clothing but comfortably draped, paying attention to modesty at every age.
- Expose the part of the body to be examined appropriately and well, or you may lose *the* vital finding.
- Keep your hands and stethoscope warm.
- Avoid using too vigorous an approach when examining tender areas.
- Talk with the patient but do not chatter. Explain as you go, anticipating the patient's concern about what comes next. Briefly state the reasons for examining an area and warn the patient of any discomfort it might incur.
- Never *order* the patient to do things. Say "please" and "thank you" (but not so endlessly so that the courtesy itself becomes obsequious). Occasionally ask if the patient is warm enough and comfortable enough or has any questions.
- Gather information from the patient's attitude, demeanor, speech, and body. It is worrisome, for example, to find the patient apathetic, disinterested, unable to respond socially, or so overwhelmed by the problem that a smile cannot be elicited. This is as true for a 3-month-old baby as it is for an adult.
- Make some assessment, at least in your own mind, about the reliability of the patient as an observer. Remember that there is much in illness and in life to put constraints on the patient's ability to observe carefully and objectively. Be objective and make no premature assumptions about what you find. Carefully describe first without diagnosing. For example, a lump in the neck may be a swollen node and not a cyst. Diagnosis can usually wait until after the examination is completed.
- Make quantitative measurements with a ruler. Do not use a coin or a piece of fruit or a nut for comparison.
- Always remember that physical findings are age oriented and that their meanings will vary according to age.
- Be reassuring only when you honestly can.
- Do not jump to conclusions and share impressions before all the information has been collected. Do not make promises that cannot be kept. Developing the composure that allows you to be reassuring without overstating the case takes practice and time.
- Do not feel that you have to do it all in one sitting. If the situation requires it, you can allow the patient a chance for rest and return later to complete the examination. You should pace your approach according to the patient's need, guided by the sense of urgency and the recognition of fatigue and frailty.

At this point, you may need to ask more questions and return to your physical examination. The clinical circumstance often requires repeated examination for you to understand the problem. You cannot assume that your initial list of clinical possibilities is all inclusive. There may be an unusual presentation of a common problem or a common presentation of a rarity. There may be more than one disease process or a confounding emotional or social problem. There may be a new illness superimposed on an existing one. You must pay attention to all clues in an effort to explain all symptoms, signs, and abnormal findings.

Finally, you need to discover where in the patient's realm you need to concentrate. To do this well, you must review all the systems and consider the entire range of pathophysiologic and psychosocial problems. You must go beyond the obvious to the obscure, always keeping probabilities in mind. Ultimately, you will have to challenge your conclusions by acting as your own devil's advocate or asking others to do so.

RELIABILITY

The health professional and the patient share responsibility for the reliability of findings and observations. The demands that you put on yourself are, of course, greater than those that you put on the patient. Take the time with open-ended questions to ensure that the patient has the opportunity to observe and to report accurately.

The Patient as Historian

There is much that can limit the patient's ability to observe well and to report accurately:

- *Sensory deprivation:* A partial or total loss of any of the senses (e.g., vision, hearing, touch, smell) is clearly constraining. Do not rely on the unaffected senses being heightened. This may be the case with some people, but not with all.
- *Emotional constraints, apparent and inapparent:* Patients who are psychotic, delirious, depressed, or in any way seriously emotionally affected may confuse you. Emphasize mental status during the history when you suspect this.
- *Language barriers:* Patients may speak a different language from yours. Translation can be difficult in the best of circumstances. Passing messages among three persons often results in changes in meaning that might have serious importance; confusion may be the result. Even using the same language may be a problem if the patient has a limited vocabulary, speaks English as a second language, or cannot read it very well.
- *Cultural barriers:* Pay attention to the possibility of cultural differences between you and the patient (see Chapter 2, Cultural Awareness). Approach the variety of life experience with candor and interested, compassionate inquiry (Box 21-4).
- *Unresponsive or comatose patient:* Refer to the section on the unresponsive patient (see Chapter 23, Emergency or Life-Threatening Situations).

BOX 21-4 **Cultural Differences Related to Life Experience**

Cultural differences manifest in many ways. While race, religion, and ethnicity are obvious, there are also meaningful separations in life experiences among the fat and the thin, the gravely ill and the well, the drug abuser and the nonuser, and the aged and the young. The recognition of these differences and the conscientious attempt to encourage the patient to talk of them and thus to educate you can build empathic bridges and eliminate, or at least minimize, doubts about each other. It is all right, for example, to ask how it feels to be markedly overweight in an airplane seat designed for a slender, short person (see Chapter 2, Cultural Awareness).

The immediate need in all of these circumstances is that you identify and understand these limitations and that you take the necessary steps to enhance reliability. Patients with a sensory impairment deserve a response from you that facilitates communication—for example, write questions; pay careful attention to the needs of a speech reader, such as good light, a slow pace to speech, and a constant visibility of your lips; and recognize that the blind cannot see your gestures.

In many circumstances, you must rely on family, friends, or an emergency medical technician for information. The rules that guide interaction with the patient guide interaction with all individuals. If possible, the patient must be aware that you are receiving information from other historians and, when possible, there must be agreement with the patient about the limits that can be placed on the sharing of information. Respect for autonomy and the rules of confidentiality remain.

There are patients, of course, who are "unreliable" because of life situations, limited intelligence, indifference, apathy, or personal emotional needs that lead to distortions, overstatements, or understatements of reality; any number of variables can get in the way. All of these possibilities require skill and sensitivity in responding to the enormous variety in the human condition. You might begin by rejecting the common use of the descriptor, "unreliable," because of its pejorative connotation.

The Professional as Observer

This topic, of course, suggests the possibility for human error. The same practitioner may palpate the same abdomen on successive days and conclude that the liver has a somewhat different span on each day. Multiple observers will palpate the same abdomen on the same day and individually decide on different liver spans. These are not unconscientious, ill-considered observations. They are demonstrations of the potential for error. Your recognition of these important considerations as you make decisions will be a measure of your reliability (Box 21-5). Remember that each of us is as subject to error as the many tests we order for a patient (Box 21-6).

BOX 21-5 The *Initial* Challenge to Reliability

There are behaviors, sometimes subtle, sometimes obvious, that may undermine our ability to communicate reliably and, therefore, our reliability as observers. There was a time when recorded histories and physical examinations contained few if any initials. After World War II, the use of initials began to proliferate. Today, it is a compulsive disease leading to misunderstanding that is at times inconvenient and at times dangerous.

Recently, at a conference in an academic hospital, the following initials were used without clarification:

- MRS (methicillin-resistant staphylococcus)
- MARS (methicillin- and aminoglycoside-resistant staphylococcus)
- MTS (methicillin-tolerant staphylococcus)
- TSS (toxic shock syndrome)
- TEN (toxic epidermal necrolysis)
- SSSS (staphylococcal scalded skin syndrome)

We are at a time when our interprofessional languages are obscured by initials; communication suffers. The obstetrician who uses ROM (rupture of membranes) talks a different language from the pediatrician who uses ROM (right otitis media) or the physiatrist's ROM (range of motion) and, these days, ROM tacked on to CD has an entirely different message. There is a temptation to initialize and to abbreviate and to get things said and written in a hurry. It should be resisted.

Every observation has a certain *sensitivity*—the assurance that if something is to be found, it will be found—and *specificity*—the assurance that if it is found, it is a true finding and not a misinterpretation or false positive. No test has 100% sensitivity and specificity (see Chapter 24, Recording Information). As a consequence, be aware of the potential for error, and to the best of your ability, guard against it. Recognize that, in all likelihood, you will not *always* be right. This potential for error increases uncertainty and reminds us that almost all decisions evolve from considerations of probabilities. A numeric value of probability can often be given, providing an idea of the degree of uncertainty. Many kinds of psychosocial, environmental, and physical considerations affect the perceptions of the same "set of facts" and have a variable impact on outcome.

BOX 21-6 **Humans Versus Machines**

There are a number of observations you can make better than machines can, including the following:
- All perceptions obtained through watching, listening, touching, and smelling
- The appearance of the patient, his or her vitality, the presence or absence of apathy, and the sense of illness
- The patient's cognitive awareness

There are, however, an almost infinite variety of diagnostic procedures that enable better understanding of patients' problems. Just as with us, these procedures are not always sensitive to potential findings or necessarily specific about them.

For example, diagnostic imaging—the use of x-ray film, nuclear medicine, ultrasonography, computed tomography (CT), and magnetic resonance imaging (MRI)—offers a powerful resource. Yet, diagnostic imaging has its limitations and penalties:
- The x-ray examination is easily available and relatively inexpensive and can give a sense of motion with the fluoroscope and cineradiograph; however, the procedure utilizes contrast agents that can be toxic, there is confusion of shadows, and the patient is exposed to radiation.
- The ultrasonograph is safe, can also provide a sense of motion, and delineates soft tissue very well; however, fat, bone, and air impede sound waves.
- CT clearly delineates anatomy, works better in the presence of obesity than does x-ray examination, and outlines soft tissues very well; however, it is expensive, does not work as well in the lean individual, and uses radiation.
- Nuclear medicine takes a step toward enhancing knowledge about the body's physiology, and it can reveal early bone infection and bone metastasis; however, it is expensive, and uses radiation.
- MRI gives excellent soft tissue contrast and precise anatomic detail without the need for contrast agents. Similar to ultrasonography, it is safe, but it is also very expensive and not always available. In addition, the machine and the process can at times intimidate patients, particularly children.

These reminders are not meant to discourage but are intended only to suggest caution and thoughtfulness in everything we do. This is particularly necessary as the newer imaging techniques that extend the reach of our presently accepted techniques come into play. Color Doppler flow imaging, a technique based on the assignment of color to the shift in ultrasound frequency associated with moving red blood cells (the Doppler effect), makes it possible to avoid venograms for the evaluation of deep vein thrombosis. Ultrasound technology has been so improved that it achieves much greater anatomic detail. It can detect acute intracranial hemorrhage, pyloric stenosis, and abdominal masses, and it can aid in the evaluation of urinary tract infection when reflux is not present. CT has become ultrafast, and is now described as "conventional." Nuclear medicinal agents, technetium-labeled dimercaptosuccinic acid (DMSA) and diethylenetriaminepentaacetic acid (DTPA), give us more information about the upper urinary tract than does intravenous urography. It will become more and more difficult to remind ourselves that no procedure occurs without cost to the human body, to emotion, and to the pocketbook.

Modified from Johns et al, 1988; Taylor, 1989.

Most of us are uncomfortable with uncertainty at the start. The diagnostic process may be initiated by thinking in a deterministic or mechanistic fashion, seeking certain and fixed knowledge, and avoiding to the extent possible anything that is subjective, a search for absolutes that are free of beliefs, attitudes, and values. However, the variables of life will not often allow this. They will not always let you express your findings in numbers.

Regardless, we often attempt to quantify data. The scales we use may require a subjective judgment: assign a number and come out with a total score. Although there is a need for constructive pseudoquantification, be cautious about accepting the "objectivity" of such scores. Rivara and Wasserman (1984), aware of our addiction to numbers, suggested that we might give more attention to psychosocial issues in our day-to-day work with people if we were able to quantify them. Tongue in cheek, they noted that one milli-Helen equals exactly that amount of beauty it takes to launch exactly one ship. Be aware of false comfort in the apparent certainty of numbers.

Because we have not yet reached that ideal state of certainty, we must continue to recognize the potential for error, the variety of interpretations of the same event, and the need to think in terms of probability. The mature observer is one who is comfortable making decisions with a certain degree of uncertainty.

EXAMINATION SEQUENCE

We remind you again that there is no one right way to put together the parts of the physical examination so that the process flows smoothly, minimizes the number of times the patient has to change positions, and conserves patient energy. The following is a suggested approach. Like any other approach, it may need to be adapted for a particular setting, patient condition, or patient disability. Box 21-7 gives a list of equipment you should have on hand.

BOX 21-7 **Equipment Supplies for Physical Examination**

Basic Materials

Cotton balls
Cotton-tipped applicator sticks
Drapes
Examining gloves
Flashlight with transilluminator
Gauze squares
Lubricant
Marking pen
Measuring tape
Nasal speculum
Odorous substances
Ophthalmoscope
Otoscope with pneumatic bulb
Penlight
Percussion hammer
Ruler
Sharp and dull testing implements

Sphygmomanometer
Stethoscope with diaphragm and bell
Taste-testing substances
Thermometer
Tongue blades
Tuning forks
Vaginal speculum
Visual acuity screening charts for near and far vision

Materials for Gathering Specimens

Culture media
Glass slides
KOH (potassium hydroxide)
Occult blood testing materials
Pap smear spatula and/or brush, fixative, and container
Saline
Sterile cotton-tipped applicators

GENERAL INSPECTION

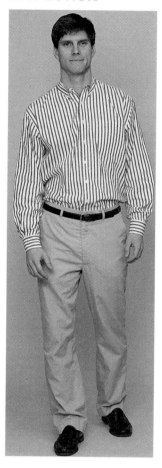

Begin the inspection as you greet the patient on entering the room, looking for signs of distress or disease. You can perform parts of your physical examination at any time as long as the patient is within your view, even in the waiting room. If you go there to invite the patient into your examining room, take a moment to see the habitus, manner of sitting, degree of relaxation, relationship with others in the room, and degree of interest in what is happening in the room. There are no blank moments when you are with the patient. On your first greeting, you can judge the alacrity with which you are met; the moistness of the palm when you shake hands; the gait as the patient walks back to the room; and the eyes, their luster, and their expression of emotion. All of this contributes to your examination, along with assessments of the following:

- Skin color
- Facial expression
- Mobility
  - Use of assistive devices
  - Gait
  - Sitting, rising from chair
  - Taking off coat
- Dress and posture
- Speech pattern, disorders, foreign language
- Difficulty hearing, assistive devices
- Stature and build
- Musculoskeletal deformities
- Vision problems, assistive devices
- Eye contact with examiner
- Orientation, mental alertness
- Nutritional state
- Respiratory problems
- Significant others accompanying patient

PATIENT INSTRUCTIONS

Respecting modesty, instruct the patient to empty the bladder, remove as much clothing as is necessary, and put on a gown. Then begin the examination. A suggested sequence follows.

MEASUREMENTS

- Measure height.
- Measure weight.
- Assess distance vision: Snellen chart.
- Document vital signs: temperature, pulse, respiration, and blood pressure in both arms.

PATIENT SEATED, WEARING GOWN

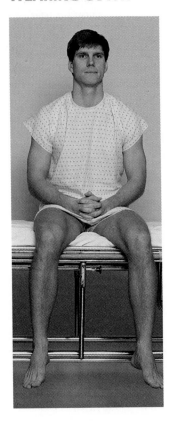

Patient is seated on examining table; examiner stands in front of patient.

Head and Face

- Inspect skin characteristics.
- Inspect symmetry and external characteristics of eyes and ears.
- Inspect configuration of skull.
- Inspect and palpate scalp and hair for texture, distribution, and quantity.
- Palpate facial bones.
- Palpate temporomandibular joint while patient opens and closes mouth.
- Palpate and percuss sinus regions; if tender, transilluminate.
- Inspect ability to clench teeth, squeeze eyes tightly shut, wrinkle forehead, smile, stick out tongue, puff out cheeks (CN V, VII).
- Test light touch sensation of forehead, cheeks, chin (CN V).

Eyes

- External examination
  - Inspect eyelids, eyelashes, palpebral folds.
  - Determine alignment of eyebrows.
  - Inspect sclera, conjunctiva, iris.
  - Palpate lacrimal apparatus.
- Near vision screening: Rosenbaum chart (CN II)
- Eye function
  - Test pupillary response to light and accommodation.
  - Perform cover-uncover test and corneal light reflex.
  - Test extraocular eye movements (CN III, IV, VI).
  - Assess visual fields (CN II).
  - Test corneal reflexes (CN V).
- Ophthalmoscopic examination
  - Test red reflex.
  - Inspect lens.
  - Inspect disc, cup margins, vessels, retinal surface.

Ears

- Inspect alignment and placement.
- Inspect surface characteristics.
- Palpate auricle.
- Assess hearing with whisper test or ticking watch (CN VIII).
- Perform otoscopic examination.
  - Inspect canals.
  - Inspect tympanic membranes for landmarks, deformities, inflammation.
- Perform Rinne and Weber tests.

Nose

- Note structure, position of septum.
- Determine patency of each nostril.
- Inspect mucosa, septum, and turbinates with nasal speculum.
- Assess olfactory function: test sense of smell (CN I).

Mouth and Pharynx
- Inspect lips, buccal mucosa, gums, hard and soft palates, floor of mouth for color and surface characteristics.
- Inspect oropharynx: note anteroposterior pillars, uvula, tonsils, posterior pharynx, mouth odor.
- Inspect teeth for color, number, surface characteristics.
- Inspect tongue for color, characteristics, symmetry, movement (CN XII).
- Test gag reflex and "ah" reflex (CN IX, X).
- Perform taste test (CN VII).

Neck
- Inspect for symmetry and smoothness of neck and thyroid.
- Inspect for jugular venous distention.
- Inspect and palpate range of motion; test resistance against examiner's hand.
- Test shoulder shrug (CN IX).
- Palpate carotid pulses, one at a time.
- Palpate tracheal position.
- Palpate thyroid.
- Palpate lymph nodes: preauricular and postauricular, occipital, tonsillar, submaxillary, submental, superficial cervical chain, posterior cervical, deep cervical, supraclavicular.
- Auscultate carotid arteries and thyroid.

Upper Extremities
- Observe and palpate hands, arms, and shoulders.
  - Skin and nail characteristics
  - Muscle mass
  - Musculoskeletal deformities
  - Joint range of motion and muscle strength: fingers, wrists, elbows, shoulders
- Assess pulses: radial, brachial.
- Palpate epitrochlear nodes.

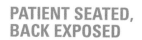

PATIENT SEATED, BACK EXPOSED

Patient is still seated on examining table. Gown is pulled down to the waist for males so the entire chest and back are exposed; for females, back is exposed, but breasts are covered. Examiner stands behind the patient.

Back and Posterior Chest
- Inspect skin and thoracic configuration.
- Inspect symmetry of shoulders, musculoskeletal development.
- Inspect and palpate scapula and spine, and percuss spine.
- Palpate and percuss costovertebral angle.

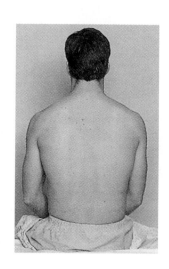

Lungs
- Inspect respiration: excursion, depth, rhythm, pattern.
- Palpate for expansion and tactile fremitus.
- Palpate scapular and subscapular nodes.
- Percuss posterior chest and lateral walls systematically for resonance.
- Percuss for diaphragmatic excursion.
- Auscultate systematically for breath sounds: note characteristics and adventitious sounds.

PATIENT SEATED, CHEST EXPOSED

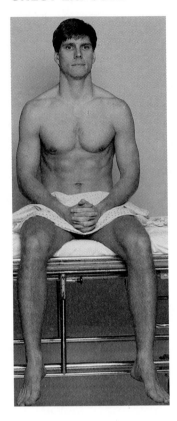

Examiner moves around to the front of the patient. The gown is lowered in females to expose the anterior chest.

Anterior Chest, Lungs, and Heart

- Inspect skin, musculoskeletal development, symmetry.
- Inspect respirations: patient posture, respiratory effort.
- Inspect for pulsations or heaving.
- Palpate chest wall for stability, crepitation, tenderness.
- Palpate precordium for thrills, heaves, pulsations.
- Palpate left chest to locate apical impulse.
- Palpate for tactile fremitus.
- Palpate nodes: infraclavicular, axillary.
- Percuss systematically for resonance.
- Auscultate systematically for breath sounds.
- Auscultate systematically for heart sounds: aortic area, pulmonic area, second pulmonic area, apical area.

Female Breasts

- Inspect in the following positions: patient's arms extended over head, pushing hands on hips, hands pushed together in front of chest, patient leaning forward.
- Palpate breasts in all four quadrants, tail of Spence, over areolae; if breasts are large, perform bimanual palpation.
- Palpate nipple, compress breasts to observe for discharge.

Male Breasts

- Inspect breasts and nipples for symmetry, enlargement, surface characteristics.
- Palpate breast tissue.

PATIENT RECLINING 45 DEGREES

Assist the patient to a reclining position at a 45-degree angle. Examiner stands to the side of the patient that allows the greatest comfort.
- Inspect chest in recumbent position.
- Inspect jugular venous pulsations and measure jugular venous pressure.

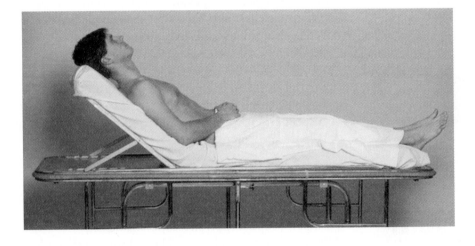

PATIENT SUPINE, CHEST EXPOSED

Assist the patient into a supine position. If the patient cannot tolerate lying flat, maintain head elevation at 30-degree angle if possible. Uncover the chest while keeping the abdomen and lower extremities draped.

Female Breasts

- Inspect and palpate using the recumbent and upright positions.
- Palpate systematically with the patient's arm over her head and also with her arm at her side.

Heart

- Palpate the chest wall for thrills, heaves, pulsations.
- Auscultate systematically; you can turn the patient slightly to the left side and repeat auscultation.

PATIENT SUPINE, ABDOMEN EXPOSED

Patient remains supine. Cover the chest with the patient's gown. Arrange draping to expose the abdomen from pubis to epigastrium.

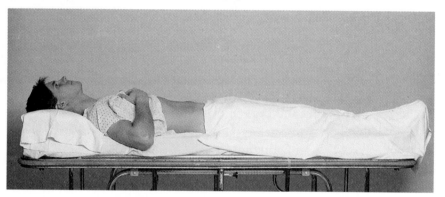

Abdomen

- Inspect skin characteristics, contour, pulsations, movement.
- Auscultate all quadrants for bowel sounds.
- Auscultate the aorta and renal, iliac, and femoral arteries for bruits or venous hums.
- Percuss all quadrants for tone.
- Percuss liver borders and estimate span.
- Percuss left midaxillary line for splenic dullness.
- Lightly palpate all quadrants.
- Deeply palpate all quadrants.
- Palpate right costal margin for liver border.
- Palpate left costal margin for spleen.
- Palpate for right and left kidneys.
- Palpate midline for aortic pulsation.
- Test abdominal reflexes.
- Have patient raise the head as you inspect the abdominal muscles.

Inguinal Area

- Palpate for lymph nodes, pulses, hernias.

External Genitalia, Males

- Inspect penis, urethral meatus, scrotum, pubic hair.
- Palpate scrotal contents.

PATIENT SUPINE, LEGS EXPOSED

Patient remains supine. Arrange drapes to cover the abdomen and pubis and to expose the lower extremities.

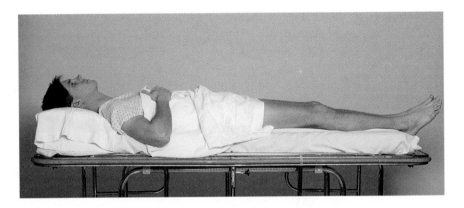

Feet and Legs

- Inspect for skin characteristics, hair distribution, muscle mass, musculoskeletal configuration.
- Palpate for temperature, texture, edema, pulses (dorsalis pedis, posterior tibial, popliteal).
- Test range of motion and strength of toes, feet, ankles, knees.

Hips

- Palpate hips for stability.
- Test range of motion and strength of hips.

PATIENT SITTING, LAP DRAPED

Assist the patient to a sitting position. The patient should have the gown on with a drape across the lap.

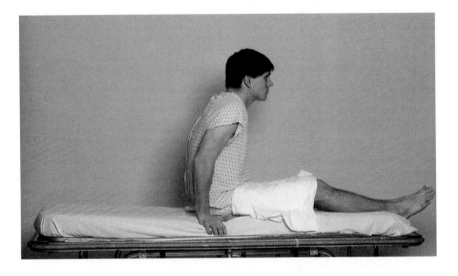

Musculoskeletal

- Observe patient moving from lying to sitting position.
- Note coordination, use of muscles, ease of movement.

Neurologic

- Test sensory function: dull and sharp sensation of forehead, paranasal sinus area, lower arms, hands, lower legs, feet.
- Test vibratory sensation of wrists, ankles.
- Test two-point discrimination of palms, thighs, back.
- Test stereognosis, graphesthesia.
- Test fine motor function and coordination. Ask the patient to perform the following tasks:
  - Touch his or her nose with alternating index fingers
  - Rapidly alternate fingers to thumb
  - Rapidly move index finger between his or her own nose and the examiner's finger
- Test fine motor function and coordination. Ask the patient to do the following:
  - Run heel down tibia of opposite leg
  - Alternately and rapidly cross leg over opposite knee
- Test position sense of upper and lower extremities.
- Test deep tendon reflexes and compare bilaterally: biceps, triceps, brachioradial, patellar, Achilles.
- Test plantar reflex bilaterally.

PATIENT STANDING

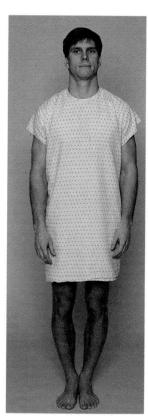

Assist patient to a standing position. Examiner stands next to patient.

Spine

- Inspect and palpate spine as patient bends over at waist.
- Test range of motion: hyperextension, lateral bending, rotation of upper trunk.

Neurologic

- Observe gait.
- Test proprioception and cerebellar function.
  - Assess Romberg test.
  - Ask the patient to walk heel to toe.
  - Ask the patient to stand on one foot, then the other, with eyes closed.
  - Ask the patient to hop in place on one foot, then the other.
  - Ask the patient to do deep knee bends.

Abdominal/Genital

- Test for inguinal and femoral hernias.

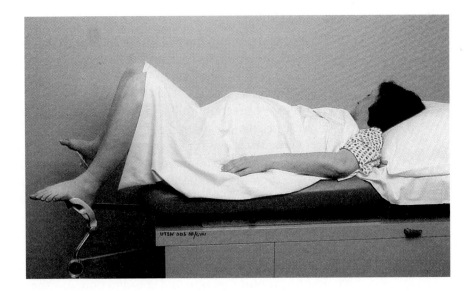

FEMALE PATIENT, LITHOTOMY POSITION

Assist female patients into lithotomy position and drape appropriately. Examiner is seated.

External Genitalia

- Inspect pubic hair, labia, clitoris, urethral opening, vaginal opening, perineal and perianal areas, anus.
- Palpate labia and Bartholin glands; milk Skene glands.

Internal Genitalia

- Perform speculum examination.
  - Inspect vagina and cervix.
  - Collect Pap smear and other necessary specimens.
- Perform bimanual palpation to assess for characteristics of vagina, cervix, uterus, adnexae.
- Perform rectovaginal examination to assess rectovaginal septum, broad ligaments.
- Perform rectal examination.
  - Assess anal sphincter tone and surface characteristics; palpate circumferentially for rectal mass.
  - Obtain rectal culture if needed.
  - Note characteristics of stool when gloved finger is removed.

MALE PATIENT, BENDING FORWARD

Assist male patients in leaning over examining table or into knee-chest position. Examiner is behind patient.

- Inspect sacrococcygeal and perianal areas.
- Perform rectal examination.
  - Palpate sphincter tone and surface characteristics; palpate circumferentially for rectal mass.
  - Obtain rectal culture if needed.
  - Palpate prostate gland and seminal vesicles.
  - Note characteristics of stool when gloved finger is removed.

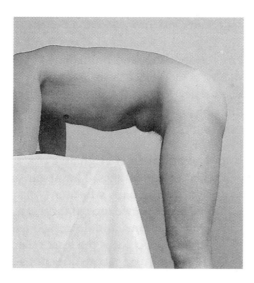

The conclusion of the examination is another point for review and reflection. It gives the patient an opportunity to hear your findings and your interpretations to the extent that you can give them, as well as to ask questions. You must be assured that the patient has a clear understanding of all aspects of the situation (Box 21-8).

BOX 21-8 | **The Stressful Moment**

There are times when what you have learned during the process of taking the history and performing the physical examination leads to a conclusion that will be unpleasant or even disastrous for the patient. Certain principles should guide you when something "bad" must be communicated. These principles apply to patients of all ages, and to the participation of a variety of family members and other persons.

- Arrange a setting that is quiet, as much as possible apart from a noisy ambience.
- If you do not know the patient well, be sure to involve in a direct manner someone who does—and who has the patient's trust—if at all possible.
- Involve family members and others essential to the emotional and practical support of the patient. Consider their base of knowledge, experience, and understanding of the situation.
- Be specific in all details.
- Provide information in a deliberate flow that is adjusted to the needs of the patient, allowing time for questions and for frequent repetition whenever necessary.
- Use jargon-free language adapted to the patient's understanding.
- Inform the patient immediately unless, for example, the sensorium is clouded. A prolonged delay in communicating needed information to which the patient is, after all, entitled does not often help and is most often inappropriate.

If the patient is examined in a hospital bed, remember to put everything back in order when you are finished. Make sure the patient is comfortably settled in an appropriate manner, with side rails up if the clinical condition warrants, and buttons and buzzers within easy reach.

INFANTS

NEWBORNS

The newborn is at greater risk but also has a better potential for health than patients of other ages. The Apgar score, taken at 1 and 5 minutes of age, provides insight to the baby's in utero, intrapartum, and immediate postnatal experience. A low score is evidence of difficulty. A depressed heart rate, respiratory difficulty, loss of muscle tone, and decreased reflex irritability all indicate trouble. Of all these observations, color is the least reliable because most new babies have blue fingers and toes. The Apgar score does not address problems that are suggested by increased irritability, tachypnea, or tachycardia. Nor should it be interpreted as an actual quantitative measure. Still, it is a readily available assessment of combined objective and subjective observations and allows communication from one observer to the next over time.

Because menstrual histories are often inaccurate, more objective means of estimating gestational age are required. The following observations are helpful in determining gestational age. Before 36 weeks, only one or two transverse creases are present on the sole of the foot, the breast nodule is less than 3 mm in diameter, no cartilage is present in the helix of the ear, and the testes are seldom in the scrotum, which has few or no rugae. By 40 weeks, many creases are present on the sole, the breast nodule exceeds 4 mm, cartilage is present in the helix of the ear, and the testes have descended into the scrotum, which is covered with rugae. Increasing muscle tone with a posture of predominantly flexed extremities is another sign of increased maturity.

The premature infant often has brief periods of apnea lasting up to 20 seconds. Respiratory distress is indicated by a sustained increased rate, grunting, retraction of intercostal and subcostal spaces and suprasternal notch, seesaw sinking of the chest with rising abdomen in contrast to the normal synchronous motions, and flaring of the nostrils.

Major congenital anomalies are usually obvious, but there are exceptions. Some life-threatening problems such as diaphragmatic hernia may not be quite readily apparent. When examining a new baby, your index of suspicion must be high and your search for clues must extend into intrauterine life, the mother's immediate perinatal and postnatal experience, and the family history. The difficulty and mode of labor and delivery will have meaning and need exploration. If the mother has fever during or after delivery or if she has herpetic lesions about the mouth or genitalia, the infant may be at risk. Her use of drugs—prescribed, nonprescribed, or illicit—will often have an impact on the baby. Most medications are safe, but some have teratogenic effects. Sedatives and anticonvulsants can have a worrisome impact on the baby's state of consciousness; frequent use of narcotics will cause the baby to go through withdrawal. Problems with earlier pregnancies may be relevant to the newborn's intrauterine life. The fate of siblings may suggest the fate of your present patient.

With a baby, as with patients at every age, it is important to look first. You can learn a lot before touching, without abruptly handling or invading with an instrument. Note the baby's degree of awareness or apathy; the posture and whether unusual flaccidity, tension, or spasticity is present; skin color; and unexpected gross deformities or distortions of facies. The responsive, eager infant with a strong suck is reassuring. Note the presence or absence of spontaneity in the baby's behavior, and always keep track of the interaction between parents and between parent and child. Observing a feeding is most informative, as is simply allowing the baby to demonstrate interest in life by latching onto your gloved finger eagerly and with strength.

When you begin the physical examination, palpate the head and fontanels, then the extremities and abdomen, and finally the rest of the baby. Use a gentle touch that will not obscure unusual findings. Chest percussion is generally of little value because of the relatively small chest, especially in the premature infant, and the examiner's relatively large hands and fingers. However, an abdomen distended from intestinal obstruction may resonate on percussion.

OLDER INFANTS

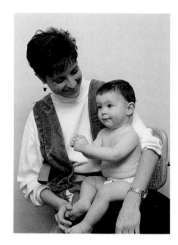

As with adults, there is no "right" sequence to the examination. From time to time, you will vary what you do depending on the age and whether the baby is awake or asleep at the start. You want to have "cooperation" for as long as possible. Again, this may be achieved by observing as much as you can before touching; for example, observe the quality and rate of respiration, flaring of the alae nasi, skin color, even the pulse (visible apical thrust), and defer anything invasive, such as examination of the ears, throat, and eyes, to the end.

Take advantage of opportunities presented throughout the examination. The sleeping infant presents a wonderful chance to auscultate the heart, lungs, and abdomen and to observe the infant's position at rest. The crying infant can be evaluated for lustiness of cry, tactile fremitus, lung excursion, and facial symmetry; the mouth and pharynx can be assessed for integrity of the soft palate and cranial nerves IX, X, and XII. Observe the infant during feeding to evaluate sucking and swallowing coordination, cranial nerve XII, and alertness and responsiveness. A crying infant may keep the eyes tightly shut, but the parent can stand and hold the infant over the shoulder while you stand behind the parent. At this point, the child will often stop crying for a moment and open the eyes. If you are poised with flashlight, you can quickly make some assessment. Similarly, the crying infant—and older children, too—will still need to take a breath, and you can be ready to listen to the heart each time a breath is taken. Over several intervals of breathing, you can hear enough of the heart and lung sounds. Seizing these advantages may mean a change in the sequence of the examination to suit the moment. Similarly, an older infant less than a year of age, given something to hold in each hand, will not always let go quickly. You may have some freedom to examine without tugs at your stethoscope.

PHYSICAL EXAMINATION SEQUENCE

The following is a guideline for the examination sequence of the newborn or young infant. The infant's temperature, weight, length, and head circumference are usually measured first. Weight, length, and head circumference are plotted on a growth curve for the infant's age. Newborns may have the Dubowitz Assessment of Gestational Age done before the examination is ordered (see Chapter 5, Growth and Measurement).

General Inspection

Inspect the undressed supine newborn on a warming table and the older infant preferably on a parent's lap.

- Assess positioning or posture at rest: symmetry and size of extremities, the newborn's assumption of in utero position, flexion of extremities, unusual flaccidity or spasticity, any difference in positioning between upper and lower extremities.
- Note voluntary movement of extremities.
- Inspect skin: color, meconium staining, and vernix in newborn; a cover glass pressed over a suspected telangiectasia will reveal pulsation.
- Note presence of tremors.
- Assess for any apparent anomalies.
- Inspect face: symmetry of features, spacing and position of features (e.g., intracanthal distance, presence of a philtrum).
- Inspect configuration and movement of the chest.
- Inspect shape of the abdomen, movement with respiration.

POSITIONING THE INFANT

When you have finished examining, it is best to place a young infant in a supine position or propped on its side. There is, contrary to long-established custom, a present concern that the prone position is not as safe as was once thought. It is a contributor to sudden infant death syndrome (SIDS).

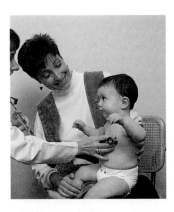

Chest, Lungs, and Heart

- Inspect the following: chest structure, symmetry of expansion with respiration; presence of retractions, heaves, or lifts.
- Note quality of respirations, count the rate.
- Inspect the breasts for nipple and tissue development.
- Palpate the chest and precordium: locate the apical impulse (point of maximal impulse), note any thrills, note tactile fremitus in crying infant.
- Auscultate entire anterior and lateral chest for breath sounds; note any bowel sounds.
- Auscultate each cardiac listening area for S_1 and S_2, splitting, murmurs.
- Count the apical pulse rate.
- Percussion may be necessary at times; not always performed.

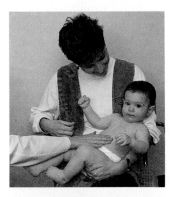

Abdomen

- Inspect shape and configuration: note scaphoid or distended appearance.
- Inspect the umbilicus, count the vessels, note oozing of blood; if the stump has fallen off, inspect the area for lesions, erythema, drainage, foul odor.
- Auscultate each quadrant for bowel sounds.
- Lightly palpate all areas: note size of liver, muscle tone, bladder, spleen tip.
- Palpate more deeply for kidneys, any masses, note any muscle rigidity or tenseness.
- Percuss each quadrant.
- Check skin turgor.
- Palpate the inguinal area for femoral pulses and lymph nodes.

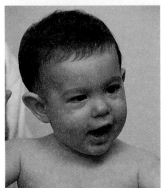

Head and Neck

Inspection and palpation can be done preceding or simultaneously with use of invasive instrument.

- Inspect shape of the head: note molding, swelling, scalp electrode site, hairline.
  - Palpate the head: fontanels, sutures, areas of swelling or asymmetry; measure fontanels in two dimensions.
  - Measure head circumference.
  - Transilluminate newborn's skull.
- Inspect ears.
  - Shape, position and alignment of auricles; patency of auditory canals; pits, sinuses
  - Otoscopic examination
- Inspect eyes: swelling of eyelids and discharge, size, shape, position, epicanthal folds, conjunctivae, pupils.
  - Pupillary response to light
  - Corneal light reflex
  - Red reflex, ophthalmoscopic examination
  - Inspection of eye movement: nystagmus, tracking a light or following a moving picture or face
- Inspect nose: flaring, discharge, size, shape.
  - Inspect nasal mucosa, alignment of septum.
  - Check patency of choanae, observe respiratory effort while alternately occluding each naris; if any doubt about patency, pass a small feeding tube through each naris to the stomach.
- Inspect mouth: lips, gums, hard and soft palates (a very high arched palate may suggest cerebral dysfunction); size of tongue; excessive secretions in the newborn, drooling in the infant; presence of teeth, lesions.

- Palpate mouth: insert gloved small finger into mouth, palpate hard and soft palates with fingerpad, evaluate suck.
  - Stimulate gag reflex.
  - Stroke each side of mouth to evaluate rooting reflex.
- Lift infant's trunk, allowing head to fall back and rest against the table, slightly hyperextended.
  - Inspect and palpate the position of the trachea.
  - Inspect for alignment of head with neck.
  - Inspect for webbing, excess skin folds.
  - Palpate for masses, thyroid, muscle tone.
  - Palpate lymph nodes: anterior and posterior cervical, preauricular, postauricular, submental, sublingual, tonsillar, supraclavicular.
  - Palpate the clavicles for integrity, crepitus.
  - Lift infant and test Moro reflex with a sudden dropping motion.
- Inspect neck with infant again supine.
  - Rotate head to each side for passive range of motion.
  - Observe tonic neck reflex for asymmetry.
  - Observe neck righting reflex in older infants.

Upper Extremities

- Inspect and palpate arms.
- Move arms through range of motion.
- Palpate brachial or radial pulses; compare quality and timing with femoral pulses.
- Open the hands: inspect nails and palmar and phalangeal creases; count fingers.
- Place a finger in infant's palms to evaluate palmar grasp reflex.
- Keeping fingers in infant's hands, pull the infant slowly to sitting position, evaluate grasp and arm strength; evaluate head control.
- Measure blood pressure.

Lower Extremities

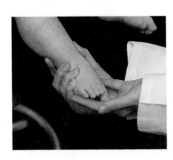

- Inspect the legs and feet for alignment and skin folds.
- Palpate the bones and muscles of each leg.
- Move legs through range of motion; adduct and abduct the hips.
- Palpate the dorsalis pedis pulses.
- Count the toes.
- Elicit the plantar, patellar, and Achilles reflexes.
- Measure blood pressure.

Genitals and Rectum

- Females: inspect external genitalia, noting size of clitoris, any discharge, hymenal opening, any ambiguity of structures.
- Males
  - Inspect placement of urethral opening without fully retracting the foreskin.
  - Inspect scrotum for rugae and presence of contents; note any ambiguity of structures.
  - Palpate scrotum for the testes, presence of hernia or hydrocele.
  - Transilluminate the scrotum when a mass other than testes is noted.
  - Observe voiding for strength of stream.
- Inspect rectum; assess sphincter tone; if newborn has not passed meconium within 24 hours of birth, evaluate rectal patency with a soft catheter.

Neurologic

Hold the infant upright facing you with your hands under the axillae.

- Observe for the sunset sign as the baby's eyes open.
- Perform the doll's eyes maneuver.
- Evaluate general body strength: without gripping the infant's chest, keep your hands under the infant's axillae, and note whether the baby begins to slip through your hands or maintains its position.
- Elicit the stepping reflex.
- Elicit the placing reflex.

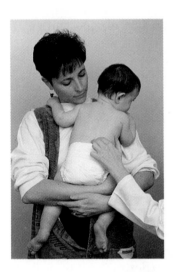

Back

Position the newborn prone on the warming table or have the parent hold the infant upright over the shoulder.

- Inspect spine: observe for alignment, symmetry of muscle development, any masses, tufts of hair, dimples, lesions, defects over lower spine.
- Palpate each spinal process for defect.
- Auscultate posterior chest for breath sounds, any heart sounds.
- Inspect symmetry of gluteal folds.

Behavior

Throughout examination of the newborn, note the alertness, ability to be quieted or consoled, and the response to handling. With the somewhat older infant, too, note the alertness, the responsiveness to the parent, and the ability of the parent to sense the infant's need for consoling and to respond.

- Note the quality of crying, presence of stridor or hoarseness.
- Note the responses to voices or noise: quieting, stopping movement, turning toward sounds.

CHILDREN

Most infants and children will be accompanied by one or more parents or parent surrogates. For children who are small enough, the parent's lap is a splendid examining table. It is helpful when taking the history to keep the child and parent together and to observe the nature of their interaction (Box 21-9). How they feel about each

---

BOX 21-9   Observing Young Children

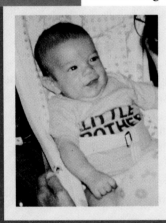

The child's ability at any age to react socially offers clues to physical and emotional well-being. It is possible to elicit responses by exploring with questions; you may also make direct observations. The classic example of a response is the "social smile"—the smile that you know is meant for you—that we learn to expect from infants by the time they are 2 to 3 months old. We can ask parents, and—as we work with the child—we can ask ourselves the following:

- Is that smile there?
- Is the child playful, alert, and responsive?
- Or is there dullness and apparent apathy?
- If the child is fearful, does he or she respond to soothing behavior?
- Does the child move around, show interest in the immediate environment, reach for toys, and ask questions?

These things matter fully as much as temperature, pulse, and respirations. A similar assessment of emotional well-being—with some adaptation to age—is obviously appropriate in the examination of adults.

> ## BOX 21-10   Why Are Children Fearful?
>
> Reasons that children may be fearful include the following:
> - They have experienced medical procedures that hurt.
> - They do not want to be separated from parents or another familiar figure.
> - They have learned that perverse behavior can get a "rise" out of adults.
> - They are abused and have great inner pain and few socially acceptable means of expression.
>
>   When a child is fearful, it is important, as always, to respect the child and parent, explain what is going to happen, and be honest, firm, unapologetic, and gently expeditious. This requires that you achieve a degree of comfort working in the presence of a sharply observant, sometimes tentative, sometimes hostile parent. Do not separate the child from the parent for the sole purpose of improving your personal comfort.

other is conveyed through the parent's touching, soothing, and reassuring gestures and the child's response. Excessive parental indulgence may indicate a smothering relationship. On the other hand, if interaction is minimal and the child does not look to the parent for help, the family dynamics may be devoid of warmth and affection. Take note of the obvious and subtle ways in which children and parents communicate with each other, and record what you learn. Ask the parent to be present when you are performing procedures, for example, venipuncture. Most will accept, and the reaction to your request gives you more information about the family's dynamics and emotional resources.

With the young of any age, you will often take a history and do a physical examination at the same time. These need not be in a rigid sequence, and the complaint and degree of illness can govern your approach to integration. In general, however, you may prefer to start with the history while making overtures to the child to establish some reassuring contact before you actually begin examination. A gentle pat (always with warm hands), a few pleasant words, or playing with the child can often win cooperation. A few relaxed moments—and patience—can break the ice. Children do not necessarily know your routine. You are often a stranger, and the environment may be frightening. Not every child will be smiling and happy about an examination (Box 21-10).

It usually does not pay to rush, and sometimes it pays not to be too persistent. It is always important to be thorough, but rarely is it necessary to be "complete" while doing a physical examination and taking a history. Unless the matter is urgent, defer some of your inquiries and observations to when the child is more relaxed and less afraid of you. It takes time, after all, to develop friendship and to establish trust.

General inspection of the toddler and preschooler may begin in the waiting room or as the child enters the examining room. The temperature, weight, and length are usually taken earlier. Offer toys or paper and pencil to entertain the child, to develop rapport, and to evaluate development, motor, and neurologic status. Use a developmental screening test such as the Denver II (see Chapter 5, Growth and Measurement) to evaluate language, motor coordination, and social skills. Evaluate mental status as the child interacts with you and with the parent.

The following sequence is intended only as a guideline to get you started. Take advantage of opportunities the child presents during the examination to make your observations. You will find that the sequence of examination may vary with each child (Box 21-11).

BOX 21-11 **Some Tips for Examining a Young Child**

Telling the child a story or asking about the child's experience, for example, about school, games, or television, can help to attract attention or, at times, to distract.

- Restraining a child with wrappings and adults looming over the examining table increases the child's apprehension and decreases cooperation. If the child's arms must be restrained and the head kept still to look at the ears, for example, it is usually better to do this on the parent's lap, using the parents' arms for restraint.
- Postpone using the tongue blade until the end of the examination. If the tongue blade must be used, ease the tendency to gag by moistening it first with warm water.
- Allow a young child to "blow out" your flashlight as one way of gaining familiarity with your instruments. Offer your flashlight, otoscope, or stethoscope as a toy (they will not break), or draw a doll's face on a tongue blade. There are times when you might get down on the floor with the child, or use your own lap as an examining table. You will not sacrifice your dignity; anything goes (within bounds of propriety) to get the information you need.
- Enlist the help of the child if he or she is ticklish. Place your hand on top of the child's hand to gently probe the abdomen or the axilla. The diaphragm of your stethoscope can also serve as a probe.
- Take the opportunity to hold and feed a young baby. This increases your understanding and helps establish rapport.
- If the child is uncomfortable or uncooperative, be patient. You can stop and come back at a later time when calm is restored to complete the examination.
- Use specific, polite directions rather than asking the child's permission at each step in the examination. It is better to say, "Please open your mouth" rather than "Do you want to open your mouth?" After all, what next if the answer is "no"?

CHILD PLAYING

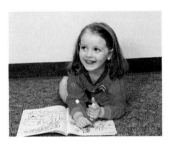

The child playing on the floor offers an opportunity to evaluate both the musculoskeletal and neurologic systems while developing a rapport with the child.
- Observe the child's spontaneous activities.
- Ask the child to demonstrate some skills: throwing a ball, building block towers, drawing geometric figures, coloring.
- Evaluate gait, jumping, hopping, range of motion.
- Muscle strength: observe the child climbing on the parent's lap, stooping, and recovering.

CHILD ON PARENT'S LAP

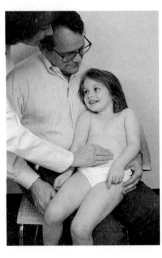

Performing the examination on the parent's lap usually enhances the child's participation. Begin with the child sitting and undressed except for the diaper or underpants.

Upper Extremities
- Inspect arms for movement, size, shape; observe use of the hands; inspect hands for number and configuration of fingers, palmar creases.
- Palpate radial pulses.
- Elicit biceps and triceps reflexes when child cooperates.
- Take blood pressure at this point or later, depending on child's attitude.

Lower Extremities
Child may stand for much or part of the examination.
- Inspect legs for movement, size, shape, alignment, lesions.
- Inspect feet for alignment, longitudinal arch, number of toes.
- Palpate dorsalis pedis pulse.
- Elicit plantar reflex and, if cooperative, the Achilles and patellar reflexes.

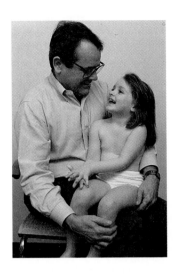

Head and Neck

- Inspect head.
  - Inspect shape, alignment with neck, hairline, position of auricles.
  - Palpate anterior fontanel for size; head for sutures, depressions; hair for texture.
- Measure head circumference.
- Inspect neck for webbing, voluntary movement.
- Palpate neck: position of trachea, thyroid, muscle tone, lymph nodes.

Chest, Heart, and Lungs

- Inspect the chest for respiratory movement, size, shape, precordial movement, deformity, nipple and breast development.
- Palpate the anterior chest, locate the point of maximal impulse, note tactile fremitus in the talking or crying child.
- Auscultate the anterior, lateral, and posterior chest for breath sounds; count respirations.
- Auscultate all cardiac listening areas for S_1 and S_2, splitting, and murmurs; count apical pulse.

CHILD RELATIVELY SUPINE, STILL ON LAP, DIAPER LOOSENED

- Inspect abdomen.
  - Auscultate for bowel sounds.
  - Palpate: identify size of the liver and any other palpable organs or masses.
  - Percuss.
- Palpate the femoral pulses, compare to radial pulses.
- Palpate for lymph nodes.
- Inspect the external genitalia.
- Males: palpate scrotum for descent of testes and other masses.

CHILD STANDING

- Inspect spinal alignment as the child bends slowly forward to touch toes.
- Observe posture from anterior, posterior, and lateral views.
- Observe gait.

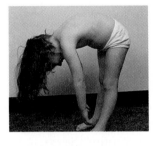

CHILD RETURNS TO PARENT'S LAP

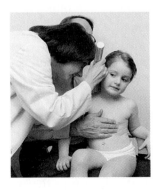

Only as a last resort should you restrain the child for the funduscopic, otoscopic, and oral examinations. Lessen the fear of this aspect of the examination by permitting the child to handle the instruments, blow out the light, or use them on a doll or the parent. Attempt to gain the child's cooperation, even if it takes more time. It will be worth the effort because future visits will be more pleasant for the child and for you. After finishing these preliminary maneuvers, perform the following:

- Inspect eyes: pupillary light reflex, red reflex, extraocular movements, funduscopic examination.
- Perform otoscopic examination.
- Inspect nasal mucosa.
- Inspect mouth and pharynx.

By the time the child is school age, it is usually possible to use an examination sequence very similar to that for adults.

PREGNANT WOMEN

The process of physical examination is the same for the pregnant woman as for the adult, with the addition of more extensive abdominal and pelvic evaluation for pregnancy status and fetal well-being. Late in pregnancy the woman may find it difficult to assume the supine position without experiencing hypotension. Therefore have her assume this position only when necessary, and provide alternative positioning by elevating the backrest or by supplying pillows for the woman to assume the side-lying position. The abdominal assessment is both more comfortable for the woman and more accurate if the bladder is empty. Remember that during pregnancy, urinary urgency and frequency are common.

OLDER ADULTS

The process of physical examination is the same for older adults as it is for younger adults. However, special considerations may be necessary. Many older patients have difficulty assuming some of the positions, particularly the lithotomy and knee-chest positions. Sometimes all that is needed is a little extra assistance and patience on your part, but otherwise you may need to use alternate positioning (see Chapter 16, Female Genitalia). The quality of clinical data is not necessarily compromised by having the patient lie on the side rather than assume a knee-chest position, for example. Your skill, thoroughness, and willingness to take whatever time is necessary are far more important in yielding accurate clinical data.

Time is a central issue in examining older patients. Time may be needed to develop the patient's trust and subsequent cooperation and to allow for any apparent degree of frailty. A hurried pace or an impatient manner can create tension that may fluster or confuse an older patient. In neurologic testing, reaction time may be longer or may require more intense stimuli.

FUNCTIONAL ASSESSMENT

Functional assessment (see p. 34) is an important part of examining the older adult (Box 21-12). Initial observation and interaction can provide a wealth of information about the individual's independent functional capacity. Watch how the patient walks, and observe the ability to follow instructions, remove clothes, and maneuver to the examining table. In doing this, you will obtain information related to mobility, balance, fine motor skills (for example, unbuttoning clothes), and range of motion (Box 21-13). In addition, you may gather some clues about perceptual abilities and mental status. Many older adults have a variety of diseases, conditions, or disorders that would seem to indicate "poor health" (Box 21-14). Yet, physical health is only one dimension of the picture, and, for many, the bottom line is not what is "wrong" with their bodies but what they are able to do and how well they are able to function.

In reality, functional assessment is simply an attempt to determine the extent to which patients can deal with the daily demands of life, that is, how well they function. This was stressed earlier (see Chapter 1, The History and Interviewing Process, p. 34) when we advised that such an assessment should be a part of every older adult's history, with attention given to self-care activities and instrumental activities such as ability to drive a car, use public transportation, and even dial a telephone.

Indeed, you will always be making this type of assessment on each patient, regardless of age. After all, an infant must be able to suck; a 6-year-old child, able to adapt to a classroom and find the way home from school; an adolescent, able to come to grips with the essentials of life in determining a sense of self and of his or her future. Thus a functional assessment underlies every history, and the judgment about each individual's ability to cope with the demands and stresses of life is an essential part of your conclusions. A functional understanding will ultimately help shape your management plans, guide the level of instruction you can provide the patient, and determine the expectation you might have about the potential fulfillment of patient needs.

| BOX 21-12 | **Geriatric Assessment** |

Geriatric assessment is a comprehensive evaluation of a frail, older person who is not succeeding in the community environment. It includes the following:
- Comprehensive history and physical examination
- Assessment of social situation

The history should include the following:
- Detailed listing of medications, for example, nonprescription drugs, especially hypnotics, sedatives, and laxatives. Try the "brown bag approach," asking the patient to bring all medications, prescribed and nonprescribed.
- Extensive review of function, including gait and activities of daily living (ADLs) and evaluation of degree of independence versus need for caretaker assistance
  - Basic ADLs: bathing, dressing, toileting, ambulation, feeding
  - Instrumental ADLs: housekeeping, grocery shopping, meal preparation, medication compliance, communication skills, money management
  - Use of assistive devices for ambulation and function: cane, walker, commode chair, hospital bed
- Systems review, particularly common geriatric problems
  - Nutritional status, evidence of malnutrition
  - Urinary incontinence
  - Early dementia
  - Depression
  - Medication-induced delirium
  - Falls, gait and balance disorders that result in fear of falling
  - Skin breakdown: decubitus ulcers
- Social situation
  - Identification of caretakers and probable caretakers, including those who maintain the home environment
  - Assessment of caretaker abilities
  - Assessment of financial resources and health insurance, with particular reference to long-term services not ordinarily covered: personal grooming, home care, medication supervision
  - Frank and open discussion of patient's wishes regarding advanced life support in the event of an irreversible condition and/or cognitive impairment, the "advance directives" in this regard (necessarily written), and the need for a Durable Power of Attorney for Health Care (the formal investment of decision-making authority for health care in a family member or other trusted person)

The physical examination should include mental status evaluation with particular attention to the following:
- Cognition
- Memory
- Mood

All of this takes time and sensitive conversation. It cannot usually be accomplished in one visit or by one person. Multiple approaches include traditional nursing and medical processes, social and dietary interventions, and rehabilitation. Nurses, physicians, social workers, and physical and occupational therapists, among others, may contribute. The evaluation is complex, but it is possible to achieve it in several brief visits.

Dr. Michele F. Bellantoni of the Gerontology Research Center, Baltimore, Md, gave considerable advice regarding geriatric assessment.

BOX 21-13 | **Examining Persons with Disabilities**

You may need to vary some aspects of the physical examination for persons with disabilities. Each disability affects each person differently. Therefore it is important for you to educate yourself about relevant facets of your patient's disability. What body system(s) is affected? What is the degree of impairment? What assistance does the patient require? What is the patient able to do without assistance? What is the communication system used by a hearing- or speech-impaired patient (e.g., sign language interpreter, word board, or talk box)? When speaking with a disabled patient, remember to speak directly to the patient. Often clinicians will inappropriately address a disabled person's friend, an attendant, or an interpreter instead of speaking directly to the patient.

Consider some variations that may facilitate the physical examination. It may not be necessary for the patient to undress fully, thereby conserving time and energy. Removing or rearranging the furnishings in an examination room will provide the space needed to maneuver a wheelchair. Some patient positions can be varied without compromising the quality of the examination (see, for example, Performing the Pelvic Examination in Chapter 16). Some patients may require only additional time and assistance in getting positioned or performing maneuvers. Some older patients, for example, may experience limitation in joint range of motion (see, for example, Examining the Musculoskeletal System in Chapter 19). Gentleness and patience are the hallmarks of a caring and sensitive examiner.

BOX 21-14 | **Factors that Influence the Perception of Persistent Symptoms**

Innumerable subjective modifications may convert disease into illness or cause illness without disease.
- Recent termination of a significant relationship because of death, divorce, or other less obvious intrusions (e.g., moving to a new city)
- Physical or emotional illness or disability in family members or other significant individuals
- Unharmonious spousal or family relationships
- School problems and stresses
- Poor self-image
- Drug and alcohol misuse
- Poor understanding of the "facts" of a physical problem
- Peer pressures: trying to keep up with the Joneses or with schoolmates
- Secondary gains from the complaints of symptoms (e.g., indulgent family response to complaints, providing extra comforts, gifts; solicitous attention from others; distraction from other intimidating problems)

At any age, circumstances such as these can modify perception and contribute to the intensity and persistence of symptoms or, quite the opposite, the denial of an insistent, objective complaint. Sometimes, as a result, the patient will be led to seek help and, at other times, to avoid it.

Adapted from Green, Stuy, 1992.

ALLIANCE AND COMPLIANCE

You cannot assume that patients will behave predictably or that they will invariably respond to your suggestions and instructions. We define adherence to our instructions as compliance. There is arrogance in the inference that when we order, the patient must respond. Still, compliance is one measure of your alliance with patients. The controlling factors include the nature of the relationship you have developed, your recognition of the patient's autonomy, your success in communicating the basics of the patient's condition, and the clarity of your instructions. Equally important factors are the patient's ability to understand the problem and the value the patient places on resolving the problem. For example, your primary concern may be a patient's hypertension,

---

BOX 21-15 | The Patient Who Is Dying

As with all patients, those who are dying, whatever their age, need your respect and attention. When we are face to face with death, we often cope by attempting to avoid it. We tend not to visit with the patient who is dying as often as with the patient we know will live. We are too often reluctant to confront the fact of dying, perhaps because of our personal fears or because we subconsciously feel we have failed in our healing role. If you learn to understand your own feelings about death, you will be better equipped to care for the dying.

Learn to accept that dying patients need you as much as other patients. Talk with them, share with them. Never hesitate to participate in chit-chat. But become comfortable with being quiet and filling the silent spaces with the touch of a hand.

Above all, do not back away from dying patients. This avoidance behavior denies them an assumptive world, the world for which they had hoped and may not have. We usually lack the wisdom to know precisely when that world will be truly denied, and backing away is a sign that hope is lost. Your attention and honest discussion offer hope without denial.

BOX 21-16 | Compassion for Those Who Are Grieving

When one of our patients dies, those who were close, family, friends or significant others, need our attention during the time they are grieving, not only in the immediate aftermath of death but also later on. Obviously, it is difficult to find words, and often the words we find may be clichés that do not seem quite appropriate for the moment. It isn't a good idea to tell people to be strong when they are really feeling utterly empty. It is all right to tell them that it is good to cry and to share feelings, and that it is permissible to talk about what has been lost and what will not be realized for the future. It is not a good idea to assure someone that time will take care of things. Your appreciation that the present moments are long and sometimes unendurable is needed. If time does heal, that may ultimately be found out. In the settings in which so many of us work, we may find ourselves minimizing a misfortune by comparing with the apparent or obvious misfortune of others. We should not allow ourselves to make such a judgment about another person's pain and loss. And, it is better not to invoke God as a being who decided that this might have been best—"It was God's will." In a moment of acute human suffering, we cannot allow our interpretations of God to be imposed on others. Theirs should prevail. In sum, we should be there. If we don't have words that seem right, our simple presence may be enough. Our words should not define someone else's feelings. We should give "permission" for the fact that it is alright to feel bad, to say so, and to share those feelings.

---

whereas the patient's main worry may be an alcoholic spouse. There are also times when a patient's refusal to comply may be appropriate. Always ask that the patient repeat the instructions to you so you can be sure he or she understands. This can also help you discover whether there may be a problem with compliance.

Obviously most interactions with patients are unique, and you must be adaptable and flexible—particularly when your first efforts may be halting. It's not always easy! You will at times be sorely tried, particularly when you are worried, rushed, and tired. If you are to be successful, you must also understand the biases you might bring to each interaction with the patient and learn how to constrain them. Because you are human, you may respond differently to people who will live and to those who are dying (Box 21-15), to children and the aged, to men and women, to blacks and whites, to rich and poor. Important also are your interactions with family members who may be suffering emotionally (Box 21-16). You must know why and how (see Chapter 2, Cultural Awareness).

Finally, you must be disciplined enough to pursue complete information, even when the solution seems obvious—because sometimes the obvious is wrong—and courageous enough to make the decision for urgency when the data are incomplete (Box 21-17).

BOX 21-17	**Assessment of the Student's Performance**

Every student's effort with patients should be observed many times by a qualified instructor. Certain behaviors will help to characterize your performance:

- At the start of the interview, did you do the following?
  - Say "hello," and greet the patient appropriately
  - Introduce yourself
  - Give appropriate attention to everyone's comfort
  - Eliminate noise and other distractions when possible
  - Outline the purposes of the interview and assess the patient's understanding
  - Begin with a comfortable, open-ended question, such as, "How can I be of help?"
- During the interview, did you do the following?
  - Encourage and facilitate further response, for example, with a head nod
  - Follow responses to open-ended questions with appropriate specific questions
  - Consistently seek clarification when a response was in some way unclear
  - Direct the course of the interview gently
  - Ask one question at a time
  - Occasionally restate what you heard to check accuracy and to ensure that you are paying attention
  - Make smooth transitions
- At the close of the interview, did you do the following?
  - Summarize and recheck for accuracy
  - Ask if there were any other questions or concerns
  - Appropriately indicate next steps
  - Say "thank you" with appreciation and with an appropriate "good-bye"
- Throughout the interview, did you do the following?
  - Maintain appropriate eye contact
  - Maintain a comfortable posture, invoking body language that shows attentiveness to the patient
  - Use appropriate silence, allowing enough time for the patient's comments, expressions, thoughts, and feelings
  - Avoid swallowing the answer to one question with the next question
  - Empathize when appropriate
  - Restate your willingness to help when appropriate
  - Confirm that you and the patient are allies, working together to find appropriate outcomes
- Did the patient do the following?
  - Appear comfortable, relaxed, and engaged, freely giving responses and discussing concerns
  - Convey a sense of understanding of your remarks

Adapted from Brown Evaluation Instrument

Serving the whole patient—the physical, emotional, and social needs—is not an easy task, but you can succeed if you follow a disciplined course and learn how to be flexible within that course, guided by it, but not imprisoned by it. You are at the point of organizing the information you have assembled into a usable whole, ready for providing care, caring, and problem solving.

More information at *Mosby* *http://www1.mosby.com/physexam_seidel*

CHAPTER 22

TAKING THE NEXT STEPS: CRITICAL THINKING

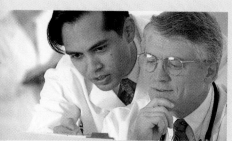

THE CLINICAL EXAMINATION

Thus far, we have been concerned with the initial interaction with the patient, the establishment of respectful rapport, and the processes by which we gather information about the patient, history, and physical examination. These together form the *clinical examination,* a necessary starting point. We then organize information, integrate it, and prepare it for the next steps. This process, which might be called "critical thinking," leads to diagnoses, the setting of priorities, and the institution of management plans (Figure 22-1). In this, we are partners with the patient all of the way.

CRITICAL THINKING

ASSESSMENT/
JUDGMENT

The first step in critical thinking is to assess what we have learned, determining its value and significance. Then priorities are assigned as to the extent to which a particular bit of information might have an impact on our diagnostic effort and on the management plans we formulate with the patient. All this requires *clinical judgment.* We form *clinical opinions.*

Further assessment depends on our preferences and those of the patient, preferences influenced by feelings, attitudes, and values. Discussion with the patient should result in mutually agreed upon decisions regarding probabilities and risks. Our clinical opinions, then, are the first step as the preferences help direct further assessment, balancing advantage and risk to the patient, increasing cost and the use of limited resources. Given this and our diagnoses based on clinical opinion, a potential management plan for the immediate and ongoing care of the patient can be formulated with the full participation of the patient.

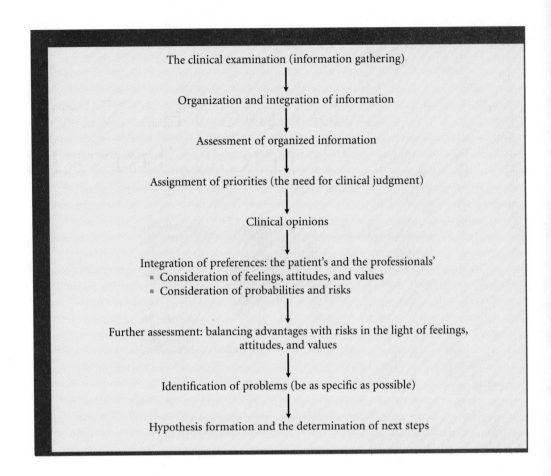

FIGURE 22-1
Steps for critical thinking.

PROBLEM IDENTIFICATION

Once both the subjective and objective information have been organized, review all findings, the expected and unexpected. Identify areas of concern for you and the patient. Frequently, the physical examination is all that is necessary to confirm problems identified during the interview.

A problem may be defined as anything that will need further evaluation and/or attention. It may be related to one or more of the following:

- An uncertain diagnosis
- New findings related to a previous diagnosis
- New findings of unknown cause
- Unusual findings revealed in the clinical examination or by laboratory tests
- Personal or social difficulties

Try to formulate problems as specifically as possible. It helps to identify and list the signs and symptoms associated with the patient's complaint. Aggregate all information, objective and subjective, related to the same body system or regions to help identify the domain of the disorder. This necessary listing of the findings, expected and unexpected, for each body system or region is a key to a clear and complete picture of a problem.

Once a particular body system or region is identified, relate the signs and symptoms to a pathologic, physical, emotional, or social process. Form hypotheses that evolve from your knowledge and experience of the full range of possible health problems, illnesses, and injuries (Box 22-1). Note the *absence* of findings that indicate health or well-being or that you might expect in support of your hypotheses. After all,

---

BOX 22-1 | **Decision Making**

There are several ways to make a diagnosis; among them are the following:

- *Recognizing patterns* (on the assumption that if he looks like Elvis, he must be Elvis)
- *Sampling the universe* (on the assumption that including everything precludes missing anything)
- Using *algorithms* (on the assumption that a rigidly defined thought process precludes error)

Although each of these may have limited use in specific situations, the broad consideration of all your findings should most often result in the development of one or more *hypotheses* needing a disciplined approach to solutions.

Guidelines to a sound decision-making process include the following:

- Always derive possibilities that are consistent with the chief complaint and your database, and with known psychosocial and pathophysiologic mechanisms.
- Remember that common problems occur commonly, and rare ones do not.
- Remember that common problems can have unusual presentations and rare ones may have a seemingly common complaint.
- But remember, too, that a rarity that has a necessary treatment available should be considered, lest harm come to a patient.
- Don't rush to a diagnosis with no available treatment, and don't pursue a line of reasoning that will not alter your course of action.
- Don't undertake procedures that are not reasonably related to your hypotheses.
- Always consider harm and cost as well as benefit when judging the need for a test or action. Consider whether the risk is worth the possible gain in information, invoking the ethical principle of nonmaleficence: do no harm.
- Recognize that your favorite hypotheses may not be valid. Remain open in your thinking and be ready to discard or modify your hypotheses when necessary; avoid the tendency to discount information that may invalidate your favorite thoughts.
- Try to have a single process explain all or most of your data, but don't be slavish in this regard. After all, a patient with many complaints and problems may have more than one disease; the chance of two common diseases occurring simultaneously is greater than the chance of one rare disease occurring.

Probability and *utility* should always be your guides to sequencing your actions unless a life-threatening situation exists. A conscientious estimate of probability is the best way to define the limits of uncertainty and utility, and the best way to establish priorities.

---

there may be no problem to be defined. Review and analyze all of your information. Reconsider the reason the patient sought care. Carefully think through the patient's nonverbal communication, attempting to determine whether there are any questions you may have neglected to ask or information you did not fully understand. When possible, seek additional information from the patient to fill in these gaps. Do not let unusual findings distort the full consideration of all you have learned.

Once a close match between the data (both subjective and objective) and a presumed diagnosis has been made, consider the laboratory tests needed to confirm the presumed diagnosis. Laboratory tests or consultation will frequently be needed for further evaluation before establishing the diagnosis. All of us need help more often than not.

VALID HYPOTHESES

Critical thinking allows you to consider and discard the variety of possible diagnoses from the common to the rare before settling on the best match between the patient's signs and symptoms and a specific disorder. As you gain experience, you will more confidently collect, analyze, evaluate, and synthesize information, relating it to the chief complaint or your initial impression of the problem. Be cautious about doing this too quickly. Do not let your first thoughts narrow the focus of your questions during the interview. In other words, do not jump to conclusions.

In the end, positive outcomes rely on the quality of your decisions, the soundness of your hypotheses, the actions they suggest, and the way in which those actions are implemented. One of your most important contributions is your ever present sensitivity. As you look for the hidden clue to a problem, stay attuned to the nuances, the slightest of variations in even the more easily recognized signs and symptoms. These may have important implications that are not at first obvious. Clinical acumen develops with that sensitivity to the meaning of events and from your ability to intermingle the precise and the probable.

One of the clichés of clinical practice is that all findings should be unified into one diagnosis. This is not always true. More than one disease process can exist in the same person, an acute illness can be imposed on a chronic one, and a chronic disease can cycle through remission and relapse endlessly. You must be sure that all of the information is logically explained by your ultimate conclusions. The laboratory and consultation can often help to validate your observations and confirm your clinical opinions.

POSSIBLE BARRIERS TO CRITICAL THINKING

Illness evolves from disease (see p. 41) and is almost always a multifaceted invasion of life. You may not be able to explain all your findings on a pathophysiologic level because the physical is inseparable from the emotional. Therefore you must not be misled into believing that, given a pathophysiologic conclusion, appropriate management will necessarily solve a problem. You must consider the full range of elements that might affect the patient's problems, from the physical to the emotional, social, and economic.

Uncritical attention to the details presented in this book may trap you into losing sight of the forest because of the trees. Actually, there is order in what may with our limited knowledge seem at times disorderly. The danger is that we may too often be lost in detail and lose the context of a broader view whether it applies to the turbulence of the flow of blood through the heart or to the expression of feelings, attitudes, and values.

Feelings, Attitudes, and Values

Complexity is intensified by emotions in both patient and provider. Feelings, attitudes and values are shared, sometimes explicitly, often implicitly. They may be so strong that our opinions may be impaired or distorted by the content of those feelings and by a consequent fear, uncertainty, anxiety, and/or resentment. If these feelings are to be given a proper context, we must know and understand ourselves. Self-analysis is a requisite for the health professional. The questioning must be relentless: "What is really happening?" "Have feelings overtaken logic?" "Have ethical concepts been ignored?" "What are the issues that matter?" "What should take precedence?" "Do I understand my contribution to the interaction?" "Do I understand the patient?"

Mechanism and Probabilism

Mechanistic (deterministic) thinking is governed by a sense that knowledge must be certain, and that it is not subject to any of the attributes of the observer (who must be detached). Knowledge is to be free of belief, attitudes, and values. There is no room for the probable, that which is likely but uncertain. And, of course, that is not so. There must be a balance between mechanism and probabilism in our decision making despite the difficulty in controlling all of the variables when we are at the patient's side. Also, we introduce variables to the decision-making process fully as much as the patient. These include, among others, our age, extent of our experience, occasional fatigue, and our worry about malpractice litigation. We are not in an isolated system uninfluenced by what we bring to it and what the patient brings to it; uncertainty in large part stems from that (see Chapter 21, Putting It All Together). Accepting the inevitability of probability does not mean skepticism. It simply recognizes that the certainty of truth, whatever that may be, is hard to achieve. Why?:

- Causes may act or interact differently at different times.
- The same effect may not always have the same cause.
- The effect of a given cause cannot be isolated with certainty.

Causes, effects, and our interpretations of them change probabilistically with time. They involve uncertainty, conjecture, and chance. Dependence on the purely "scientific" and the "technical" offers an unrealistic comfort; certainty can often be more apparent than real (Box 22-2).

Acknowledging uncertainty and accepting probabilistic critical thinking may be viewed as gambling. True, but it is gambling with the justification (?faith) that there is order in the world and that our effort to validate what we do is constant. That puts limits on uncertainty, and probability can be quantified. A high probability diminishes uncertainty; a low probability does not.

We cannot be dominated by the mechanistic assumption that there is a precise and discoverable cause for every event. That can be a trap leading to excessive invasion of the patient. Making judgments on the basis of well-informed probabilities recognizes the complexity and saves the patient and ourselves pain and cost, both physical and emotional. Comfort with uncertainty and complexity permits considered judgment of the information gleaned from the clinical examination.

BOX 22-2   **The Computer: A Reprise**

The computer is a remarkable resource. It is helpful in recording and providing of information. It can remind us about possibilities in diagnosis that we may not have considered and can place at our fingertips, if we have entered it all correctly, the information we have about the patient. Still, it poses a threat. There is an unacceptable temptation to substitute the computer at times for critical thinking. The computer has no sense of the subtleties of the human dimension. It poses a serious threat to confidentiality; it must be used with discretion. Confidentiality can be breached not only by random, inadvertent accidental intrusion by any of many users, but also by purposeful invasion. Although it is our responsibility to provide information appropriately and with the knowledge of the patient, we must remain the guardian of what after all belongs to the patient.

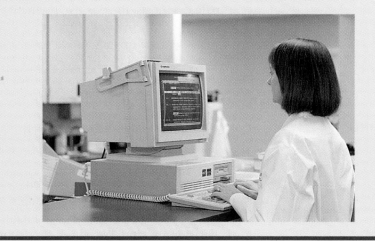

Thus, critical thinking does not require a compulsive listing of all of the possible options directed toward diagnosis and management. Rather, it is dominated by hypothesis formation, asking whether a particular diagnosis should be made at all depending on its probability, or whether a test or other technical modality may be indicated, depending at least in part on the probability suggested by its sensitivity and specificity.

VALIDITY OF THE CLINICAL EXAMINATION

We are in a time when there is considerable effort to reduce the cost of health care. If we recognize that the great majority of diagnoses can be achieved with the information gleaned from a competent clinical examination, we can limit the indiscriminate use of expensive technology. This requires some assurance of the reliability of our observations so that, with demonstrated greater sensitivity and specificity, we can relieve potential uncertainty. Unfortunately, there is not yet a mass of information that allows widespread quantification of the information learned on clinical examination. Laboratory tests are easier to evaluate in this way. Nevertheless, with accumulating experience, we can learn more of the sensitivity and specificity of our findings and begin to assign such values. Some observations are so reliable that we must be compulsive in ensuring that we do not miss them. Such an effort provides a discipline that might lend itself to the reporting of accumulated experience in the future so that we can share experience with others.

Keep the following definitions in mind:
- *Sensitivity:* the ability of an observation to identify correctly those who have a disease
- *Specificity:* the ability of an observation to identify correctly those who do not have the disease
- *True positive:* an expected observation that is found when the disease characterized by that observation is present
- *True negative:* an expected observation that is not found when the disease characterized by that observation is not present
- *False positive:* an observation made that suggests a disease when that disease is not present
- *False negative:* a disease is present, the observation is there to be made, and it is not appreciated
- *Positive predictive value:* the proportion of persons with an observation characteristic of a disease who have it (i.e., when an observation is made 100 times and 95 of those times that observation proves to be consistent with the ultimate diagnosis, the positive predictive value of the observation is 95%)
- *Negative predictive value:* the proportion of persons with an expected observation who ultimately prove not to have the expected condition (i.e., if 100 observations are made expecting a disease, and 95 times that observation is not found and the condition proves not to have been the diagnosis, the negative predictive value of the observation is 95%)

BAYES' FORMULA

As a critical thinker, you will discover that the likelihood of your diagnosis being related to your findings depends on the probability of those findings being associated with that diagnosis, and the prevalence of both that particular diagnosis and that combination of findings in the community you are serving. Patterns prevail. It is not common that just one observation ensures a diagnosis. These considerations have been formalized as *Bayes' formula*. This juggling of probabilities is implicit during diagnostic decision making. We do not think consciously of Bayes' formula most of the time, but we are at some level using it all of the time.

We have stressed that diagnostic decision making is generally best served by the development of hypotheses that will provide a disciplined approach to solutions. If you are uncertain about an observation, never hesitate to recheck its validity. That is vital to critical thinking. To limit uncertainty, the ratio of fact to conjecture must be positive, and it must be achieved within the emotional and social context of your patient. Quite obviously, much as we strive to be "scientific," basing what we do on the disciplined principles of science, at times we will make undeniable intuitive judgments. Intuition, however, must be as fully subject to critical thinking as is any other aspect of our effort.

THE MANAGEMENT PLAN/SETTING PRIORITIES

We decide what we think is going on (the diagnosis) and what we are going to do about it (the management plan). We often need to investigate further, deciding on which of the available laboratory and imaging techniques we might use and who might help us with it. Having thought critically and always with the patient, we can arrive at a jointly considered approach that may include some of the following:

■ Laboratory studies to be obtained
■ Consultation requested
■ Medications or appliances prescribed
■ Special care to be provided (e.g., nursing, physical therapy, respiratory therapy)
■ Surgery
■ Diet modification
■ Activity modification
■ Follow-up visit schedule
■ Patient education needs

In addition, we need to decide the degree of urgency of each of these items and what it is that underlies the issues in terms of the social, economic, and pathophysiologic considerations. Priorities must be set. There is much to think about. The following is only a partial guide:

■ What is the patient's physical condition?
  • Is something going on that overrides every other consideration, for example, a problem with the central nervous system, the heart, the kidneys, a degree of pain, a distressing change in mental status?
  • Are there abnormal laboratory values that need immediate attention?
■ What is the patient's social circumstance?
  • Will a job be threatened if there is prolonged absence from work?
  • Are there small children at home for whom no other caretaker is available?
  • Is there available and convenient transportation to and from services and care?
■ What is the patient's economic circumstance?
  • Is there adequate insurance coverage?
  • Is the cost of care going to compromise other areas of the patient's life?

These are but a few of the considerations. They suggest the kind of critical thinking that must address the setting of priorities and the development of a management plan, which may be modified to meet a particular circumstance. Perhaps, without risk, there can be delay in tests, in treatments, in therapies; perhaps there might be a sequence of steps that meets priority needs, some needing to be done now, some that might await the information gleaned from an earlier step or the result of a first therapeutic attempt.

The entire process must be recorded, thoughtfully and completely (see Chapter 24, Recording Information).

Remember to check   *http://www1.mosby.com/physexam_seidel*

CHAPTER 23

EMERGENCY OR LIFE-THREATENING SITUATIONS

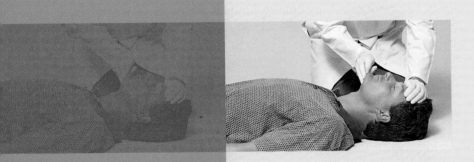

An emergency situation, whether unresponsiveness, an acute medical condition, drug intoxication, or trauma, demands alterations in the usual sequence of history taking and examination. Life-threatening conditions must be rapidly identified and managed (Table 23-1). The steps to achieve this should take seconds, not minutes. Patients are assessed and treatment priorities established based on the physiologic condition and the stability of vital signs, rather than on a specific diagnosis. A logical, sequential priority system must be implemented to provide an overall assessment of the patient. The Committee on Trauma of the American College of Surgeons and, in particular, its Subcommittee on Advanced Trauma Life Support have defined an approach for treating trauma patients that is applicable in other emergency situations. It is presented here in modified form as follows.

The patient's vital functions must be determined quickly and efficiently through a rapid *primary assessment* with resuscitation of vital functions as necessary, followed by a more detailed *secondary assessment*. Finally, the initiation of *definitive care* is begun. A primary survey involves a rapid assessment of the patient's physiologic status performed in a sequence known as the ABCs.

THE ABCs OF PRIMARY ASSESSMENT

During the *primary assessment*, life-threatening conditions are identified, and simultaneous management is begun:

A: Airway maintenance with cervical spine (C-spine) control is performed.
B: Breathing (ventilatory ability) is assessed.
C: Circulation is assessed and hemorrhage controlled.

TABLE 23-1 Signs and Symptoms of Certain Life-Threatening Conditions

	Definition	Causes	Signs and Symptoms
Upper airway obstruction	Compromise of airway space, resulting in impaired respiratory exchange	Foreign body Infection (e.g., epiglottitis) Tumor (e.g., goiter) Trauma Smoke inhalation Aspiration of chemicals (e.g., hydrocarbons)	Patient grasps neck Fatigue Severe dyspnea Tachypnea Stridor Hoarseness Dysphagia Sore throat Drooling Extreme anxiety Tripod positioning

Hypovolemic shock	Loss of fluid from intravascular space, resulting in inadequate tissue perfusion	Gastrointestinal bleeding
		Hemorrhage (trauma)
		Dehydration
		  Gastrointestinal fluid loss
		  Renal fluid loss
		  Cutaneous fluid loss (burns, perspiration)
		Internal fluid loss
		Ascites
			Anxiety
			Pallor
			Diaphoresis
			Oliguria
			Coma (alteration in mental status)
			Circulatory collapse
			Tachycardia
			Hypotension
			Delayed capillary refill

Hypoxemia	Severely reduced blood oxygen levels in major organs resulting from respiratory distress, poor tissue perfusion, ventilatory failure, or severe lung injury with increased permeability of alveoli	Aspiration
		Trauma (CNS)
		Increased intracranial pressure
		Drug overdose
		Disseminated intravascular coagulation
		Infection
		Toxins
		  Oxygen
		  Smoke
		  Volatile chemicals
		Shock
		Severe trauma
		Inadequate ventilation
		Upper airway obstruction
		Lower airway obstruction
		  Asthma
		  Chronic infection
		  Emphysema
		  Cystic fibrosis
			Severe dyspnea
			Cyanosis (pallor, mottling)
			Altered mental status (lethargy to coma; anxiety, combativeness may precede lethargy)
			Tachypnea
			Tachycardia

Status epilepticus	Seizures of any type that are protracted and recurrent without recovery of consciousness	Associated with a variety of epilepsies of uncertain cause: Convulsive types of every variety, generalized or partial Nonconvulsive types of every variety, petit mal or absence, psychomotor, or complex partial	Obvious convulsive movements with unresponsiveness when prolonged as much as 60 minutes Hypotension Cardiac dysrhythmias Fever

Continued

TABLE 23-1   Signs and Symptoms of Certain Life-Threatening Conditions—cont'd

	Definition	Causes	Signs and Symptoms
Status asthmaticus	A severe and prolonged asthma attack resisting usual therapeutic approaches; asthma itself characterized by dyspnea and wheezing, the result of widespread narrowing of the intrapulmonary airways; airways then defined as hyperreactive	A wide variety of physical, chemical, and pharmacologic stimuli	History of dyspnea and increasing use of medication over a period of many days Ability to get only a few words out between breaths Tachycardia (often more than 130 beats/min) Tachypnea (may be variable) Hypertension Dyspnea Hypoxemia Wheezing (unless airflow is so diminished that it obscures wheezing) Pulsus paradoxus greater than 20 mm Hg
Increased intracranial pressure	The skull, a closed space, limits expansion of brain tissue or fluid volume (blood or CSF), resulting in rising pressure with trauma or disease processes	Tumor or head trauma } Increased brain volume or mass Subdural or epidural hematoma Hypoxia Hypercapnia Vasodilators } Increased blood volume Tumor Infection Seizures Anatomic defect } Increased CSF volume (hydrocephalus)	Headache (be especially wary with a child younger than age 10 or 11); watch for Cushing's triad, a drop in pulse rate, rising blood pressure, and a widened pulse pressure Changes in mental status Lethargy Irritability Slowed responsiveness In severe circumstance, somnolence, stupor, coma Seizures Syncope Meningismus Retinal hemorrhages Cranial nerve palsy, particularly VI (abducens paralysis)

Ventilatory failure (i.e., hypercapnic respiratory failure)	Compromised exhalation of carbon dioxide because of alveolar hypoventilation	Upper airway obstruction
		Neurologic disorders
		  CNS
		  Drug overdose
		  Increased intracranial pressure
		  Upper cervical spinal cord involving third to fifth nerve roots serving diaphragm
		  Injury
		Phrenic nerve paralysis
		Neuromuscular disease
		  Guillain-Barré disease (acute polyneuritis)
		Chest wall compromise
		  Severe kyphoscoliosis
		  Trauma with "flail chest"
		  Pulmonary contusion
			Apprehension, confusion
			Headache, occasionally; somnolence to coma (may be quite subtle if the process is chronic)
			Patient complaint of respiratory distress
			Slowed respiratory rate
			Paradoxic respiration

D: Disability (neurologic status) is assessed in terms of the patient's degree of responsiveness.

E: Exposure—undress the patient as much as possible when trauma is apparent or suspected to identify all injuries. Do not hesitate to cut clothing away.

The immediate goal is to identify such threatening conditions as an airway obstruction, impaired ventilation and hypoxemia, hypovolemic shock, and hemorrhage. The primary assessment is interrupted to manage a life-threatening condition as soon as it is detected. Once the condition is stabilized, the primary assessment is continued. This should be repeated every 5 minutes during an emergency, because physiologic status may change rapidly.

A *secondary assessment* is an in-depth, head-to-toe examination to identify anatomic problems, additional conditions that are potentially life-threatening, and the patient's previously diagnosed condition. This assessment begins only after all life-threatening conditions have been stabilized. The assessment is also interrupted for repeated primary assessment and if any life-threatening condition develops. The assessment for an acute medical condition is not too different from a screening medical examination. In cases of trauma the assessment is intended to identify the full range of injuries, with particular focus on body systems affected by the mechanism of injury.

Special procedures required for patient assessment, such as peritoneal lavage, radiologic evaluation, and laboratory studies, are also conducted during this secondary phase. Assessment of the eyes, ears, nose, mouth, rectum, and pelvis should not be neglected. This examination requires "tubes and fingers in every orifice."

PRIMARY ASSESSMENT

The primary assessment should be completed very rapidly and, with a stable patient, may take only 30 seconds. It may, however, take several minutes when the mechanism of injury leads you to suspect underlying critical conditions. The historical information obtained during the primary assessment is generally limited to the chief complaint.

Airway and Cervical Spine

The patency of the upper airway is assessed at the start by asking the patient a question. If the patient answers, this is a sign that the airway is open *at this time* (Box 23-1). It also gives some assurance at this point about the level of responsiveness. If the patient does not respond, place your ear close to the patient's nose and mouth to detect any air movement (Figure 23-1). Look for any blood, vomitus, teeth, or other foreign bodies that may be obstructing the airway. If the patient is supine, use a chin lift or jaw thrust to raise the tongue (the most common cause of airway obstruction) out of the oropharynx (Figure 23-2). Remove blood, vomitus, or foreign bodies from the airway by suction.

In cases of actual or suspected trauma above the clavicle, it is necessary to control the cervical spine when performing any airway maneuvers or patient movement. Excessive movement of the cervical spine can convert a fracture or dislocation without neurologic damage to one with neurologic injury. The patient's head and neck, therefore, should never be hyperextended or hyperflexed to establish or maintain an airway. Control the cervical spine by manually maintaining the neck in a neutral position, in alignment with the body (Figure 23-3). Neurologic examination alone does not eliminate the possibility of cervical spine injury. Ultimately, appropriate x-ray films of all seven cervical vertebrae must be obtained.

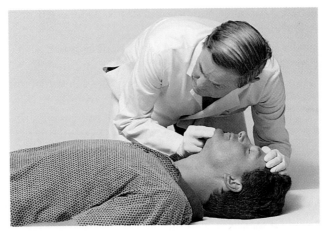

FIGURE 23-1

Look, listen, and feel for adequate breathing to assess patency of the upper airway.

BOX 23-1 | **Assessment of Airway Patency**

Sources of Obstruction

- Foreign body
- Trauma: blunt or penetrating
- Infection: epiglottitis, croup, peritonsillar abscess, retropharyngeal abscess
- Inflammation: burn, smoke inhalation
- Tumor: thyroid, hemangioma, hematoma, squamous cell carcinoma, edema
- Neurologic lesion: vocal cord paralysis
- Congenital abnormalities: laryngeal web, tracheomalacia

Symptoms of Obstruction

- Respiratory distress: dyspnea, tachypnea
- Anxiety: tense, deeply worried facies (may signal epiglottitis)
- Difficulty swallowing
- Pain, sometimes related directly to area of difficulty, sometimes diffuse
- Cough and associated "strain" or change in voice
- Restless behavior: inability to find a comfortable position
- Lethargy at times

Signs of Obstruction

- Hoarse voice and/or cough, sometimes characterized as a "bark"
- Stridor: severity related to extent of obstruction and the patient's respiratory effort
- Inspiratory: obstruction at the glottis, epiglottis
- Expiratory: obstruction below the glottis
- Retraction
  - Suprasternal notch: obstruction at or above trachea
  - Intercostal and subcostal, below suprasternal notch: obstruction in bronchial tree or below
- Drooling (difficulty swallowing): obstruction at glottis or above
- Bleeding: hemoptysis, hematoma, particularly with trauma
- Subcutaneous emphysema, particularly with trauma
- Fracture, often palpable

Breathing

Expose the patient's chest to assess ventilatory effort. Note the *approximate* rate and depth of respirations. Taking the time to count the respiratory rate is not generally appropriate during the primary survey. Bilateral chest movement should be synchronized with breathing. Use the stethoscope to assess the presence of breath sounds. Note any signs of respiratory distress, such as retractions, tachypnea, and cyanosis. Provide ventilatory assistance with oxygen, if needed, before continuing with the primary assessment.

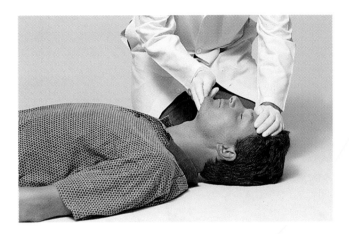

FIGURE 23-2
Use a chin lift to ensure an open airway.

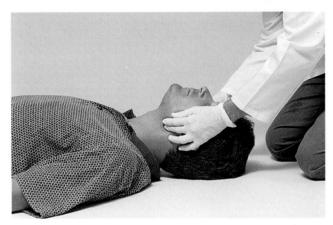

FIGURE 23-3
Properly position both hands to maintain the head and neck in a neutral position, in alignment with the body.

In cases of trauma, look for bruising, paradoxic chest movement, and open chest wounds. Palpate the upper chest and neck for crepitation, a sign of air leakage into soft tissue. Bruising should alert you to the possibility of pulmonary contusion, which often results in a spontaneous pneumothorax. Open chest wounds must be immediately sealed, because they often cause a tension pneumothorax. Paradoxic chest movement may be associated with fractured ribs or a *flail chest*. This fracture should be stabilized immediately.

Circulation

Adequate circulation is needed to oxygenate the brain. Circulation can be impaired because of cardiac conditions, hemorrhage, dehydration, and other medical conditions. To assess peripheral perfusion and detect hypovolemic shock, note the skin color, presence and quality of pulses in and the temperature of the extremities, and the capillary refill time, as there may not be enough time for an adequate blood pressure determination.

Pulses should be detected in the distal extremities (radial, dorsalis pedis, or posterior tibial). If no pulses are detected at these sites, check the brachial and popliteal sites and then the femoral and carotid sites (Figure 23-4). Diminished pulses in the distal sites indicate poor perfusion and hypovolemic shock. Generally, if the radial pulse is palpable, the systolic pressure will be greater than 80 mm Hg; if the femoral or carotid pulse is palpable, the systolic pressure will be greater than 70 mm Hg. To assess capillary refill, press firmly over a nail bed or bony prominence (chin, forehead, or sternum) until the skin blanches. Count the seconds it takes for color to return. A capillary refill time in excess of 2 seconds indicates poor perfusion.

A REMINDER FOR RESUSCITATION

Airway maintenance, assisted ventilation and chest compression, and other life-saving modalities for patient care should be initiated when the problem is identified, rather than *after* completion of the primary assessment.

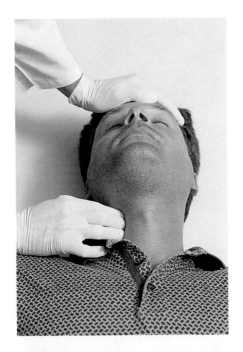

FIGURE 23-4
Check the carotid pulse to confirm circulation, one side at a time.

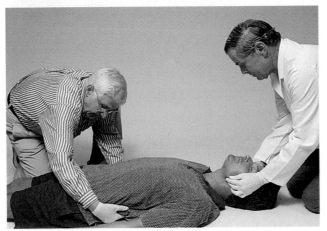

FIGURE 23-5
Quickly assess the entire body for bleeding sites.

Make a quick total body appraisal for bleeding sites, being especially careful to look and feel for dampness in dark clothing that may obscure hemorrhage (Figure 23-5). Control bleeding before continuing the primary assessment, and estimate the amount of blood loss. Significant amounts of blood, enough to cause hypovolemic shock, can also be lost into the thoracic and abdominal cavities. Do not assume that there has not been hemorrhage simply because no blood is seen.

Disability

A brief neurologic evaluation is performed, primarily to determine the patient's responsiveness or level of consciousness. (A more detailed neurologic evaluation is performed during the secondary assessment.) However, it is appropriate at this time to determine whether the patient is at one of these levels of responsiveness (the mnemonic *AVPU*): *a*lert, responsive to *v*erbal stimuli, responsive to *p*ainful stimuli, or *u*nresponsive. A decrease in the level of consciousness may indicate hypoxemia or hypovolemic shock, necessitating a reevaluation of the patient's ABCs.

MNEMONICS

PATIENT'S LEVEL OF RESPONSIVENESS: AVPU

A *A*lert

V *V*erbal stimuli: responsive to

P *P*ainful stimuli: responsive to

U *U*nresponsive

SECONDARY ASSESSMENT

Exposure

In cases of trauma, the patient should be as completely undressed as possible to facilitate a brief body search for major injuries that may have been missed during the ABCs.

Check the vital signs before beginning the head-to-toe survey of the body in the search for additional injuries. Determine the heart rate, respiratory rate, and blood pressure. (In effect, this is a recheck. Initial observations of pulses and respirations are obviously part of the primary assessment.) Compare these values with those expected for the patient. It is important to recognize that vital sign values above or below those expected for the person's age are indicative of particular problems.

It is also appropriate at this time to quantify the patient's level of consciousness with the Glasgow Coma Scale (see Box 4-3). This score can be used for comparison with those computed during periodic reassessments to determine changes in the patient's level of consciousness.

History

Usually someone other than the examiner obtains an abbreviated history from the patient, family, emergency medical technicians, or scene bystanders. Pertinent information is then shared with the examiner during the assessment process. This abbreviated history should focus on information relevant to the emergency condition. A useful mnemonic is *AMPLE*, reflecting the individual sections of the history.

Head and Neck

Inspect and palpate the head and scalp, looking for any depressions, bone instability, crepitus, lacerations, penetrating injuries, or drainage from the ears or nose. Clear or amber-colored drainage from the nose or ears may indicate a basilar skull fracture. Note any bruising around the eyes (raccoon eyes) or behind the ears (Battle sign), indicating a skull fracture (Box 23-2).

Examine the eyes for pupillary size and responsiveness to light. Examine the retinas and conjunctivae for hemorrhage and the lens for dislocation. A quick visual examination of both eyes is performed by asking a conscious patient to read the words on the side of any container.

MNEMONICS

SECTIONS OF THE HEALTH HISTORY: AMPLE

A *Allergies*

M *Medications or drugs of any kind currently being taken by the patient*

P *Past illnesses, such as diabetes, epilepsy, hypertension*

L *Last meal*

E *Events preceding the precipitating event*

BOX 23-2   Signs of Injury

There are certain signs that will alert you to serious problems in the emergency situation associated with trauma. They include the following:

Battle sign: Ecchymotic discoloration and swelling behind either or both ears after a head injury, indicating a possible basilar skull fracture.

Cullen sign: A bluish "halo" surrounding the umbilicus, indicating bleeding into the tissues, associated with intraabdominal bleeding and trauma, ectopic pregnancy, pancreatitis.

Grey-Turner sign: Subcutaneous bruising around the flanks and umbilicus, suggestive of a retroperitoneal hematoma.

Hamman crunch: A crunching sound synchronous with the heartbeat and heard on auscultation of the precordium, suggestive of hemothorax, pneumothorax, respiratory failure.

Kehr sign: Pain in the subscapular region of the shoulder, usually on the left, referred from an irritated phrenic nerve, the result of rupture of the spleen, or possibly ectopic pregnancy or gastrointestinal disease.

Raccoon eyes: Ecchymotic discoloration and swelling around either or both eyes, associated with head trauma, suggestive of basilar skull fracture or facial bone fracture.

Modified from Revere, Hasty, 1993.

Inspect the neck for penetrating injury, bruising, and tracheal deviation, and palpate for deformity and crepitus. Be certain that the neck is manually maintained in neutral position until radiographic documentation confirming the absence of cervical injury has been obtained.

If a patient wearing any type of sports helmet does *not* exhibit respiratory distress, a lateral cervical spine film should be obtained *before* the helmet is removed. Otherwise, the patient's neck should be held in a neutral position while the helmet is removed. During this two-person procedure, in-line manual stabilization of the neck is applied from below and the helmet is expanded laterally. In-line manual stabilization of the neck is then reestablished from above, and the patient is adequately immobilized.

Chest

Inspect the chest for bruising or obvious signs of deformity. Palpate the sternum, each rib, and clavicle. Blunt sternal pressure will be painful if any attached ribs are fractured. Patterns of bruising may indicate the mechanism of injury and may signal a possible pulmonary contusion.

Auscultate breath sounds at the apex, base, and midaxillary areas. Note any diminished or absent breath sounds, which may indicate a pneumothorax or hemothorax. Auscultate the heart for clarity of heart sounds. Distant muffled heart sounds and distended neck veins may indicate cardiac tamponade, a life-threatening condition. In a noisy emergency department, heart sounds may be difficult to hear and hypovolemia may prevent distention of neck veins; therefore a narrow pulse pressure may be the only reliable indicator of cardiac tamponade.

Abdomen

Inspect the abdomen for bruising and distention. Gently palpate the abdomen, noting guarding and pain. Hollow organs in the abdomen are often ruptured with blunt trauma and result in occult hemorrhage; pain and distention may indicate an underlying hemorrhage.

Back

The back is briefly inspected for signs of injury. The patient must be log-rolled to maintain cervical spine stabilization.

Extremities

Inspect and palpate all extremities for signs of fractures or deformities, crepitus, pain, and lack of spontaneous movement. Palpation of the bones with rotational or three-point pressure along the shaft helps identify fractures where alignment has been maintained. Note any wounds over the site of a suspected fracture, the possible indication of an open fracture. Palpate all peripheral pulses. It is particularly important to document skin temperature, capillary refill time, and the presence of a pulse in extremities with a suspected fracture.

Pelvic fractures are detected by placing downward pressure with the heels of the hands on both anterior superior iliac spines and on the symphysis pubis. Pelvic fractures are associated with occult hemorrhage, which may become a life-threatening condition.

Rectum and Perineum

A rectal and perineal examination is essential to assess abdominal, pelvic, and neurologic injuries. The rectal examination is performed to detect blood within the bowel lumen, a high-riding prostate, pelvic fractures, the integrity of the abdominal wall, and the quality of sphincter tone.

Neurologic Examination

A more complete neurologic evaluation is performed once the patient's condition has been stabilized. Reassess the patient's Glasgow Coma Scale score. Then perform a more detailed motor and sensory evaluation. Note any paralysis or paresis, which suggests major injury to the spinal column or peripheral nervous system.

Reevaluate the Patient

The patient must be reevaluated frequently so that any new signs and symptoms are not overlooked. A primary survey should be performed every 5 minutes and the results compared with those obtained in previous surveys. Vital signs must be monitored continuously. As life-threatening conditions are managed, other equally life-threatening problems may develop and less severe conditions may become evident. A high index of suspicion and constant alertness facilitate early recognition and management.

Urgent or Emergent Threat

Sometimes there may be no obvious trauma, and the reason for a medical emergency may not be readily evident. On other occasions, the message is clear. Regardless, any situation (such as odor, Box 23-3), however subtle, that suggests a patient's increased vulnerability may indicate an urgent or emergent threat. Table 23-2 defines eight primary symptoms that may be associated with a life-threatening condition.

PEDIATRIC PRIORITIES

Priorities for the infant and child are basically the same as for adults. Although blood volume, fluid requirements, and size may be smaller, and associated disease or the mechanism of injury may be different, the assessment sequence is the same. Remember, too, to keep the patient warm and to involve the parents as much as possible every step of the way.

BOX 23-3	Smell the Breath

Sometimes, when a situation is urgent, the patient's breath may have a distinctive odor, a clue to the source of difficulty, a possible ingestion or poisoning.

Odor	Possible Source
Sweet, fruity	Chloroform, lacquer, salicyclates
Fruity, alcohol	Ethyl alcohol, phenol
Pear-like, acrid	Chloral hydrate, paraldehyde
"Halitosis"	Amphetamine
Wintergreen	Methyl salicylate
Bitter almond	Cyanide, jetberry bush
Camphor	Mothballs (naphthalene)
Garlic	Phosphorus, arsenic, tellurium, parathion, malathion
Coal gas	Coal gas (associated with odorless but toxic carbon monoxide poisoning)
Metallic	Iodine
Rotten eggs	Hydrogen sulfide mercaptans
Shoe polish	Nitrobenzene
Stale tobacco	Nicotine
Burned rope	Marijuana
"Cloret's sign"	Lozenges (to cover up telltale odors!)

Adapted from Wilson, 1997, and McMillan et al, 1977.

TABLE 23-2   **Symptoms and Risks of Life-Threatening Conditions**

Primary Symptoms	Possible Accompanying Symptoms	Possible Diagnosis	Risk
Sudden onset of unexplained shortness of breath	Persistent chest pain, sharp and stabbing, that worsens with breathing or coughing Faintness or actual fainting spell Cough with bloody sputum Swelling and pain in leg Cyanosis around the mouth Recently having been bed-bound for a long period Having sat in one position for a prolonged time, as in an overseas flight	Pulmonary embolism, usually from a site in the leg or pelvis	Two thirds of patients with a massive embolism die; intensive treatment of smaller embolism can limit the amount of damage to lung tissue
Vomiting blood or black or dark brown material that resembles coffee grounds	Recurrent bouts of gnawing pain in the upper part of the abdomen Black or tarlike stool Loss of appetite Unexplained weight loss Weakness Paleness Progressive fatigue Increased awareness of the heartbeat (palpitations)	Bleeding ulcer of the stomach or duodenum, bleeding from esophageal varices	Possibly fatal hemorrhage
Crushing pain in the center of the chest	Radiation of the pain to the arm(s), neck, or jaw Sweating Nausea and vomiting Shortness of breath Fainting Feeling of impending doom	Myocardial infarction	Mortality figures vary with the age of the patient and the location and extent of damage to the heart. Since most deaths occur within minutes or hours of the attack, the speed of treatment is crucial; rapid administration of anticlotting drugs may limit some damage
Severe throbbing pain in and around one bloodshot eye	Blurred vision in the affected eye Eyeball is both tender and firm to the touch Abnormal sensitivity to light Fixed and dilated pupil	Acute glaucoma	Delayed treatment can result in complete and permanent blindness in affected eye

Modified from *The Johns Hopkins Medical Letter*, 1990.

INJURY ASSESSMENT

If trauma is the root of the problem, a history of the injury or examination of the injury-producing mechanism may be helpful. Injury can be divided into two basic types: *blunt* and *penetrating*. Each can be further classified according to the direction of energy force for blunt trauma and the degree of severity for penetrating trauma.

BLUNT TRAUMA

The severity of injury will vary according to the amount of energy transferred from an object to the human body. The direction of impact determines the pattern of injuries. The automobile accounts for the majority of severe blunt trauma cases and is therefore used as an example here. The emergency medical technicians or other first responders who were present at the scene should describe the appearance of the vehicle and the damage sustained to the passenger compartment.

On the basis of this information, the examiner can identify the portions of the body that absorbed the greatest transfer of energy. The following are some examples:

- A bent steering wheel and a bull's-eye fracture of the windshield should alert to the potential for C-spine injuries, central flail chest, myocardial contusion, fractured spleen or liver, and posterior fracture or dislocation of the hip.

TABLE 23-2	Symptoms and Risks of Life-Threatening Conditions—cont'd		
Primary Symptoms	**Possible Accompanying Symptoms**	**Possible Diagnosis**	**Risk**
Flashes of light in the field of vision of one eye	Absence of pain in the affected eye Black cobweb-like floating spots Partial loss of vision spreading as a curtain-like shadow from the top or one side of the eye	Retinal detachment	Delayed treatment can result in further detachment extending to the area of most detailed vision (macula); permanent loss of central vision may result without treatment, detachment can cause blindness in the affected eye
Sudden and progressively more severe abdominal pain	Nausea and vomiting Swollen or tender abdomen Severe constipation Temperature above 100° F (38° C)	Acute (surgical) abdomen (appendicitis, obstruction)	Delayed treatment can result in rupture or ischemic destruction of the involved organ and peritonitis
Sudden feeling of weakness and unsteadiness that may result in momentary loss of consciousness	Loss of movement of arm(s) or leg(s) Numbness and/or tingling in any part of the body Excruciating headache Confusion Difficulty speaking Blurred or double vision, or loss of vision in one eye	Transient ischemic attack (TIA) or stroke (CVA)	TIA: although short-lived, it may signal an impending stroke; risk can be diminished with appropriate therapy. Stroke: the outcome depends on the location and extent of the interruption of the blood supply. Overall, one third of strokes are fatal; one third leave some degree of permanent damage; one third have no long-lasting effect
Difficult breathing that occurs suddenly (often in the middle of the night) and worsens rapidly	Restlessness, anxiety, and sense of doom Swollen ankles Cough producing frothy pink or brownish, blood-flecked sputum Audible bubbling sound when breathing Bluish lips and nail beds Profuse sweating	Pulmonary edema, related to a sudden left-sided heart failure	Delayed treatment can be fatal, although timely and appropriate therapy usually results in dramatic relief of acute symptoms

- A side impact may cause contralateral neck sprain, lateral flail chest, ruptured spleen or liver (depending on the side of impact), and fractured pelvis or acetabulum.
- Rear impact collision can result in neck injuries (that is, cervical strain or "whiplash").
- Persons ejected from a vehicle can sustain multiple injuries, including a cervical spine fracture, depending on the part of the body that strikes first.
- An airbag injury commonly results in abrasions, sometimes severe, over arms, face and neck; less commonly, particularly in small individuals, the force may cause life-threatening internal injuries.

PENETRATING TRAUMA

The following two factors determine the type of injury and subsequent management:

- The *region* of the body sustaining the injury will anatomically determine the potential for specific organ injury.
- The *transfer* of energy is determined by the *force* of the penetrating object on impact. The amount of force is further measured by the *velocity* of the missile and the *distance* from the source (for example, a 0.38 caliber handgun has a

muzzle velocity of 850 feet per second). Energy transfer is also determined by the *rate* or change in *speed* once the missile is inside the patient's body and also by the *frontal projection* of the missile. In most penetrating injuries, the most important factor in determining energy is the speed of the missile.

BURNS

Burns should alert the examiner to the possibilities of smoke, heat, and chemical inhalation and carbon monoxide poisoning. Blunt trauma and fractures may also be associated with thermal injuries as a result of an explosion, falling debris, or the individual's attempts to escape the fire.

INFANTS AND CHILDREN

A smaller anatomy and differing physiologic responses to injury and acute illness by infants and children are important considerations when examining them during an emergency (Box 23-4). For example, cardiac arrest is rarely a primary event in chil-

---

BOX 23-4   Findings that Indicate a Sense of Urgency in Infants and Children

Airway and Breathing

- Respiratory distress indicated by nasal flaring, retractions
- Respiratory rate >60, sustained, especially with oxygen administration
- Respiratory rate <20, especially in the presence of acute illness or with injury to the chest or abdomen
- Cyanosis: a late sign in respiratory failure, first seen in the mucous membranes of the mouth
- Stridor indicates upper airway obstruction
- Head bobbing indicates impending respiratory failure
- Prolonged expiration indicates reactive airway disease
- Grunting indicates alveolar collapse or loss of lung volume

Circulation

- Heart rate >180 or <80 (<5 years old)
- Heart rate >160 (>5 years old)
- Sinus tachycardia, sustained
- Bradycardia: sign of impending cardiac arrest
- Hypotension: late sign of hypovolemia that indicates decompensation. A fall of 10 mm Hg is significant
- Absence of peripheral pulses indicates poor tissue perfusion
- Absent central pulse is an ominous sign
- Capillary refill time: >2 seconds indicates poor tissue perfusion, hypothermia, constricted blood flow (perhaps the result of a tight cast)
- Mottling, pallor, and peripheral cyanosis are indicators of poor tissue perfusion, respiratory distress
- Diminished urinary output may indicate poor renal perfusion

Neurologic Disability

- Diminished level of consciousness (see Glasgow Coma Scale, Box 4-3)
- Agitation, anxiety
- Lethargy
- Irritability to passivity
- Unresponsiveness
- Failure to recognize parents
- Muscles: hypotonia and/or lost deep tendon reflexes may indicate hypoperfusion of the brain
- Generalized convulsions may indicate a seizure disorder, drug ingestion, hypoglycemia, hypertensive encephalopathy, severe renal dysfunction
- Pupil dilation may indicate increased intracranial pressure

dren as it is in adults. The child usually experiences respiratory and ventilatory failure that progresses to respiratory arrest first. Without rapid and appropriate intervention, a cardiac arrest occurs as a secondary event. Because a cardiac arrest in children is complicated by prolonged hypoxemia and/or acidosis, resuscitation is seldom successful, even when expeditious.

For this reason, repeated primary assessment of the child with respiratory distress is critical if deterioration is to be detected in time to allow adequate intervention. During respiratory failure, carbon dioxide is not sufficiently expired (blown off), with hypoxia being the result. In the event of shock (poor tissue perfusion), blood is shunted to the vital organs, allowing the child a short period of physiologic compensation. Failure to reverse the hypoxia and to clear metabolites by improving perfusion will result in hypoxemia, acidemia (low blood pH), and tissue acidosis. Early intervention usually prevents progression to cardiac arrest.

ASSESSMENT IN CHILDREN

Given the primary assessment, a secondary one may be somewhat more deliberate if the situation allows. Additional information may be sought and further judgments made.

- Parents usually know the child's weight in pounds. The conversion factor is 2.2 lb = 1 kg. If the weight is not known, estimate in kilograms: 8 + (2 × child's age in years).
- The approximate expected systolic blood pressure for a child older than 1 year: 80 + (2 × child's age in years).
- A crying child has, at that moment, a patent airway
- Capillary refill is a marker for circulatory perfusion. A time greater than 2 seconds or greater than the time it takes to say, slowly, "capillary refill," suggests a problem.
- The AVPU mnemonic (p. 848) is helpful with children as well as with adults.
- The aspects of physical examination in children discussed throughout the book are applicable in the emergency or life-threatening situation. Be mindful of the expected ways in which children differ physically from adults (Box 23-5).

Intervention, of course, must begin immediately in the event of a life-threatening situation but, given time and the opportunity, do the following:

- Attempt to establish rapport with the child consistent with the situation.
- Using the mnemonic AMPLE (p. 849) as a base for history taking, add questions about the mother's pregnancy and delivery, for example, due date, hypertension, vaginal bleeding, if the infant is still in the first few weeks of life.
- Consistent with age and condition, get as much information as possible from the child. For example, "Please show me with one finger where it hurts."
- Evaluate the meaning of signs and symptoms with deliberate speed (Box 23-6).

The Febrile Infant or Child: Really Sick or Reasonably Well?

The Yale Observation Scales (Table 23-3) are a guide *if* you recognize the subjectivity and, hence, the possible variability in some of the observations, and *if* you recognize that the well-appearing infant or child may not be all that well. *The higher the score, the more likely the child is ill, particularly when the sum approaches or is greater than 10.* These observations are also helpful when a child is not febrile. As always, measures like this can aid but not dictate final judgments.

BOX 23-5 Ways in Which Children Differ Physically From Adults

Although children differ physically from adults, the closer they are in age to an adult, the more like an adult they become (Figure 23-6).

Skin

- By age 10, the surface area relative to body mass is greater, more nearly approximating the adult relationship.
- The skin is thinner, with less subcutaneous fat, and is less protective against burns and more likely to develop hypothermia.

Head

- To about age 4 years, the head is larger and heavier relative to the rest of the body.
- The bones of the skull are softer and are separated by fibrous tissue and cartilage until about age 5 years; this is somewhat protective against increased intracranial pressure, at least for a short time.
- The developing brain, particularly to age 5 years, is more vulnerable to injury, infection, and poisons.
- The dura, very firmly attached to the skull, is more apt to tear and bleed with injury.

Airway

- Nasal passages are relatively smaller and more easily obstructed with discharges or foreign bodies. Since newborns and young infants are obligate nose breathers, they are particularly vulnerable.
- The tongue is relatively larger and more easily able to obstruct the upper airway.
- The trachea is relatively much narrower and its cartilage more elastic and collapsible, thus it is more vulnerable to edema, pressure, and inflammation; hyperextension or flexion can "crimp" and obstruct.
- The larynx is higher and more anterior, more "available" for aspiration.

Chest and Lungs

- The rib cage is more elastic and flexible, less vulnerable to injury, more apt to allow retraction during increased respiratory distress.
- Lung tissue is fragile and more easily contused.
- The mediastinum is more mobile and more vulnerable to tension pneumothorax.
- Chest muscles are not well developed. Their use, in addition to the expected diaphragmatic effort, suggests respiratory distress; they tire more easily with prolonged effort.
- The higher metabolic rate and greater oxygen requirement increase vulnerability to hypoxemia.

Heart and Circulation

- Infants and children have a relatively smaller total circulating blood volume but will lose as much blood as will an adult from a similar laceration.
- When a significant blood or fluid volume is lost, children maintain their blood pressure longer than adults do.
- Bradycardia, usually the initial response to hypoxemia in neonates, may herald cardiac arrest.

Abdomen

- The liver and spleen are relatively larger and more vascular; thus they are less protected by the ribs and more susceptible to injury.

Extremities

- The not yet fully calcified bones of children are softer than those of adults until puberty and are more vulnerable to fracture.

Nervous System

- An infant is able to feel pain anywhere in the body, but cannot localize or isolate it.
- Children who appear passive in stressful situations and do not seek comforting reassurance from parents may have an altered, depressed level of consciousness, or, if alert, may be providing a clue to child abuse.

Modified from Eichelberger et al, 1998.

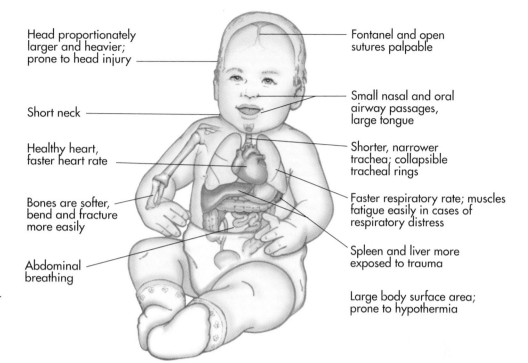

FIGURE 23-6

The unique anatomic and physiologic features of infants and young children.

Redrawn from Eichelberger et al, 1998.

BOX 23-6 | **Classic Signs of Physiologic Problems in Children**

Pain

Shallow breathing
Irritable crying
Splinting
Facial expression change when touched or moved
Resists movement
Rigid posturing

Early Shock

Tachycardia >130 beats/min
Capillary refill >2 sec
Pale, cool skin
Altered level of consciousness
Normal systolic blood pressure

Moderate Dehydration

Sunken fontanel
Pallor
Doughy skin texture
Dry mucous membranes

Respiratory Distress

Nasal flaring
Mottled, dusky skin color
Tachypnea, shallow breathing
Altered level of consciousness
Sounds—stridor, hoarseness, muffled voice, wheezing
Tripod positioning
Retractions
Asymmetric chest movement
"See-saw" respirations

Late Shock

Tachycardia >130 beats/min
Capillary refill >5 sec
Pallor, cold extremities
Altered level of consciousness
Systolic BP <80 mm Hg (except infants, whose systolic BP is often normally lower); sometimes, even in late shock, the pressure may be normal

Severe Dehydration

Sunken fontanel
Signs of shock
Parched mucous membranes
No tears (dry cry)
Sunken eyeballs

Altered Level of Consciousness

Combative
Decreased responsiveness
Lethargy
Weak cry, moaning
Personality change

Increased Intracranial Pressure

Bulging fontanel (in infant)
Altered level of consciousness
High-pitched cry
Change in vital signs
Irritable cry, impossible to distract or console child

From Eichelberger et al, 1998.

TABLE 23-3	Yale Observation Scales for Children		
	Score of observation*		
Observation Item	Reassuring (1)	Worrisome (3)	Ominous (5)
Quality of cry	Strong, with expected tone OR Content and not crying	Whimpering OR Sobbing	Weak OR Moaning OR High pitched
Reaction to parental stimulation	Cries briefly then stops OR Content and not crying	Cries off and on	Continual cry OR Hardly responds
Awake or asleep	If awake, stays awake OR If asleep and stimulated, awakens quickly	Eyes close briefly, then awakens OR Awakens with prolonged stimulation	Falls asleep OR Will not rouse
Color	Pink	Pale extremities OR Acrocyanosis	Pale OR Cyanotic OR Mottled OR Ashen
Hydration	Appropriate skin turgor AND Eyes and mucous membranes moist	Appropriate skin turgor, eyes moist AND Mouth slightly dry	Skin doughy OR Tented AND Dry mucous membranes AND/OR Sunken eyes
Response (talk, smile) to social overtures	Smiles OR Consistently alert (≤2 mo)	Brief smile OR Briefly alert (≤2 mo)	No smile OR Face anxious, dull, expressionless OR Not alert (≤ 2 mo)

Modified from McCarthy et al, 1985

*The higher the score, the more likely the child is ill, particularly when the score approaches or is greater than 10.

RECORDS AND LEGAL CONSIDERATIONS

RECORDS

Meticulous record keeping is very important. Often more than one person cares for the patient; therefore precise records are essential to evaluate the patient's needs and clinical status. Do not rely solely on your memory. The patient record becomes a *legal document* in the sense that it can be used in legal proceedings. It is a record of what you observed, evaluated, ordered, and performed, and conversely, what you did not: "If you didn't document it, you didn't do it." So be thorough but concise; be clear and accurate. Pertinent negatives are as important as pertinent positives, and it is as important to document their absence as it is to document their presence.

Medical and legal problems frequently arise during emergency situations, and precise records are of aid to all concerned. Chronologic reports using flow sheets help in the quick recording of assessment of changes in the patient's condition. Legibility is always essential. Write so that others can read; if that is not possible, print or type. Do not erase a mistake, draw a line through the error so that it remains legible. Do not use any but the most conventional abbreviations. Initial any corrections and date them.

CONSENT FOR TREATMENT

Consent is usually obtained before treatment. In life-threatening emergencies, the needed treatment should most often be given and formal consent obtained later. If forensic trauma is suspected, the personnel caring for the patient must preserve evidence. All items, such as bullets and clothing, must be saved for law enforcement personnel, with a documented chain of possession by health professionals.

ADVANCE DIRECTIVES, LIVING WILLS, AND DURABLE POWER OF ATTORNEY FOR HEALTH CARE

It is necessary to make a conscientious effort to learn whether a patient has left a formal statement of wishes in the event of an accident or illness that results in a cognitive impairment that prevents adequate participation in medical decision making. A central concern involves the vigor with which life maintenance measures should be instituted. There is legal provision in most states for such statements, *advance directives,* usually in writing. There may also be a close relative or other trusted person to whom decision-making authority can be legally delegated in the form of a *durable power of attorney for health care.* Clearly, advance documentation of the patient's wishes in a so-called *living will* or even in a prior entry in a medical record can be helpful to those giving care, and to those persons with durable power of attorney.

Advance Directives

The purpose of an advance directive is to ensure that legally competent adult patients, generally those 18 or older who are not mentally ill or under guardianship, may express their wishes regarding the extent of their care in end-of-life circumstances. It is now common practice to offer to all patients the possibility of an advance directive and to ensure a reasonable effort to discover if such a directive exists in writing; these directives should be placed in the patient's medical record. Precise documentation is protective of the patient and provider and is essential. If there has not been a written advance directive, the patient's wishes as told to a health care provider, validated by a witness, and entered in the patient's record can be considered legally competent.

Living Wills

Such advance directives can be considered *living wills.* Living wills must have been completed voluntarily and, in general, must have been witnessed by two competent persons unrelated to the patient either directly or by marriage, without financial interest to be derived from the patient or the patient's estate, and without financial or other responsibilities for the patient's care either directly or indirectly.

The provisions of a living will may become applicable when the patient is in a terminal condition, which usually is validated by two physicians, both of whom have personally examined the patient. To be considered terminal, a condition must be incurable to a reasonable degree of certainty and, despite the application of life-sustaining procedures, give no evidence of a potential for recovery.

Although it is the patient's responsibility to bring attention to a living will, this is of course not always possible. Health care providers must make every effort to discover the patient's intentions and to abide by them. Certainly, if the provider cannot in conscience follow the patient's directive, it becomes a responsibility then to arrange for care with another provider.

The patient always has the right to revoke the declaration of a living will. This, too, is best done in writing and with witnesses.

Durable Power of Attorney for Health Care

The durable power of attorney gives a person selected by the patient the power to make health care decisions in the event that the patient's cognition is lost. That representative or "agent" then has the authority to decide with the provider what if any measures may be taken to sustain life or prolong dying artificially (e.g., tube feeding, antibiotics, and respirators). Again, it is generally required that two physicians validate that a condition is or is likely to be terminal. It is important to note that the durable power of attorney for health care does not give authority for the patient's representative to handle other matters (e.g., financial or property). These can be left in the hands of yet another person. At times it is appropriate to suggest that a lawyer help the patient in the preparation of directives.

Clearly, advance documentation of a patient's wishes can be enormously helpful to those giving care and to those persons with durable power of attorney for health care. It imposes a grave responsibility complicated by the variety of possible ethical interpretations. Clearly stated wishes and candid, respectful involvement of everyone concerned smooths the way.

SUMMARY

Notably, diagnosis is not necessarily made before the initiation of treatment. Life-threatening physiologic indicators of disease or trauma are identified rapidly, leading to immediate management. The causes underlying these physiologic indicators—the diagnosis—can be determined after the condition of the patient is stabilized, and a thorough examination can then be performed.

Evaluation and care are divided into the following four phases:
1. Primary assessment: assessment of ABCs
   *A*irway and C-spine control is performed.
   *B*reathing is assessed.
   *C*irculation is assessed, with hemorrhage control or shock management.
   *D*isability: neurologic function is briefly evaluated.
   *E*xposure: completely undress the patient whenever possible.
2. Resuscitation
   The management of life-threatening problems identified in the primary survey is continued.
   Mechanical monitoring is implemented.
3. Secondary assessment
   Develop the history, guided by the mnemonic *AMPLE.* Total evaluation of the patient is performed in the following areas: head and skull, neck, chest, abdomen, rectum and perineum, and extremities (for fractures).
   Complete neurologic examination is performed, along with appropriate x-ray examinations, laboratory tests, and special studies.
   "Tubes and fingers" are in every orifice.
4. Definitive care
   After identifying and ascertaining the patient's injuries, managing life-threatening problems, and obtaining special studies, diagnosis and treatment specific to the condition can begin.
   Heart rate, respiratory rate, level of consciousness, capillary refill time and the assessment of central versus distal pulses all need a return to comfortable levels before you can relax; 100% oxygen, cervical immobilization, and the maintenance of core temperature are essential until the clinical situation stabilizes.

Check it out— *http://www1.mosby.com/physexam_seidel*

CHAPTER 24

RECORDING INFORMATION

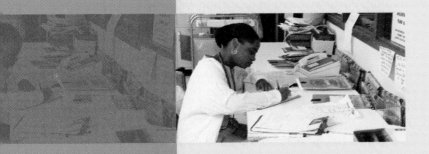

After collecting the history and completing the physical examination, the health care practitioner must condense, organize, and record the collected raw data along with the problems identified and plan of care. The information in the patient's record enables you and your colleagues to care for the patient by identifying health problems, making diagnoses, planning appropriate care, and monitoring the patient's responses to treatment.

Appropriate medical terminology and a traditional organizational style make the record more readily understood by your colleagues. The patient's record is only as good as the accuracy, depth, and detail provided.

A customary organization of information from the interview and physical examination is used by most health professionals. Health agencies often incorporate the information in standardized forms or systems of recording. Following this customary outline of information enables all health professionals in the agency to find and use the patient information more efficiently. The Problem-Oriented Medical Record is one such system.

Remember that the patient's record is a legal document, and any information contained in it may be used in court and in other legal proceedings, as well as to make health care payment determinations. It is your responsibility to present the data legibly, accurately, and in a manner that is representative of the examination. Recorded information should not be erased. Make necessary changes by lining out data, leaving crossed-out data legible. Initial and date the changes. Any portion of the examination that has been deferred or omitted should be so noted, rather than neglecting to mention particular findings. It is appropriate in some circumstances to defer a portion of an examination, and stating the reason for that deferral is useful. A clear, exact record of your assessment, analysis of the problem, and a management plan are vital to your protection should there ever be a question relevant to your care of the patient.

Concerns about the privacy of health data have grown with the development of computer-based health data systems and the ease with which electronic data can be accessed and transferred. The health agency should have policies that control access to both paper and electronic patient record databases, so data can only be used for the legitimate purposes of direct care, utilization review, quality assessment, public health, and research.

GENERAL GUIDELINES

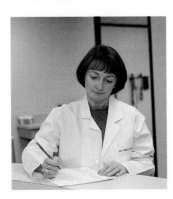

It is certainly permissible to take brief notes about the patient's concerns and your findings during the course of the interview and physical examination. You should record certain data as you obtain it, specifically the vital signs and any measurements. However, do not try to record all the data during the visit, because writing must not distract your attention from the patient.

New information related to a previously discussed topic may emerge later in the interview or examination. Postponement of recording will sharpen your interviewing skills, but it also enables you to gather, reflect, and organize all the data appropriately before making the record final.

Your recall of information is limited, however, so recording should be completed as soon as possible after the examination. Resist going on to other patients before completing the first patient's record. Although this is sometimes unavoidable, you can easily become confused about which patient had a particular finding or even forget to record an important finding.

It is important to be concise because of the volume of information collected during the examination. Use an outline form to avoid the repetition of phrases such as, "Patient states . . .". Abbreviations and symbols may be used judiciously and sparingly, but take care to use only those acceptable in your setting. Inappropriate abbreviations may be confusing to other health professionals. Similarly, avoid the use of words such as *normal, good, poor,* and *negative,* because these words are open to various interpretations by other examiners.

Document what you observe and what the patient tells you, rather than the conclusions you interpret or infer. Use direct quotes from the patient when a description is particularly vivid. Keep subjective and symptomatic data in the history, making sure none gets woven into the physical findings. Physical examination findings should be the result of your observation and interpretation of the patient's description. For example, when a patient complains of pain (a symptom) during palpation, you should note "tenderness" (a sign) in the record or report the patient's reaction to pain, such as crying, withdrawal, rigid posturing, or facial expression.

DESCRIPTION OF FINDINGS

MNEMONICS

RECORDING THE HISTORY OF THE PRESENT ILLNESS

Use the OLDCARTS mnemonic to make sure all characteristics of a problem are described in the history of present illness to assure a comprehensive presentation. The order of recording these characteristics does not need to be consistent.

O *Onset*

L *Location*

D *Duration*

C *Character*

A *Aggravating/associated factors*

R *Relieving factors*

T *Temporal factors*

S *Severity of symptoms*

It is as important to record expected findings, both what the patient tells you and what you observe, as it is to record the unexpected. Any physical finding that can change with age, disease, or pathologic condition should be described in its present state. Detectable changes can then be better compared and documented in the future. If details of a patient's history and examination are not recorded, clues about health changes over time are lost.

Subjective Data

One way to record expected findings is to indicate the absence of symptoms—for example, "no vomiting, diarrhea, or constipation."

Unexpected findings should be described by their quality or character. Indicating the presence of pain without providing characteristics (timing, location, severity, quality) is not useful, either for future comparison or for determining the extent of the present problem. The severity of pain may be recorded on a scale of 1 to 10, with 0 indicating no pain and 10 representing the most pain ever felt by the patient. The severity of pain may also be described by its interference with activity. Note whether the patient is able to continue regular activity in spite of pain, or if it is necessary to decrease or stop all activity until pain subsides (see Appendix A).

Objective Data

Relate physical findings to the processes of inspection, palpation, auscultation, and percussion, making clear the process of detection so confusion does not occur. For example, "no masses on palpation" may be stated when recording abdominal findings. Details about expected objective findings should be included as well, such as, "tympanic membranes pearly gray, translucent, light reflex and bony landmarks present, mobility to positive and negative pressure bilaterally." Accurate description of unexpected objective findings should also be provided. Suggestions for recording the character and quality of objective findings follow.

Location of findings. Use topographic and anatomic landmarks to add precision to your description of findings. Indicating the liver span measurement at the midclavicular line enables future comparison, since measurement at this location can be replicated. The location of the apical impulse is commonly described by both a topographic landmark (the midsternal line) and an anatomic landmark (a specific intercostal space)—for example, "the apical impulse is 4 cm from the midsternal line at the fifth intercostal space."

In some cases, location of a finding on or near a specific structure (tympanic membrane, rectum, vaginal vestibule) may be described by its position on a clock. It is important that others recognize the same landmarks for the 12 o'clock reference point. For rectal findings use the anterior midline, and for vaginal vestibule findings (Bartholin glands, episiotomy scar) use the clitoris.

Incremental grading. Findings that vary by degrees are customarily graded or recorded in an incremental scale format. Pulse amplitude, heart murmur intensity, muscle strength, and deep tendon reflexes are findings often recorded in this manner. In addition, retinal vessel changes and prostate size are sometimes graded similarly. See the chapters in which these examination techniques are discussed for the grading system used to describe the findings.

Organs, masses, and lesions. For organs or any type of mass, such as an enlarged lymph node, or skin lesion, the following characteristics, which are noted through inspection and palpation, are described:

- Texture or consistency: smooth, soft, firm, nodular, granular, fibrous, matted
- Size: recorded in centimeters on two diameters, plus height if the lesion is elevated; future changes in the lesion size can then be accurately detected. (This is more precise than comparing the lesion's size to fruit or nuts, which have different dimensions.)
- Shape or configuration: annular, linear, tubular, elliptical
- Mobility: moves freely under skin or fixed to overlying skin or underlying tissue
- Tenderness
- Induration
- Heat
- Color: hyperpigmentation or hypopigmentation, redness or erythema, or the specific color of the lesion
- Location
- Other characteristics may include oozing, bleeding, discharge, scab formation, scarring, excoriation

Discharge. Regardless of the orifice, discharge is described by color and consistency (clear, serous, mucoid, white, green, yellow, purulent, bloody or sanguinous), odor, and amount (minimal, moderate, copious).

Teeth. The American Dental Association sequential numbering system is used to designate missing, filled, and carious teeth (Figure 24-1). Numbers for 1 to 32 are used,

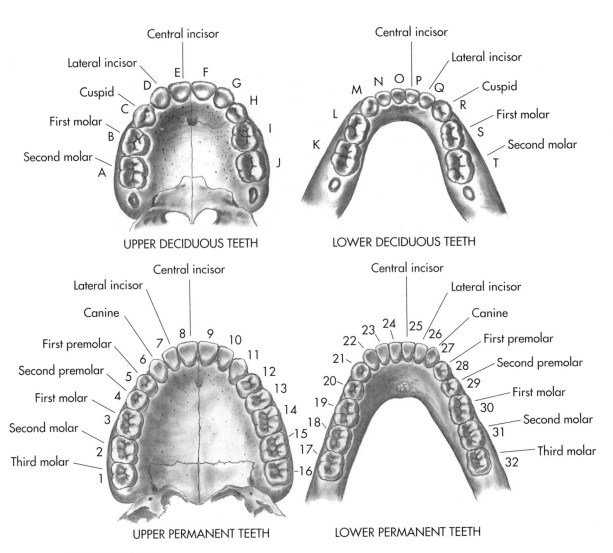

FIGURE 24-1
Tooth identification using either name or American Dental Association numbering system; letters for deciduous teeth, numbers for permanent teeth.

FIGURE 24-2
Illustration of the location of a breast mass.

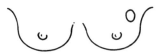

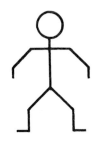

FIGURE 24-3
Illustration of a stick person.

with number 1 being the third molar in the patient's right maxilla. Numbering is sequential around the entire maxilla and then continues in the left mandible third molar. Letters are used for deciduous teeth. If preferred, the tooth name may also be used for recording dental information.

Illustrations. Drawings can sometimes provide a better description than words and should be used when appropriate. You do not have to be an artist to communicate information. Illustrations are particularly useful in describing the origin of pain and where it radiates and the size, shape, and location of a lesion (Figure 24-2). Stick figures are useful to compare findings in extremities, such as pulse amplitude and deep tendon reflex response (Figure 24-3).

PROBLEM-ORIENTED MEDICAL RECORD

The Problem-Oriented Medical Record (POMR) is one format commonly used to organize patient data for long-term health care management. The POMR format provides a well-organized record that reflects and facilitates sound clinical thinking and decision making. It documents the problem assessment process, describes plans made and actions taken to address these problems, lists the information and education provided to the patient, and describes the patient's response to care provided. The consistent recording format enables more effective communication and coordination among professionals caring for the patient.

There are six components of the POMR:

- Comprehensive health history
- Complete physical examination
- Problem list
- Assessment and plan
- Baseline and problem-directed laboratory and radiologic studies
- Progress notes

COMPREHENSIVE HEALTH HISTORY AND PHYSICAL EXAMINATION

The comprehensive health history must include all data collected, both positive and negative, that contribute directly to your assessment. Arrange the history in chronologic order, starting with the current episode and then filling in relevant background information. Arrange the physical examination findings in the order and style preferred by the health agency. Follow a consistent order. This allows future readers, and you, to find specific points of information. It also enables you to quickly remember key components for assessment on each encounter.

Make your headings clear, using indentations and spacing to accentuate your organization. Underline important points. Use short phrases for descriptions, saving time and space by omitting superfluous words. Use only those common abbreviations and symbols approved by the health care agency. (See Appendix H for some commonly used abbreviations).

PROBLEM LIST

The problem list is created after the subjective and objective information have been organized. All pertinent data and positive examination findings, laboratory data, and prior diagnoses are reviewed to develop a problem list in the form of a running log with the following information: problem number, date of onset, description of problem, and date problem was resolved or became an inactive concern.

A problem may be defined as anything that will require further evaluation or attention. A problem may be related to any of the following:

- A firmly established diagnosis (e.g., diabetes mellitus, hypertension)
- A new symptom or physical finding of unknown etiology or significance (e.g., right knee effusion)
- Unexpected and new findings revealed by laboratory tests (e.g., cardiomegaly on chest radiograph)
- Personal or social difficulties (e.g., unemployment, homelessness)
- Risk factors for serious conditions (e.g., smoking, family history of coronary artery disease)
- Factors crucial to remember long term (e.g., allergy to penicillin)

This list enables all health professionals to quickly assess the patient's history by the summary presented on this list. Problems may be listed in chronological order, according to the severity of problem, or in the order of presentation over time. Once problems are numbered, that numbering is not changed. When a problem is resolved, a line may be drawn through the row on the chart and the date of resolution is added to the last column. Surgical correction of a condition is one example of a resolved problem.

ASSESSMENT

Develop an assessment for each problem on the Problem List. Begin the process of making a differential diagnosis by discussing and giving priority to possible causes and contributing factors for a problem or symptom. Present the rationale for the potential causes and validate the assessment from data contained in the comprehensive health history, physical examination, consultations, and any laboratory data available. Explain why a serious potential cause is no longer under consideration.

Describe any pertinent negative information when other portions of the history or physical examination suggest that an abnormality might exist or develop in an area. Avoid the use of words such as *normal* or *within normal limits,* because they do not describe what is inspected, palpated, percussed, or auscultated. Be as objective as possible. Assessment may include anticipated potential problems such as complications or progression of the disease.

PLAN

Develop a plan for each problem on the Problem List. The plan is divided into three sections: diagnostics (Dx), therapeutics (Rx), and patient education (Pt. Ed.).
- Dx: list the diagnostic tests to be performed or ordered.
- Rx: describe the therapeutic treatment plan; provide a rationale for any change or addition to an established treatment plan.
- Pt. Ed.: describe health education provided or planned. Include materials dispensed and evidence of the patient's understanding or lack thereof. List any referrals initiated with purpose and to whom the referral is made. State the target date for reevaluating the plan.

PROGRESS NOTES

MNEMONICS

FOLLOW-UP VISIT NOTE
Carefully review all SOAP notes on a regular basis to detect the emergence of a condition that accounts for many or all of the patient's complaints.

S *Subjective*

O *Objective*

A *Assessment*

P *Plan*

Follow-up visits for problems identified in the POMR are recorded with the progress notes. After the database has been completed through the construction of the POMR, subsequent visits are much briefer. The patient is known to you and the facility, so recording is primarily updated information.

Each problem is addressed by number and name. An interval history, including subjective status of the problem, current medications, and review of systems related to the problem are presented in the subjective portion of the note. The objective portion includes vital signs, a record of any physical examination performed at the time of the visit, and results of laboratory data or radiographic studies performed since the last visit.

The assessment section includes your assessment of the problem status. If the problem was formerly a symptom, such as shortness of breath, you may have enough data to make a diagnosis. The rationale for the diagnosis is presented in this section, and the problem list is updated accordingly.

Plans are presented in the three components: diagnostics, therapeutics, and patient education.

PROBLEM-ORIENTED MEDICAL RECORD FORMAT

THE HISTORY

The patient's history, especially for an initial visit, provides a comprehensive data base. Information should be recorded appropriately in specific categories, usually in a particular sequence. The following organized sequence, which includes the appropriate information to record, will guide you in writing a POMR.

Identifying Information

The patient's name, date of birth, and an assigned history number are the first items of information recorded. Most health agencies have forms with headings for each category of information to be recorded.

Problem List

Although the problem list itself is added to the record after the subjective and objective information have been organized, the printed POMR form provides space for this information at the beginning of the record where it can be reviewed at a glance by medical personnel. The problem list is an ongoing record of a patient's medical problems that is added to, as appropriate, after each visit.

Each problem is given a number. The date of onset is recorded along with a brief description of the problem, and space is also provided to record the date that the problem was resolved or became an inactive concern.

General Patient Information

Additional identifying information for each patient includes address, home phone number, social security number, employer, position or title, business address and phone number, sex, marital status, and health insurance company name and member identification number.

Source and Reliability of Information

Document the historian's identity, that is, the patient or the person's relationship to the patient. Indicate when the old record is used. State your judgment about the reliability of the historian's information.

Chief Complaint

The chief complaint is a brief description of the patient's main reason(s) for seeking care, stated verbatim in quotation marks. Include duration of problem.

History of Present Illness

This section contains a detailed description of the problem. It includes a description of all symptoms that may be related to the chief complaint, and it describes the problem chronologically, dating events and symptoms. When describing the present illness, it is important for the examiner to record the absence of certain symptoms commonly associated with the particular area, or system, involved. Also inquire about anyone in the household with the same symptoms or possible exposure to infection or toxic agents. If pertinent to the present illness, include relevant information from the review of systems, family history, and personal/social history. When more than one problem is identified, address each problem in a separate paragraph. Include the following details of each symptom's occurrence, described in narrative form by categories:

- Onset: when problem or symptom first started; setting and circumstances (while exercising, sleeping, working, etc.); manner of the onset (sudden vs. gradual)
- Location: exact location of pain (localized, generalized, radiation patterns)
- Duration: length of problem or episode; if intermittent, include the duration of each episode
- Character: nature of pain (stabbing, burning, sharp, dull, gnawing)
- Aggravating and associated factors: food, activity, rest, certain movements; nausea, vomiting, diarrhea, fever, chills

- Relieving factors: food, rest, activity, position; prescribed and/or self remedies; effect on the problem
- Temporal factors: frequency of occurrence (single attack, intermittent, chronic); describe typical attack; change in symptom improvement or worsening over time
- Severity of the symptoms: (0-10 scale), effect on lifestyle, work performance

Past Medical History

The past medical history includes general health and strength over the patient's lifetime as the patient perceives it. List and describe each of the following with dates of occurrence and any specific information available:

- Hospitalizations and/or surgery: dates, hospital, diagnosis, complications; injuries and disabilities
- Major childhood illnesses: measles, mumps, whooping cough, chickenpox, smallpox, scarlet fever, rheumatic fever, diphtheria, polio
- Adult illnesses: tuberculosis, hepatitis, diabetes mellitus, hypertension, myocardial infarction, tropical or parasitic diseases, other infections
- Immunizations: polio, diphtheria, pertussis, tetanus toxoid, hepatitis, measles, mumps, rubella, hemophilus influenza, influenza, cholera, typhus, typhoid, BCG, last PPD or other skin tests, unusual reaction to immunizations
- Medications: past, current, and recent medications (dosage, home remedies, nonprescription medications)
- Allergies: drugs, foods, environmental allergens,
- Transfusions: reason, date, and number of units transfused; reaction
- Emotional status: mood disorders, psychiatric attention or medications

Family Medical History

Include a genogram (with at least 3 generations). If it is not part of the genogram, include a family history of major health or genetic disorders (hypertension, cancer, cardiac, respiratory, kidney, strokes, or thyroid disorders; asthma or other allergic manifestations; blood dyscrasias; psychiatric difficulties; tuberculosis; rheumatologic diseases; diabetes mellitus; hepatitis; or other familial disorders). Spontaneous abortions and stillbirths suggest genetic problems.

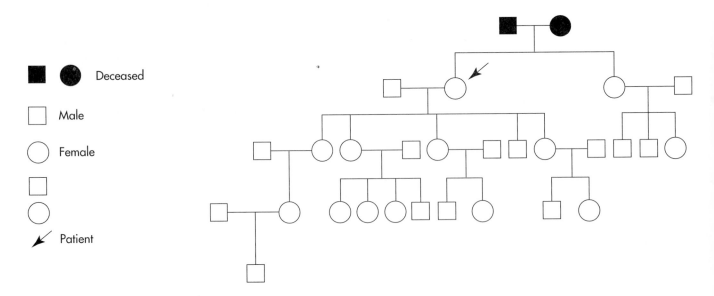

Personal/Social History

The information included in this section varies according to the concerns of the patient and the influence of the health problem on the patient's life.

- Cultural background and practices, birthplace, where raised, home environment as youth, education, position in family, marital status, general life satisfaction, hobbies, interests, sources of stress; religious preference: determine any religious proscriptions concerning medical care
- Economic condition, housing, number in household
- Occupation: usual work and present work if different, list of job changes, work conditions and hours, physical or mental strain, duration of employment, present and past exposure to heat and cold, industrial toxins, protective devices required or used
- Environment: home, school, work, structural barriers if handicapped, community services utilized; travel and other exposure to contagious diseases, residence in tropics, water and milk supply, other sources of infection when applicable
- Current health habits and/or risk factors: exercise; smoking (packs per day/duration); salt intake; obesity/weight control; alcohol intake: beer, wine, hard liquor (amount/day), duration; CAGE question responses; blackouts, seizures, or DTs; drug or alcohol treatment program or support group; recreational drugs used (e.g., marijuana, cocaine, heroin, LSD, PCP, etc.) and methods (injection, sniffing, smoking, or use of shared needles).
- Exposure to chemicals, toxins, poisons, asbestos, or radioactive material at home or work and duration; caffeine use: cups/glasses/day.
- Sexual activity: contraceptive or barrier protection method used; past sexually transmitted disease (syphilis, gonorrhea, chlamydia, PID, herpes, warts, other); treatment.

REVIEW OF SYSTEMS

- General constitutional symptoms: fever, chills, malaise, easily fatigued, night sweats, weight (average, preferred, present, change)
- Diet: appetite, likes and dislikes, restrictions (because of religion, allergy, or other disease), vitamins and other supplement, caffeine-containing beverages (coffee, tea, cola); food diary or daily listing of food intake as needed
- Skin, hair, and nails: rash or eruption, itching, pigmentation or texture change; excessive sweating, unusual nail or hair growth
- Head and neck: frequent or unusual headaches, their location, dizziness, syncope, severe head injuries; loss of consciousness (momentary or prolonged)
- Eyes: visual acuity, blurring, double vision, light sensitivity, pain, change in appearance or vision; use of glasses/contacts, eye drops or other medication used; history of trauma, glaucoma, or familial eye disease
- Ears: hearing loss, pain, discharge tinnitus, vertigo
- Nose: sense of smell, frequency of colds, obstruction, nose bleeds, postnasal discharge, sinus pain
- Throat and mouth: hoarseness or change in voice; frequent sore throats, bleeding or swelling of gums; recent tooth abscesses or extraction; soreness of tongue or buccal mucosa, ulcers; disturbance of taste
- Endocrine: Thyroid enlargement or tenderness, heat or cold intolerance, unexplained weight change, polydipsia, polyuria, changes in facial or body hair, increased hat and glove size, skin striae
  - Males: puberty onset, erections, emissions, testicular pain, libido, infertility

- Females: onset of menses, regularity, duration, and amount of flow; dysmenorrhea; last period; intermenstrual discharge or bleeding; itching; date of last Pap smear; age at menopause; libido; frequency of intercourse; sexual difficulties; infertility; gravidity and parity (G = # of pregnancies, T = # of term pregnancies, P = # of preterm pregnancies, A = # of abortions/miscarriages, L = # of living children); number and duration of each pregnancy, delivery method; complications during any pregnancy or postpartum period; use of oral or other contraceptives.
- Breasts: pain, tenderness, discharge, lumps, galactorrhea, mammograms (screening or diagnostic), frequency of breast self-examination
- Chest and lungs: pain related to respiration, dyspnea, cyanosis, wheezing, cough, sputum (character and quantity), hemoptysis, night sweats, exposure to tuberculosis; last chest x-ray
- Heart and blood vessels: chest pain or distress, precipitating causes, timing and duration, relieving factors, palpitations, dyspnea, orthopnea (number of pillows), edema, claudication, hypertension, previous myocardial infarction, exercise tolerance, past cardiac tests
- Hematologic: anemia, tendency to bruise or bleed easily, thromboses, thrombophlebitis, any known blood cell disorder, transfusions
- Lymphatic: enlargement, tenderness, suppuration
- Gastrointestinal: appetite, digestion, intolerance of any foods, dysphagia, heartburn, nausea, vomiting, hematemesis, bowel regularity, constipation, diarrhea, change in stool color or contents (clay, tarry, fresh blood, mucus, undigested food), flatulence, hemorrhoids, hepatitis, jaundice, dark urine; history of ulcer, gallstones, polyps, tumor; previous radiographic studies (where, when, findings)
- Genitourinary: dysuria, flank or suprapubic pain, urgency, frequency, nocturia, hematuria, polyuria, hesitancy, dribbling, loss in force of stream, passage of stone; edema of face, stress incontinence, hernias, sexually transmitted disease
- Musculoskeletal: joint stiffness, pain, restriction of motion, swelling, redness, heat, bony deformity
- Neurologic: syncope, seizures, weakness or paralysis, problems with sensation or coordination, tremors
- Psychiatric: depression, mood changes, difficulty concentrating, nervousness, tension, suicidal thoughts, irritability, sleep disturbances

PHYSICAL EXAMINATION FINDINGS

The objective data are usually recorded by body systems and anatomic location. Begin with a general statement about the overall health status of the patient. All observations of physical signs should be described in the appropriate body system or region, usually organized in sequence from head to toe. Take care to describe findings in detail rather than make diagnostic statements.

List each anatomic location or body system as a separate category, using the groupings customary for your institution. The findings generally included in each category are listed below.

General Statement

- Age, race, sex, general appearance
- Weight, height, frame size, body mass index
- Vital signs: temperature, pulse rate, respiratory rate, blood pressure (2 arms, 2 positions)

Mental Status

- Physical appearance and behavior
- Cognitive: consciousness level, response to questions, reasoning, arithmetic ability, memory, attention span; specific mental test scores
- Emotional stability: depression, anxiety, disturbance in thought content, hallucinations
- Speech and language: voice quality, articulation, coherence, comprehension

Skin

- Color, uniformity, integrity, texture, temperature, turgor, hygiene, tattoos, scars
- Presence of edema, moisture, excessive perspiration, unusual odor, mobility
- Presence and description of lesions (size, shape, location, configuration, blanching, inflammation, tenderness, induration, discharge), parasites, trauma
- Hair texture, distribution, color, quality
- Nail configuration, color, texture, condition, nail base angle, ridging, beading, pitting, peeling, nail plate firmness, adherence to nail bed

Head

- Size and contour of head, scalp appearance, head position
- Symmetry and spacing of facial features, tics, characteristic facies
- Presence of edema or puffiness
- Temporal arteries: thickening, hardness, tenderness, bruits

Eyes

- Visual acuity (near, distant, peripheral)
- Appearance of orbits (edema, sagging tissue, puffiness), firmness of eyeball, conjunctivae, sclerae, eyelids (redness, flakiness, fasciculations, ptosis), eyebrows
- Extraocular movements, corneal light reflex, cover-uncover test, nystagmus
- Pupillary shape, consensual response to light and accommodation, depth of anterior chamber
- Ophthalmoscopic findings of cornea, lens, retina, red reflex, optic disc and macula characteristics, retinal vessel size, caliber, and arteriovenous (AV) crossings

Ears

- Configuration, position, and alignment of auricles, nodules, tenderness of auricles or in mastoid area
- Otoscopic findings of canals (cerumen, lesions, discharge, foreign body) and tympanic membranes (integrity, color, landmarks, mobility)
- Hearing: Weber and Rinne tests, other stimuli

Nose

- Appearance of external nose, nasal patency
- Presence of discharge, crusting, flaring, polyp
- Appearance of turbinates, alignment of septum
- Presence of sinus tenderness (by palpation or percussion), swelling
- Discrimination of odors

Throat and Mouth

- Number, occlusion, and condition of teeth; missing teeth; presence of dental appliances

- Characteristics of lips, tongue, buccal and oral mucosa, and floor of mouth (color, moisture, surface characteristics, symmetry, induration)
- Appearance of oropharynx, tonsils, palate
- Symmetry and movement of tongue, soft palate, and uvula; gag reflex
- Discrimination of taste

Neck

- Fullness, mobility, suppleness, and strength
- Position of trachea, tracheal tug, movement of hyoid bone and cartilages with swallowing
- Thyroid size, shape, nodules, tenderness, bruits
- Presence of masses, webbing, skin folds

Chest

- Size and shape of chest, anteroposterior versus transverse diameter, symmetry of movement with respiration, superficial venous patterns
- Presence of retractions, use of accessory muscles
- Diaphragmatic excursion

Lungs

- Respiratory rate, depth, regularity, quietness or ease of respiration
- Palpation findings: symmetry and quality of tactile fremitus
- Percussion findings: quality and symmetry of percussion notes
- Auscultation findings: characteristics of breath sounds, (intensity, pitch, duration, quality, vesicular, bronchial, bronchovesicular, adventitious breath sounds), phase and location where audible
- Characteristics of cough
- Presence of friction rub, egophony, bronchophony, whispered pectoriloquy, vocal resonance

Breasts

- Size, contour, symmetry, supernumerary nipples, venous patterns
- Tissue consistency, presence of masses, scars, tenderness, thickening, retractions or dimpling
- Characteristics of nipples and areolae (inversion, eversion, retraction), discharge

Heart

- Anatomic location of apical impulse
- Heart rate, rhythm, contour and symmetry of apical impulse and pulse in extremities
- Palpation findings: pulsations, thrills, heaves, or lifts
- Auscultation findings: characteristics of S_1 and S_2 (location, intensity, pitch, timing, splitting, systole, diastole)
- Presence of murmurs, clicks, snaps, S_3 or S_4. Description by timing, location, radiation, intensity, pitch, quality, variation with respiration

Blood Vessels

- Amplitude, symmetry of pulses in extremities
- Jugular vein pulsations and distension, pressure measurement; jugular vein and carotid artery pulse waves

- Presence of bruits over carotid, temporal, renal, iliac, and femoral arteries, abdominal aorta
- Temperature, color, hair distribution, skin texture, muscle atrophy, nail beds of lower extremities
- Presence of edema, swelling, vein distention, varicosities, Homans sign, tenderness of lower extremities or along superficial vein

Abdomen

- Shape, contour, visible aorta pulsations, surface motion, venous patterns, hernia or separation of muscles
- Auscultation findings: presence and character of bowel sounds in all quadrants, friction rub over liver or spleen
- Palpation findings: aorta, organs, feces, masses; location, size, contour, consistency, tenderness, muscle resistance
- Percussion findings: tone in each quadrant, areas of different percussion notes, costovertebral angle (CVA) tenderness, liver span

Male Genitalia

- Appearance of external genitalia, penis (symmetry, circumcision status, unusual thickening, smegma, color, texture, location and size of urethral opening, discharge), urethral discharge with stripping, lesions, distribution of pubic hair
- Palpation findings: penis, testes, epididymides, vasa deferentia, contour, consistency, tenderness
- Presence of hernia or scrotal swelling, transillumination findings

Female Genitalia

- Appearance of external genitalia and perineum, distribution of pubic hair, tenderness, scarring, discharge, inflammation, irritation, lesions, caruncle, polyps
- Internal examination findings: appearance of vaginal mucosa, cervix (color, position, surface characteristics, shape of os), discharge, odor
- Bimanual examination findings: size, contour, and position of uterus, tenderness and mobility of cervix, uterus, adnexae, and ovaries (size, shape, consistency, tenderness)
- Recto vaginal examination findings
- Urinary incontinence when patient bears down

Anus and Rectum

- Sphincter tone and control, presence of hemorrhoids, fissures, skin tags, pilonidal dimpling, hair tufts, inflammation, excoriation
- Rectal wall contour, tenderness
- Prostate size, contour, consistency, mobility
- Color and consistency of stool

Lymphatic System

- Presence of lymph nodes in head, neck, clavicular, epitrochlear, axillary, or inguinal areas
- Size, shape, warmth, tenderness, mobility, consistency (matted or discreteness of nodes)
- Redness or streaks in localized area

Musculoskeletal System

- Posture: alignment of extremities and spine, symmetry of body parts

- Symmetry of muscle mass, tone, strength, grading of strength; fasciculation, spasms
- Range of motion (active and passive), presence of pain with movement
- Appearance of joints: presence of deformities, tenderness, crepitus, swelling

Neurologic System

- Cranial nerves: specific findings for each or specify those tested, if findings are recorded in head and neck sections
- Gait (posture, rhythm, sequence of stride and arm movements)
- Balance, coordination with rapid alternating motions
- Sensory function: presence and symmetry of response to pain, touch, vibration, temperature stimuli; monofilament test
- Superficial and deep tendon reflexes: symmetry, grade; ankle clonus

ASSESSMENT (FOR EACH PROBLEM ON PROBLEM LIST)

The diagnosis with rationale, derived from the subjective and objective data, is stated. If a diagnosis cannot yet be made, differential diagnoses are prioritized. Assessment includes anticipated potential problems, if appropriate (complications, progression of disease, sequelae, etc.).

PLAN (FOR EACH PROBLEM ON PROBLEM LIST)

- Diagnostic tests performed or ordered
- Therapeutic treatment plan, including changes or additions to the established treatment plan with rationale
- Patient education: health education provided or planned; materials such as handouts/pamphlets dispensed; evidence of patient's understanding (or lack or understanding); counseling
- Referrals initiated (including to whom the patient is referred to and the purpose)
- Target dates for reevaluating the results of the plan

INFANTS

The organizational structure for recording the history and physical examination of newborns and infants is the same as for adults. The recorded information varies from the adult's primarily because of the developmental status of the infant. With newborns the focus is on their transition to extrauterine life and the detection of any congenital anomalies. *Specific additions to the history and physical examination are listed below.*

History

Present problem. For older infants, record information as for adults; however, for newborns include the details of the mother's pregnancy and any events occurring since birth.

Details of pregnancy. Weeks of gestation, prenatal care, mother's illnesses, x-ray exposure, drugs taken, bleeding, hypertension, diabetes, weight gained, planned pregnancy, complications of pregnancy.

Infant's status at birth. Respiratory status, color, Apgar scores if known; nutrition; nursery care needed.

Past medical history. There is no past medical history for newborns. Older infants should have prenatal and neonatal events added to this category, unless this information is directly related to the present problem.

Family history. Focus on congenital anomalies and hereditary disorders in the family.

Personal/social history. Focus on the newborn's and infant's family structure, number of siblings, presence of both parents, stresses of new infant in family, arrangements for infant care, and mother's plans to return to work.

Growth and development. Placement of this information is variable by agency or according to the purpose of the examination. For the infant with no growth or development problems, it may be recorded as either history or review of systems, or it may be a separate category. When a problem with growth or development is apparent, the information will be recorded in the section for the present problem. Passing or failing of the Denver II would be recorded with objective data.

Developmental milestones. List developmental milestones with the age at which they are attained.

Current motor and interaction abilities. Specify current attainments unless the Denver II is used, in which case this information is repetitive.

Injury prevention. List parents' efforts to consistently prevent injuries.

Diet. Placement of this information varies by institution; it may appear in the present illness or review of systems, or it may be a separate category.

Breast-fed infants. Note the frequency; use of supplemental feedings and vitamins; mother's diet, fluid intake, concern with milk supply, and any problems with nipple soreness, cracking, or infections.

Formula-fed infants. Note the specific formula and preparation method, concentration and amount of water added, frequency of feeding, amount per feeding, total ounces per day, and whether juice, water, or vitamins are given.

Solid foods. Note the age at which cereal and other foods were introduced; specifics about feeding methods, amount, food preparation; and the response of infant to foods.

Physical Examination Findings

General
- Age in hours, days, weeks, or months; gender; race
- Gestational age
- Length, weight, and head circumference with percentiles; for newborns note percentiles for gestational age
- Infant state during examination (irritable, crying, sleeping, alert, quiet)

Skin
- Color, texture, presence of lanugo or vernix, Mongolian spot, nails
- Presence of hemangiomas, nevi, telangiectasia, milia

Lymphatic
- Visible or palpable lymph nodes

Head
- Shape, molding, forceps or electrode marks
- Fontanel sizes, swelling
- Transillumination

Eyes
- Red reflex, corneal light reflex, follows object with eyes
- Swelling of lids, discharge

Ears
- Shape and alignment of auricles, presence of skin tags or pits
- Startle to noise or response to voice

Nose
- Patency of nares, nasal flaring, discharge

Mouth
- Palate and lip integrity
- Presence and number of teeth
- Strength of sucking, coordinated sucking and swallowing

Neck
- Head position, neck control
- Presence of masses, webbing, excess skinfolds

Chest and lungs
- Symmetry of shape, circumference
- Breast swelling or discharge
- Abdominal or thoracic breathing
- Presence of retractions (intercostal, supraclavicular, substernal), presence of grunting or stridor
- Quality of cry

Heart and blood vessels
- No variations in manner of recording; however, peripheral vascular findings are often integrated in this section

Abdomen
- Number of umbilical arteries and veins, stump dryness, color, odor
- Any bulging or separation of abdominal wall
- Apparent peristaltic waves

Male genitalia
- Appearance of penis, scrotum; position of urethra
- Location of testes: descended, descendable, do not descend, not palpable
- Urinary stream
- Presence of hernia or hydrocele

Female genitalia
- Appearance of labia, presence of discharge

Anus, rectum
- Perforate, sphincter control
- Character of meconium or stool, if observed
- Presence of pilonidal dimple

Musculoskeletal system
- Alignment of limbs and spine
- Presence of joint deformity, fixed or flexible; integrity of clavicles
- Symmetry of movement in all extremities, hip abduction
- Number of fingers and toes, webbing or extra digits, palmar creases

Neurologic system
- Presence and symmetry of primitive reflexes
- Consolability, presence of tremors or jitteriness
- Gross and fine motor development

CHILDREN & ADOLESCENTS

As during infancy, some adaptations in recorded history reflect the developmental progress of the child. *Such modifications in recording the child's history are discussed next.*

History

Past medical history. Prenatal and neonatal history is less important as the child gets older. Birth weight and major neonatal problems are generally included in the history of an initial examination until the child reaches school age. If a health problem can be related to birth events, more detail is recorded, often summarized from old records, because the mother's recall may not be as accurate as time elapses.

Personal/social history. Record how the child gets along with parents, siblings, and other children; his or her behavior in group situations; and any evidence of family problems. Describe prevention strategies used by child and family.

For older children, record school performance: grade level, progress, adjustment to school, and the parents' attitude toward education. Note any habits of the child, such as nail biting or thumb sucking, and hobbies, sports participation, clubs, and temperament.

For adolescents, add peer group activities, conflicts, sexual activity, concerns with identity and independence, self-esteem, and favorite activities.

Growth and development

For toddlers and young children, list motor skills and language milestones attained, age toilet trained, and age weaned from bottle.

Physical examination findings. The physical findings are recorded in the same format used for adults and infants. Some additional notations related to development include the following:

Breasts. For females, record the Tanner stage of breast development.

Genitalia. Record the Tanner stage of pubic hair and genital development as appropriate. Record the sexual maturity rating.

Neurologic system. Findings should indicate developmental expectations of mental status, cerebellar function, cranial nerves, and deep tendon reflexes.

PREGNANT WOMEN

The organizational structure of the record does not vary from that of other adults. *However, information about the pregnancy is added, and some aspects of the examination are modified.*

History

Identifying information. List the gravidity and parity along with other routinely recorded information.

Obstetric history. This additional history category should provide information on previous pregnancies and their outcomes.

Personal/social history. In addition to the information usually obtained, include the adjustment to the pregnancy by the woman and her significant others, information about whether pregnancy was planned, acceptance by the father and family, any history of abuse, and support available to the mother and child after delivery.

Physical Examination Findings

Abdomen
- Status of the pregnancy, fundal height in relation to dates
- Fetal heart rate, position, well-being, fetal movement

Pelvic region
- Pelvic measurements
- Uterine size

During late pregnancy and labor. Note the centimeters of dilation and effacement, the station of the fetus, and the position of the fetal head or presenting part.

OLDER ADULTS

The organizational structure, again, does not vary from that recorded for other adults. *A few modifications in aspects of the history and physical examination are made, as described next.*

History

Personal/social history. Describe the community and family support systems. Add the functional assessment of ability to prepare meals, manage personal affairs, and engage in social and other meaningful activities.

Physical Examination Findings

General assessment
- Extra time to assume positions for physical examination
- Position modifications needed for specific systems

Skin
- Presence of common lesions of older age
- Character and color of hair, baldness patterns

Chest and lungs
- Change in chest shape and percussion tones
- Effect of chest shape on respiratory status

Heart and blood vessels
- Location of the apical pulse
- Characteristics of superficial vessels and distal pulses

Musculoskeletal system
- Posture and muscle mass changes
- Functional assessment of mobility, muscle strength, and fine motor movements

Neurologic system
- Functional assessment of cognitive function, memory, and reasoning and calculation
- Gait and balance

SAMPLE RECORDS

Information must be recorded as precisely as possible. Colorful language or expressive metaphors can be used, but select words for the patient's history carefully, because some words may have different implications. Health professionals have commonly used the term "denies" when a patient reports that no symptom has occurred. The term "denies" may imply a confrontational or unproductive relationship. It is better to write either "reports no" or "indicates no" symptoms, statements that more positively record the patient's cooperation in providing needed information.

AMBULATORY ADULT

See the sample record for the ambulatory adult on pp. 879-884.

Progress Notes

Follow-up visits for problems identified in the POMR are recorded via progress notes. After the data base has been completed through the construction of the POMR, recording of subsequent visits is much briefer. The patient is known to you or the facility, so recording is primarily updating information.

Each problem is addressed by number and name. An interval history, including subjective status of the problem, current medications, and the review of systems related to the problem, are presented in the subjective portion of the note. The objective portion includes vital signs and a record of any physical examination performed at the time of the visit and results of laboratory data or radiographic studies performed since the last visit.

The assessment section includes your assessment of the status of the problem. If the problem was formerly a symptom, i.e., shortness of breath, and you now have determined that the patient is asthmatic, your rationale for this diagnosis is presented in this section and the problem list is updated accordingly.

Plans are presented for each problem with the three components: diagnostics, therapeutics, and patient education.

Text continued on p. 885.

Name: Martha Smith   **Date:** 11-30-98

Date of Birth: 5-22-43

History Number: 54970B

PROBLEM LIST:

Problem #	Onset (date)	Problem	Inactive/resolved (date)
1	5/98	Pain and stiffness hands bilat	
2	1988	Seasonal rhinitis	
3	1983	s/p Total abd. hysterectomy with oophorectomy	
4		Family history diabetes	
5		Family history Alzheimer disease	
6		Family history glaucoma	

General Patient Information

Address: 841 Foxtrail Drive
St. Louis, MO 63146

Home phone: 555-6423
Social security number: 111-11-1111

Employer: Memorial Hospital

Position/title: Registered Nurse

Business address: 1050 Randolph Ctr.
Hometown, MO 66666

Business phone: 747-0000

Age: 55

Martial status: Married

Sex: Female

Health insurance provider: Aetna

Member # X45789

SOURCE AND RELIABILITY OF INFORMATION

Self—very reliable historian
Old record

CHIEF COMPLAINT

Time for annual examination. Has noticed pain in hands when doing needlework.

PRESENT PROBLEM

Pain and stiffness in fingers and hands, began about 6 months ago but seems to be increasing in severity and with shorter time of activity. Dull, aching pain now occurs after 15 minutes of needlepoint or crocheting, right hand more than left hand. Pain ranges between 2 and 4 on a 10-point severity scale. Usually resolves with rest. Some stiffness in morning but does not currently interfere with ability to perform all job and household activities. Uses aspirin (650 mg q 4 hr) when pain does not resolve with rest; effective relief. Has not tried heat or ice. No other systematic symptoms such as fatigue, fever, or weight loss. No other joints affected.

PAST MEDICAL HISTORY

Generally healthy

Hospitalizations, Illnesses, and Injuries. *Hysterectomy for fibroids in 1983, usual childhood illnesses, no major adult illnesses, auto accident 1988 without major injury.*

Previous Health Care. *Annual physical, hepatitis B vaccine × 32 years ago, Td booster 5 years ago, oral polio vaccine series in 1972, dental care q 4 months, vision exam q year. Pap smear and mammogram 6 months ago with no problems detected, 2 pregnancies (1965 and 1969), both vaginal delivery without complications.*

Allergies. *Hay fever in spring, no food or drug allergies known, no reaction to blood transfusion in 1983 (type A + blood).*

Family History. *See genogram below. No history of cancer, tuberculosis, blood dyscrasias, or respiratory, renal, thyroid, or psychiatric disorders.*

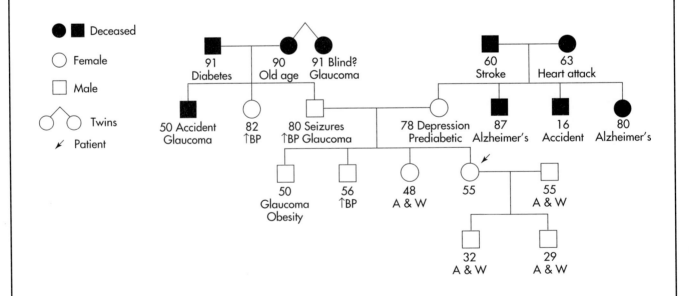

PERSONAL/SOCIAL HISTORY

Lives with husband, a psychologist in private practice, in 3-bedroom home in well-maintained neighborhood. Works as RN in hospital clinic 3 days a week. Has 2 sons, both married with 2 children each. Visits each at least once a month. Both parents still living, in retirement home in town, visits them 2 to 3 times a week. Active in church and local arts and crafts group. Needlepoint and crocheting main hobbies.

Current Health Habits. *Walks dog daily about 1/2 mile; 15 lb weight gain in last 2 years, tries dieting, loses a few pounds and then stops; no smoking or recreational drug use, 2 to 3 glasses wine on weekends, 2 to 3 cups coffee and 1 glass iced tea daily.*

Diet/Nutrition. *Would like to lose 15 lbs; currently 150 lbs, 5'5"; diets sporadically; uses 1200 calorie diabetic exchange lists, usually has desired results when she persists, losing approximately 8 lb in 4 weeks; does own grocery shopping and cooking; rarely fries foods; binges on ice cream when traveling.*

REVIEW OF SYSTEMS

General Constitutional Symptoms. *No fever, chills, malaise; would like to lose 15 lbs gained over past 2 years.*

Skin, Hair, and Nails. *Several flat nevi, no change in appearance noted; bathes daily without special skin preparations; washes hair once a week, permanent and colored; nails short, crack and split frequently.*

Head and Neck. *Periodic headaches, no more than once a month, related to tension, pain up neck and back of head, relieved by aspirin. No neck tenderness or stiffness currently, has had muscle spasm in past, some pain with auto accident 6 years ago, no enlarged lymph nodes noted.*

Eyes. *Wears glasses for reading; no pain, swelling, tearing, or halos around lights. Sees optometrist yearly.*

Ears. *No change in hearing noted; no dizziness, sensitivity to noise, or pain; some pressure and popping in ears when hay fever symptoms occur, resolves with Allerest.*

Nose and Sinuses. *Hay fever in spring, postnasal drip, no problem with sense of smell. Uses Allerest for hay fever as needed.*

Mouth and Throat. *No sore throats, hoarseness, change in voice, no dental appliances, no difficulty eating or chewing food, brushes and flosses daily.*

Breasts. *No pain, tenderness, or nipple discharge; breast self-exam done when she remembers, about every 2 months; mammogram 6 months ago revealed no masses; no history of masses.*

Cardiovascular. *No difficulty performing regular activities, no shortness of breath or chest pain, last BP 126/82, no pain, tenderness, discoloration, temperature change, or swelling in extremities; wears support hose for work, some varicose veins.*

Chest and Lungs. *No history of asthma, bronchitis, or pneumonia; no breathing difficulties, cough, or pain. PPD at work 3 months ago, negative.*

Endocrine. *No history of changes in thyroid, skin, hair, or temperature preference; no polydipsia or polyuria; takes no estrogen replacement therapy.*

Hematologic. *No bleeding, excess bruising, anemia.*

Lymphatic. *No known lymph node enlargement.*

Gastrointestinal. *No diarrhea, constipation, blood in stool, or emesis; has bowel movement every other day, brown, formed, no pain; hemorrhoids during pregnancies only; indigestion occasionally after eating fried or rich foods, resolves with Gelusil. Uses no laxatives, tries to add bulk to daily food intake.*

Genitourinary. *Voids five to six times a day, light yellow; no change in odor or color, no complaint of nocturia or dysuria, good control of stream, no stress incontinence; no history of sexually transmitted disease; no known genital lesions, discharge, pain, itching, dyspareunia; satisfied with sexual activity, about twice a month.*

Musculoskeletal. No weakness, twitching, or pain other than in hands; no history of backache, fracture.

Neurologic. No problems with walking, balance, or sensations; no known changes in cognitive functioning; expresses concern with family history of Alzheimer disease and her possibility of developing the disorder.

Mental Status and Psychiatric. Coping well with stress of older parents requiring increasing care; no history of long-term depression; gets depressed and anxious occasionally about growing old, but feels this does not interfere with her ability to work or lead a productive life.

PHYSICAL EXAMINATION

General. 55-year-old white female, alert, cooperative, well groomed, communicates well, makes eye contact, and expresses appropriate concern throughout history.

> T 98.4° F, P 72, R 18
>
> BP 130/76 sitting L arm, 134/80 supine L arm, 132/78 sitting R arm
>
> Wt. 66.2 kg (150 lb), Ht. 165 cm (5¢5¢¢), about 50th percentile weight for height, medium
>   frame, BMI = 25.0

Mental Status. Oriented to time, place, and person; reasoning and arithmetic calculations intact. Memory intact, Mini-mental score 5 30; speech clear, smoothly enunciated; comprehends directions.

Skin, Hair, and Nails. Pink, soft, moist, turgor with instant recoil, no lesions, tenderness, or edema; nail beds pink without clubbing, uniform thickness; nails smooth, firmly adhered to nail bed, brisk capillary refill; hair with silky texture, thinning on crown, female distribution.

Head. Head erect and midline; scalp pink, freely movable without lesions or tenderness; well-spaced symmetric facial features. Temporal arteries soft, nontender, no bruits.

Eyes. Brows, lids, and lashes evenly distributed; no tearing; conjunctivae pink without discharge; pupils react equally to light and accommodation; extraocular movements intact, no lid lag, no nystagmus; visual field equals examiner's, corneal light reflex equal bilaterally, red reflex present, discs cream colored with well-defined border bilaterally; arterial-venous ratio 2:5, no crossing changes noted; cornea, lens, and vitreous clear; retina pink, no hemorrhages or exudates; macula yellow; Snellen 20/20 each eye without glasses; near vision 20/40 each eye without glasses, 20/20 with glasses.

Ears. Auricles in proper alignment, without lesions, masses, or tenderness; canals with small amount dry cerumen; tympanic membranes gray, translucent; light reflex and bony landmarks present; no perforations. Rinne—air conduction > bone conduction bilaterally; Weber—no lateralization, repeats whispered words at 2 ft bilaterally.

Nose and Sinuses. No flaring of nares, septum slightly to left of midline, patent bilaterally, mucosa pink and moist, no polyps or discharge; correctly identified coffee, chocolate, and orange odors bilaterally; no frontal or maxillary sinus tenderness with palpation or percussion.

Throat and Mouth. Buccal mucosa pink and moist, no lesions, salivary glands nontender; 28 teeth in good repair, no movement; 1,16,17, and 32 missing; gingivae slightly erythematous and spongy; tongue in midline without fibrillation, no lesions; uvula midline with elevation of soft palate; gag reflex intact; pharynx without erythema; no hoarseness; correctly identified sweet, salty, and sour tastes bilaterally.

Neck. Trachea midline, no tracheal tug, thyroid and cartilages move with swallowing, thyroid lateral borders palpable, no enlargement or nodules noted, lymph nodes nonpalpable, full range of motion and appropriate strength.

Chest and Lungs. AP diameter < lateral with 1:2 ratio; muscle and respiratory effort symmetric without use of accessory muscles; inspiration = expiration; tactile fremitus symmetric; resonant percussion throughout; 4 cm excursion bilaterally; vesicular breath sounds throughout without adventitious sounds; even, quiet breathing.

Breasts. *Moderate size, L slightly > R nodular, granular consistency bilaterally; nipples erect without discharge; areolas symmetric with Montomery tubercles; no palpable axillary nodes; no dimpling, venous patterns symmetric.*

Heart. *Apical impulse barely palpable at 5th intercostal space, 4 cm from midsternal line, no heaves, lifts or thrills, S_1 and S_2 heard without splitting, no murmurs, S_1 heard best at apex, S_2 heard best at base, apical impulse timed with radial pulse, no visible pulsations, no audible S_3, S_4 or murmur.*

Blood Vessels. *Pulse regular rhythm, smooth contour, no pulse deficit; jugular venous pulsation visible at sternal angle with 30-degree elevation; no carotid, renal, or abdominal bruits; no edema, swelling, or tenderness in lower extremities; Homans sign negative; lower extremities warm, pink with symmetric hair distribution; superficial varicosities in lower extremities, L > R.*

PULSE AMPLITUDE

	C	B	R	F	P	DP
L	2+	2+	2+	2+	2+	1+
R	2+	2+	2+	2+	2+ +	1+

Abdomen. *Soft, rounded, faded 12-cm scar from umbilicus to symphysis pubis; aorta midline with no visible pulsation, no bruit; bowel sounds heard in all quadrants; tympanic percussion tones over epigastrium, remainder dull to percussion; liver span 6 cm at R midclavicular line by percussion; spleen percussed at L midaxillary line; liver, spleen, and kidney not palpable; no tenderness on palpation; no CVA tenderness; superficial abdominal reflexes intact.*

Genital/Rectal. *Deferred. Gyn exam 6 months ago.*

Lymphatic. *No palpable lymph nodes in neck, supraclavicular, axillary, epitrochlear, or inguinal areas.*

Musculoskeletal. *Heberden nodes at distal interphalangeal joints on both hands; good mobility of hands but tenderness when making a tight fist bilaterally; no swelling, heat, or erythema noted. Remainder of muscles appear symmetric, muscle strength appropriate and equal bilaterally, full range of active and passive motion, spine and extremities in good alignment, slight kyphosis.*

Neurologic. *Coordinated, smooth gait; negative Romberg sign; balance, rapid alternating movements, sensory functioning, and cranial nerves I-XII grossly intact; plantar flexion of toes bilaterally with plantar reflex, no clonus.*

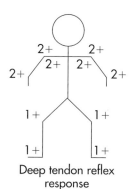

Deep tendon reflex
response

ASSESSMENT PLAN

Problem #1: Pain and stiffness in both hands

Assessment: Degenerative arthritis is the most likely diagnosis. This is supported by presence of Heberden nodes bilaterally and lack of systemic signs and that could suggest an inflammatory process. Pain is well controlled with aspirin. Since noninflammatory symptoms are evident, analgesia could be achieved with acetaminophen with less risk of gastrointestinal side effects.

Dx: None at present

Rx: Acetaminophen 325 mg, 2 tabs q 4 hr prn

Pt. Ed.: Discuss suspected pathophysiologic process of degenerative joint disease (DJD). Reassure that DJD pain can usually be successfully controlled with mild analgesics. Recommend trials of heat and ice to augment analgesia. Return to clinic if increased signs/symptoms, any associated redness, swelling or heat.

Problem #2: Seasonal rhinitis

Assessment: Mild nasal stuffiness q spring secondary to pollen exposure. Well controlled on nonprescription antihistamine/decongestant preparation

Dx: None at present

Rx: None at present

Pt. Ed.: Stay indoors as much as possible when pollen counts are elevated. If nonprescription agent does not control signs/symptoms, may try nonsedating antihistamine. Warned about sedating properties of many nonprescription preparations. Discussed increased risk of sinusitis when turbinates swell. To return to clinic if fever, facial pain, purulent nasal discharge develops.

Problem #3: s/p Total abdominal hysterectomy (TAH)

Assessment: TAH with bilateral oophorectomy performed 1983 for fibroids per patient. Patient never supplemented with estrogen replacement therapy (ERT). There are no apparent contraindications to ERT. Pt not symptomatic with hot flashes, but is at increased risk for osteoporosis and coronary heart disease (CHD). Will complete baseline evaluations and develop plan with patient.

Dx: Baseline bone densometry of hips and L-spine
      Fasting cholesterol and lipid profile

Rx: Ca supplement (nonprescription) as augment to diet to ensure 1500 mg Ca/day.
      Vit D 400 mg po qd

Pt. Ed.: Discuss increased risk of CHD and osteoporosis secondary to early surgical menopause. Explain risks and advantages of ERT. Describe alternatives to ERT. Increase weight bearing exercise.
Will discuss individual plan after obtaining baseline studies.

Problem #4: Family history of diabetes

Assessment: No symptomatic evidence of hyperglycemia. Slightly obese.

Dx: Fasting serum glucose, U/A

Rx: None at present

Pt. Ed.: Benefit of weight loss, goal to reach ideal body weight to avoid insulin insensitivity. Moderate exercise 3 to 4 times/week.

Problem #5: Family history of Alzheimer disease

Assessment: No evidence of cognitive deficit at present.

Dx: None

Rx: None

Pt. Ed.: Return to clinic if memory or other cognitive difficulties develop.

Problem #6: Family history of glaucoma

Assessment: Sees optometrist on yearly basis. Will obtain latest tonometry screening values. No visual changes or objective signs of increased eye pressures.

Dx: None

Rx: None

Pt. Ed.: Discuss important yearly glaucoma screening as glaucoma a preventable cause of blindness. To report visual changes, eye pain immediately.

Progress Note Sample Write-Up

The patient in the previous POMR returns 2 months later (see the sample of a progress note below).

SUBJECTIVE

cc: Pain in hands increasing

Since last seen in clinic, patient has noted more stiffness in hands q am and pain with needlework after only 10 minutes. Pain relieved with acetaminophen but stiffness lasts several hours. This is interfering with fine motor skills. She still states there is no other joint involvement, fever, weight loss, swelling, redness, or heat of involved joints. No analgesic used today.

OBJECTIVE

T 98.2° F, P 88 reg, R 12 unlabored, BP 130/78, L arm supine

Extremities: Heberden nodes in distal interphalangeal joints bilaterally. Bouchard nodes in proximal interphalangeal joints right hand. No swelling or heat present. Mild tenderness to palpation of joints of 2nd digits bilat. Limitation of flexion in R hand, cannot make fist without pain. No tenderness, heat, limited motion of other joints.

ASSESSMENT

Degenerative arthritis both hands, exacerbated by needle working. Will attempt to decrease symptoms with NSAID and rest of affected joints for 2 weeks. No contraindications to nonsteroidals evident.

PLAN

Dx: None

Rx: Ibuprofen 400 mg qid × 2 wks.

Pt. Ed: Medication schedule, warn possibility of GI upset. May take meds with food. To defer needlework until symptoms better controlled. Encouraged to try nonpharmacologic therapies (ice, heat) as degenerative joint disease is a chronic process. Return to clinic if no improvement or if symptoms worsen.

INFANT

See the sample record for an infant on pp. 886-888.

EPISODIC ILLNESS VISIT

Patients often seek care for acute problems such as common colds or minor injuries, which are rapidly resolved. There are three ways to incorporate these problems into the record.

1. List the problem as an acute problem within the ongoing patient record and do not give it a number in the complete problem list. This avoids complicating the ongoing problem list.
2. Each acute minor problem can be given a number and included with the ongoing problem list. A line is drawn through each problem as it is resolved.
3. Another method is to use a specially designed form for each acute problem. These forms are kept in a special section of the patient record and are not included in the problem list.

Text continued on p. 890.

Name: Tom Mitchell   **Date:** 11-3-98

Date of Birth: 3-25-98

History Number: 49076M

PROBLEM LIST:

Problem #	Onset (date)	Problem	Inactive/resolved (date)

General Patient Information

Address: 749 Delta Circle, Apt. 5   **Home phone:** 555-9307
Baltimore, MD 21205   **Social security number:** 222-22-2222

Parent/Guardian's name: Anne Mitchell

Age: 7 months   **Sex:** Male

Health insurance provider: Kaiser Permanente   **Member #:** M57143

SOURCE AND RELIABILITY OF INFORMATION
Mother, reliable historian

CHIEF COMPLAINT
Needs immunizations.

PRESENT PROBLEM
No illnesses or concerns at present. Cold last month resolved without fever or sequelae. Overdue for third shot.

PAST MEDICAL HISTORY
Prenatal. Full-term infant, birth weight 7 lb 9 oz, 21 in, mother healthy throughout pregnancy, no x-ray examinations, prescription drugs, or health problems. Began care in third month, vaginal vertex delivery after 10 hours labor, spinal anesthesia, awake for delivery, baby breathed immediately, in regular nursery, home with mother on next day.

Health Care. Has attended well baby clinic since birth, goes to Dr. Green or hospital clinic for illness. DPT 6-1-98, 8-8-98; IPV 6-1-98, 8-8-98; HIB 6-1-98, 8-8-98; HBV 4-10-98, 6-1-98.

DIET/NUTRITION

Breast-fed since birth, feeds 3 times a day, uses supplemental feeding of Similac, 8 oz, 2 times a day in effort to begin weaning, seems content. Started cereal and fruit at 4 months of age, vegetables at 6 months of age, now introducing meat. Takes about 2 Tbsp each of cereal and fruit in am and 2 Tbsp each of vegetable and meat in pm. Takes 3 oz juice and 3 oz water and teething cookies a day. Eats eagerly. Gives ADC vitamins with iron.

PERSONAL/SOCIAL

Lives with parents and 4-year-old brother in 2-bedroom apartment, inner city neighborhood but parents concerned about increasing violence, father employed as machinist, mother worked as secretary
until Tom's birth, to return to work part time next week in temporary secretarial pool. Maternal GM to care for Tom during day while mother works. Lives close to grandparents, many family events, attends church fairly regularly. Money has been tight for last few months, but family has met major expenses. Tom was planned child, has been pleasure to family, some sibling rivalry with older son, father helps occasionally in care of infant, more in care of older son.

FAMILY HISTORY

Grandparents all living: maternal GF 55 years with hypertension, maternal GM 51 years A & W, paternal GF 60 years with myocardial infarction 2 years ago, paternal GM 58 with hypertension; mother 32 years and father 34 years, both healthy; aunts and uncles A & W, 1 brother 4 years old with asthma. No known diabetes, cancer, tuberculosis, renal, seizure, psychiatric, or hereditary disorders.

GROWTH AND DEVELOPMENT

Sitting without support for 2 weeks, reaches for objects, passes object hand to hand, babbles and coos, uses walker, has started scooting on floor, rolled over at 3 months.

REVIEW OF SYSTEMS

General. Happy infant, easy temperament, cries only when hungry or wet.
Skin, Hair, and Nails. Slight jaundice after birth, never enough to be treated; birthmark on back; fingernails fully formed.
Head and Neck. Holds head up well, turns head in all directions.
Eyes. Seems to follow mother around room with eyes; no crossed eyes noted; no tearing, redness, or discharge noted.
Ears. No infections, turns head toward loud noise or family member speaking.
Nose. One cold with clear to whitish discharge from nose, lasted 1 week, saw doctor, given nose drops and Triaminic Syrup.
Mouth and Throat. 2 front teeth, no difficulty sucking or swallowing.
Chest and Lungs. No problems breathing, noisy breathing with cold.
Cardiovascular. No known heart murmur, has never turned blue, does not tire easily with feeding, no excess perspiration.
Hematologic/Immunologic. No bleeding, bruises, no known anemia, has had only 1 cold, no swollen glands.
Gastrointestinal. No vomiting or diarrhea; spits up small amount of milk after feeding formula; bowel movement 2 times a day, light brown, mushy.
Genitourinary. Circumcised; strong urine stream, 10 wet or dirty diapers a day, no odor to urine; had hydrocele at birth, not noted 2 months ago.
Musculoskeletal. Moves all extremities, stands with support, left foot turned in at birth, seems straight now, ready to buy first hard-sole shoes.
Neurologic. No seizures or tremors noted.

PHYSICAL EXAMINATION FINDINGS

General. *7-month-old black male, alert, happy, playful, responsive, and easily consoled by mother.*

T 37.1° C, P 100, R 26, BP 90/62 L arm

Wt 9.0 kg, 75%; length 70 cm, 50%; head circ. 45 cm, 50%

Skin. *Soft, smooth, light brown, good turgor, Mongolian spot over buttocks, cafe au lait spot 2 × 4 cm over R scapula, no lesions, nail beds pink.*

Head. *Normocephalic, anterior fontanel 1 × 2 cm, flat, posterior fontanel closed, scalp without lesions, sparse fine hair, facial features symmetric, well spaced.*

Eyes. *Conjunctivae pink without discharge, no excess tearing, PERRLA, follows object with eyes 180 degrees, no epicanthal folds, blinks to bright light, corneal light reflex symmetric, red reflex present bilaterally, discs visualized with clear margins, retina pink.*

Ears. *Auricles well formed, appropriate alignment with outer eye canthus; tympanic membranes pink, light reflex and bony landmarks present, mobile bilaterally; turns head to noise and mother's voice.*

Nose. *No discharge, nasal mucosa pink, nares patent bilaterally.*

Mouth and Throat. *Buccal mucosa pink and moist; 2 lower incisors present, 2 upper incisors erupting; palate intact, uvula midline and soft palate rises symmetrically with crying, pharynx without erythema; drooling saliva, sucks and swallows well.*

Neck. *Trachea midline; thyroid not palpable; supple, full passive range of motion; no palpable masses.*

Chest and Lungs. *Symmetric shape and expansion with respiration, no retractions, equal fremitus with crying, lungs clear to auscultation, even smooth respirations.*

Heart and Blood Vessels. *Apical impulse at 4th ICS, 3 cm from midsternal line; no heaves or thrills; S_1 heard loudest at apex, S_2 heard loudest at base, splitting of S_2 with inspiration, no murmurs; radial and femoral pulses strong and equal.*

Abdomen. *Soft, nontender, rounded, umbilical ring open 2 cm with hernia, bowel sounds heard all quadrants, liver palpable 1 cm below right costal margin at R midclavicular line, spleen and kidney not palpable, no other masses palpable, tympany percussed at epigastrium, dullness over remainder of abdomen.*

Genitalia. *Circumcised, urethral opening on tip of glans, both testes descended, no hernia or hydrocele noted, voids with good stream, urine pale yellow.*

Anus and Rectum. *Adequate sphincter control, no fissures or cracks.*

Lymphatic. *Few shotty anterior cervical lymph nodes, 1 cm in diameter, no other lymph nodes palpable.*

Musculoskeletal. *Spine and extremities in alignment, full hip abduction bilaterally, muscle development symmetric, slight inward twisting of tibia bilaterally, weight bearing with support, 5 digits each hand and foot, all palmar creases present.*

Neurologic. *Strong grasp, suck, head control; patellar and biceps deep tendon reflexes 2+ and plantar reflex toes ⬆⬆ bilaterally, no clonus, cranial nerves II-XII intact.*

ASSESSMENT

Healthy 7-month-old needing immunizations.

Mild internal tibial torsion, bilateral.

Umbilical hernia.

MANAGEMENT PLAN

DPT # 3, HIB # 3, HBV # 3

Hematocrit and hemoglobin

Anticipatory guidance: nutrition, safety, fostering growth and development, shoes

Reevaluate tibial torsion and umbilical hernia at 12 months of age

Name: Mary Jones   **Date:** 12/07/98

ID: 6789

Patient identification: 21-year-old white female

SUBJECTIVE

cc. "Cold for two weeks"

HPI. Patient was well until 2 weeks ago when she developed intermittent nasal congestion and clear watery nasal discharge while at work during the day. Four days later a dry cough developed, which became productive of small amounts of yellow sputum 1 week ago. Her cough is more productive and copious on awakening in the am. Nasal congestion clears within 1 hour of awakening. She has not taken any nonprescription medications or attempted other therapeutic measures to relieve her symptoms. The patient states no shortness of breath, dyspnea on exertion, hemoptysis, wheezing, facial pain, sore throat ear pain, ear congestion, fever, chills, myalgias, arthralgias.

Current Medications. Oral contraceptives × 4 years, daily multivitamin with iron

PMH. No history of asthma, heart disease, diabetes, seasonal allergies or frequent URIs, T & A age 3 for "frequent strep throats"

Social History. Full-time nursing student, lives in dorm with smoking roommate, patient has never smoked or used illicit drugs. Drinks 1 to 2 beers q weekend. CAGE (-).

OBJECTIVE

T 99.2°F, P 92 reg, R 12 unlabored, BP 118/68, L arm supine, no acute distress

Head. No sinus tenderness elicited with palpation

Eyes. Conjunctiva clear, no injection or exudate

Ears. Canals clear. TMs pearly gray, intact, with normal light reflex. Bony landmarks visible; there is no injection, exudate, or retraction evident. Negative tragus.

Nose. Turbinates, red and moderately edematous. Discharge clear.

Throat. Pharynx mildly injected, tonsils surgically absent, there is no exudate.

Neck. No palpable adenopathy in anterior, posterior triangles, submental, postauricular, or supraclavicular regions.

Chest. Chest symmetrical without deformities, percussion is resonant in all lung fields. Tactile fremitus equal bilaterally, diaphragm moves 4 cm with deep inspiration. There are scattered rhonchi bilaterally that clear completely with cough leaving vesicular breath sounds all fields. There are no crackles or wheezes audible.

ASSESSMENT

Viral bronchitis: There is no evidence of respiratory compromise or systemic symptoms (fever, chills). Patient has no history or asthma and is a nonsmoker. She will therefore be treated symptomatically unless symptoms worsen or purulent sputum production lasts in excess of 3 weeks. Chest x-ray is not indicated at this time.

PLAN

Dx: None

Rx: Increase hydration to a minimum of 10 glasses noncaffeinated liquids/day

Pt. Ed: Discuss pathophysiology of assessed disease process. Promote respiratory hygiene: avoid smoke-filled environments.

Call or return to clinic if symptoms do not improve in 1 week, if develops fever, chills, myalgias, ear pain, facial pain.

Regardless of the method chosen. A brief SOAP note is written in the chart to address each acute problem. It is not necessary to repeat the entire comprehensive health history, but do include pertinent information such as smoking, allergies, or other information that would increase your usual level of concern regarding the problem presented.

EPISODIC ILLNESS NOTES

In certain facilities, such as urgent care centers or the emergency department, you may see a patient who is new to you and the facility, so there is no POMR to refer to. An episodic illness note, which is more extensive, is then required. It includes identifying information and a complete present problem, pertinent past medical history, family history, and personal/social history, as well as a relevant review of systems. The remainder of the note follows the SOAP format.

EPISODIC NOTE SAMPLE WRITE-UP

In the sample of the episodic note write-up on p. 889, the patient is not known to you or the facility.

SUMMARY

As you begin to examine patients, it is often difficult to determine how to cluster information that will lead to a diagnosis. As a result, all collected information is initially part of the puzzle. With experience, you will be able to identify appropriate groupings of information, enabling you to better organize and synthesize the raw data. Your first attempts to write a complete history and physical examination will be lengthy and perhaps disorganized, but clinical experience will eventually lead to a more concise and organized record.

http://www1.mosby.com/physexam_seidel

PHOTO AND ILLUSTRATION CREDITS

American College of Rheumatology: *Clinical slide collection on the rheumatic diseases,* Atlanta, 1991, American College of Rheumatology.

Andrews JS: Making the most of the sports physical, *Contemporary Pediatrics* 14(3):196-197, 1997.

Baran R et al: *Color atlas of the hair, scalp, and nails,* St Louis, 1990, 1992, Mosby.

Barkauskas VH et al: *Health and physical assessment,* ed 2, St Louis, 1998, Mosby.

Barkauskas VH et al: *Health and physical assessment,* St Louis, 1994, Mosby.

Battaglia FC, Lubchenco LC: The practical classification of newborn infants by weight and gestational age, *J Pediatr* 71:159, 1967.

Belcher A: *Cancer nursing,* St Louis, 1993, Mosby.

Berne RM, Levy MN: *Principles of physiology,* ed 2, St Louis, 1996, Mosby.

Bingham BJG, Hawke M, Kwok P: *Atlas of clinical otolaryngology,* St Louis, 1992, Mosby.

Bull TR: *A colour atlas of ENT diagnosis,* London, 1974, Wolfe Medical Publications.

Burke B: The dietary history as a tool in research, *J Am Dietic Assoc* 23:1044-1046, 1947.

Canobbio MM: *Cardiovascular disorders,* St Louis, 1990, Mosby.

Chernick V, editor: *Kendig's disorders of the respiratory tract in children,* ed 5, Philadelphia, 1990, WB Saunders.

Cohen BA: *Atlas of pediatric dermatology,* St Louis, 1993, Mosby.

Crouch JE: *Functional human anatomy and physiology,* ed 4, New York, 1985, Lea & Febiger.

Crouch JE, McClintic JR: *Human anatomy and physiology,* ed 2, New York, 1976, John Wiley & Sons.

DePalma AF: *Surgery of the shoulder,* ed 3, Philadelphia, 1983, JB Lippincott.

Des Jardin T, Burton GG: *Clinical manifestations and assessment of respiratory disease,* ed 3, St Louis, 1995, Mosby.

Diagnostic picture tests in clinical medicine, St Louis, 1984, Mosby.

Donaldson DD: *Atlas of the eye: the crystalline lens,* vol V, St Louis, 1976, Mosby.

Doughty DB, Jackson DB: *Gastrointestinal disorders,* St Louis, 1993, Mosby.

Dubowitz L, Dubowitz V, Goldberg C: Clinical assessment of gestational age in newborn infant, *J Pediatr* 77:1, 1970.

Dyken PR, Miller MD: *Facial features of neurologic syndromes,* St Louis, 1980, Mosby.

Edge V, Miller M: *Women's health care,* St Louis, 1994, Mosby.

Ezrein D, Godden JO, Volpe R: *Systematic endocrinology,* ed 2, New York, 1979, Harper & Row.

Farrar WE et al: *Infectious diseases,* ed 2, London, 1992, Gower.

Folstein M et al: The meaning of cognitive impairment in the elderly, *J Am Geriatr Soc* 33:228, 1985.

Food and Nutrition Board, Institute of Medicine, 1992.

400 more self assessment picture tests in clinical medicine, St. Louis, 1988, Mosby International.

Gallager HS et al: *The breast,* St Louis, 1978, Mosby.

Gardner HL: Cervical endometriosis, a lesion of increasing importance, *Am J Obstet Gynecol* 84:170, 1962.

Gardner HL, Kaufman RH: *Benign diseases of the vulva and vagina,* St Louis, 1969, Mosby.

Giddens JF: *Student workbook and laboratory manual to accompany Health Assessment for Nursing Practice* St Louis, 1998, Mosby.

Goldman MP, Fitzpatrick RE: *Cutaneous laser surgery: the art and science of selective photothemolysis,* St Louis, 1994, Mosby.

Goodman RM, Gorlin RJ: *Atlas of the face in genetic orders,* ed 2, St Louis, 1977, Mosby.

Grimes D: *Infectious diseases,* St Louis, 1991, Mosby.

Grossman SA et al: A comparison of the Hopkins Pain Rating Instrument with standard visual analogue and verbal descriptor scales in patients with cancer pain, *Pain Symptom Manage* 7:196-203, 1992.

Guzzetta CD, Dossey BM: *Cardiovascular nursing: holistic practice,* St Louis, 1992, Mosby.

Habif TP: *Clinical dermatology,* ed 3, St Louis, 1996, Mosby.

Halstead CL et al: *Physical evaluation of the dental patient,* St Louis, 1982, Mosby.

Harris JA et al: *The measurement of man,* Minneapolis, 1930, University of Minnesota Press.

Hughes JG: *Synopsis of pediatrics,* ed 6, St Louis, 1984, Mosby.

Iliff A, Lee VA: *Child Devel* 23: 1952.

Jolly H: *Diseases of children,* ed 4, Oxford, 1981, Blackwell Scientific Publications.

Kaufman RH, Faro S: *Benign diseases of the vulva and vagina,* ed 4, St Louis, 1994, Mosby.

Korones SB: *High-risk newborn infants: the basis for intensive nursing care,* ed 4, St Louis, 1986, Mosby.

Lawrence CM, Cox NH: *Physical signs in dermatology: color atlas and text,* St Louis, 1993, Mosby.

Lloyd-Davies RW et al: *Color atlas of urology,* ed 2, London, 1994, Mosby.

Lowdermilk DL, Perry SE, Bobak IM: *Maternity and women's health care,* ed 6, St Louis, 1997, Mosby.

Lubchenco LC et al: Intrauterine growth in length and head circumference as estimated from live births at gestational ages from 26 to 42 weeks, *Pediatrics* 37:403, 1966.

Mann RA, Coughlin MJ: *Surgery of the foot,* ed 6, vol 2, St Louis, 1993, Mosby.

Mansel R, Bundred N: *Color atlas of breast disease,* St Louis, 1995, Mosby.

Marks JG, DeLeo VA: *Contact and occupational dermatitis,* St Louis, 1992, Mosby.

Mazzaferri EL: *Endocrinology case studies,* ed 2, Flushing, NY, 1975, Medical Examination Publishing.

McCance KM, Huether SE: *Pathophysiology: the biologic basis for disease in adults and children,* ed 3, St Louis, 1998, Mosby.

McKusick VA: *Heritable disorders of connective tissues,* ed 4, St Louis, 1972, Mosby.

Medcom: Selected topics in ophthalmology. *Medcom clinical lecture guides,* Garden Grove, Calif, 1983, Medcom.

Meheus A, Ursi JP: *Sexually transmitted diseases,* Kalamazoo, Mich, 1982, The Upjohn Co.

Miyasaki-Ching CM: *Chasteen's essentials of clinical dental assisting,* ed 5, St Louis, 1997, Mosby.

Moore KL: *The developing human: clinically oriented embryology,* ed 2, Philadelphia, 1977, WB Saunders.

Morison M, Moffatt C: *A colour guide to the assessment and management of leg ulcers,* ed 2, St Louis, 1994, Mosby.

Morse SA, Moreland AA, Holmes KK: *Atlas of sexually transmitted diseases and AIDS,* ed 2, St Louis, 1996, Mosby.

Nellhaus G: Head circumference from birth to eighteen years, *Pediatrics* 41:106, 1968.

Newell FW: *Ophthalmology: principles and concepts,* ed 6, St Louis, 1986, Mosby.

Newell FW: *Ophthalmology: principles and concepts,* ed 8, St Louis, 1996, Mosby.

Owen GM: Measurement, recording, and assessment of skin-fold thickness in childhood and adolescence: a report of a small meeting, *Am J Clin Nutr* 35:629, 1982.

Palay DA, Krachmer JH: *Ophthalmology for primary care physician,* St Louis, 1997, Mosby.

Prior JA et al: *Physical diagnosis: the history and examination of the patient,* ed 6, St Louis, 1981, Mosby.

Ross Laboratories: *Nutrition screening initiative,* Washington, DC.

Rudy EB: *Advanced neurological and neurosurgical nursing,* St Louis, 1984, Mosby.

Saunders WH et al: *Nursing care in eye, ear, nose, and throat disorders,* ed 4, St Louis, 1979, Mosby.

Schneider HA et al: *Nutritional support of medical practice,* ed 2, New York, 1977, Harper & Row.

Sigler BA, Schuring LT: *Ear, nose, and throat disorders,* St Louis, 1993, Mosby.

Smith DW: *Growth and its disorders,* Philadelphia, 1977, WB Saunders.

Stein HA, Slatt BJ, Stein RM: *The ophthalmic assistant: fundamentals and clinical practice,* ed 5, St Louis, 1988, Mosby.

Stein HA, Slatt BJ, Stein RM: *The ophthalmic assistant: fundamentals and clinical practice,* ed 6, St Louis, 1994, Mosby.

Stewart WD, Danto JL, Maddin S: *Dermatology: diagnosis and treatment of cutaneous disorders,* St Louis, 1978, Mosby.

Swaiman KF, Wright FS: *The practice of pediatric neurology,* ed 2, St Louis, 1982, Mosby.

Symonds EM, Macpherson MBA: *Color atlas of obstetrics and gynecology,* St Louis, 1994, Mosby.

Tanner JM, Davis PSW: Clinical longitudinal standards for height and height velocity for North American children, *J Pediatr* 107:317, 1985.

Thibodeau GA, Patton KT: *Anatomy & physiology,* ed 3, St Louis, 1996, Mosby.

Thompson JM et al: *Mosby's clinical nursing,* ed 2, St Louis, 1989, Mosby.

Thompson JM et al: *Mosby's clinical nursing,* ed 3, 1993, St. Louis, Mosby.

Thompson JM et al: *Mosby's clinical nursing,* ed 4, St Louis, 1997, Mosby.

Thompson JM, Wilson SF: *Health assessment for nursing practice,* St Louis, 1996, Mosby.

Trevor-Roper PD, Curran PV: *The eye and its disorders,* ed 2, Oxford, 1984, Blackwell Scientific Publications.

Van Wieringen et al: Growth diagrams 1965 Netherlands. Second national survey on 0-24-year-olds, 1971, Netherlands, Wolters-Noordhoff.

Weston WL, Lane AT: *Color textbook of pediatric dermatology,* St Louis, 1991, Mosby.

Weston WL, Lane AT, Morelli JG: *Color textbook of pediatric dermatology,* ed 2, St Louis, 1996, Mosby.

White GM: *Color atlas of regional dermatology,* St Louis, 1994, Mosby.

Willson JR, Carrington ER, Ledger WJ: *Obstetrics and gynecology,* ed 8, St Louis, 1987, Mosby.

Wilson JD, Walsh PC. In Harrison JH et al: *Campbell's urology,* ed 4, Philadelphia, 1979, WB Saunders.

Wilson SF, Thompson JM: *Respiratory disorders,* St Louis, 1990, Mosby.

Wong DL: *Whaley and Wong's nursing care of infants and children,* ed 5, St Louis, 1995, Mosby.

Wood NK, Goaz PW: *Differential diagnosis of oral lesions,* ed 4, St Louis, 1991, Mosby.

Yannuzzi LA, Guyer DR, Green WR: *The retina atlas,* St Louis, 1995, Mosby.

Zitelli BJ, Davis HW: *Atlas of pediatric physical diagnosis,* ed 3, St Louis, 1997, Mosby.

References

Acute Pain Management Guideline Panel: *Acute pain management: operative or medical procedures and trauma,* AHCPR pub. no. 92-0032, Rockville, Md, 1992, Agency for Health Care Policy and Research, Public Health Service, US Department of Health and Human Services.

Adams MS, Niswander JD: Birth weight of North American Indians: a correlation and amplification, *Hum Biol* 45:351, 1973

Alagaratnam TT, Wong J: Limitations of mammography in Chines females, *Clin Radiol* 36:175, 1985.

American Academy of Ophthalmology: *Comprehensive pediatric eye evaluation, preferred practice pattern,* San Francisco, 1992, American Academy of Ophthalmology.

American Academy of Pediatrics: Sports preparticipation examination. In Dyment PG, editor: *Sports medicine: health care for young athletes,* ed 2, Elk Grove Village, Ill., 1991, American Academy of Pediatrics.

American Academy of Pediatrics, Committee on Sports Medicine and Fitness: Medical conditions affecting sports participation, *Pediatrics* 94(5):757, 1994.

American Cancer Society: Breast Cancer Information, http://www.cancer.org/bcn/brrisk.html, Sept. 16, 1997.

American Cancer Society: Prostate Cancer Information: http://www.cancer.org/prostate/prearly.html, Sept. 16, 1997.

American Cancer Society: *Fibrocystic breasts: a non-disease,* code 534, 1992, American Cancer Society.

American College of Allergy, Asthma & Immunology (ACAAI) Latex Allergies: http://pw2.netcom.com/~nam1/latex_allergy/Qanda.htm, October 6, 1997.

American College of Obstetrics and Gynecology: *Hypertension in pregnancy,* ACOG Technical Bulletin, 219, January 1996.

American Heart Association: Jones criteria (revised) for guidance in the diagnosis of rheumatic fever, *Circulation* 69:204A, 1984.

American Journal of Nursing Company: Carpal-tunnel syndrome, *Am J Nurs* 93:64, 1993.

American Medical Association, Group on Science and Technology: Athletic preparticipation examinations for adolescents: report of the Board of Trustees, *Arch Pediatr Adolesc Med* 148:93, 1994.

American Medical Student Association Standing Committee on Lesbian, Gay, and Bisexual People in Medicine: *Taking a sensitive sexual history with the gay patient in mind,* 1991.

American Psychiatric Association: *Diagnostic and statistical manual of mental disorders,* ed 4, Washington, DC, 1994, Association.

Andrews JS: Making the most of the sports physical, *Contemporary Pediatrics* 14(3):182, 1997.

Angell M: Privilege and health: what is the connection, *N Engl J Med* 329:126, 1993.

Augustyn M, et al: Silent victims: children who witness violence, *Contemp Pediatr* 12:35, 1995.

Autotte PA: Folk medicine, *Arch Pediatr Adolesc Med* 149:949, 1995.

Axelson G, Gedegard B: Torus mandibularis among Icelanders, *Am J Phys Anthropol* 54:383, 1981.

Babian R et al: Diagnostic testing for prostate cancer detection: less is best, *Urology* 41:5, 1993.

Ballock RT, Richards BS: Hip dysplasia: early diagnosis makes a difference, *Contemp Pediatr* 14:108, 1997.

Bamjo M et al: Palpable lymph nodes in healthy newborns and infants, *Pediatrics* 78:573, 1986.

Barkauskus VH et al: *Health and physical assessment,* ed 2, St Louis, 1998, Mosby.

Barness LA: *Manual of pediatric physical diagnosis,* ed 6, Chicago, 1991, Mosby.

Berenson A et al: Inadequate weight gain among pregnant adolescents: risk factors and relationship to infant birth weight, *Am J Obstet Gynecol* 176:1220, 1997.

Berger SE: *Horizontal woman,* New York, 1996, Houghton Mifflin.

Binns HJ et al: Growth of Chicago-area infants 1985 through 1987: not what the curves predict. *Arch Pediatr Adolesc Med* 150:842, 1996.

Blackhall LJ et al: Ethnicity and attitudes toward patient autonomy, *JAMA* 274:820, 1996.

Bluestone CD, Klein JO: *Otitis media in infants and children,* ed 2, Philadelphia, 1995, WB Saunders.

Bluestone CD, Shurin PA: Middle ear disease in children: pathogenesis, diagnosis, and management, *Pediatr Clin North Am* 21:379, 1974.

Boekeloo BO et al: Young adolescents' comfort with discussion about sexual problems with their physicians, *Arch Pediatr Adolesc Med* 150:1146, 1996.

Bowers AC, Thompson JM: *Clinical manual of health assessment,* ed 4, St. Louis, 1992, Mosby.

Bradford BJ: Don't let our youth go down tobacco road, *Contemp Pediatr* 9:96, 1992.

Brothwell DR, Carbonell VM, Goose DH: Congenital absence of teeth in human populations. In Brothwell DR, editor: *Dental anthropology,* Tarrytown, NY, 1963, Pergamon Press.

Brown MS, Hurlock JT: Preparation of the breast for breast feeding, *Nurs Res* 24:448, 1975.

Brown-Jones LC, Orr OP: Enlisting parents as allies against depression, *Contemp Pediatr* 13:67, 1996.

Burrow GN: Thyroid diseases. In Burrow GN, Ferris TF, editors: *Medical complications during pregnancy,* ed 4, Philadelphia, 1995, WB Saunders.

Butz AM et al: Infant health care utilization predicted by pattern of prenatal care, *Pediatrics* 92:50, 1993.

Callahan CM: The benefit of the doubt, *JAMA* 264:341, 1990.

Caputo GM et al: Assessment and management of foot disease in patients with diabetes, *N Engl J Med* 331:854, 1994.

Carrese JA, Rhodes LA: Western bioethics on the Navajo reservation: benefit or harm? *JAMA* 274:826, 1995.

Caufield C: A developmental approach to hearing screening in children, *Pediatr Nurs* 4:39, 1978.

Chernick V, editor: *Kendig's disorders of the respirator tract in children,* ed 5, Philadelphia, 1990, WB Saunders.

Christianson RE et al: Incidence of congenital anomalies among white and black live births with long-term follow-up, *Am J Public Health* 71:1333, 1981.

Chrzastek-Spruch H, Wolanski N, Wrebiakowski H: Socioeconomic and endogenous factors in growth of 11 year old children from Lublin, *Collegium Anthropologium* 8:57, 1984.

Churgay CA: Diagnosis and treatment of pediatric foot deformities, *Am Fam Physician* 47:883, 1993.

Coles R: *The call of stories: teaching and the moral imagination,* Boston, 1989, Houghton Mifflin.

Collins JW Jr, David RJ: Differential survival rates among low birth weight black and white infants in a tertiary care hospital, *Epidemiology* 1:16, 1990.

Connelly JE: Emotions and clinical decisions, *SGIM News* 13:1, 1990.

Cooper-Patrick L, Crum RM, Ford DE: Identifying suicidal ideation in general medical patients. *JAMA* 272:1757, 1994.

Crigger N, Forbes W: Assessing neurologic function in older adults, *Am J Nurs* 97:37, 1997.

Crowell DH et al: Race, ethnicity and birth-weight: Hawaii 1983 to 1986, *Hawaii Med J* 51:242, 1992.

Cugell DW: Lung sound nomenclature, *Am Rev Respir Dis* 136:1016, 1987.

Curative Health Services: *The curative footsense 5.07 monofilament,* East Setauket, NJ, 1996, Author.

Dahlberg AO: Analyses of the American Indian dentition. In Brothwell DR, editor: *Dental anthropology,* Tarrytown, NY, 1963, Pergamon Press.

Dains J, Baumann L, Scheibel P: *Advanced assessment and clinical diagnosis in primary care,* St Louis, 1998, Mosby.

Daniels SR, Khoury PR, Morrison JA: The utility of body mass index as a measure of body fatness in children and adolescents: differences by face and gender, *Pediatrics* 99:804, 1997.

Davies R: *World of wonders,* New York, 1977, Penguin.

Davies T, Mills C: Personal communication, 15 September 1997.

DeSwiet MD: The respiratory system. In Hytten F, Chamberlain G, editors: *Clinical physiology in obstetrics,* ed 2, Boston, 1991, Blackwell Scientific Publications.

Dewey KG et al: Height and weight of Southeast Asian preschool children in northern California, *Am J Public Health* 76:806, 1986.

DiFrancesco E: Getting teens to talk to you, *Pediatric News* August 19, 1992.

Dillon MJ: Investigation and management of hypertension in children: a personal perspective, *Pediatr Nephrol* 1:59, 1987.

Donnelly WJ: Medical language as symptoms: doctor talk in teaching hospitals, *Perspectives in Biology and Medicine* 30:81, 1986.

Drolett B et al: The hair collar sign: marker for cranial dysraphism, Pediatrics 96:309, 1995.

Dubowitz L, Dubowitz V, Goldberg C: Clinical assessment of gestational age in the newborn infant, *J Pediatr* 77:1, 1970.

Eddy DM: The anatomy of a decision, *JAMA* 263:441, 1990.

Edge V, Miller M: *Women's health care,* St. Louis, 1994, Mosby.

Education for Latex Allergy Support Team & Information Coalition (elastic) Physician Information, http://www.latexallergyhelp.com/latex.htm, October 6, 1997.

Eichelberger MR et al: *Pediatric emergencies: a manual for prehospital care providers,* Englewood Cliffs, NJ, 1998, Brady.

Emanuel EJ, Emanuel LL: Four models of the physician-patient relationship, *JAMA* 267:2221, 1992.

Ewing JA: Detecting alcoholism, the CAGE questionnaire, *JAMA* 252:1905, 1984.

Fai FV et al: Assessment of fetal health should be based on maternal perception of clusters rather than episodes of fetal movements, *J Obstet Gynecol Res* 22:299, 1996.

Falkner G, Tanner J: *Human growth I: principles and prenatal growth,* New York, 1978, Plenum Press.

Ferreyra S, Hughes K: *Table manners: a guide to the pelvic examination for disabled women and health care providers,* Alameda/San Francisco, 1982, Planned Parenthood.

Ferris TF: Hypertension and pre-eclampsia. In Burrow GN, Ferris TF, editors: *Medical complications of pregnancy,* ed 4, Philadelphia, 1995, WB Saunders.

Folstein M et al: The meaning of cognitive impairment in the elderly, *J Am Geriatr Soc* 33:228, 1985.

Folstein MF, Folstein SE, McHugh PR: "Mini-Mental State:" a practical method for grading the cognitive state of patients for the clinician, *J Psychiatric Res* 12:189, 1975.

Ford CA, Millstein SG: Delivery of confidentiality assurances to adolescents by primary care physicians. *Arch Pediatr Adolesc Med* 151:505, 1997.

Foster TA et al: Anthropometric and maturation measurements of children, ages 5 to 14 years, in a biracial community: the Bogalusa Heart Study, *Am J Clin Nutr* 30:582, 1977.

Fox G: *J Fam Pract* 21:400, 1985.

Freeman JM: The three-cent neurologic exam and other tools for an era of managed care, *Contemp Pediatr* 14:153, 1997.

Fried LP: Functional assessment: the role of the clinician. Presented as part of Annual Geriatrics Symposium at The Johns Hopkins Medical Institutions, February 3-8, 1992.

Frisancho A: New norms of upper limb fat and muscle areas for assessment of nutritional status, *Am J Clin Nutr* 34:2540, 1981.

Frisancho AR: New standards of weight and body composition by frame size and height for assessment of nutritional status of adults and the elderly, *Am J Clin Nutr* 40:808, 1984.

Gallagher-Allred CR, *Implementing nutrition screening and intervention strategies,* Washington, DC, 1993, Nutrition Screening Initiative.

Gallo AM: Osteoporosis and children at risk with genetic hypercalciuria, *IMAGE: J Nurs Sch* 28:368, 1996.

Gans B: Breast and nipple pain in early stages of lactation, *Br Med J* 5100:830, 1958.

Garn SM, Clark DC, Guire KE: Level of fatness and size attainment, *Am J Phys Anthropol* 40:447, 1974.

Garner J: Guideline for isolation precautions in hospitals, *Am J Infect Control* 24:24, 1996.

Garner JS, Hospital Infection Control Practices Advisory Committee: Guideline for isolation precautions in hospitals, *Infect Control Hosp Epidemiol* 17:53, 1996

Garner JS, Hospital Infection Control Practices Advisory Committee: Guideline for isolation precautions in hospitals, *Am J Infect Control* 24:24-52, 1996.

Garrick JG: Sports medicine, *Pediatr Clin North Am* 24:737, 1977.

Gladman DD, Urowitz MB: Rheumatic diseases in pregnancy. In Burrow GN, Ferris TF, editors: *Medical complications of pregnancy,* ed 4, Philadelphia, 1995, WB Saunders.

Goldberg B et al: Preparticipation sports assessment: an objective evaluation, *Pediatrics* 66(5):736, 1980.

Goldenring JM, Cohen G: Getting into adolescent heads. *Contemp Pediatr* 5:75, 1988.

Goodenough-Harris Drawing Test, Psychological Corporation, 757 Third Ave., New York, NY 10017.

Grant A: Nutritional assessment guidelines, ed 2, Seattle, 1979, Author.

Green M: The 10-minute visit: anything but routine, *Contemp Pediatr* 9:53, 1992.

Green M, Stuy MZ: Persistent symptoms: how to end the frustration, *Contemp Pediatr* 9:104, 1992.

Griffith LSC, Seidel HM: *Clinical history and physical examination,* Baltimore, 1986, Johns Hopkins School of Medicine.

Gross RH: The pediatric orthopaedic examination. In Morrissy RT, Weinstein SL, editors: *Lovell & Winter's Pediatric Orthopaedics,* ed 4, Philadelphia, 1996, Lippincott-Raven.

Grossman SA et al: A comparison of the Hopkins rain rating instrument with standard visual analogue and verbal descriptor scales in patients with cancer pain, *J Pain Symptom Manage* 7:196, 1992.

Guzzetta CD, Dossey BM: *Cardiovascular nursing: holistic practice,* St Louis, 1982, Mosby.

Hahn BA: Children's health: racial and ethnic differences in the use of prescription medications, *Pediatrics* 95:727, 1995.

Haka-Ikse K, Mian M: Sexuality in children, *Pediatr Rev* 14:10, 1993.

Halffman CM, Scott CR, Pedersen PO: Palatine torus in Greenlandic Norse, *Am J Phys Anthropol* 88:145, 1992.

Hall ET: *The hidden dimension,* Garden City, NY, 1969 Anchor Books, Doubleday and Co.

Hamill PV, et al: Physical growth: National Center for Health Statistics percentiles, *Am J Clin Nutr* 32: 607, 1979.

Hamill PV, Johnston FE, Lemeshow S: Body weight, stature, and sitting height: white and Negro youths 12-17 years, *Vital Health Stat* 11:1, 1973.

Hammer A: *Essentials of the orthopaedic examination,* London, 1995, Oxford University Press.

Harvey AM et al: *The principles and practice of medicine,* ed 22, Norwalk Conn/San Mateo, Calif, 1988, Appleton & Lange.

Hays AM, Borger F: A test in time, *Am J Nurs* 85:1107, 1985.

Herman-Giddens ME, et al: Secondary sexual characteristics and menses in young girls seen in office practice: a study from the pediatric research in office setting network. *Pediatrics* 99:505, 1997.

Herzog LW: Prevalence of lymphadenitis of the head and neck in infants and children, *Clin Pediatr* 22:485, 1983.

Hirsch ED Jr: *Cultural literary: what every American needs to know,* Boston 1987, Houghton Mifflin.

Hitchcock JM, Wilson HS: Personal risking: lesbian self-disclosure of sexual orientation to professional health care providers, *Nurs Res* 41:178 1992.

Hughes JD: *Synopsis of pediatrics,* ed 6, St. Louis, 1984, Mosby.

Hulsey TC, Levkoff AH, Alexander GR: Birth weights of infants of black and white mothers without pregnancy complications, *Am J Obstet Gynecol* 164(part 1):1299, 1991.

Ibraimov IA: Brief communication: cerumen phenotypes in certain populations of Eurasia and Africa, *Am J Phys Anthropol* 84:209, 1991.

Ikegami N: Functional assessment and its place in health care, *N Engl J Med* 332:598, 1995.

Isaacson G: Sinusitis in childhood, *Pediatr Clin North Am* 43:1297, 1996.

James WD, Carter JM, Rodman OG: Pigmentary demarcation lines: a population survey: *J Am Acad Dermatol* 16(3, part 1):584, 1987.

Jantz JW, Blosser CD, Fruechting LA: A motor milestone change noted with a change in sleep position, *Arch Pediatr Adolesc Med* 151:565, 1997.

Jarvis A, Gorlin RJ: Minor orofacial abnormalities in an Eskimo population, *Oral Surg* 33:417, 1972.

Jecker NS, Carrese JA, Pearlman RA: Caring for patients in cross-cultural settings, *Hastings Center Report* 25:6, 1995.

Jellinck MS et al: Psychosocial aspects of ambulatory pediatrics, *Curr Probl Pediatr* 20:623, 1990.

Jellinck MS et al: The difficult parent—and the difficult physician, *Contemp Pediatr* 8:118, 1991.

Johns RJ, Fortuin NJ, Wheeler PS: The collection and evaluation of clinical information. In Harvey AM et al, editors: *Principles and practice of medicine,* ed 22, Norwalk, Conn, 1988, Appleton & Lange.

Jones AK: Primary care management of acute low back pain, *Nurse Pract* 22:50, 1997.

Judge R, Zuidema G, Fitzgerald F: *Clinical diagnosis,* ed 5, Boston, 1988, Little, Brown.

Kain CD, Reilly N, Schultz ED: The older adult: a comparative assessment, *Nurs Clin North Am* 25:833, 1990.

Keith NM, Wagner HP, Barker NW: Some different types of essential hypertension: their course and prognosis, *Am J Med Sci* 197:337, 1939.

Keller C, Stevens KR: Childhood obesity: measurement and risk assessment, *Pediatr Nurs* 22:494, 1996.

Kemp CH et al: *Current pediatric diagnosis and treatment,* ed 9, Stamford, Conn., 1987, Appleton & Lange.

Kemper KJ, Rivara FP: Parents in jail, *Pediatrics* 92:261, 1993.

Klebanoff MA et al: Pre-term and small for gestational-age birth across generations, *Am J Obstet Gynecol* 176:521, 1997.

Klein JD et al: Adolescents' risky behavior and mass media use, *Pediatrics* 92:24, 1993.

Kleinman A, Eisenberg L, Good B: Clinical lessons from anthropological and cross-cultural research, *Ann Intern Med* 88:251, 1978.

Kluckholn C: *Culture and behavior,* New York, 1962, The Free Press.

Kluckholn F: Dominant and variant value orientation. In Brink P, editor: *Transcultural nursing: a book of readings,* Englewood Cliffs, NJ, 1976, Prentice-Hall.

Koop CE: *The Surgeon General's letter on child sexual abuse,* Rockville, Md, 1988, US Department of Health and Human Services, Public Health Service.

Koutures CG, Landry GL: The acutely injured knee, *Pediatr Ann* 26:50, 1997.

Krajicek MJ, Tomlinson AT: *Detection of developmental problems in children,* ed 2, Baltimore, 1983, University Park Press.

Lembo NJ et al: Bedside diagnosis of systolic murmurs, *N Engl J Med* 318:1572, 1988.

Levin J: When doctors question kids (letter to editor), *N Engl J Med* 323:1569, 1990.

Lin WS: Physical growth of Chinese school children 7-18 years, in 1985, *Ann Hum Biol* 19:41, 1992.

Lowdermilk DL, Perry SE, Bobak IM: *Maternity and women's health care,* ed 6, St. Louis, 1997, Mosby.

Lowrey GH: *Growth and development of children,* ed 8, Chicago, 1986, Mosby.

Lurie N et al: Preventive care for women: does the sex of the physician matter? *N Engl J Med* 329:478. 1993.

Mace JW et al: Clinical pediatrics 15:58, 1976. In McMillan JA, Nieburg PL, Oski FA: *The whole pediatrician catalog,* Philadelphia, 1977, WB Saunders.

Magann EF, Evans SF, Newnham JP: Employment, exertion, and pregnancy outcome: assessment by kilocalories expended each day, *Am J Obstet Gynecol* 175: 182, 1996.

Malina RM, Hamill PV, Lemeshow S: Body dimensions and proportions, white and Negro children 6-11 years, *Vital Health Stat* 11:1, 1974.

Malina RM, Zavaleta AN, Little BB: Body size, fatness, and leanness of Mexican American children in Brownsville, Texas: changes between 1972 and 1983, *Am J Pub Health* 77:573, 1987.

Manning ML: Health assessment of the early adolescent, *Nurs Clin North Am* 25:923, 1990.

Margileth AM, Hadfield TL: A new look at old cat-scratch, *Contemp Pediatr* 7:25, 1990.

Martin JL, Crump EP: Leukoedema of the buccal mucosa in Negro children and youth, *Oral Surg* 34:49, 1972.

Matsunaga E: The dimorphism in human normal cerumen, *Ann Hum Genet* 25:273, 1962.

Mays RM, Gillon JE: Autism in young children: an update, *J Pediatr Health Care* 7:17, 1993.

McCance KL, Huether SE: *Pathophysiology: the biologic basis for disease in adults and children,* ed 3, St Louis, 1998, Mosby.

McCarthy PL et al: History and observation variables in assessing febrile children, *Pediatrics* 65:1090, 1985.

McCarty DJ: *Arthritis and allied conditions: a textbook of rheumatology,* ed 2, Philadelphia, 1993, Lea & Febiger.

McMillan JA, Neiburg PL, Oski FA: *The whole pediatrician catalogue,* vol 1, Philadelphia, 1977, WB Saunders.

McMillan JA, Stockman JA, Oski FA: *The whole pediatric catalogue,* vol 3, Philadelphia, 1982, WB Saunders.

Merz ML et al: Tooth diameters and arch perimeters in a black and white population, *Am J Orthod Dentofacial Orthop* 100:53, 1991.

Meskin LH, Gorlin RJ, Isaacson RJ: Abnormal morphology of the soft palate: the prevalence of cleft uvula, *Cleft Palate* 1:342, 1965.

Meuller DH, Burke F: Vitamin and mineral therapy. In Morrison G, Hark L, editors: *Medical nutrition and disease,* Cambridge, 1996, Blackwell Science.

Migliori ME, Gladstone GJ: Determination of the normal range of exophthalmometric values for black and white adults, *Am J Ophthalmol* 98:438, 1984.

Molitch ME: Pituitary, thyroid, adrenal, and parathyroid disorders. In Barron WM, Lindheimer MD, editors: *Medical disorders during pregnancy,* ed 2, St. Louis, 1995, Mosby.

Najjar M: Anthropometric reference data and prevalence of overweight, United States, 1976-1980, *Vital Health Stat Series* 11, no. 238, 1987.

National Cancer Institute: NCAB issues mammography screening recommendations (3/97), http://rex.nci.nih.gov/INTRFCE_GIFS/MASSMED_INTR_DOC.htm, June 22, 1998.

National Cancer Institute: Questions and answers about mammography screening (3/97), http://www.icic.nci.nih.gov/clinpdq/detec; answers_about_mammography_screening.hml#1, Sept 16, 1997.

National Center for Health Statistics: Advance report of final natality statistics, 1979, *Monthly Vital Statistics Report* 30:1, 1981.

National Center for Infectious Diseases: Epidemiology and prevention of viral hepatitis a to e, on-line slide set, http://www.cdc.gov/ncidod/diseases/hepatitis/slideset/httoc.htm, August 22, 1997.

National Center for Infectious Diseases: hepatitis fact sheets, http/WWW.cdc.gov/ncidod/diseases/hepatitis/hepatitis.htm, August 22, 1997.

National Cholesterol Education Program Coordinating Committee: *National cholesterol education program highlights of the report of the expert panel on blood cholesterol levels in children and adolescents,* Bethesda, 1991, NHLBI Information Center.

National Institutes of Health: *Detection, evaluation, and treatment of high cholesterol in adults,* NIH Publication No. 93-3096, Washington, DC, 1993, NIH.

National Institutes of Health: *Second report of the Expert Panel on detection, evaluation, and treatment of high blood cholesterol in adults,* NIH publication no. 93-3096: Washington, DC, September 1993, NIH.

National Institute for Occupational Safety and Health (NIOSH) Alert: *Preventing allergic reaction to natural rubber latex in the workplace, June 1997, DHHS (NIOSH),* Publication No. 97-135.

National Institute for Occupational Safety and Health (NIOSH) Latex Allergy Facts, June 1997 Document #705006, http://www.cdc.gov//niosh/latexfs.html, August 12, 1997.

Office of Disease Prevention and Health Promotion, Public Health Service, US Department of Health and Human Services: *Clinician's handbook of preventive services: put prevention into practice,* Washington, DC, 1994, Government Printing Office.

Ostgaard HC: Assessment and treatment of low back pain in working pregnant women, *Semin Perinatol* 20:61, 1996.

Papiernik E et al: Ethnic differences in duration of pregnancy, *Ann Hum Biol* 13:259, 1986.

Pappas G et al: The increasing disparity in mortality between socioeconomic groups in the United States, 1960 and 1986, *N Engl J Med* 329:103, 1993.

Pawson EG, Petrakis NL: Comparisons of breast pigmentation among women of different racial groups, *Hum Biol* 47:441, 1975.

Peck EB, Ullrich HD: *Children and weight: a changing perspective,* Berkley, Calif, 1985, Nutrition Communications Associates.

Penninger J: Urinary incontinence: new approaches to age-old problems, *Greater Houston Nursing* 1:2, 1993.

Petit J, Barkhaus PE: Evaluation and management of polyneuropathy: a practical approach, *Nurse Pract* 22:131, 1997.

Petrakis NL: Cerumen genetics and human breast cancer, *Science* 173:347, 1971.

Plant SM: Boundary violations in professional-client relationships: overview and guidelines for prevention, *Sexual and Marital Therapy* 12:79, 1997.

Prazor GE, Friedman SB: An office-based approach to adolescent psychosocial issues, *Contemporary Pediatr* 14:59, 1997.

Priddy KD: Immunological adaptations during pregnancy, *J Obstet Gynecol Neonat Nurs* 26:338, 1997.

Quill TE: Recognizing and adjusting to barriers in doctor-patient communication, *Ann Intern Med* 112:51, 1989.

Rampen FHJ: Nevocytic nevi and skin complexion, *Dermatologia* 176:111, 1988.

Rampen FHJ, de Wit PEJ: Racial differences in mole proneness, *Acta Derm Venereol* 69:234, 1989.

Ravussin E, Tataranni PA: Dietary fat and human obesity, *J Am Diet Assoc* 97:S42, 1997.

Ravussin E, Tataranni PA: Dietary fat and human obesity. In Williams CL, Williams GM, editors: *Reducing dietary fat: putting theory into practice,* Chicago, 1997, American Dietetic Association.

Resnick MB et al: Effect of birth weight, race, and sex on survival of low birth weight infants in neonatal intensive care, *Am J Obstet Gynecol* 161:184, 1989.

Revere C, Hasty R: Diagnostic and characteristic signs of illness and injury, clinical notebook (Halpern J, editor) *J Emerg Nurs* 19:2, 1993.

Richardson JL et al: Relationship between after school care of adolescents and substance abuse, risk taking, depressed mood, and academic achievement, *Pediatrics* 92:22, 1993.

Riggs SR, Alario A: *RAFFT questions: Project ADEPT Manual,* Providence RI, 1987, Brown University.

Risser AL, Mazur LJ: Use of folk remedies in a Hispanic population, *Arch Pediatr Adolesc Med* 149:978, 1995.

Rivara FP, Wasserman AL: Teaching psychosocial issues to pediatric house officers, *J Med Educ* 59:45, 1984.

Robinson CH et al: *Normal and therapeutic nutrition,* ed 17, New York, 1986, Macmillan.

Robinson CH, Weigley ES, Mueller DH, editors: *Basic nutrition and diet therapy,* ed 7, Upper Saddle River, NJ, 1993, Prentice Hall.

Roche AF et al: Reference data for weight/stature in Mexican Americans from the Hispanic Health and Nutrition Survey (HHANES 1982-1984), *Am J Clin Nutr* 51:917S, 1990.

Rosenberg D: *Fascinating rhythm: George and Ira Gershwin,* New York, 1991, Dutton (Penguin Books).

Rudy EB: *Advanced neurological and neurosurgical nursing,* St. Louis, 1984, Mosby.

Ryan AS et al: Median skinfold thickness distributions and fat-wave patterns in Mexican-American children from the Hispanic Health and Nutrition Survey (HHANES 1982-1984), *Am J Clin Nutr* 51:925S, 1990.

Samiy AH, Douglas RG Jr, Barondess JA: *Textbook of diagnostic medicine,* Philadelphia, 1987, Lea & Febiger.

Sapar JR: *Headache disorders: current concepts and treatment strategies,* Boston, 1983, PSG Publishing.

Second Report of the Expert Panel on Detection, Evaluation, and Treatment of High Blood Cholesterol in Adult (Adult Treatment Panel II), Executive Summary, NIH, NHLBI, September 1993, NIH.

Schaumann BF, Peagler FD, Gorlin RJ: Minor orofacial anomalies among a Negro population, *Oral Surg* 29:566, 1970.

Schuman AJ: New products for pediatrics: 1995, *Contemp Pediatr* 12:49, 1995.

Schutta HS: Intervertebral disc disorders and other spondyloarthropathies. In Joynt RJ, Griggs RC, editors: *Clin Neurol* 1996.

Schutte JE: Growth differences between lower and middle income black male adolescents, *Hum Biol* 52:193, 1980.

Seidel HM: On paternalism, *Pediatr Ann* 21:295, 1992.

Selfridge J, Sanning SS: The accuracy of the tympanic membrane thermometer in detecting fever in infants aged 3 months and younger in the emergency department setting, *J Emerg Nurs* 19:2, 1993.

Shapiro J, Roper J, Schulzinger J: Managing delirious patients, *Nursing* 93:78, 1993.

Shipman JJ: *Mnemonics and tactics in surgery and medicine,* ed 2, Chicago, 1984, Mosby.

Simel DL: The clinical examination: an agenda to make it more rational. *JAMA* 277:572, 1997.

The Sixth Report of the Joint National Committee on Prevention, Detection, Evaluation, and Treatment of High Blood Pressure, National Institutes of Health, National Heart, Lung, and Blood Institute, NIH Publication No. 98-4080, November 1997.

Smith AC III, Kleinman S: Managing emotions in medical school: students' contacts with the living and the dead, *Soc Psychol Q* 52:56, 1989.

Smith DM et al: *Preparticipation physical evaluation,* ed 2, Minneapolis, 1997, McGraw-Hill.

Smith DW: *Growth and its disorders,* Philadelphia, 1977, WB Saunders.

Smith RD, McNamara JJ: The neurologic examination of children with school problems, *J Sch Health* 54(7):231-234, 1984.

Sokol RJ, Martier SS, Ager JW: The TACE questions: practical prenatal detection of risk drinking, *Am J Obstet Gynecol* 160:863, 1989.

Southworth K, Gilham B: *Clinical nutrition and dietetics pocket reference,* Austin, Tex, 1992, Abel's Copies, University of Texas at Austin.

Sprague J: Vision screening. In Krajicek M, Tomlinson AIT, editors: *Detection of developmental problems in children,* ed 2, Baltimore, 1983, University Park Press.

Stashwick C: When you suspect an eating disorder, *Contemp Pediatr* 13:124, 1996.

Strauss KF: American Indian school children height and weight survey, *The Provider* 18:1, 1993.

Stule DM: The family as a bearer of culture. In Cookfair JM, editor: *Nursing process and practice in the community,* St. Louis, 1991, Mosby.

Subcommittee on the Tenth Edition of the RDAs, Food and Nutrition Board: *Recommended Dietary Allowances,* ed 10, Washington, DC, 1989, National Academy Press.

Tachdjian MO: *Clinical pediatric orthopedics: the art of diagnosis and principles of management,* Stamford, Conn, 1997, Appleton & Lange.

Tanner JM: *Foetus into man: physical growth from conception to maturity,* ed 2, Cambridge, Mass, 1990, Harvard University Press.

Tanner JM, Davis PSW: Clinical longitudinal standards for height and height velocity for North American children, *J Pediatr* 107:317, 1985.

Taylor GA: Neuroimaging techniques in pediatrics, lecture, Baltimore, 1989, The Johns Hopkins Medical Institutions.

Teasdale G, Jennete B: Assessment of coma and impaired consciousness: a practical scale, *Lancet* 2:81, 1974.

Thibodeau GA, Patton KT: *Anatomy & physiology,* ed 3, St Louis, 1996, Mosby.

Thompson JM et al: *Mosby's clinical nursing,* ed 4, St Louis, 1997, Mosby.

Thomson M: Heavy birthweight in Native Indians of British Columbia, *Can J Public Health* 81:443, 1990.

Trauner DA: *Childhood neurological problems: A textbook for health professionals,* Chicago, 1979, Mosby.

Update on Task Force Report on High Blood Pressure in Children, *Pediatrics* 98:649, 1996.

U.S. Centers for Disease Control: http://www.cdc.gov/ncidod/hip/isolat/isopart2.htm, Feb. 18, 1997.

Veille JC, Kitzman DW, Bacevice AF: Effects of pregnancy on the electrocardiogram in healthy subjects during exercise, *Am J Obstet Gynecol* 175:1360, 1996.

Wagley PF: Counselling the patient contemplating suicide, *Hum Med* 8:317, 1992.

Walsh S: Cardiovascular disease in pregnancy: a nursing approach, *J Cardiovasc Nurs* 2:53, 1998.

Wardlaw GM, Insel PM, Seyler MF: *Contemporary nutrition,* ed 2, St. Louis, 1994, Mosby.

Waring WW, Jeansonne LO: *Practical manual of pediatrics,* ed 2, St Louis, 1982, Mosby.

Wasserman HP: *Ethnic pigmentation: historical, physiological and chemical aspects,* New York, 1974, American Elsevier.

Wharton P, Mowrer DE: Prevalence of cleft uvula among school children in kindergarten through grade five, *Cleft Palate J* 29:10, 1992.

Whittle J et al: Racial differences in the use of invasive cardiovascular procedures in the Department of Veterans Affairs Medical System, *N Engl J Med* 329:621, 1993.

Wiens L et al: Chest pain in otherwise healthy children and adolescents, *Pediatrics* 90:350, 1992.

Williams CL, Bollella M, Wynder EL: A new recommendation for dietary fiber in childhood. In Williams CL, editor: The role of dietary fiber in childhood, *Pediatrics* 96(suppl), 1995.

Wilson HS, Kneisl CR: *Psychiatric Nursing,* ed 3, Redwood City, Menlo Park, Calif, 1988, Addison-Wesley Publishing Co.

Wilson MEH: Odor (unusual body and urine). In Hoekelman RA et al, editors: *Primary pediatric care,* ed 3, St Louis, 1997, Mosby.

Wong DL: *Whaley and Wong's Nursing Care of Infant and Children,* ed 5, 1995, St Louis, Mosby.

World Health Organization: *Energy and protein requirements: report of a Joint FAO/WHO/UNU expert consultation,* Technical Report Series 724, Geneva, 1985, WHO.

Yip R, Li Z, Chong WH: Race and birth weigh: the Chinese example, *Pediatrics* 87:688, 1991.

Zhang J, Savitz DA: Preterm birth subtypes among blacks and whites, *Epidemiology* 3:428, 1992.

GLOSSARY

abduction Movement of the limbs toward the lateral plane or away from the axial line of a limb.

abruptio placenta Premature separation of the placenta during pregnancy or labor before delivery of the fetus.

accommodation Adjustment of the eye for various distances through modification of the lens curvature; negative accommodation is adjustment for far vision by relaxation of ciliary muscle; positive accommodation is adjustment for near vision by contraction of ciliary muscle.

acini cells Milk-producing alveoli located in the glandular tissue of the breast.

adduction Movement of the limbs toward the medial plane of the body or toward the axial line of a limb.

adenitis Inflammation of a lymph node or a group of lymph nodes.

adnexae Appendages (e.g., adnexae uteri are the structures adjacent to the uterus, including the ovaries, fallopian tubes, and uterine ligaments).

adventitious Accidental or acquired, not natural or hereditary; located away from the usual place.

alveolar ridge Bony prominence of the maxilla and mandible that supports the teeth or dentures.

amblyopia Reduced vision in an eye that appears structurally normal and without detectable cause when examined, including inspection with an ophthalmoscope.

amenorrhea Absence of menses.

anacrotic The upstroke of the pulse, which also implies a "notch" or "shoulder" on the upstroke.

anesthesia Partial or complete loss of sensation.

aneurysm A balloon-like swelling of the wall of an artery, vein, or heart; generally the result of a congenital defect in the wall or degenerative disease or infection (e.g., atherosclerosis or syphilis); dissecting aneurysm is longitudinal splitting of the arterial wall from hemorrhage.

angle of Louis (Sternal angle) the angle between the manubrium and the body of the sternum.

annulus A ring or circular structure; e.g., tympanic annulus is a fibrous ring around the tympanic membrane that looks whiter and denser than the membrane itself.

anosmia Absence of the sense of smell.

anthropometry Measurement of the size, weight, and proportions of the human body.

apex beat The visible or palpable pulsation made by the apex of the left ventricle as it strikes the chest wall in systole; usually located in the fifth left intercostal space, several centimeters to the left of the median line (midsternal line).

aphakia A condition in which part or all of the crystalline lens of the eye is absent, usually because of surgical removal for the treatment of cataracts.

aphasia Impairment of language function in which speech or writing is not understood (receptive or sensory), words cannot be formed (expressive), or a combination of both.

apical Pertaining to the apex or the area of the apex (top or tip) of a body, organ, or part.

appropriate for gestational age A weight classification of newborns associated with better health outcomes, the weight falling between the 10th and 90th percentiles on the intrauterine growth curve for the newborn's calculated gestational age.

apnea A temporary halt to breathing.

apraxia Inability to execute a skilled or learned motor act, not related to paralysis or lack of comprehension; caused by a lesion in the cerebral cortex.

arrhythmia (see dysrhythmia) A deviation from the expected rhythm of the heart.

arteriovenous fistula A pathologic direct communication between an artery and a vein without an intervening capillary bed.

arteriovenous shunt The passage of blood directly from an artery to a vein, without an intervening capillary network.

articulation The ability to pronounce speech sounds, words, and thoughts clearly and fluently; the junction of two or more bones; contact of the occlusal surfaces of the teeth.

ascites Abnormal intraperitoneal accumulation of serous fluid.

asterixis Postural tremor characterized by nonrhythmic, flapping movements of wide amplitude; extended wrist or fingers suddenly and briefly flex and then return to their original position.

astigmatism An abnormal condition in which the light rays cannot be focused clearly in a point on the retina because of an irregular curvature of the cornea or lens.

ataxia Impaired ability to coordinate muscular movement, usually associated with staggering gait and postural imbalance.

atelectasis Incomplete expansion of the lung, either congenital or acquired.

athetosis Slow, twisting, writhing movements, with larger amplitude than chorea, that commonly involve the hands.

atrioventricular valve Refers to the tricuspid or mitral valves.

Austin Flint murmur A presystolic murmur, not unlike that of mitral stenosis, best heard at the apex of the heart; caused by aortic insufficiency.

autonomic nervous system The portion of the nervous system that regulates involuntary functions supporting life; divided into the sympathetic and parasympathetic nervous systems.

baroreceptor Sensory nerves within the walls of the atria, vena cava, aortic arch, and carotid sinus that monitor blood pressure change.

barrel chest Increased anteroposterior diameter of the chest, often with some degree of kyphosis; commonly seen with COPD.

Bartholin glands (Vestibular glands) mucus-secreting glands located posterolaterally to the vaginal opening.

biferious pulse An arterial pulse with two palpable peaks, the second stronger than the first, but not markedly so; detected in instances of decreased arterial tension.

bifurcated Having two branches, tines, or prongs.

begiminal pulse A pulse in which two beats occur in rapid succession so that they seem coupled and distinct from the succeeding set of two. Each set is separated by a longer interval.

bisferiens pulse The double-peaked systolic pulse.

borborygmi Rumbling, gurgling, tinkling noises heard on auscultation of the abdomen as a result of hyperactive intestinal peristalsis.

bossing Bulging of the frontal areas of the skull; associated with prematurity and rickets.

boutonnière deformity Fixed flexion of the proximal interphalangeal joint associated with hyperextension of the distal interphalangeal joint.

bradycardia A heart rate less than 60 beats per minute.

bradypnea Slower than expected respiratory rate.

bronchial breathing Harsh breathing characterized by prolonged high-pitched expiration with a tubular quality; often heard when lung tissue is consolidated.

bronchial fremitus Adventitious pulmonary or voice sounds palpable over the chest or audible to the ear.

bronchiectasis Persistent dilation of bronchi or bronchioles as a consequence of inflammatory disease, obstruction, or congenital abnormality.

bronchiolitis (Bronchopneumonia) inflammation of the bronchioles, caused by bacteria or viruses.

bronchogenic Originating from the bronchi.

bronchophony An exaggeration of vocal resonance emanating from a bronchus surrounded by consolidated lung tissue.

bronchopulmonary dysplasia A form of chronic lung disease of uncertain cause sometimes seen in children who have had intensive respiratory support during the neonatal period.

bronchovesicular Pertaining to bronchial tubes and alveoli.

bruit An unexpected audible swishing sound or murmur over an artery or vascular organ.

bruxism Compulsive unconscious grinding of the teeth.

bubo Inflammation and swelling of one or a group of lymph nodes, particularly in the groin or axilla, often accompanied by suppuration.

buccal mucosa Mucous membrane inside the mouth.

bundle of His A small band of modified heart muscle fibers that originates at the atrioventricular node and passes through the right atrioventricular junction to the interventricular septum, where the fibers divide into right and left branches and enter the respective ventricles; this bundle carries the atrial contractual rhythm to the ventricles; an interruption results in some degree of heart block.

bunion Unexpected prominence of the medial aspect of the first metatarsal head, with bursa formation, resulting in lateral or valgus deviation of the great toe.

bursa Disk-shaped, fluid-filled synovial sacs that develop at points of friction around joints, between tendons, cartilage, and bone; they decrease friction and promote ease of motion.

canthus The angle at the medial or lateral margin of the eyelid; the medial canthus opens into a small space containing openings to the lacrimal duct.

caput succedaneum An edematous swelling of the scalp of the newborn resulting from labor.

cardiac cycle The complete sequence of cardiac action occurring from one heartbeat to the next, including both systole and diastole.

cardiac impulse The thrust of the ventricles against the chest wall as a result of cardiac contraction.

cardiac output The amount of blood ejected by the heart, usually stated in liters per minute, calculated by stroke volume × number of heartbeats per unit of time.

cardiac reserve The heart's ability to respond to demands that exceed ordinary circumstances.

carrying angle The angle at which the humerus and radius articulate.

cellulitis Inflammation of soft or connective tissue that causes a watery exudate to spread through the tissue spaces.

cephalhematoma A subperiosteal hemorrhage, usually benign, along one of the cranial bones; it generally results from birth trauma.

cheilitis Inflammation and cracking of the lips.

chemoreceptor Any cell that is activated by a change in its chemical milieu and thereby originates a flow of nervous impulses; nerve cells sensitive to changes in the composition of the blood or cerebrospinal fluid.

choanae A pair of posterior openings between the nasal cavity and the nasopharynx.

chordee Ventral curvature of the penis caused by a fibrous band of tissue, often associated with hypospadias or gonorrhea.

chorea Purposeless, involuntary rapid movements associated with muscle weakness and behavioral change; these are not tics, athetosis, or hyperkinesis. Chorea is often a delayed manifestation of rheumatic fever and may be confused with manifestations of Huntington chorea, systemic lupus erythematosis, Wilson disease, and drug reactions.

choreiform movements Brief, rapid, jerky, irregular, and involuntary movements that occur at rest or interrupt normal coordinated movements; most often involve the face, head, lower arms, and hands.

choroid The thin, highly vascular membrane covering the posterior five sixths of the eye between the retina and sclera.

cicatricial Composed of scar tissue that is avascular, pale, and contracted.

ciliary body The thickened part of the vascular tunic of the eye that joins the iris with the anterior portion of the coroid.

circumcorneal Around the cornea.

circumduction Circular movement of a limb (e.g., the shoulder) or the eye.

circumlocution The use of pantomime, nonverbal expressions, or word substitutions to avoid revealing that a word has been forgotten.

claudication The condition resulting from muscle ischemia due to decreased arterial blood flow to an area and characterized by intermittent pain and limping.

clonus Rapidly alternating involuntary contraction and relaxation of skeletal muscles.

coarctation Constriction, stricture, stenosis, or narrowing, as of the aorta.

cochlea A coiled bony structure within the inner ear; it contains the organ of Corti and perforations for the passage of the cochlear division of the auditory nerve.

cognition The mental process of knowing, thinking, learning, and judging.

colic Gradual onset of pain that increases in crescendo fashion until it reaches a peak of severity, then slowly subsides.

colostrum Yellow, milky secretion from the breast that precedes the onset of true lactation; composed primarily of serum and white blood cells.

concha A structure that is shell-shaped; the deep cavity in the auricle of the external ear containing the auditory canal meatus.

conductive hearing loss Reduction in hearing acuity relating to interference of sound being transmitted through the outer and middle ear.

confabulation Fabrication of detailed, plausible experiences and events to cover gaps in memory.

conjunctivitis Inflammation of the conjunctiva caused by infectious agents or by allergies.

consolidation Solidification of part of the lung into a firm, dense mass, particularly when the alveoli fill with fluid as a result of inflammation.

contracture Permanent fixed flexion of a joint resulting from atrophy and shortening of muscles or from loss of skin elasticity.

coryza Rhinitis; inflammation of the nasal mucous membranes, accompanied by swelling of the mucosa and nasal discharge.

crackle A general term for an unexpected sound heard on auscultation of the chest; sometimes used to describe crepitus heard on auscultation (see Box 12-7).

craniotabes An unusual softness of the skull in infants with hydrocephalus and rickets; the skull feels brittle and has a Ping Pong ball–snapping sensation when firmly pressed.

crepitus A crinkly, crackling, grating feeling or sound in the joints, skin, or lungs; the quality of sound is simulated by Rice Krispies in milk; the quality of touch is somewhat simulated by rubbing hair between the fingers.

croup An inflammation of the larynx, causing swelling of the vocal chords and sometimes severe obstruction; characterized by harsh, difficult breathing, stridor, and a hoarse cough; usually occurs in young children.

cryptorchidism Failure of one or both testicles to descend into the scrotum.

cyanosis A bluish or purplish color (may range from slight to intense) of the skin and mucous membranes because of insufficient oxygen levels in the blood.

deafness Partial or complete loss of hearing.

decerebrate posturing Rigid extension of all four extremities with hyperpronation of the forearms and plantar flexion of the feet.

dermatome The area of skin innervated by a single posterior spinal nerve.

development The process of growth and differentiation; the acquisition of function associated with cell differentiation and maturation of individual organ systems.

dextrocardia Location of the heart in the right hemithorax, either by displacement from disease or congenital mirror-image reversal.

diastole That time between two contractions of the heart when the muscles relax, allowing the chambers to fill with blood; diastole of the atria precedes that of the ventricles; diastole alternates, usually in a regular rhythm, with systole.

dicrotic notch The notch in a pulse tracing between two elevations for each pulse beat.

dicrotic pulse The double-peaked pulse; the second peak is usually weaker than the first and diastolic in timing.

diplopia Double vision caused by defective function of the extraocular muscles or a disorder of the nerves that innervate the muscles.

dizziness (Vertigo) sensation of an inability to maintain normal balance in a standing or sitting position.

dorsiflexion Backward bending or flexion of a joint.

dysarthria Defective articulation secondary to a motor deficit involving the lips, tongue, palate, or pharynx.

dysfunctional uterine bleeding (DUB) Abnormal uterine bleeding not associated with tumor, inflammation, pregnancy, trauma, or hormonal imbalance; a diagnosis is given only after these causes are ruled out.

dyspareunia Difficult or painful sexual intercourse.

dysphagia Difficulty in swallowing.

dyspnea Difficult and labored breathing, shortness of breath.

dysrhythmia Unexpected variation in the regular rhythm of the heart.

ecchymosis (Bruise) discoloration of the skin or mucous membrane as the result of hemorrhage into subcutaneous tissue.

echolalia Automatic and meaningless repetition of another's words or phrases.

edema Excessive accumulation of fluid in the cells, tissues, or serous cavities of the body.

edentulous Without teeth.

effacement The shortening of the vaginal portion of the cervix and thinning of its walls as it is stretched and dilated during labor.

effusion Loss of fluid from the blood vessels or lymphatics into the tissues or a body cavity.

ejection murmur A diamond-shaped systolic murmur occupying most but not necessarily all of systole; produced by the ejection of blood into the aorta or pulmonary artery.

electrocardiogram (ECG) A graphic record of the heart's electrical currents obtained with an electrocardiograph.

embolism Obstruction of an artery by a blood clot or foreign matter.

emphysema Pathologic accumulation of air in tissue or organs, especially the lungs.

encephalocele A congenital gap in the skull, usually with herniation of the brain or meninges.

endocardium The innermost membrane lining the heart cavities that is continuous with the lining of the blood vessels; its slippery surface eases the flow of blood.

epicardium The inner visceral layer of the serous pericardium lying directly on the heart, forming the outermost layer of the heart wall.

epigastrium The upper central region of the abdomen between the costal margins and a line drawn horizontally across the lowest costal margin.

epispadias A congenital defect resulting in the urethra opening on the dorsum of the penis.

epulis A tumor on the gingiva.

erythema marginatum A distinctive evanescent pink rash, a rare manifestation of rheumatic fever. The erythematous areas have pale centers and round or serpiginous margins; they vary in size and appear mainly on the trunk and extremities, never on the face. The erythema is transient and migratory and may be induced by application of heat.

esotropia (Cross-eye) the inward or nasal deviation of an eye.

eustachian tube The cartilaginous and bony passage between the nasopharynx and the middle ear that allows equalization of air pressure between the inner ear and external pressure.

exotrophia (Walleye) the outward or temporal deviation of an eye.

extension Movement that increases the angle between two adjoining bones to 180 degrees, bringing a limb toward a straight line.

external rotation Lateral turning of a limb.

exudate Fluid that has escaped from tissue or capillaries, usually after injury or inflammation, typically containing protein and white blood cells.

facies Expression or appearance of the face; often used to describe characteristic expressions of disease states or congenital anomalies.

fasciculation A localized, uncoordinated twitching of a single muscle group innervated by a single motor nerve filament; it is visible or palpable.

fibrosis The formation of excessive connective tissue as an attempt to repair damage or as a reaction to foreign material, resulting in scarring and thickening.

flaccid Muscles that are weak, soft, and flabby, lacking expected muscle tone.

flail chest A flapping, unfixed chest wall caused by loss of stability of the thoracic cage after fractures of the sternum and/or ribs.

flank The posterior part of the body below the ribs and above the ilium.

flatulence The presence of excessive air or gases in the stomach or intestines, causing abdominal distention and resulting in rectal passage.

flexion Movement that decreases the angle between two articulating bones, bending the limb.

floater One or more spots that appear to drift in front of the eye; caused by a shadow cast on the retina by vitreous debris or separation of the vitreous humour from the retina.

fluctuant A wavelike motion that is felt when a structure containing liquid is palpated.

flutter A rapid vibration or pulsation that impedes appropriate function.

fontanels Membranous spaces at the juncture of an infant's cranial bones that later ossify.

foramen ovale The communication between the two atria of the fetal heart; if it remains patent, blood shunts between the atria after birth, usually from left to right.

Fordyce spots Ectopic sebaceous glands of the buccal mucosa appearing as small yellow-white raised lesions.

fornix Arched structure (e.g., the vaginal fornix is the recess between the cervix and the vaginal wall); although one continuous structure, the vaginal fornix is anatomically divided into the anterior, posterior, and lateral fornices.

fourchette Ridges of tissue formed by the fusion of the labia minora at the posterior aspect of the vulva.

fovea centralis A tiny pit in the center of the macula lutea that is the area of clearest vision, permitting light to fall on the cones; it appears as an oval yellow spot on the retina and is free of blood vessels.

fremitus A tremor vibration in any part of the body, detectable on palpation.

frenulum, lingual Band of tissue that attaches the ventral surface of the tongue to the floor of the mouth.

friction rub A sound audible through the stethoscope, resulting from the rubbing of opposed, inflamed serous surfaces.

functional assessment Measurement of the abilities and activities used to perform the activities of daily living necessary for survival, vocational and social pursuits, and leisure activities.

galea aponeurotica The fibrous sheet or tendonous material connecting the frontalis and occipitalis muscles over the skull.

gaussian distribution A frequency distribution of observations and/or events that results in a plotted curve having the shape of a bell, reasonable symmetry, and the potential for infinite extent in either direction.

gestational age Fetal age of a newborn, calculated from the number of completed weeks since the first day of the mother's last menstrual period to the date of birth.

gingivae Gums of the mouth.

glaucoma An abnormal condition of elevated pressure within an eye resulting from obstruction of the outflow of aqueous humor.

glottis Pertaining to the vocal apparatus of the larynx, the true vocal cords, and the opening between them.

goiter Cystic or fibrous enlargement of the thyroid gland, often related to thyroid dysfunction.

Graham Steell murmur An early diastolic murmur of pulmonic insufficiency secondary to pulmonary hypertension.

graphesthesia The ability to recognize symbols, shapes, numbers, and letters traced on the skin.

helix The prominent outer rim of the auricle of the ear.

hemangioma A benign tumor of newly formed blood vessels that may occur anywhere in the body, most readily noticed in the skin and subcutaneous tissues.

hemianesthesia Loss of sensation on one side of the body.

hemiplegia Loss of motor function and sensation (paralysis) on one side of the body.

hemodynamic Pertaining to the movement of blood and other aspects of the circulation.

hemoptysis Coughing up blood or blood-stained sputum from the respiratory tree.

hernia Protrusion of an organ or tissue through an opening in the muscle wall.

hilus of the lung A hollow depression on the mediastinal surface of each lung, which is the point of entry of the bronchus, blood vessels, nerves, and lymphatics.

hirsutism Excessive hair growth, especially an adult male pattern of hair distribution in women; usually related to heredity, hormonal dysfunction, porphyria, or medications.

holodiastolic Occupying all of diastole.

holosystolic Occupying all of systole.

Homans sign Pain or discomfort behind the knee or in the calf when the ankle is gently dorsiflexed while the knee is flexed; it suggests thrombosis of the leg veins.

homonymous hemianopia Defective vision in half of the visual field, occurring on the same side in each eye.

hydramnios A condition of pregnancy characterized by an excess of amniotic fluid.

hydrocephaly Enlargement of the head by an excessive accumulation of fluid dilating the cerebral ventricles, thinning the cerebral cortex, and causing separation of the cranial bones.

hyperesthesia Unusual increased sensitivity to sensory stimuli, such as touch or pain.

hyperextension A position of maximum extension.

hyperkeratosis Overgrowth of the cornified layer of the skin or the cornea.

hyperkinesia Excessive muscular activity; hyperactivity.

hypermenorrhea Excessive bleeding during a menstrual period of usual duration.

hyperopia (Farsightedness) a refractive error in which light rays entering the eye are focused behind the retina.

hyperpnea Respiration that is deeper and more rapid than expected.

hyperresonance Greater than expected resonance that is lower pitched in response to percussion of the chest wall or abdomen.

hyperthyroidism Excessive activity of the thyroid gland with an increase in thyroid secretion.

hyperventilation A state in which an increased amount of air enters the lungs, usually a result of deep and rapid breathing; if severe, it leads to alkalosis with the excessive loss of carbon dioxide.

hypesthesia Decreased sensitivity to sensory stimuli such as touch and pain.

hypokinesia Unusually diminished muscular activity.

hypomenorrhea Decreased amount of menstrual flow.

hypospadias A congenital defect in which the urethra opens on the ventral surface of the penis rather than on the glans.

hypotension A condition in which arterial blood pressure is lower than expected.

hypothyroidism Diminished activity of the thyroid gland with consequent reduction of thyroid hormone.

incus One of the three ossicles of the middle ear, lying between the malleus and stapes.

induration Excessive hardening or firmness of any body site.

infarction An acute interruption to the blood supply of a part of the body by thrombi, emboli, extrinsic pressure, or twisting of blood vessels resulting in tissue death at the involved site.

infrapatellar fat pad The soft tissue palpable in front of the joint space on either side of the patellar tendon.

intermittent claudication Cramping pain and limping commonly in the calf brought on by walking; caused by ischemia of the muscles, usually from atheroma that narrows the leg's arteries.

internal rotation Medial turning of a limb.

intertriginous An area where opposing skin surfaces touch and may rub, such as skin folds in the axillae, groin, inner thighs, and beneath large breasts.

introitus The vaginal opening.

isthmus A narrow band of tissue connecting the two lateral lobes of the thyroid.

Janeway lesions (spots) Tiny hemorrhagic spots, a bit raised or nodular, occurring principally on the palms and soles, suggesting subacute bacterial endocarditis.

joint instability An unusual increase in joint mobility.

jugular pulse A pulsation in the jugular vein resulting from waves transmitted from the right side of the heart via circulating blood.

keratin A scleroprotein that is the primary constituent of epidermis, hair, and nails.

Kiesselbach plexus A convergence of small, fragile arteries and veins located superficially on the anterosuperior portion of the nasal septum.

Koplik spots Small red spots with bluish-white centers on the buccal mucosa opposite the molar teeth, appearing in the prodromal stage of measles.

kyphosis An increased convex curvature of the thoracic spine.

lactation The production and secretion of milk from the breasts.

large for gestational age (LGA) A weight classification of newborns associated with poorer health outcomes, the weight falling above the 90th percentile on the intrauterine growth curve for the infant's calculated gestational age.

leukoplakia Circumscribed, firmly attached, thick white patches on the tongue and other mucous membranes, often occurring as a precancerous growth.

lobule A small lobe; the soft, lower, pendulous portion of the auricle of the ear.

locking Inability to fully extend the joint, or stiffness after being in one position for an extended time.

log-rolling Keeping the body of the patient rigid, that is, similar to a log, while being turned.

lordosis Accentuation of the lumbar curvature of the spine.

lymphangioma A tumor composed of lymphatic vessels that vary in size and are often dilated.

lymphangitis Inflammation of lymph vessels from bacterial infection of an extremity, characterized by fine red streaks running from the area of infection toward the groin or axilla.

lymphedema Swelling, particularly of subcutaneous tissues, caused by obstruction of the lymphatic system and accumulation of interstitial fluid.

macroglossia Excessively large tongue.

malleus One of the three ossicles of the middle ear, connected to the tympanic membrane.

malocclusion Inappropriate contact between the teeth of the upper and lower jaws.

McBurney point In acute appendicitis, extreme sensitivity over the appendix, approximately 2 inches above the right anterosuperior iliac spine, on a line between that spine and the umbilicus.

meconium First stools of the newborn; viscous, sticky, dark green, usually sterile and odorless.

mediastinum The space in the thoracic cavity behind the sternum and between the two pleural sacs; contains the remaining thoracic organs and structures.

medulla oblongata The lowest subdivision of the brainstem, immediately adjacent to the spinal cord.

menarche The first menstruation and initiation of cyclic menstrual function.

meninges One of three membrane layers (dura mater, pia mater, and arachnoid) that enclose the brain and spinal cord.

meningomyelocele A protrusion of the meninges and spinal cord through a defect in the vertebral column.

menorrhagia Excessive bleeding during a menstrual period that is longer in duration than usual.

metrorrhagia Menstrual bleeding at irregular intervals, sometimes prolonged, but of expected amount.

microcephaly An unusually small head of a newborn.

midaxillary line A vertical line drawn midway between the anterior and posterior axillary folds.

midclavicular line A vertical line drawn through the midpoint of the clavicle.

midsternal line A vertical line drawn through the middle of the sternum.

miosis Contraction of the pupil to less than 2 mm in diameter.

mitral valve The heart valve between the left atrium and left ventricle consisting of two cusps; it allows blood to flow into the ventricle and prevents backflow.

Montgomery tubercles Enlarged sebaceous glands located on the areola of the breast.

mucopurulent An exudate that contains both pus and mucus.

murmur A heart sound audible with the stethoscope, generated by disruptions in the passage of blood within the heart or blood vessels.

Murphy sign Pain on inspiration during palpation of the liver and gallbladder that causes the patient to stop inspiration; usually a sign of gallbladder disease.

muscle tone Level of tension or consistency of muscle mass.

myalgia Tenderness or pain in muscle.

myocardium The middle and thickest of the three layers of the wall of the heart, consisting of cardiac muscle.

myopia (Nearsightedness) a condition resulting from a refractive error in which light rays entering the eye are brought into focus in front of the retina.

myxedema A condition caused by hypothyroidism characterized by dry, waxy skin, coarse hair, intolerance to cold, cognitive impairment, and slowing of the relaxation phase of deep tendon reflexes.

nasal polyp Boggy, dependent mucosa that is rounded and elongated, and projects into the nasal cavity.

nasopharynx The portion of the pharynx extending from the posterior nares to the level of the soft palate.

neurogenic Arising from or caused by the nervous system.

nevus A circumscribed skin lesion that is presumed to be genetic; the excess or deficient tissue may involve epidermal or connective tissue, nerve elements, or vascular elements; the nevus may be pigmented or nonpigmented.

nocturia Urination at night; the individual is awakened from sleep by the need to void.

nuchal rigidity Resistance to flexion of the neck, seen in individuals with meningitis.

nystagmus Involuntary rhythmic movements of the eyes; the oscillations may be horizontal, vertical, rotary, or mixed.

oligomenorrhea Infrequent menstruation.

oncotic pressure The pressure difference between the osmotic pressure of blood and that of tissue fluid or lymph; an important force in maintaining balance between blood and surrounding tissues.

onycholysis The loosening of the nails starting at the border.

oropharynx Division of the pharynx extending from behind the soft palate dorsally to the upper edge of the epiglottis.

orthostatic Referring to an upright body position; orthostatic edema develops after standing; orthostatic hypotension occurs when the patient stands erect.

Osler nodes Small, tender, swollen areas, varying in color from pink or red to bluish, generally in the fleshy pads of fingers or toes, or in the thenar or hypothenar prominences; findings indicating subacute bacterial endocarditis.

ossification The formation of bone.

otorrhea Discharge, especially a purulent one, from the ear.

pack-years of smoking An index risk for cardiac and pulmonary problems; calculated by multiplying number of years of smoking by number of packs smoked each day.

palpebral fissures The elliptical opening between the upper and lower eyelids.

palpitation Beating of the heart so vigorous that the patient is aware of it; causes include exertion, emotional stress, hyperthyroidism, and various heart diseases.

papillae Small nipple-shaped projections; papillae on the dorsal portion of the tongue contain the taste buds.

papilledema Edema of the optic disc resulting in loss of definition of the disc margin; the cause often is increased intracranial pressure.

paradoxic pulse Variation in systolic pressure with respiration, diminishing with inspiration and increasing with expiration; also known as *pulsus paradoxus.*

parasternal Situated close to or beside the sternum.

parasympathetic nervous system The division of the autonomic nervous system responsible for the protection, conservation, and restoration of body resources.

parenchyma The functional cells of an organ, as distinguished from the supporting connective tissue framework.

paresthesia Unusual sensation such as numbness, tingling, or burning.

parietal Referring to inner walls of any body cavity.

paroxysm A sudden sharp spasm, convulsion, or attack; a sudden relapse of disease.

peak height velocity The time during pubescence at which the tempo of growth is greatest.

peau d'orange Dimpling of the skin that gives it the appearance of the skin of an orange.

pectoriloquy A striking transmission of voice sounds through the pulmonary structures, so that they are clearly audible through the stethoscope; commonly occurs from lung consolidation.

pectus carinatum (Pigeon chest) forward protrusion of the sternum.

pectus excavatum (Funnel chest) depression of the sternum.

pedunculated Having a stalk or stem that acts as a means of connection.

pericardium The fibroserous membrane covering the heart and roots of the great vessels.

perineum The region between the thighs, in the female between the vulva and the anus and in the male between the scrotum and the anus.

peristalsis The wavelike motion by which the alimentary tract propels its contents.

petechiae Purple or red pinpoint spots on the skin, the result of minute hemorrhages into the dermal or submucosal layers.

Peyer patches Collections of closely packed lymphoid follicles, forming elevations on the mucous membrane of the small intestine.

philtrum The vertical groove in the midline above the upper lip.

photophobia Increased sensitivity to light; the condition is prevalent in albinism and disorders of the conjunctiva and cornea.

pica A craving to eat nonfood substances such as dirt, clay, or starch; may occur with some nutritional deficiency states, pregnancy, or mental disorders.

pilonidal Pertaining to the sacrococcygeal area.

pitch A quality of sound that typifies its highness or lowness of tone, as determined by the frequency of vibrations.

plantar flexion Extension of the foot so that the forepart is lower than the ankle.

pleura The serous membranes covering the lungs (visceral pleura) and lining the inner aspect of the pleural cavity (parietal pleura).

pleural cavity The potential space between the usually closely opposed parietal and visceral layers of the pleura.

pleurisy Inflammation of the pleura, often associated with pneumonia.

plumbism Lead poisoning.

pneumothorax Accumulation of air or gas in the pleural space.

polydactyly Extra digits on the hands or feet.

polymenorrhea Increased frequency of menstruation not consistently associated with ovulation.

postauricular Behind the auricle of the ear.

posterior axillary line A vertical line drawn inferiorly from the posterior axillary fold.

postmenopausal bleeding Menstrual bleeding occurring 1 year or more after menopause.

postterm infant An infant born after 41 completed weeks of gestation.

postural hypotension (Orthostatic hypotension) the presence of low blood pressure when the patient stands erect.

preauricular In front of the auricle of the ear.

precordium That area of the thorax situated over the heart.

prepuce The foreskin of the penis.

presbyopia Hyperopia and impaired near vision from loss of lens elasticity, generally developing during middle age.

preterm infant An infant born before 37 weeks' gestation.

prodromal event An early sign or warning of a developing disorder.

prognathism Protrusion of the jaws, causing malocclusion of the teeth.

pronate The act of assuming a prone position; applied to the hand, the act of turning the palm backward or downward by medially rotating the forearm; applied to the foot, turning the medial edge of the foot lower and outward by eversion and abduction of the tarsal and metatarsal joints.

proprioception The sensation of position and muscular activity originating from within the body, which provides awareness of posture, movement, and changes in equilibrium.

proptosis, proptotic Bulging or protrusion of an organ, such as the eyes.

pruritus An itching sensation producing the urge to scratch.

ptosis Prolapse of an organ or part; drooping of the upper eyelid.

pubarche Beginning growth of pubic hair, breasts, and genitals.

pulmonary pressure The blood pressure in the pulmonary artery.

pulmonary valve The valve at the junction of the pulmonary artery and right ventricle consisting of three half-moon–shaped cusps; it prevents blood from regurgitating into the ventricle.

pulse The palpable, rhythmic expansion and contraction of an artery, the result of an increased thrust of blood into the circulation each time the heart contracts; it is readily felt in the arterial component of the systemic circulation and also occurs in veins (e.g., jugular vein) and highly vascular organs (e.g., liver).

punctum The tiny aperture in the margin of each eyelid that opens into a lacrimal duct.

purpura Brownish-red or purple discolorations on the skin as the result of hemorrhage into the tissue; also a group of disorders characterized by purpura.

pyrosis Epigastric burning sensation; heartburn.

QRS complex The central deflections of the electrocardiogram representing the activity of the ventricles.

rale (See *crackle*) a general term for an unexpected sound heard on auscultation of the chest; sometimes used to denote crepitus heard on ausculation.

regurgitation A backward flowing (e.g., the blood between the chambers of the heart or between the great vessels and the heart).

retrognathia Position of the jaws behind the frontal plane of the forehead.

rhonchus A dry, coarse sound in the bronchial tubes heard on auscultation of the chest, the result of partial obstruction; a sonorous rhonchus is low pitched; a sibilant rhonchus is high pitched and squeaky.

rigidity A condition of hardness and inflexibility.

saccular Pouched; shaped like a sac.

scapular line A vertical line drawn through the inferior angle of the scapula.

sclerosis Hardening or induration of body tissues, which can be the result of inflammation, particularly when it is prolonged.

scoliosis Lateral curvature of the spine.

scotoma A loss of vision in a defined area in one or both eyes; shimmering film appearing as an island in the visual field, often occurring as a prodromal symptom.

scrotal raphe The line of union of the two halves of the scrotum; often more highly pigmented than the surrounding tissue.

sebum A thick substance secreted by the sebaceous glands that consists of fat and epithelial debris.

semilunar valve Refers to the pulmonic or aortic valves.

sensorineural hearing loss Reduction in hearing acuity related to a defect in the inner ear or damage to the eighth cranial nerve.

sessile Attached by a base rather than a stalk; a sessile lesion adheres closely to the surface of the skin or mucosa (see *pedunculated*).

shunt, left to right Referring to a diversion of blood from the left side of the heart to the right (e.g., from a septal defect) or from the systemic circulation to the pulmonary circulation (e.g., from a patent ductus arteriosus).

sibilant Having the character of a hiss or whistle.

sign An objective finding perceived by the examiner.

simian crease A single palmar crease associated with Down syndrome.

sinus dysrhythmia An increase in heart rate with inspiration. It is a physiologic response to decreased left ventricular volume during inspiration producing a cyclic irregularity with each inspiration.

sinus rhythm The expected regular cardiac rhythm stimulated by the sinoatrial node.

situs inversus The inversion or transposition of the body viscera so that the heart is on the right and the liver on the left; the chest and abdominal contents become mirror images of the usual.

Skene glands (Paraurethral glands) mucus-secreting glands that open onto the vestibule on each side of the urethra.

small for gestational age (SGA) A weight classification of newborns associated with poorer health outcomes, the weight falling below the 10th percentile on the intrauterine growth curve for the infant's calculated gestational age.

smegma Sebaceous material secreted by the glans penis and epithelial cells desquamated from the prepuce; it appears as a cheesy white material.

spasm Involuntary contraction of a muscle or group of muscles, interfering with usual function of that particular muscle group.

spastic Increased muscle tone, spasms, or uncontrolled contractions of skeletal muscles causing stiff, awkward movements.

spotting Small amounts of intermenstrual bloody vaginal discharge ranging from pink to dark brown.

sprain Traumatic injury to the tendons, muscles, or ligaments around a joint.

stapes One of the three ossicles of the middle ear, connected to the inner ear.

steatorrhea Frothy, foul-smelling fecal matter that floats because of its high fat content; associated with malabsorption syndromes.

stellate Shaped like a star; arranged in a rosette.

stereognosis The ability to recognize objects by the sense of touch.

striae Streaks or lines; skin striae result from weakening of the elastic tissue associated with pregnancy, weight gain, rapid growth periods, and high levels of corticosteroids.

stridor A harsh, high-pitched sound during respiration caused by laryngeal or tracheal obstruction.

stroke Common term indicating a sudden neurologic impairment of varying degree usually related to a more or less sudden interruption of blood flow to the brain as from hemorrhage, thrombosis, or embolism.

stroke volume The amount of blood pumped out of one ventricle of the heart as the result of a single contraction.

stroma The supportive connective tissue framework of an organ as distinguished from the functional tissue (parenchyma).

sty A purulent infection of a meibomian gland of the eyelid, often caused by a staphylococcal organism.

subaortic stenosis Congenital narrowing of the outflow tract of the left ventricle caused by a ring of fibrous tissue or hypertrophy of the muscular septum just below the aortic valve.

subcutaneous emphysema The presence of air or gas beneath the skin.

subcutaneous nodules Firm and painless nodules discovered in the presence of acute rheumatic fever. These nodules occur only rarely and, when they do, usually in the presence of carditis. They appear over the extensor surfaces of certain joints, particularly the elbows, knees, and wrists; over the spinous processes of the thoracic and lumbar vertebrae; and in the suboccipital area. The skin over these nodules moves freely and is not inflamed.

subgaleal The area underlying the galea aponeurotica.

subjective data That information collected during the interview with the patient or a significant other.

subluxation Partial or incomplete dislocation.

sulcus A shallow groove or depression on the surface of an organ (e.g., the median sulcus of the prostate gland separating the two lateral lobes).

supernumerary nipples Extra nipples usually not associated with underlying glandular tissue located along the embryonic mammary ridge.

supinate To assume a supine position; applied to the arm, the act of turning the palm forward or upward by laterally rotating the forearm; applied to the foot, the act of raising the medial margin of the foot.

sutures A fibrous joint in which the bones are closely approximated, as between the infant's cranial bones, permitting expansion of the skull for brain growth.

swan neck deformity Hyperextension of the proximal interphalangeal joint with fixed flexion of the distal interphalangeal joint.

sympathetic nervous system The division of the autonomic nervous system that activates responses to physiologic or psychologic stress.

symptom The subjective indication of disease perceived by the patient.

syndactyly Webbing between the digits of the hands or feet.

systole The part of the cardiac cycle during which the heart contracts, particularly the ventricles, resulting in a forceful flow of blood into both the systemic and pulmonary circulations.

tachycardia Rapid heart rate greater than 100 beats per minute.

tachypnea Rapid, usually shallow, breathing.

tactile fremitus A tremor or vibration in any part of the body detected on palpation.

tail of Spence Upper outer tail of the breast that extends into the axilla.

term infant An infant born between 37 and 41 weeks' gestation.

terminal hair The pigmented coarse hair that grows on the scalp, axilla, pubis, and in males, the face.

thelarche The beginning of female pubertal breast development.

thrill A palpable vibration or tremor resulting from a cardiac murmur or a disruption in vascular blood flow.

thrombophlebitis Inflammation of the wall of a vein associated with thrombus formation.

thrombosis The formation or presence of a blood clot within a blood vessel or within one of the cavities of the heart.

thyrotoxicosis A disease caused by excessive quantities of thyroid hormones.

tic An involuntary movement or spasm of a small group of muscles that may be aggravated by stress or anxiety; sometimes momentarily controllable.

tinnitus An auditory sensation in the absence of sound heard in one or both ears, such as ringing, buzzing, hissing, or clicking.

tocolysis Suppression of premature labor with drugs.

tonus Expected state of muscle tone, maintained by partial contraction or alternate contraction and relaxation of neighboring muscle fibers in a group of muscles.

tophus A chalky deposit of uric acid crystals around joints or on the external ear; associated with gout.

tragus The cartilaginous projection of the ear anterior to the auditory canal meatus.

transient ischemic attack (TIA) A transient episode of cerebral dysfunction, rapid (within minutes) in onset; usually due to vasospasm, hypotension, or a variety of events producing an ischemia which resolves usually in less than 24 hours; most often referable to the areas served by carotid and/or vertebrobasilar arteries.

transient tachypnea of the newborn A self-limited neonatal respiratory problem characterized by a rapid respiratory rate and associated with maternal treatment with narcotics or analgesics during labor, premature labor and, at times, Caesarean delivery.

tremor Rhythmic, purposeless, quivering movements resulting from involuntary alternate contraction and relaxation of opposing muscle groups.

tricuspid valve A heart valve between the right atrium and right ventricle, consisting of three cusps, that allows blood to flow to the ventricle and prevents backflow.

turbinates Extensions of the ethmoid bone located along the lateral wall of the nose, covered by erectile mucous membrane.

tympanic membrane (Eardrum) a membranous structure separating the external ear from the middle ear.

umbo Landmark on the tympanic membrane created by the attachment of the tympanic membrane to the malleus.

valgus A position in which part of a limb is twisted outward away from the midline.

Valsalva maneuver Forced expiratory effort against a closed airway (i.e., closed mouth and nose or glottis).

varicosity An unnaturally swollen, often tortuous, blood or lymph vessel.

varus A position in which part of a limb is twisted inward toward the midline.

vascular Referring to blood vessels.

vasoconstriction A narrowing in the caliber of a blood vessel.

vasomotor Referring to control over the dilation and constriction of blood vessels.

vasopressor Stimulating contraction of the muscular tissues of the capillaries and arteries, causing a rise in blood pressure.

vellus hair The soft, nonpigmented hair that covers the body.

velocity of growth The rate of growth or change in growth measurements over a period of time.

venous hum A continuous musical murmur heard on auscultation over the major veins at the base of the neck, particularly when a patient is anemic, upright, and looking to the contralateral side; also heard in the healthy individual, particularly the young.

venous thrombosis Formation or presence of a blood clot within a vein.

ventilation The movement of air into and out of the lungs, resulting in the exchange of gases between the lungs and the air.

vertigo Sensation of dizziness, either of spinning oneself or of external objects whirling around oneself.

vesicular breath sounds Expected breathing sounds when the patient is healthy and free of respiratory embarrassment.

vestibular function Balance.

vestibule The almond-shaped area enclosed by the labia minora laterally, extending from the clitoris to the fourchette anteroposteriorly.

Virchow node (Signal or sentinel node) a firm supra-clavicular lymph node, particularly on the left, so enlarged that it is palpable.

virilization The process by which a female acquires male secondary sexual characteristics, usually as a result of adrenal dysfunction.

vulva (Pudendum) the visible external female genitalia consisting of the mons pubis, labia, clitoris, vaginal orifice, vestibule, and vestibular glands.

water-hammer pulse Full, forcible impulse and immediate collapse, providing a jerking sensation; characteristic of aortic regurgitation.

webbing Skin folds in the neck from the acromion to the mastoid; associated with chromosomal anomalies.

whispered pectoriloquy The transmission of a whisper in the same way as that of more readily audible speech, commonly detected when the lung is consolidated by pneumonia (see *pectoriloquy*).

whoop The noisy spasm of inspiration that terminates the paroxysms of coughing characteristic of pertussis (whooping cough); caused by a sudden, sharp increase in tension of the vocal chords.

winged scapula An outward prominence of the scapula caused by disruption of its nerves or muscles.

xanthelasma Xanthoma located on the eyelids.

xanthoma Small, flat, yellowish skin plaques, the result of lipid deposition in histiocytes (cells of the reticuloendothelial system).

xiphodynia Pain in the cartilage of the xiphoid process.

ASSESSMENT OF PAIN

Pain is a common and uncomfortable sensation and emotional experience associated with actual or potential tissue damage. Acute pain is sudden and of short duration, usually associated with surgery, injury, or an acute illness episode. Chronic pain is persistent, lasting many months or longer, usually associated with a prolonged disease process.

Persons have individualized responses to pain because it is a physiologic, behavioral, and emotional phenomenon. The threshold at which pain is perceived and the tolerance level for pain vary widely among individuals. Because of the subjective nature of pain, assessment is based mostly on history and patient responses to various scales that evaluate pain intensity and quality. When the patient experiences an injury, surgery, or illness that causes pain, you may be able to observe behavioral and physiologic cues of pain.

When the patient's chief complaint is pain, the location and related symptoms may assist in the diagnosis of a patient's condition. If the pain is related to a diagnosed condition, for example, trauma, surgery, or cancer, assessment of its character and intensity is necessary for pain control.

Unfortunately, it is often poorly controlled because there is inadequate determination of the intensity, uncertainty about the etiologic factors, and sometimes misplaced concern about the potential of addiction, tolerance, or other side effects relative to medications for pain. Patients, as well as health professionals, share many of these concerns, and if they are worried about this, they may not fully express or at times even admit the intensity of discomfort they are experiencing. That possibility, often strong, requires a direct approach to inquiry about the possible presence of pain and its intensity and character.

ANATOMY AND PHYSIOLOGY

Peripheral pain receptors transmit sensation to the spinal cord through sensory nerve-fibers. Sensory fibers are specialized for rapidly transmitted, sharp, well-localized pain and for more slowly transmitted, dull, burning, diffusely localized pain. The sensory nerve cell bodies are located in the dorsal root ganglia.

If the pain sensation is not blocked by physiologically produced interceptors, opioids, or stimulation, it is relayed from the spinal cord to the brain through the spinothalamic and spinoreticular nerve pathways. Emotions, cultural background, sleep deprivation, previous pain experience, and age are among those factors that have an impact on the perception and interpretation of pain.

Neonates are capable of perceiving pain, because the nervous system is adequately developed for pain perception by the twentieth week of gestation.

907

REVIEW OF RELATED HISTORY

Present Problem

- Onset: date of onset, sudden or slow, time of day, duration, variation, rhythm
- Quality: throbbing, shooting, stabbing, sharp, cramping, gnawing, hot or burning, aching, heavy, tender, splitting, tiring or exhausting, sickening, fear producing, punishing or cruel
- Intensity: may range from slight to severe
- Precipitating factors: what increases or decreases pain
- Location
- Effect of pain on daily activities: limitation of activity, interruption of sleep, increased need for rest periods, change in appetite
- Effect of pain on psyche: change in mood or social interactions, poor concentration, can think only about pain; irritability
- Pain control measures: distraction, relaxation, heat, electrical stimulation
- Medications: opioids, anxiolytics, nonsteroidal antiinflammatories; nonprescription

Personal and Social History

- Previous experiences with pain and its effect; typical coping strategies for pain control
- Family's concerns and cultural beliefs about pain: expect or tolerate pain in certain situations
- Attitude toward the use of opioids, anxiolytics, and other pain medications for pain control; fear of addiction
- Current or past use of illicit substances

CHILDREN

- Word(s) the child uses for pain, such as "ouch" or "hurt"
- The child's response when suddenly hurt (e.g., falling down)
- The child's response with longer lasting pain (e.g., an earache)
- How the child or parent rates pain

PHYSICAL EXAMINATION

Throughout your examination of the patient, be alert to signs of pain, which may include any combination on the following list. In cases in which communication is a problem, as with young children and elderly adults, have a family member describe known cues to the patient's expression of pain.

- Guarding, protective behavior, hands over painful area, distorted posture
- Facial mask of pain: lackluster eyes, "beaten look," wrinkled forehead, tightly closed or opened eyes, fixed or scattered movement, grimace or other distorted expression
- Vocalizations: grunting, groaning, crying, talkative patient becomes quiet
- Body movements such as head rocking, pacing, or inability to keep the hands still
- Changes in vital signs: blood pressure, pulse, respiratory rate and depth, with acute exacerbations of pain; fewer changes in vital signs found in cases of chronic pain
- Pallor and diaphoresis
- Pupil dilation
- Dry mouth
- Decreased attention span

There are a number of classic pain patterns that provide valuable clues to underlying conditions:

- Heavy, throbbing, and aching pain may be associated with a tumor pressing on a cavity.
- Burning, shocklike pain may indicate nerve tissue damage.
- A clenched fist over the chest with diaphoresis and grimacing is the classic picture of myocardial infarction.

Pain Assessment Scales

A variety of scales and instruments have been developed to obtain and measure a patient's perception of pain intensity and quality; only a sample is presented here (Figures A-1 through A-4). Very few of the instruments widely used include the patient's emotional response to pain. Remember that the patient's perception may not compare with expected pain intensity identified by other individuals. It is that perception, however, that should be the "gold standard," the controlling variable. The use of scales also permits the very important day-to-day documentation of the response to therapy.

FIGURE A-1
Descriptive Pain Intensity Scale

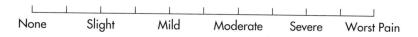

None   Slight   Mild   Moderate   Severe   Worst Pain

FIGURE A-2
Numeric Pain Intensity Scale

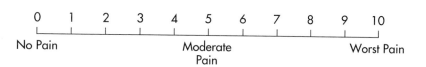

FIGURE A-3
Visual Analogic Scale

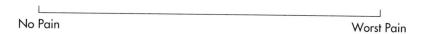

No Pain   Worst Pain

FIGURE A-4
Self-contained, portable, pain-rating instrument that can provide an immediate assessment of pain. It is a 5×20-cm plastic visual analogue scale with a sliding marker that moves within a 10-cm groove. The side facing the patient (**A**) resembles a traditional visual analogue scale, whereas the opposite side (**B**) is marked in centimeters to quantify pain intensity. The scale has been shown to be a valid tool to measure pain intensity. It facilitates the documentation of pain and the monitoring of pain relief interventions.

From Grossman et al, 1992.

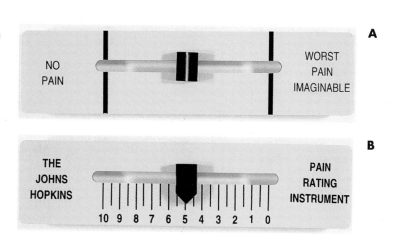

Ask the patient to identify the pain scale he or she prefers to use. Document the selection and use it consistently in all subsequent assessments of pain intensity.

When assessing pain, remember that intensity may vary in different sites. Use body drawings to have the patient identify sites of pain. Pain intensity may also vary with routine activity such as moving, coughing, or deep breathing. Be sure to link pain intensity reported with location and activity.

CHILDREN

The history and physical examination will provide much information about a child's pain. Some children as young as 3 years of age have adequate communication skills to respond to pediatric pain assessment scales. Be sure a child understands concepts of higher/lower and more/less in order to use the scales. Children do best when given an opportunity to practice the chosen scale using selected examples of past painful experiences, such as a finger prick, earache, or skinned knee.

The Wong/Baker Faces Rating Scale (Figure A-5) and the Oucher Scale (Figures A-6, A-7, and A-8) are examples of pain scales that are reliable and valid for children.

Using Figures A-6, A-7, and A-8, ask the child to select the face that fits his or her level of pain. Use the version that best fits the child's cultural identity (Caucasian, African-American, or Hispanic).

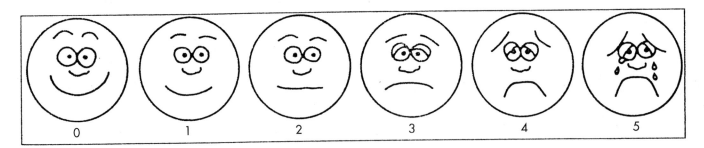

FIGURE A-5

Wong/Baker Faces Rating Scale. Explain to the patient that each face is for a person who feels happy because he has no pain (hurt) or sad because he has some or a lot of pain. **Face 0** is very happy because the person doesn't hurt at all. **Face 1** hurts just a little bit. **Face 2** hurts a little more. **Face 3** hurts a little more. **Face 4** hurts a whole lot. **Face 5** hurts as much as you can imagine, although you don't have to be crying to feel this bad. Ask the patient to choose the face that best describes how he or she is feeling. *Recommended for persons 3 years and older.*

Originally published by Whaley L and Wong D: *Nursing care of infants and children,* ed 3, 1987, Mosby. Reprinted by permission. Research reported in Wong D and Backer C: Pain in children: comparison of assessment scales, *Pediatric Nursing* 14(1):9-17, 1988.

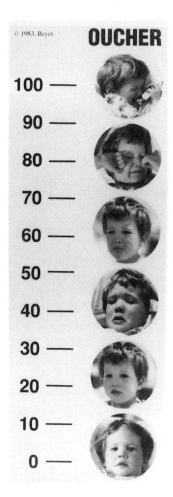

FIGURE A-6
Oucher Scale (Caucasian).

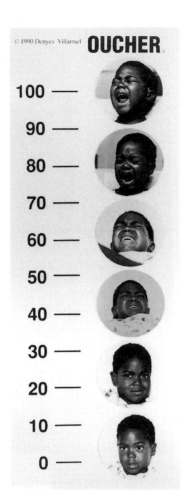

FIGURE A-7
Oucher Scale (African-American).

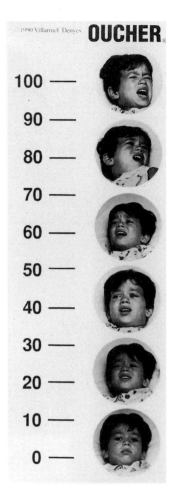

FIGURE A-8
Oucher Scale (Hispanic).

Sports Preparticipation Evaluation

Each year millions of children and youth who participate in organized sports seek a health care provider's signature on a preparticipation evaluation (PPE) (American Academy of Pediatrics, 1991). States and local school districts require young athletes to obtain "medical clearance" before participation in sports. Moreover, rare high-profile cases of death and serious injury on the playing field, usually among big-time college and professional athletes, keep concerns about the risks of sports participation in the public eye.

Whether athletes receive the PPE in the context of an ongoing primary care relationship or as a focused preseason check-up, certain goals of the evaluation are universal:

- To identify conditions that may interfere with a person's ability to participate in a sport
- To identify health problems that increase the risk of injury or death during sports participation
- To help select an appropriate sport for a person's particular abilities and physical status

The ultimate goal of the PPE is to ensure safe participation in an appropriate physical activity. Sports and disciplined physical effort enhance fitness and coordination, increase self-esteem, and provide positive social experiences. Ultimately, relatively few persons undergoing PPEs have conditions that might limit participation, and most of these conditions are known before the PPE takes place.

A PPE may be performed in many settings, but ideally it occurs in the office of a regular provider in the context of an ongoing primary care relationship. This takes advantage of a medical history that may already exist in the provider's records. It is individualized and tailored to the specific needs of the particular patient, and discussion of important issues that may be unrelated to sports participation is feasible and expected. Coordination of follow-up care should be efficient.

Another approach to the PPE is the *stations method,* in which a large number of patients are evaluated in a single session by providers from many disciplines, including physicians, nurses, trainers, and physical therapists. Each provider takes responsibility for a specific aspect of the evaluation at a station dedicated to that purpose. Athletes move from one station to the next, accumulating historical and objective information on a standard form. A check-out station is critical to the success of this approach. The person in charge of this station reviews the data collected during the

This appendix contributed by John S. Andrews, MD, Johns Hopkins Children's Center, Baltimore, Maryland.

evaluation and coordinates any necessary follow-up action, communicating directly with the athlete (and parents if appropriate) and generating a written report. If the PPE is not itself a comprehensive service that addresses issues unrelated to sports participation, the need for routine primary care remains. This point should be emphasized at the check-out station.

The PPE should be completed well enough in advance of the projected sports participation so that rehabilitation or therapy of any problems identified can be completed before participation begins. As a rule, 6 weeks before participation is appropriate. Once an initial, thorough PPE has been completed, subsequent PPEs can be more brief and give attention to interim problems.

The only proven benefit of the PPE is recognition of athletes at risk for later orthopedic injury by identifying recent or poorly rehabilitated injuries that can become worse with sports participation (American Medical Association, Group on Science and Technology, 1994). Most of these injuries are detected by a careful history. In fact, over 75% of all problems affecting athletes are detected by history alone (Goldberg et al, 1980; American Medical Association, Group on Science and Technology, 1994). Asthma is a good example. Unless a patient is in respiratory distress at the time of the evaluation, physical examination is unlikely to lead to recognition of this condition. However, a history should lead quickly to the diagnosis. Sudden cardiac death on the playing field is a source of great concern. Conditions leading to this very uncommon event are rarely associated with detectable physical findings. They may, however, be associated with symptoms or family history revealed by a careful history at the time of the PPE.

The physical examination component of the PPE should center on high-yield areas, particularly those related to sports participation and those identified by the history. Items such as auscultation of the lung fields and otoscopy are low-yield—unless the patient is symptomatic at the time of the evaluation—and can distract from more fruitful areas such as the cardiac and orthopedic examinations.

Recommended components of the PPE are shown in Table B-1. Elements of the history and physical examination are organized by system, with physical examination items in italics. The orthopedic component of the physical examination is the one with which most primary care providers are unfamiliar. Garrick has developed a "2-minute" screening orthopedic examination that is useful for this purpose (Figure B-1) (Garrick, 1977). Having undergone several revisions since its publication in 1977, the 14-step examination consists of observing the athlete in a variety of positions and postures that highlight asymmetries in range of motion, strength, and muscle bulk. These differences serve to identify acute or old, poorly rehabilitated injuries.

Once a PPE has been completed, the information gathered must be used to guide sport selection, to plan therapy or rehabilitation of illnesses or injuries detected during the evaluation, and in rare instances, to limit participation or disqualify a child (Figures B-2 and B-3). These decisions are individual, but there are resources available to guide them (Tables B-2, B-3, and B-4). There is nothing legally binding about a health care provider's recommendation to limit participation.

The 14-step screening orthopedic examination

The athlete should be dressed so that the joints and muscle groups included in the examination are easily visible—usually gym shorts for males, gym shorts and a T-short for females. Keep in mind that one of the most important points to look for in the orthopedic screening examination is symmetry. (Adapted from *Preparticipation Physical Evaluation, ed 2*.)

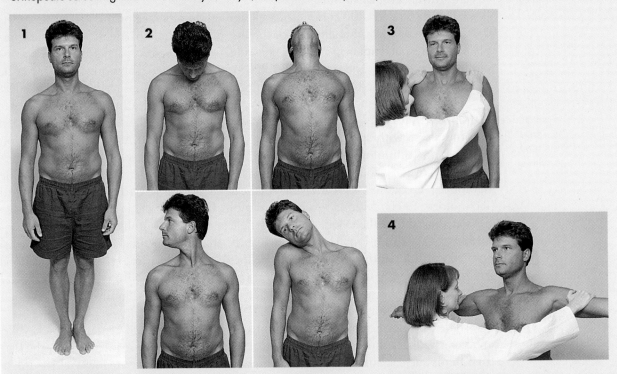

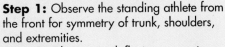

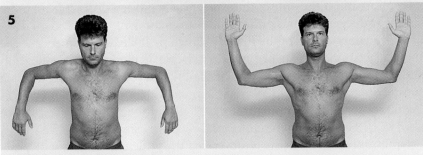

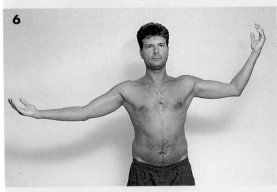

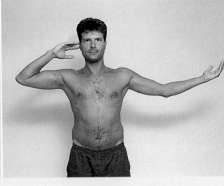

Step 1: Observe the standing athlete from the front for symmetry of trunk, shoulders, and extremities.

Step 2: Observe neck flexion, extension, lateral flexion on each side, and rotation to evaluate range of motion and the cervical spine.

Step 3: Have the athlete shrug the shoulders against resistance from the examiner to evaluate trapezius strength.

Step 4: Have the athlete perform shoulder abduction against resistance from the examiner to assess deltoid strength.

Step 5: Observe internal and external rotation of the shoulder to evaluate range of motion of the glenohumeral joint.

Step 6: Observe extension and flexion of the elbow to assess range of motion.

FIGURE B-1

The 14-step screening orthopedic examination

From Andrews, 1997.

Step 7: Observe pronation and supination of the forearm to evaluate elbow and wrist range of motion.

Step 8: Have the athlete clench the fist, then spread the fingers to assess range of motion in the hand and fingers.

Step 9: Observe the standing athlete from the rear for symmetry of trunk, shoulders, and extremities.

Step 10: Have the athlete stand with the knees straight and bend backward from the waste. Discomfort with extension of the lumbar spine may be associated with spondylolysis and spondylolisthesis.

Step 11: Have the athlete stand with the knees straight and flex forward at the waist, first away from the examiner, then toward the examiner, to assess for scoliosis, spine range of motion, and hamstring flexibility.

Step 12: Have the athlete stand facing the examiner with quadriceps flexed to observe symmetry of leg masculature.

Step 13: Have the athlete duck walk four steps to assess hip, knee, and ankle range of motion, strength, and balance.

Step 14: Have the athlete stand on the toes, then the heels to evaluate calf strength, symmetry, and balance.

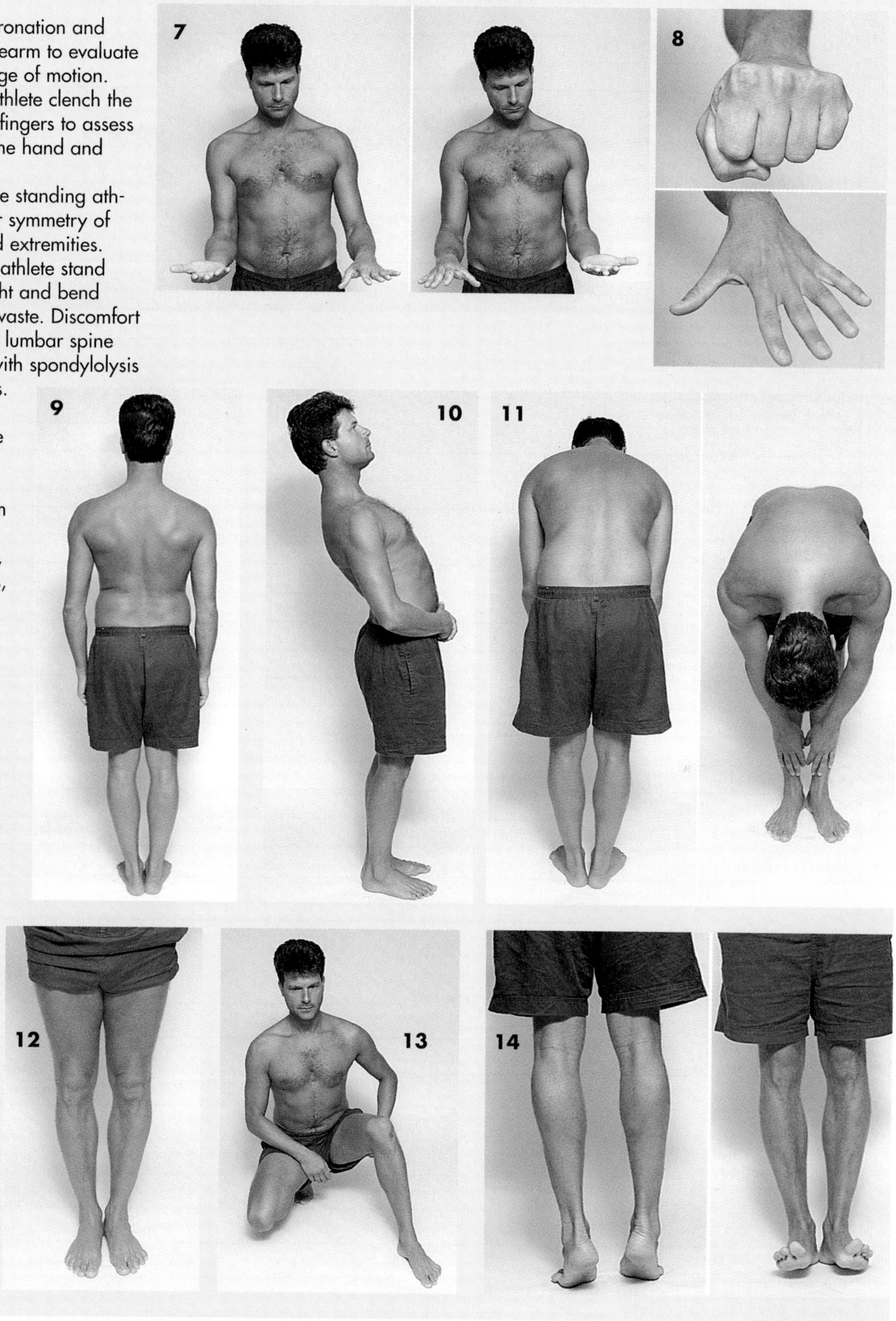

FIGURE B-1—cont'd

Preparticipation Physical Evaluation

PHYSICAL EXAMINATION

Name _____ Date of birth _____

Height _____ Weight _____ % Body fat (optional) _____ Pulse _____ BP___/____ (___/___ , ___/___)

Vision R 20/ _____ L 20/ _____   Corrected: Y N   Pupils: Equal _____   Unequal _____

	NORMAL	ABNORMAL FINDINGS	INITIALS*
MEDICAL			
Appearance			
Eyes/Ears/Nose/Throat			
Lymph Nodes			
Heart			
Pulses			
Lungs			
Abdomen			
Genitalia (males only)			
Skin			
MUSCULOSKELETAL			
Neck			
Back			
Shoulder/arm			
Elbow/forearm			
Wrist/hand			
Hip/thigh			
Knee			
Leg/ankle			
Foot			

* Station-based examination only

CLEARANCE

❑ Cleared

❑ Cleared after completing evaluation/rehabilitation for: _____

_____

_____

_____

❑ Not cleared for: _____   Reason: _____

Recommendations: _____

_____

_____

_____

Name of physician (print/type) _____ Date _____

Address _____ Phone_____

Signature of physician _____, MD or DO

FIGURE B-2

Preparticipation Physical Evaluation

HISTORY

DATE OF EXAM _____

Name_____ Sex _____ Age _____ Date of birth_____

Grade____ School _____ Sport(s) _____

Address _____ Phone_____

Personal physician_____

In case of emergency, contact

Name _____ Relationship _____ Phone (H) _____ (W) _____

Explain "Yes" answers below.
Circle questions you don't know the answers to.

	Yes	No
1. Have you had a medical illness or injury since your last check up or sports physical?	☐	☐
Do you have an ongoing or chronic illness?	☐	☐
2. Have you ever been hospitalized overnight?	☐	☐
Have you ever had surgery?	☐	☐
3. Are you currently taking any prescription or nonprescription (over-the-counter) medications or pills or using an inhaler?	☐	☐
Have you ever taken any supplements or vitamins to help you gain or lose weight or improve your performance?	☐	☐
4. Do you have any allergies (for example, to pollen, medicine, food, or stinging insects)?	☐	☐
Have you ever had a rash or hives develop during or after exercise?	☐	☐
5. Have you ever passed out during or after exercise?	☐	☐
Have you ever been dizzy during or after exercise?	☐	☐
Have you ever had chest pain during or after exercise?	☐	☐
Do you get tired more quickly than your friends do during exercise?	☐	☐
Have you ever had racing of your heart or skipped heartbeats?	☐	☐
Have you had high blood pressure or high cholesterol?	☐	☐
Have you ever been told you have a heart murmur?	☐	☐
Has any family member or relative died of heart problems or of sudden death before age 50?	☐	☐
Have you had a severe viral infection (for example, myocarditis or mononucleosis) within the last month?	☐	☐
Has a physician ever denied or restricted your participation in sports for any heart problems?	☐	☐
6. Do you have any current skin problems (for example, itching, rashes, acne, warts, fungus, or blisters)?	☐	☐
7. Have you ever had a head injury or concussion?	☐	☐
Have you ever been knocked out, become unconscious, or lost your memory?	☐	☐
Have you ever had a seizure?	☐	☐
Do you have frequent or severe headaches?	☐	☐
Have you ever had numbness or tingling in your arms, hands, legs, or feet?	☐	☐
Have you ever had a stinger, burner, or pinched nerve?	☐	☐
8. Have you ever become ill from exercising in the heat?	☐	☐
9. Do you cough, wheeze, or have trouble breathing during or after activity?	☐	☐
Do you have asthma?	☐	☐
Do you have seasonal allergies that require medical treatment?	☐	☐

	Yes	No
10. Do you use any special protective or corrective equipment or devices that aren't usually used for your sport or position (for example, knee brace, special neck roll, foot orthotics, retainer on your teeth, hearing aid)?	☐	☐
11. Have you had any problems with your eyes or vision?	☐	☐
Do you wear glasses, contacts, or protective eyewear?	☐	☐
12. Have you ever had a sprain, strain, or swelling after injury?	☐	☐
Have you broken or fractured any bones or dislocated any joints?	☐	☐
Have you had any other problems with pain or swelling in muscles, tendons, bones, or joints?	☐	☐

If yes, check appropriate box and explain below.

☐ Head	☐ Elbow	☐ Hip
☐ Neck	☐ Forearm	☐ Thigh
☐ Back	☐ Wrist	☐ Knee
☐ Chest	☐ Hand	☐ Shin/calf
☐ Shoulder	☐ Finger	☐ Ankle
☐ Upper arm		☐ Foot

	Yes	No
13. Do you want to weigh more or less than you do now?	☐	☐
Do you lose weight regularly to meet weight requirements for your sport?	☐	☐
14. Do you feel stressed out?	☐	☐

15. Record the dates of your most recent immunizations (shots) for:

Tetanus _____   Measles _____

Hepatitis B _____   Chickenpox _____

FEMALES ONLY

16. When was your first menstrual period? _____

When was your most recent menstrual period? _____

How much time do you usually have from the start of one period to the start of another? _____

How many periods have you had in the last year?_____

What was the longest time between periods in the last year? _____

Explain "Yes" answers here:_____

_____

_____

_____

_____

_____

_____

_____

_____

_____

I hereby state that, to the best of my knowledge, my answers to the above questions are complete and correct.

Signature of athlete _____ Signature of parent/guardian _____ Date _____

FIGURE B-2—cont'd

Preparticipation Physical Evaluation

CLEARANCE FORM

❑ **Cleared**

❑ **Cleared after completing evaluation/rehabilitation for:** _____

_____

_____

_____

❑ **Not cleared for:** _____ **Reason:** _____

Recommendations: _____

_____

_____

_____

Name of physician (print/type) _____ **Date** _____

Address _____ **Phone** _____

Signature of physician _____ **, MD or DO**

FIGURE B-3

Table B-1: Recommended Components of the PPE

Medical History

Illnesses or injuries since the last check-up or PPE

Hospitalizations or surgeries

Medications used by the athlete (including those he or she may be taking to enhance performance)

Use of any special equipment or protective devices during sports participation

Allergies, particularly those associated with anaphylaxis or respiratory compromise and those provoked by exercise

Immunization status including hepatitis B and varicella

Height and weight*

Cardiac

Symptoms of syncope, dizziness, or chest pain during exercise

History of high blood pressure or heart murmurs

Family history of heart disease

Previous history of disqualification or limited participation in sports because of a cardiac problem

Blood pressure

Heart rate and rhythm

Pulses

Auscultation for murmurs

Respiratory

Asthma, coughing, wheezing, or dyspnea with exercise

Neurology

History of a significant head injury or concussion

Numbness or tingling in the extremities

Severe headaches

Vision

Visual problems

Corrective lenses

Visual acuity

Orthopedic

Previous injuries that have limited sports participation

Injuries that have been associated with pain, swelling, or the need for medical intervention

Screening orthopedic examination

Psychosocial

Weight control and body image

Stresses at home or in school

Use or abuse of drugs and alcohol

Attention to signs of eating disorders including oral ulcerations, decreased tooth enamel, edema

Genitourinary

Age at menarche, last menstrual period, regularity of menstrual periods, number of periods in the last year, and longest interval between periods

Palpation of the abdomen

Palpation of the testicles

Examination of inguinal canals

From Andrews, 1997.

*Italics indicate physical exam items

Table B-2: Classification of Sports by Contact

CONTACT/COLLISION	LIMITED CONTACT	NONCONTACT
Basketball	Baseball	Archery
Boxing*	Bicycling	Badminton
Diving	Cheerleading	Body building
Field hockey	Canoeing/kayaking	Bowling
Football	(white water)	Canoeing/kayaking
Flag	Fencing	(flat water)
Tackle	Field	Crew/rowing
Ice hockey	High jump	Curling
Lacrosse	Pole vault	Dancing
Martial arts	Floor hockey	Field
Rodeo	Gymnastics	Discus
Rugby	Handball	Javelin
Ski jumping	Horseback riding	Shot put
Soccer	Racquetball	Golf
Team handball	Skating	Orienteering
Water polo	Ice	Power lifting
Wrestling	Inline	Race walking
	Roller	Riflery
	Skiing	Rope jumping
	Cross-country	Running
	Downhill	Sailing
	Water	Scuba diving
	Softball	Strength training
	Squash	Swimming
	Ultimate Frisbee	Table tennis
	Volleyball	Tennis
	Windsurfing/surfing	Track
		Weight lifting

From American Academy of Pediatrics, 1994.
*Participation not recommended

Table B-3: Medical Conditions and Sports Participation

This table is designed to be understood by medical and nonmedical personnel. In the "Explanation" section below, "Needs evaluation" means that a physician with appropriate knowledge and experience should assess the safety of a given sport for an athlete with the listed medical condition. Unless otherwise noted, this is because of the variability of the severity of the disease or of the risk of injury among the specific sports in Table B-2, or both.

CONDITION	MAY PARTICIPATE?
Atlantoaxial instability (instability of the joint between cervical vertebrae 1 and 2) *Explanation:* Athlete needs evaluation to assess risk of spinal cord injury during sports participation.	Qualified Yes
Bleeding disorder *Explanation:* Athlete needs evaluation.	Qualified Yes
Cardiovascular diseases	
Carditis (inflammation of the heart) *Explanation:* Carditis may result in sudden death with exertion.	No
Hypertension (high blood pressure) *Explanation:* Those with significant essential (unexplained) hypertension should avoid weight and power lifting, body building, and strength training. Those with secondary hypertension (hypertension caused by a previously identified disease), or severe essential hypertension, need evaluation.	Qualified Yes
Congenital heart disease (structural heart defects present at birth) *Explanation:* Those with mild forms may participate fully; those with moderate or severe forms, or who have undergone surgery, need evaluation.	Qualified Yes
Dysrhythmia (irregular heart rhythm) *Explanation:* Athlete needs evaluation because some types require therapy or make certain sports dangerous, or both.	Qualified Yes
Mitral valve prolapse (abnormal heart valve) *Explanation:* Those with symptoms (chest pain, symptoms of possible dysrhythmia) or evidence of mitral regurgitation (leaking) on physical examination need evaluation. All others may participate fully.	Qualified Yes
Heart murmur *Explanation:* If the murmur is innocent (does not indicate heart disease), full participation is permitted. Otherwise the athlete needs evaluation (see congenital heart disease and mitral valve prolapse above).	Qualified Yes
Cerebral palsy *Explanation:* Athlete needs evaluation.	Qualified Yes
Diabetes mellitus *Explanation:* All sports can be played with proper attention to diet, hydration, and insulin therapy. Particular attention is needed for activities that last 30 minutes or more.	Yes
Diarrhea *Explanation:* Unless disease is mild, no participation is permitted, because diarrhea may increase the risk of dehydration and heat illness. See "Fever" below.	Qualified No
Eating disorders Anorexia nervosa Bulimia nervosa *Explanation:* These patients need both medical and psychiatric assessment before participation.	Qualified Yes
Eyes Functionally one-eyed athlete Loss of an eye	Qualified Yes

From American Academy of Pediatrics, 1994.

Continued

Table B-3: Medical Conditions and Sports Participation—cont'd

CONDITION	MAY PARTICIPATE?
Eyes, cont'd	
Detached retina	
Previous eye surgery or serious eye injury	
Explanation: A functionally one-eyed athlete has a best corrected visual acuity of <20/40 in the worse eye. These athletes would suffer significant disability if the better eye was seriously injured as would those with loss of an eye. Some athletes who have previously undergone eye surgery or had a serious eye injury may have an increased risk of injury because of weakened eye tissue. Availability of eye guards approved by the American Society for Testing Materials (ASTM) and other protective equipment may allow participation in most sports, but this must be judged on an individual basis.	
Fever	No
Explanation: Fever can increase cardiopulmonary effort, reduce maximum exercise capacity, make heat illness more likely, and increase orthostatic hypotension during exercise. Fever may rarely accompany myocarditis or other infections that may make exercise dangerous.	
Heat illness, history of	Qualified Yes
Explanation: Because of the increased likelihood of recurrence, the athlete needs individual assessment to determine the presence of predisposing conditions and to arrange a prevention strategy.	
HIV infection	Yes
Explanation: Because of the apparent minimal risk to others, all sports may be played that the state of health allows. In all athletes, skin lesions should be properly covered, and athletic personnel should use universal precautions when handling blood or body fluids with visible blood.	
Kidney: absence of one	Qualified Yes
Explanation: Athlete needs individual assessment for contact/collision and limited contact sports.	
Liver: enlarged	Qualified Yes
Explanation: If the liver is acutely enlarged, participation should be avoided because of risk of rupture. If the liver is chronically enlarged, individual assessment is needed before collision/contact or limited contact sports are played.	
Malignancy	Qualified Yes
Explanation: Athlete needs individual assessment.	
Musculoskeletal disorders	Qualified Yes
Explanation: Athlete needs individual assessment.	
Neurologic	
History of serious head or spine trauma, severe or repeated concussions, or craniotomy.	Qualified Yes
Explanation: Athlete needs individual assessment for collision/contact or limited contact sports, and also for noncontact sports if there are deficits in judgment or cognition. Recent research supports a conservative approach to management of concussion.	
Convulsive disorder, well controlled	Yes
Explanation: Risk of convulsion during participation is minimal	
Convulsive disorder, poorly controlled	Qualified Yes
Explanation: Athlete needs individual assessment for collision/contact or limited contact sports. Avoid the following noncontact sports: archery, riflery, swimming, weight or power lifting, strength training, or sports involving heights. In these sports, occurrence of a convulsion may be a risk to self or others.	
Obesity	Qualified Yes
Explanation: Because of the risk of heat illness, obese persons need careful acclimatization and hydration.	

Table B-3: Medical Conditions and Sports Participation—cont'd

CONDITION	MAY PARTICIPATE?
Organ transplant recipient	Qualified Yes
Explanation: Athlete needs individual assessment.	
Ovary: absence of one	Yes
Explanation: Risk of severe injury to the remaining ovary is minimal.	
Respiratory	
Pulmonary compromise including cystic fibrosis	Qualified Yes
Explanation: Athlete needs individual assessment, but generally all sports may be played if oxygenation remains satisfactory during a graded exercise test. Patients with cystic fibrosis need acclimatization and good hydration to reduce the risk of heat illness.	
Asthma	Yes
Explanation: With proper medication and education, only athletes with the most severe asthma will have to modify their participation.	
Acute upper respiratory infection	Qualified Yes
Explanation: Upper respiratory obstruction may affect pulmonary function. Athlete needs individual assessment for all but mild disease. See "Fever" above.	
Sickle cell disease	Qualified Yes
Explanation: Athlete needs individual assessment. In general, if status of the illness permits, all but high exertion, collision/contact sports may be played. Overheating, dehydration, and chilling must be avoided.	
Sickle cell trait	Yes
Explanation: It is unlikely that individuals with sickle cell trait (AS) have an increased risk of sudden death or other medical problems during athletic participation except under the most extreme conditions of heat, humidity, and possibly increased altitude. These individuals, like all athletes, should be carefully conditioned, acclimatized, and hydrated to reduce any possible risk.	
Skin: boils, herpes, simplex, impetigo, scabies, molluscum contagiosum	Qualified Yes
Explanation: While the patient is contagious, participation in gymnastics with mats, martial arts, wrestling, or other collision/contact or limited contact sports is not allowed. Herpes simplex virus probably is not transmitted via mats.	
Spleen, enlarged	Qualified Yes
Explanation: Patients with acutely enlarged spleens should avoid all sports because of risk of rupture. Those with chronically enlarged spleens need individual assessment before playing collision/contact or limited contact sports.	
Testicle: absent or undescended	Yes
Explanation: Certain sports may require a protective cup.	

Table B-4: Classification of Sports by Strenuousness

HIGH TO MODERATE INTENSITY		
HIGH TO MODERATE DYNAMIC AND STATIC DEMANDS	**HIGH TO MODERATE DYNAMIC AND LOW STATIC DEMANDS**	**HIGH TO MODERATE STATIC AND LOW DYNAMIC DEMANDS**
Boxing*	Badminton	Archery
Crew/rowing	Baseball	Auto racing
Cross-country skiing	Basketball	Diving
Cycling	Field hockey	Equestrian
Downhill skiing	Lacrosse	Field events (jumping)
Fencing	Orienteering	Field events (throwing)
Football	Ping Pong	Gymnastics
Ice hockey	Race walking	Karate or judo
Rugby	Racquetball	Motorcycling
Running (sprint)	Soccer	Rodeoing
Speed skating	Squash	Sailing
Water polo	Swimming	Ski jumping
Wrestling	Tennis	Water skiing
	Volleyball	Weight lifting

LOW INTENSITY (LOW DYNAMIC AND LOW STATIC DEMANDS)
Bowling
Cricket
Curling
Golf
Riflery

From American Academy of Pediatrics, 1994.
*Participation not recommended

CONVERSION TABLES

Length

IN	CM	CM	IN
1	2.54	1	0.4
2	5.08	2	0.8
4	10.16	3	1.2
6	15.24	4	1.6
8	20.32	5	2.0
10	25.40	6	2.4
20	50.80	8	3.1
30	76.20	10	3.9
40	101.60	20	7.9
50	127.00	30	11.8
60	152.40	40	15.7
70	177.80	50	19.7
80	203.20	60	23.6
90	228.60	70	27.6
100	254.00	80	31.5
150	381.00	90	35.4
200	508.00	100	39.4

1 in = 2.54 cm
1 cm = 0.3937 in

Weight

LB	KG	KG	LB
1	0.5	1	2.2
2	0.9	2	4.4
4	1.8	3	6.6
6	2.7	4	8.8
8	3.6	5	11.0
10	4.5	6	13.2
20	9.1	8	17.6
30	13.6	10	22
40	18.2	20	44
50	22.7	30	66
60	27.3	40	88
70	31.8	50	110
80	36.4	60	132
90	40.9	70	154
100	45.4	80	176
150	66.2	90	198
200	90.8	100	220

1 lb = 0.454 kg
1 kg = 2.204 lb

TEMPERATURE EQUIVALENTS

CELSIUS*	FAHRENHEIT†	CELSIUS*	FAHRENHEIT†
34.0	93.2	38.6	101.4
34.2	93.6	38.8	101.8
34.4	93.9	39.0	102.2
34.6	94.3	39.2	102.5
34.8	94.6	39.4	102.9
35.0	95.0	39.6	103.2
35.2	95.4	39.8	103.6
35.4	95.7	40.0	104.0
35.6	96.1	40.2	104.3
35.8	96.4	40.4	104.7
36.0	96.8	40.6	105.1
36.2	97.1	40.8	105.4
36.4	97.5	41.0	105.8
36.6	97.8	41.2	106.1
36.8	98.2	41.4	106.5
37.0	98.6	41.6	106.8
37.2	98.9	41.8	107.2
37.4	99.3	42.0	107.6
37.6	99.6	42.2	108.0
37.8	100.0	42.4	108.3
38.0	100.4	42.6	108.7
38.2	100.7	42.8	109.0
38.4	101.1	43.0	109.4

From Hoekelman, 1992.

*To convert Celsius to Fahrenheit: $(9/5 \times \text{Temperature}) + 32$).

†To convert Fahrenheit to Celsius: $5/9 \times (\text{Temperature} - 32)$.

GROWTH CURVE CHARTS FOR CHILDREN AND ADOLESCENTS

Growth curves are needed to determine the appropriateness of an infant's or a child's height, weight, and head circumference for age. Clues to significant health problems are sometimes revealed because the child is not growing as expected. These growth curves can be used for a one-time assessment, but they become more valuable if used over time to plot the child's growth pattern.

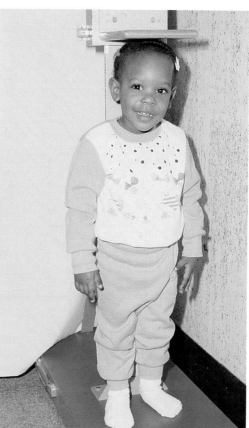

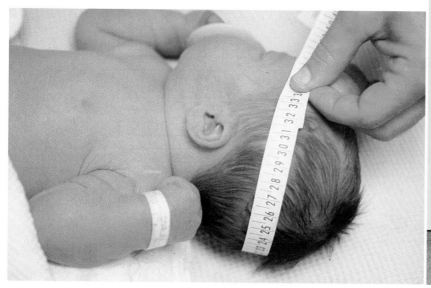

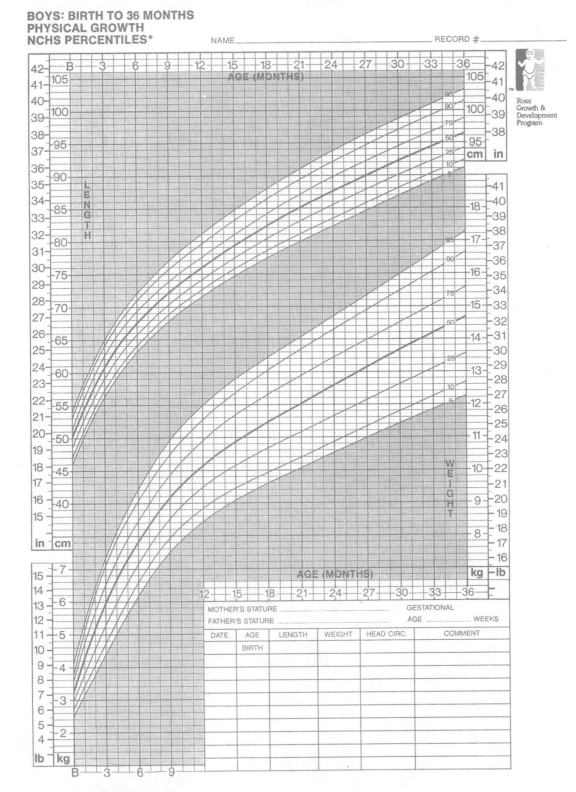

FIGURE E-1, A

Physical growth curves for children: birth to 36 months. **A,** Boys.

Courtesy Ross Laboratories, Columbus, Ohio.

BOYS: BIRTH TO 36 MONTHS
PHYSICAL GROWTH
NCHS PERCENTILES*

NAME_____   RECORD #_____

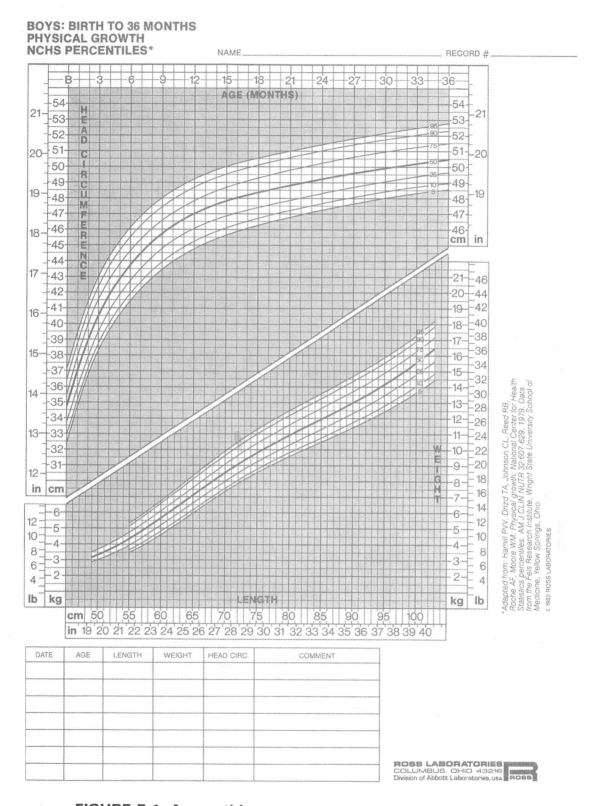

*Adapted from: Hamill PVV, Drizd TA, Johnson CL, Reed RB, Roche AF, Moore WM. Physical growth: National Center for Health Statistics percentiles. AM J CLIN NUTR 32:607-629, 1979. Data from the Fels Research Institute, Wright State University School of Medicine, Yellow Springs, Ohio.
© 1982 ROSS LABORATORIES

DATE	AGE	LENGTH	WEIGHT	HEAD CIRC.	COMMENT

ROSS LABORATORIES
COLUMBUS, OHIO 43216
Division of Abbott Laboratories, USA

FIGURE E-1, A—cont'd

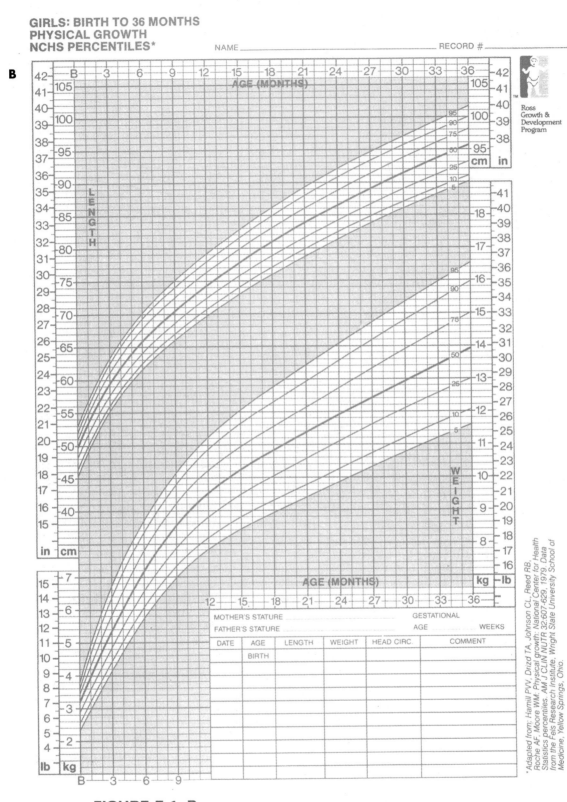

GIRLS: BIRTH TO 36 MONTHS
PHYSICAL GROWTH
NCHS PERCENTILES*

NAME _____ RECORD # _____

Ross
Growth &
Development
Program

*Adapted from: Hamill PVV, Drizd TA, Johnson CL, Reed RB, Roche AF, Moore WM. Physical growth: National Center for Health Statistics percentiles. AM J CLIN NUTR 32:607-629, 1979. Data from the Fels Research Institute, Wright State University School of Medicine, Yellow Springs, Ohio.

© 1982 ROSS LABORATORIES

MOTHER'S STATURE _____ GESTATIONAL
FATHER'S STATURE _____ AGE _____ WEEKS

DATE	AGE	LENGTH	WEIGHT	HEAD CIRC.	COMMENT
	BIRTH				

FIGURE E-1, B
Physical growth curves for children: birth to 36 months. **B,** Girls.

Courtesy Ross Laboratories, Columbus, Ohio.

GIRLS: BIRTH TO 36 MONTHS
PHYSICAL GROWTH
NCHS PERCENTILES*

NAME_____ RECORD #_____

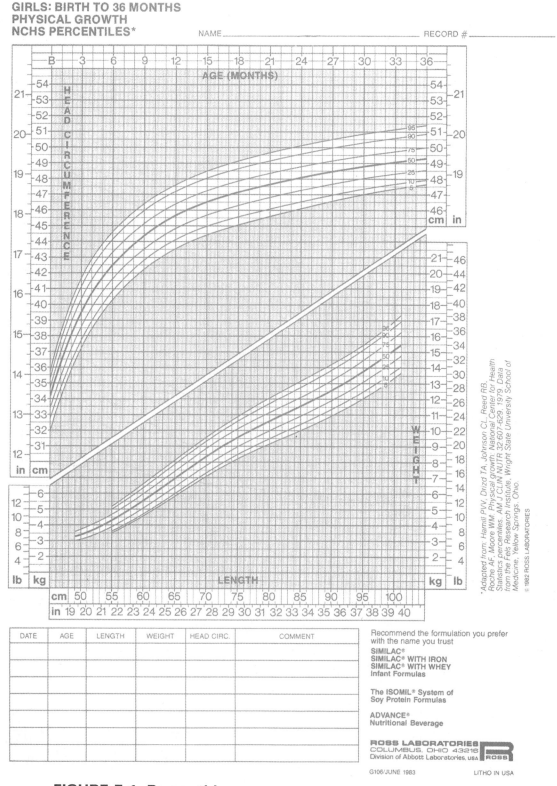

*Adapted from: Hamill PVV, Drizd TA, Johnson CL, Reed RB, Roche AF, Moore WM. Physical growth: National Center for Health Statistics percentiles. AM J CLIN NUTR 32:607-629, 1979. Data from the Fels Research Institute, Wright State University School of Medicine, Yellow Springs, Ohio.

© 1982 ROSS LABORATORIES

DATE	AGE	LENGTH	WEIGHT	HEAD CIRC.	COMMENT

Recommend the formulation you prefer
with the name you trust

SIMILAC®
SIMILAC® WITH IRON
SIMILAC® WITH WHEY
Infant Formulas

The ISOMIL® System of
Soy Protein Formulas

ADVANCE®
Nutritional Beverage

FIGURE E-1, B—cont'd

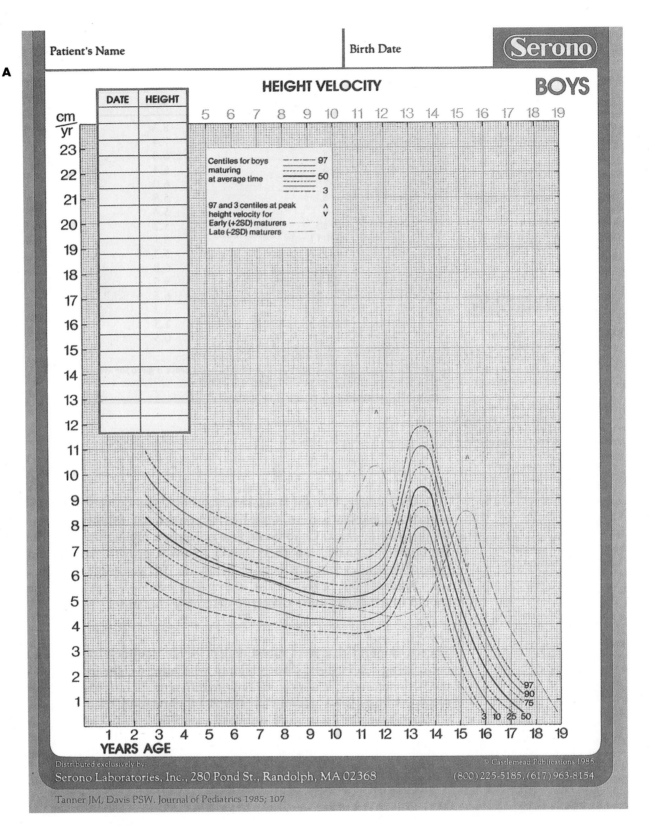

FIGURE E-2

Height velocity growth curves. **A,** Boys.

From Tanner, Davis, 1985.

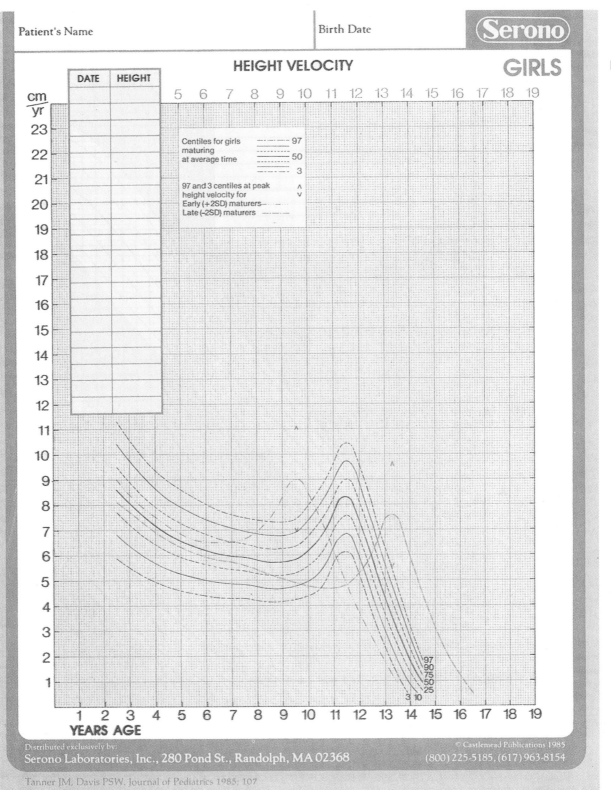

FIGURE E-2—cont'd
Height velocity growth curves. **B,** Girls.
From Tanner, Davis, 1985.

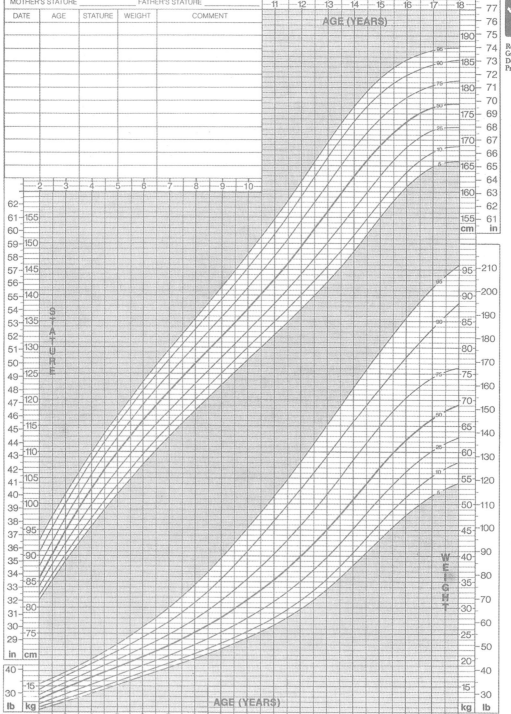

FIGURE E-3

Physical growth curves for children, ages 2 through 18 years, for height and weight. **A,** Boys.

Courtesy Ross Laboratories, Columbus, Ohio.

GIRLS: 2 TO 18 YEARS
PHYSICAL GROWTH
NCHS PERCENTILES*

NAME_____   RECORD #_____

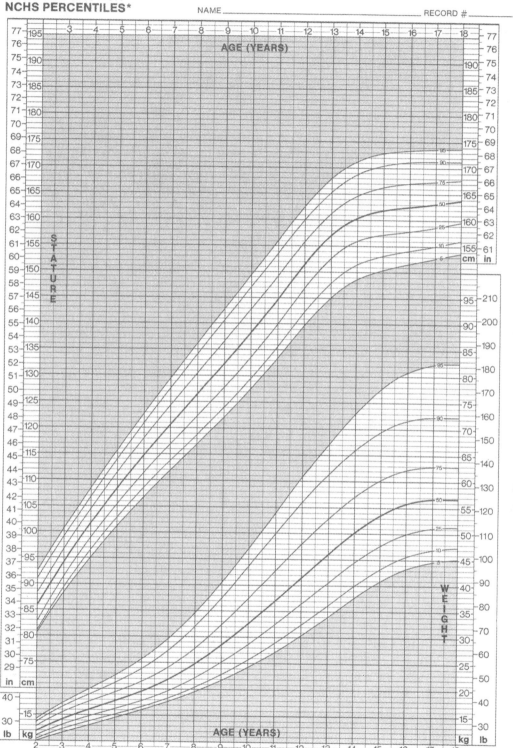

FIGURE E-3—cont'd

Physical growth curves for children, ages 2 through 18 years, for height and weight. **B,** Girls.

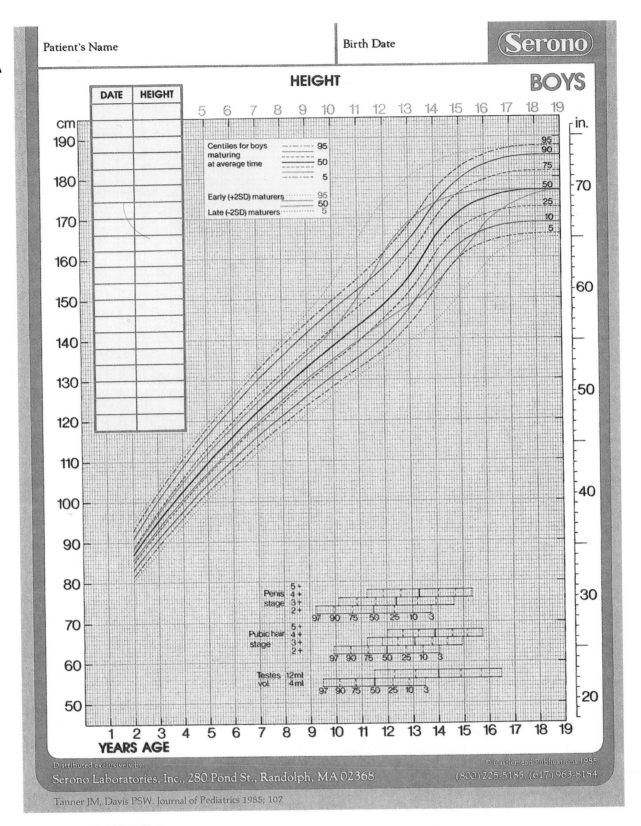

FIGURE E-4
Physical growth curves for children and adolescents, ages 2 through 19 years, for height and sexual development. **A,** Boys.

From Tanner, Davis, 1985.

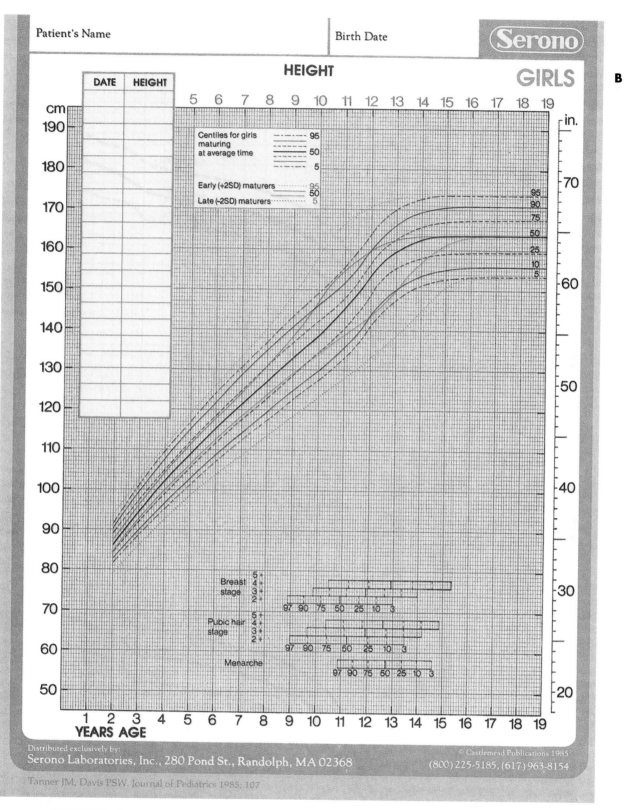

FIGURE E-4—cont'd
Physical growth curves for children and adolescents, ages 2 through 19 years, for height and sexual development. **B,** Girls.
From Tanner, Davis, 1985.

DENVER II DEVELOPMENTAL SCREENING TOOL

The Denver II Developmental Screening Tool is a standardized screening tool widely used to assess an infant's or a child's development between birth and 6 years of age. Fine and gross motor skills, language, and personal-social skills are all assessed. Recording the screening results can be done repeatedly on the same Denver II form for a child, enabling the examiner to mark the child's developmental progress over time.

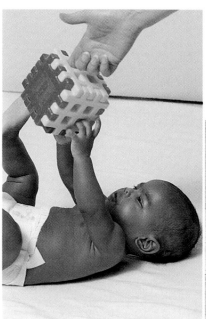

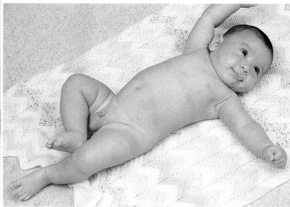

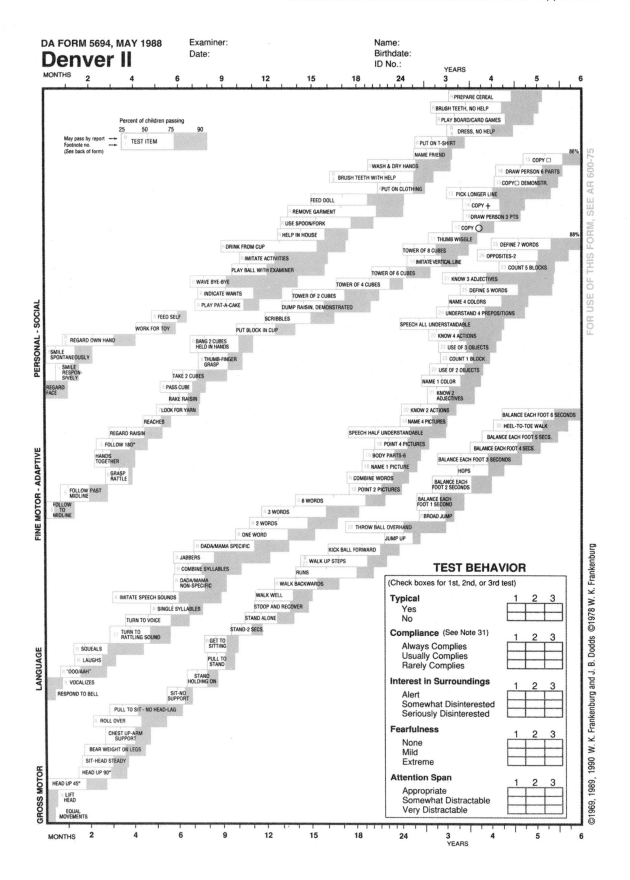

DA FORM 5694, MAY 1988   Examiner: Name:
Denver II   Date: Birthdate:
                                                     ID No.:

DIRECTIONS FOR ADMINISTRATION

1. Try to get child to smile by smiling, talking or waving. Do not touch him/her.
2. Child must stare at hand several seconds.
3. Parent may help guide toothbrush and put toothpaste on brush.
4. Child does not have to be able to tie shoes or button/zip in the back.
5. Move yarn slowly in an arc from one side to the other, about 8" above child's face.
6. Pass if child grasps rattle when it is touched to the backs or tips of fingers.
7. Pass if child tries to see where yarn went. Yarn should be dropped quickly from sight from tester's hand without arm movement.
8. Child must transfer cube from hand to hand without help of body, mouth, or table.
9. Pass if child picks up raisin with any part of thumb and finger.
10. Line can vary only 30 degrees or less from tester's line.
11. Make a fist with thumb pointing upward and wiggle only the thumb. Pass if child imitates and does not move any fingers other than the thumb.

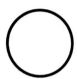 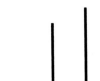 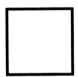

12. Pass any enclosed form. Fail continuous round motions.
13. Which line is longer? (Not bigger.) Turn paper upside down and repeat. (pass 3 of 3 or 5 of 6)
14. Pass any lines crossing near midpoint.
15. Have child copy first. If failed, demonstrate.

When giving items 12, 14, and 15, do not name the forms. Do not demonstrate 12 and 14.

16. When scoring, each pair (2 arms, 2 legs, etc.) counts as one part.
17. Place one cube in cup and shake gently near child's ear, but out of sight. Repeat for other ear.
18. Point to picture and have child name it. (No credit is given for sounds only.)
    If less than 4 pictures are named correctly, have child point to picture as each is named by tester.

 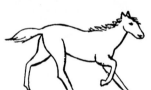 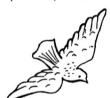 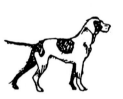 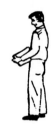

19. Using doll, tell child: Show me the nose, eyes, ears, mouth, hands, feet, tummy, hair. Pass 6 of 8.
20. Using pictures, ask child: Which one flies?... says meow?... talks?... barks?... gallops? Pass 2 of 5, 4 of 5.
21. Ask child: What do you do when you are cold?... tired?... hungry? Pass 2 of 3, 3 of 3.
22. Ask child: What do you do with a cup? What is a chair used for? What is a pencil used for?
    Action words must be included in answers.
23. Pass if child correctly places <u>and</u> says how many blocks are on paper. (1, 5).
24. Tell child: Put block **on** table; **under** table; **in front of** me, **behind** me. Pass 4 of 4.
    (Do not help child by pointing, moving head or eyes.)
25. Ask child: What is a ball?... lake?... desk?... house?... banana?... curtain?... fence?... ceiling? Pass if defined in terms of use, shape, what it is made of, or general category (such as banana is fruit, not just yellow). Pass 5 of 8, 7 of 8.
26. Ask child: If a horse is big, a mouse is __? If fire is hot, ice is __? If the sun shines during the day, the moon shines during the __? Pass 2 of 3.
27. Child may use wall or rail only, not person. May not crawl.
28. Child must throw ball overhand 3 feet to within arm's reach of tester.
29. Child must perform standing broad jump over width of test sheet (8 1/2 inches).
30. Tell child to walk forward, ⚬⚬⚬⚬⚬⚬➤ heel within 1 inch of toe. Tester may demonstrate.
    Child must walk 4 consecutive steps.
31. In the second year, half of normal children are non-compliant.

OBSERVATIONS:

NUTRITION SCREENING FORMS

The following forms are included in this appendix:

- *Level I Screen*, a nutritional screen, which can be used for adults or healthy older adults. It includes a *BMI nomogram* for determining body mass index.
- *Level II Screen*, a more detailed nutritional screen that can be used with older adults or those at nutritional risk.
- *Determine Your Nutritional Health*, a quick and easy screening form to determine whether an individual is at nutritional risk. It discusses the warning signs of nutritional risk and can be used for patient education.
- *Medications Use Checklist*, to identify factors and medications that may cause adverse food/nutrient/medication interactions.
- *A One-Day (24-Hour) Record of Food Intake* and a *Food Diary*, both of which can be used to obtain an individual's food intake to allow estimation of the adequacy of the diet (see also p. 142 in the text).

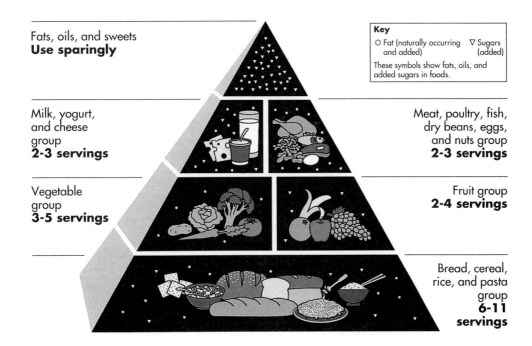

FOOD GUIDE PYRAMID
A Guide to Daily Food Choices

Fats, oils, and sweets **Use sparingly**

Key
○ Fat (naturally occurring and added)   ▽ Sugars (added)
These symbols show fats, oils, and added sugars in foods.

Milk, yogurt, and cheese group **2-3 servings**

Meat, poultry, fish, dry beans, eggs, and nuts group **2-3 servings**

Vegetable group **3-5 servings**

Fruit group **2-4 servings**

Bread, cereal, rice, and pasta group **6-11 servings**

Level I Screen

Body Weight

Measure height to the nearest inch and weight to the nearest pound. Record the values below and mark them on the Body Mass Index (BMI) scale to the right. Then use a straight edge (ruler) to connect the two points and circle the spot where this straight line crosses the center line (body mass index). Record the number below.

Healthy adults should have a BMI between 22 and 27.

Height (in):_____
Weight (lbs):_____
Body Mass Index:_____
(number from center column)

Check any boxes that are true for the individual:

☐ Has lost or gained 10 pounds (or more) in the past 6 months.

☐ Body mass index <22

☐ Body mass index >27

For the remaining sections, please ask the individual which of the statements (if any) is true for him or her and place a check by each that applies.

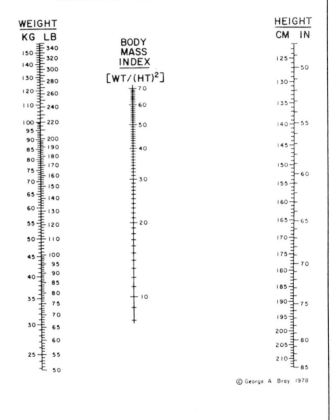

NOMOGRAM FOR BODY MASS INDEX

© George A Bray 1978

Eating Habits

☐ Does not have enough food to eat each day

☐ Usually eats alone

☐ Does not eat anything on one or more days each month

☐ Has poor appetite

☐ Is on a special diet

☐ Eats vegetables two or fewer times daily

☐ Eats milk or milk products once or not at all daily

☐ Eats fruit or drinks fruit juice once or not at all daily

☐ Eats breads, cereals, pasta, rice, or other grains five or fewer times daily

☐ Has difficulty chewing or swallowing

☐ Has more than one alcoholic drink per day (if woman); more than two drinks per day (if man)

☐ Has pain in mouth, teeth, or gums

Reprinted with permission of the Nutrition Screening Initiative, a project of the American Academy of Family Physicians, the American Dietetic Association, and the National Council on the Aging, Inc., and funded in part by a grant from Ross Products Division, Abbott Laboratories.

A health care provider should be contacted if the individual has gained or lost 10 pounds unexpectedly or without intending to during the past 6 months. A health care provider should also be notified if the individual's body mass index is above 27 or below 22.

Living Environment

- ☐ Lives on an income of less than $6000 per year (per individual in the household)

- ☐ Lives alone

- ☐ Is housebound

- ☐ Is concerned about home security

- ☐ Lives in a home with inadequate heating or cooling

- ☐ Does not have a stove and/or refrigerator

- ☐ Is unable or prefers not to spend money on food (<$25-30 per person spent on food each week)

Functional Status

Usually or always needs assistance with (check each that apply):

- ☐ Bathing

- ☐ Dressing

- ☐ Grooming

- ☐ Toileting

- ☐ Eating

- ☐ Walking or moving about

- ☐ Traveling (outside the home)

- ☐ Preparing food

- ☐ Shopping for food or other necessities

If you have checked one or more statements on this screen, the individual you have interviewed may be at risk for poor nutritional status. Please refer this individual to the appropriate health care or social service professional in your area. For example, a dietitian should be contacted for problems with selecting, preparing, or eating a healthy diet, or a dentist if the individual experiences pain or difficulty when chewing or swallowing. Those individuals whose income, lifestyle, or functional status may endanger their nutritional and overall health should be referred to available community services: home-delivered meals, congregate meal programs, transportation services, counseling services (alcohol abuse, depression, bereavement, etc.), home health care agencies, day care programs, etc.

Please repeat this screen at least once each year--sooner if the individual has a major change in his or her health, income, immediate family (e.g., spouse dies), or functional status.

Level II Screen

Complete the following screen by interviewing the patient directly and/or by referring to the patient chart. If you do not routinely perform all of the described tests or ask all of the listed questions, please consider including them but do not be concerned if the entire screen is not completed. Please try to conduct a minimal screen on as many older patients as possible, and please try to collect serial measurements, which are extremely valuable in monitoring nutritional status. Please refer to the manual for additional information.

Anthropometrics

Measure height to the nearest inch and weight to the nearest pound. Record the values below and mark them on the Body Mass Index (BMI) scale to the right. Then use a straight edge (paper, ruler) to connect the two points and circle the spot where this straight line crosses the center line (body mass index). Record the number below; healthy older adults should have a BMI between 22 and 27; check the appropriate box to flag an abnormally high or low value.

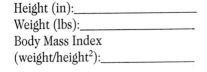

Height (in):_____
Weight (lbs):_____
Body Mass Index
(weight/height^2):_____

Please place a check by any statement regarding BMI and recent weight loss that is true for the patient.

❑ Body mass index <22

❑ Body mass index >27

❑ Has lost or gained 10 pounds (or more) of body weight in the past 6 months

Record the measurement of mid-arm circumference to the nearest 0.1 centimeter and of triceps skinfold to the nearest 2 millimeters.

Mid-Arm Circumference (cm):_____
Triceps Skinfold (mm):_____
Mid-Arm Muscle Circumference (cm):_____

Refer to the table and check any abnormal values:

❑ Mid-arm muscle circumference <10th percentile

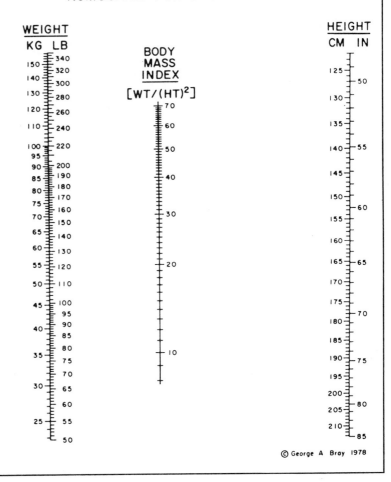

NOMOGRAM FOR BODY MASS INDEX

WEIGHT
KG LB

BODY MASS INDEX
$[WT/(HT)^2]$

HEIGHT
CM IN

© George A Bray 1978

❑ Triceps skinfold <10th percentile

❑ Triceps skinfold >95th percentile

Note: mid-arm circumference (cm) - {0.314 x triceps skinfold (mm)}= mid-arm *muscle* circumference (cm)

For the remaining sections, please place a check by any statements that are true for the patient.

Laboratory Data

❑ Serum albumin below 3.5 g/dl

❑ Serum cholesterol below 160 mg/dl

❑ Serum cholesterol above 240 mg/dl

Drug Use

❑ Three or more prescription drugs, OTC medications, and/or vitamin/mineral supplements daily

Reprinted with permission of the Nutrition Screening Initiative, a project of the American Academy of Family Physicians, the American Dietetic Association, and the National Council on the Aging, Inc., and funded in part by a grant from Ross Products Division, Abbott Laboratories.

Clinical Features

Presence of (check each that apply):

- ❑ Problems with mouth, teeth, or gums
- ❑ Difficulty chewing
- ❑ Difficulty swallowing
- ❑ Angular stomatitis
- ❑ Glossitis
- ❑ History of bone pain
- ❑ History of bone fractures
- ❑ Skin changes (dry, loose, nonspecific lesions, edema)

Percentile	Men 55-65 y	Men 65-75 y	Women 55-65 y	Women 65-75 y
Arm circumference (cm)				
10th	27.3	26.3	25.7	25.2
50th	31.7	30.7	30.3	29.9
95th	36.9	35.5	38.5	37.3
Arm muscle circumference (cm)				
10th	24.5	23.5	19.6	19.5
50th	27.8	26.8	22.5	22.5
95th	32.0	30.6	28.0	27.9
Triceps skinfold (mm)				
10th	6	6	16	14
50th	11	11	25	24
95th	22	22	38	36

From: Frisancho AR. New norms of upper limb fat and muscle areas for assessment of nutritional status. Am J Clin Nutr 1981; 34:2540-2545. © 1981 American Society for Clinical Nutrition.

Eating Habits

- ❑ Does not have enough food to eat each day
- ❑ Usually eats alone
- ❑ Does not eat anything on one or more days each month
- ❑ Has poor appetite
- ❑ Is on a special diet
- ❑ Eats vegetables two or fewer times daily
- ❑ Eats milk or milk products once or not at all daily
- ❑ Eats fruit or drinks fruit juice once or not at all daily
- ❑ Eats breads, cereals, pasta, rice, or other grains five or fewer times daily
- ❑ Has more than one alcoholic drink per day (if woman); more than two drinks per day (if man)

Living Environment

- ❑ Lives on an income of less than $6000 per year (per individual in the household)
- ❑ Lives alone
- ❑ Is housebound
- ❑ Is concerned about home security

- ❑ Lives in a home with inadequate heating or cooling
- ❑ Does not have a stove and/or refrigerator
- ❑ Is unable or prefers not to spend money on food (<$25-30 per person spent on food each week)

Functional Status

Usually or always needs assistance with (check each that apply):

- ❑ Bathing
- ❑ Dressing
- ❑ Grooming
- ❑ Toileting
- ❑ Eating
- ❑ Walking or moving about
- ❑ Traveling (outside the home)
- ❑ Preparing food
- ❑ Shopping for food or other necessities

Mental/Cognitive Status

- ❑ Clinical evidence of impairment, e.g. Folstein<26
- ❑ Clinical evidence of depressive illness, e.g. Beck Depression Inventory>15, Geriatric Depression Scale>5

Patients in whom you have identified one or more major indicator (see pg 944) of poor nutritional status require immediate medical attention; if minor indicators are found, ensure that they are known to a health professional or to the patient's own physician. Patients who display risk factors of poor nutritional status should be referred to the appropriate health care or social service professional (dietitian, nurse, dentist, case manager, etc.).

The Warning Signs of poor nutritional health are often overlooked. Use this checklist to find out if you or someone you know is at nutritional risk.

Read the statements below. Circle the number in the yes column for those that apply to you or someone you know. For each yes answer, score the number in the box. Total your nutritional score.

DETERMINE YOUR NUTRITIONAL HEALTH

	YES
I have an illness or condition that made me change the kind and/or amount of food I eat.	2
I eat fewer than 2 meals per day.	3
I eat few fruits or vegetables, or milk products.	2
I have 3 or more drinks of beer, liquor or wine almost every day.	2
I have tooth or mouth problems that make it hard for me to eat.	2
I don't always have enough money to buy the food I need.	4
I eat alone most of the time.	1
I take 3 or more different prescribed or over-the-counter drugs a day.	1
Without wanting to, I have lost or gained 10 pounds in the last 6 months.	2
I am not always physically able to shop, cook and/or feed myself.	2
TOTAL	

Total Your Nutritional Score. If it's ---

0-2   **Good!** Recheck your nutritional score in 6 months.

3-5   **You are at moderate nutritional risk.** See what can be done to improve your eating habits and lifestyle. Your office on aging, senior nutrition program, senior citizens center or health department can help. Recheck your nutritional score in 3 months.

6 or more   **You are at high nutritional risk.** Bring this checklist the next time you see your doctor, dietitian or other qualified health or social service professional. Talk with them about any problems you may have. Ask for help to improve your utritional health.

Remember that warning signs suggest risk, but do not represent diagnosis of any condition. Turn the page to learn more about the Warnings Signs of poor nutritional health.

These materials developed and distributed by the Nutrition Screening Initiative, a project of:

 AMERICAN ACADEMY OF FAMILY PHYSICIANS

 THE AMERICAN DIETETIC ASSOCIATION

 NATIONAL COUNCIL ON THE AGING, INC.

DISEASE

Any disease, illness or chronic condition which causes you to change the way you eat, or makes it hard for you to eat, puts your nutritional health at risk. Four out of five adults have chronic diseases that are affected by diet. Confusion or memory loss that keeps getting worse is estimated to affect one out of five or more of older adults. This can make it hard to remember what, when or if you've eaten. Feeling sad or depressed, which happens to about one in eight older adults, can cause big changes in appetite, digestion, energy level, weight and well-being.

EATING POORLY

Eating too little and eating too much both lead to poor health. Eating the same foods day after day or not eating fruit, vegetables, and milk products daily will also cause poor nutritional health. One in five adults skip meals daily. Only 13% of adults eat the minimum amount of fruit and vegetables needed. One in four older adults drink too much alcohol. Many health problems become worse if you drink more than one or two alcoholic beverages per day.

TOOTH LOSS/ MOUTH PAIN

A healthy mouth, teeth and gums are needed to eat. Missing, loose or rotten teeth or dentures which don't fit well or cause mouth sores make it hard to eat.

ECONOMIC HARDSHIP

As many as 40% of older Americans have incomes of less than $6,000 per year. Having less--or choosing to spend less--than $25-30 per week for food makes it very hard to get the foods you need to stay healthy.

REDUCED SOCIAL CONTACT

One-third of all older people live alone. Being with people daily has a positive effect on morale, well-being and eating.

MULTIPLE MEDICINES

Many older Americans must take medicines for health problems. Almost half of older Americans take multiple medicines daily. Growing old may change the way we respond to drugs. The more medicines you take, the greater the chance for side effects such as increased or decreased appetite, change in taste, constipation, weakness, drowsiness, diarrhea, nausea, and others. Vitamins or minerals when taken in large doses act like drugs and can cause harm. Alert your doctor to everything you take.

INVOLUNTARY WEIGHT LOSS/GAIN

Losing or gaining a lot of weight when you are not trying to do so is an important warning sign that must not be ignored. Being overweight or underweight also increases your chance of poor health.

NEEDS ASSISTANCE IN SELF CARE

Although most older people are able to eat, one of every five have trouble walking, shopping, buying and cooking food, especially as they get older.

ELDER YEARS ABOVE AGE 80

Most older people lead full and productive lives. But as age increases, risk of frailty and health problems increase. Checking your nutritional health regularly makes good sense.

 The Nutrition Screening Initiative • 1010 Wisconsin Avenue, NW • Suite 800 • Washington, DC 20007
The Nutrition Screening Initiative is funded in part by a grant from Ross Laboratories, a division of Abbott Laboratories.

The Warning Signs of poor nutritional health are often overlooked. Use this checklist to find out if you or someone you know is at nutritional risk because of factors related to over-the-counter drugs or prescribed medications.

MEDICATIONS USE CHECKLIST

Read the statements below. Circle the number in the yes column for those that apply to you or someone you know. For each yes answer, add the number in the box. Write the total in the last box.

	YES
I do not know if I should take my medications before or after eating.	1
I take 3 or more medications each day.	2
I have gained or lost more than 10 lbs. since I started taking my medications.	1
I go to more than one pharmacy or drugstore to get my prescriptions filled.	2
I do not always ask my doctor about the safety of taking prescribed medications or vitamins and minerals.	2
I take one or more of the following medications: (Check the ones you take.) ( ) Digoxin ( ) Lithium ( ) Theophylline ( ) Phenytoin (Dilantin) and my doctor does not check my blood level.	2
I drink 2 or more alcoholic beverages on a daily basis.	2
I take insulin or pills for the control of diabetes and I sometimes skip my supper and/or bedtime snack.	2
I cannot read the labels on my medication.	2
TOTAL	

Total Your Medications Used Score.

If it's more than 2, you may have a problem with your health because of your medications and diet. Talk with your doctor or pharmacist. Bring this checklist the next time you see them. Remember that warning signs suggest risk, but do not represent diagnosis of any condition.

These materials developed and distributed by the Nutrition Screening Initiative, a project of:

 AMERICAN ACADEMY OF FAMILY PHYSICIANS

 THE AMERICAN DIETETIC ASSOCIATION

 NATIONAL COUNCIL ON THE AGING

The Nutrition Screening Initiative is funded in part by a grant from Ross Products Division of Abbott Laboratories.

 The Nutrition Screening Initiative
1010 Wisconsin Avenue, NW, Suite 800
Washington, DC 20007

Reprinted with permission of the Nutrition Screening Initiative, a project of the American Academy of Family Physicians, the American Dietetic Association, and the National Council on the Aging, Inc., and funded in part by a grant from Ross Products Division, Abbott Laboratories.

A One-Day (24-Hour) Record of Food Intake

NAME_____ DATE OF RECORD _____

BREAKFAST   Time Eaten _____

Food/Beverage	Type and/or Method of Preparation (List Ingredients)	Amount
MILK		
FRUIT Fresh, canned, sweetened, etc.		
CEREAL _____ with milk _____ with sugar _____ other	Brand_____	
BREAD _____ margarine/butter _____ mayonnaise _____ other	White_____ Brown_____	
EGGS		
MEAT or OTHER PROTEIN		
BEVERAGE _____ with milk _____ with sugar _____ other		
OTHER FOODS		

Did you eat a mid-morning snack?   Yes _____   No _____   If yes, time? _____
(list foods and beverages eaten)

_____

_____

Adapted from Burke, 1947; reprinted from Giddens, 1998.

NOON MEAL   Time Eaten _____

Food/Beverage	Type and/or Method of Preparation (List Ingredients)	Amount
SOUP		
BREAD _____ margarine/butter _____ mayonnaise _____ other	White _____ Brown _____	
_____ MEAT _____ EGG _____ FISH _____ CHEESE		
VEGETABLES _____ cooked _____ raw _____ topping/seasoning (butter, white sauce, cheese sauce, etc.)		
SALAD _____ dressing (brand, etc.)		
FRUIT Fresh, canned, sweetened, etc.		
MILK		
BEVERAGE _____ with milk _____ with sugar _____ other		
DESSERT		
OTHER FOODS		

Did you eat an afternoon snack?   Yes _____   No _____   If yes, time? _____
(list foods and beverages eaten)

_____

EVENING MEAL   Time Eaten _____

Food/Beverage	Type and/or Method of Preparation (List Ingredients)	Amount
MAIN DISH _____ meat _____ cheese _____ poultry _____ other protein _____ pasta _____ rice		
VEGETABLES _____ cooked _____ raw _____ topping/seasoning (butter, white sauce, cheese sauce, etc.)		
SALAD _____ dressing (brand, etc.)		
BREAD _____ margarine/butter _____ mayonnaise _____ other	White _____ Brown _____	
FRUIT Fresh, canned, sweetened, etc.		
MILK		
BEVERAGE _____ with milk _____ with sugar _____ other		
DESSERT		
OTHER FOODS		

Did you eat an evening snack?   Yes _____   No _____   If yes, time? _____
(list foods and beverages eaten)

_____

_____

Food Diary

Name _____ **Date** _____

Time	Food type and amount	Where eaten and with whom	Other activity while eating	How you feel before eating (e.g., anxious, bored, tired, angry, depressed)

ABBREVIATIONS

A & P	Anterior and posterior; auscultation and percussion
A & W	Alive and well
abd	Abdomen; abdominal
a̅c̅	Before meals
ADL	Activities of daily living
AJ	Ankle jerk
AK	Above knee
ANS	Autonomic nervous system
AP	Anteroposterior
bid	Twice a day
BK	Below knee
BP	Blood pressure
BPH	Benign prostatic hypertrophy
BS	Bowel sounds; breath sounds
c̅	With
CAD	Coronary artery disease
CC	Chief complaint
CHD	Childhood disease; congenital heart disease; coronary heart disease
CHF	Congestive heart failure
CNS	Central nervous system
c/o	Complains of
COPD	Chronic obstructive pulmonary disease
CV	Cardiovascular
CVA	Costovertebral angle; cerebrovascular accident
CVP	Central venous pressure
Cx	Cervix
D & C	Dilation and curettage
D/C	Discontinued
DM	Diabetes mellitus
DOB	Date of birth
DOE	Dyspnea on exertion
DTRs	Deep tendon reflexes
DUB	Dysfunctional uterine bleeding
Dx	Diagnosis
ECG, EKG	Electrocardiogram; electrocardiograph
EENT	Eye, ear, nose, and throat

ENT	Ear, nose, and throat
EOM	Extraocular movement
FB	Foreign body
FH	Family history
FROM	Full range of motion
FTT	Failure to thrive
Fx	Fracture
GB	Gallbladder
GE	Gastroesophageal
GI	Gastrointestinal
GU	Genitourinary
GYN	Gynecologic
HA	Headache
HCG	Human chorionic gonadotropin
HEENT	Head, eyes, ears, nose, and throat
HPI	History of present illness
Hx	History
ICS	Intercostal space
IOP	Intraocular pressure
IUD	Intrauterine device
IV	Intravenous
JVP	Jugular venous pressure
KJ	Knee jerk
KUB	Kidneys, ureters, and bladder
lat	Lateral
LCM	Left costal margin
LE	Lower extremities
LLL	Left lower lobe (lung)
LLQ	Left lower quadrant (abdomen)
LMD	Local medical doctor
LMP	Last menstrual period
LOC	Loss of consciousness; level of consciousness
LS	Lumbosacral; lumbar spine
LSB	Left sternal border
LUL	Left upper lobe (lung)
LUQ	Left upper quadrant (abdomen)
M	Murmur
MAL	Midaxillary line
MCL	Midclavicular line
MGF	Maternal grandfather
MGM	Maternal grandmother
MSL	Midsternal line
MVA	Motor vehicle accident
NA	No answer; not applicable
N & T	Nose and throat
N & V	Nausea and vomiting
NKA	No known allergies
NPO	Nothing by mouth
NSR	Normal sinus rhythm
OD	Oculus dexter; right eye

OM	Otitis media
OS	Oculus sinister; left eye
OTC	Over the counter
OU	Oculus uterque; both eyes
p̄	After
P & A	Percussion and auscultation
p̄c	After meals
PE	Physical examination
PERRLA	Pupils equal, round, react to light and accommodation
PGF	Paternal grandfather
PGM	Paternal grandmother
PI	Present illness
PID	Pelvic inflammatory disease
PMH	Past medical history
PMI	Point of maximum impulse; point of maximum intensity
PMS	Premenstrual syndrome
prn	As necessary
Pt	Patient
PVC	Premature ventricular contraction
q	Every
qd	Every day
qh	Every hour
qod	Every other day
RCM	Right costal margin
REM	Rapid eye movement
RLL	Right lower lobe (lung)
RLQ	Right lower quadrant (abdomen)
RML	Right middle lobe (lung)
ROM	Range of motion
ROS	Review of systems
RSB	Right sternal border
RUL	Right upper lobe (lung)
RUQ	Right upper quadrant (abdomen)
s̄	Without
SCM	Sternocleidomastoid
SQ	Subcutaneous
Sx	Symptoms
T & A	Tonsillectomy and adenoidectomy
TM	Tympanic membrane
TPR	Temperature, pulse, and respiration
UE	Upper extremities
URI	Upper respiratory infection
UTI	Urinary tract infection
WD	Well developed
WN	Well nourished

WORD PARTS

Word Parts Commonly Used as Prefixes

WORD PART	MEANING	WORD PART	MEANING
a-	Without, not	inter-	Between
af-	Toward	intra-	Within
an-	Without, not	iso-	Same, equal
ante-	Before	macro-	Large
anti-	Against; resisting	mega-	Large; million(th)
auto-	Self	mes-	Middle
bi-	Two; double	meta-	Beyond, after
circum-	Around	micro-	Small; millionth
co-, con-	With; together	milli-	Thousandth
contra-	Against	mono-	One (single)
de-	Down from, undoing	neo-	New
dia-	Across, through	non-	Not
dipl-	Twofold, double	oligo-	Few, scanty
dys-	Bad; disordered; difficult	ortho-	Straight; correct, normal
ectop-	Displaced	para-	By the side of; near
ef-	Away from	per-	Through
em-, en-	In, into	peri-	Around; surrounding
endo-	Within	poly-	Many
epi-	Upon	post-	After
eu-	Good	pre-	Before
ex-, exo-	Out of, out from	pro-	First; promoting
extra-	Outside of	quadr-	Four
hapl-	Single	re-	Back again
hem-, hemat-	Blood	retro-	Behind
hemi-	Half	semi-	Half
hom(e)o-	Same; equal	sub-	Under
hyper-	Over; above	super-, supra-	Over, above, excessive
hypo-	Under; below	trans-	Across; through
infra-	Below, beneath	tri-	Three; triple

From Thibodeau G, Patton K, 1993.

Word Parts Commonly Used as Suffixes

WORD PART	MEANING	WORD PART	MEANING
-al, -ac	Pertaining to	-malacia	Softening
-algia	Pain	-megaly	Enlargement
-aps, -apt	Fit; fasten	-metric, -metry	Measurement, length
-arche	Beginning; origin	-oid	Like; in the shape of
-ase	Signifies an enzyme	-oma	Tumor
-blast	Sprout; make	-opia	Vision, vision condition
-centesis	A piercing	-oscopy	Viewing
-cide	To kill	-ose	Signifies a carbohydrate (especially a sugar)
-clast	Break; destroy		
-crine	Release; secrete	-osis	Condition, process
-ectomy	A cutting out	-ostomy	Formation of an opening
-emesis	Vomiting	-otomy	Cut
-emia	Refers to blood condition	-penia	Lack
-flux	Flow	-philic	Loving
-gen	Creates; forms	-phobic	Fearing
-genesis	Creation; production	-phragm	Partition
-gram	Something written	-plasia	Growth, formation
-graph(y)	To write, draw	-plasm	Substance, matter
-hydrate	Containing H_2O (water)	-plasty	Shape; make
-ia, -sia	Condition; process	-plegia	Paralysis
-iasis	Abnormal condition	-pnea	Breath, breathing
-ic, -ac	Pertaining to	-(r)rhage, -(r)rhagia	Breaking out, discharge
-in	Signifies a protein	-(r)rhaphy	Sew, suture
-ism	Signifies "condition of"	-(r)rhea	Flow
-itis	Signifies "inflammation of"	-some	Body
-lemma	Rind; peel	-tensin, -tension	Pressure
-lepsy	Seizure	-tonic	Pressure, tension
-lith	Stone; rock	-tripsy	Crushing
-logy	Study of	-ule	Small, little
-luna	Moon; moonlike	-uria	Refers to urine condition

From Thibodeau G, Patton K, 1993.

Word Parts Commonly Used as Roots

WORD PART	MEANING	WORD PART	MEANING
acro-	Extremity	hist-	Tissue
aden-	Gland	hydro-	Water
alveol-	Small hollow cavity	hyster-	Uterus
angi-	Vessel	iatr-	Treatment
arthr-	Joint	kal-	Potassium
asthen-	Weakness	kary-	Nucleus
bar-	Pressure	kerat-	Cornea
bili-	Bile	lact-	Milk; milk production
brachi-	Arm	lapar-	Abdomen
brady-	Slow	leuk-	White
bronch-	Air passage	lig-	To tie, bind
capn-	Smoke	lip-	Lipid (fat)
carcin-	Cancer	lys-	Break apart
card-	Heart	mal-	Bad
cephal-	Head, brain	melan-	Black
cerv-	Neck	men-, mens-, (menstru-)	Month (monthly)
chem-	Chemical	muta-	Change
chol-	Bile	my-, myo-	Muscle
chondr-	Cartilage	myc-	Fungus
corp-	Body	myel-	Marrow
cortico-	Pertaining to cortex	nat-	Birth
crani-	Skull	natr-	Sodium
crypt-	Hidden	nephr-	Nephron, kidney
cusp-	Point	neur-	Nerve
cut(an)-	Skin	noct-, nyct-	Night
cyan-	Blue	ocul-	Eye
cyst-	Bladder	odont-	Tooth
cyt-	Cell	onco-	Cancer
dactyl-	Fingers, toes (digits)	ophthalm-	Eye
dendr-	Tree; branched	orchid-	Testis
dent-	Tooth	osteo-	Bone
derm-	Skin	oto-	Ear
diastol-	Relax; stand apart	ov-, oo-	Egg
dips-	Thirst	oxy-	Oxygen
ejacul-	To throw out	path-	Disease
electr-	Electrical	ped-	Children
enter-	Intestine	phag-	Eat
eryth(r)-	Red	pharm-	Drug
esthe-	Sensation	phleb-	Vein
febr-	Fever	photo-	Light
gastr-	Stomach	physio-	Nature (function) of
gingiv-	Gums	plex-	Twisted; woven
glomer-	Wound into a ball	pneumo-	Air, breath
gloss-	Tongue	pneumon-	Lung
gluc-	Glucose, sugar	pod-	Foot
glutin-	Glue	poie-	Make; produce
glyc-	Sugar (carbohydrate); glucose	presby-	Old
		proct-	Rectum
hepat-	Liver	pseud-	False

From Thibodeau, Patton, 1993.

Word Parts Commonly Used as Roots—cont'd

WORD PART	MEANING	WORD PART	MEANING
psych-	Mind	syn-	Together
pyel-	Pelvis	systol-	Contract; stand together
ren-	Kidney		
rhino-	Nose	tachy-	Fast
rigor-	Stiffness	therm-	Heat
sarco-	Flesh; muscle	thromb-	Clot
scler-	Hard	tox-	Poison
semen-, semin-	Seed; sperm	troph-	Grow; nourish
sept-	Contamination	tympan-	Drum
sin-	Cavity; recess	varic-	Enlarged vessel
son-	Sound	vas-	Vessel, duct
spiro-, spire-	Breathe	vesic-	Bladder; blister
stat-, stas-	A standing, stopping		

ENGLISH-TO-SPANISH TRANSLATION GUIDE: KEY MEDICAL QUESTIONS

The following is a guide to help you complete the history and examination of Spanish-speaking patients. Initial questions presented are general ones used at the beginning of the examination. Questions for pain assessment follow. The remainder of the translations are arranged in order of the body systems. Each system's section contains basic vocabulary, questions used for history taking, and instructions that would facilitate examination. The intent of this guide is to offer an array of questions and phrases from which the examiner can choose as appropriate for assessment.

HINTS FOR PRONUNCIATION OF SPANISH WORDS

1. *h* is silent.
2. *j* is pronounced as *h*.
3. *ll* is pronounced as a *y* sound.
4. *r* is pronounced with a trilled sound, and *rr* is trilled even more.
5. *v* is pronounced with a *b* sound.
6. A *y* by itself is pronounced with a long *e* sound.
7. Accent marks over the vowel indicate the syllable that is to be stressed.

INTRODUCTORY

I am _____.	Soy _____.
What is your name?	¿Cómo se llama usted?
I would like to examine you now.	Quisiera examinarlo(a) ahora.

GENERAL

How do you feel?	¿Cómo se siente?
Good	Bien
Bad	Mal
Do you feel better today?	¿Se siente mejor hoy?
Where do you work?	¿Dónde trabaja? (¿Cuál es su profesión o trabajo?) (¿Qué hace usted?)
Are you allergic to anything?	¿Tiene usted algerias?
Medications, foods, insect bites?	¿Medicinas, alimentos, picaduras de insectos?
Do you take any medications?	¿Toma usted algunas medicinas?
Do you have any drug allergies?	¿Es usted alérgico(a) algún médicamento?

Do you have a history of	¿Padece usted enfermedad
heart disease?	del corazón?
diabetes?	del diabetes?
epilepsy?	la epilepsia?
bronchitis?	de bronquitis?
emphysema?	de enfisema?
asthma?	de asma?

PAIN

Have you any pain?	¿Tiene dolor?
Where is the pain?	¿Dónde está el dolor?
Do you have any pain here?	¿Tiene usted dolor aquí?
How severe is the pain?	¿Qué tan fuerte es el dolor?
Mild, moderate, sharp, or severe?	¿Ligero, moderado, agudo, severo?
What were you doing when the pain started?	¿Qué haciá usted cuando le comenzó el dolor?
Have you ever had this pain before?	¿Ha tenido este dolor antes?
	(¿Ha sido siempre así?)
Do you have a pain in your side?	¿Tiene usted dolor en el costado?
Is it worse now?	¿Está peor ahora?
Does it still pain you?	¿Le duele todavía?
Did you feel much pain at the time?	¿Sintió mucho dolor entonces?
Show me where.	Muéstreme dónde.
Does it hurt when I press here?	¿Le duele cuando aprieto aquí?

HEAD

Vocabulary

Head	La cabeza
Face	La cara

History

How does your head feel?	¿Cómo siente la cabeza?
Have you any pain in the head?	¿Le duele la cabeza?
Do you have headaches?	¿Tiene usted dolores de cabeza?
Do you have migranes?	¿Tiene usted migrañas?
What causes the headaches?	¿Qué le causa los dolores de cabeza?

Examination

Lift up your head.	Levante la cabeza.

EYES

Vocabulary

Eye	El ojo

History

Have you had pain in your eyes?	¿Ha tenido dolor en los ojos?
Do you wear glasses?	¿Usa usted anteojos/gafas/lentes/ espejuelos?
Do you wear contact lenses?	¿Usa usted lentes de contacto?
Can you see clearly?	¿Puede ver claramente?

Better at a distance?	¿Mejor a cierta distancia?
Do you sometimes see things double?	¿Ve las cosas doble algunas veces?
Do you see things through a mist?	¿Ve las cosas nubladas?
Were you exposed to anything that could have injured your eye?	¿Fue expuesto a cualquier cosa que pudiera haberle dañado el ojo?
Do your eyes water much?	¿Le lagrimean mucho los ojos?

Examination

Look up.	Mire para arriba.
Look down.	Mire para abajo.
Look toward your nose.	Mírese la nariz.
Look at me.	Míreme.
Tell me what number it is.	Digame qué número es éste.
Tell me what letter it is.	Digame qué letra es ésta.

EARS/NOSE/THROAT

Vocabulary

Ears	Los oídos
Eardrum	El tímpano
Laryngitis	La laringitis
Lip	El labio
Mouth	La boca
Nose	La naríz
Tongue	La lengua

History

Do you have any hearing problems?	¿Tiene usted problemas de oir?
Do you use a hearing aid?	¿Usa usted un audífono?
Do you have ringing in the ears?	¿Le zumban los oídos?
Do you have allergies?	¿Tiene alergias?
Do you use dentures?	¿Usa usted dentadura postiza?
Do you have any loose teeth, removable bridges, or any prosthesis?	¿Tiene dientes flojos, dientes postizos, o cualquier prostesis?
Do you have a cold?	¿Tiene usted un resfriado/resfrío?
Do you have sore throats frequently?	¿Le duele la garganta con frecuencia?
Have you ever had a strep throat?	¿Ha tenido alguna vez (infección de la garganta)?

Examination

Open your mouth.	Abra la boca.
I want to take a throat culture. This will not hurt.	Quiero hacer un cultivo de la garganta. Esto no le va a doler.

CARDIOVASCULAR

Vocabulary

Heart	El corazón
Heart attack	El ataque al corazón
Heart disease	La enfermedad del corazón
Heart murmur	El soplo del corazón
High blood pressure	Alta presión

History

Have you ever had any chest pain?	¿Ha tenido alguna vez dolor de pecho?
Where?	¿Dónde?
Do you notice any irregularity of heart beat or any palpitations?	¿Nota cualquier latido o palpitación irregular?
Do you get short of breath?	¿Tiene usted problemas con la respiracion?
When?	¿Cuándo?
Do you take medicine for your heart?	¿Toma medicina para el corazón?
How often?	¿Con qué frecuencia?
Do you know if you have high blood pressure?	¿Sabe usted si tiene la presión alta?
Is there a history of hypertension in your family?	¿En su familia se encuentron varias personas con alta presión?
Are any of your limbs swollen?	¿Están hinchados algunos de sus miembros?
Hands, feet, legs?	¿Manos, pies, piernas?
How long have they been swollen like this?	¿Desde cuándo están hinchados así? (¿Qué tanto tiempo tiene usted con esta inchason?)

Examination

Let me feel your pulse.	Déjeme tomarle el pulso.
I am going to take your blood pressure now.	Le voy a tomar la presión ahora.

RESPIRATORY

Vocabulary

Chest	El pecho
Lungs	Los pulmones

History

Do you smoke?	¿Fuma usted?
How many packs a day?	¿Cuántos paquetes al día?
Have you any difficulty in breathing?	¿Tiene dificultad al respirar?
How long have you been coughing?	¿Desde cuándo tiene tos?
Do you cough up phlegm?	¿Al toser, escupe usted flema(s)?
What is the color of your expectorations?	¿Cuándo usted escupe, qué color es?
Do you cough up blood?	¿Al toser, arroja usted sangre?
Do you wheeze?	¿Le silba a usted el pecho?

Examination

Take a deep breath.	Respìre profundo.
Breathe normally.	Respìre normalmente.
Cough.	Tosa.
Cough again.	Tosa otra vez.

GASTROINTESTINAL

Vocabulary

Abdomen	El abdomen
Intestines/bowels	Los intestinos/ las entrañas

Liver	El hígado
Nausea	Náusea
Gastric ulcer	La úlcera gástrica
Stomach	El estomago, la panza, la barriga
Stomachache	El dolor de estómago

History

What foods disagree with you?	¿Qué alimentos le caen mal?
Do you get heartburn?	¿Suele tener ardor en el pecho?
Do you have indigestion often?	¿Tiene indigestión con frecuencia?
Are you going to vomit?	¿Va a vomitar (arrojar)?
Do you have blood in your vomit?	¿Tiene usted vómitos con sangre?
Do you have abdominal pain?	¿Tiene dolor en el abdomen?
How are your stools?	¿Cómo son sus defecaciones?
Are they regular?	¿Son regulares?
Have you noticed their color?	¿Se ha fijado en el color?
Are you constipated?	¿Está estreñido?
Do you have diarrhea?	¿Tiene diarrea?

GENITOURINARY

Vocabulary

Genitals	Los genitales
Kidney	El riñón
Penis	El pene, el miembro
Urine	La orina

History

Have you any difficulty passing water?	¿Tiene dificultad en orinar?
Do you pass water involuntarily?	¿Orina sin querer?
Do you have a urethral discharge?	¿Tiene descho de la uretra?
Do you have burning with urination?	¿Tiene ardor al orinar?

MUSCULOSKELETAL

Vocabulary

Ankle	El tobillo
Arm	El brazo
Back	La espalda
Bones	Los huesos
Elbow	El codo
Finger	El dedo
Foot	El pie
Fracture	La fractura
Hand	La mano
Hip	La cadera
Knee	La rodilla
Leg	La pierna
Muscles	Los músculos
Rib	La costilla
Shoulder	El hombro
Thigh	El muslo

History

Did you fall and how did you fall?	¿Se cayó, y cómo se cayó?
How did this happen?	¿Cómo sucedío esto?
How long ago?	¿Cuanto tiempo hace?

Examination

Raise your arm.	Levante el brazo.
Raise it more.	Más alto.
Now the other.	Ahora el otro.
Stand up and walk.	Parese y camine.
Straighten your leg.	Enderece la pierna.
Bend your knee.	Doble la rodilla.
Push	Empuje
Pull	Jale
Up	Arriba
Down	Abajo
In/out	Adentro/afuera
Rest	Descanse
Kneel	Arrodíllese

NEUROLOGIC

Vocabulary

Brain	El cerebro
Dizziness	El vértigo, el mareo
Epilepsy	La epilepsia
Fainting spell	El desmayo
Unconscious	La insensibilidad (inconsiente)

History

Have you ever had a head injury?	¿Ha tenido alguna vez daño a la cabeza?
Do you have convulsions?	¿Tiene convulsiones?
Do you have tingling sensations?	¿Tiene hormigueos?
Do you have numbness in your hands, arms, or feet?	¿Siente entumecidos las manos, los brazos, o los pies?
Have you ever lost consciousness?	¿Perdió alguna vez el sentido? (inconsiente)
For how long?	¿Por cuánto tiempo?
How often does this happen?	¿Con qué frecuencia ocurre esto?

Examination

Squeeze my hand.	Apriete mi mano.
Can you not do it better than that?	¿No puede hacerlo más fuerte?
Turn on your left/right side.	Voltéese al lado izquiedo/ al lado derechos.
Roll over and sit up over the edge of the bed.	Voltéese y siéntese sobre el borde del la cama.
Stand up slowly. Put your weight only on your right/left foot.	Párese despacio. Ponga peso sólo en la pierna derecha/izquierda.
Take a step to the side.	Dé un paso al lado.

Turn to your left/right.

Doble a la izquierda/derecha.

Is this hot or cold?

¿Está frío o caliente esto?

Am I sticking you with the point or the head of the pin?

¿Le estoy pinchando con la cabeza del alfiler?

ENDOCRINE/ REPRODUCTIVE

Vocabulary

Uterus

El útero, la matríz

Vagina

La vagina

History

Have you had any problems with your thyroid?

¿Ha tenido alguna vez problemas con tiroides?

Have you noticed any significant weight gain or loss?

¿Ha notado pérdida o aumento de peso?

What is your usual weight?

¿Cuál es su peso usual?

How is your appetite?

¿Qué tal su apetito?

Women:

How old were you when your periods started?

¿Cuántos años tenía cuando tuvo la primera regla?

How many days between periods?

¿Cuántos días entre las reglas?

When was your last menstrual period?

¿Cuándo fue su última regla?

Have you ever been pregnant?

¿Ha estado embarazada?

How many children do you have?

¿Cuántos hijos tiene?

When was your last Pap smear?

¿Cuándo fue su última prueba de Papanicolado?

Would you like information on birth control methods?

¿Quiere usted información sobre los métodos del control de la natalidad?

Do you have a vaginal discharge?

¿Tiene descho vaginales?

INDEX

To help us publish the most useful materials for students, we would appreciate your comments on this book. Please take a few moments to complete the form below, then tear it out and mail it back to us. Thank you in advance for your input!

Book Title: _____

Author Name: _____

1. Did the content of this textbook help you meet the requirements for passing this course? Explain: _____
_____

2. What do you like most about this product? _____
_____

   What do you like least? _____
_____

3. Which chapters were most helpful? Which were least helpful? _____
_____

4. If you could change one thing about this book, what would it be? _____
_____

5. If applicable, did you purchase/use the student learning guide accompanying the text? If so, did you purchase the student learning guide on your own or at the direction of the instructor? _____
_____

6. Was the book a good value for the price? _____
_____

7. Are you planning to keep this text? Why or why not? _____
_____

Are you interested in doing in-depth reviews of our nursing textbooks? If so, please fill out the information below:

Name: _____ Telephone: _____

Address: _____

Thank you!

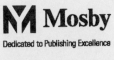

Mosby
Dedicated to Publishing Excellence

A Times Mirror Company

tape shut here

BUSINESS REPLY MAIL
FIRST-CLASS MAIL   PERMIT NO. 135   SAINT LOUIS MO

POSTAGE WILL BE PAID BY ADDRESSEE

NO POSTAGE
NECESSARY
IF MAILED
IN THE
UNITED STATES

JANET BLANNER
NURSING MARKETING
MOSBY INC
11830 WESTLINE INDUSTRIAL DR
SAINT LOUIS MO 63146-9987

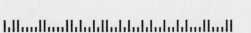

tape shut here

LIFESPAN CONTENTS